W9-AAS-781

Clinical Neurology
for Psychiatrists

Clinical Neurology for Psychiatrists

SIXTH EDITION

David Myland Kaufman, M.D.

Departments of Neurology and Psychiatry
Montefiore Medical Center
Albert Einstein College of Medicine
Bronx, New York

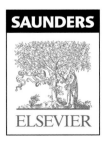

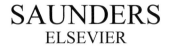

SAUNDERS
ELSEVIER

1600 John F. Kennedy Blvd.
Ste 1800
Philadelphia, PA 19103-2899

CLINICAL NEUROLOGY FOR PSYCHIATRISTS   ISBN-13: 978-1-4160-3074-4
Sixth Edition   ISBN-10: 1-4160-3074-3

Copyright © 2007 by Saunders, an imprint of Elsevier Inc.

All rights reserved. No part of this publication may be reproduced or transmitted in any form or by any means, electronic or mechanical, including photocopying, recording, or any information storage and retrieval system, without permission in writing from the publisher. Permissions may be sought directly from Elsevier's Health Sciences Rights Department in Philadelphia, PA, USA: phone: (+1) 215 239 3804, fax: (+1) 215 239 3805, e-mail: healthpermissions@elsevier.com. You may also complete your request on-line via the Elsevier homepage (http://www.elsevier.com), by selecting 'Customer Support' and then 'Obtaining Permissions'.

Notice

Knowledge and best practice in this field are constantly changing. As new research and experience broaden our knowledge, changes in practice, treatment and drug therapy may become necessary or appropriate. Readers are advised to check the most current information provided (i) on procedures featured or (ii) by the manufacturer of each product to be administered, to verify the recommended dose or formula, the method and duration of administration, and contraindications. It is the responsibility of the practitioner, relying on their own experience and knowledge of the patient, to make diagnoses, to determine dosages and the best treatment for each individual patient, and to take all appropriate safety precautions. To the fullest extent of the law, neither the Publisher nor the Author assumes any liability for any injury and/or damage to persons or property arising out or related to any use of the material contained in this book.

The Publisher

Previous editions copyright (2001, 1995, 1990, 1985, 1982, 1981)

Library of Congress Cataloging-in-Publication Data

Kaufman, David Myland.
   Clinical Neurology for Psychiatrists / David Myland Kaufman. – 6th ed.
     p. ; cm.
   Includes bibliographical references and index.
   ISBN 1-4160-3074-3
    1. Nervous system–Diseases. 2. Neurology. 3. Psychiatrists. I. Title.
   [DNLM: 1. Nervous System Diseases–diagnosis. 2. Diagnosis, Differential.
3. Psychiatry–methods. WL 141 K21c 2007]
RC346.K38 2007
616.8–dc22

                                 2006050035

Editor: Susan Pioli
Editorial Assistant: Joan Ryan
Project Manager: David Saltzberg
Marketing Manager: Laura Meiskey

Printed in China.

Last digit is the print number: 9 8 7 6 5 4 3 2 1

Working together to grow libraries in developing countries

www.elsevier.com | www.bookaid.org | www.sabre.org

ELSEVIER   BOOK AID International   Sabre Foundation

This book is dedicated to the ones I love—Rita, my wife of 35 years, whose love has made everything possible, and our children, Rachel and Bob, Jennifer and William, and Sarah and Josh.

Acknowledgments

In addition to being my wife and best friend, Rita acted as my muse by originally suggesting writing this book by expanding the syllabus for my course, "Clinical Neurology for Psychiatrists," and then giving me numerous ideas for each future edition. Our daughter, Jennifer, with tremendous literary sensibility, added clarity with style. Dr. Eliezer Schnall, my scholarly adviser for this edition, has not only been knowledgeable, sensitive, and meticulous, but always a fine teacher and mensch. For all the previous editions, Mr. Michael Lipton offered similar generous advice. Ms. Meryl Ranzer, Mr. Barry Morden, and Ms. Ann Mannato captured the sense of neurology in their wonderful illustrations.

My attorneys, Mr. Jeffrey A. Lowin, of Morris Cohen LLP, and Mr. H. Joseph Mello, of Thelen Reid & Priest, provided excellent counsel. My students, housestaff, and colleagues at Montefiore Medical Center/Albert Einstein College of Medicine have reviewed each chapter and question-and-answer set. The staff of Montefiore Medical Center and the D. Samuel Gottesman Library of the Albert Einstein College of Medicine have graciously provided me with information and the technology to get more.

I came to Montefiore Medical Center as an intern in 1968 and have remained here to this day. Drs. Spencer Foreman (President of the Medical Center), Byram Karasu (Chair of Psychiatry), Herbert Schaumburg (Chair Emeritus of Neurology), Mark Melher (Chair of Neurology), and Michael Swerdlow (my partner at Neurologic Associates) have created a vibrant, world-renowned medical center that has provided me the framework and encouragement to pursue writing this book and undertake other academic work. At the same time, they have greatly expanded Montefiore into a major, patient-centered, multifaceted, urban academic medical center.

I thank my colleagues who have generously offered reviews of the medical and stylistic aspects of the book: Drs. Andrew Brown, Koshi Cherian, Brian Grosberg, Howard Geyer, Jayson Lerner, Adi Loebl, Mark Milstein, John Nogueira, Irfan Qureshi, Amy Sanders, Gail Solomon, and Jessica Zwerling.

I also thank my editors at Elsevier, Ms. Susan Pioli and Ms. Joan Ryan, who have opened the doors and generated many improvements for this edition. Finally, my thanks goes to Amanda Hellenthal and the team at SPi for their hard work and dedication to this project.

Notes About References

Most chapters provide specific references from the neurologic and general medical literature. In addition, several standard, well-written textbooks contain relevant information about many topics:

1. Biller J: *Practical Neurology DVD Review.* Philadelphia, Lippincott Williams & Wilkins, 2005.
2. Blumenfield M, Strain J (eds): *Psychosomatic Medicine in the 21st Century.* Philadelphia, Lippincott Williams & Wilkins, 2005.
3. Cummings JL, Mega MS: *Neuropsychiatry and Behavioral Neuroscience.* Oxford, Oxford University Press, 2003.
4. Ellison D, Love S, Chimelli L, et al: *Neuropathology: A Reference Text of CNS Pathology,* ed 2. Philadelphia, Mosby, 2004.
5. Feinberg TE, Farah MJ: *Behavioral Neurology and Neuropsychology,* ed 2. New York, McGraw-Hill, 2003.
6. Goetz CG: *Textbook of Clinical Neurology,* ed 2. Philadelphia, WB Saunders, 2003.
7. Heilman KM, Valenstein E: *Clinical Neuropsychology,* ed 4. New York, Oxford University Press, 2003.
8. Pfeffer CR, Solomon GE, Kaufman DM (eds): Neurologic disorders: Developmental and behavioral sequelae. In *Child and Adolescent Psychiatric Clinics of North America.* Philadelphia, WB Saunders, 1999.
9. Pincus J, Tucker G: *Behavioral Neurology,* ed 4. New York, Oxford University Press, 2003.
10. Rizzo M, Eslinger PJ: *Principles and Practice of Behavioral Neurology and Neuropsychology.* Philadelphia, WB Saunders, 2004.
11. Samuels MA, Feske SK (eds): *Office Practice of Neurology,* ed 2, Philadelphia, Churchill Livingstone, 2003.
12. Scheiber SC, Kramer TAM, Adamowski SE (eds): *Core Competencies for Psychiatric Practice: What Clinicians Need to Know. A Report of the American Board of Psychiatry and Neurology, Inc.* Washington, D.C., American Psychiatric Publishing, Inc., 2003.
13. Sirven JI, Malamut BL: *Clinical Neurology of the Older Adult.* Philadelphia, Lippincott Williams & Wilkins, 2002.

Web Sites That Offer Information About Several Areas

(Sites relevant to single areas are listed in each chapter's references and in Appendix 1.)

American Academy of Neurology's Practice Guidelines: *http://www.aan.com/professionals/practice/guideline/index.cfm*

Grateful Med: http://igm.nlm.nih.gov

National Institute of Health: http://info.nih.gov

Physician-Readers, Please Note

Clinical Neurology for Psychiatrists discusses medications, testing, procedures, and other aspects of medical care. Despite their purported effectiveness, many are fraught with side effects, other adverse outcomes, and a low benefit-risk ratio. Discussions in this book are neither recommendations nor medical advice, and they are not intended to apply to individual patients. The physician, who should consult the package insert and the medical literature, must remain responsible for medications' indications, dosage, contraindications, precautions, side effects, and alternatives, including doing nothing. Some aspects of medical care that this book discusses are widely and successfully used for particular purposes but not approved by the Food and Drug Administration (FDA) or other review panel. As regards these unorthodox or "off-label" treatments, as well as conventional ones, this book merely reports their prescription by neurologists and other physicians.

Preface

PURPOSE

I have written *Clinical Neurology for Psychiatrists* from my perspective as a neurologist at a major academic medical center, as a collegial, straightforward guide. In a format combining traditional neuroanatomic correlations with symptom-oriented discussions, the book should assist psychiatrists in learning about modern neurology. It emphasizes neurologic conditions that are frequently occurring, common to psychiatry and neurology, illustrative of a scientific principle, or accompanied by psychiatric comorbidity.

ORGANIZATION AND CONTENT

The organization and content of *Clinical Neurology for Psychiatrists* arose from my experience as Professor of Neurology and Psychiatry at the Albert Einstein College of Medicine, co-founder of a large faculty practice at Montefiore Medical Center, and supervisor of numerous residents; consultation with my colleagues, many of whom are world renowned physicians; and feedback from many of the 15,000 psychiatrists who have attended my course and 42,000 who have purchased previous editions of this book. Learning the material in this book should help readers prepare for examinations, perform effective consultations, and improve their practice and teaching.

Section 1 (Chapters 1–6) reviews classic anatomic neurology and describes how to approach patients with a suspected neurologic disorder, identify central or peripheral nervous system disease, and correlate physical signs. Section 2 (Chapters 7–22) discusses common and otherwise important clinical areas, emphasizing aspects a psychiatrist may encounter. Topics include neurologic illnesses, such as multiple sclerosis, brain tumors, and strokes; common symptoms, such as headaches, chronic pain, and seizures; and conditions with many different manifestations, such as involuntary movement disorders and traumatic brain injury. For each topic, chapters describe the relevant history, neurologic and psychiatric comorbidity, easily performed office and bedside examinations, appropriate laboratory tests, differential diagnosis, and management options. I have located and discussed overarching concepts that correlate basic science with neurologic illnesses and link various illnesses.

Many chapters contain outlines for a bedside examination; reproductions of standard bedside tests, such as the Mini-Mental Status Examination (MMSE), hand-held visual acuity card, and Abnormal Involuntary Movement Scale (AIMS); and references to recent articles and reviews. Appendices, which contain information pertaining to most chapters, include Patient and Family Support Groups (Appendix 1); Costs of Tests and Treatments (Appendix 2); Diseases Transmitted by Chromosome Abnormalities, Mitochondria Abnormalities, and Excessive Trinucleotide Repeats (Appendix 3); and Chemical and Biological Neurotoxins (Appendix 4).

The book also reviews neurologic conditions that have entered the public arena. Psychiatrists are liable to be drawn into debates involving their own patients or the medical community as a whole and should be well-versed in the intricacies of the following conditions that this book describes:

- Amyotrophic lateral sclerosis and multiple sclerosis as battlegrounds of assisted suicide
- Meningomyelocele with Arnold-Chiari malformation as an indication for late term abortion and the value of spending limited resources on this fatal or severely limiting condition
- Cancer (malignant) pain as the fulcrum for legalizing marijuana and heroin
- Opioid (narcotic) treatment for chronic benign pain, such as low back pain
- Parkinson's disease, spinal cord injury, and other disorders amenable to research and treatment with stem cells
- Persistent vegetative state and continuing life-support technology

ADDITIONS AND OTHER CHANGES FOR THE SIXTH EDITION

The first five editions of *Clinical Neurology for Psychiatrists* have enjoyed considerable success in the United States, Canada, and abroad. The book has been translated into Japanese, Italian, and Korean. In the sixth edition, rewritten 5 years after the previous one, I have clarified my presentations, discussed recent developments in many areas of neurology, and added computer generated graphics and clinical-anatomic illustrations. For the question-and-answer sections, I have increased the number of questions, refined them, expanded the discussions, and provided more illustrations to give these sections greater didactic power.

This edition also references the definitions from the Diagnostic and Statistical Manual of Mental Disorder, 4th Edition, Text Revision (DSM-IV-TR) that pertain to various neurologic disorders. Along the same line, it points out occasional discrepancies and omissions.

In addition to the updates, this edition adds many new subjects:

- Descriptions of altered mental status, including the minimally responsive state and minimal cognitive impairment
- Neurotoxins, including industrial toxins and marine poisons, and pseudoneurotoxic disease
- Nutritional deficiencies and errors of metabolism, especially involving homocysteine
- Psychiatric comorbidity of epilepsy, migraine, multiple sclerosis, Parkinson's disease, stroke, Tourette's disease, and other neurologic illnesses
- Standard clinical assessment tools, such as the Alzheimer's Disease Assessment Scale Cognitive Section (ADAS-Cog) and the Epworth Sleepiness Scale
- Treatments for common neurologic illnesses
  - Deafness: cochlear implant
  - Epilepsy: antiepileptic drugs, deep brain stimulation, and vagus nerve stimulation
  - Involuntary movements: deep brain stimulation
  - Multiple sclerosis: immunomodulators and their complications
  - Chronic pain: stimulators, opioid maintenance, adjuvant medications
  - Uses of psychiatric medications for neurologic illnesses, such as antidepressants for migraine, chronic pain, and peripheral neuropathy; and antipsychotic agents for dementia, epilepsy, and other conditions

DIDACTIC DEVICES: THE VISUAL APPROACH AND QUESTION-AND-ANSWER SECTIONS

The book—like much of the practice of neurology—relies on a visual approach. It provides abundant illustrations, including numerous sketches of "patients," that personify or reinforce clinical descriptions, correlate the basic science with clinical findings, and serve as the basis for question-and-answer learning. This approach conforms to neurologists' predilection to "diagnose by inspection." For example, they rely on their observations for the diagnoses of gait abnormalities, psychogenic neurologic deficits, neurocutaneous disorders, strokes, and involuntary movements. In addition, the book reproduces neurologic test results, which are also visual records, such as those of computed tomography (CT), magnetic resonance imaging (MRI), and electroencephalography (EEG).

Clinical Neurology for Psychiatrists also complements the text with question-and-answer sections at the end of most chapters and at the conclusion of the book. Sections at the end of chapters refer to material discussed within that chapter, whereas those questions at the book's conclusion tend to require comparison of neurologic disorders that have appeared under different headings. In Chapter 4, before the question-and-answer review of the preceding chapters' material, the book offers a guide for preparing for standardized tests.

The Albert Einstein College of Medicine and many other medical schools have come to rely on similar "problem-based interactive studying"—question-and-answer or problem solving—as meaningful and efficient. The book's questions do not merely quiz the reader, but form an integral part of the learning experience. In fact, many readers find that these question-and-answer sections are the single most informative portion of the book and term them "high yield." In keeping with the visual emphasis of the book, many of the questions are based on sketches of patients and reproductions of MRIs, CTs, and EEGs.

Readers should be cautioned that, for educational purposes, I have highlighted certain aspects of cases and disregarded others. Thus, unencumbered by many real-world complexities, cases may appear more straightforward than those physicians encounter in practice.

ONE CAVEAT

Clinical Neurology for Psychiatrists expects well-educated and thoughtful readers. It demands attention and work, and asks them to follow a rigorous course in order to master difficult material. Readers should find the book, like the practice of medicine, complex and challenging, but at the same time rich and fulfilling.

Despite the additions of text, illustrations, and questions, the sixth edition of *Clinical Neurology for Psychiatrists* remains manageable in size, depth, and scope. It is still succinct enough for psychiatrists to read and enjoy from cover to cover.

David Myland Kaufman, M.D.

Contents

First Encounter with a Patient: Examination and Formulation

Despite the ready availability of sophisticated tests, the "hands on" neurologic examination remains the fundamental aspect of the specialty. Beloved by neurologists, this examination provides a vivid portrayal of both function and illness. When neurologists say they have seen a case of a particular illness, they mean that they have really *seen* it.

When a patient's history suggests a neurologic illness, the neurologic examination may unequivocally demonstrate it. Even if they themselves will not actually be examining patients in the physical sense, psychiatrists should appreciate certain neurologic signs and be able to assess a neurologist's conclusion.

Physicians should examine patients systematically. They should test interesting areas in detail during a sequential evaluation of the nervous system's major components. Physicians should try to adhere to the routine while avoiding omissions and duplications. Despite obvious dysfunction of one part of the nervous system, physicians should evaluate all major areas. A physician can complete an initial or screening neurologic examination in about 20 minutes and return to perform special testing of particular areas, such as the mental status.

EXAMINATION

Physicians should note the patient's age, sex, and handedness and then review the primary symptom, present illness, medical history, family history, and social history. They should include detailed questions about the primary symptom, associated symptoms, and possible etiologic factors. If a patient cannot relate the history, the physician might interrupt the process to look for language, memory, or other cognitive deficits. Many chapters in Section 2 of this book contain outlines of standard questions related to common symptoms.

After obtaining the history, physicians should anticipate the patient's neurologic deficits and be prepared to look for disease, primarily of the central nervous system (CNS) or the peripheral nervous system (PNS). At this point, without yielding to rigid preconceptions, the physician should have developed some insight about the problem at hand.

Then physicians should look for the site of involvement (i.e., "localize the lesion"). A hallowed goal of the examination and "localization" is useful in most cases. However, it is often somewhat of an art and inapplicable in several important neurologic illnesses.

The examination, which overall remains irreplaceable in diagnosis, consists of a functional neuroanatomy demonstration: mental status, cranial nerves, motor system, reflexes, sensation, and cerebellar system (Table 1-1). This format should be followed during every examination. Until it is memorized, a copy should

---

TABLE 1-1 ■ Neurologic Examination

Mental status
  Cooperation
  Orientation (to month, year, place, and any physical or mental deficits)
  Language
  Memory for immediate, recent, and past events
  Higher intellectual functions: arithmetic, similarities/differences
Cranial nerves
  I Smell
  II Visual acuity, visual fields, optic fundi
  III, IV, VI Pupil size and reactivity, extraocular motion
  V Corneal reflex and facial sensation
  VII Strength of upper and lower facial muscles, taste
  VIII Hearing
  IX-XI Articulation, palate movement, gag reflex
  XII Tongue movement
Motor system
  Limb strength
  Spasticity, flaccidity, or fasciculations
  Abnormal movements (e.g., tremor, chorea)
Reflexes
  DTRs
    Biceps, triceps, brachioradialis, quadriceps, Achilles
  Pathologic reflexes
    Extensor plantar response (Babinski sign), frontal release
Sensation
  Position, vibration, stereognosis
  Pain
Cerebellar system
  Finger-to-nose and heel-to-shin tests
  Rapid alternating movements
  Gait

DTRs, deep tendon reflexes.

be taken to the patient's bedside to serve both as a reminder and a place to record neurologic findings.

The examination usually starts with an assessment of the mental status because it is the most important neurologic function, and impairments may preclude an accurate assessment of other neurologic functions. The examiner should consider specific intellectual deficits, such as language impairment (see Aphasia, Chapter 8), as well as general intellectual decline (see Dementia, Chapter 7). Tests of cranial nerves may reveal malfunction of nerves either individually or in groups, such as the *ocular motility nerves* (III, IV, and VI) and the *cerebellopontine angle nerves* (V, VII, and VIII) (see Chapter 4).

The examination of the motor system is usually performed more to detect the pattern than the severity of weakness. Whether weakness is mild to moderate (*paresis*) or complete (*plegia*), the pattern, rather than severity, offers more clues to localization. On a practical level, of course, the severity of the paresis determines whether a patient will remain able to walk, require a wheelchair, or stay bedridden.

Three common important patterns of paresis are easy to recognize. If the lower face, arm, and leg on one side of the body are paretic, the pattern is called *hemiparesis* and it indicates damage to the contralateral cerebral hemisphere or brainstem. Both legs being weak, *paraparesis*, usually indicates spinal cord damage. Paresis of the distal portion of all the limbs indicates PNS rather than CNS damage.

Eliciting two categories of reflexes assists in determining whether paresis or another neurologic abnormality originates in the CNS or PNS. *Deep tendon reflexes (DTRs)* are normally present with uniform reactivity (speed and forcefulness) in all limbs, but neurologic injury often alters their activity or symmetry. In general, with CNS injury that includes corticospinal tract damage, DTRs are hyperactive, whereas with PNS injury, DTRs are hypoactive.

In contrast to DTRs, *pathologic reflexes* are not normally elicitable beyond infancy. If found, they are a sign of CNS damage. The most widely recognized pathologic reflex is the famous *Babinski sign*. Current medical conversations justify a clarification of the terminology regarding this sign. After plantar stimulation, the great toe normally moves downward (i.e., it has a flexor response). With brain or spinal cord damage, plantar stimulation typically causes the great toe to move upward (i.e., to have an extensor response). This reflex extensor movement, which is a manifestation of CNS damage, is the Babinski sign (see Fig. 19-3). It and other signs may be "present" or "elicited," but they are never "positive" or "negative." Just as a traffic stop sign may be either present or absent but never positive or negative, a Babinski sign is either present or elicited.

Frontal release signs, which are other pathologic reflexes, reflect frontal lobe injury. They are helpful in indicating an "organic" basis for a change in personality. In addition, to a limited degree, they are associated with intellectual impairment (see Chapter 7).

The sensory system examination is long and tedious. Moreover, unlike abnormal DTRs and Babinski signs, which are reproducible, objective, and virtually impossible to mimic, the sensory examination relies almost entirely on the patient's report. Its subjective nature has led to the practice of disregarding the sensory examination if it varies from the rest of the evaluation. Under most circumstances, the best approach is to test the major sensory modalities in a clear anatomic order and tentatively accept the patient's report.

Depending on the nature of the suspected disorder, the physician may test sensation of position, vibration, and stereognosis (appreciation of an object's form by touching it)—all of which are carried in the posterior columns of the spinal cord. Pain (pinprick) sensation, which is carried in the lateral columns, should be tested carefully with a nonpenetrating, disposable instrument, such as a cotton swab.

Cerebellar function is evaluated by observing the patient for intention tremor and incoordination during several standard maneuvers that include the *finger-to-nose test* and rapid repetition of *alternating movement test* (see Chapter 2). If at all possible, physicians should watch the patient walk because a normal gait requires intact CNS and PNS motor pathways, coordination, proprioception, and balance. Moreover, all these systems must be well integrated.

Examining the gait is probably the single most valuable assessment of the motor aspects of the nervous system. Physicians should watch not only for cerebellar-based incoordination (*ataxia*), but also for hemiparesis and other signs of corticospinal tract dysfunction, involuntary movement disorders, apraxia (see Table 2-3), and even orthopedic conditions. In addition, physicians will find that certain cognitive impairments are associated with particular patterns of gait impairment. Whatever its pattern, gait impairment is not merely a neurologic or orthopedic sign, but a condition that routinely leads to fatal falls and permanent incapacity for numerous elderly people each year.

FORMULATION

Although somewhat ritualistic, a succinct and cogent *formulation* remains the basis of neurologic problem solving. The classic formulation consists of an appraisal of the four aspects of the examination: symptoms, signs, localization, and differential diagnosis. The clinician might also have to support a conclusion that neurologic disease is present or, equally important, absent. For this step, psychogenic signs must be separated, if only tentatively, from neurologic ("organic") ones.

Evidence must be demonstrable for a psychogenic or neurologic etiology while acknowledging that neither is a diagnosis of exclusion. Of course, as if to confuse the situation, patients often manifest grossly exaggerated symptoms of a neurologic illness (see Chapter 3).

Localization of neurologic lesions requires the clinician to determine at least whether the illness affects the CNS, PNS, or muscles (see Chapters 2 through 6). Precise localization of lesions within them is possible and generally expected. The physician must also establish whether the nervous system is affected diffusely or in a discrete area. The site and extent of neurologic damage will indicate certain diseases. A readily apparent example is that cerebrovascular accidents (strokes) and tumors generally involve a discrete area of the brain, but Alzheimer's disease usually causes widespread, symmetric changes.

Finally, the differential diagnosis is the disease or diseases—up to three—most consistent with the patient's symptoms and signs. In addition, the list should include illnesses that, although unlikely, would be life threatening if present. When specific diseases cannot be suggested, major categories, such as "structural lesions," should be offered.

A typical formulation might be as follows: "Mr. Jones, a 56-year-old man, has had left-sided headaches for 2 months and had a generalized seizure on the day before admission. He is lethargic. He has papilledema, a right hemiparesis with hyperactive DTRs, and a Babinski sign. The lesion seems to be in the left cerebral hemisphere. Most likely, he has a tumor, but a stroke is possible." This formulation briefly recapitulates the crucial symptoms, positive and negative elements of the history, and physical findings. It tacitly assumes that neurologic disease is present because of the obvious, objective physical findings. The localization is based on the history of seizures, the right-sided hemiparesis, and abnormal reflexes. The differential diagnosis is based on the high probability of these conditions being caused by a discrete cerebral lesion.

To review, the physician should present a formulation that answers *The Four Questions of Neurology:*

- What are the *symptoms* of *neurologic* disease?
- What are the *signs* of *neurologic* disease?
- *Where* is the lesion?
- *What* is the lesion?

RESPONDING TO CONSULTATIONS

Psychiatry residents in many programs rotate through neurology departments where they are expected to provide neurology consultations solicited by physicians working in the emergency department, medical clinic, and other referring services. When responding to a request for a neurology consultation, the psychiatry resident must work with a variation of the traditional summary-and-formulation format. The response should primarily or exclusively answer the question posed by the referring physician. Moreover, the consultant should not expect to follow the patient throughout the illness, much less establish a long-term doctor-patient relationship. Rather, attention should be directed to the referring physician, who is shouldering the burden of primary care and may or may not accept the consultant's suggestions.

Before beginning the consultation, both the referring physician and consultant should be clear about the reason for it. The consultation may concern a single aspect of the case, such as the importance of a neurologic finding, the significance of a computed tomography report, or whether a given treatment would be best. The consultant should insist on a specific question and ultimately answer that question. Eventually, the differential diagnosis should contain no more than three possible etiologies—starting with the most likely. Even at tertiary care institutions, common conditions arise commonly. Just as "hoof beats are usually from horses, not zebras," patients are more likely to have hemiparesis from a stroke than from an unwitnessed seizure.

Consultants should be helpful by ordering routine tests not by merely suggesting them. At the same time, consulting psychiatry residents should not suggest hazardous tests or treatments without obtaining a second opinion.

Finally, consultants should develop an awareness of the entire situation, which often contains incomplete and conflicting elements. They should also be mindful of the position of the referring physician and patient.

Central Nervous System Disorders

Lesions in the two components of the central nervous system (CNS)—the brain and the spinal cord—typically cause paresis, sensory loss, and visual deficits (Table 2-1). In addition, lesions in the cerebral hemispheres (the cerebrum) cause neuropsychologic disorders. Symptoms and signs of CNS disorders must be contrasted to those resulting from peripheral nervous system (PNS) and psychogenic disorders. Neurologists tend to rely on the physical rather than mental status evaluation, thereby honoring the belief that "one Babinski sign is worth a thousand words."

SIGNS OF CEREBRAL HEMISPHERE LESIONS

Of the various signs of cerebral hemisphere injury, the most prominent is usually *contralateral hemiparesis* (Table 2-2): weakness of the lower face, trunk, arm, and leg opposite to the side of the lesion. It results from damage to the *corticospinal tract,* which is also called the *pyramidal tract* (Fig. 2-1). During the corticospinal tract's entire path from the cerebral cortex to the anterior horn cells of the spinal cord, it is considered the *upper motor neuron (UMN)* (Fig. 2-2). The anterior horn cells, which are part of the PNS, are the beginning of the *lower motor neuron (LMN).* The division of the motor system into upper and lower motor neurons is a basic tenet of clinical neurology.

Cerebral lesions that damage the corticospinal tract are characterized by **signs of UMN injury** (Figs. 2-2, 2-3, 2-4, and 2-5):

- Paresis with muscle spasticity
- Hyperactive deep tendon reflexes (DTRs)
- Babinski signs

In contrast, peripheral nerve lesions, including anterior horn cell or motor neuron diseases, are associated with **signs of LMN injury**:

- Paresis with muscle flaccidity and atrophy
- Hypoactive DTRs
- No Babinski signs

Cerebral lesions are not the only cause of hemiparesis. Because the corticospinal tract has such a long course (Fig. 2-1), lesions in the brainstem and spinal cord as well as the cerebrum may produce hemiparesis and other signs of UMN damage. Signs pointing to injury in various regions of the CNS can help identify the origin of hemiparesis, that is, localize the lesion.

Another indication of a cerebral lesion is loss of certain sensory modalities over one half of the body, that is, *hemisensory loss* (Fig. 2-6). A patient with a cerebral lesion characteristically loses contralateral position sensation, two-point discrimination, and the ability to identify objects by touch (stereognosis). Loss of those modalities is often called a "cortical" sensory loss.

Pain sensation, a "primary" sense, is initially received by the thalamus. Because the thalamus is just above the brainstem, pain perception is retained with cerebral lesions. For example, patients with

TABLE 2-1 ■ Signs of Common CNS Lesions

Cerebral hemisphere*
  Hemiparesis with hyperactive deep tendon reflexes, spasticity, and Babinski sign
  Hemisensory loss
  Homonymous hemianopsia
  Partial seizures
  Aphasia, hemi-inattention, and dementia
  Pseudobulbar palsy
Basal ganglia*
  Movement disorders: parkinsonism, athetosis, chorea, and hemiballismus
Brainstem
  Cranial nerve palsy with contralateral hemiparesis
  Internuclear ophthalmoplegia (MLF syndrome)
  Nystagmus
  Bulbar palsy
Cerebellum
  Tremor on intention^
  Impaired rapid alternating movements (dysdiadochokinesia)^
  Ataxic gait
  Scanning speech
Spinal cord
  Paraparesis or quadriparesis
  Sensory loss up to a "level"
  Bladder, bowel, and sexual dysfunction

CNS, central nervous system; MLF, medial longitudinal fasciculus.
*Signs contralateral to lesions.
^Signs ipsilateral to lesions.

TABLE 2-2 ■ Signs of Common Cerebral Lesions

Either hemisphere*
    Hemiparesis with hyperactive DTRs and a Babinski sign
    Hemisensory loss
    Homonymous hemianopsia
    Partial seizures: simple, complex, or secondarily generalized
Dominant hemisphere
    Aphasias: fluent, nonfluent, conduction, isolation
    Gerstmann's syndrome: acalculia, agraphia, finger agnosia, and left-right
        confusion
    Alexia without agraphia
Nondominant hemisphere
    Hemi-inattention
    Anosognosia
    Constructional apraxia
Both hemispheres
    Dementia
    Pseudobulbar palsy

DTRs, deep tendon reflexes.
*Signs contralateral to lesions.

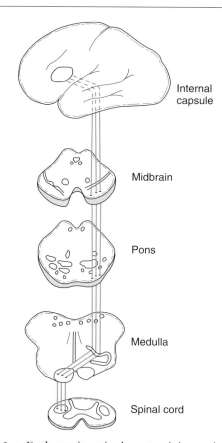

FIGURE 2-1 ■ Each corticospinal tract originates in the cerebral cortex, passes through the internal capsule, and descends into the brainstem. It crosses in the pyramids, which are long protuberances on the inferior portion of the medulla, to descend in the spinal cord as the *lateral corticospinal tract.* It terminates by forming a synapse with the *anterior horn cells* of the spinal cord, which give rise to peripheral nerves. The corticospinal tract is sometimes called the *pyramidal* tract because it crosses in the pyramids. A complementary tract, which originates in the basal ganglia, is called the *extrapyramidal* tract.

cerebral infarctions may be unable to specify a painful area of the body but will still feel the pain's intensity and discomfort. Also, patients in intractable pain did not obtain relief when they underwent experimental surgical resection of the cerebral cortex. The other aspect of the thalamus' role in sensing pain is seen when patients with thalamic infarctions develop spontaneous, disconcerting, burning pains over the contralateral body (see thalamic pain, Chapter 14).

Visual loss of the same half-field in each eye, *homonymous hemianopsia* (Fig. 2-7), is a characteristic sign of a contralateral cerebral lesion. Other equally characteristic visual losses are associated with lesions involving the eye, optic nerve, or optic tract (see Chapters 4 and 12). Because they would be situated far from the visual pathway, lesions in the brainstem, cerebellum, or spinal cord do not cause visual field loss.

Another conspicuous sign of a cerebral hemisphere lesion is *partial seizures* (see Chapter 10). The major varieties of partial seizures—elementary, complex, and secondarily generalized—result from cerebral lesions. In fact, about 90% of partial complex seizures originate in the temporal lobe.

Although hemiparesis, hemisensory loss, homonymous hemianopsia, and partial seizures may result from lesions of either cerebral hemisphere, several neuropsychologic deficits are referable to either the dominant or nondominant hemisphere. Because approximately 95% of people are right-handed, unless physicians know otherwise about an individual patient, they should assume that the left hemisphere serves as the dominant hemisphere.

Signs of Damage of the Dominant, Nondominant, or Both Cerebral Hemispheres

Lesions of the dominant hemisphere usually cause language impairment, *aphasia,* a prominent and frequently occurring neuropsychologic deficit (see Chapter 8). In addition to producing aphasia, dominant hemisphere lesions typically produce an accompanying right hemiparesis because the corticospinal tract sits adjacent to the language centers (see Fig. 8-1).

When the *non*dominant parietal lobe is injured, patients often have one or more characteristic neuropsychologic deficits that comprise the "nondominant syndrome" as well as left-sided hemiparesis or homonymous hemianopsia. For example, patients may

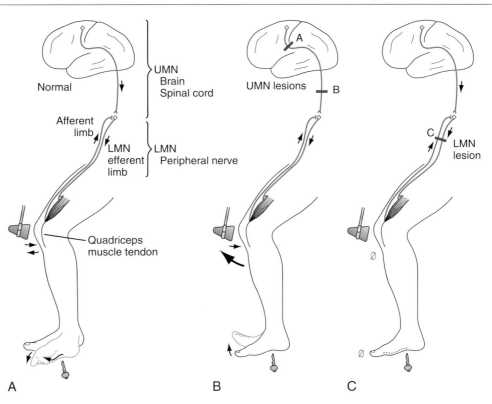

FIGURE 2-2 ■ *A,* Normally, when the quadriceps tendon is struck with the percussion hammer, a deep tendon reflex (DTR) is elicited. In addition, when the sole of the foot is stroked to elicit a plantar reflex, the big toe bends downward (flexes). *B,* When brain or spinal cord lesions involve the corticospinal tract and cause upper motor neuron (UMN) damage, the DTR is hyperactive, and the plantar reflex is extensor (i.e., a Babinski sign is present). *C,* When peripheral nerve injury causes lower motor neuron (LMN) damage, the DTR is hypoactive and the plantar reflex is absent.

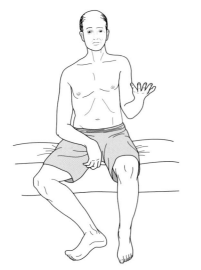

FIGURE 2-3 ■ This patient with severe right hemiparesis typically has weakness of the right arm, leg, and lower face. The right-sided facial weakness causes the widened palpebral fissure and flat nasolabial fold; however, the forehead muscles are normal (see Chapter 4 regarding this discrepancy). The right arm is limp, and the elbow, wrist, and fingers are flexed. The right hemiparesis also causes the right leg to be externally rotated and the hip and knee to be flexed.

neglect or ignore left-sided visual and tactile stimuli (*hemi-inattention,* see Chapter 8). Patients often fail to use their left arm and leg more because they neglect

their limbs than because of paresis. When they have left hemiparesis, patients may not even acknowledge it (*anosognosia*). Many patients lose their ability to arrange matchsticks into certain patterns or copy simple forms (*constructional apraxia,* Fig. 2-8).

All signs discussed so far are referable to unilateral cerebral hemisphere damage. Bilateral cerebral hemisphere damage produces several important disturbances. One of them, *pseudobulbar palsy,* best known for producing emotional lability, results from bilateral *corticobulbar tract* damage (see Chapter 4). The corticobulbar tract, like its counterpart the corticospinal tract, originates in the motor cortex of the posterior portion of the frontal lobe. It innervates the brainstem motor nuclei that in turn innervate the head and neck muscles. Head trauma and many illnesses, including cerebral infarctions (strokes) and frontotemporal dementia (see Chapter 7), are apt to strike the corticobulbar tract and the surrounding frontal lobes and thereby cause pseudobulbar palsy.

Damage of both cerebral hemispheres—from large or multiple discrete lesions, degenerative diseases, or metabolic abnormalities—also causes dementia (see Chapter 7). In addition, because CNS damage that causes dementia must be extensive and severe, it usually produces at least subtle neurologic findings, such as hyperactive DTRs, Babinski signs, mild gait impairment, and frontal lobe release reflexes. Many illnesses that cause dementia, such as Alzheimer's

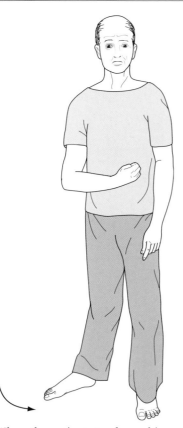

FIGURE 2-4 ■ When the patient stands up, his weakened arm retains its flexed posture. His right leg remains externally rotated, but he can walk by swinging it in a circular path. This maneuver is effective but results in *circumduction* or a *hemiparetic gait.*

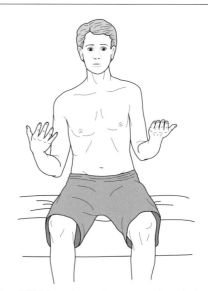

FIGURE 2-5 ■ Mild hemiparesis may not be obvious. To exaggerate a subtle hemiparesis, the physician has asked this patient to extend both arms with his palms held upright, as though each outstretched hand were holding a water glass or both hands were supporting a pizza box (the "pizza test"). After a minute, a weakened arm slowly sinks (drifts), and the palm turns inward (pronates). The imaginary glass in the right hand would spill the water inward and the imaginary pizza would slide to the right. This arm's drift and pronation represent a *forme fruste* of the posture seen with severe paresis (Fig. 2-3).

disease, do not cause overt findings, such as hemiparesis. In acute care hospitals, the five conditions most likely to cause discrete unilateral or bilateral cerebral lesions are strokes, primary or metastatic brain tumors, trauma, complications of acquired immune deficiency syndrome (AIDS, see Chapter 7), and multiple sclerosis (MS, see Chapter 15). (Section 2 offers detailed discussions of these conditions.)

SIGNS OF BASAL GANGLIA LESIONS

The basal ganglia, located subcortically in the cerebrum, are composed of the globus pallidus and the putamen (the striatum), the substantia nigra, and the subthalamic nucleus (corpus of Luysii) (see Fig. 18-1). They give rise to the *extrapyramidal* tract, which modulates the corticospinal (pyramidal) tract. The extrapyramidal tract controls muscle tone, regulates motor activity, and generates the postural reflexes through its efferent fibers that play on the cerebral cortex, thalamus, and other CNS structures. However, the extrapyramidal tract's efferent fibers are confined to the brain and do not act directly on the spinal cord or LMNs.

Signs of basal ganglia injury include a group of fascinating, often dramatic, *involuntary movement disorders* (see Chapter 18):

- *Parkinsonism* is the combination of resting tremor, rigidity, bradykinesia (slowness of movement) or akinesia (absence of movement), and postural abnormalities. Minor features include micrographia and festinating gait (Table 2-3). Parkinsonism usually results from substantia nigra degeneration (Parkinson's disease and related illnesses), dopamine-blocking antipsychotic medications, or toxins.
- *Athetosis* is the slow, continuous, writhing movement of the fingers, hands, face, and throat. Kernicterus or other perinatal basal ganglia injury usually causes it.
- *Chorea* is intermittent, randomly located, jerking of limbs and the trunk. The best-known example occurs in *Huntington's* disease (previously called "Huntington's chorea"), in which the caudate nuclei characteristically atrophy.
- *Hemiballismus* is the intermittent flinging of the arm and leg on one side of the body. It is classically associated with small infarctions of the contralateral subthalamic nucleus, but similar lesions in other basal ganglia may be responsible.

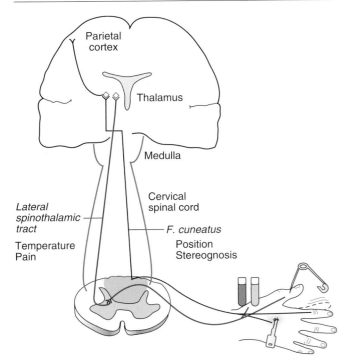

FIGURE 2-6 ■ Peripheral nerves carry pain and temperature sensations to the spinal cord. After a synapse, these sensations cross and ascend in the *contralateral lateral spinothalamic tract* (*blue*) to terminate in the thalamus. From there, other tracts relay the sensations to the limbic system and brainstem as well as the cerebral cortex. In contrast, the peripheral nerves also carry position sense (tested by movement of the distal finger joint) and stereognosis (tested by tactile identification of common objects) to the *ipsilateral f. cuneatus* and *f. gracilis*, which together constitute the spinal cord's *posterior columns* (*light blue*) (Fig. 2-15). Unlike pain and temperature sensation, these sensations rise in ipsilateral tracts (*black*). They cross in the decussation of the medial lemniscus, which is in the medulla, synapse in the thalamus, and terminate in the parietal cortex. (To avoid spreading blood-borne illnesses, examiners should not use a pin when testing pain.)

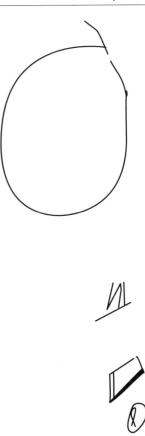

FIGURE 2-8 ■ With constructional apraxia from a right parietal lobe infarction, a 68-year-old woman was hardly able to complete a circle (*top figure*). She could not draw a square on request (*second highest figure*) or even copy one (*third highest figure*). She spontaneously tried to draw a circle and began to retrace it (*bottom figure*). Her constructional apraxia consists of the rotation of the forms, perseveration of certain lines, and the incompleteness of the second and lowest figures. In addition, the figures tend toward the right-hand side of the page, which indicates that she has neglect of the left-hand side of the page, that is, left hemi-inattention.

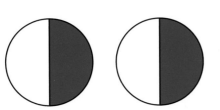

FIGURE 2-7 ■ In homonymous hemianopsia, the same half of the visual field is lost in each eye. In this case, a right homonymous hemianopsia is attributable to damage to the left cerebral hemisphere. This sketch portrays the standard visual field losses from the patient's perspective (see Figs. 4-1 and 12-9).

TABLE 2-3 ■ Gait Abnormalities Associated with CNS Disorders

Gait	Associated Illness	Figure
Apraxic	Normal pressure hydrocephalus	7-7
Astasia-Abasia	Psychogenic disorders	3-4
Ataxic	Cerebellar damage	2-13
Festinating (*marche à petits pas*)	Parkinson's disease	18-9
Hemiparetic	Cerebrovascular accidents	
Circumduction		2-4
Spastic hemiparesis		13-3
Steppage	Tabes dorsalis (CNS syphilis) Peripheral neuropathies	2-20
Waddling	Duchenne's dystrophy and other myopathies	6-4

CNS, central nervous system.

In general, when damage is restricted to the extra-pyramidal tract, as in many cases of hemiballismus and athetosis, patients have no paresis, DTR abnormalities, or Babinski signs—signs of corticospinal (pyramidal) tract damage. More important, in many of these conditions, patients have no cognitive impairment or other neuropsychologic abnormality. On the other hand, several involuntary movement disorders, in which the cerebrum as well as the basal ganglia is affected, are notoriously associated with dementia, depression, or psychosis. Noteworthy examples of this clinical combination include Huntington's disease, Wilson's disease, and advanced Parkinson's disease (see Table 18-4).

Unlike illnesses that affect the cerebrum, most basal ganglia diseases progress slowly, cause bilateral damage, and result from biochemical abnormalities rather than discrete structural lesions. With unilateral basal ganglia damage, signs develop contralateral to the damage. For example, hemiballismus results from infarction of the contralateral subthalamic nucleus, and unilateral parkinsonism ("hemiparkinsonism") results from degeneration of the contralateral substantia nigra.

SIGNS OF BRAINSTEM LESIONS

The brainstem contains the cranial nerve nuclei, the corticospinal tracts and other "long tracts" that travel between the cerebral hemispheres and the limbs, cerebellar afferent (inflow) and efferent (outflow) tracts, and several largely self-contained systems. Combinations of cranial nerve and long tract signs indicate the presence and location of a brainstem lesion. The localization should be supported by the *absence* of signs of cerebral injury, such as visual field cuts and neuropsychologic deficits. For example, brainstem injuries cause *diplopia* (double vision) because of cranial nerve impairment, but visual acuity and visual fields remain normal because the visual pathways, which pass from the optic chiasm to the cerebral hemispheres, do not travel within the brainstem (see Fig. 4-1). Similarly, a right hemiparesis associated with a left third cranial nerve palsy indicates that the lesion is in the brainstem and that neither aphasia nor dementia will be present.

Massive brainstem injuries, such as extensive infarctions or barbiturate overdoses, cause coma, but otherwise brainstem injuries do not impair consciousness or mentation. With the exception of MS and metastatic tumors, few illnesses simultaneously damage the brainstem and the cerebrum.

Several brainstem syndromes are important because they illustrate critical anatomic relationships, such as the location of the cranial nerve nuclei or the course of the corticospinal tract; however, none of them involves neuropsychologic abnormalities. Although each syndrome has an eponym, for practical purposes it is only necessary to identify the clinical findings and, if appropriate, attribute them to a lesion in one of *three divisions of the brainstem* (Fig. 2-9):

- Midbrain
- Pons
- Medulla

Whichever the division, most brainstem lesions consist of an occlusion of a small branch of the basilar or vertebral arteries.

In the midbrain, where the oculomotor (third cranial) nerve passes through the descending corticospinal tract, both pathways can be damaged by a single small infarction. Patients with oculomotor nerve paralysis and contralateral hemiparesis typically have a midbrain lesion ipsilateral to the paretic eye (see Fig. 4-9).

Patients with abducens (sixth cranial) nerve paralysis and contralateral hemiparesis likewise have a pons lesion ipsilateral to the paretic eye (see Fig. 4-11).

Lateral medullary infarctions create a classic but complex picture. Patients have paralysis of the ipsilateral palate because of damage to cranial nerves IX through XI; ipsilateral facial numbness (*hypalgesia*) (Greek, decreased sensitivity to pain) because of damage to cranial nerve V, with contralateral anesthesia of the body (*alternating hypalgesia*) because of ascending spinothalamic tract damage; and ipsilateral ataxia because of ipsilateral cerebellar dysfunction. Fortunately, it is unnecessary to recall all the features of this syndrome: physicians need only to realize that those cranial nerve palsies and the alternating hypalgesia, without cognitive impairment, characterize a lower brainstem (medullary) lesion (Fig. 2-10).

Although these particular brainstem syndromes are distinctive, the most frequently observed sign of brainstem dysfunction is *nystagmus* (repetitive jerk-like eye movements, usually simultaneously of both eyes). Resulting from any type of injury of the brainstem's large vestibular nuclei, nystagmus can be a manifestation of various disorders, including intoxication with alcohol, phenytoin (Dilantin), or barbiturates; ischemia of the vertebrobasilar artery system; MS; Wernicke-Korsakoff syndrome; or viral labyrinthitis. Among individuals who have ingested phencyclidine (PCP), characteristically course vertical and horizontal (three directional) nystagmus accompanies an agitated delirium and markedly reduced sensitivity to pain and cold temperatures. Unilateral nystagmus may be a component of *internuclear ophthalmoplegia,* a disorder of ocular motility in which the brainstem's medial longitudinal fasciculus (MLF) is damaged. The usual cause is MS or a small infarction (see Chapters 4 and 15).

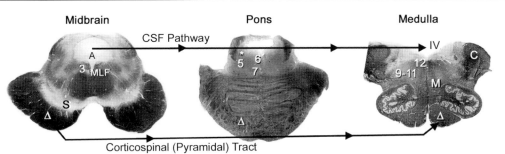

FIGURE 2-9 ■ Myelin-stains of the three divisions of the brainstem—midbrain, pons, and medulla—show several clinically important tracts, the cerebrospinal fluid (CSF) pathway, and motor nuclei of the cranial nerves. *Midbrain,* The midbrain (Greek, *meso,* middle) is identifiable by its distinctive silhouette and gently curved (unstained) substantia nigra (S). The aqueduct of Sylvius (A) is surrounded by the periaqueductal gray matter. Below the aqueduct, near the midline, lie the oculomotor (3) and trochlear (not pictured) cranial nerve nuclei. The nearby medial longitudinal fasciculus (MLF), which ascends from the pons, terminates in the oculomotor nuclei. The large, deeply stained cerebral peduncle, inferior to the substantia nigra, contains the corticospinal (pyramidal [Δ]) tract. Originating in the cerebral cortex, the corticospinal tract descends through the midbrain, pons, and medulla. It crosses in the medulla's pyramids to continue within the contralateral spinal cord. CSF flows downward from the lateral ventricles through the aqueduct of Sylvius into the fourth ventricle (IV), which overlies the lower pons and medulla. CSF exits from the fourth ventricle into the subarachnoid space. (Also see the drawing [Fig. 4-5], computer-generated rendition [Fig. 18-2], and sketch [Fig. 21-1].) *Pons,* The pons (Latin, bridge) houses the trigeminal motor division (5), abducens (6), facial (7), and acoustic/vestibular (not shown) cranial nerve nuclei and, inferior and lateral to the fourth ventricle, the locus ceruleus (*). In addition to containing the descending corticospinal tract, the basilar portion of the pons, the "basis pontis," contains large criss-crossing cerebellar tracts. (Also see the drawing [Fig. 4-7] and an idealized sketch [Fig. 21-2].) *Medulla,* The medulla (Latin, marrow), readily identifiable by the pair of unstained scallop-shaped inferior olivary nuclei, includes the cerebellar peduncles (C), which contains afferent and efferent cerebellar tracts; the corticospinal tract (Δ); and the floor of the fourth ventricle (IV). It also contains the decussation of the medial lemniscus (M), the nuclei for cranial nerves IX–XI grouped laterally and XII situated medially, and the trigeminal sensory nucleus (not pictured) that descends from the pons to the cervical-medullary junction. (Also see a functional drawing [Fig. 2-10].)

SIGNS OF CEREBELLAR LESIONS

The cerebellum (*Latin,* diminutive of cerebrum) is composed of two hemispheres and a central portion, the *vermis.* Each hemisphere controls coordination of the ipsilateral limbs, and the vermis controls coordination of "midline structures": the head, neck, and trunk. Because the cerebellum controls coordination of the limbs on the *same side of the body,* it is unique—a quality captured by the aphorism, "Everything in the brain, except for the cerebellum, is contralateral." Another unique feature of the cerebellum is that when one hemisphere is damaged, the other will eventually assume the functions for both. Thus, although loss of one cerebellar hemisphere will cause incapacitating ipsilateral incoordination, the disability improves as the remaining hemisphere compensates almost entirely. For example, patients who lose one cerebellar hemisphere to a stroke or trauma typically regain their ability to walk, although they may never dance or perform other activities requiring both cerebellar hemispheres. Young children who sustain such an injury are more resilient and often can learn to ride a bicycle, dance, and perform various athletic activities.

In addition to incoordination, cerebellar lesions cause subtle motor changes, such as muscle hypotonia and pendular DTRs. However, they do not cause paresis, hyperactive DTRs, or Babinski signs.

Although a few studies suggest that the cerebellum plays a role in cognition, it does not play an obvious one for everyday clinical purposes. For example, unless they simultaneously involve the cerebrum, cerebellar lesions do not lead to dementia, language impairment, or other cognitive impairment. A good example is the normal intellect of children and young adults who have undergone resection of a cerebellar hemisphere for removal of an astrocytoma (see Chapter 19).

A characteristic sign of cerebellar dysfunction is *intention tremor.* Both the finger-to-nose (Fig. 2-11) and heel-to-shin tests (Fig. 2-12) can demonstrate this tremor. It is present when the patient moves willfully but absent when the patient rests. In a classic contrast, Parkinson's disease causes a *resting tremor* that is present when the patient sits quietly and is reduced or even abolished when the patient moves (see Chapter 18).

Another sign of a cerebellar lesion that reflects incoordination of the limbs is impaired ability to perform rapid alternating movements, *dysdiadochokinesia.* When asked to slap the palm and then the back of the hand rapidly and alternately on his or her own knee, for example, a patient with dysdiadochokinesia will

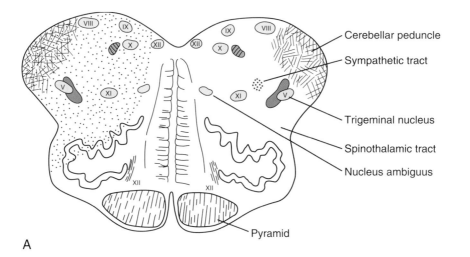

A

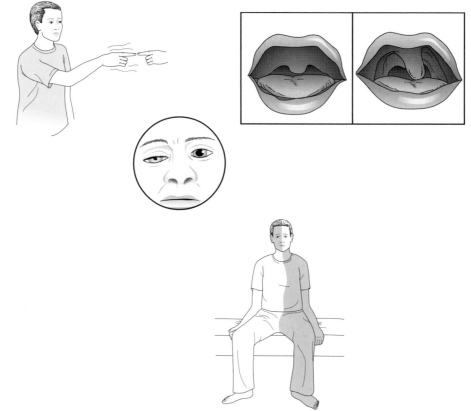

B

FIGURE 2-10 ■ *A,* If the posterior inferior cerebellar artery (PICA) were occluded, the lateral portion of the medulla may suffer an infarction. This infarction damages important lateral structures: the cerebellar peduncle, the trigeminal nerve (V) sensory tract, the spinothalamic tract (which arose from the contralateral side of the body), the nucleus ambiguus (cranial nerves IX to XI motor nuclei), and poorly delineated sympathetic fibers. However, it spares medial structures: the corticospinal tract, medial longitudinal fasciculus (MLF), and hypoglossal nerve (XII) nucleus. The stippled area represents the right lateral medulla, which suffered an infarction when the right PICA or its parent artery, the vertebral artery, was occluded. *B,* This patient, who suffered such an infarction of the right lateral medulla, has a right-sided Wallenberg syndrome. He has a right-sided Horner's syndrome (ptosis and miosis) because of damage to the sympathetic fibers (also see Fig. 12-16B). He has right-sided ataxia because of damage to the ipsilateral cerebellar tracts. He has an alternating hypalgesia: diminished pain sensation on the *right* side of his face, accompanied by loss of pain sensation on the *left* trunk and extremities. Finally, he has hoarseness and paresis of the right soft palate because of damage to the right nucleus ambiguus. Because of the right-sided palate weakness, the palate deviates upward toward his left on voluntary phonation (saying "ah") or in response to the gag reflex.

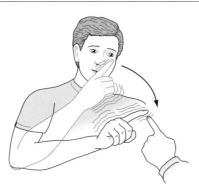

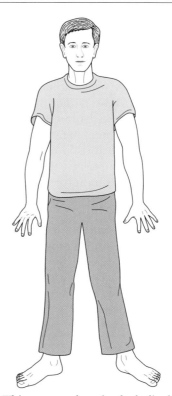

FIGURE 2-11 ■ This young man, who has a multiple sclerosis (MS) plaque in the right cerebellar hemisphere, has a right-sided *intention tremor*. During repetitive *finger-to-nose* movements, as his right index finger approaches his own nose and then the examiner's finger, it develops a coarse and irregular path. This irregular rhythm is called *dysmetria*.

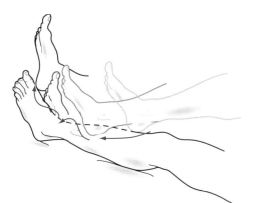

FIGURE 2-12 ■ In the *heel-to-shin test*, the patient with the right-sided cerebellar lesion in Figure 2-11 displays limb *ataxia* as his right heel wobbles when he pushes it along the crest of his left shin.

FIGURE 2-13 ■ This man, a chronic alcoholic, has developed diffuse cerebellar degeneration. He has a typical *ataxic gait*: broad-based, unsteady, and uncoordinated. To steady his stance, he stands with his feet apart and pointed outward.

use uneven force, move irregularly, and lose the alternating pattern.

Damage to either the entire cerebellum or the vermis alone causes incoordination of the trunk (*truncal ataxia*). It forces patients to place their feet widely apart when standing and leads to a lurching, unsteady, and wide-based pattern of walking (*gait ataxia*) (Table 2-3 and Fig. 2-13). A common example is the staggering and reeling of people intoxicated by alcohol or phenytoin.

Extensive damage of the cerebellum also causes *scanning speech*, a variety of dysarthria. Scanning speech, which reflects incoordination of speech production, is characterized by poor modulation, irregular cadence, and inability to separate adjacent sounds. Dysarthria—whether from cerebellar injury, bulbar or pseudobulbar palsy, or other neurologic conditions—should be distinguishable from aphasia, which is a language disorder that stems from dominant cerebral hemisphere injury (see Chapter 8).

Before considering the illnesses that damage the cerebellum, physicians must appreciate that the cerebellum undergoes age-related changes that appear between ages 50 and 65 years in the form of mildly impaired functional ability and abnormal neurologic test results. For example, as people age beyond 50 years, they walk less rapidly and less sure-footedly. They begin to lose their ability to ride a bicycle and to stand on one foot while putting on socks. During a neurologic examination they routinely tend to topple when walking heel-to-toe, that is, performing the "tandem gait" test.

Illnesses that Affect the Cerebellum

The illnesses that are responsible for most *cerebral* lesions—strokes, tumors, trauma, AIDS, and MS—also cause most *cerebellar* lesions. The cerebellum is also particularly vulnerable to toxins, such as alcohol, toluene (see Chapters 5 and 15), and organic mercury; medications, such as phenytoin; and deficiencies of certain vitamins, such as thiamine and vitamin E. Some conditions damage the cerebrum as well as the cerebellum and may cause a combination of cognitive impairment and incoordination.

Genetic abnormalities underlie numerous cerebellar illnesses. Most of them follow classic autosomal dominant or recessive patterns. Several result from unstable trinucleotide repeats in chromosomal DNA or abnormalities in mitochondrial DNA (see Chapter 6 and Appendix 3). For example, *Friedreich's ataxia*, the most common hereditary ataxia, results from excessive trinucleotide repeats. Some hereditary ataxias cause cognitive impairment and characteristic non-neurologic manifestations, such as kyphosis, cardiomyopathy, and pes cavus (Fig. 2-14), in addition to cerebellar signs.

One large, heterogenous group of genetic illnesses, the *spinocerebellar ataxias (SCAs)*, damages the spinal cord, the cerebellum, and its major connections. In general, the SCAs consist of progressively severe gait ataxia, scanning speech, and incoordination of hand and finger movements. Depending on the SCA variety, patients may also show cognitive impairment, sensory loss, spasticity, or ocular motility problems.

Another genetic cerebellar disorder is deficiency of vitamin E, a fat-soluble antioxidant. Although the SCAs cannot be treated, vitamin E deficiency ataxia responds to replenishing the vitamin.

Cerebellar dysfunction has been suspected in autism because several magnetic resonance imaging

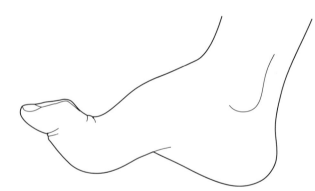

FIGURE 2-14 ■ The *pes cavus* foot deformity consists of a high arch, elevation of the dorsum, and retraction of the first metatarsal. When pes cavus occurs in families with childhood-onset ataxia and posterior column sensory deficits, it is virtually pathognomonic of Friedreich's ataxia.

and autopsy studies have detected cerebellar hemisphere hypoplasia and a reduction of more than 50% of its Purkinje cells, one of its basic elements. However, most of those abnormalities are inconsistent, do not correlate with the clinical findings, and are found in other conditions.

SIGNS OF SPINAL CORD LESIONS

A broad **H**-shaped, gray matter structure composed largely of neurons that transmit nerve impulses in a horizontal plane occupies the center of the spinal cord. It is surrounded by white matter, composed of myelinated tracts that convey information in a vertical direction (Fig. 2-15). Because most signs of spinal cord injury are due to interruption of the myelinated tracts, spinal cord injury is often called "myelopathy." The pattern of the spinal cord anatomy—gray matter on the inside with white outside—is opposite that of the cerebrum.

The major descending pathway is the *lateral corticospinal tract*.

The major ascending pathways, which are virtually all sensory, include the following:

- *Posterior columns*, composed of the *fasciculi cuneatus* and *gracilis*, carry position and vibration sensations to the thalamus.
- *Lateral spinothalamic tracts* carry temperature and pain sensations to the thalamus.
- *Anterior spinothalamic tracts* carry light touch sensation to the thalamus.
- *Spinocerebellar tracts* carry joint position and movement sensations to the cerebellum.

Conditions that Affect the Spinal Cord

Discrete Injuries

The site of a spinal cord injury—cervical, thoracic, or lumbosacral—determines the nature and distribution of the motor and sensory deficits. Cervical spinal cord

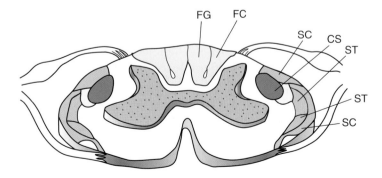

FIGURE 2-15 ■ In this sketch of the spinal cord, the centrally located gray matter is stippled. The surrounding white matter contains myelin-coated tracts that ascend and descend within the spinal cord. Clinically important ascending tracts are the spinocerebellar tracts (SC) (light blue), the lateral spinothalamic tract (ST) (light blue), and the posterior column (fasciculus cuneatus [FC], from the upper limbs, and fasciculus gracilis [FG], from the lower limbs) (gray). The most important descending tract is the lateral corticospinal (CS) tract (dark blue).

transection, for example, blocks all motor from descending and sensory perception from arising through the neck. This lesion will cause paralysis of the arms and legs (*quadriparesis*) and, after 1 to 2 weeks, spasticity, hyperactive DTRs, and Babinski signs. In addition, it will prevent the perception of all limb, trunk, and bladder sensation. Similarly, a midthoracic spinal cord transection will cause paralysis of the legs (*paraparesis*) with similar reflex changes and sensory loss of the trunk below the nipples and the legs (Fig. 2-16). In general, all spinal cord injuries disrupt bladder control and sexual function, which rely on delicate, intricate systems (see Chapter 16).

Even with devastating spinal cord injury, however, cerebral function is preserved. In a frequently occurring and tragic example, soldiers surviving a penetrating gunshot wound of the cervical spinal cord, although quadriplegic, retain intellectual, visual, and verbal facilities. Those surviving spinal cord injuries are often beset with depression from isolation, lack of social support, and physical impairment. They have a high divorce rate, and their suicide rate is about five times greater than that of the general population. In addition, several patients with quadriplegia have requested withdrawal of mechanical life support not only immediately after the injury, when their decision may be attributed to depression, but also several years later when they are clearheaded and not overtly depressed.

Of the various spinal cord lesions, the most instructive is the *Brown-Séquard syndrome*. This classic disturbance results from an injury that transects the lateral half of the spinal cord (Fig. 2-17). It is characterized by the combination of corticospinal tract damage that causes paralysis of the ipsilateral limb(s) and by adjacent lateral spinothalamic tract damage that causes loss of pain sensation (hypalgesia) in the contralateral limb(s). Simply put, one leg is weak and the other is numb.

The cervical region of the spinal cord is particularly susceptible to common nonpenetrating trauma because in most accidents, sudden and forceful hyperextension of the neck crushes the cervical vertebrae. Approximately 50% of civilian spinal cord injuries result from motor vehicle crashes; 20% from falls; 15%

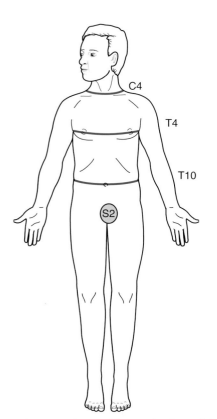

FIGURE 2-16 ■ In a patient with a spinal cord injury, the "level" of hypalgesia indicates the site of the damage. The clinical landmarks are C4, T4, and T10. C4 injuries cause hypalgesia below the neck; T4 injuries, hypalgesia below the nipples; T10 injuries, hypalgesia below the umbilicus.

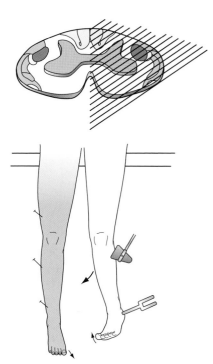

FIGURE 2-17 ■ In this case of hemitransection of the patient's spinal cord (Brown-Séquard syndrome), the left side of the thoracic spinal cord has been transected, as by a knife wound. Injury to the left lateral corticospinal tract results in the combination of left-sided leg paresis, hyperactive deep tendon reflexes (DTRs), and a Babinski sign; injury to the left posterior column results in impairment of left leg vibration and position sense. Most striking, injury to the left spinothalamic tract causes loss of temperature and pain sensation in the right leg. The loss of pain sensation contralateral to the paresis is the signature of the Brown-Séquard syndrome.

from gunshot wounds and other violence; and 15% from diving accidents and other sports injuries. The other dangerous sports are football, skiing, surfing, trampoline work, and horseback riding. Hanging by the neck dislocates or fractures cervical vertebrae. It crushes the cervical spinal cord and cuts off the air supply. Survivors are likely to be quadriplegic as well as brain damaged.

Another notable cervical spinal cord injury consists of the great expansion of its *central canal*. This canal is essentially a minute tube that runs vertically within the gray matter. For unclear reasons, in teenagers and young adults, the canal may spontaneously expand to form a cavity filled with cerebrospinal fluid (CSF), a *syringomyelia* or *syrinx* (Greek, *syrinx,* pipe or tube + *myelos* marrow). Spinal cord trauma can cause a syrinx by bleeding within the canal, a *hematomyelia.*

The clinical findings of a syrinx are distinctive and reflect the underlying neuroanatomy (Fig. 2-18). As a syrinx expands, its pressure rips apart the lateral spinothalamic tracts as they cross from one to the other side of the spinal cord. It also compresses on the anterior horn cells of the anterior gray matter. The expansion not only causes neck pain, but also loss in the arms

and hands of pain and temperature sensation, muscle bulk, and DTRs. Because these findings are restricted to the arms, patients are said to have a *cape-like* or *suspended sensory loss.* Moreover, the sensory deficit is characteristically restricted to loss of pain and temperature sensation because the posterior columns, merely displaced, remain functional.

Neurologic Illnesses

MS, the most common CNS demyelinating illness, typically causes myelopathy alone or in combination with cerebellar, optic nerve, or brainstem damage (see Chapter 15). Tumors of the lung, breast, and other organs that spread to the vertebral bodies often compress the spinal cord and cause myelopathy. Similarly, regions of degenerative spine disease, such as cervical spondylosis, can narrow the spinal canal enough to compress the spinal cord (see Fig. 5-10).

Several illnesses damage only specific spinal cord tracts (Fig. 2-19). The posterior columns—*fasciculus gracilis* and *f. cuneatus*—seem particularly vulnerable. For example, tabes dorsalis (syphilis), combined

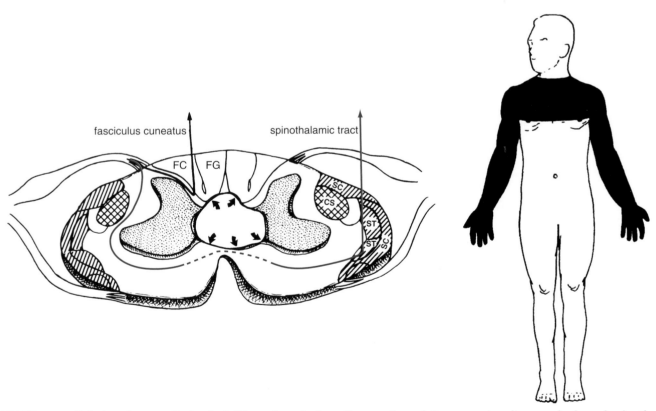

FIGURE 2-18 ■ *Left,* A syringomyelia (syrinx) dilates the spinal cord's central canal. Its expansion disrupts the lateral spinothalamic tract (blue) as it crosses and compresses the anterior horn cells of the gray matter. Unless the syrinx is large, it only presses on the posterior columns and corticospinal tracts and does not impair their function. *Right,* The classic finding is a *suspended sensory loss* (loss of only pain and temperature sensation in the arms and upper chest [in this case, C4-T4]) that is accompanied by weakness, atrophy, and deep tendon reflex (DTR) loss in the arms.

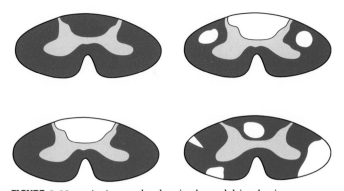

FIGURE 2-19 ■ *A,* A standard spinal cord histologic preparation stains normal myelin (white matter) black and leaves the central H-shaped column gray. *B,* In combined system disease (vitamin B$_{12}$ deficiency), posterior column and corticospinal tract damage causes their demyelination and lack of stain. *C,* In tabes dorsalis (tertiary syphilis), damage to the posterior column leaves them unstained. *D,* Multiple sclerosis (MS) leads to asymmetric, irregular, demyelinated unstained plaques.

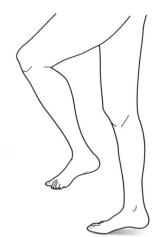

FIGURE 2-20 ■ The steppage gait consists of each knee being excessively raised when walking. This maneuver compensates for a loss of position sense by elevating the feet to ensure that they will clear the ground, stairs, and other obstacles. It is a classic sign of posterior column spinal cord damage from tabes dorsalis. However, peripheral neuropathies more commonly impair position sense and lead to this gait abnormality.

system disease (B$_{12}$ deficiency, see Chapter 5), Friedreich's ataxia, and the SCAs, each damages the posterior columns alone or in combination with other tracts. In these conditions, impairment of the posterior columns leads to a loss of position sense that prevents affected people from being able to stand with their eyes closed (*Romberg's sign*). When they walk, this sensory loss produces a *steppage gait* (Fig. 2-20). In another example, human T-lymphotropic virus type 1 (HTLV–1) myelopathy (see Chapter 15), a common illness in which an infective agent predominantly attacks the lateral columns, patients develop spastic paraparesis that resembles MS.

Most important, myelopathy is associated with dementia because of concomitant cerebral damage in several illnesses. Examples of this association include tabes dorsalis, combined system disease, AIDS, and, when disseminated throughout the cerebrum, MS.

Psychogenic Neurologic Deficits

Classic studies of hysteria, conversion reactions, and related conditions included patients who had only rudimentary physical examinations and minimal, if any, laboratory testing. Studies that re-evaluated the same patients after many years reported that as many as 20% of them eventually had specific neurologic conditions, such as movement disorders, multiple sclerosis (MS), or seizures, that had probably been responsible for the original symptoms. In addition, some patients had systemic illnesses, such as anemia or congestive heart failure, that could have contributed to their initial symptoms. Another interesting aspect of these studies is that many illnesses assumed to be entirely "psychogenic" in the first two thirds of the 20th century are now acknowledged to be "neurologic," such as Tourette's disorder, writer's cramp and other focal dystonias, erectile dysfunction, migraines, and trigeminal neuralgia. To be fair, the medical community has still not reached a consensus on the etiology of several conditions, such as fibromyalgia, chronic fatigue syndrome, and some aspects of chronic pain. Also unexplained, in many patients, is their persistent weakness and disability for more than a decade after their physicians seem to have established a psychogenic basis for their symptoms.

Although today's physicians still fail to reach 100% accuracy in diagnosis, they skillfully diagnose psychogenic deficits. Their greater accuracy does not mean that they are more astute than their classic counterparts. Rather, today's physicians usually have received formal training, attend continuing medical education, and must apply relatively strict diagnostic criteria. When uncertain, they can consult with readily available colleagues. Moreover, these physicians commonly have at their disposal an arsenal of high-tech tests, including computed tomography (CT), magnetic resonance imaging (MRI), electroencephalography (EEG), and closed circuit television (CCTV) monitoring.

THE NEUROLOGIST'S ROLE

Even in the face of flagrant psychogenic signs, neurologists must confirm the absence of neurologic disease. Although aware of risk factors for psychogenic illness—abuse in childhood, multiple somatic symptoms, a symptom model, prior psychogenic deficits, and secondary gain—neurologists tend to treat each new symptom as possibly organic. In this context, the adage "All hypochondriacs eventually die of a real illness" seems to drive multiple re-evaluations.

Neurologists generally test for conditions that could explain all of the patient's symptoms, particularly for those illnesses that would be serious or life threatening. In addition, although observing the course of the illness regularly proves most informative of its origin, neurologists instead usually request extensive testing during the initial evaluation to obtain objective evidence of disease or its absence as soon as possible.

Typically, neurologists disregard the distinction between conscious and unconscious disorders. For example, their examinations do not allow them to distinguish between patients with "blindness" due to an unconscious conflict from those deliberately pretending to be blind to gain insurance money.

In addition to diagnosing the purely psychogenic deficit, neurologists consider gross exaggerations of a deficit, *embellishment,* as psychogenic. For various reasons, they merge all psychiatrically based impairments into the category of "psychogenic neurologic deficits."

Within the framework of this potential oversimplification, neurologists reliably diagnose psychogenic seizures (see Chapter 10), diplopia and other visual problems (see Chapter 12), and tremors and other movement disorders (see Chapter 18). In addition, they acknowledge the psychogenic aspects of pain (see Chapter 14), sexual dysfunction (see Chapter 16), posttraumatic headaches and whiplash injuries (see Chapter 22), and many other neurologic disorders. Although they do not distinguish between the various psychiatric diagnoses associated with deficits, a neurologic examination can show signs that the patient is, at some level, actively mimicking the disorder. Some neurologists even concede a psychogenic component to every neurologic illness.

When consulting on patients who have been shown to have a psychogenic disturbance, neurologists usually offer reassurances, strong suggestions that the deficits will resolve by a certain date, and a referral for psychiatric consultation. Sometimes they allow patients acceptable exits by prescribing placebos or nonspecific treatment, such as physical therapy. They avoid ordering invasive diagnostic procedures, surgery, and medications, especially habit-forming or otherwise potentially dangerous ones.

Patients often have mixtures of neurologic and psychogenic deficits, disproportionate posttraumatic disabilities, and minor neurologic illnesses that preoccupy them. As long as serious, progressive physical illness has been excluded, physicians can consider some symptoms to be chronic illnesses. For example, chronic low back pain can be treated as a "pain syndrome" with empiric combinations of antidepressant medications, analgesics, rehabilitation, and psychotherapy, without expecting to either cure the pain or determine its exact cause (see Chapter 14).

Psychiatrists, abiding by the *Diagnostic and Statistical Manual of Mental Disorders, 4th edition, Text Revision (DSM-IV-TR)*, often classify psychogenic deficits that have originated in unconscious processes as manifestations of a *somatoform disorder*, particularly *somatization* or *conversion disorders*. In listing the diagnostic criteria for somatization disorder, the DSM-IV-TR allows certain pseudoneurotic symptoms, including impaired coordination, loss of balance, paralysis, double vision, and seizures, but not movement disorders (see Chapter 18). When an unconscious psychiatric disturbance underlies a conscious imitation of a neurologic deficit, the DSM-IV-TR would apply the diagnosis of *factitious disorder*. However, when individuals deliberately mimic neurologic deficits to obtain compensation or another tangible or intangible commodity, the DSM-IV-TR would diagnose no psychiatric illness but instead describe the action as *malingering*.

PSYCHOGENIC SIGNS

What general clues prompt a neurologist to suspect a psychogenic disturbance? When a deficit violates the *laws of neuroanatomy*, neurologists almost always deduce that it has a psychogenic origin. For example, if temperature sensation is preserved but pain perception is "lost," the deficit is *nonanatomic* and therefore likely to be psychogenic. Likewise, tunnel vision, which clearly violates these laws, is a classic psychogenic disturbance (see Fig. 12-8).

Another clue to a psychogenic basis is a changing deficit. For example, if someone who appears to have hemiparesis either walks when unaware of being observed or walks despite seeming to have paraparesis while in bed, neurologists conclude that the paresis has a psychogenic basis. Another noted example occurs when someone with a psychogenic seizure momentarily "awakens" and stops convulsive activity but resumes it when assured of being observed. The

psychogenic nature of a deficit can be confirmed if it is reversed during an interview under hypnosis or barbiturate infusion.

Motor Signs

One indication of psychogenic weakness is a nonanatomic distribution of deficits, such as loss of strength in the arm and leg accompanied by blindness in one eye, and deafness in one ear—all on the same side of the body. Another indication is the absence of functional impairment despite the appearance of profound weakness, such as ability to walk even though manual testing seems to show marked paraparesis.

Deficits that are intermittent also suggest a psychogenic origin. For example, a "give-way" effort, in which the patient offers a brief (several seconds) exertion before returning to an apparent paretic position, indicates an intermittent condition that is probably psychogenic. Similarly, the *face-hand test*, in which the patient momentarily exerts sufficient strength to deflect his or her falling hand from hitting his or her own face (Fig. 3-1), also indicates a psychogenic paresis.

A reliable indication of unilateral psychogenic leg weakness is *Hoover's sign* (Fig. 3-2). Normally, when someone attempts to raise a genuinely paretic leg, the other leg presses down. The examiner can feel the downward force at the patient's normal heel and can use the straightened leg, as a lever, to raise the entire leg and lower body. In contrast, Hoover's sign consists of the patient unconsciously pressing down with a "paretic" leg when attempting to raise the unaffected leg and failing to press down with the unaffected leg when attempting to raise the "paretic" leg.

A similar test involves abduction (separating) the legs. Normally, when asked to abduct one leg, a person reflexively and forcefully abducts both of them. Someone with genuine hemiparesis will abduct the normal leg but will be unable to abduct the paretic one. In contrast, someone with psychogenic weakness will reflexively abduct the "paretic" leg when abducting the normal leg (*abductor sign*) (Fig. 3-3).

Gait Impairment

Many psychogenic gait impairments closely mimic neurologic disturbances, such as tremors in the legs, ataxia, or weakness of one or both legs. The most readily identifiable and psychogenic gait impairment is *astasia-abasia* (lack of station, lack of base). In this disturbance, patients stagger, balance momentarily, and appear to be in great danger of falling; however,

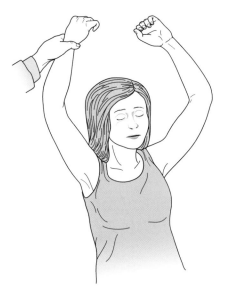

FIGURE 3-1 ■ In the face-hand test, a young woman with psychogenic right hemiparesis inadvertently demonstrates her preserved strength by deflecting her falling "paretic" arm from striking her face as the examiner drops it.

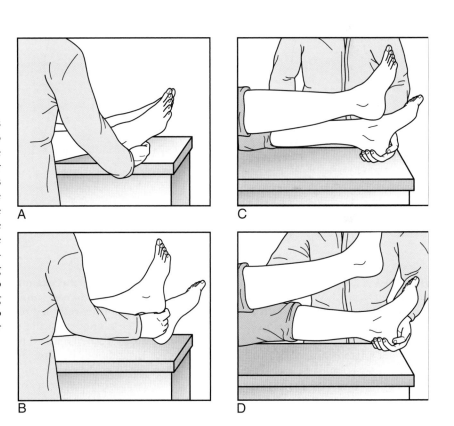

FIGURE 3-2 ■ A neurologist demonstrates Hoover's sign in a 23-year-old man who has a psychogenic left hemiparesis. *A,* She asks him to raise his left leg as she holds her hand under his right heel. *B,* Revealing his lack of effort, the patient exerts so little downward force with his right leg that she easily raises it. *C,* When she asks him to raise his right leg while cupping his left heel, the patient reveals his intact strength as he unconsciously forces his left, "paretic" leg downward. *D,* As if to carry the example to the extreme, the patient forces his left leg downward with enough force to allow her to use his left leg as a lever to raise his lower torso.

catching themselves at "the last moment" by grabbing hold of railings, furniture, and even the examiner, they never actually injure themselves (Fig. 3-4).

Another blatant psychogenic gait impairment occurs when patients drag a "weak" leg as though it was a completely lifeless object apart from their body. In contrast, patients with a true hemiparetic gait (as previously discussed [see Fig. 2-4]) swing their paretic leg outward with a circular motion (i.e., "circumduct" their leg).

Sensory Deficits

Although the sensory examination is the least reliable portion of the neurologic examination, several sensory

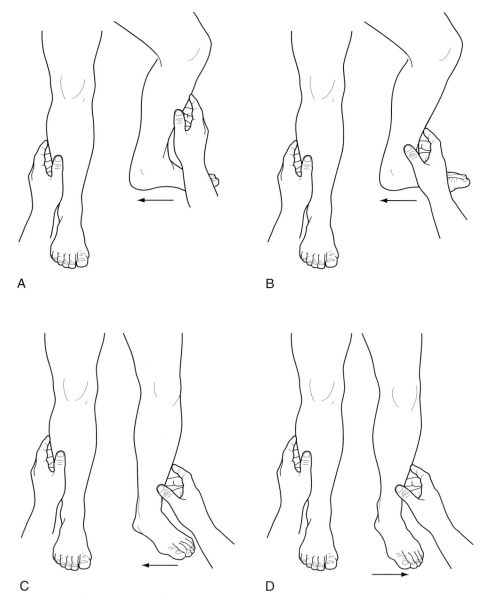

A

B

C

D

FIGURE 3-3 ■ Upper series: Left hemiparesis from a stroke with the examiner's hands pushing the legs together, that is, adducting them. *A,* When asked to abduct the left leg, that leg's weakness cannot resist a physician's pressure, which moves the leg toward the midline (adducts it). At the same time, the normal right leg reflexively abducts. *B,* When asked to abduct the normal right leg, it abducts forcefully. The paretic left leg cannot resist the examiner's pressure, and the examiner pushes the leg inward. Lower series: Psychogenic left hemiparesis. *C,* When asked to abduct both legs, the left leg fails to resist the examiner's hand pushing it inward (adducting it). In addition, because of the patient's failure to abduct the right leg, the examiner's hand also presses it inward. *D,* When asked to abduct the normal right leg, the patient complies and abducts it forcefully; however, the left leg, which has psychogenic weakness, reflexively resists the physician's inward pressure and abducts—*the abductor sign.* (Courtesy of Sonoo Masahiro, MD, Department of Neurology, Teikyo University School of Medicine.)

abnormalities indicate a psychogenic basis. For example, loss of sensation to pinprick* that stops abruptly at the middle of the face and body is the classic *splitting the midline.* This finding suggests a psychogenic loss

*Neurologists now use pins cautiously, if at all, to avoid blood-borne infections. Testing for pain is performed with nonpenetrating, disposable instruments, such as cotton sticks.

because the sensory nerve fibers of the skin normally spread across the midline (Fig. 3-5). Likewise, because vibrations naturally spread across bony structures, loss of vibration sensation over half of the forehead, jaw, sternum, or spine strongly suggests a psychogenic disturbance.

A similar abnormality is loss of sensation of the entire face but not of the scalp. This pattern is

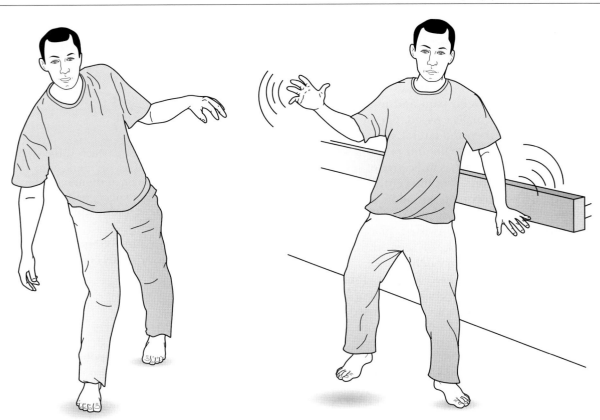

FIGURE 3-4 ■ A young man demonstrates astasia-abasia by seeming to fall when walking but catching himself by balancing carefully. He even staggers the width of the room to grasp the rail. He sometimes clutches physicians and pulls them toward himself and then drags them toward the ground. While dramatizing his purported impairment, he actually displays good strength, balance, and coordination.

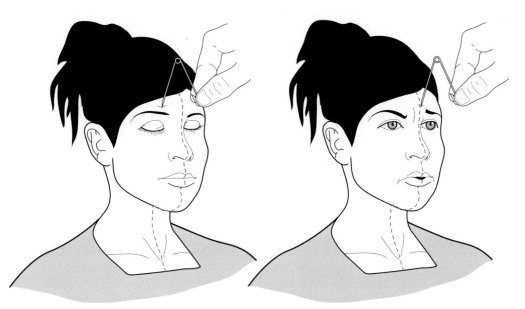

FIGURE 3-5 ■ A young woman with psychogenic right hemisensory loss appears not to feel a pinprick until the pin, which is used only for illustrative purposes, reaches the midline of her forehead, face, neck, or sternum (i.e., she splits the midline). When the pin is moved across the midline, she appears to feel a sharp stick.

inconsistent with the anatomic distribution of the trigeminal nerve, which innervates the face and scalp anterior to the vertex but not the angle of the jaw (see Fig. 4-12).

A psychogenic sensory loss, as already mentioned, can be a discrepancy between pain and temperature sensations, which are normally carried together by the peripheral nerves and then the lateral spinothalamic tracts. (Discrepancy between pain and position sensations in the fingers, in contrast, is indicative of syringomyelia [syrinx]. In this condition the central fibers of the spinal cord, which carry pain sensation, are ripped apart by the expanding central canal.) Testing for sensory loss when the arms are twisted, placed out of sight behind the patient's back, or seen in a mirror may expose psychogenic sensory deficits.

Finally, because sensory loss impairs function, patients with genuine sensory loss in their feet or hands cannot perform many tasks if their eyes are closed. Also, those with true sensory loss in both feet—from severe peripheral neuropathy or injury of the spinal cord posterior columns, usually from vitamin B_{12} deficiency, tabes dorsalis, or MS—tend to fall when standing erect with their eyes shut (i.e., they have *Romberg's sign*, see Chapter 2). In contrast, patients with psychogenic sensory loss can still generally button their shirts, walk short distances, and stand with their feet together with their eyes closed.

Special Senses

When cases of blindness, tunnel vision, diplopia, or other disorders of vision violate the laws of neuroanatomy, which are firmly based on the laws of optics, neurologists diagnose them as psychogenic. Neurologists and ophthalmologists can dependably separate psychogenic and neurologic visual disorders (see Chapter 12).

A patient with psychogenic deafness usually responds to unexpected noises or words. Unilateral hearing loss in the ear ipsilateral to a hemiparesis is highly suggestive of a psychogenic etiology because extensive auditory tract synapses in the pons ensure that some tracts reach the upper brainstem and cerebrum despite central nervous system (CNS) lesions (see Fig. 4-16). If doubts about hearing loss remain, neurologists often request audiometry, brainstem auditory evoked responses, and other technical procedures.

Patients can genuinely lose the sense of smell (anosmia) from a head injury (see Chapter 22) or advanced age; however, these patients can usually still perceive noxious volatile chemicals, such as ammonia or alcohol, which irritate the nasal mucosa endings of the trigeminal nerve rather than the olfactory nerve. This

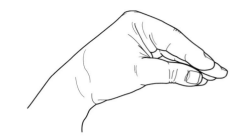

FIGURE 3-6 ■ Carpopedal spasm, which is the characteristic neurologic manifestation of hyperventilation, consists of flexion of the wrist and proximal thumb and finger joints. Also, although the thumb and fingers remain extended, they are drawn together and tend to overlap.

distinction is usually unknown to individuals with psychogenic anosmia, who typically claim inability to smell any substance.

Miscellaneous Conditions

A distinct but common psychogenic disturbance, the *hyperventilation syndrome*, occurs in people with an underlying anxiety disorder, including panic disorder. It leads to lightheadedness and paresthesias around the mouth, fingers, and toes, and, in severe cases, to *carpopedal spasm* (Fig. 3-6). Although the disorder seems distinctive, physicians should be cautious before diagnosing it because partial complex seizures and transient ischemic attacks (TIAs) produce similar symptoms.

In this syndrome, hyperventilation first causes a fall in carbon dioxide tension that leads to respiratory alkalosis. The rise in blood pH from the alkalosis produces hypocalcemia, which induces the tetany of muscles and paresthesias. To demonstrate the cause of the spasms, physicians may re-create them by having a patient hyperventilate. This procedure may also induce giddiness, anxiety, or confusion. If so, the physician should abort the demonstration by having the patient continually rebreathe expired air from a paper bag cupped around the mouth.

POTENTIAL PITFALLS

The neurologic examination of a patient suspected of having a psychogenic deficit requires particular sensitivity. It can be undertaken in conjunction with a psychiatric evaluation, need not follow the conventional format, and can be completed in two or more sessions. A threatening, embarrassing, or otherwise inept evaluation may obscure the diagnosis, harden the patient's resolve, or precipitate a catastrophic reaction.

Despite their general usefulness, guidelines to identify a psychogenic problem are fallible. Patients may display psychogenic signs to emphasize a neurologic deficit that they feel may go unnoticed. Another unreliable indication is lack of affect concerning a deficit, often termed *la belle indifference*. In particular, it is a well-known manifestation of hemi-inattention, Anton's syndrome, and frontal lobe injury.

Although the neurologic examination itself seems rational and reliable, some findings are potentially misleading. For example, many anxious or "ticklish" individuals, with or without psychogenic hemiparesis, have brisk deep tendon reflexes and extensor plantar reflexes. Another potentially misleading finding is a right hemiparesis unaccompanied by aphasia. In actuality, a stroke might cause this situation if the patient were left-handed, or if the stroke were small and located in the internal capsule or upper brainstem (i.e., a subcortical motor stroke). With a suspected psychogenic left hemiparesis, physicians must assure themselves that the problem does not actually represent left-sided inattention or neglect (see Chapter 8).

Neurologists tend to misdiagnose several types of disorders as psychogenic when they are unique or bizarre, or when their severity is greater than expected. This error may simply reflect an individual neurologist's lack of experience. They also may misdiagnose disorders as psychogenic when a patient has no accompanying objective physical abnormalities. This determination might be faulty in illnesses in which objective signs are often transient or subtle, such as MS, partial complex seizures, and small strokes. With an incomplete history, neurologists may not appreciate transient neurologic conditions, such as transient hemiparesis induced by migraines, postictal paresis, or TIAs and transient mental status aberrations induced by alcohol, medications, seizures, or other conditions (see Table 9-3).

Another potential pitfall is dismissing an entire case because a patient is grossly exaggerating a deficit. Patients may feel that they must overstate a genuine medical problem to gain the necessary attention. In addition, the prospect of having developed a neurologic disorder may trigger overwhelming anxiety. For example, patients with a persistent headache may so fear a brain tumor that they embellish their history with additional symptoms to obtain a MRI.

Possibly the single most common error is failure to recognize MS because its early signs may be evanescent, exclusively sensory, or so disparate as to appear to violate several laws of neuroanatomy. Neurologists can usually make the correct diagnosis early and reliably—even in ambiguous cases—with MRIs, visual evoked response testing, and cerebrospinal fluid analysis (see Chapter 15). On the other hand, trivial sensory or motor symptoms that are accompanied by normal variations in these highly sensitive tests may lead to false-positive diagnoses of MS.

Neurologists are also prone to err in diagnosing involuntary movement disorders as psychogenic. These disorders, in fact, often have some stigmata of psychogenic illness (see Chapter 2). For example, they can appear bizarre, precipitated or exacerbated by anxiety, or apparently relieved by tricks, such as when a dystonic gait can be alleviated by walking backward. Also, barbiturate infusions usually temporarily reduce or even abolish involuntary movements. Because laboratory tests are not available for many disorders—chorea, tics, tremors, and focal dystonia—the diagnosis rests on the neurologist's clinical evaluation. As a general rule, movement disorders should first be considered neurologic (see Chapter 18).

Epileptic and psychogenic seizures are often misdiagnosed in both directions (see Chapter 10). In general, psychogenic seizures are clonic and unaccompanied by incontinence, tongue biting, or loss of body tone (Fig. 3-7). Furthermore, although exceptions occur, patients generally regain awareness and have no retrograde amnesia. On the other hand, frontal lobe seizures and mixtures of epileptic and psychogenic seizures notoriously mimic pure psychogenic seizures. CCTV monitoring for EEG changes during and between episodes is the standard diagnostic test.

In the past, individuals with changes in their mental status have often been misdiagnosed—often by default—with a psychogenic disturbance. Some of them were eventually found to be harboring meningiomas

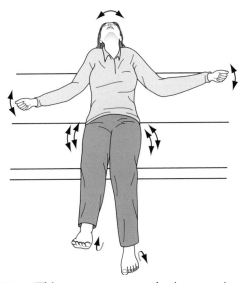

FIGURE 3-7 ■ This young woman, who is screaming during an entire 30-second episode, is having a psychogenic seizure. Its non-neurologic nature is revealed in several typical features. In addition to verbalizing throughout the episode rather than only at its onset (as in an epileptic cry), she maintains her body tone, which is required to keep her sitting upright. She has alternating flailing limb movements rather than organized bilateral clonic jerks. She has subtle but suggestive pelvic thrusting.

or other tumors in the frontal lobe. These tumors notoriously escape early detection because they can produce affective or thought disorders without accompanying physical defects. Now, with the ready availability of CT and MRI, physicians rarely overlook any tumor.

REFERENCES

1. Baker GA, Hanley JR, Jackson HF, et al: Detecting the faking of amnesia: Performance differences between simulators and patients with memory impairments. J Clin Exp Neuropsychol 15:668–684, 1993.
2. Caplan LR, Nadelson T: Multiple sclerosis and hysteria: Lessons learned from their association. JAMA 243:2418–2421, 1980.
3. Eisendrath SJ, McNiel DE: Factitious disorders in civil litigation: Twenty cases illustrating the spectrum of abnormal illness-affirming behavior. J Am Acad Psychiatry Law 30:391–399, 2002.
4. Feldman MD, Eisendrath SJ: The Spectrum of Factitious Disorders. Washington, D.C., American Psychiatric Press, 1996.
5. Glatt SL, Kennedy D, Barter R, et al: Conversion hysteria: A study of prognosis with long-term follow-up. Neurology 41(Suppl 1):120, 1991.
6. Hayes MW, Graham S, Heldorf P, et al: A video review of the diagnosis of psychogenic gait. Move Disord 14:914–921, 1999.
7. Hurst LC: What was wrong with Anna O? J R Soc Med 75:129–131, 1982.
8. Letonoff EJ, Williams TR, Sidhu KS: Hysterical paralysis: A report of three cases and a review of the literature. Spine 27:E441–445, 2002.
9. Mace CJ, Trimble MR: Ten-year prognosis of conversion disorder. Br J Psychiatry 169:282–288, 1996.
10. Richtsmeier AJ: Pitfalls in diagnosis of unexplained symptoms. Psychosomatics 25:253–255, 1984.
11. Sonoo M: Abductor sign: A reliable new sign to detect unilateral non-organic paresis of the lower limb. J Neurol Neurosurg Psychiatry 75:121–125, 2004.
12. Stone J, Sharpe M, Rothwell PM, et al: The 12 year prognosis of unilateral functional weakness and sensory disturbance. J Neurol Neurosurg Psychiatry 74:591–596, 2003.
13. Teasell RW, Shapiro AP: Misdiagnosis of conversion disorders. Am J Phys Med Rehabil 81:236–240, 2002.
14. Therapeutics and Technology Assessment Subcommittee, American Academy of Neurology: Assessment: Neuropsychological testing of adults. Neurology 47:592–599, 1996.
15. Wolf M, Birger M, Ben Shoshan J, et al: Conversion deafness. Ann Otol Rhinol Laryngol 102:349–352, 1993.

Cranial Nerve Impairments

Individually, in pairs, or in groups, the cranial nerves are vulnerable to numerous conditions. Moreover, when a nerve seems to be impaired, the underlying problem might not be damage to the cranial nerve itself but rather a cerebral injury, neuromuscular junction problem, or psychogenic disturbance. Following custom, this chapter reviews the 12 cranial nerves according to their Roman numeral designations, which can be recalled with the classic mnemonic device, "On old Olympus' towering top, a Finn and German viewed some hops."

I	Olfactory	VII	Facial
II	Optic	VIII	Acoustic
III	Oculomotor	IX	Glossopharyngeal
IV	Trochlear	X	Vagus
V	Trigeminal	XI	Spinal accessory
VI	Abducens	XII	Hypoglossal

OLFACTORY (FIRST)

Olfactory nerves transmit the sensation of smell to the brain. As the work that led to the 2004 Nobel Prize in Physiology or Medicine has shown, olfaction begins with highly complex, genetically determined specific G protein-coupled odorant receptors. Odoriferous molecules bind onto one or more receptors, which leads to their identification. Rats, who live by their sense of smell, have about 1400 olfactory receptor genes. Humans have about 350 olfactory receptor genes, which comprise almost 1.5% of their total genome.

From the olfactory receptors located deep in the nasal cavity, branches of the pair of olfactory nerves pass upward through the multiple holes in the cribriform plate of the skull to several areas of the brain. Some terminate on the undersurface of the frontal cortex, home of the olfactory sensory areas. Others terminate deep in the hypothalamus and amygdala—cornerstones of the limbic system (see Fig. 16-5). The olfactory nerves' input into the limbic system, at least in part, accounts for the influence of smell on psychosexual behavior and memory.

To test the olfactory nerve, the patient is asked to identify certain substances by smelling through one nostril while the examiner compresses the other nostril. Testing must be done with readily identifiable and odoriferous but innocuous substances, such as coffee. Volatile and irritative substances, such as ammonia and alcohol, are not suitable because they may trigger intranasal trigeminal nerve receptors and bypass a possibly damaged olfactory nerve. For detailed testing, physicians might use a commercial set of "scratch and sniff" odors.

When disorders impair both olfactory nerves, patients, who are then said to have *anosmia*, cannot perceive smells or appreciate the aroma of food. Anosmia has potentially life-threatening consequences, as when people cannot smell escaping gas. More commonly, food without a perceptible aroma is left virtually tasteless. Thus, people with anosmia, to whom food is completely bland, tend to have a decreased appetite.

One-sided anosmia may result from tumors adjacent to the olfactory nerve, such an olfactory groove meningioma. In the classic Foster-Kennedy syndrome, a meningioma compresses the olfactory nerve and the nearby optic nerve. The damage to those two nerves causes the combination of unilateral blindness and anosmia. If the tumor grows into the frontal lobe, it can also produce personality changes, dementia, or seizures.

In most cases of bilateral anosmia, the underlying disturbance is mundane. Anosmia is routine in anyone with nasal congestion and those who regularly smoke cigarettes. Head trauma, even from minor injuries, can shear off the olfactory nerves as they pass through the cribriform plate and cause anosmia (see Head Trauma, Chapter 22).

With advancing age, otherwise normal individuals begin to lose their sense of smell. Studies have shown that more than 50% of individuals older than 65 years and 75% of those older than 80 years have some degree of anosmia. Patients with Alzheimer's disease, Parkinson's disease, or other neurodegenerative diseases have even a higher incidence of anosmia. Some researchers have even proposed that testing smell can detect Alzheimer's disease before cognitive function overtly deteriorates. Schizophrenic patients also have an increased incidence of anosmia but not to the degree of those with the neurodegenerative diseases.

Studies have also shown that loss of olfactory acuity—inability to identify smells—is a risk factor for Alzheimer's disease. In both older age and neurodegenerative illnesses, particularly Alzheimer's and Parkinson's diseases, anosmia reflects degeneration of the olfactory tracts rather than the brain's olfactory center. In Alzheimer's disease, portions of the olfactory bulb have the same plaques and tangles that characterize the changes in the cerebral cortex. Similarly, in Creutzfeldt-Jakob disease, the olfactory nerves contain the same spongiform changes found in the cerebral cortex (see Chapter 7).

Humans with genetic defects in their G protein-coupled receptor complex have anosmia for one or more specific odors.

Anosmia may, of course, be psychogenic. A psychogenic origin can be revealed when a patient reports being unable to smell either irritative or innocuous, aromatic substances. Such a complete sensory loss would be possible only if an illness completely obliterated both pairs of trigeminal and olfactory nerves.

Olfactory hallucinations may represent the first phase or *aura* (Latin, breeze) of partial complex seizures that originate in the medial-inferior surface of the temporal lobe. These auras usually consist of several second episodes of ill-defined and unpleasant, but often sweet or otherwise pleasant, smells superimposed on impaired consciousness and behavioral disturbances (see Chapter 10). Also, although most migraine auras are visual hallucinations, some individuals experience an olfactory migraine aura (see Chapter 9).

On the other hand, olfactory hallucinations can be purely psychogenic. In contrast to smells induced by uncinate seizures, psychogenic "odors" are almost always foul smelling, are continuous, and not associated with impaired consciousness. However, most abnormal smells, which are typically putrid, originate in sinusitis and other cranial, dental, and cervical infections.

OPTIC (SECOND)

Unique among the cranial nerves, the optic nerves (and a small proximal portion of the acoustic nerves) are actually projections of the brain coated by myelin derived from *oligodendrocytes*. In other words, they are extensions of the central nervous system (CNS). Thus, CNS illnesses, particularly childhood-onset metabolic storage diseases, migraines (see Chapter 9), and multiple sclerosis (MS)-induced optic neuritis (see Chapter 15), are apt to attack the optic nerves and, to a lesser extent, the acoustic nerves.

In contrast, *Schwann cells* produce the myelin coat of both the remaining cranial nerves and all nerves of the peripheral nervous system (PNS). These nerves are susceptible to diseases that strike the PNS, such as Guillain-Barré syndrome.

The optic nerves and their tracts have two main functions that reflect a common initial path that splits, with one path projecting to the cerebral cortex and the other projecting to the midbrain:

- In the cortex path, the optic nerves, after a complex reconfiguring, convey patterns of light to the occipital cortex. While the patterns are perceived as visual information, additional projections convey information to other areas of the cerebral cortex for further processing, such as reading and tracking moving objects.
- In the midbrain path, optic nerves also serve as the afferent limb of the pupillary light reflex, conveying the degree of light intensity to the midbrain. Depending on the brightness, the efferent limb, situated in the oculomotor nerve, constricts the pupils.

The optic nerves originate in visual receptors in the retina and project posteriorly to the otic chiasm. At the chiasm, nasal fibers of the nerves cross, but temporal fibers continue uncrossed (Fig. 4-1). Temporal fibers of one *nerve* join the nasal fibers of the other to form the optic *tracts*. The tracts pass through the temporal and parietal lobes to terminate in the calcarine cortex of the occipital lobe. Thus, each occipital lobe receives its visual information from the contralateral visual field.

Visual field abnormalities are considered among the most important, reliable, and classic findings in neurology. Almost all of them reliably localize a lesion (see Fig. 12-9). Many reflect specific conditions, such as optic neuritis, pituitary adenomas, migraines, and psychogenic impairments. In addition, several visual field abnormalities are closely associated with other clinical disturbances, such as left homonymous hemianopsia associated with anosognosia, right homonymous hemianopsia with alexia, and a unilateral scotoma with paraparesis.

In their other function, the optic nerves and tracts form the afferent limb of the *pupillary light reflex* by sending small branches containing information about light intensity to the midbrain. After a single synapse, the oculomotor nerves (the third cranial nerves) form the efferent limb. The light reflex adjusts pupil size in response to the intensity of light striking the retina. Simply put, the light reflex constricts the pupils when a bright light is shown into one or both eyes (Fig. 4-2).

The neuroanatomy explains the important distinction between vision and the pupils' reacting to light. At the midbrain, the light reflex and visual system

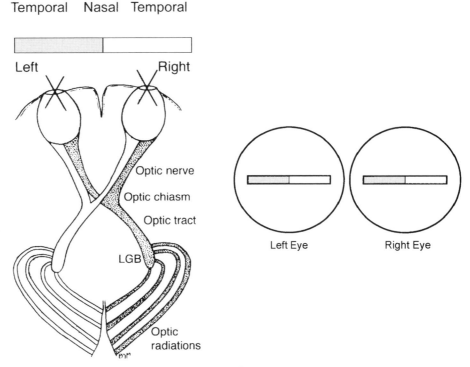

FIGURE 4-1 ■ *Left,* The optic nerves originate in the retinae. Their medial portions cross at the optic chiasm while the temporal portions continue uncrossed. The optic nerves form the optic tracts that synapse at the lateral geniculate bodies (LGB). The optic tracts sweep through the posterior cerebral hemispheres to terminate at the occipital cortex, which is often called the "visual cortex." One primary consequence of this system is that the impulses from each visual field are brought to the contralateral occipital lobe cortex. In this sketch, impulses conveying the shaded half of the bar, which is in the patient's left visual field, are conveyed to the right occipital cortex. *Right,* As in this case, medical illustrations typically present a patient's visual fields from the patient's perspective. In this illustration, the bar is portrayed in the left visual field of each eye.

diverge. The light reflex remains a brainstem function, but the visual system constitutes a higher level, cortical system. Thus, devastating cerebral cortex injuries—from trauma, anoxia, or degenerative illnesses—produce blindness ("cortical blindness"). No matter how terrible the cerebral cortex damage—even to the point of patients being severely demented, bedridden, and blind—the pupils continue to react normally to light.

Routine testing of the optic nerve includes examination of (1) visual acuity (Fig. 12-2), (2) visual fields (Fig. 4-3), and (3) the ocular fundi (Fig. 4-4). Because the visual system is important, complex, and subject to numerous ocular, neurologic, iatrogenic, and psychogenic disturbances, this book dedicates an entire chapter to visual disturbances particularly relevant to psychiatry (see Chapter 12).

OCULOMOTOR, TROCHLEAR, ABDUCENS NERVES (THIRD, FOURTH, SIXTH)

The oculomotor, trochlear, and abducens nerves constitute the "extraocular muscle system" because, acting in unison, they move the eyes in parallel to provide normal *conjugate gaze.* Damage of any of these nerves causes *dysconjugate* gaze, which results in *diplopia* (double vision). Extraocular muscle nerve damage leads to characteristic patterns of diplopia. In addition, with oculomotor nerve damage, patients also lose their pupillary constriction to light and strength of the eyelid muscle.

The oculomotor nerves (third cranial nerves) originate in the midbrain (Fig. 4-5) and eventually supply the pupil constrictor, eyelid, and adductor and elevator muscles of each eye (medial rectus, inferior oblique, inferior rectus, and superior rectus). Oculomotor nerve impairment, a common condition, thus leads to a distinctive constellation: a dilated pupil, ptosis, and outward deviation (abduction) of the eye (Fig. 4-6). As just discussed, oculomotor nerve impairment also impairs the efferent limb of the light reflex. In addition, it impairs the efferent limb of the *accommodation reflex,* in which the visual system adjusts the shape of the lens to focus on near or distant objects. (Impaired focusing ability in older individuals, *presbyopia* [Greek, *presbys,* old man; *opia,* eye], results from the aging lens losing its flexibility not from oculomotor nerve impairment.)

The trochlear nerves (fourth cranial nerves) also originate in the midbrain. They supply only the superior oblique muscle, which is responsible for depression of the eye when it is adducted (turned inward). To compensate for an injured trochlear nerve, patients tilt their head away from the affected side. Unless the physician sees a patient with diplopia perform this telltale maneuver, a trochlear nerve injury is difficult to diagnose.

Unlike the third and fourth cranial nerves, the abducens nerves (sixth cranial nerves) originate in the pons (Fig. 4-7 and see Fig. 2-9). Like the fourth cranial nerves, the abducens nerves have only a single function and innervate only a single muscle. The abducens nerves abduct the eyes by innervating lateral

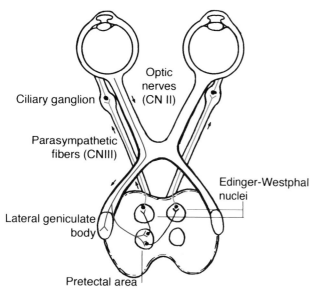

FIGURE 4-2 ■ The light reflex, which is more complex than a deep tendon reflex, begins with its afferent limb in the optic nerve (cranial nerve II). The optic nerve transmits light impulses from the retinas to two neighboring midbrain structures: (1) In conveying vision, axons synapse on the *lateral geniculate body.* Then postsynaptic tracts convey visual information to the occipital lobe's visual cortex. (2) In conveying the light reflex, optic nerve axons also synapse in the *pretectal region.* Postsynaptic neurons travel a short distance to both the ipsilateral and contralateral *Edinger-Westphal nuclei,* which are the parasympathetic divisions of the oculomotor (third cranial nerve) nuclei. Those nuclei give rise to parasympathetic oculomotor nerve fibers, which constitute to the reflex's efferent limb (see Fig. 12-17 Top). Their fibers synapse in the ciliary ganglia and postsynaptic fibers terminate in the iris constrictor (sphincter) muscles. Thus, light shone in one eye constricts the pupil of that eye (the "direct" [ipsilateral] light reflex) and the contralateral eye (the "consensual" [indirect or contralateral] light reflex). This figure also indicates how oculomotor nerve injuries, because they usually include damage to the parasympathetic component, lead to pupil dilation. Similarly, it illustrates how damaged sympathetic nervous innervation with unopposed parasympathetic innervation, as in the lateral medullary and Horner's syndromes, produces pupil constriction (*miosis*). Finally, it shows how ciliary ganglion damage produces a dilated but extremely sensitive "Adie's pupil" (see Fig. 12-17 Bottom).

rectus muscles. Abducens nerve impairment, which is also relatively common, causes inward deviation (adduction) of the eye, but no ptosis or pupil changes (Fig. 4-8). To review: the lateral rectus muscle is innervated by the sixth cranial (abducens) nerve and the superior oblique by the fourth (trochlear), but all the others by the third (oculomotor). A mnemonic device, "LR$_6$SO$_4$" captures this relationship.

To produce conjugate eye movements, the oculomotor nerve on one side works in tandem with the abducens nerve on the other. For example, when an individual looks to the left, the left sixth nerve and right third nerve activate their respective muscles to produce conjugate leftward eye movement. Such complementary innervation is essential for conjugate gaze. If both third nerves were simultaneously active, the eyes would look toward the nose; if both sixth nerves were simultaneously active, the eyes would look toward opposite walls.

Diplopia is most often attributable to a lesion in the oculomotor nerve on one side or the abducens nerve on the other. For example, if a patient has diplopia when looking to the left, then either the left abducens nerve or the right oculomotor nerve is paretic. Diplopia on right gaze, of course, suggests a paresis of either the right abducens or left oculomotor nerve. Although elaborate diagnostic tests may be performed, the presence or absence of other signs of oculomotor nerve palsy (a dilated pupil and ptosis) usually indicates whether that nerve is responsible.

The ocular cranial nerves may be damaged by lesions in the brainstem, in the nerves' course from the brainstem to the ocular muscles, or in their neuromuscular junctions but not in the cerebral hemispheres (the cerebrum). Because cerebral lesions do not injure these cranial nerves, conjugate gaze is preserved. Thus, patients with advanced Alzheimer's disease and those who have sustained cerebral anoxia have devastating cerebral lesions but normal, full conjugate ocular motility. These patients typically exist in a persistent vegetative state while retaining normal eye movements.

For learning purposes, physicians might best consider ocular cranial nerves lesions according to their brainstem level (midbrain, pons, and medulla) and correlate the clinical features with the admittedly complex anatomy. Because the anatomy is so compact, brainstem lesions that damage cranial nerves typically produce classic combinations of injuries of the ocular nerves and the adjacent corticospinal (pyramidal) tract or cerebellar outflow tracts. These lesions cause diplopia accompanied by contralateral hemiparesis or ataxia. The pattern of the diplopia is the signature of the lesion's location. The etiology in almost all cases is an occlusion of a small branch of the basilar artery causing a small brainstem infarction (see Chapter 11).

Most important, despite producing complex neurologic deficits, brainstem lesions generally do not impair cognitive function. However, certain exceptions to this dictum bear mentioning. *Wernicke's encephalopathy,* one well-known exception, consists of memory impairment (amnesia) accompanied by nystagmus and oculomotor or abducens nerve impairment (see Chapter 7). Another exception is *transtentorial herniation,* in which a cerebral mass lesion, such as a subdural hematoma, squeezes the anterior tip of the temporal lobe

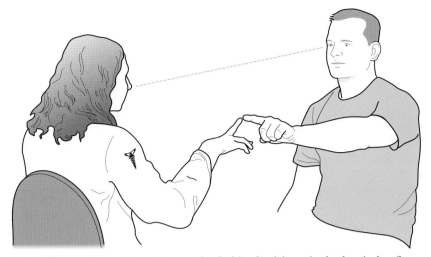

FIGURE 4-3 ■ In testing visual fields by the confrontation method, this physician wiggles her index finger as the patient points to it without diverting his eyes from her nose. She should test the four quadrants of each eye's visual field. (Only by testing each eye individually will she detect a bitemporal quadrantanopia, which is the visual field defect characteristic of pituitary adenomas.) Young children and others unable to comply with this testing method may be examined in a more superficial but still meaningful manner. In this case, the physician might assess the response to an attention-catching object introduced to each visual field. For example, a dollar bill, toy, or glass of water should capture a patient's attention. If the patient does not respond, the physician should consider visual field deficit(s) including blindness, but also psychogenic visual loss (see later) and inattention or neglect (see Chapter 8).

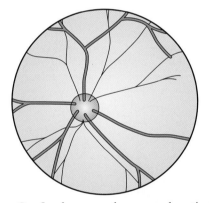

FIGURE 4-4 ■ On funduscopy, the normal optic fundus or disk appears yellow, flat, and clearly demarcated from the surrounding red retina. The retinal veins, as everywhere else in the body, are larger than their corresponding arteries. The retinal veins can normally be seen to pulsate except when intracranial pressure is elevated.

through the tentorial notch. In this situation, the mass compresses the oculomotor nerve and brainstem to cause coma and a dilated pupil (see Fig. 19-3).

With a right-sided midbrain infarction a patient would have a right oculomotor nerve palsy, which would cause right ptosis, a dilated pupil, and diplopia, accompanied by left hemiparesis (Fig. 4-9). With a slightly different right-sided midbrain infarction, a patient might have right oculomotor nerve palsy and left tremor (Fig. 4-10).

MIDBRAIN

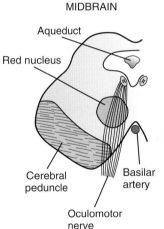

FIGURE 4-5 ■ The oculomotor (third cranial) nerves arise from nuclei in the dorsal portion of the midbrain (see Fig. 2-9). Each descends through the red nucleus, which carries cerebellar outflow fibers to the contralateral limbs. Then each passes through the cerebral peduncle, which carries the corticospinal tract destined to innervate the contralateral limbs.

A right-sided pons lesion translates into a right abducens nerve paresis and left hemiparesis (Fig. 4-11). Notably, in each of these brainstem injuries, mental status remains normal because the cerebrum is unscathed.

Another common site of brainstem injury that affects ocular motility is the *medial longitudinal fasciculus*

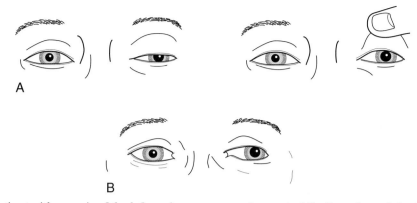

A

B

FIGURE 4-6 ■ *A,* The patient with paresis of the left oculomotor nerve has typical findings: lateral deviation of the left eye; the left pupil dilated and unreactive to light; and the upper eyelid covering a portion of the pupil constituting *ptosis. B,* In a milder case, close inspection reveals subtle ptosis, lateral deviation of the eye, and dilation of the pupil. In both cases, patients have diplopia that increases when looking to the right because this movement requires adducting the left eye; however, the paretic left medial rectus muscle cannot participate and the gaze becomes dysconjugate (also see Fig. 12-14).

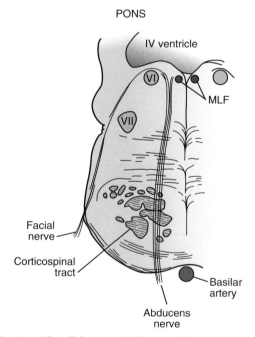

FIGURE 4-7 ■ The abducens (sixth cranial) nerves arise from nuclei located in the dorsal portion of the pons. These nuclei are adjacent to the medial longitudinal fasciculus (MLF; see Fig. 15-3). As the abducens nerves descend, they pass medial to the facial nerves, and then between the (UMN) neurons of the corticospinal tract.

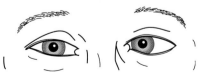

FIGURE 4-8 ■ The patient with paresis of the left abducens nerve has medial deviation of the left eye. There will be diplopia on looking ahead and toward the left, but not when looking to the right (see Fig. 12-15).

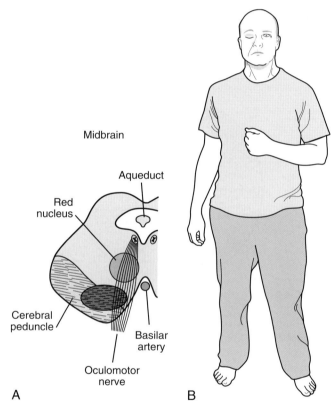

A   B

FIGURE 4-9 ■ *A,* A right midbrain infarction damages the oculomotor nerve that supplies the ipsilateral eye and the adjacent cerebral peduncle, which contains the corticospinal tract that subsequently crosses in the medulla, ultimately supplying the contralateral arm and leg. *B,* The patient has right-sided ptosis from the right oculomotor nerve palsy and left hemiparesis from the corticospinal tract injury. Also note that the ptosis elicits a compensatory unconscious elevation of the eyebrow to uncover the eye. (Similar eyebrow elevations can be seen in other conditions that cause ptosis, including cluster headache, myasthenia gravis, and lateral medullary syndrome.)

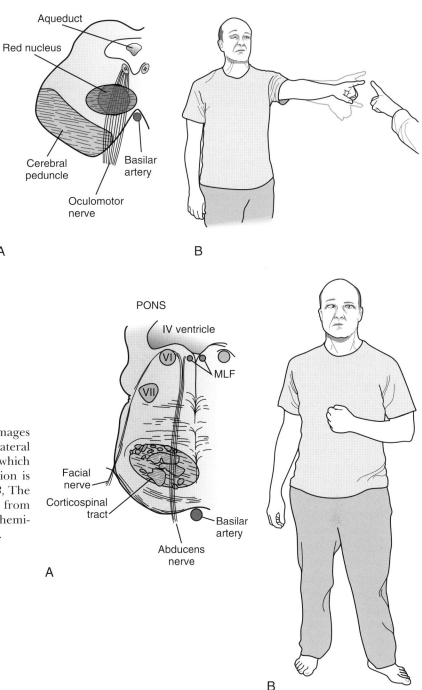

MIDBRAIN

FIGURE 4-10 ■ *A*, The *red nucleus* is the intermediate step in conveying cerebellar outflow from the cerebellum to the ipsilateral arm and leg. Each cerebellar hemisphere innervates the contralateral red nucleus that, in turn, innervates the contralateral arm and leg. Because this pattern involves two contralateral steps, it is often called a "double cross." In this case, a right midbrain infarction damages the oculomotor nerve and adjacent red nucleus, which innervates the left arm and leg. *B*, The patient has right ptosis from the oculomotor nerve palsy and left arm ataxia from the damage to the cerebellar outflow tract.

FIGURE 4-11 ■ *A*, A right pontine infarction damages the abducens nerve, which supplies the ipsilateral eye, and the adjacent corticospinal tract, which supplies the contralateral limbs. (This situation is analogous to midbrain infarctions; Fig. 4-9.) *B*, The patient has inward deviation of the right eye from paresis of the right abducens nerve and left hemiparesis from right corticospinal tract damage.

(MLF). This structure is the heavily myelinated midline tract, between the pons and the midbrain, that links the nuclei of the abducens and oculomotor nerves (see Figs. 2-9, 4-11, 15-3, and 15-4). Its interruption produces the *MLF syndrome*, also called *internuclear ophthalmoplegia (INO)*, which consists of nystagmus of the abducting eye and failure of the adducting eye to cross the midline. This disorder is best known as a characteristic finding of MS.

The oculomotor or abducens nerves are particularly vulnerable to injury in their long paths between their brainstem nuclei and ocular muscles. Lesions in those nerves produce simple, readily identifiable clinical pictures: extraocular muscle impairment without hemiparesis, ataxia, or mental status impairment. *Diabetic infarction*, the most frequent lesion of the oculomotor nerves, produces a sharp headache and paresis of the affected muscles. Although otherwise typical of oculomotor nerve infarctions, diabetic infarctions characteristically spare the pupil. In other words, diabetic infarctions cause ptosis and ocular abduction, but the pupil remains normal in size, equal to its counterpart, and reactive to light.

Ruptured or expanding aneurysms of the posterior communicating artery may compress the oculomotor nerve, just as it exits from the midbrain. In this case, oculomotor nerve palsy—which would be the least of the patient's problems—is just one manifestation of a life-threatening subarachnoid hemorrhage that usually renders patients prostrate with a severe headache. Children occasionally have migraine headaches accompanied by temporary oculomotor nerve paresis (see Chapter 9). By way of contrast, in the motor neuron diseases, amyotrophic lateral sclerosis (ALS) and poliomyelitis, the oculomotor and abducens nerves retain normal function despite destruction of large numbers of motor neurons. Patients may have full, conjugate eye movements despite being unable to breathe, lift their limbs, or move their head.

Disorders of the neuromuscular junction—the nervous system's furthest extent—also produce oculomotor or abducens nerve paresis. In myasthenia gravis (see Fig. 6-3) and botulism, for example, impairment of acetylcholine neuromuscular transmission leads to combinations of ocular and other cranial nerve paresis. These deficits may be perplexing to physicians because the muscle weakness is often subtle and variable in severity and pattern. These disorders are always important, especially in their extremes. In severe cases, respiratory impairment may ensue, and mild cases may be either overlooked or misdiagnosed as psychogenic.

A related condition, congenital dysconjugate or "crossed" eyes, *strabismus*, does not cause double vision because the brain suppresses one of the images. If uncorrected in childhood, strabismus leads to blindness of the deviated eye, *amblyopia*.

People can usually feign ocular muscle weakness only by staring inward, as if looking at the tip of their nose. Children often do this playfully; however, physicians diagnose adults with their eyes in such a position as displaying voluntary, bizarre activity. Another disturbance, found mostly in health care workers, comes from surreptitiously instilling eye drops that dilate the pupil to mimic ophthalmologic or neurologic disorders.

TRIGEMINAL (FIFTH)

In contrast to the exclusively sensory function of cranial nerves I and II and the exclusively motor functions of cranial nerves III, IV, and VI, the trigeminal nerves have both sensory and motor functions. The trigeminal (Latin, *threefold*) nerves convey sensation from the face and innervate the large, powerful muscles that protrude and close the jaw. Because these muscles' main function is to chew, they are often called the "muscles of mastication."

The trigeminal nerves' motor nucleus is situated in the pons, but the sensory nucleus extends from the midbrain through the medulla. The nerves leave the brainstem at the side of the pons, together with the facial and acoustic nerves, to become the three cranial nerves—V, VII, and VIII—that pass through the *cerebellopontine angle*.

Examination of the trigeminal nerve begins by testing sensation in its three sensory divisions (Fig. 4-12). The examiner touches the side of the patient's forehead, cheek, and jaw. Areas of reduced sensation, *hypalgesia*, should conform to anatomic outlines.

Assessing the *corneal reflex* is useful, especially in examining patients whose sensory loss does not conform to neurologic expectations. The corneal reflex is a "superficial reflex" that is essentially independent of upper motor neuron (UMN) status. It begins with stimulation of the cornea by a wisp of cotton or a breath of air that triggers the trigeminal nerve's V_1 division, which forms the reflex's afferent limb. A brainstem synapse stimulus innervates both facial (seventh cranial) nerves, which form the efferent limb.

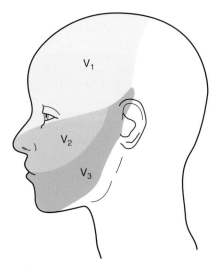

FIGURE 4-12 ■ The three divisions of the trigeminal nerve convey sensory innervation of the face. The first division (V_1) supplies the forehead, the cornea, and the scalp up to the vertex; the second (V_2) supplies the malar area; and the third (V_3) supplies the lower jaw, except for the angle. These distributions have more than academic importance. These dermatomes may be mapped by *herpes zoster* infections (shingles), trigeminal neuralgia (see Chapter 9), and facial angioma in the Sturge-Weber syndrome (see Fig. 13-13). In contrast, patients with psychogenic disturbances do not restrict their sensory loss to these boundaries.

The synapse innervates both sets of orbicularis oculi muscles.

Normally, because of the synapse, stimulating one cornea will provoke bilateral blinking. However, if the cotton tip is first applied to the *right* cornea and *neither* eye blinks, and then to the *left* cornea and *both* eyes blink, *the right trigeminal nerve* (afferent limb) is impaired. On the other hand, if cotton stimulation on the *right* cornea fails to provide a right eye blink but succeeds in provoking a *left* eye blink, the *right facial nerve* (efferent limb) is impaired.

In testing the motor component, jaw muscle strength is performed by asking the patient to clench and then protrude the jaw. The *jaw jerk reflex*, which is similar to a deep tendon reflex, consists of a prompt but not overly forceful closing after a tap (Fig. 4-13). A hyperactive response indicates an UMN (corticobulbar tract) lesion, and a hypoactive response indicates a lower motor neuron (LMN) or cranial nerve lesion. The physician should test the jaw jerk in patients with dysarthria, dysphagia, and emotional lability—mostly to assess the likelihood of pseudobulbar palsy (see later).

Injury of a trigeminal nerve causes facial hypalgesia, afferent corneal reflex impairment, jaw jerk hypoactivity, and deviation of the jaw toward the side of the lesion. A variety of conditions—nasopharyngeal tumors, gunshot wounds, and tumors of the cerebellopontine angle, such as acoustic neuromas (see Fig. 20-27)—may cause trigeminal nerve injury.

In the opposite situation, *trigeminal neuralgia* (tic douloureux) results from trigeminal nerve irritation by an aberrant vessel or other lesion in the cerebellopontine angle. Instead of having hypalgesia, patients with trigeminal neuralgia have bursts of lancinating face pain in the distribution of the third or other division of the nerve (see Chapter 9). Another common trigeminal nerve problem is *herpes zoster* infection, which causes a rash followed by excruciating pain (*postherpetic neuralgia*) in one division of the nerve (see Chapter 14).

Finally, a psychogenic sensory loss involving the face will usually encompass the entire face or be included in a sensory loss of one half of the body. In almost all cases, the following three nonanatomic features will be present: (1) the sensory loss will not involve the scalp (although the portion anterior to the vertex is supplied by the trigeminal nerve), (2) the corneal reflex will remain intact, and (3) when only one half the face is affected, sensation will be lost sharply rather than gradually at the midline (i.e., the midline will be split) (see Fig. 3-5).

FACIAL (SEVENTH)

The facial nerves' major functions, like the trigeminal nerves' major functions, are both sensory and motor: to convey taste sensation and to innervate the facial muscles. Their motor and sensory nuclei are in the pons, and the nerves exit through the side of the brainstem with the other cerebellopontine angle nerves.

Just as the trigeminal nerves supply the muscles of mastication, the facial nerves supply the "muscles of facial expression." In a unique and potentially confusing arrangement in their neuroanatomy, cerebral impulses innervate both the contralateral and ipsilateral facial nerve motor nuclei. Each facial nerve supplies its ipsilateral temporalis, orbicularis oculi, and orbicularis oris muscles—those responsible for a frown, raised eyebrows, wink, smile, and grimace. In the classic explanation, because of their crossed and uncrossed supply, the upper facial muscles are ultimately innervated by both cerebral hemispheres, whereas the lower facial muscles are innervated by only the contralateral cerebral hemisphere (Fig. 4-14). In an alternative explanation, interneurons link the facial nerve nuclei. This theory postulates that the "crossing" takes place in the brainstem rather than in the cerebrum.

Whatever the actual underlying neuroanatomy, facial nerve injuries cause ipsilateral paresis of both upper and lower face muscles. This pattern is termed a "peripheral facial" or "lower motor neuron weakness." Injuries of the cerebral cortex or upper brainstem, which affect the corticobulbar tract, cause

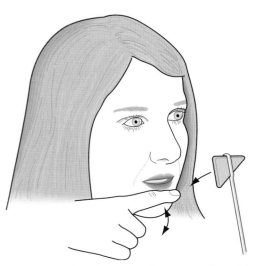

FIGURE 4-13 ■ Tapping the normal, open, relaxed jaw will move it slightly downward. The jaw jerk reflex is the soft rebound. Abnormalities are mostly a matter of rapidity and strength. In a hypoactive reflex, as found in bulbar palsy and other lower motor neuron (LMN) injuries, there is little or no rebound. In a hyperactive reflex, as in pseudobulbar palsy and other upper motor neuron (UMN) (corticobulbar tract) lesions, there is a quick and forceful rebound.

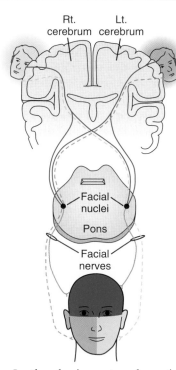

Rt.   Lt.
cerebrum cerebrum

Facial
nuclei

Pons

Facial
nerves

FIGURE 4-14 ■ In the classic portrayal, corticobulbar tracts originating in the ipsilateral, as well as in the contralateral, cerebral hemisphere supply each facial nerve nucleus. Each facial nerve supplies the ipsilateral muscles of facial expression. Because the upper half of the face receives cortical innervation from both hemispheres, cerebral injuries lead to paresis only of the lower half of the contralateral face. In contrast, facial nerve injuries lead to paresis of both the upper and lower half of the ipsilateral side of the face.

contralateral paresis of only the lower face. That pattern is termed "central" or "upper motor neuron weakness."

Taste sensation is more straightforward. The facial nerves convey impulses from taste receptors of the anterior two thirds of the tongue, and the glossopharyngeal nerves (the ninth cranial nerve) convey those from the posterior third. A remarkable aspect of this sensation is that, despite the extraordinary variety of foods, taste perceptions are limited, even with the rediscovery of an additional one. According to conventional wisdom, taste receptors detect only four fundamental sensations: bitter, sweet, sour, and salty. However, reconsideration of an idea proposed 100 years ago by a Japanese researcher confirmed that people were able to perceive a fifth taste sensation, originally labeled *umami,* that people often describe as "richness." This taste is based on detecting L-glutamate, which is an amino acid abundant in high protein foods and a constituent of the flavoring, monosodium glutamate (MSG). Further research showed that H^+, K^+, and Na^+ trigger salty and sour tastes, and G-protein receptors trigger the other tastes.

Food actually derives most of its flavor from its aroma, which is detected by the olfactory nerve. Moreover, the olfactory nerve, not the facial nerve, has extensive connections with the frontal lobe and limbic system.

Routine facial nerve testing involves examining the strength of the facial muscles and, at certain times, assessing taste. An examiner observes the patient's face, first at rest and then during a succession of maneuvers that use various facial muscles: looking upward to furrow the forehead, closing the eyes, and smiling. When weakness is present, the examiner should try to ascertain whether it involves both the upper and lower, or only the lower, facial muscles. Upper and lower face paresis suggests a lesion of the facial nerve itself. (As previously mentioned, this pattern of paresis may be termed a peripheral or LMN weakness.) In this case, the lesion also probably impairs taste sensation.

With unilateral or even bilateral facial nerve injuries, of course, patients have no congnitive impairment. In contrast, paresis of only the lower facial muscles suggests a lesion of the contralateral cerebral hemisphere, which may be associated with mental changes and hemiparesis. In addition, with weakness of the right lower face, aphasia may be present. In these cases, taste sensation will be preserved.

To test taste, the examiner applies either a dilute salt or sugar solution to the anterior portion of each side of the tongue, which must remain protruded to prevent the solution from spreading. A patient will normally be able to identify the fundamental taste sensations, but not those "tastes" that depend on aroma, such as onion and garlic.

Facial nerve damage produces paresis of the ipsilateral upper and lower face muscles with or without loss of taste sensation. Sudden onset, idiopathic facial paralysis, usually with loss of taste sensation, generically labeled *Bell's palsy,* has traditionally been attributed to an inflammation or infection (Fig. 4-15). In many of these cases, *herpes simplex* virus or less often *Borrelia burgdorferi,* a tick-borne spirochete that causes *Lyme disease* (see Chapters 5 and 7), has been the culprit. Destructive injuries, including lacerations, cerebellopontine angle tumors, and carcinomatous meningitis, damage not only the facial nerve but usually its neighboring cerebellopontine angle nerves as well.

Lesions that stimulate the nerve have the opposite effect. For example, aberrant vessels in the cerebellopontine angle can irritate the facial nerve and produce intermittent, completely involuntary, prolonged contractions of the muscles of the ipsilateral side of the face. This disorder, *hemifacial spasm* (see Chapter 18), which might be misdiagnosed as a "nervous tic," represents the facial nerve counterpart of trigeminal neuralgia.

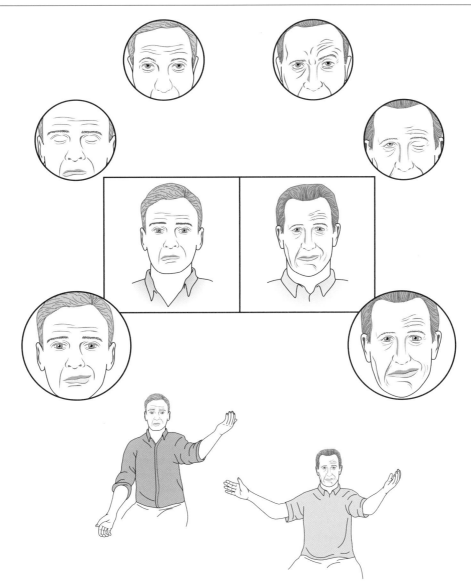

FIGURE 4-15 ■ The patient on the left has weakness of his right lower face from thrombosis of the left middle cerebral artery. He might be said to have a "central" (central nervous system [CNS]) facial paralysis. The patient on the right has right-sided weakness of both his upper and lower face from a right facial nerve injury (Bell's palsy). He might be said to have a "peripheral" facial (cranial nerve) paralysis. In the *center boxed sketches*, the man with the central palsy *(left)* has flattening of the right nasolabial fold and sagging of the mouth downward to the right. This pattern of weakness indicates paresis of only the lower facial muscles. The man with the peripheral palsy *(right)*, however, has right-sided loss of the normal forehead furrows in addition to flattening of his nasolabial fold. This pattern of weakness indicates paresis of the upper as well as the lower facial muscles. In the *circled sketches at the top*, the patients have been asked to look upward—a maneuver that would exaggerate upper facial weakness. The man with central weakness has normal upward movement of the eyebrows and furrowing of the forehead. The man with peripheral weakness has no eyebrow or forehead movement, and the forehead skin remains flat. In the *circled sketches second from the top*, the men have been asked to close their eyes—a maneuver that also would exaggerate upper facial weakness. The man with the central weakness has widening of the palpebral fissure, but he is able to close his eyelids and cover the eyeball. The man with the peripheral weakness is unable to close the affected eyelids, although his genuine effort is made apparent by the retroversion of the eyeball (Bell's phenomenon). In the *lowest circled sketches*, the men have been asked to smile—a maneuver that would exaggerate lower facial weakness. Both men have strength only of the left side of the mouth, and thus it deviates to the left. If tested, the man with Bell's palsy would have loss of taste on the anterior two thirds of his tongue on the affected side. The *bottom sketches* show the response when both men are asked to elevate their arms. The man with the central facial weakness also has paresis of the adjacent arm, but the man with the peripheral weakness has no arm paresis. In summary, the man on the left with the left middle cerebral artery occlusion has paresis of his right lower face and arm. The man on the right with right Bell's palsy has paresis of his right upper and lower face and loss of taste on the anterior two thirds of his tongue.

People cannot mimic unilateral facial paresis. Some people who refuse to be examined, particularly children, might forcefully close their eyelids and mouth. The willful nature of this maneuver is evident when the examiner finds resistance on opening the eyelids and jaw and observes, when the eyelids are pried open, that the eyeballs retrovert (Bell's phenomena).

Although impairment of taste, *dysgeusia* (Greek, *geusis*, taste), usually occurs along with facial muscle weakness, as in Bell's palsy and other facial nerve injuries, it might occur with large brainstem lesions, such as MS plaques. However, such lesions would also produce problems that would overshadow impaired taste. On the other hand, dysgeusia might develop in isolation. It might be medication-induced. For example, tricyclic antidepressants, acetazolamide (for treatment of pseudotumor cerebri), levodopa (Parkinson's disease), and several antiepileptic drugs all can diminish or distort taste. Chemotherapy, especially with radiotherapy directed at the head and neck, causes loss of taste through a combination of salivary secretion loss and tongue damage.

Normal age-related changes lead to a loss of taste sensation. Older individuals routinely lose taste sensitivity and discrimination. In addition, both age-related decrease in salivary secretions and several medications lead to "dry mouth," which markedly impairs taste function and the enjoyment of eating. Many older individuals require enhanced flavors and special preparations to make food desirable.

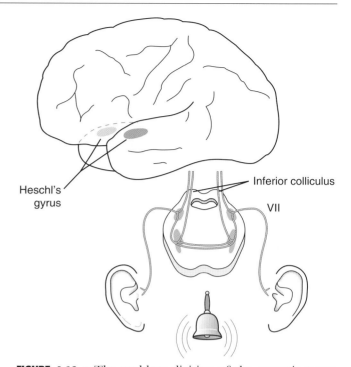

FIGURE 4-16 ■ The cochlear division of the acoustic nerve synapses extensively in the pons. Crossed and uncrossed fibers pass upward through the brainstem to terminate in the ipsilateral and contralateral auditory (Heschl's gyrus) cortex of each temporal lobe; however, Heschl's gyri, which sit in the planum temporale, receive auditory stimuli predominantly from the contralateral ear. In addition, the dominant hemisphere Heschl's gyrus almost abuts Wernicke's language area (see Fig. 8-1) and has a role in language function.

ACOUSTIC (EIGHTH)

Each acoustic nerve is actually composed of two divisions with separate courses and functions: hearing and balance. The *cochlear nerve,* one of the two divisions, transmits auditory impulses from the middle and inner ear mechanisms to the superior temporal gyri of both cerebral hemispheres (Fig. 4-16). This bilateral cortical representation of sound explains the clinical finding that damage to the acoustic nerve or ear itself may cause deafness in that ear, but unilateral lesions of the brainstem or cerebral hemisphere—CNS damage—will not cause hearing impairment. For example, cerebral lesions, such as tumors or strokes, that involve the temporal lobes, may cause aphasia and hemiparesis, but they do not impair hearing.

During the routine examination, the examiner initially tests hearing by whispering into one of the patient's ears while covering the other. Acoustic nerve injury may result from medications, such as aspirin or streptomycin; by skull fractures severing the nerve; or by cerebellopontine angle tumors, particularly acoustic neuromas associated with neurofibromatosis (see Chapter 13). *In utero* rubella infections or kernicterus (see Chapter 13) commonly cause congenital deafness accompanied by mental retardation.

On the other hand, when patients seem to mimic deafness, the examiner may attempt to startle them with a loud sound or may watch for an *auditory-ocular reflex* (involuntarily looking toward a noise). The diagnosis of psychogenic hearing loss may be confirmed by testing brainstem auditory evoked responses (BAERs; see Chapter 15).

About 25% of people older than 65 years develop hearing impairment from degeneration of the acoustic nerve or the cochlea and other middle ear structures. Hearing loss associated with older age, *presbycusis* (Greek, *presbys*, old man; *acusis*, hearing), typically begins with loss of high frequency and eventually progressing to involve all frequencies. Early in its course, presbycusis impairs the ability to distinguish between consonants, for example, *b* and *v*. One of the first and generally always the most troublesome problem for individuals with presbycusis is impaired speech discrimination in rooms crowded with talking people, such as restaurants and cocktail parties. Characteristically, their inability to hear conversational speech is disproportionately greater than their hearing loss.

As with many age-related impairments, presbycusis results more from degeneration of the special sensory organ than the cranial nerve itself (Table 4-1). In this case, the cochlear mechanism, rather than the acoustic nerve itself, withers. Similarly, loss of elasticity of the ocular lens leads to visual impairments associated with advanced age (presbyopia) and atrophy of the taste follicles of the tongue leads to loss of taste perception.

Not surprisingly, presbycusis thus potentially leads to inattention and social isolation. In addition, when hearing impairments accompany visual impairments, sensory deprivation may precipitate hallucinations. Such impairments may overwhelm someone with minimal cognitive impairment (see Chapter 7) or lead to misdiagnoses of dementia and psychosis. For the limited problem of age-related hearing impairment in the elderly, as a general rule, physicians should dispense hearing aids readily and even on a trial basis.

Another problem common among the elderly consists of hearing incessant ringing, buzzing, hissing, or whistling. This condition, *tinnitus,* is often accompanied by mild to moderate hearing impairment. Medications, particularly aspirin, which damage the inner ear, or ischemia, from atherosclerotic cerebrovascular disease, may cause tinnitus. If it develops unilaterally in a young or middle-aged adult, tinnitus might be a symptom of an acoustic neuroma. Otherwise, it is usually only a nuisance. Psychiatric medications have not been implicated as a cause. In fact, possibly because of a comorbidity of tinnitus and depression, tricyclic antidepressants can reduce tinnitus.

Sometimes the sounds are rhythmic. This variation, *pulsatile tinnitus,* although often the result of heightened sensitivity, may be a manifestation of atherosclerotic cerebrovascular or cardiac disease.

Auditory evaluations are necessary in patients suspected of having a psychogenic hearing impairment;

in children with autism, cerebral palsy, mental retardation, or speech impediments, and poor school performance; and in most older adults.

In a unique, life-improving innovation, surgically implanting acoustic nerve stimulators (*cochlear implants*) has allowed hearing-impaired infants and children to develop hearing and speaking abilities, such that most of them can enter mainstream education. In addition, cochlear implants have allowed adults with hearing loss uncorrected by hearing aides to regain useful hearing.

The other division of the acoustic nerve, the *vestibular nerve,* transmits impulses from the labyrinth governing equilibrium, orientation, and change in position. The most characteristic symptom of vestibular nerve damage is *vertigo,* a sensation that one is spinning within the environment or that the environment itself is spinning. Unfortunately, patients casually say "dizziness" when they mean lightheadedness, anxiety, weakness, or unsteadiness.

The most common cause of *vertigo* is vestibular injury, such as viral infections of the inner ear, *labyrinthitis,* or ischemia. When the vertigo is induced by an otherwise normal patient placing the head in certain positions or merely changing positions, the disorder is called *benign positional vertigo.* One theory suggests that in this disorder, which is relatively common among middle-aged and older individuals, free-floating debris comprised of stone-like material, *otoliths,* disturbs the semicircular canals. In any case, exercises that place the head in certain positions alleviate the symptom in some individuals, presumably by securing the debris in innocuous places.

Ménière's disease, which deserves special attention, is a relatively common chronic vestibular disorder of unknown etiology that causes attacks of unequivocal vertigo, unilateral tinnitus, and nystagmus. More prevalent in women than in men, it also leads to progressive hearing loss. Although most attacks of Ménière's disease are obvious, they may be indistinguishable from basilar artery transient ischemic attacks (TIAs), basilar artery migraines, and mild hyperventilation.

TABLE 4-1 ■ Age-Related Special Sense Impairments*	
Smell	Some degree of anosmia in 75% of individuals older than 80 years
Vision	Presbyopia: mostly inability to accommodate to see closely held or small objects; cataracts (see Chapter 12)
Taste	Loss of taste sensitivity and discrimination, as well as anosmia for aroma
Hearing	Presbycusis: loss of speech discrimination, especially for consonants; poor high-pitched sound detection, tinnitus

*The impairment stems more from degeneration of the sensory organ than the cranial nerve.

BULBAR: GLOSSOPHARYNGEAL, VAGUS, SPINAL ACCESSORY NERVES (NINTH, TENTH, ELEVENTH)

The *bulbar* cranial nerves (IX through XII)—the last of the three cranial nerve groups—arise from nuclei in the brainstem caudal to the ocular (III, IV, and VI) and the cerebellopontine (V, VII, and VIII) cranial nerve groups. The bulb is technically equivalent to the medulla. However, from a clinical viewpoint, it also includes the pons (see Figs. 20-1 and 20-17).

In addition to containing the nuclei and initial portions of cranial nerves IX through XII, the bulb contains several important tracts: the descending corticospinal tract, ascending sensory tract, and sympathetic nervous system. The bulbar cranial nerves innervate the muscles of the soft palate, pharynx, larynx, and tongue. They implement speaking and swallowing.

As for afferent functions of the bulbar cranial nerves, the glossopharyngeal nerve brings taste sensations from the posterior third of the tongue to the brain; the vagus nerve brings autonomic nervous system impulses to the medulla, from where they are relayed to cephalad regions of the brainstem and the cerebral cortex. The lateral medullary infarction, the most common brainstem stroke, has already illustrated the bulbar cranial nerves' relationship to several CNS tracts (see Wallenberg syndrome, Fig. 2-10).

Although the bulbar cranial nerves originate in the caudal end of the brainstem, located nowhere near the cerebral cortex, and execute only simple and mechanical functions, they are involved in several neurologic conditions that have psychiatric aspects. For example, in *vagus nerve stimulation,* a pacemaker-like device stimulates the vagus nerve as it rises through the neck toward the brainstem. Originally found effective in suppressing epilepsy (see Chapter 10), vagus nerve stimulation has been proposed as an ancillary treatment for depression and chronic pain.

Another example is the famous *bulbar/pseudobulbar* distinction: Impairment of the bulbar cranial nerves leads to bulbar palsy, but frontal lobe impairment leads to pseudobulbar palsy. Although pseudobulbar palsy shares some physical characteristics with its bulbar palsy counterpart, it induces unprovoked outbursts of laughing, crying, or both (see later). Likewise, the *locked-in syndrome,* which is itself important, may be contrasted with the persistent vegetative state (see Chapter 11), in which cognitive function is obliterated but vegetative functions—respiration, sleeping, and swallowing—persist.

Finally, bulbar nerve overactivity leads to certain seemingly bizarre disorders, such as spasmodic dysphonia and spasmodic torticollis, which until recently have been considered psychogenic and untreatable (see Chapter 18).

Bulbar Palsy

Bulbar cranial nerve injury within the brainstem or along the course of the nerves leads to bulbar palsy. This commonly occurring disorder is characterized by *dysarthria* (speech impairment), *dysphagia* (swallowing impairment), and hypoactive jaw and gag reflexes (Table 4-2).

TABLE 4-2 ■ Comparison of Bulbar and Pseudobulbar Palsy

	Bulbar	Pseudobulbar
Dysarthria	Yes	Yes
Dysphagia	Yes	Yes
Movement of palate		
Voluntary	No	No
Gag reflex	No	Yes
Respiratory impairment	Yes	No
Jaw jerk	Hypoactive	Hyperactive
Emotional lability	No	Yes
Intellectual impairment	No	Yes

To assess bulbar nerve function, the examiner should listen to the patient's spontaneous speech during casual conversation and while eliciting the history. The patient should be asked to repeat syllables that require lingual ("la"), labial ("pa"), and guttural or pharyngeal ("ga") speech mechanisms. Most patients with bulbar palsy speak with a thick, nasal intonation. Some remain mute. Even if a patient's speech is not strikingly abnormal during casual conversation, repetition of the guttural consonant, "ga...ga...ga...," will typically evoke thickened, nasal sounds, uttered "gna...gna...gna...." In addition, when saying "ah," a patient with bulbar palsy will have completely impaired or asymmetric palate elevation because of paresis.

In contrast, the speech of patients with cerebellar dysfunction is characterized by an irregular rhythm (scanning speech), which is akin to ataxia (see Chapter 2). The speech of patients with spasmodic dysphonia has a "strained and strangled" quality, often with a superimposed tremor (see Chapter 18). Unlike aphasic patients (see Chapter 8), those with bulbar palsy have normal comprehension and can express themselves in writing.

In addition to causing dysarthria, impaired palatal and pharyngeal movement in bulbar palsy causes dysphagia. Food tends to lodge in the trachea or go into the nasopharyngeal cavity. Liquids tend to regurgitate through the nose. When patients attempt to eat, they tend to aspirate food and saliva and develop aspiration pneumonia.

Impairment of palate sensation or movement leads to the characteristic loss of the gag reflex (Fig. 4-17). Finally, extensive bulbar damage will injure the medulla's respiratory center or its cranial nerves that innervate respiratory muscles. For example, the bulbar form of poliomyelitis (polio) forced its childhood victims into "iron lungs" to support their respiration. Even today, many patients with bulbar palsy from Guillain-Barré syndrome, myasthenia gravis, and similar conditions must undergo tracheostomy for respiratory support.

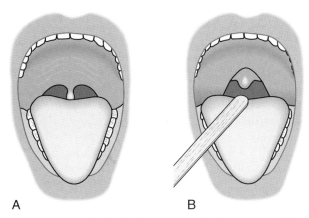

A   B

FIGURE 4-17 ■ *A,* The soft palate normally forms an arch from which the uvula seems to hang. *B,* When the pharynx is stimulated, the gag reflex elicits pharyngeal muscle contraction; the soft palate rises with the uvula remaining in the midline. With bulbar nerve injury (bulbar palsy)—lower motor neuron (LMN) injury—the palate has little, no, or asymmetric movement. With corticobulbar tract injury (pseudobulbar palsy)—upper motor neuron (UMN) injury—the reaction is brisk and forceful. Unfortunately, it often precipitates retching, coughing, or crying. (If the purpose of the examination is to assess the patient's ability to swallow, a more reliable decision can be reached by simply observing the patient attempt to swallow a few sips of water.)

Depending on its cause, bulbar palsy is associated with still other physical findings. When the jaw muscles are involved, the jaw jerk reflex will be depressed (Fig. 4-13). If a brainstem lesion also damages the corticospinal tract, patients develop hyperactive deep tendon reflexes (DTRs) and Babinski signs. However, as in other conditions that strike only the brainstem, bulbar palsy is associated with neither cognitive impairment nor emotional abnormalities.

Illnesses that commonly cause bulbar palsy by damaging the cranial nerves within the brainstem are ALS, poliomyelitis, and the lateral medullary infarction. Those that damage the nerves after they have emerged from the brainstem—a subtle distinction—include the Guillain-Barré syndrome, chronic meningitis, and tumors that grow along the base of the skull or within the adjacent meninges. In a more substantial difference, myasthenia gravis and botulism cause bulbar palsy by impairing neuromuscular junction transmission (see Chapter 6). Most important, none of these conditions *directly* changes cognitive function or emotional stability because their damage does not involve the cerebrum.

PSEUDOBULBAR PALSY

When frontal lobe damage causes dysarthria and dysphagia, the condition is termed pseudobulbar palsy.

This condition is better known than bulbar palsy because of its associated, nonphysical manifestations that overshadow all of its other aspects. Most important, pseudobulbar palsy causes prominent, unprovoked episodes of emotional outbursts, which are its hallmark. In turn, pseudobulbar palsy is often accompanied by aphasia or dementia.

Dysarthria in pseudobulbar palsy is characterized by variable rhythm and intensity with an "explosive" cadence. For example, when asked to repeat the consonant "ga," patients might blurt out "GA... GA... GA... ga... ga... ga." The dysphagia often results in inadequate nutrition and aspiration. Although these complications might be circumvented by surgical placement of gastrostomy tubes, installing these mechanical devices has created almost as much controversy as the use of respirators in artificially prolonging life.

From an admittedly narrow neurologic perspective, another distinguishing characteristic of pseudobulbar palsy is hyperactivity of certain reflexes because of damage to the corticobulbar tracts (Fig. 4-18); thus, it is sometimes called *supra*bulbar palsy. As in bulbar palsy, patients with pseudobulbar palsy have little or no palatal or pharyngeal movement in response to voluntary effort, as when attempting to say "ah." However, when the gag reflex is tested, these patients have brisk elevation of the palate and contraction of the pharynx, often overreacting with coughing, crying, and retching (Fig. 4-17). Likewise, the jaw jerk reflex, depressed in bulbar palsy, is hyperactive in pseudobulbar palsy because of UMN corticobulbar tract damage.*

In addition, in pseudobulbar palsy, damage to the frontal lobes is so common that it almost always leads to signs of bilateral corticospinal tract damage, such as hyperactive DTRs and Babinski signs. Frontal lobe damage also leads to corticobulbar tract damage that makes the face sag and impairs expression (Fig. 4-19).

The most notorious feature of pseudobulbar palsy has been termed *emotional lability*—a tendency to burst into tears or, less often, laughter, but not in response to underlying emotions. Patients who appear to alternate unexpectedly between euphoria and depression often describe themselves as being awash with emotions. Amitriptyline and some selective serotonin reuptake inhibitors, given in relatively low doses, may suppress the unwarranted *pathologic laughing* and *crying*, apart from their antidepressant effect.

Although pseudobulbar palsy has become the commonly accepted explanation for unwarranted emotional states in people with brain damage, tearfulness

---

*A theory recently offered as an alternative to UMN damage causing pseudobulbar palsy proposes that the disorder stems from disruption of a cerebral-brainstem-cerebellum circuit that coordinates emotion, its expression, and the social context.

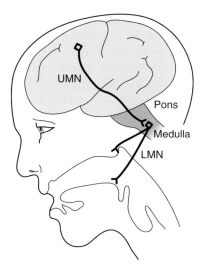

FIGURE 4-18 ■ Damage to the bulbar cranial nerves (bulbar palsy) abolishes the jaw jerk and gag reflexes, both of which are characteristic of lower motor neuron (LMN) injury (see Fig. 2-2C). Although mental changes may be the most conspicuous feature of pseudobulbar palsy, corticobulbar tract damage leads to hyperactive reflexes, which are characteristic of upper motor neuron (UMN) injury (see Fig. 2-2B).

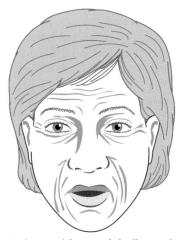

FIGURE 4-19 ■ Patients with pseudobulbar palsy, such as this woman who has sustained multiple cerebral infarctions, often sit with a slack jaw, furrowed forehead, and vacant stare.

should not always be ascribed exclusively to brain damage. A great deal of true sadness can be expected with neurologic illness. Many patients obviously have both depression and pseudobulbar palsy.

Because of the extensive cerebral damage usually underlying it, pseudobulbar palsy is associated with dementia as well as emotional lability. Likewise, when the left cerebral hemisphere is heavily damaged, pseudobulbar palsy may be associated with aphasia, usually of the nonfluent variety (see Chapter 8). This association also might account for aphasic patients crying at minimal provocation, even in frustration at naming

objects. In any case, patients with pseudobulbar palsy should be evaluated for both dementia and aphasia.

Damage to both frontal lobes or, more often, the entire cerebrum by any of a wide variety of degenerative, structural, or metabolic disturbances causes pseudobulbar palsy. Its most common causes are Alzheimer's disease, multiple cerebral infarctions, head trauma, and MS. Congenital cerebral damage (i.e., cerebral palsy) causes pseudobulbar palsy along with bilateral spasticity and choreoathetotic movement disorders. Finally, because ALS causes both UMN and LMN damage, it leads to a mixture of bulbar and pseudobulbar palsy; however, because ALS is exclusively a motor neuron disorder, it is not associated with either dementia or aphasia (see Chapter 5).

HYPOGLOSSAL (TWELFTH)

The hypoglossal nerves originate from paired nuclei near the midline of the medulla and descend through the base of the medulla (see Fig. 2-9). They pass through the base of the skull and travel through the neck to innervate the tongue muscles. Each nerve innervates the ipsilateral tongue muscles. These muscles move the tongue within the mouth, protrude it when people eat and speak, and push it to the contralateral side. Because of the muscle contractions, each side is balanced, and the tongue protrudes in the midline.

If one hypoglossal nerve is injured, that side of the tongue will become weak and, with time, atrophic. When protruded, the partly weakened tongue deviates toward the weakened side (Fig. 4-20), which illustrates the adage, "the tongue points toward the side of the lesion." If both nerves are injured, as in bulbar

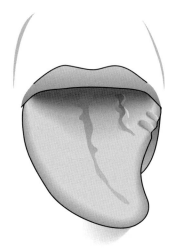

FIGURE 4-20 ■ With (left) hypoglossal nerve damage, the tongue deviates toward the weaker side and its affected (left) side undergoes atrophy.

palsy, the tongue will become immobile. Patients with hypoglossal LMN dysfunction from ALS have tongue fasciculations, as well as atrophy (see Fig. 5-9).

The most frequently occurring conditions in which one hypoglossal nerve is damaged are medial medullary infarctions, penetrating neck wounds, and nasopharyngeal tumors. Guillain-Barré syndrome, myasthenia gravis, and ALS usually simultaneously damage hypoglossal and other bulbar cranial nerves.

Questions and Answers

PREPARING FOR STANDARDIZED TESTS

When studying for a standardized test, such as the one offered by the American Board of Psychiatry and Neurology (ABPN), many readers rely on *Clinical Neurology for Psychiatrists*. This book offers, at a level expectable of psychiatrists, a reliable survey of neurologic basic science and current practice. In particular, the question-and-answer sections provide a realistic review of the relevant material.

Undoubtedly readers have successfully navigated numerous standardized tests and are already familiar with the format. Nevertheless, professionals may grow rusty and perhaps resentful. Some may also feel out of their element fielding questions pertaining to neurology and concerned by the failure rate on Part 1 of the ABPN examination, which has typically ranged between 30% to 35%. In that vein, let me offer several guidelines:

1. Try to extract the question's underlying idea even if a question-and-answer set does not explicitly state one.
2. Because test-takers answer incorrectly most often because they have misread the question, read each question twice, do not analyze it, reword unclear questions, and chose the simplest answer.
3. Mentally underline key words and phrases, such as "never," "except," and "always." Because these "mind-set altering" terms often define the situation, rereading the question based on the key word may clarify it.
4. Test-takers can usually simplify potential answers to bite-sized "true-false" statements. To give an example of this and the previous point: If the question asks, "Which of the following symptoms is never a feature of disease X?" the reader might approach the question as, "Is *a* ever a feature of X?" "Is *b* ever a feature of X?" "Is *c* ever a feature of X?"
5. Narrow the choices as much as possible and then select the answer with the greatest likelihood of being correct. Even if the test administrators deduct a small amount of credit for incorrect answers, the "odds" turn in the favor of the test-taker who eliminates even a single incorrect answer.
6. When approaching a lengthy question, skim the introductory material—returning to it after reading the actual question. The test-taker might ask, just like the psychiatrist might ask of a patient, boss, or lover, "What do they want from me?" The following is an example of a time-consuming and potentially frustrating question that initially hides the main idea: "Bus fare is $2, and the cost of a transfer $1. A bus begins its route with 5 passengers. At North Street, 3 additional passengers board and 2 depart. At Mechanic Street, 8 board and 3 depart. One requests a transfer before leaving, 2 board, and 5 depart when the bus stops at Tulip Street. How many stops did the bus make?"
7. Candidates for the ABPN and other standardized tests might consider forming study groups that meet on a weekly basis or more frequently. Individual study should include sitting isolated for stretches of 3.5 hours answering practice questions. Prospective test-takers should build up their physical and mental endurance until they can spend 8 hours, including a 1-hour lunch break, in a day answering questions.

QUESTIONS AND ANSWERS

1–7: Match the description with the visual field pattern (a–f):

1. Right homonymous hemianopsia
2. Bilateral superior nasal quadrantanopia
3. Right homonymous superior quadrantanopia
4. Blindness of the right eye
5. Left homonymous superior quadrantanopia
6. Bilateral inferior nasal quadrantanopia
7. Visual field deficit produced by a protuberant nose

Answers: b, d, c, f, a, e, e

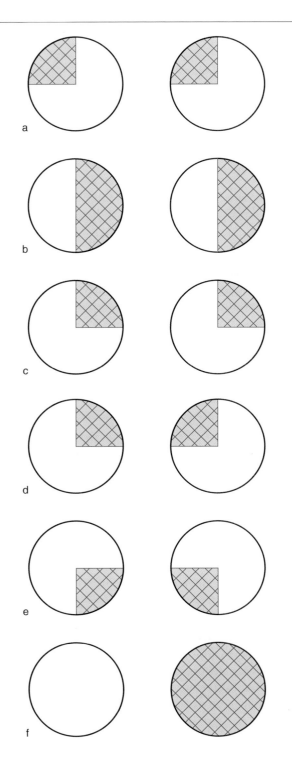

8. A 68-year-old man has sudden, painless onset of paresis of the right upper and lower face, inability to abduct the right eye, and paresis of the left arm and leg. Where is the lesion?
a. Cerebrum (cerebral hemispheres)
b. Cerebellum
c. Midbrain
d. Pons
e. Medulla
f. None of the above

Answer: d. The damaged structures include the right-sided abducens (VI) and facial (VII) nerves and the corticospinal tract destined to supply the left limbs. The corticospinal tract has a long course during which an injury would produce left hemiparesis; however, cranial nerves VI and VII originate in the pons and have a relatively short course. A small lesion, such as a stroke, in the right side of the pons could damage all these structures. (If the lesion pictured in Fig. 4-11 extended more laterally, it would create these deficits.)

9. An elderly man has left ptosis and a dilated and unreactive left pupil with external deviation of the left eye; right hemiparesis; right-sided hyperactive DTRs; and right-sided Babinski sign. He does not have either aphasia or hemianopsia. Where is the lesion?
a. Cerebrum
b. Cerebellum
c. Midbrain
d. Pons
e. Medulla
f. None of the above

Answer: c. Because the patient has only a left oculomotor nerve palsy and right hemiparesis, the lesion must be in the left midbrain. He does not have a language or visual field deficit because the lesion is in the brainstem, nowhere near the cerebrum.

10. In which two locations might a lesion cause a left superior homonymous quadrantanopia?
a. Frontal lobe
b. Parietal lobe
c. Occipital lobe
d. Temporal lobe
e. None of the above

Answers: c, d. This visual field loss is usually found with destruction of the right temporal or inferior occipital lobe. The most likely etiology would be a brain tumor or occlusion of the posterior cerebral artery. Rarely, an optic tract lesion would be responsible.

11. A 20-year-old woman reports having lost all vision in her right eye, right hemiparesis, and right hemisensory loss. Pupil and deep tendon reflexes are normal. She does not press down with her left leg while attempting to lift her right leg. Where is the lesion?
a. Cerebrum
b. Cerebellum
c. Midbrain
d. Pons
e. Medulla
f. None of the above

Answer: f. The symptoms cannot be explained by a single lesion, cannot be confirmed by objective signs, and lack the usual accompanying symptom of right hemiparesis, aphasia. If she had a left cerebral lesion, the visual impairment would have been a right homonymous hemianopsia. Moreover, she fails to exert maximum effort with one leg while "trying" to lift the other against resistance (Hoover's sign, see Chapter 3). Neurologic disease is probably absent.

12. A 50-year-old woman describes having many years of gait impairment and right-sided decreased hearing. The right corneal reflex is absent. The entire right side of her face is weak. Auditory acuity is diminished on the right. There are left-sided hyperactive DTRs with a Babinski sign, and right-sided difficulty with rapid alternating movements. What structures are involved?
    a. Optic nerves
    b. Cerebellopontine angle structures
    c. Extraocular motor nerves
    d. Bulbar cranial nerves
    e. None of the above

Answer: b. The right-sided corneal reflex loss, facial weakness, and hearing impairment indicate damage to the trigeminal, facial, and acoustic cranial nerves, respectively. These nerves (V, VII, VIII) emerge together from the brainstem at the cerebellopontine angle. The right-sided dysdiadochokinesia reflects right-sided cerebellar damage. The left-sided DTR abnormalities are caused by compression of the pons. Common cerebellopontine lesions are meningiomas and acoustic neuromas, which are often manifestations of neurofibromatosis (particularly the NF2 variant).

13. A 60-year-old man has interscapular back pain, paraparesis with hyperreflexia, loss of sensation below the umbilicus, and incontinence. Where is the lesion?
    a. C7
    b. T4
    c. T10
    d. L1
    e. S2
    f. None of the above

Answer: c. The lesion affects the thoracic spinal cord at the T10 level. The umbilicus is the landmark for T10.

14. After a minor motor vehicle crash, a young man describes having visual loss, paralysis of his legs, and loss of sensation to pin and position below the waist; however, sensation of warm versus cold is intact. He can see only 2 m^2 at every distance. He

is unable to raise his legs or walk. He has brisk DTRs, but his plantar responses are flexor. Where is the lesion?
    a. C7
    b. T4
    c. T10
    d. L1
    e. S2
    f. None of the above

Answer: f. Many features of the examination indicate that the basis of his symptoms and signs is not neurologic: (1) the constant area (2 m^2) of visual loss at all distances—tunnel vision—is contrary to the optics of vision, in which a greater area of vision is encompassed at greater distances from the eye; (2) the sensory loss to pain (pin) is inconsistent with preservation of temperature sensation because pain and temperature sensory systems are contained in the same pathway; and (3) despite his apparent paraparesis, the normal plantar response indicates that both the upper motor neurons (UMNs) and lower motor neurons (LMNs) are intact. His DTRs are likely brisk because of anxiety.

15. A 50-year-old man with mild dementia has absent reflexes, loss of position and vibration sensation, and ataxia. Which areas are affected?
    a. Cerebrum only
    b. The entire central nervous system (CNS)
    c. The entire CNS and peripheral nervous system (PNS)
    d. The cerebrum and the spinal cord's posterior columns
    e. Autonomic nervous system

Answer: d. Conditions that cause dementia and dysfunction of the posterior columns of the spinal cord and the cerebellar system are combined system disease (pernicious anemia), tabes dorsalis, some spinocerebellar degenerations, and heavy metal intoxication. The posterior columns seem to be especially vulnerable to environmental toxins and are frequently damaged by hereditary illnesses.

16. After she has suffered with increasing severe depression for 3 years, physicians find that a 55-year-old woman has right-sided optic atrophy and left-sided papilledema. Where is the lesion?
    a. Frontal lobe
    b. Parietal lobe
    c. Occipital lobe
    d. Temporal lobe
    e. None of the above

Answer: a. This woman has the classic Foster-Kennedy syndrome. In her case, a right frontal lobe tumor probably compresses the underlying right optic nerve, causing optic atrophy. Raised intracranial pressure causes papilledema of the left optic nerve. If the physicians had performed the appropriate testing, they would have found that she has anosmia on at least her right side.

17. After enjoying excellent health, except for hypertension, a middle-aged man becomes distraught when he develops impotence. A neurologic examination reveals that he has orthostatic hypotension and lightheadedness, but no other abnormalities. Which neurologic system is most likely impaired?
    a. Cerebrum only
    b. The entire CNS
    c. The entire CNS and PNS
    d. The cerebrum and the spinal cord's posterior columns
    e. Autonomic nervous system

Answer: e. Impotence in the presence of orthostatic hypotension is likely to be the result of autonomic nervous system dysfunction. In this patient, antihypertensive medications may be responsible.

18. A 60-year-old man with right upper lobe pulmonary carcinoma has the rapid development of lumbar spine pain, weak and areflexic legs, loss of sensation below the knees, and urinary and fecal incontinence. Where is the lesion?
    a. Cerebrum
    b. Brainstem
    c. Spinal cord
    d. Peripheral nervous system
    e. Neuromuscular junction

Answer: d. The lumbar spine pain and absent DTRs suggest that the lesion is in the cauda equina. This structure is composed of lumbosacral nerve roots, which are part of the peripheral nervous system.

19. Subsequently, the man in Question 18 develops a flaccid, areflexic paresis of the right arm and a right Horner's syndrome. Where is the lesion?
    a. Cerebrum
    b. Brainstem
    c. Spinal cord
    d. Peripheral nervous system
    e. Neuromuscular junction
    f. None of the above

Answer: d. His problem is now a lesion of the right C4-6 nerve roots and the thoracic sympathetic chain. He has a Pancoast tumor. He should have computed tomography (CT) of the chest.

20. Of the following, which two structures comprise the posterior columns of the spinal cord?
    a. Lateral spinothalamic tract
    b. Fasciculus cuneatus
    c. Fasciculus gracilis
    d. Posterior horn cells
    e. Lateral spinothalamic tract

Answers: b, c.

21. Of the structures listed in Question 20, which one carries temperature sensation?

Answer: e.

22. A 40-year-old man has interscapular spine pain, paraparesis with hyperactive DTRs, bilateral Babinski signs, and a complete sensory loss below his nipples. What is the location of the lesion?
    a. C7
    b. T4
    c. T10
    d. L1
    e. S2
    f. None of the above

Answer: b. The lesion clearly affects the spinal cord at the T4 level. The nipples represent the T4 landmark. Common causes include benign and malignant mass lesions (a herniated thoracic intervertebral disk or an epidural metastatic tumor), infection (abscess or tuberculoma), and inflammation (transverse myelitis or multiple sclerosis [MS]). Human immunodeficiency virus (HIV) infection itself does not produce such a discrete lesion; however, complications of acquired immunodeficiency syndrome (AIDS), such as lymphoma, toxoplasmosis, and tuberculosis, might create a mass lesion that would compress the spinal cord. Magnetic resonance imaging (MRI) is routinely performed to rule out mass lesions compressing the spinal cord.

23. Which cranial nerves are covered totally or partly by CNS-generated myelin?
    a. Optic and acoustic
    b. Facial, acoustic, and trigeminal
    c. Bulbar
    d. All
    e. None

Answer: a. The entire optic and a small, proximal portion of the acoustic cranial nerves are covered with CNS-generated myelin.

24. An elderly, hypertensive man develops vertigo, nausea, and vomiting. He has a right-sided Horner's syndrome, loss of the right corneal reflex, and dysarthria because of paresis of the

palate. The right face and left limbs and left side of the trunk are relatively hypalgesic. Which way does the palate deviate?
a. Right
b. Left
c. Up
d. Down

Answer: b. The patient has a right-sided lateral medullary (Wallenberg's) syndrome. This syndrome includes crossed hypalgesia (right-facial and left-"body," in this case), ipsilateral ataxia, and ipsilateral palate weakness. His palate deviates to the left because of right-sided palatal muscle weakness. Because the cerebrum is spared, patients do not have emotional or cognitive impairment or physical signs of cerebral damage, such as visual field cuts or seizures.

25. In her last trimester of a normal pregnancy, a 28-year-old physician developed pain in her lower back. Immediately before delivery, the pain spread down her right anterolateral thigh. That quadriceps muscle was slightly weak and its DTR was reduced. By 2 weeks postpartum, after delivery of a healthy 11-pound baby girl, all signs and symptoms resolved. Which of the following was the most likely diagnosis?
a. A herniated disk with sciatic nerve compression
b. Compression of the lateral femoral cutaneous nerve (meralgia paresthetica)
c. Compression of the femoral nerve or its nerve roots
d. Multiple sclerosis

Answer: c. An enlarged uterus can compress the lumbosacral plexus in the pelvis or the femoral nerve as it exits from the inguinal area. Meralgia paresthetica, which results from nerve compression in the inguinal region, is painful but not associated with weakness or DTR loss. Herniated disks occur in pregnancy because of weight gain, hyperlordosis, and laxity of ligaments; however, sciatica usually causes low back pain that radiates to the posterior portion of the leg. The distribution of the pain and hypoactive DTRs exclude multiple sclerosis.

26. Where is the primary damage in Wilson's disease, Huntington's chorea, and choreiform cerebral palsy?
a. Pyramidal system
b. Extrapyramidal system
c. Entire CNS
d. Cerebellar outflow tracts

Answer: b. These diseases, like Parkinson's disease, damage the basal ganglia, which are the foundation of the extrapyramidal motor system. Basal ganglia

dysfunction can cause tremor, chorea, athetosis, rigidity, and bradykinesia. In contrast, corticospinal (pyramidal) tract dysfunction can cause spasticity, DTR hyperreflexia, clonus, and Babinski signs.

27. What of the following are termed "frontal release" reflexes?
a. Babinski sign
b. Parachute reflex
c. Cremasteric reflex
d. Anal reflex
e. Moro reflex
f. Romberg sign
g. Clonus
h. None of the above

Answer: h. The frontal release reflexes involve the face (snout, suck, and rooting reflex), jaw (jaw-jerk), and palm (palmomental and grasp reflexes). Almost all frontal release signs are normally present in infants. In adults, none of the frontal release reflexes reliably indicates the presence of a pathologic condition. However, the presence of several of them suggests a congenital cerebral injury, frontal lobe lesion, or neurodegenerative condition, including frontotemporal dementia. In contrast, Babinski signs and clonus are signs of upper motor neuron (corticospinal tract) damage. The parachute and Moro reflexes are normal responses in infants to change in position or posture. The cremasteric and anal reflexes are normally occurring superficial reflexes that depend on the integrity of the nerves of the lumbosacral plexus and the CNS. The Romberg sign develops if either the posterior columns of the spinal cord or the peripheral nerves of the lower extremities are damaged enough to interrupt sensory information passing to the brain.

28–39. Match the condition with its description (a–l):
28. Anosognosia
29. Aphasia
30. Astereognosis
31. Athetosis
32. Bradykinesia
33. Chorea
34. Dementia
35. Dysdiadochokinesia
36. Gerstmann's syndrome
37. Dysarthria
38. Ataxia
39. Dysmetria
a. Slowness of movement, which is a manifestation of many basal ganglia diseases, is characteristic of parkinsonism.
b. An involuntary movement disorder characterized by slow writhing, sinuous movement of the

arm(s) or leg(s) that is more pronounced in the distal part of the limbs. It usually results from basal ganglia damage from perinatal jaundice, anoxia, or prematurity.

c. Impairment in speech production that may result from lesions in the cerebrum, brainstem, cranial nerves, or even vocal cords.

d. A disorder of verbal or written language rather than simply speech production. It almost always results from discrete lesions in the dominant cerebral hemisphere's perisylvian language arc. However, occasionally degenerative conditions, including Alzheimer's disease, may cause aspects of it.

e. An impairment of memory and judgment, abstract thinking, and other cognitive functions of a degree sufficient to impair social activities or interpersonal relationships.

f. An involuntary movement characterized by intermittent, random jerking of the limbs, face, or trunk. Medications, such as L-dopa and typical neuroleptics, and many basal ganglia diseases may cause it.

g. Inability to identify objects by touch. It is a variety of cortical sensory loss that is found with lesions of the contralateral parietal lobe.

h. Incoordination of voluntary movement. It is often a sign of cerebellar injury and associated with intention tremor, hypotonia, and impaired rapid alternating movements.

i. Impairment of rapid alternating movements that is characteristic of cerebellar injury but may be result of red nucleus damage.

j. Failure to recognize a deficit or disease. The most common example is ignoring a left hemiparesis—not the hemiparesis itself—because of a right cerebral infarction. Another example is denial of blindness—again, not the blindness itself—from occipital lobe infarctions (Anton's syndrome).

k. Irregularities on performing rapid alternating movements. The term does not refer to a measure of distance, but to rhythm.

l. Combination of agraphia, finger agnosia, dyscalculia, and inability to distinguish right from left.

Answers: 28-j; 29-d; 30-g; 31-b; 32-a; 33-f; 34-e; 35-i; 36-l; 37-c; 38-h; 39-k.

40. A 65-year-old neurologist was attending a party when a colleague described a patient with PD (Parkinson's disease); however, he thought that she had said TD (tardive dyskinesia) and proceeded to discuss iatrogenic illness. When speaking with someone in a quiet room, he almost never

misunderstood. However, he conceded that mistakes in public been happening frequently during the previous year. Which of the following is least likely to be the cause of the neurologist's problem?
a. Inability to distinguish between "T" and "P"
b. Mild cognitive impairment
c. Diminished ability to hear high tones
d. Impaired speech discrimination

Answer: b. His hearing impairment is normal age-related presbycusis, which typically begins with loss of high-frequency hearing and inability to distinguish between closely sounding consonants. Individuals with presbycusis characteristically describe impaired speech discrimination in rooms crowded with talking people but not in one-to-one conversations. Elderly individuals with hearing impairment often withdraw. They may appear to have depression or, because they frequently misunderstand, cognitive impairment.

41. Three months after a young man sustained closed head injury, he has insomnia, fatigue, cognitive impairment, and personality changes. He also reports that food is tasteless. What is the most specific origin of his symptoms?
a. Post-traumatic stress disorder
b. Frontal lobe, head, and neck trauma
c. Partial complex seizures
d. Frontal lobe and olfactory nerve trauma

Answer: d. He probably has had a contusion of both frontal lobes resulting in a postconcussion syndrome manifested by changes in mentation and personality. The anosmia results from shearing of the thin fibers of the olfactory nerve in their passage through the cribriform plate.

42. A middle-aged woman has increasing blindness in the right eye, where the visual acuity is 20/400 and the optic disc is white. The right pupil does not react either directly or consensually to light. The left pupil reacts directly, although not consensually. All motions of the right eye are impaired. In which area is the lesion?
a. Neuromuscular junction
b. Orbit
c. Retro-orbital structures
d. Cerebrum

Answer: c. She evidently has right-sided optic nerve damage. She has right-sided impaired visual acuity, optic atrophy, and loss of direct light reflex in that eye with loss of the indirect (consensual) light reflex in the other. In addition, the complete extraocular muscle paresis indicates oculomotor, trochlear, and abducens nerve damage. Only a lesion located immediately behind the orbit, such as a sphenoid wing meningioma, would be able to damage all these nerves.

43. In which of the following conditions do pupils usually accommodate but not react to light?
a. Psychogenic disturbances
b. Oculomotor nerve injuries
c. Midbrain lesions
d. Argyll-Robertson

Answer: d. In Argyll-Robertson, which is a sign of syphilis, pupils accommodate but do not react.

44. In which of the following conditions is a patient in an agitated, confused state with abnormally large pupils?
a. Heroin overdose
b. Multiple sclerosis
c. Atropine, scopolamine, or sympathomimetic intoxication
d. Hyperventilation

Answer: c.

45. In what condition is a patient typically comatose with respiratory depression and pinpoint-sized pupils?
a. Heroin overdose
b. Multiple sclerosis
c. Atropine, scopolamine, or sympathomimetic intoxication
d. Hyperventilation

Answer: a. Heroin, morphine, barbiturate, and other overdoses are the most common cause of the combination of coma and miosis. Infarctions and hemorrhages in the pons also produce the same picture. Narcotic overdoses are also often complicated by respiratory depression and pulmonary edema.

46. Match the reflex limb (a–f) with the cranial nerve (1–9) that carries it.
a. Afferent limb of the light reflex
b. Efferent limb of the light reflex
c. Afferent limb of the corneal reflex
d. Efferent limb of the corneal reflex
e. Afferent limb of the accommodation reflex
f. Efferent limb of the accommodation reflex
1. Optic nerve
2. Oculomotor nerve
3. Trochlear nerve
4. Trigeminal nerve
5. Abducens nerve
6. Facial nerve
7. Acoustic nerve
8. Olfactory nerve
9. Hypoglossal nerve

Answers: a-1, b-2, c-4, d-6, e-1, f-2.

47. What is the name of the object that hangs down from the soft palate toward the back of the throat?
a. Hard palate
b. Soft palate
c. Vallecula
d. Uvula

Answer: d.

48. On looking to the left, a patient has horizontal diplopia without nystagmus. Which nerve or region is affected?
a. Left III or right VI
b. Right III or left VI
c. Left medial longitudinal fasciculus
d. Right medial longitudinal fasciculus

Answer: b.

49. Which nerve is responsible when the left eye fails to abduct fully on looking to the left?
a. Left III
b. Right III
c. Left VI
d. Right VI

Answer: c.

50. The patient's right eyelid has ptosis, the eye is abducted, and its pupil is dilated. Which nerve or region is injured?
a. Left III
b. Right III
c. Left VI
d. Right VI

Answer: b.

51. After returning home from a party, a 15-year-old girl was lethargic and disoriented. On examination, she walks with an ataxic gait and has slurred speech. She also has bilateral, horizontal, and vertical nystagmus. What is the most likely cause of her findings?
a. Multiple sclerosis
b. A cerebellar tumor
c. A psychogenic disturbance
d. None of the above

Answer: d. She may be intoxicated with alcohol, barbiturates, or other drugs. A cerebellar tumor is an unlikely possibility without headache or signs of raised intracranial pressure or corticospinal tract damage.

Multiple sclerosis is unlikely because of her lethargy, disorientation, and young age. Nystagmus can be a congenital abnormality, a toxic-metabolic aberration, or a manifestation of a structural brainstem lesion, but it cannot be a psychogenic sign.

52. A young man has suddenly developed vertigo, nausea, vomiting, and left-sided tinnitus. He has nystagmus to the right. What is the lesion?
    a. Multiple sclerosis
    b. A cerebellar tumor
    c. A psychogenic disturbance
    d. Labyrinthine dysfunction

Answer: d. The unilateral nystagmus, hearing abnormality, nausea, and vomiting are most likely caused by left-sided inner ear disease, such as labyrinthitis, rather than by neurologic dysfunction.

53. A 21-year-old soldier has vertical and horizontal nystagmus, mild spastic paraparesis, and ataxia of finger-to-nose motion bilaterally. Which region of the CNS is not affected?
    a. Cerebrum
    b. Brainstem
    c. Cerebellum
    d. Spinal cord

Answer: a. This patient has lesions in the brainstem causing nystagmus; in the cerebellum causing ataxia; and in the spinal cord causing paraparesis. This picture of scattered or "disseminated" lesions is typical of but not diagnostic of multiple sclerosis.

54. What is the most caudal (lowermost) level of the CNS?
    a. Foramen magnum
    b. Slightly caudal to the thoracic vertebrae
    c. The sacrum
    d. None of the above

Answer: b. The spinal cord, which is one of the two major components of the CNS, has a caudal extent to the T12-L1 vertebrae. Gunshot wounds, tumors, or other injuries below that level can be devastating because they can disrupt the cauda equina, but they do not damage the spinal cord.

55. A 35-year-old man, who has been shot in the back, has paresis of the right leg and loss of position and vibration sensation at the right ankle. Pinprick sensation is lost in the left leg. Where is the lesion?
    a. Right side of the cervical spinal cord
    b. Left side of the cervical spinal cord
    c. Right side of the thoracic spinal cord
    d. Left side of the thoracic spinal cord
    e. Right side of the lumbosacral spinal cord
    f. Left side of the lumbosacral spinal cord
    g. One or both lumbar plexuses

Answer: c. The gunshot wound has caused hemi-transection of the right side of the thoracic spinal cord (the Brown-Séquard syndrome, see Fig. 2-17). Occasionally, to alleviate intractable pain, neurosurgeons purposefully sever the lateral spinothalamic tract.

56.

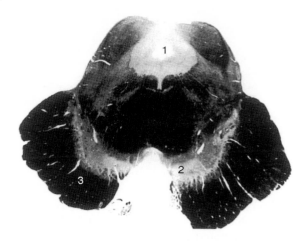

1. What is the name of the entire structure?
2. Which regions of the brain does structure "1" connect?
3. What is the region that surrounds structure "1"?
4. Where do most of the axons terminate that originate in structure "2"?
5. What is the termination of most of the axons that pass through structure "3"?

Answers:

1. This is the midbrain, which is the rostral (uppermost) region of the brainstem. The midbrain is identifiable by its silhouette, particularly the wide ventral cleft; unstained semilunar region, which contains the substantia nigra; and the upper, central aqueduct of Sylvius.
2. This is the aqueduct of Sylvius, which is the channel for cerebrospinal fluid (CSF) to flow from the third to fourth ventricles.
3. Periaqueductal gray matter
4. Structure "2" is the substantia nigra. Its neurons form the nigrostriatal tract, which terminates in the striatum (caudate and putamen).

5. Structure "3" is the cerebral peduncle, which carries the corticospinal tract. Most of its axons descend, cross in the pyramids, and synapse with the contralateral anterior horn cells of the spinal cord.

6. Structure "3," the basis pontis, contains the descending corticospinal tracts and the crossing pontocerebellar tracts.

58.

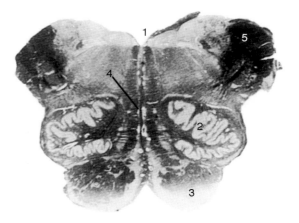

57.

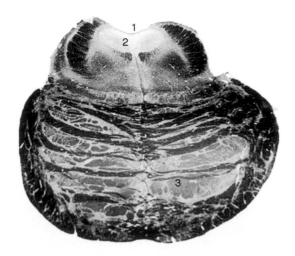

1. What is the name of the entire structure?
2. What is the name of the fluid-filled structure designated structure "1"?
3. Which structure lies dorsal to structure "1"?
4. Which cranial nerve nucleus is located at structure "2"?
5. Which white matter tract that connects the third and sixth cranial nerve nuclei lies near structure "2"?
6. In which two structures do axons passing through structure "3" terminate?

Answers:

1. This is the pons. The bulbous ventral portion, the *basis pontis*, characterizes its configuration.
2. The fourth ventricle lies dorsal to the pons and medulla.
3. The cerebellum forms the roof of the fourth ventricle (see Fig. 21-2 and Chapter 20).
4. The nuclei of the abducens nerves (cranial nerves VI) are located as a pair of midline, dorsal structures in the pons. The nuclei of the other cranial nerves involved in ocular motility, the third and fourth cranial nerves, are similarly located as paired midline dorsal structures but in the midbrain.
5. The MLF, a heavily myelinated tract, connects the sixth and contralateral third cranial nerve nuclei. It is essential for conjugate vision.

1. What is the name of the entire structure?
2. What is the name of the fluid-filled structure designated structure "1"?
3. Which structure lies dorsal to structure "1"?
4. What is the name of the pair of scalloped nuclei designated structure "2"?
5. Which structure, which transmits proprioception, is shown in structure "4"?
6. What is the common name of structure "5," which is also called the restiform body?

Answers:

1. This is the medulla, which is readily identified by the unique pair of scalloped nuclei (see later).
2. The fourth ventricle lies dorsal to both the pons and medulla.
3. The cerebellum forms the roof of the fourth ventricle.
4. They are the inferior olivary nuclei. Although conspicuous and complex, they seem to be involved in only a few neurologic illnesses, such as olivopontocerebellar degeneration and palatal myoclonus.
5. Structure "4" is the decussation of the medial lemniscus where ascending proprioception and vibration sensation tracts cross to terminate in the contralateral thalamus.
6. The cerebellar peduncles are located in the lateral medulla and contain afferent and efferent (inflow and outflow) cerebellar tracts.

59. Match the gait abnormalities (1–6), which are important neurologic signs, with their descriptions (a–f).

1. Apraxic
2. Astasia-abasia
3. Ataxic
4. Festinating
5. Hemiparetic
6. Steppage

a. Short-stepped, narrow-based with a shuffle but tendency to accelerate
b. Impaired alternation of feet and inconsistently shifting weight to the forward foot
c. Broad-based and lurching
d. Seeming to be extraordinarily unbalanced, but without falling
e. Stiffness of one leg and swinging it outward with excessive wear on the inner sole
f. Excessively lifting the knees to raise the feet

Answers: 1-b, 2-d, 3-c, 4-a, 5-e, 6-f.

60. Match the neurologic conditions (a–f) with the gait abnormalities (1–6) they induce.
    a. Cerebral infarction
    b. Cerebellar degeneration
    c. Parkinsonism
    d. Normal pressure hydrocephalus
    e. Psychogenic inability to walk
    f. Tabes dorsalis
    1. Apraxic
    2. Astasia-abasia
    3. Ataxic
    4. Festinating
    5. Hemiparetic
    6. Steppage

Answers: a-5; b-3; c-4; d-1; e-2; f-6. Normal pressure hydrocephalus is characterized by dementia, incontinence, and, most strikingly, apraxia of gait. Gait apraxia is characterized by an inability to alternate leg movements and inappropriately attempting to lift the weight-bearing foot. The feet are often immobile because the weight is not shifted to the forward foot, and the patient attempts to lift the same foot twice. The feet seem magnetized to the floor (see Fig. 7-8).

Astasia-abasia is a psychogenic pattern of walking in which the patient seems to alternate between a broad base for stability and a narrow, tightrope-like stance, with contortions of the chest and arms that give the appearance of falling (see Fig. 3-4).

Ataxia of the legs and trunk in cerebellar degeneration force the feet widely apart (in a broad base) to maintain stability. Because coordination is also impaired, the gait has an uneven, unsteady, lurching pattern (see Fig. 2-13).

Festinating gait, also called *marche à petits pas*, a feature of Parkinson's disease, is a shuffling, short-stepped gait with a tendency to accelerate.

Hemiparesis and increased tone (spasticity) from cerebral infarctions force patients to swing (circumduct) a paretic leg from the hip. Circumduction permits hemiparetic patients to walk if they can extend their hip and knee. The weak ankle drags the inner front surface of the foot (see Fig. 2-4).

Patients with tabes dorsalis have impairment of position sense. To prevent their toes from catching, especially when climbing stairs, patients raise their legs excessively.

61. In the development of syringomyelia (syrinx), which tract is most vulnerable to injury?
    a. Lateral spinothalamic
    b. Corticospinal
    c. Spinocerebellar
    d. Fasciculus cuneatus

Answer: a. As a syrinx expands within the center of the spinal cord, it stretches—and eventually lyses—lateral spinothalamic fibers as they cross. Thus, a syrinx, which typically develops in the cervical spinal cord, usually severs the upper extremities' pain and temperature-carrying tracts.

62–67. This patient is looking slightly to her right and attempting to raise both arms. Her left eye deviates across the midline to the right, but her right eye cannot abduct. (The answers are provided after question 67.)

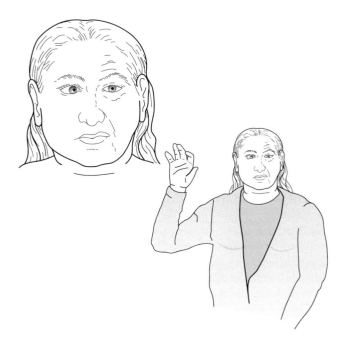

62. Paresis of which extraocular muscle prevents the right eye from moving laterally?
a. Right superior oblique
b. Right abducens
c. Left abducens
d. Left lateral rectus
e. Right lateral rectus

63. The left face does not seem to be involved by the left hemiparesis. Why might the left side of the face be uninvolved?
a. It is. The left forehead and mouth are contorted.
b. The problem is in the right cerebral hemisphere.
c. The corticospinal tract is injured only after the corticobulbar tract has innervated the facial nerve.
d. The problem is best explained by postulating two lesions.

64. On which side of the body would a Babinski sign most likely be elicited?
a. Right
b. Left
c. Both
d. Neither

65. What is the most likely cause of this disorder?
a. Bell's palsy
b. Hysteria
c. Cerebral infarction
d. Medullary infarction
e. Pontine infarction
f. Midbrain infarction

66. With which conditions is such a lesion associated?
a. Homonymous hemianopsia
b. Diplopia
c. Impaired monocular visual acuity
d. Nystagmus
e. Various nondominant hemisphere syndromes

67. Sketch the region of the damaged brain, inserting the damaged structures and the area of damage.

Answers: 62-e; 63-c; 64-b; 65-e; 66-b. This patient has weakness of the right lateral rectus muscle, which prevents the eye from moving laterally; weakness of the right upper and lower face; and paresis of the left arm. Because of the right eye's inability to abduct, she would have diplopia on right lateral gaze. The proper clinical assessment would be that she has injury of the right abducens and facial cranial nerves and the corticospinal tract before it crosses in the medulla. The lesion is undoubtedly located in the base of the pons. The most likely etiology is an occlusion of a small branch of the basilar artery.

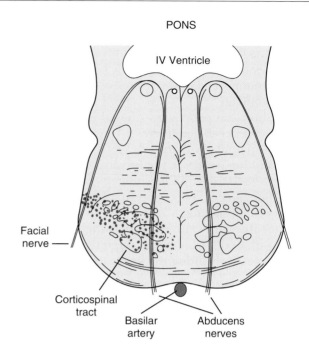

PONS

IV Ventricle

Facial nerve —

Corticospinal tract

Basilar artery

Abducens nerves

68. Where does the corticospinal tract cross as it descends?
a. Internal capsule
b. Base of the pons
c. Pyramids
d. Anterior horn cells

Answer: c. Because the corticospinal tracts cross in the medulla's pyramids, they are often called the "pyramidal tract."

69. Which artery supplies Broca's area and the adjacent corticospinal tract?
a. Anterior cerebral
b. Middle cerebral
c. Posterior cerebral
d. Basilar
e. Vertebral

Answer: b. The left middle cerebral artery

70. Which illnesses are suggested by the presence of spasticity, clonus, hyperactive deep tendon reflexes, and Babinski signs?
a. Poliomyelitis, cerebrovascular accidents, spinal cord trauma
b. Bell's palsy, cerebrovascular accidents, psychogenic disturbances
c. Spinal cord trauma, cerebrovascular accidents, congenital cerebral injuries
d. Brainstem infarction, cerebellar infarction, spinal cord infarction

e. Parkinson's disease, cerebrovascular accidents, cerebellar infarction

Answer: c. The common denominator is UMN injury.

71. Which group of illnesses is suggested by the presence of muscles that are paretic, atrophic, and areflexic?
    a. Poliomyelitis, diabetic peripheral neuropathy, traumatic brachial plexus injury
    b. Amyotrophic lateral sclerosis, brainstem infarction, psychogenic disturbance
    c. Spinal cord trauma, cerebrovascular accidents, congenital cerebral injuries
    d. Brainstem infarction, cerebellar infarction, spinal cord infarction
    e. Parkinson's disease, cerebrovascular accidents, cerebellar infarction
    f. Guillain-Barré syndrome, multiple sclerosis, and uremic neuropathy

Answer: a. The common denominator is LMN injury.

72. Match the location of the nerve, nucleus, or lesion (a–k) with its brainstem location (1–3):
    a. Cranial nerve nucleus III
    b. Cranial nerve nucleus IV
    c. Cranial nerve nucleus VI
    d. Cranial nerve nucleus VII
    e. Cranial nerve nucleus IX
    f. Cranial nerve nucleus X
    g. Cranial nerve nucleus XI
    h. Abducens paresis and contralateral hemiparesis
    i. Abducens and facial paresis and contralateral hemiparesis
    j. Palatal deviation to one side, contralateral Horner's syndrome, and ataxia
    k. Miosis, ptosis, anhidrosis
    1. Midbrain
    2. Pons
    3. Medulla

Answers: a-1, b-1, c-2, d-2, e-3, f-3, g-3, h-2, i-2, j-3, k-3.

73. During "Spring Break," a college student dove into the shallow end of a swimming pool. He struck his forehead firmly against the bottom. His friends noted that he was unconscious and resuscitated him. On recovery in the hospital several days later, he noticed that he had weakness in both hands. A neurologist finds that the intrinsic muscles of the hands are weak and DTRs in the arms are absent. Also, pain sensation is diminished, but position and vibration sensations are preserved. He has mild, aching neck pain. The legs are strong and have normal sensation, but their DTRs are brisk. Plantar reflexes are equivocal. There is a large, tender ecchymotic area on the forehead. Which of the following is the most likely cause of the hand weakness?
    a. Cerebral concussion
    b. Intoxication
    c. Syringomyelia
    d. Herniated intervertebral disk

Answer: c. Striking a forehead against the bottom of a swimming pool produces a forceful hyperextension (extreme backward bending) injury to the neck, as well as head trauma. In this case, the spinal cord developed a hematomyelia or syringomyelia (syrinx) because of bleeding into the center of the spinal cord. With a syrinx, the cervical spinothalamic tracts, as they cross within the spinal cord, are ripped by the hematoma as it expands the spinal cord's central canal. The corticospinal tracts destined for the legs are compressed but not interrupted. In this type of swimming pool accident, victims should be evaluated for alcohol and drug intoxication, as well as for sequelae of head trauma. Similar situations occur in motor vehicle crashes where the victim's forehead strikes the dashboard or inside of the windshield, and in sports accidents in which the athlete's head and neck are snapped backward.

74. A 65-year-old man describes many problems, but his most bothersome is loss of hearing in both ears during the previous 6 to 12 months. This problem began with his being unable to distinguish his dinner partner's conversation in restaurants. It progressed to his being unable to hear telephone conversations. He started to withdraw from social occasions. Audiometry shows bilateral high tone hearing loss. In addition to the hearing impairment, he has difficulty recalling names of recent acquaintances, impaired vibratory sense in his toes, and mild bilateral anosmia. However, he does not have dementia. What should the physician do first?
    a. Obtain an MRI of the head
    b. Do a spinal tap
    c. Obtain a serum B_{12} level
    d. Advise him to obtain a hearing aid

Answer: d. All his symptoms are attributable to "normal changes of old age." The initial manifestation of age-related hearing loss, *presbycusis*, is loss of speech discrimination, especially in situations with competing conversations. It interferes with social and cognitive function. It is severe enough at times to give the false impression of depression or dementia. In presbycusis, audiometry initially shows loss of high frequencies but eventually loss of all frequencies. Without delay, he should be fitted for a hearing aid.

75. In the examination of a patient, which maneuver reveals most about the function of the patient's motor system?
    a. Testing plantar reflexes
    b. Manual muscle testing
    c. Deep tendon reflex testing
    d. Observation of the patient's gait

Answer: d. To walk normally a person must have normal corticospinal tracts and LMNs, coordination, proprioception, and balance.

76. Which structure separates the cerebrum from the cerebellum?
    a. CSF
    b. Foramen magnum
    c. Falx
    d. Tentorium

Answer: d. The tentorium lies above the cerebellum (see Fig. 20-18).

77. Which of the structures in question 76 separate the two cerebral hemispheres?

Answer: c. The falx cerebri, which often gives rise to meningiomas, separates the cerebral hemispheres.

78. Which two cranial nerves convey taste sensation from the tongue to the brain?
    a. V and VII
    b. VII and IX
    c. IX and X
    d. IX and XI

Answer: b. The facial nerve (VII) conveys taste sensation from the anterior two thirds of the tongue and the glossopharyngeal nerve (IX) from the posterior one third.

79. Which will be the pattern of a myelin stain of the cervical spinal cord's ascending tracts several years after a thoracic spine gunshot wound?
    a. The entire cervical spinal cord will be normal.
    b. The myelin will be unstained.
    c. The fasciculus cuneatus will be stained black, and the f. gracilis will be unstained.
    d. The f. gracilis will be stained black, and the f. cuneatus will be unstained.

Answer: c. Because the f. cuneatus arises from the arms and upper trunk, it will be uninjured and

normally absorb stain: that tract, being normal, will be stained black. In contrast, the f. gracilis will be unstained because its myelin will be lost distal (downstream) from the lesion. As for the other major tracts, the corticospinal tract, which is descending, will be normally stained black because it originates proximal to the lesion. However, the portion of the spinothalamic tract that originates in the legs and lower trunk will remain unstained. Overall, the loss of staining reflects *Wallerian degeneration,* in which injury to axons leads to loss of their myelin and axons distal (downstream) from the injury, whether the axons are flowing toward or away from the brain.

80. A 20-year-old man has become progressively dysarthric during the previous 2 years. He has no mental impairments or cranial nerve abnormalities. His legs have mild weakness and Babinski signs but poorly reactive DTRs. All his limbs are ataxic and his speech is scanning. He has impaired position and vibration sensation in his hands and feet. His feet have a high arch, elevated dorsum, and retracted first metatarsal. A cardiac evaluation reveals hypertrophic cardiomyopathy. His two younger brothers seem to have developed the same problem. His parents, three aunts and uncles, and two older siblings have no neurologic symptoms or physical abnormalities. Which of the following genetic features will probably be found on further evaluation of the patient?
    a. Excessive trinucleotide repeats on both alleles of chromosome 9
    b. Excessive trinucleotide repeats on only one allele of chromosome 6
    c. Two Y chromosomes, giving him an XYY karyotype
    d. Two X chromosomes, giving him an XXY karyotype

Answer: a. The patient and his two younger brothers have Friedreich's ataxia, which is characterized by posterior column sensory abnormalities, Babinski signs, limb ataxia, scanning speech, and the characteristic foot deformity, "pes cavus." Friedreich's ataxia is an autosomal recessive condition resulting from excessive trinucleotide repeats on chromosome 9. Spinocerebellar ataxia (SCA), which has at least six common varieties, is usually an autosomal dominant disorder with predominantly cerebellar dysfunction.

81. A man with diabetic neuropathy is unable to stand erect with feet together and eyes closed. When attempting this maneuver, he tends to topple, but he catches himself before falling. What is the

name of this sign (a–d), and to which region of the nervous system (1–5) is it referable in this patient?
a. Hoover's
b. Babinski's
c. Chvostek's
d. Romberg's
1. Cerebrum
2. Cerebellum
3. Spinal cord
4. Labyrinthine system
5. Peripheral nerves

Answers: d, 5. He has a Romberg's sign, but it results from PNS rather than CNS disease. Falling over when standing erect and deprived of visual sensory input suggests a loss of joint position sense from the legs. When deprived of vision and joint position sense, people must rely on labyrinthine (vestibular) input, but that input is important only with rapid or relatively large changes in position. For example, it comes into play when people start to fall and prevents their tumbling over.

Romberg's sign was classically attributed to injury of the spinal cord's posterior columns when position sense from the feet could not be conveyed to the brain. It is a classic sign of combined system disease and tabes dorsalis—conditions in which the posterior columns are destroyed. Romberg's sign is now detected most often in people with peripheral neuropathy who have lost position sense, as well as other sensations, in their feet and ankles.

82. In which conditions would Romberg's sign be detectable?
a. Tabes dorsalis
b. Multiple sclerosis
c. Combined system disease
d. Alcoholism
e. Diabetes
f. Uremia
g. Cerebellar disease
h. Blindness

Answers: a–f. Impairment of either the peripheral nerves (d–f) or the posterior columns of the spinal cord (a–c) can cause Romberg's sign. However, closing the eyes will not make a person more unstable with either cerebellar disease or blindness.

83. A 25-year-old man who has had diabetes mellitus since childhood develops erectile dysfunction. He has been found previously to have retrograde ejaculation during an evaluation for sterility. Examination of his fundi reveals hemorrhages and exudates. He has absent DTRs at the wrists and ankles, loss of position and vibration sensation at the ankles, and no demonstrable anal or cremasteric reflexes. Which three other conditions are likely to be present?
a. Urinary bladder hypotonicity
b. Bilateral Babinski signs
c. Gastroenteropathy
d. Dementia
e. Anhidrosis

Answers: a, c, e. He has a combination of peripheral and autonomic system neuropathy because of diabetes mellitus. A peripheral neuropathy is suggested by the distal sensory and reflex loss and the absent anal and cremasteric reflexes. Autonomic neuropathy is suggested by the retrograde ejaculation. Common manifestations of autonomic neuropathy are erectile dysfunction, urinary bladder hypotonicity, gastroenteropathy, and anhidrosis.

84. Where in the CNS do the vagus nerves' afferent fibers terminate?
a. Temporal lobe
b. Diencephalon
c. Midbrain
d. Pons
e. Medulla

Answer: e. The vagus nerves' afferent fibers originate in the thoracic and abdominal viscera. The vagus nerves travel upward through the neck, where they are readily accessible to surgeons, and terminate in the solitary nucleus of the medulla. From there, their neurons project widely to the cortex, as well as to more rostral portions of the brainstem. The relationship of the vagus nerves to the brainstem and the cerebral cortex comes into effect when vagus nerve stimulation is used in antiepileptic treatment.

85. How would a sympathetic nervous system injury from a lateral medullary infarction or an upper lobe lung cancer change the pupils?
a. Miosis (constricted pupil) ipsilateral to the lesion
b. Miosis contralateral to the lesion
c. Mydriasis (dilated pupil) ipsilateral to the lesion
d. Mydriasis contralateral to the lesion

Answer: a. Interruption of the pupil's sympathetic innervation causes ipsilateral miosis and usually ptosis and anhidrosis, that is, a Horner's syndrome.

86. Which two of the following would result from ciliary ganglia damage?
a. Miosis
b. Mydriasis
c. Hypersensitivity to mydriatic agents (medications that dilate the pupil)

d. Hypersensitivity to miotic agents (medications that constrict the pupil)

Answers: b, d. Damage to the ciliary ganglion will interrupt parasympathetic innervation of the pupil's sphincter muscles. Then, unopposed sympathetic innervation will dilate the pupil. Also, because of denervation hypersensitivity, the pupillary sphincter muscles will be unusually sensitive to miotic agents. This is the situation with an *Adie's pupil,* which is characteristically dilated because of ciliary ganglion damage, but constricts readily when dilute solutions of miotics are applied to the eye.

87. A 20-year old waitress has developed neck pain and difficulty writing. The neurologist finds that she has atrophy as well as weakness of intrinsic hand muscles. The biceps, triceps, and brachioradialis DTRs are markedly hypoactive, but those in her legs are normal. Plantar reflexes are flexor. She has decreased sensation to pain and temperature in both arms and hands and from approximately C4 to T2; however, vibration and position sensations are preserved. Of the following, which is the most likely diagnosis?
    a. Occupational muscle strain
    b. Multiple sclerosis
    c. Brown-Séquard syndrome
    d. Syringomyelia
    e. Herniated intervertebral disk

Answer. d. She has a syringomyelia (syrinx). This disorder may follow trauma, but it typically develops spontaneously in the cervical spinal cord of teenagers and young adults. She presents with classic symptoms and signs: neck pain, areflexic weakness and atrophy of the upper extremity muscles, and a *suspended* sensory loss to pain but not position. Multiple sclerosis would have caused hyperactive DTRs and other upper motor neuron signs and sensory loss to all modalities. Brown-Séquard syndrome, which results from a lateral transection of the spinal cord at any level, consists of weakness and position sense loss of the limbs on the side ipsilateral to the injury and loss of pain and temperature sensation on the contralateral side.

88. A 29-year-old woman, with a long history of depression with multiple somatic complaints, reports that when she awoke she was unable to rise from bed. During the examination, she failed to move her left arm and leg either spontaneously or on request, but raised her arm to catch a ball. She denied that she was paralyzed on the left. She ignored attractive objects, such as a $1 bill brought into her left visual field. Her left nasolabial fold was flatter on her left than right side when she attempted to smile. Which is the most likely explanation for the left arm and leg immobility?
    a. Left hemiparesis from multiple sclerosis, stroke, or other right cerebral lesion
    b. A conscious attempt to mimic hemiparesis
    c. An unconscious process producing the appearance of hemiparesis
    d. Hemi-inattention and anosognosia from a right cerebral lesion

Answer: d. She probably has sustained a right cerebral lesion in view of the left visual field cut and flattened (paretic) left lower face as well as the neuropsychologic symptoms, hemi-inattention (hemineglect) and anosognosia. Parietal lobe lesions can spare some motor function but still produce the neuropsychologic deficits.

89. Neurologists suspect that a 29-year-old man has psychogenic left-hemiparesis. On examination, when asked to abduct his legs against the examiner's hands, the right leg abducts against the force of the examiner's hand. At the same time, the examiner's hand meets considerable resistance when trying to push the left leg medially. Then, the patient is asked to abduct his left leg against the examiner's hand. That leg fails to abduct and, at the same time, the right leg exerts so little force that the examiner easily pushes it medially. Which one of the following statements concerning this case is false?
    a. This patient's abductor test suggests a psychogenic basis
    b. The patient will probably display a Hoover sign
    c. This patient might also have a sensory "loss" that stops abruptly at the midline
    d. Recent studies have confirmed that psychogenic hemiparesis much more often affects the left than right side

Answer: d. Recent studies have *failed* to confirm earlier observations that psychogenic hemiparesis much more often affects the left than right side. A left-sided predominance of psychogenic hemiparesis had been observed in small series and based on the rationale that, given the choice, individuals would garner the same primary and secondary gains but endure less impairment with a left than right hemiparesis. This patient's examination illustrated major elements of the abductor sign, which indicates a psychogenic basis of a hemiparesis involving the legs. The Hoover sign, which also involves reflexive or unconscious movement of the legs, is another reliable sign of psychogenic hemiparesis. In general, these and other motor signs are more reliable than sensory findings in detecting psychogenic neurologic deficits.

90. Which of the following statements is untrue regarding cochlear implants in children with congenital deafness?
   a. Postoperative meningitis and other complications are rare.
   b. Cochlear implants are effective in restoring useful hearing.
   c. Cochlear implants will allow most deaf children to receive mainstream education.
   d. The benefits of cochlear implants in most children are equal or better than their learning sign language.
   e. They are suitable treatment for presbycusis.

Answer: e. Cochlear implants have been a major advance in correcting deafness in infants and young children. However, one obstacle for cochlear implants in many adults is that they cannot decode the implant's electronic signals into words and language. Their inability results from a different set of stimuli than the ones they learned reaching their auditory cortex. Advances in computer science, audiology, and surgical technique will shortly overcome many of the end-organ problems. At the very least, cochlear implant technology will point the way toward replacing other damaged sensory organs, such as congenitally damaged eyes.

91. Which of the following is not a taste perceived by humans?
   a. L-glutamate
   b. Umami
   c. Success
   d. Sweet
   e. Sour
   f. Salty

Answer: c. Umami, which is perception of L-glutamate, lends food a "rich" taste. It has joined the four basic tastes: sweet, salty, sour, and bitter.

92. Which of the following tastes are triggered by small cations?
   a. L-glutamate
   b. Umami
   c. Salty
   d. Sweet
   e. Bitter

Answer: c. H^+, K^+, and Na^+ trigger salty and sour tastes. G-protein receptors trigger umami, sweet, and bitter tastes.

93. After campus police bring an incoherent, agitated college student to the emergency room, the physicians see that he is wearing only light clothing with no coat despite freezing outdoor temperatures. He seems oblivious to frostbite on his nose and fingertips. He is hypervigilant and possibly hallucinatory, but disoriented and completely uncooperative to examination. The physicians could determine only that he has course vertical and horizontal (three-directional) nystagmus. Which is the most likely intoxicant?
   a. Beer
   b. Vodka
   c. Heroin
   d. Phencyclidine (PCP)
   e. Phenytoin (Dilantin)

Answer: d. Wernicke-Korsakoff syndrome or simply alcohol intoxication leads to nystagmus that is fine and rarely three-directional. Moreover, it is usually associated with depressed sensorium. Similarly, phenytoin intoxication causes fine nystagmus and depressed sensorium. Although heroin intoxication causes stupor, it also causes respiratory depression and small pupils, but no nystagmus. PCP causes agitated delirium and, because it is an anesthetic agent, insensitivity to pain and cold. Its hallmark is course, three-directional nystagmus.

Peripheral Nerve Disorders

By relying on clinical findings, physicians can distinguish peripheral nervous system (PNS) from central nervous system (CNS) disorders. In PNS disorders, damage to one, a group, or all peripheral nerves causes readily observable patterns of paresis, deep tendon reflex (DTR) loss, and sensory impairments. Some PNS disorders are characteristically associated with mental changes, systemic illness, or a fatal outcome.

ANATOMY

The spinal cord's *anterior horn cells* form the motor neurons of the peripheral nerves—the PNS starting point. The peripheral nerves are also the final link in the neuron chain that transmits motor commands from the brain through the spinal cord to muscles (Fig. 5-1). Nerve roots emerging from the anterior spinal cord mingle within the brachial or lumbosacral plexus to form the major peripheral nerves, such as the radial and femoral. Although peripheral nerves are quite long, especially in the legs, they faithfully conduct electrochemical impulses over considerable distances. Because *myelin,* the lipid-based sheath generated by Schwann cells, surrounds peripheral nerves and acts as insulation, the impulses are preserved.

When stimulated, motor nerves release packets of acetylcholine (ACh) from storage vesicles at the neuromuscular junction. The ACh packets traverse the junction and bind onto specific ACh receptors on the muscle end plate. The interaction between ACh and its receptors depolarizes the muscle membrane and initiates a muscle contraction (see Chapter 6). Neuromuscular transmission culminating in muscle depolarization is a discrete, quantitative action: ACh does not merely seep out of the presynaptic terminal as loose molecules and drift across the neuromuscular junction to trigger a muscle contraction.

Peripheral nerves also transmit sensory information, but in the reverse direction: from the PNS to the CNS. For example, pain, temperature, vibration, and position receptors—which are located in the skin, tendons, and joints—send impulses through peripheral nerves to the spinal cord.

MONONEUROPATHIES

Disorders of single peripheral nerves, *mononeuropathies,* are characterized by flaccid paresis, DTR loss (*areflexia*), and reduced sensation, particularly for pain (*hypalgesia* [Greek *hypo,* under + *algos,* pain] or *analgesia* [Greek, insensitivity to pain]) (Table 5-1). Paradoxically, mononeuropathies and other peripheral nerve injuries sometimes lead to spontaneously occurring sensations, *paresthesias* (Greek *para,* near + *aisthesis,* sensation) that may be painful, *dysesthesias.* They also convert stimuli that ordinarily do not cause pain, such as a light touch or cool air, into painful sensations, *allodynia*; exaggerate painful responses to mildly noxious stimuli, such as the point of a pin, *hyperalgesia*; or delay but then exaggerate and prolong pain from noxious stimuli, *hyperpathia.*

Several mononeuropathies are common, important, and readily identifiable. They usually result

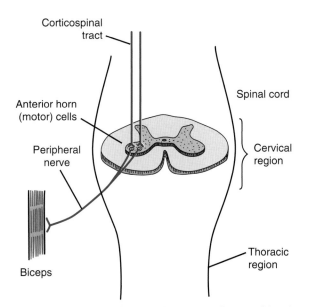

FIGURE 5-1 ■ The corticospinal tracts, as discussed in Chapter 2 and as their name indicates, consist of upper motor neurons (UMNs) that travel from the motor cortex to the spinal cord. They synapse on the spinal cord's *anterior horn cells,* which give rise to the lower motor neurons. These neurons join sensory fibers to form peripheral nerves.

TABLE 5-1 ■ Major Mononeuropathies

Nerve	Motor Paresis	DTR Lost	Pain or Sensory Loss	Examples
Median	Thumb abduction with thenar atrophy	None	Thumb, 2nd and 3rd fingers, and lateral ½ of 4th	Carpal tunnel syndrome
Ulnar	Finger and thumb adduction ("claw hand")	None	5th and medial ½ of 4th fingers	
Radial	Wrist, thumb, and finger extensors ("wrist drop")	Brachioradialis*	Dorsum of hand	Saturday night palsy
Femoral	Knee extensors	Quadriceps (knee)	Anterior thigh, medial calf	
Sciatic	Ankle dorsi flexors and plantar flexors ("flail ankle")	Achilles (ankle)	Buttock, lateral calf, and most of foot	Sciatica from a herniated disk
Peroneal	Ankle dorsiflexors and evertors ("foot drop")	None	Dorsum of foot and lateral calf	Foot drop from lower knee injury

DTR, deep tendon reflex.

*When the radial nerve is damaged by compression in the spiral groove of the humerus, the triceps DTR is spared.

from penetrating or blunt trauma, compression, diabetic infarctions, or other damage to single nerves.

Compression, especially of nerves protected only by overlying skin and subcutaneous tissue rather than by bone, viscera, or thick layers of fat, is especially common. People most susceptible are diabetics; those who have rapidly lost weight, thereby depleting nerves' protective myelin covering; workers in certain occupations, such as watchmakers; and those who have remained in disjointed positions for long periods, often because of drug or alcohol abuse. One of the most common compressive mononeuropathies—"Saturday night palsy"—affects the radial nerve, which is vulnerable at the point where it winds around in the spiral grove of the humerus. Thus, people in alcohol-induced stupor who lean against their upper arm for several hours are apt to develop a *wrist drop* (Fig. 5-2). *Foot drop,* its lower extremity counterpart, often results from common peroneal nerve compression from prolonged leg crossing or a constrictive lower-leg cast pushing against the nerve as it winds around the head of the fibula.

Carpal tunnel syndrome, another mononeuropathy, results from damage of the median nerve as it travels through the carpal tunnel of the wrist (Fig. 5-3, left). Forceful and repetitive wrist movements can traumatize the nerve in that confined passage. Meat and fish processing, certain assembly-line work, and carpentry are all closely associated with carpal tunnel syndrome. However, despite initial claims, word processing and other keyboarding actually have a weak association with the disorder. In another mechanism, fluid retention during pregnancy or menses entraps the median nerve in the carpal tunnel. Similarly, inflammatory tissue changes in the wrist from rheumatoid arthritis can compress the median nerve.

Whatever the mechanism, carpal tunnel syndrome causes paresthesias and pains that shoot from the wrist to the palm, thumb, and adjacent two or sometimes

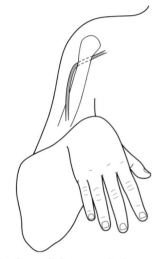

FIGURE 5-2 ■ As the radial nerve winds around the humerus, it is vulnerable to compression and other forms of trauma. Radial nerve damage leads to the readily recognizable *wrist drop* that results from paresis of the extensor muscles of the wrist, finger, and thumb.

three fingers (see Fig. 5-3, right). Symptoms worsen at night and awaken the victims, who shake their hands in an attempt to find relief. The syndrome's characteristic *Tinel's sign* may be elicited by percussing the wrist, which generates electric sensations that shoot from the wrist into the palm and fingers. With chronic carpal tunnel syndrome, median nerve damage leads to thenar (thumb) muscle weakness and atrophy. Most patients respond to rest and, sometimes, splints. Diuretics and anti-inflammatory drugs are also helpful. In refractory cases, a surgeon might inject steroids into the carpal tunnel or resect the transverse carpal ligament to decompress the tunnel.

In another example of damage to a major nerve of the upper extremity, trauma and compression can injure the ulnar nerve, particularly as it passes through the ulnar grove of the elbow (the "funny bone") or more distally in the cubital tunnel. When

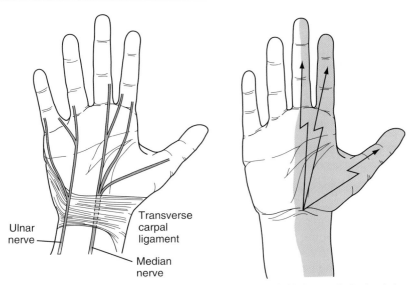

FIGURE 5–3 ■ *Left,* The median nerve passes through the carpal tunnel, which is a relatively tight compartment. In it, the median nerve is vulnerable to trauma from repetitive movement and compression by fluid accumulation. The ulnar nerve, in contrast, passes above and medial to the *transverse carpal ligament,* which is the roof of the tunnel, and escapes damage from such trauma and compression. *Right,* The usual sensory distribution of the median nerve is the palm, thenar eminence (thumb base), thumb, and adjacent two fingers. In carpal tunnel syndrome, pain that spontaneously shoots distally from the wrist is superimposed on this area. The Tinel's sign, a reliable indication of carpal tunnel syndrome, can be elicited by a physician's tapping the palmar wrist surface and producing pain or paresthesias in the median nerve distribution.

FIGURE 5-4 ■ *Left,* With ulnar nerve injuries, the palmar view shows that intrinsic muscles of the hand, particularly those of the hypothenar eminence (fifth finger base), undergo atrophy. The fourth and fifth fingers are flexed and abducted. When raised, the hand and fingers assume the "benediction sign." In addition, the medial two fingers and palm are anesthetic. *Right,* Ulnar nerve injuries also produce a "claw hand" because of atrophy of the muscles between the thumb and adjacent finger (first dorsal interosseous and adductor pollicis), as well as of those of the hypothenar eminence.

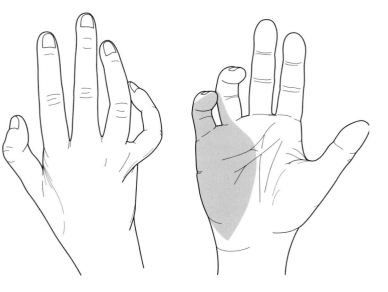

individuals rest their arms' weight on their elbows, the pressure often damages the ulnar nerve. These individuals develop atrophy and weakness of their hand muscles (Fig. 5-4). The ulnar nerve damage also leads to loss of sensation of the fourth and fifth fingers and the medial surface of the hand. This disorder had been so common among watchmakers that it was once dubbed "watchmakers' palsy."

Mononeuropathies can result from systemic illnesses, such as diabetes mellitus, vasculitis (e.g., lupus erythematosus, polyarteritis nodosa), and lead intoxication (see later)—as well as from trauma. In most of the

systemic conditions, pain, weakness, and other symptoms have an abrupt onset, in contrast to the slow onset of compressive and repetitive stress nerve injuries. Additionally, systemic illnesses often cause stroke-like CNS insults along with the mononeuropathies.

MONONEURITIS MULTIPLEX

Mononeuritis multiplex is a serious, complex PNS condition that consists of simultaneous or stepwise development of multiple peripheral injuries often accompanied by cranial injuries. For example, a patient might suddenly develop left radial, right sciatic, and right third cranial nerve deficits. Mononeuritis multiplex is usually a manifestation of a systemic illness, such as vasculitis, diabetes mellitus, or, in Africa and Asia, leprosy.

POLYNEUROPATHIES (NEUROPATHIES)

The most frequently occurring PNS disorder, *polyneuropathy* or, for short, *neuropathy*, is generalized, symmetric involvement—to either a greater or lesser extent—of all peripheral nerves. Some neuropathies also attack cranial nerves. Neurologists usually divide neuropathies into those that damage predominantly either the myelin (demyelinating neuropathies) or axons (axonopathies).

Neuropathies can produce both sensory and motor impairment, but in general one or the other is more of a problem. Patients with *sensory neuropathy* usually experience numbness and paresthesias in the distal part of their arms or legs and typically describe burning or numbness in their fingers and toes (i.e., *stocking-glove hypalgesia,* Fig. 5-5). Sometimes the paresthesias are so disconcerting that they provoke involuntary leg movements, such as in *restless leg syndrome* (see Chapter 17).

Patients with motor neuropathy usually have distal limb weakness that impairs fine, skilled movements, such as buttoning a shirt. In addition, because patients' ankle and toe muscles are typically much weaker than their hip muscles, they will have difficulty raising their feet when they walk or climb stairs. Their neuropathy usually leads to muscle atrophy and flaccidity, as well as weakness. It also diminishes DTRs because of lower motor neuron (LMN) injury (see Fig. 2-2C), with the wrist and ankle DTRs lost first and the more proximal ones lost later.

Neuropathies: Mental Status Usually Unaffected

Neuropathies are common and exemplify general neurologic principles. In addition, several are associated with dementia and other mental status changes (Table 5-2).

Guillain-Barré Syndrome

Acute inflammatory demyelinating polyradiculoneuropathy (AIDP) or postinfectious demyelinating polyneuropathy, commonly known as Guillain-Barré syndrome, is both the quintessential PNS illness and the primary example of a demyelinating neuropathy.

Although often idiopathic, this syndrome typically follows an upper respiratory or gastrointestinal illness. Cases following a week's episode of watery diarrhea are apt to be associated with a gastrointestinal *Campylobacter jejuni* infection and be more extensive and severe than idiopathic cases. Many other cases seem to be a complication of other infectious illnesses, including human immunodeficiency virus (HIV) infection, Lyme disease, mononucleosis, hepatitis, cytomegalovirus (CMV), and West Nile virus.

In general, young and middle-aged adults first develop paresthesias and numbness in the fingers and toes and then areflexic, flaccid paresis of their feet and legs. Weakness, which then becomes a much greater problem than numbness, ascends to involve the hands and arms. Many patients progress to develop respiratory insufficiency from involvement of the phrenic and intercostal nerves and require intubation for respirator assistance. If weakness ascends still further, patients develop cranial nerve involvement that may lead to dysphagia and other aspects of bulbar

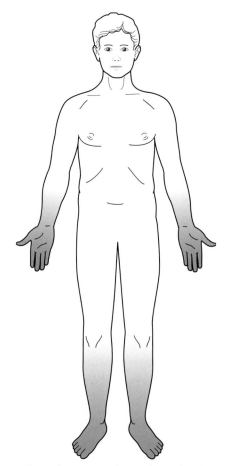

FIGURE 5-5 ■ In polyneuropathy, pain and other sensations are typically lost symmetrically, more severely in the distal than proximal portions of the limbs, and more severely in the legs than the arms. This pattern of sensory loss is termed *stocking-glove hypalgesia.*

TABLE 5-2 ■ Important Causes of Neuropathy

Endogenous toxins
    Acute intermittent and variegate porphyria*
    Diabetes mellitus
    Uremia*
Nutritional
    Deficiencies
        Combined system disease*
        Starvation, malabsorption, alcoholism*
        Celiac disease
    Excessive intake
        Vitamin B_6 (pyridoxine)
Medicines
    Antibiotics:
        Anti-HIV (ddI, ddC)
        Dapsone
        Isoniazid (INH)*
        Nitrofurantoin
    Antineoplastic agents
    Vitamin B_6 (pyridoxine), in high doses
Industrial or chemical toxins
    Metals: arsenic, lead, mercury, thallium
    Nitrous oxide N_2O^+
    Organic solvents: n-hexane^, toluene^*
    Ciguatera fish poisoning*
Infectious/inflammatory conditions
    Mononucleosis, hepatitis, Lyme disease*, leprosy, syphilis*, AIDS*
    Guillain-Barré syndrome
    Vasculitides: systemic lupus erythematosus, polyarteritis*
Genetic diseases
    Adrenoleukodystrophy*
    Friedreich's ataxia and spinocerebellar ataxias
    Metachromatic leukodystrophy*

HIV, human immunodeficiency virus.
*Associated with mental status abnormalities.
^May be substances of abuse.

palsy (see Chapter 4). Still further involvement causes facial weakness and then sometimes even ocular immobility. Nevertheless, possibly because optic and acoustic nerves are protected by myelin generated by the CNS—not the PNS—patients continue to see and hear.

Even if the illness worsens to the point of total paralysis, patients usually remain conscious with a normal mental status—allowing for anxiety and depressive symptoms from enduring a life-threatening illness. Patients who are completely paralyzed and unable to speak are said to be in a *locked-in syndrome* (see Chapter 11). Cerebrospinal fluid (CSF) exhibits an elevated protein concentration but with few white cells (i.e., the classic *albumino-cytologic dissociation*) (see Table 20-1).

The illness usually resolves almost completely within 3 months as the PNS myelin is regenerated. By way of treatment, plasmapheresis (plasma exchange), which extracts circulating inflammatory mediators, particularly autoantibodies, but also compliment and cytokines, reduces the severity and duration of the paresis. Alternatively, administration of intravenous human immunoglobulin (IVIG), which "blocks" the antibodies at the neuromuscular junction, also restores patients' strength.

Not only is Guillain-Barré syndrome a life-threatening illness but it also epitomizes the distinction between PNS and CNS diseases. Although paraparesis or quadriparesis might be a feature common to PNS and CNS illnesses, different patterns of muscle weakness, changes in reflexes, and sensory distribution characterize PNS and CNS illnesses (Table 5-3). Also, in Guillain-Barré syndrome, as in most neuropathies other than diabetic neuropathy (see later), bladder, bowel, and sexual functions are preserved. In contrast, patients with spinal cord disease usually have incontinence and impotence at the onset of the injury.

Another contrast arises from the difference between demyelinating diseases of the CNS and PNS. Despite performing a similar insulating function, CNS and PNS myelin differ in chemical composition, antigenicity, and cells of origin. Oligodendrocytes produce CNS myelin, and Schwann cells produce PNS myelin. In other words, oligodendrocytes are to Schwann cells as the CNS is to the PNS. Also, each oligodendrocyte produces myelin that covers many nearby CNS axons, but each Schwann cell produces myelin than covers only one portion of a single PNS axon. From a clinical viewpoint, Schwann cells regenerate damaged PNS myelin and Guillain-Barré patients usually recover. In contrast, because oligodendrocytes do not regenerate damaged CNS myelin, impairments are permanent in patients who have lost CNS myelin to toxins and infections. For example, the CNS demyelination that results from toluene use represents a permanent loss.

TABLE 5-3 ■ Differences Between Central (CNS) and Peripheral Nervous System (PNS) Signs

	CNS	PNS
Motor system	Upper motor neuron	Lower motor neuron
Paresis	Patterns*	Distal
Tone	Spastic^	Flaccid
Bulk	Normal	Atrophic
Fasciculations	No	Sometimes
Reflexes		
DTRs	Hyperactive+	Hypoactive
Plantar	Babinski sign(s)	Absent
Sensory loss	Patterns*	Hands and feet

*Examples: motor and sensory loss of one side or lower half of the body (e.g., hemiparesis or paraparesis), and hemisensory loss.
^May be flaccid initially.
+May be absent initially.

Multiple sclerosis (MS) appears to be an exception. In this illness, episodes of demyelination of several CNS areas, including the optic nerves, partially or even completely resolve (see Chapter 15). However, the improvement results from resolution of myelin inflammation rather than regeneration. When MS finally encompasses large areas of cerebral CNS myelin, it often results in dementia and other mental status changes.

From another perspective, patients with uncomplicated cases of Guillain-Barré syndrome, despite profound motor impairment, should not have a changed mental status because it is a disease of the PNS. Nevertheless, mental changes develop in patients who have complications involving the CNS, which include cerebral hypoxia from respiratory insufficiency, "steroid psychosis" from high-dose steroid treatment (now outdated), hydrocephalus from impaired reabsorption of CSF that has an elevated protein concentration, hyponatremia from inappropriate antidiuretic hormone secretion (SIADH), or sleep deprivation. Guillain-Barré syndrome patients with the most pronounced impairments—quadriparesis, dependency on artificial ventilation, and multiple cranial nerve involvement—are the ones most apt to experience a psychotic episode. Thus, psychiatric consultants should look first for hypoxia and then other medical complications in Guillain-Barré patients who develop mental aberrations. Also, unless the patient is already on a respirator, psychiatrists should avoid prescribing medications that might depress respirations.

Diabetes

Although rigid treatment of diabetes may delay or even prevent diabetic neuropathy, most patients who have diabetes for more than 10 years lose sensation in the classic stocking-glove distribution. Although their strength remains relatively normal, they lose the DTRs in their ankles then knees. With long-standing diabetic neuropathy, sensation in the fingertips is impaired, preventing blind diabetics from reading Braille. In addition to the distal symmetric sensory loss, diabetic patients suffer from suddenly occurring painful mononeuropathies and mononeuritis multiplex. By a different mechanism—damaging blood vessels—diabetes can lead to cerebrovascular disease that eventually may cause multi-infarct (vascular) dementia.

Diabetic neuropathy often causes painful paresthesias. Patients typically feel an intense burning painful sensation in their feet, which is especially distressing at night and prevents sleep. Three groups of medicines suppress the pain of diabetic neuropathy and other neuropathies. Of the various analgesics, however, only narcotics (opioids) help. The antiepileptic drugs, gabapentin and its congener, pregabalin, reduce pain and promote sleep. In addition, although usually to a lesser extent, several conventional antiepileptics are useful. The third group, tricyclic antidepressants, in doses too low to relieve depression, reduces pain and promotes sleep. In contrast, selective serotonin reuptake inhibitors (SSRIs) provide little analgesia; however, serotonin-norepinephrine reuptake inhibitors, such as duloxetine, are beneficial. In an alternative, local approach, a skin cream containing capsaicin, which depletes substance P, the putative neurotransmitter for pain, can provide some analgesia, along with numbness, to limited areas. However, nonsteroidal anti-inflammatory drugs (NSAIDs) provide little benefit.

Patients with diabetic neuropathy can also have autonomic nervous system involvement that causes gastrointestinal immobility, bladder muscle contraction, and sexual dysfunction. In fact, erectile dysfunction is occasionally the first or most disturbing symptom of diabetic autonomic neuropathy (see Chapter 16).

Toxic-Metabolic Disorders

Numerous toxins, metabolic derangements, and medications frequently cause neuropathy. For example, renal insufficiency is a common cause of neuropathy that is almost universal in patients undergoing maintenance hemodialysis. Also, medications used for chemotherapy of neoplasms and various infections, including tuberculosis and HIV disease (see later), routinely cause neuropathy; however, antipsychotics, antidepressants, and most antiepileptic drugs, except for phenytoin (Dilantin), do not cause it. When medications, chemicals, or other substances cause CNS or PNS damage, neurologists label them *neurotoxins*.

Several heavy metals cause combinations of PNS and CNS problems. For example, lead poisoning causes a neuropathy in adults and other problems in children. Pica (craving for unnatural foods), mostly from hunger, in young children prompts them to eat lead-pigment paint chips from toys or decaying tenement walls. (Lead paint on interior walls has been illegal in most cities for decades.) Even at low concentrations lead is neurotoxic in children. It is associated with inattention, learning disabilities, and poor school performance. High concentrations are associated with seizures and mental retardation. Because lead has a different deleterious effect on the mature nervous system, adults with lead poisoning develop mononeuropathies, such as a foot drop or wrist drop, rather than cerebral impairments. Adults most often develop lead poisoning from industrial exposure, drinking homemade alcohol distilled in equipment with lead pipes ("moonshine"), or burning car batteries for heat.

Chronic, low-level intoxication by several other heavy metals causes polyneuropathy, dermatologic abnormality, and mental changes. However, acute poisoning with them typically leads to fatal gastrointestinal symptoms and cardiovascular collapse. Arsenic, which is tasteless and odorless, is a popular poison used in murder. With chronic, low-level, deliberate, accidental, or industrial intoxication, arsenic causes anorexia, malaise, and a distal neuropathy that might be so severe as to mimic Guillain-Barré syndrome. It also causes several characteristic dermatologic abnormalities: Mees' lines on the fingernails (Fig. 5-6), hyperpigmentation, and hyperkeratosis.

Chronic mercury intoxication is more complex than arsenic poisoning. Organic mercury compounds, such as methylmercury, can enter the food chain at the lowest level and progress upward to saturate edible fish. Eating fish exposed to a massive industrial discharge of mercury can poison individuals. (However, without eating overtly contaminated fish or having a continual, high-level industrial exposure, people rarely develop mercury poisoning.) Individuals with mercury poisoning develop prominent CNS deficits, such as ataxia, dysarthria, and visual field changes. They also develop a neuropathy and a telltale dark line along the gums (Fig. 5-7). In contrast to poisoning with organic mercury, poisoning with inorganic mercury, widely used in industry, causes kidney damage, but only mild cognitive impairment.

At one time, mercury-based dental amalgams ("fillings") had been suspected of causing Alzheimer's disease and other neurodegenerative illnesses because they were thought to emit a mercury vapor or allow mercury to dissolve into the blood or saliva. Also, because ethyl mercury was a major component of the common vaccine preservative, *thimerosal,* routine childhood vaccinations were suspected of causing autism and other childhood illnesses (see Chapter 13). However, statistically powerful epidemiologic studies disproved both of those suspicions.

Thallium, another heavy metal, is the active ingredient of some rodenticides. Murderers occasionally lace food with it. Like other chronic heavy metal intoxications, chronic thallium intoxication causes a neuropathy that might be painful. Its characteristic dermatologic sign is hair loss (alopecia).

Aging Related Changes

Although the condition is not yet considered a neuropathy and has not yet received a name, as people age they develop sensory loss from peripheral nerve degeneration. Almost all people who are older than 80 years have lost some joint position and a great deal of vibratory sensation in their feet. This sensory

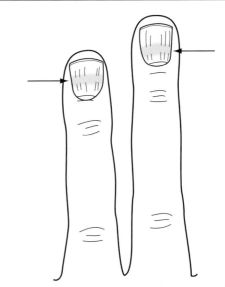

FIGURE 5-6 ■ Mees' lines, white bands *(arrows)* that stretch across the fingernails, characteristically indicate arsenic poisoning. However, poisoning by other heavy metals and trauma can also cause them.

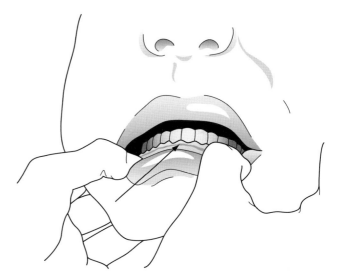

FIGURE 5-7 ■ Individuals with chronic mercury poisoning develop a dark blue or back line *(arrow)* along the gum line. Individuals with this mercury-induced gum line usually also have neuropathy and central nervous system (CNS) signs, such as ataxia and dysarthria.

neuropathy, which is accompanied by absent ankle DTRs, prevents them from standing with their feet placed closely together, impairs their gait, does not allow them to walk heel-to-toe (*tandem gait*), and predisposes them to falling. In addition, age- and work-related degenerative changes in the lumbar spine compress the lumbar nerve roots as they exit their neural foramina (see later, lumbar spondylosis).

Neuropathies: Mental Status Usually Affected

Although most neuropathies, as described in the previous section, may be painful, incapacitating, or even devastating to the PNS, they generally do not cause mental aberrations in adults. For example, most people who are old, diabetic, on hemodialysis, or receiving chemotherapy, remain intelligent, thoughtful, and competent even though beset by pain, sensory loss, and weakness. In contrast, only a few disease categories (Table 5-2) cause the combination of dementia and neuropathy, which would reflect both cerebral cortex and peripheral nerve damage. An analogous combination would be dementia and movement disorders, which would indicate cerebral cortex and basal ganglia damage (see Table 18-4).

Nutritional Deficiencies

Deficiencies of thiamine (vitamin B_1), niacin (nicotinic acid, B_3), or vitamin B_{12} each produce a predominantly sensory neuropathy accompanied by dementia or other mental status abnormality (Table 5-4). From a worldwide perspective, starvation has been the most common cause of deficiencies of vitamins, their carrier-fats, minerals, and other nutrients. For example, *beriberi* was the starvation-induced neuropathy attributable to thiamine deficiency endemic in eastern Asia. In the United States, alcoholism, bariatric surgery, and malabsorption syndromes are the most common causes of nutritional neuropathies. On the other hand, few patients with anorexia nervosa or self-imposed extreme diets develop a neuropathy. Their protection may lie in a selective, possibly secret, intake of food or vitamins.

Alcohol-induced neuropathy has been virtually synonymous with thiamine deficiency because most cases are found in alcoholics who typically subsist on alcohol and carbohydrate-rich foods that are devoid of thiamine. However, studies seem to show that alcohol itself may cause a neuropathy and that thiamine deficiency is not present in all cases of neuropathy.

Whatever the cause, thiamine deficiency leads to absent DTRs and loss of position sensation. In fact, until patients walk in the dark when they must rely on position sense generated in the legs and feet, their deficits may remain asymptomatic. In the well-known *Wernicke-Korsakoff syndrome*, amnesia, dementia, cerebellar degeneration, and, in the acute illness, nystagmus and ocular-motor paresis (see Chapter 7) accompany the neuropathy associated with alcoholism.

In another example of vitamin deficiency causing neuropathy, niacin deficiency is associated with or causes *pellagra* (Italian, rough skin). This starvation-induced disorder consists of dementia, dermatitis, and diarrhea—the "three Ds." Despite pellagra's status as a classic illness, the role of niacin deficiency has been challenged: deficiencies of other nutrients either coexist with or are more likely to be the actual cause.

Because vitamin B_{12} serves, among many functions, to sustain CNS and PNS myelin, B_{12} deficiency leads to the combination of CNS and PNS damage—*combined system disease*. Its manifestations include a neuropathy, but cognitive impairment and sensory loss reflecting demyelination of the posterior columns of the spinal cord (see Fig. 2-19B) are more prominent symptoms. Also, patients may develop a characteristic megaloblastic anemia. Most important, this disease is best known as a "correctable cause of dementia" because B_{12} injections can reverse the cognitive impairment and other CNS and PNS manifestations. The usual causes of B_{12} deficiency include pernicious anemia, malabsorption, a pure vegetarian diet, or prolonged exposure to nitrous oxide (N_2O), a gaseous dental anesthetic.

TABLE 5-4 ■ Neurologic Aspects of the Vitamins			
Vitamin	**Diseases Associated with a Deficiency**	**Diseases Associated with an Excess**	**Miscellaneous Actions**
A (e.g., retinol)	Night blindness	Pseudotumor cerebri	
B_1 Thiamine	Wernicke-Korsakoff syndrome* Beriberi^		
B_2 Riboflavin			
B_3 Niacin	Pellagra^		
B_6 Pyridoxine	Seizures, psychosis	Neuropathy	
B_9 Folic acid/folate	Neural tube defects		Reduces elevated homocysteine levels
B_{12} Cobalamine	Combined system disease^		
C Ascorbic acid	Scurvy		
E Alpha-tocopherol	Ataxia, neuropathy		Scavenges free radicals

*Includes neuropathy as part of the illness.
^Associated with neuropathy.

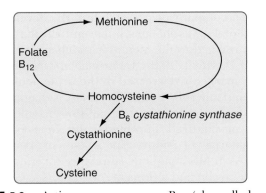

FIGURE 5-8 ■ Acting as a coenzyme, B_{12} (also called *cobalamine*), along with folate, facilitates the conversion of homocysteine to methionine. Other enzymes complete the cycle by converting methionine back to homocysteine. The absence of B_{12} leads to the accumulation of both methionine and homocysteine. Nitrous oxide (N_2O) poisons this cycle and creates B_{12} deficiency because it oxidizes the cobalt in B_{12} (not pictured) to an inactive form. Whatever the cause, an elevated homocysteine level has been established as a risk factor for neural tube defects, cerebrovascular and cardiovascular disease, and other neurologic conditions.

The screening test for B_{12} deficiency consists of determining the serum B_{12} level. In equivocal cases, especially when mental or spinal cord abnormalities are not accompanied by anemia, determining the serum homocysteine and methylmalonic acid levels can corroborate the diagnosis: in B_{12} deficiency, both homocysteine and methylmalonic acid levels will be elevated (Fig. 5-8). Intrinsic factor antibodies, a classic finding in pernicious anemia, will be detectable in only about 60% of cases. The standard confirmatory test is the Schilling test.

A variation on nutritional deficiencies causing neuropathy is celiac disease. In this condition, foods containing wheat gluten or similar protein constituents of rye and barley trigger an autoimmune response. Patients develop not only malabsorption, which is not always readily apparent, but also neuropathy and sometimes ataxia. Severely affected patients develop cancer, osteoporosis, and cardiac disease.

In contrast to neuropathy resulting from malnutrition, *excessive intake* of certain vitamins is also deleterious. Several food faddists once developed a profound sensory neuropathy from deliberately taking excessive vitamin B_6 (pyridoxine). Although the normal adult daily requirement of this vitamin is only 2 to 4 mg, the faddists had been consuming several grams. Similarly, high vitamin A intake may cause pseudotumor cerebri (see Chapter 9) or induce fetal abnormalities.

Infectious Diseases

Several common organisms have a predilection for infecting the peripheral nerves and sparing the CNS.

For example, *herpes zoster* infects a single nerve root or a branch of the trigeminal nerve, usually in people older than 65 years or those with an impaired immune system. It causes an ugly, red, painful, vesicular eruption ("shingles") that may remain excruciating long after the skin infection has resolved (see Postherpetic Neuralgia, Chapter 14). As another example, leprosy, infection with *Mycobacterium leprae* (Hansen's disease), causes anesthetic, hypopigmented patches of skin, anesthetic fingers and toes, and palpable nerves. It particularly affects the cool portions of the body, such as the nose, ear lobes, and digits; however, sometimes the infection strikes the ulnar or another large nerve either singly or along with others.

Some infections involve the CNS as well as the PNS. Named for the town in Connecticut where it was discovered, *Lyme disease* has risen to endemic levels in New England, Westchester, eastern Long Island, Wisconsin, Minnesota, and the Pacific Northwest. *Borrelia burgdorferi*, a spirochete whose vector is a certain tick, causes Lyme disease. The illness' peak incidence occurs in June through September, when people spend time in tick-infested wooded areas.

Acute Lyme disease typically produces multiple problems, such as arthritis, malaise, low-grade fever, cardiac arrhythmias, and a pathognomonic bull's-eye-shaped rash, *erythema migrans* (moving red rash), surrounding the tick bite. In addition, Lyme disease frequently causes a facial nerve paresis, similar to Bell's palsy, either unilaterally or bilaterally (see Fig. 4-15). Its PNS manifestations range from a mild neuropathy causing only paresthesias to a severe Guillain-Barré-like illness.

With CNS involvement, patients typically have headache, delirium (see Chapter 7), and other signs of meningitis or encephalitis. Their CSF may show a pleocytosis, elevated protein and decreased glucose concentrations, and Lyme antibodies. Serologic tests for Lyme disease remain unreliable. Another confusing aspect of the diagnosis is that patients may have a biologic false-positive test for syphilis because *B. burgdorferi* is a spirochete (see Chapter 7).

Numerous individuals and physicians attribute years of symptoms—cognitive impairment, weakness, fatigue, and arthralgias—after an attack of adequately treated Lyme disease to a persistent Lyme infection or disordered immunologic response to it. This condition, "chronic Lyme disease," meets with skepticism in the neurologic community because it lacks consistent clinical criteria, pathology, and test results and does not respond to additional treatment.

Even though Lyme disease is common, the most widespread infection of the CNS and PNS is *acquired immunodeficiency syndrome (AIDS)*. Although direct HIV infection probably causes neuropathy associated with AIDS, alternative potential etiologies include opportunistic infectious agents and HIV medicines, such as nucleoside reverse transcriptase inhibitors (ddI [didanosine, Videx] and ddC [zalcitabine]). The most common AIDS-associated peripheral nerve disorder is an insidiously developing and long-standing neuropathy that is distal, symmetrical, and predominantly sensory. Its main symptoms consist of painful dysesthesias, which can be agonizing, and numbness of the soles of the feet. Motor symptoms are less pronounced, debilitating, or bothersome: patients only have mild ankle and foot weakness and loss of ankle DTRs.

HIV-associated polyneuropathy generally develops late in the course of the illness when many other problems overshadow the neuropathy, the viral titer is elevated, and the CD4 count is low. It is often accompanied by depression and decreased physical function. In general, treatments for diabetic neuropathy are appropriate for painful AIDS neuropathy: opioids, tricyclic antidepressants, and certain antiepileptics.

Inherited Metabolic Illnesses

Although numerous genetically determined illnesses cause neuropathy, two are notorious because they also cause psychosis.

Acute intermittent porphyria (AIP), the classic autosomal dominant genetic disorder of porphyrin metabolism, causes dramatic attacks of quadriparesis and colicky abdominal pain. In about 25% to 50% of attacks, AIP patients develop any of a variety of psychiatric symptoms, including agitation, delirium, depression, and psychosis. During attacks, excess porphyrins color the urine red. New quantitative tests that replace the classic Watson-Schwartz test show urinary excretion of porphobilinogen and amino levulinic acid during an attack. Although barbiturates may exacerbate an attack, phenothiazines are relatively safe. Despite its prominence as a standard examination question, AIP is rare in the United States.

Metachromatic leukodystrophy (MLD), an autosomal recessive illness, is named for the colored granules that accumulate in the brain, peripheral nerves, and many non-neurologic organs, such as the gallbladder, testicles, and retinae. Most important, MLD, like MS, causes a demyelination process in the CNS white matter (*leuko*dystrophy), and, to a lesser extent, the PNS (see Chapter 15).

MLD symptoms usually first appear in infants and children but occasionally do so in young adults. In those older than 16 years, MLD causes progressively severe personality and behavioral changes, psychosis that can mimic schizophrenia, and cognitive impairment. MLD-induced mental disturbances are often termed "frontal dementia" (see Chapter 7). Peripheral neuropathy and signs of CNS demyelination—spasticity and ataxia—typically accompany or closely follow the development of the mental status changes, but eventually the physical deficits overshadow the mental status changes.

In MLD, activity of the lysosomal enzyme arylsulfatase A is markedly decreased in the urine, leukocytes, serum, and amniotic fluid. The illness is diagnosed by demonstrating reduced activity of this enzyme in leukocytes or cultured fibroblasts and metachromatic lipid material in biopsy specimens of peripheral nerves. As in MS, magnetic resonance imaging (MRI) shows demyelinated lesions in the brain (see Chapters 15 and 20). Despite the clear-cut pathology, no treatment arrests the illness.

Volatile Substance Exposure

Industrial organic solvents, which are generally lipophilic and volatile at room temperature, enter the body through inhalation, absorption through the skin, or occasionally by ingestion. Particularly vulnerable workers are those exposed to metal-part degreasing agents, paint and varnish, and shoe manufacturing chemicals; however, toxic exposures are related more to poor ventilation or inadequate safety barriers than to particular industries.

Because of their lipophilic properties, industrial solvents, such as *n*-hexane, toluene, ethylene oxide, and carbon disulfide, penetrate or dissolve the lipid-based myelin insulating the nervous system. Although these neurotoxins readily damage the PNS, CNS, or both, industrial solvents primarily cause a neuropathy. In addition, they sometimes also cause various neuropsychologic symptoms—cognitive impairment, personality changes, inattention, depression, headaches, fatigue, and even psychosis—together termed *solvent-induced encephalopathy*.

In addition to workers developing neurotoxicity from industrial exposure, other individuals self-inflict it by substance abuse. Recreational inhaling of certain volatile substances, "huffing," also damages the one or both components of the nervous system. For example, in "glue sniffing," where the intoxicating component is the common hydrocarbon solvent *n*-hexane, sensation-seekers typically develop polyneuropathy and other PNS complications. In contrast, toluene, a component of spray paint and glue, is also a recreational volatile drug; however, it damages CNS rather than PNS myelin. Occasionally inhaling toluene initially produces an uncomplicated euphoria, but, whether deliberate or accidental, chronic overexposure can cause personality changes, psychosis, or cognitive impairment that can reach the severity of dementia. When toluene-induced dementia occurs, it falls into the category of subcortical dementia, in which language function is relatively spared (see Chapter 7). Chronic overexposure to toluene also causes widespread physical signs of comparable severity, including spasticity, ataxia, and visual impairment. Severe toluene-induced cerebral demyelination (leukoencephalopathy) can be seen on MRI (see Chapter 15). Thus, the clinical findings and MRI abnormalities mimic those of MS.

Nitrous oxide, the dental anesthetic, is also a potentially toxic. It is readily available in both gas cartridges that are used to make whipped cream and large, safeguarded medical containers. As with toluene, individuals who inhale nitrous oxide experience a few minutes of euphoria as well as anesthesia. Frequently inhaling nitrous oxide, even intermittently for several weeks, may induce a profound neuropathy. In addition, this exposure may cause a B_{12} deficiency that damages the spinal cord (see previous). Succumbing to nitrous oxide abuse, with its neurologic consequences, is an occupational hazard for dentists.

Pseudoneurotoxic Disease

Neurologists often implicate an occupational neurotoxin when a group of workers has similar objective symptoms and signs, environmental tests detect elevated concentrations of neurotoxins in the workplace, the neurotoxin is an established cause of the problem in animals or humans, and laboratory testing shows abnormalities consistent with the symptoms. To be fair, symptoms of solvent-induced encephalopathy and other alleged neurotoxic states are usually nonspecific, largely subjective, and beyond the realm of neurologic testing. Moreover, the relevant psychologic tests are often unreliable, generally accepted diagnostic criteria often do not exist, and safe exposure limits to many neurotoxins are unknown.

Sometimes workers' disorders have an explanation other than exposure to a neurotoxin. In *pseudoneurotoxic disease,* individuals attributing an illness to a neurotoxin have actually suffered the emergence or worsening of a neurologic or psychiatric disorder—alone or in combination—coincident with a neurotoxin exposure. In other words, despite their symptoms, they have no ill effects from the neurotoxin. To attribute the problem to the neurotoxin is a post hoc fallacy.

The symptoms in some cases may actually be manifestations of a neurologic illness, such as Parkinson's disease or MS, that has emerged or worsened following the exposure. Similarly, patients may attribute aged-related changes and variations in normal neurologic function to a neurotoxin exposure. Alternatively, the patients may have a somatic disorder, mood disorder, alcohol abuse, or other psychiatric disturbance whose manifestations mimic solvent-induced encephalopathy or other neurotoxic disorder.

The *multiple chemical sensitivity syndrome* serves as a prime example of pseudoneurotoxic disease originating from a psychiatric disturbance. This disorder consists of miniscule exposures to environmental chemicals, ones usually volatile and unavoidable in day-to-day life, such as commercial cleaning agents or air fresheners, allegedly producing multiple but variable symptoms. According to affected individuals, exposure to innumerable chemicals is followed by attacks, which are often incapacitating, consisting of headache, alterations in level of consciousness, paresis, or various physical problems. Despite their dramatic and compelling histories and remaining psychiatrically asymptomatic between episodes, scientific analysis has shown that the symptoms are unrelated to chemical exposure and no physiologic disorder underlies them.

Marine Toxicology

Shellfish and free-swimming fish produce a completely different category of toxins. *Ciguatera fish poisoning,* the best-understood and most commonly occurring example of "marine toxicology," has unique symptoms and a clear-cut underlying pathology. Their toxin reaches humans by moving up the food chain from toxin-producing dinoflagellates to large, edible reef fish, particularly grouper, red snapper, and barracuda. Unlike other toxins, ciguatoxin causes a prolonged opening of voltage-gated sodium channels in nerves and muscles.

Individuals who ingest ciguatera toxin first have nausea and vomiting, as with most food poisonings, but then many develop symptoms of an acute painful neuropathy with paresthesias, pain, and lack of sensation in their limbs. Victims also experience a unique symptom: "cold reversal," in which they misperceive cold objects as feeling hot. Although they eventually recover, malaise, depression, and headaches complicate their recuperation.

MOTOR NEURON DISORDERS

Amyotrophic Lateral Sclerosis

Amyotrophic lateral sclerosis (ALS) was known for decades as "Lou Gehrig's disease" because the famous baseball player Lou Gehrig succumbed to this dreadful illness. Among neurologists, ALS is known as the classic *motor neuron disease* because both upper motor neurons (UMNs) and LMNs degenerate while other neurologic systems—notably mental faculties—are spared.

The etiology of ALS remains an enigma, but several genetic, environmental, and pathologic clues hold some promise. One finding is that 5% to 10% of patients seem to have inherited ALS in an autosomal dominant pattern. Some of them—2% of the total ALS patients—carry a mutation of a gene on chromosome 21 (Cu, Zn superoxide dismutase [SOD1]) that normally assists in detoxifying superoxide free radicals.

Also, an 18% increase in ALS among U.S.—Army and Air Force but not Navy or Marine—veterans of the First Persian Gulf War initially implicated a war-related environmental exposure. In an extensive study of United Kingdom veterans, who had no increase in ALS risk, almost all reported having had contact with pesticides, diesel fuel and other common chemicals, pyridostigmine (prophylactic treatment for nerve gas attacks [see Chapter 6]), anthrax vaccinations, or numerous other potential toxins. More than 90% of them reported one or more symptoms, including muscle and joint pain (39%) and memory problems (24%). However, clinical and electrophysiologic studies have shown no consistent clinical syndrome and no specific physiologic impairment in the peripheral nerves, skeletal muscles, or their junction. In contrast, tobacco use, representing an unequivocal environmental factor, carries a dose-response increase in ALS risk to almost four-fold.

The pathology of ALS, characterized by an absence of a cellular reaction surrounding degenerating motor neurons, weighs against inflammatory and infectious conditions. Many ALS patients do respond, albeit modestly, to blocking glutamate, the excitatory neurotransmitter (see Chapter 21). Putting together these clues—the lack of a cellular response and a beneficial response to glutamate blocking—suggests that *glutamate excitotoxicity* leads to cell death from *apoptosis* (see Chapters 18 and 21).

People develop ALS at a median age of 66 years. Their first symptoms consist of weakness, atrophy, and subcutaneous muscular twitching (*fasciculations*)—a sign of degenerating anterior horn cells—in one arm or leg (Fig. 5-9). Surprisingly, even from these atrophic muscles, physicians can elicit brisk DTRs and Babinski signs—signs of upper motor degeneration—because undamaged LMNs are supplied by damaged UMNs. The weakness, atrophy, and fasciculations spread asymmetrically to other limbs and also to the face, pharynx, and tongue. Dysarthria and dysphagia (bulbar palsy) eventually develop in most patients. When pseudobulbar palsy superimposes itself on bulbar palsy, patients' speech becomes unintelligible and interrupted by "demonic" or "pathologic" laughing and crying (see Chapter 4). Despite their extensive paresis, patients' ocular muscle control and bladder and bowel function, as well as their cognitive capacity, remain normal.

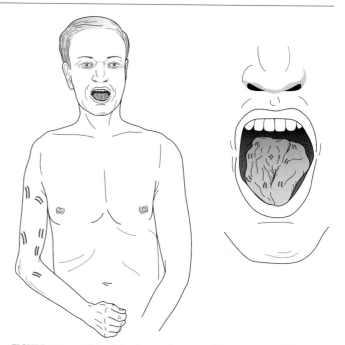

FIGURE 5-9 ■ This elderly gentleman with amyotrophic lateral sclerosis (ALS) has typical (right arm) asymmetric limb atrophy, paresis, and fasciculations. His tongue, which also has fasciculations, has undergone atrophy, as indicated by clefts and furrows.

No treatment cures or even arrests ALS. However, riluzole (Rilutek) seems to slow progression, delaying the time until tracheostomy or death. By inhibiting presynaptic glutamate release and possibly also blocking postsynaptic receptors, riluzole presumably reduces glutamate excitotoxicity and thereby preserves motor neuron function.

The outstanding clinical feature of ALS is that patients, except for a small group (approximately 5%), remain tragically alert, mentally competent, and completely aware of their plight throughout the course of their illness. That group of ALS patients usually has coexisting frontotemporal dementia, in which behavioral changes and language impairment, as well as dementia, accompany bulbar palsy (see Chapter 7).

As consulting psychiatrists who are drawn into this painful situation will find, almost all ALS patients have the cognitive capacity to chose their medical care and make other important decisions. In particular, many patients confronting their situation refuse resuscitation measures, mechanical ventilation, and other life-support devices. After litigation or legislation, several patients have hastened the inevitable process of ALS. About 80% of ALS patients receiving standard medical care die, usually from respiratory complications or sepsis, within 5 years from the time of diagnosis. Because patients remain lucid, competent, and usually free of sedating medications, but follow a relatively rapid untreatable fatal disease, ALS has become the archetypical illness for discussions concerning end-of-life care, patients' right-to-die, physician-assisted suicide, and euthanasia.

Several other motor neuron diseases also cause extensive loss of anterior horn cells (LMNs) while sparing UMNs and extraocular muscle movement. For example, hereditary motor neuron diseases in infants (Werdnig-Hoffmann disease) and children (Kugelberg-Welander disease)—varieties of spinal muscular atrophy—are characterized exclusively by LMN involvement: flaccid quadriplegia with atrophic, areflexic muscles, and fasciculations. Both are autosomal recessive illnesses carried on chromosome 5.

Poliomyelitis

Poliomyelitis (polio) had been the most frequently occurring motor neuron disease until Jonas Salk and his coworkers developed the vaccine. Polio, which has almost been entirely eradicated, is a viral infection of the anterior horn (motor neuron) cells of the spinal cord and lower brainstem (the bulb). Polio patients, who were mostly children, developed an acute, febrile illness with ALS-type LMN signs: paresis that was typically asymmetric, muscle fasciculations, and absent DTRs. Patients with the bulbar variety of polio had throat and chest muscle paralysis that forced them to be placed in the "iron lung" to support their respirations. (The iron lung was essentially an approximately 3 feet in diameter and 5 feet long, airtight metal tube that extended from the patient's neck, which was surrounded by an airtight rubber seal, to the feet. A pump would withdraw air from the inside of the iron lung to create negative pressure that forced room air into the patient's lungs.)

In polio, as in ALS, oculomotor, bladder, bowel, and sexual functions are normal (see Chapters 12 and 16). Likewise, polio patients, no matter how devastating their illness, retain normal mental function. For example, Franklin Roosevelt, handicapped by polio-induced paraplegia, served as president of the United States. Unfortunately, some middle-aged individuals who had poliomyelitis in childhood tend to develop further weakness and fasciculations of muscles initially affected or spared. An ALS-like condition, the *post-polio syndrome* has been postulated to explain this late deterioration; however, if this syndrome exists at all, it is rare. In actuality, the deterioration can almost always be readily attributed to common non-neurologic conditions, such as lumbar spine degeneration.

Benign Fasciculations

Fasciculations are commonplace, innocuous muscle twitches that are usually precipitated by excessive physical exertion, psychologic stress, drinking strong coffee, or exposure to some insecticides. Diagnosis may be difficult because benign fasciculations mimic ALS-induced fasciculations and are sometimes associated with fatigue and hyperactive DTRs. The clinical guidelines would be that, in contrast to ALS-induced fasciculations, benign fasciculations are unaccompanied by weakness, atrophy, or pathologic reflexes, and they usually last for only several days to weeks. They will help calm fears of medical students and others acquainted with ALS.

Sometimes the fasciculations are confined to the eyelid muscles (orbicularis oculi) and create annoying twitching or jerking movements. In a different situation—if the movements are bilateral, forceful enough to close the eyelids, or exceed a duration of 1 second—they may represent a facial dyskinesia, such as blepharospasm, hemifacial spasm, or tardive dyskinesia (see Chapter 18).

Orthopedic Disturbances

Cervical spondylosis is the age- and occupation-related degenerative condition, osteoarthritis, in which bony encroachment leads to narrowing (stenosis) of the vertebral foramina and spinal canal (Fig. 5-10). In this disorder, cervical spine "wear and tear" narrows the nerve and spinal cord passages or tunnels. Stenosis of the neural foramina can constrict ("pinch") cervical nerve roots and cause neck pain with arm and hand paresis, atrophy, hypoactive DTRs, and fasciculations—signs of LMN injury. In addition, spinal canal stenosis can compress the spinal cord and cause leg spasticity, hyperreflexia, and Babinski signs—signs of UMN injury.

As with cervical spondylosis, *lumbar spondylosis* produces lumbar nerve compression and low back pain. Although patients could not have spinal cord compression (because the spinal cord terminates at the first lumbar vertebra [see Fig. 16-1]), they will have signs of lumbar peripheral nerve damage: leg and feet paresis, atrophy, fasciculations, sensory loss, and paresthesias. Sometimes patients with lumbar stenosis have symptoms of pain and weakness in their legs only when they walk (*neurogenic claudication*).

In addition to being common, disabling, and painful, cervical and lumbar spondylosis, by causing both PNS and CNS signs, mimics ALS. The distinguishing features of spondylosis are neck or low back pain, sensory loss, and absence of abnormalities in the facial, pharyngeal, and tongue muscles.

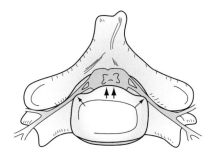

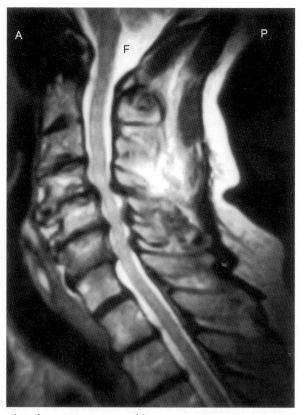

FIGURE 5-10 ■ *Left,* In cervical spondylosis, bony proliferation damages upper and lower motor neurons. Intervertebral ridges of bone *(double arrows)* compress the cervical spinal cord (blue). At the same time, narrowing of the foramina *(single arrows)* constrict cervical nerve roots (blue). *Right,* The magnetic resonance imaging (MRI) shows the lateral view of cervical spondylosis. The cerebrospinal fluid (CSF) in the foramen magnum (F) and surrounding the spinal cord is bright white. The spinal cord is gray. In the mid- to low cervical spine, bony protrusions compress the spinal cord and its surrounding CSF to give the spinal column a "wash-board" appearance.

Gelatinous intervertebral disks, which are shaped like checkers, normally cushion adjacent vertebral bodies. Sometimes trauma, strain, poor posture, or obesity forcefully extrudes (herniates) a portion of a disk. Herniated disk material can press against the adjacent nerve roots and other structures. The compression typically causes pain, sensory loss, weakness, and, when severe and in the lumbar area, incontinence and sexual dysfunction. Almost all herniated disks develop in the cervical or lumbosacral spine.

More than 90% of lumbosacral disk herniations occur at either the L4–5 or L5-S1 intervertebral space (Fig. 5-11). Lumbar herniated disks usually cause low back pain that radiates to the buttocks and down the leg along the compressed nerve root. The pain in the buttock and leg, as well as in the low back, is characteristically increased by coughing, sneezing, or elevating the straightened leg because these maneuvers press the herniated disk more forcefully against

the nerve root (Fig. 5-12). Pain that radiates in the distribution of the sciatic nerve, *sciatica,* is indicative of a lumbar herniated disk and distinguishes it from other causes of low back pain, such as aortic aneurysms, endometriosis, and degenerative spine disease.

Cervical intervertebral disks typically cause weakness of arm or hand muscles, pain that radiates down the arm as well as neck pain, and loss of an upper extremity DTR. Injuries confined to the soft tissues of the neck or degenerative spine disease would not cause the radiating pain or reflex loss. "Whiplash" automobile injuries and other trauma are the most common cause of cervical intervertebral disks.

However, neither cervical nor lumbar disks are usually responsible for all the pain, disability, sexual dysfunction, and multitudinous other symptoms blamed on them. In fact, herniated disks may be an innocuous, chance finding in many individuals: MRI studies have revealed a herniated disk in about 20% of asymptomatic individuals younger than 60 years. Even more so,

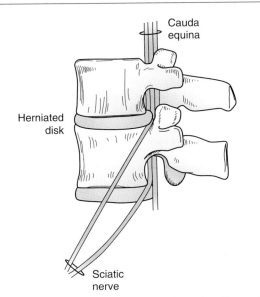

FIGURE 5-11 ■ The *cauda equina* (Latin, horse's tail) consists of the bundle of lumbar and sacral nerve roots in the spinal canal. The nerve roots leave the spinal canal through foramina. Herniated disks might compress the nerve roots in or near those narrow passages. Compressed nerve roots usually cause pain in the low back that radiates along the distribution of the sciatic nerve. Common movements that momentarily further herniate the disk, such as coughing, sneezing, or straining at stool, intensify the pain.

bulging and desiccated disks, which do not compress nerve roots, cannot be held responsible for these symptoms.

For acute low back pain, nonopioid analgesics, anti-inflammatory drugs, and reduction in physical activity are usually helpful. Opinion varies as to whether the most effective approach is at most a 2-day course of bed rest, continuing routine activities when physically tolerable, or performing certain exercises. Epidural injections of steroids improve acute pain from herniated disks but do not alter the outcome. Whatever the particular treatment, conservative measures help 90% of acute low back pain cases.

Nevertheless, patients who recover from low back pain are subject to recurrences. Chronic, persistent low back pain is another matter. Physicians should consider it a variety of chronic pain rather than a prolonged bout of herniated disk symptoms (see Chapter 14).

WEB SITES

Agency for Toxic Substances and Disease Registry: http://atsdr1.atsdr.cdc.gov:8080/cx.html

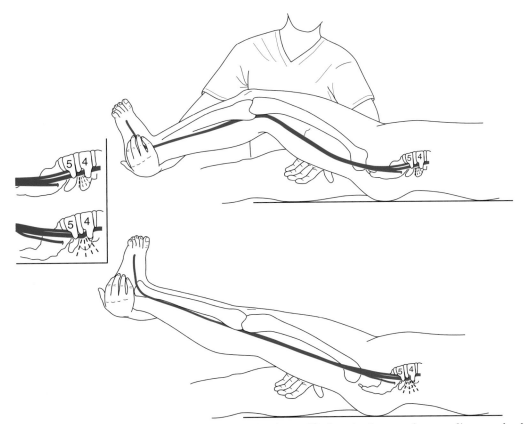

FIGURE 5-12 ■ With herniated disks, the low back pain is also intensified and often made to radiate to the buttocks if an examiner raises the patient's *straightened* leg (Lasègue's sign). In this maneuver the nerve root is compressed and irritated because it is drawn taut against the edge of the herniated disk.

REFERENCES

1. Alao AO, Soderberg MG, Geller G: Psychiatric symptoms in acute intermittent porphyria. Resident Staff Physician 50:28–32, 2004.
2. Albert SM, Rabkin JG, Del Bene ML, et al: Wish to die in end-stage ALS. Neurology 65:68–74, 2005.
3. Aubourg P, Adamsbaum C, Lavallard-Rousseau MC, et al: A two-year trial of oleic and erucic acids ("Lorenzo's oil") as treatment for adrenomyeloneuropathy. N Engl J Med 329:745–752, 1993.
4. Berger JR: The neurologic complications of bariatric surgery. Arch Neurol 61:1185–1189, 2004.
5. Black DN, Taber KH, Hurley RA: Metachromatic leukodystrophy: A model for the study of psychosis. J Neuropsychiatry Clin Neurosci 15:289–293, 2003.
6. Clarkson TW, Magos L, Myers GL: The toxicology of mercury—current exposures and clinical manifestations. N Engl J Med 349:1731–1736, 2003.
7. Estrov Y, Scaglia F, Bodamer OA: Psychiatric symptoms of inherited metabolic disease. J Inherit Metab Dis 23:2–6, 2000.
8. Filley CM, Halliday W, Kleinschmidt-DeMasters BK: The effects of toluene on the central nervous system. J Neuropathol Exp Neurol 63:1–12, 2004.
9. Filley CM, Kleinschmidt-DeMasters BK: Toxic leukoencephalopathies. N Engl J Med 345:425–432, 2001.
10. Ganzini L, Johnston WS, Silveira MJ: The final months of life in patients with ALS. Neurology 59:428–431, 2002.
11. Gonzalez-Arriaza HL, Bostwick JM: Acute porphyrias. Am J Psychiatry 160:450–458, 2003.
12. Henderson DA: Mercury in vaccines—Reassuring news. Lancet 360:1711–1712, 2002.
13. Hyde TM, Ziegler JC, Weinberger DR: Psychiatric disturbances in metachromatic leukodystrophy. Arch Neurol 49:401–406, 1992.
14. Jeha LE, Sila CA, Lederman RJ, et al: West Nile virus infection. A new paralytic illness. Neurology 61:55–59, 2003.
15. Katz JN, Simmons BP: Carpal tunnel syndrome. N Engl J Med 346:1807–1812, 2002.
16. Prass K, Brück W, Schröder NWJ, et al: Adult-onset leukoencephalopathy with vanishing white matter presenting with dementia. Ann Neurol 50:665–668, 2001.
17. Quality Standards Subcommittee of the American Academy of Neurology: Practice advisory on the treatment of amyotrophic lateral sclerosis with riluzole. Neurology 49:657–659, 1997.
18. Quecedo E, Sanmartin O, Febrer MI, et al: Mees' lines: A clue to the diagnosis of arsenic poisoning. Arch Dermatol 132:349–350, 1996.
19. Reinvang I, Borchgrevink HM, Aaserud O, et al: Neuropsychological findings in a non-clinical sample of workers exposed to solvents. J Neurol Neurosurg Psychiatry 57:614–616, 1994.
20. Rowland LP, Shneider NA: Amyotrophic lateral sclerosis. N Engl J Med 344:1688–1700, 2001.
21. Saito M, Kumano H, Yoshiuchi K, et al: Symptoms profile of multiple chemical sensitivity in actual life. Psychosom Med 67:318–325, 2005.
22. Schaumburg HH, Albers JW: Pseudoneurotoxic disease. Neurology 65:22–26, 2005.
23. Schifitto G, McDermott MP, McArthur JC, et al: Incidence of and risk factors for HIV-associated distal sensory polyneuropathy. Neurology 54:1764–1768, 2002.
24. Schnorf H, Taurarii M, Cundy T: Ciguatera fish poisoning. Neurology 58:873–880, 2002.
25. Sharief MK, Priddin J, Delamont RS, et al: Neurophysiologic analysis of neuromuscular symptoms in UK Gulf War veterans: a controlled study. Neurology 59:1518–1525, 2002.
26. Sindrup SH, Jensen TS: Pharmacologic treatment of pain in polyneuropathy. Neurology 55:915–920, 2000.
27. Staudenmayer H, Selner JC, Buhr MP: Double-blind provocations chamber challenges in 20 patients presenting with "multiple chemical sensitivity." Regul Toxicol Pharmacol 18:44–53, 1993.
28. Strong MJ, Lomen-Hoerth C, Caselli RJ, et al: Cognitive impairment, frontotemporal dementia, and the motor neuron disease. Ann Neurol 54(Suppl 5):S20–23, 2003.
29. Thaisetthawatkul P, Collazo-Clavell ML, Sarr MG, et al: A controlled study of peripheral neuropathy after bariatric surgery. Neurology 63:1462–1470, 2004.
30. Triebig G, Nasterlack M, Hacke W, et al: Neuropsychiatric symptoms in active construction painters with chronic solvent exposure. Neurotoxicology 21:791–794, 2000.
31. Vroomen PCAJ, De Krom MCTFM, Wilmink JT: Lack of effectiveness of bed rest for sciatica. N Engl J Med 340:418–423, 1999.
32. Weiss H, Rastan V, Mullges W, et al: Psychotic symptoms and emotional distress in patients with Guillain-Barré symptoms. Eur Neurol 47:74–78, 2002.
33. White RF, Proctor SP: Solvents and neurotoxicity. Lancet 340:1239, 1997.

Questions and Answers

1. After recovering from an overdose, a 21-year-old heroin addict has paresis of his right wrist, thumb, and finger extensor muscles. All DTRs are normal except for a depressed right brachioradialis reflex. Where is the lesion?
   a. Cerebral hemisphere
   b. Spinal cord
   c. Radial nerve
   d. Median nerve

   Answer: c. The patient has a wrist drop from compression of the radial nerve as it winds around the humerus. This is a common problem for drug addicts and alcoholics who lean against their arm while stuporous. Drug addicts are also liable to develop brain abscesses, AIDS, and cerebrovascular accidents—but these are all diseases of the CNS that cause hyperactive DTRs, a different pattern of weakness, and, usually when the dominant cerebrum is involved, aphasia.

2. An 18-year-old waiter who had 8 days of watery diarrhea has developed profound Guillain-Barré syndrome. Which is the most likely cause of her illness?
   a. Lyme disease
   b. Mononucleosis
   c. A viral respiratory tract infection
   d. *Campylobacter jejuni*

   Answer: d. All of these infectious illnesses can cause Guillain-Barré syndrome. However, *Campylobacter jejuni* infections, which cause diarrhea, characteristically lead to the most severe, extensive, and slowly resolving deficits.

3. A 24-year-old woman has the sudden onset of low back pain with inability to dorsiflex and evert her right ankle. She also has some mild weakness of ankle inversion. Raising her straightened right leg produces back pain that radiates down the lateral leg. Sensation is diminished on the dorsum of her right foot. No alteration in DTRs is detectable. What is the most likely lesion?
   a. Peroneal nerve diabetic infarction
   b. Polyneuropathy
   c. Femoral nerve compression
   d. L4-5 herniated intervertebral disk

   Answer: d. The dorsiflexion and eversion paresis of her right ankle, pain on straight leg raising (Lasègue's

sign), and sensory loss on the dorsum of her right foot indicate that the low back pain involves nerve root injury rather than merely muscle strain, degenerative spine disease, or retroperitoneal conditions, such as endometriosis. In particular, those findings indicate a L5 nerve root lesion. In view of the sudden onset and statistical likelihood in a young woman, she probably has an L4-5 herniated intervertebral disk compressing the L5 nerve root. A peroneal nerve injury would not cause the ankle invertor weakness.

4. A 54-year-old man with pulmonary carcinoma has had 2 weeks of midthoracic back pain. He describes the sudden onset of abnormal sensation in his legs and difficulty walking. He has weakness of both legs, which are areflexic, and hypalgesia from the toes to the umbilicus. What process is evolving?
   a. Cervical spinal cord compression
   b. Thoracic spinal cord compression
   c. Lumbar spinal cord compression
   d. Guillain-Barré syndrome

   Answer: b. He has acute thoracic spinal cord compression from a metastatic tumor that is causing paraparesis, sensory loss below T10, and areflexia from "spinal shock." His problem is not a neuropathy because of the absence of symptoms in the upper extremities, the presence of a sensory level (rather than a stocking-glove sensory loss), and his localized back pain.

5. After recovering consciousness, while still sitting on a toilet, a 27-year-old drug addict is unable to walk. He has paresis of the knee flexor (hamstring) muscles and all ankle and toe muscles. His knee DTRs are normal, but the ankle DTRs and plantar reflexes are absent. Sensation is absent below the knees. Where is the lesion(s)?
   a. Bilateral anterior cerebral artery occlusions
   b. Lumbar spinal cord injury
   c. Bilateral sciatic nerve compression
   d. Ankle or foot injuries

   Answer: c. He has sustained bilateral sciatic nerve injury, which often happens to drug addicts who take an overdose when sitting on a toilet. This injury, the "toilet seat neuropathy," is the lower extremity counterpart of the wrist drop (see question 1).

6. A 58-year-old carpenter reports weakness of his right arm and hand. He has fasciculations and

atrophy of the hand and triceps muscles and no triceps reflex. There is mild sensory loss along the medial surface of his right hand. What process is occurring?
a. Amyotrophic lateral sclerosis (ALS)
b. Cervical spondylosis
c. Polyneuropathy
d. Cervical spinal cord syrinx

Answer: b. He has symptoms and signs of cervical spondylosis with nerve root compression, which is an occupational hazard among laborers. Cervical spondylosis resembles ALS because of the atrophy and fasciculations, but the sensory loss precludes that diagnosis. In cervical spondylosis, depending on the degree of foraminal compression, DTRs may be either hyperactive or hypoactive. In ALS, despite the loss of anterior horn cells, DTRs are almost always hyperactive. A syrinx can mimic cervical spondylosis, but the syrinx causes pronounced sensory loss and, in the absence of an acute severe injury, develops in adolescence. Also, an MRI would easily distinguish a syrinx from spondylosis.

7. A 30-year-old computer programmer describes painful tingling in both of her palms and first three fingers on both hands that often wakes her from sleep. In addition, she frequently drops small objects. She has mild paresis of her thumb (thenar) flexor and opposition muscles. Percussion of the wrist re-creates the paresthesias. DTRs are normal. What is the cause?
a. Cervical spondylosis
b. Carpal tunnel syndrome
c. Toxic neuropathy
d. Fatigue

Answer: b. Despite the mild and indefinite symptoms, she has bilateral carpal tunnel syndrome (i.e., median nerve compression at the wrist). She has typical sensory disturbances and an almost pathognomonic Tinel's sign (percussion of the flexor surface of the wrist creates a tingling sensation in the median nerve distribution). The carpal tunnel syndrome frequently occurs when fluid accumulates in the carpal tunnel, such as during pregnancy and before menses. Acromegaly or hypothyroidism also leads to tissue or fluid accumulation in the carpal tunnel. It also occurs after trauma to the wrist, including wrist fractures and occupational "repetitive stress injuries," such as assembly-line handwork, word processing, and carpentry. The clinical diagnosis in this case, and in most others, can be based on the occupation, sensory symptoms, and Tinel's sign. Weakness and atrophy of the thenar muscles develop inconsistently and only late in carpal tunnel syndrome. Nerve conduction velocity studies demonstrating focal slowing across the wrist can confirm the diagnosis.

8. A young woman has developed marked confusion and hallucinations, flaccid paresis, and abdominal pain. Her urine has turned red. Which test on the urine should be performed?
a. Cocaine metabolites
b. Narcotic metabolites
c. Watson-Schwartz
d. Myoglobin

Answer: c. She has acute intermittent porphyria. The classic Watson-Schwartz test has been supplanted by quantitative tests for urinary porphobilinogen and amino levulinic acid. Phenothiazines may be used to treat the psychotic symptoms, but barbiturates are contraindicated.

9. A 31-year-old neurosurgery resident has the sudden onset of inability to elevate and evert her right ankle. Her DTR and plantar reflexes are normal, but she has hypalgesia on the lateral aspect of the calf and dorsum of the foot. What is the most likely diagnosis?
a. Spinal cord compression
b. Sciatic nerve injury
c. Peroneal nerve injury
d. Polyneuropathy

Answer: c. She has had the sudden, painless onset of a peroneal nerve injury. This injury commonly results from peroneal nerve compression from crossing the legs, leaning against furniture, or wearing a cast. The nerve is injured at the lateral aspect of the knee where it is covered only by skin and subcutaneous tissue. When patients lose weight, the nerve is vulnerable to compression because subcutaneous fat is depleted. Sometimes diabetes, Lyme disease, or a vasculitis causes this or other mononeuropathy. An L4-L5 herniated disk is unlikely because the onset was painless and the sensory loss is too lateral.

10. Several workers in a chemical factory describe tingling of their fingers and toes and weakness of their feet. Each worker has a stocking-glove hypalgesia and absent ankle DTRs. Of the following, which is the most common cause of such symptoms in the industrial setting?
a. Psychogenic disturbances
b. Repetitive stress injury
c. Exposure to an industrial toxin
d. Drug abuse

Answer: c. The loss of ankle DTRs is objective. Although the hypalgesia and other symptoms and signs can be mimicked, areflexia cannot. The stocking-glove hypalgesia and absent ankle DTRs indicate a neuropathy. The lack of back pain almost entirely excludes lumbar spondylosis and other repetitive stress injuries.

Heavy metals, organic solvents, *n*-hexane, and other hydrocarbons are industrial toxins that cause neuropathies.

11. A 29-year-old woman, recently diagnosed with hypertension, rapidly develops a paresis of the dorsiflexors and evertors of the right foot, paresis of the extensors of the wrist and thumb of the left hand, and paresis of abduction of the right eye. What is the most likely cause of her deficits?
    a. Guillain-Barré syndrome
    b. Alcohol abuse
    c. Drug abuse
    d. Mononeuritis multiplex

Answer: d. Because several geographically separated nerves—the right common peroneal, left radial, and right abducens—are simultaneously affected, she has mononeuritis multiplex. This disorder usually results from a systemic illness, such as vasculitis. Although Wernicke-Korsakoff syndrome can cause abducens nerve palsy, it would also cause ataxia and mental status changes, but not isolated nerve injuries in the limbs.

12. A 17-year-old man, after a (losing) fist fight, states that he has inability to walk or feel anything below his waist. He has complete inability to move his legs, which have normally active DTRs and flexor plantar responses. He has no response to noxious (pinprick) stimulation below his umbilicus, but sensation of position, vibration, and temperature is preserved. Where is the lesion?
    a. Spinal cord
    b. Cauda equina
    c. Peripheral nerves
    d. None of the above

Answer: d. There is neither a peripheral nor central nervous system lesion, such as a spinal cord lesion, because he has no objective sign of neurologic disease, such as changes in the DTRs or the presence of Babinski signs. Moreover, he is able to feel temperature change but not pinprick, although the same neurologic pathway carries both sensations.

13. A 68-year-old diabetic man has the sudden onset of pain in the anterior right thigh. He has right-sided weakness of knee extension, absent quadriceps DTR, and hypalgesia of the anterior thigh. What is the etiology?
    a. Polyneuropathy
    b. Mononeuritis multiplex
    c. Spinal cord injury or tumor
    d. Sciatic nerve infarction
    e. Femoral nerve infarction
    f. Peroneal nerve infarction

Answer: e. The knee weakness and especially the loss of its DTR indicate that the femoral nerve, rather than any CNS injury, has led to his deficits. A sciatic nerve infarction would have lead to ankle weakness and areflexia of the Achilles DTR. Diabetes causes infarctions most often of the femoral, sciatic, peroneal, oculomotor, and abducens nerves.

14. A 34-year-old man with chronic low back pain has a sudden exacerbation while raking leaves. He has difficulty walking and pain that radiates from the low back down the left posterior thigh to the lateral ankle. He has paresis of plantar flexion of the left ankle and an absent ankle DTR. He has an area of hypalgesia along the left lateral foot. What is the etiology of his condition?
    a. Cauda equina syndrome
    b. L4-L5 herniated disk
    c. L5-S1 herniated disk
    d. Femoral nerve infarction
    e. Sciatic nerve infarction
    f. None of the above

Answer: c. He probably has a herniated L5-S1 intervertebral disk that compresses the S1 root on the left. The radiating pain, paresis, and loss of an ankle DTR characterize an S1 nerve root compression that usually results from a herniated disk. In contrast, compression of the L5 nerve root does not lead to an absent ankle DTR. His symptoms and signs, although quite bothersome, are not as extensive as would be found with a cauda equina syndrome, which would cause incontinence as well as bilateral leg weakness and areflexia.

15. A 62-year-old man has the onset over three months of weakness of both arms and then the left leg. On examination he is alert and oriented but has dysarthria. His jaw-jerk is hyperactive and his gag reflex is absent. The tongue is atrophic and has fasciculations. The muscles of his arms and left leg have atrophy and fasciculations. All DTRs are hyperactive, and Babinski signs are present. Sensation is intact. What is the etiology of his illness?
    a. ALS
    b. Cervical syrinx
    c. Multiple sclerosis
    d. Multiple strokes

Answer: a. He obviously has ALS with both bulbar and pseudobulbar palsy and wasting of his limb muscles as well as cranial muscles. Although fasciculations are commonplace and usually benign, when they occur in multiple limbs and are associated with muscle weakness, muscle atrophy, and hyperactive DTRs, they indicate ALS. Moreover, the corticobulbar and corticospinal tracts, brainstem nuclei, and spinal anterior horn cells are all involved. Characteristically, he has normal ocular movements and mental faculties. A syrinx would have a characteristic sensory loss and both multiple sclerosis and multiple strokes would have exclusively UMN signs.

16. A 47-year-old watchmaker has become gradually unable to move his thumbs and fingers of both hands. He has sensory loss of the fifth and medial aspect of the fourth fingers, but no change in reflexes. What is the cause of his weakness?
   a. ALS
   b. Syrinx
   c. Cervical spondylosis
   d. Ulnar nerve palsies

   Answer: d. His symptoms and signs are confined to the ulnar nerves, which are vulnerable to pressure at the elbows. His diagnosis is bilateral "tardy" (late or slowly developing) ulnar nerve palsy, which is an injury caused by pressure on the ulnar nerves at the elbows. Tardy ulnar palsy is an occupational hazard of old-time watchmakers, draftsmen, and other workers who must continuously lean on their elbows. (See question 7 for occupations that predispose to median nerve compression [carpal tunnel syndrome]).

17. Which one of the follow characteristics renders industrial volatile solvents dangerous to the nervous system?
   a. Hydrophilia
   b. Lipophilia
   c. Ability to block neuromuscular transmission
   d. Tendency to generate free radicals

   Answer: b. Volatile solvents are generally hydrocarbons, relatively odorless, and lipophilic. Several of them, such as *n*-hexane, cause inhalation chemical dependency. Because they are lipophilic, which is why they are useful as a solvent, these substances readily permeate and seem to dissolve CNS and PNS myelin. Those solvents that permeate the CNS cause multiple sclerosis (MS)-like physical deficits as well as cognitive and personality changes. Those that permeate the PNS cause neuropathy.

18. Which one of the following is an effect of superoxide free radicals?
   a. Accelerates aging and death of neurons
   b. Alzheimer's disease
   c. Diabetes
   d. Hypoxia

   Answer: a. Superoxide free radicals are toxic by-products of normal metabolism that are usually neutralized by superoxide dismutase. They accelerate aging and promote premature death of neurons. They tend to accumulate in elderly people and those with certain diseases when superoxide dismutase fails. Excess superoxide free radicals have been postulated to cause Parkinson's disease and familial cases of ALS.

19. On awakening from a binge, a 24-year-old alcoholic man finds that he cannot extend his right wrist, thumb, and fingers. He is not aphasic and has no visual field cut. His DTRs remain intact except for a depression of the right brachioradialis. What is the etiology of his weakness?
   a. A left cerebral infarction
   b. Drug abuse
   c. Heavy metal intoxication
   d. Radial nerve compression

   Answer: d. He has sustained a "wrist drop" from a radial nerve injury. During a drunken stupor, he probably compressed his radial nerve as it winds around the humerus.

20. Pat, a 25-year-old anxious medical student who is in psychotherapy, describes fasciculations in the limb muscles, calf cramps at night, and muscle aches during the day. A classmate found that Pat's strength was normal and that no muscle was atrophic; however, all DTRs were brisk. Pat's father, who had been a house painter, had developed arm muscle weakness and fasciculations before he died of pulmonary failure. Which is the most likely cause of Pat's fasciculations?
   a. ALS
   b. Psychotropic medications
   c. Anxiety and fatigue
   d. Cervical spondylosis

   Answer: c. In view of the lack of atrophy and weakness, the fasciculations are probably benign fasciculations. This commonly occurring disorder in young adults, which strikes fear into the heart of almost every medical student, may be accompanied by aches, cramps, and hyperactive DTRs. Also, Pat is much too young to have contracted ALS. The father probably had cervical spondylosis, which is an occupational hazard of painters who must daily, for many hours, extend their head and neck. As for Pat's fasciculations, hearing a diagnosis of benign fasciculations epitomizes the medical adage that the three greatest words in the English language are not "I love you" but "It is benign."

21–25. Match the cause with the illness.

21. White lines of the nails (Mees' lines)
22. Lyme disease
23. Nitrous oxide neuropathy
24. *n*-Hexane neuropathy

25. Metachromatic leukodystrophy (MLD)
   a. Genetic abnormality
   b. Glue sniffing
   c. Spirochete infection
   d. Dental anesthetic abuse
   e. Arsenic poisoning

Answers: 21-e, 22-c, 23-d, 24-b, 25-a.

26–36. Which conditions are associated with fasciculations? (Yes or No)
26. Acute inflammatory demyelinating polyradiculoneuropathy (AIDP)
27. Spinal cord compression
28. ALS
29. Insecticide poisoning
30. Spinal muscular atrophy
31. Fatigue
32. Porphyria
33. Psychologic stress
34. Cervical spondylosis
35. Post-polio syndrome
36. Poliomyelitis

Answers: 26-No, 27-No, 28-Yes, 29-Yes, 30-Yes, 31-Yes, 32-No, 33-Yes, 34-Yes, 35-Yes, 36-Yes.

37. Found with a suicide note, a 42-year-old man is brought to the hospital in coma with cyanosis, bradycardia, and miosis; flaccid, areflexic quadriplegia; and pronounced muscle fasciculations. How had he attempted suicide?
   a. Arsenic ingestion
   b. Carbon monoxide inhalation
   c. Strangulation
   d. Insecticide ingestion

Answer: d. He has most likely swallowed an anticholinesterase-based insecticide. Most of them block neuromuscular transmission (see Chapter 6), which causes an acute generalized flaccid paralysis accompanied by fasciculations. In addition, the increased parasympathetic activity causes miosis and bradycardia. The bradycardia and other manifestations of abnormally increased parasympathetic activity can be reversed by atropine.

38. Which of the following conditions are associated with sexual dysfunction? (Yes or No)
   a. Peroneal nerve palsy
   b. Carpal tunnel syndrome
   c. Diabetes
   d. Poliomyelitis
   e. MS
   f. Post-polio syndrome
   g. ALS
   h. Myasthenia gravis

Answers: a-No, b-No, c-Yes, d-No, e-Yes, f-No, g-No, h-No.

39. A 40-year-old man with rapidly advancing Guillain-Barré syndrome develops confusion, overwhelming anxiety, and agitation. Which one of the following statements is correct?
   a. He should be treated with a benzodiazepine while further evaluation is undertaken.
   b. He may be developing hypoxia, hypercapnia, or both because of chest and diaphragm muscle paresis.
   c. He probably has "ICU psychosis."
   d. Hypokalemia, which is a frequent complication, can cause these symptoms.

Answer: b. Guillain-Barré syndrome, also called AIDP, is not associated directly with CNS dysfunction. However, respiratory insufficiency, a common manifestation, might cause anxiety and agitation. Other complications that can induce mental changes are metabolic aberrations, pain, sleep deprivation, or an adverse reaction to a medication. However, hypokalemia is not a frequent complication and, when it does occur, it does not cause mental aberrations. In contrast, severe hyponatremia can complicate Guillain-Barré syndrome and cause mental aberrations. Of course, investigations should be initiated for porphyria, Lyme disease, and other conditions that might mimic Guillain-Barré syndrome. Treatment with a benzodiazepine for the psychosis, whatever its cause, is contraindicated because it might completely suppress respirations. The term "ICU psychosis" is a misnomer and should be avoided because it implies that psychosis results from the psychologic stress of a life-threatening illness. Instead, almost all cases of psychosis complicating Guillain-Barré syndrome result from serious medical illnesses.

40. Two days after admission to the hospital for several months of weight loss and neuropathy, a 43-year-old man suddenly developed belligerence and physical agitation. Then he developed a seizure. Of the following, which was the most likely cause of his neuropathy?
   a. Guillain-Barré syndrome
   b. B_{12} deficiency
   c. Nutritional deficiency
   d. Leprosy

Answer: c. Alcoholic neuropathy, which is probably due to thiamine deficiency, is associated with delirium tremens (DTs) when hospitalized alcoholic patients are deprived of their usual alcohol consumption. DTs are often accompanied by alcohol withdrawal seizures.

41. Which structure comprises the roof of the carpal tunnel?

a. The median nerve
b. The ulnar nerve
c. Transverse carpal ligament
d. Plantar fascia

Answer: c. The transverse carpal ligament underlies the skin of the palmar surface of the wrist and forms the roof of the carpal tunnel. The median nerve passes through the carpal tunnel, but the ulnar nerve passes above and medial to it.

42–45. A 60-year-old man who has had mitral valve stenosis and atrial fibrillation suddenly developed quadriplegia with impaired swallowing, breathing, and speaking. He required tracheostomy and a nasogastric feeding tube during the initial part of his hospitalization. Four weeks after the onset of the illness, although quadriplegic with oculomotor pareses, hyperactive DTRs, and Babinski signs, he appears alert and blinks appropriately to questions. The vision is intact when each eye is tested separately.

42. What findings indicate that the problem is caused by CNS injury?
43. Is the lesion within the cerebral cortex or the brainstem?
44. Does the localization make a difference?
45. Which neurologic tests would help distinguish brainstem from extensive cerebral lesions?

Answer: 42. The hyperactive DTRs and Babinski signs indicate that there is CNS rather than PNS damage.

Answer: 43. Although quadriparesis could have several explanations, oculomotor pareses and apnea indicate a brainstem injury. The lesion spared his cerebral functions, such as mentation and vision, as well as his upper brainstem functions, such as blinking. He has the well-known "locked-in syndrome" (see Chapter 11) and should not be mistaken for being comatose, demented, or vegetative.

Answer: 44. If a lesion is confined to the brainstem, as in this case, intellectual function is preserved. With extensive cerebral damage, he would have had irreversible dementia.

Answer: 45. Although CT might be performed to detect or exclude a cerebral lesion, only an MRI would be sensitive enough to detect his brainstem lesion. An EEG in this case would be a valuable test because, with his cerebral hemispheres intact, it would show a relatively normal pattern. Visual evoked responses (VERs) would determine the integrity of the entire visual system, which is not part of the brainstem. Brainstem

auditory evoked responses (BAERs) would determine the integrity of the auditory circuits, which are predominantly based in the brainstem. Positron emission tomography (PET) and single photon emission computed tomography (SPECT) can also be helpful.

46–60. Which conditions are associated with multiple sclerosis, Guillain-Barré syndrome, both, or neither?
a. MS
b. Guillain-Barré syndrome
c. Both
d. Neither

46. Areflexic DTRs
47. Typically follows an upper respiratory tract infection
48. Unilateral visual loss
49. Paresthesias
50. Internuclear ophthalmoplegia
51. Paraparesis
52. Cognitive impairment early in the course of the illness
53. Produced by Lyme disease
54. A demyelinating polyneuropathy
55. Recurrent optic neuritis
56. Leads to pseudobulbar palsy
57. Leads to bulbar palsy
58. An axonal polyneuropathy
59. A monophasic illness that typically lasts several weeks to several months
60. Sexual dysfunction can be the only or primary persistent deficit

Answers: 46-b, 47-b, 48-a, 49-c, 50-a, 51-c, 52-d, 53-b, 54-b, 55-a, 56-a, 57-b, 58-d, 59-b, 60-a.

61. A 19-year-old waitress, who describes subsisting on minimal quantities of food and megavitamin treatments, develops paresthesias of her fingers and toes. She is gaunt and pale. She has marked sensory loss and areflexia of her distal limbs. Which is the least likely cause of her symptoms?
a. Nutritional deficiency
b. Multiple sclerosis
c. Substance abuse
d. Nutritional supplement toxicity

Answer: b. In view of the distal limb sensory symptoms and areflexia, the problem is not a CNS disorder but a neuropathy or other PNS disorder. In teenagers who develop a neuropathy, several conditions might be given special consideration. Lyme disease and mononucleosis, a common condition of young adults, may be complicated by the development of a neuropathy. Substance abuse—alcohol, glue, paint thinners, or N_2O—might be responsible, particularly when neuropathy develops concurrently in a group of risk-taking friends. Even abuse of supposedly nutritious foods, such as pyridoxine (vitamin B_6), should be considered as a potential cause of a sensory neuropathy. Also, teenagers sometimes develop alcoholism and suffer its complications.

62. One year after successful gastric partitioning for morbid obesity, a 30-year-old man seems depressed and has signs of neuropathy. Which condition is least likely to be responsible?
   a. Thiamine deficiency
   b. B_{12} deficiency
   c. Toxic neuropathy

Answer: c. Surgical resection of the stomach or duodenum, whether for morbid obesity or peptic ulcer disease, may be complicated in the acute period by Wernicke-Korsakoff syndrome (thiamine deficiency) or electrolyte imbalance. After 6 months, when their stores of vitamin B_{12} are depleted, patients may develop combined-system disease. Thus, a change in mental status following gastric surgery for obesity may be a manifestation of a potentially fatal metabolic aberration.

63. A 29-year-old lifeguard at Cape Cod developed profound malaise, an expanding rash, and then bilateral facial weakness (facial diplegia). Blood tests for Lyme disease, mononucleosis, AIDS, and other infective illnesses were negative. Of the following, which should be ordered?
   a. Lumbar puncture
   b. MRI of the head
   c. MRI of the spine
   d. Electrophysiologic studies (e.g., nerve conduction velocities and EMGs)

Answer: a. The patient has a typical history, dermatologic signature (erythema migrans), and neurologic findings for Lyme disease, which is endemic on Cape Cod and other areas of the Northeast coast. Serologic tests are notoriously inaccurate for Lyme disease. Blood tests are frequently negative early in the illness and even throughout its course. Another possibility is that she has Guillain-Barré syndrome that began, as in a small fraction of cases, with involvement of the cranial nerves rather than with the lower spinal nerves. Myasthenia gravis is a possibility, but it is unlikely because of the absence of oculomotor paresis. Sarcoidosis is a rare cause of facial diplegia. The next step would be to perform a lumbar puncture to test the CSF. In Guillain-Barré syndrome, the CSF protein is characteristically elevated and the cell count has little or no increase. However, when Lyme disease causes a Guillain-Barré-like syndrome, the CSF has increased cells as well as an elevated protein concentration. MRI studies will not help in cases of PNS disease. Electrophysiologic studies might only indicate a demyelinating rather than an axonal neuropathy. If the diagnosis remains unclear, the best course might be to treat for Lyme disease.

64. In which ways are CNS and PNS myelin similar?
   a. The same cells produce CNS and PNS myelin.
   b. CNS and PNS myelin possess the same antigens.
   c. CNS and PNS myelin insulate electrochemical transmissions in the brain and peripheral nerves, respectively.
   d. They are both affected by the same illnesses.

Answer: c.

65. Which is the correct relationship?
   a. Oligodendrocytes are to glia cells as CNS is to PNS
   b. Oligodendrocytes are to Schwann cells as PNS is to CNS
   c. Oligodendrocytes are to Schwann cells as CNS is to PNS
   d. Oligodendrocytes are to neurons as CNS is to PNS

Answer: c.

66. Which of the following statements is false concerning the neuropathy that affects otherwise normal people older than 75 years?
   a. It includes loss of ankle DTRs.
   b. It contributes to their tendency to fall.
   c. Position sensation is lost more than vibration sensation.
   d. The peripheral nerves' sensory loss is greater than their motor loss.

Answer: c. The normal elderly often develop a subtle neuropathy that causes loss of ankle DTRs and impairs vibration sensation to a greater degree than position sensation. The neuropathy contributes to the elderly individual's gait impairment and lack of stability. Nevertheless, the neuropathy does not reduce their strength. In addition, elderly people without neuropathy cannot perform tandem gait, but they are still considered normal.

67–70. Match the illness (a–d) with the skin lesion (67–70):
   a. Pellagra
   b. Lyme disease
   c. Herpes zoster
   d. Leprosy

67. Erythema migrans

68. Dermatitis

69. Depigmented anesthetic areas on ears, fingers, and toes

70. Vesicular eruptions in the first division of the trigeminal nerve

Answers: 67-b, 68-a, 69-d, 70-c.

71. The wife of a homicidal neurologist enters psychotherapy because of several months of fatigue and painful paresthesias. She also describes numbness in a stocking-glove distribution, darkening of her skin, and the appearance of white lines across her nails. In addition to a general medical evaluation, which specific test should be performed?
a. Thyroid function and other endocrinology tests
b. Mononucleosis
c. Lyme titer
d. Heavy metal blood levels

Answer: d. The astute psychiatrist suspected arsenic poisoning and ordered analysis of hair and nail samples. While many illnesses induce fatigue, the white lines across her nails (Mees' lines) pointed to the correct diagnosis.

72. Which is the most common PNS manifestation of AIDS?
a. Guillain-Barré syndrome
b. Myopathy
c. Neuropathy
d. Myelopathy

Answer: c. Although neuropathy is the most common complication of AIDS, the other conditions frequently occur in AIDS patients.

73. Regarding low back pain, which one of the following statements is true?
a. If an MRI shows a herniated disk, the patient should have surgery.
b. MMPI results will be a reliable guide to recommending surgery.
c. Work-related low back pain is relatively resistant to treatment.
d. A traditional 7- to 10-day course of bed rest, despite its simplicity, is more effective than a 2-day course.

Answer: c. In about of 20% of asymptomatic individuals, an MRI will show a herniated disk. Most patients with a herniated disk will improve spontaneously with conservative treatment. Although surgery will improve patients in the immediate postoperative period, at 4 years and longer, patients who have surgery and those who have had conservative treatment

will have a similar status. Work-related and litigation-related low back pain is resistant to both conservative and surgical treatment. A 2-day course of bed rest is beneficial, but longer periods of bed rest are not more effective. In fact, merely continuing with a modified schedule may be the best treatment in most cases of low back pain.

74–77. Match the vitamin deficiency with the illness that it causes:
a. Ascorbic acid (vitamin C)
b. Cobalamine (vitamin B_{12})
c. Niacin (vitamin B_3)
d. Thiamine (vitamin B_1)
e. Riboflavin

74. Wernicke-Korsakoff syndrome

75. Pellagra

76. Combined system disease

77. Scurvy

Answers: 74-d, 75-c, 76-b, 77-a.

78. A 35-year-old man with AIDS presents with very painful burning of his feet. He has slight lower leg weakness and absent ankle DTRs. He has no history of diabetes, use of medications, or problem other than AIDS that might cause the symptom. Which of the following is not likely to be found?
a. Loss of sensation on his soles
b. High viral load
c. High CD4 count
d. Depression and functional impairment

Answer: c. He has the typical, symmetric, predominantly sensory neuropathy that complicates the late stage of AIDS. Patients with this complication are apt to have depression and limited functional ability. Because the sensory neuropathy is a complication of the late stage of AIDS, he is likely to have a high viral load but also a low CD4 count.

79. In the previous question, which medication would not be a reasonable option for treatment of the painful burning of his feet?
a. Isoniazid (INH)
b. Nortriptyline
c. Gabapentin
d. A long-acting morphine preparation
e. Capsaicin cream

Answer: a. Except for isoniazid (INH), all the medicines listed represent classes of analgesics useful in painful neuropathies, such as tricyclic antidepressants, antiepileptics, narcotics, and topically applied substance P depletors. INH, which is an anti-tuberculosis (anti-TB) drug, interferes with pyridoxine (B$_6$) metabolism. Excessive INH treatment can lead to seizures and psychosis.

80–82. Which of the following illnesses are associated with autosomal dominant (AD), autosomal recessive (AR), or sex-linked (SL) inheritance?

80. Acute intermittent porphyria (AIP)

81. Metachromatic leukodystrophy (MLD)

82. ALS with the superoxide dismutase (SOD1) gene abnormality

Answers: 80. AIP-AD; 81. MLD-AR; 82. ALS/SOD1-AD.

83–85. Match the dermatologic abnormality, found with a neuropathy, with its cause:

83. Alopecia

84. Mees' lines

85. Dark blue gum line
a. Arsenic poisoning
b. Lead poisoning
c. Thallium poisoning
d. Mercury poisoning

Answers: 83-c, 84-a, 85-d.

86. Which of the following statements is false?
a. A major component of thimerosal is ethyl mercury.
b. Thimerosal had been used as a vaccine preservative.
c. Organic mercury poisoning causes ataxia, dysarthria, and cognitive impairments.
d. Childhood vaccines have been proven to cause autism.

Answer: d. Large-scale, statistically powerful studies have disproved the widespread suggestion that the thimerosal (ethyl mercury), which had been used as a vaccine preservative, caused autism. Although ingestion of organic mercury can cause ataxia, dysarthria, and cognitive impairments, far insufficient amounts are absorbed from the vaccines or from dental fillings to cause such problems.

Muscle Disorders

The clinical evaluation can distinguish disorders of muscle from those of the central nervous system (CNS) and peripheral nervous system (PNS) (Table 6-1). It can then divide muscle disorders into those of the neuromuscular junction and those of the muscles themselves, *myopathies* (Table 6-2). Surprisingly, considering their physiologic distance from the brain, several muscle disorders are associated with mental retardation, cognitive decline, personality changes, or use of psychotropic medications.

NEUROMUSCULAR JUNCTION DISORDERS

Myasthenia Gravis

Neuromuscular Transmission Impairment

Normally, discrete amounts—packets or *quanta*—of *acetylcholine (ACh)* are released across the neuromuscular junction to trigger a muscle contraction (Fig. 6-1). Afterward, acetylcholinesterase (AChE) (or simply "cholinesterase") inactivates the ACh.

In myasthenia gravis, the classic neuromuscular junction disorder, *ACh receptor antibodies* block, impair, or actually destroy ACh receptors (Fig. 6-2). These antibodies are selective in that they attack ACh receptors located predominantly in the extraocular, facial, neck, and proximal limb muscles. When binding to antibody-inactivated receptors, ACh produces only weak, unsustained muscle contractions. Another characteristic of the ACh receptor antibodies is that they attack only *nicotinic ACh*—not muscarinic ACh—receptors. Moreover, they do not penetrate the blood–brain barrier and do not interfere with CNS function. In contrast, they readily pass through the placenta and cause transient myasthenia symptoms in neonates of mothers with myasthenia gravis.

In approximately 80% of myasthenia gravis cases, the serum contains ACh receptor antibodies. In one half of the remainder, the serum has antibodies to anti*muscle-specific kinase* (MuSK).

Standard medicines for myasthenia gravis attempt to either increase ACh concentration at the neuromuscular junction or restore the integrity of ACh receptors. To increase ACh concentration, neurologists typically first prescribe *anticholinesterases* or simply *cholinesterase inhibitors*, such as edrophonium (Tensilon) and pyridostigmine (Mestinon). These medicines inactivate cholinesterase that would normally metabolize ACh. Prolonging ACh activity increases strength in myasthenia gravis.

To restore the integrity of ACh receptors, neurologists administer steroids, other immunosuppressive medications, plasmapheresis, or intravenous infusions of immunoglobulins (IVIG). (They also use IVIG in Guillain-Barré syndrome [see Chapter 5], another inflammatory PNS illness, to remove hostile antibodies or directly repair the receptors.)

Changes in ACh neuromuscular transmission may be caused by other illnesses or may be purposefully induced by medications. For example, *botulinum toxin*, as both a naturally occurring food poison and a medication, blocks the release of ACh packets from the presynaptic membrane and causes paresis (see later).

At the postsynaptic side of the neuromuscular junction, *succinylcholine* binds to the ACh receptors. With their ACh receptors inactivated, muscles weaken to the point of flaccid paralysis. Succinylcholine, which resists cholinesterases, has a paralyzing effect that lasts for hours. It facilitates major surgery and electroconvulsive therapy (ECT).

ACh, unlike dopamine and serotonin, serves as a transmitter at both the neuromuscular junction and the CNS. Also, its action is terminated almost entirely by metabolism instead of reuptake. Antibodies

TABLE 6-1 ■ Signs of CNS, PNS, and Muscle Disorders

	CNS	PNS	Muscle
Paresis	Pattern*	Distal	Proximal
Muscle tone	Spastic	Flaccid	Sometimes tender or dystrophic
DTRs	Hyperactive	Hypoactive	Normal or hypoactive
Babinski signs	Yes	No	No
Sensory loss	Hemisensory	Stocking-glove	None

CNS, central nervous system; DTRs, deep tendon reflexes; PNS, peripheral nervous system.
*Hemiparesis, paraparesis, etc.

TABLE 6-2 ■ Common Neuromuscular Junction and Muscle Disorders

NEUROMUSCULAR JUNCTION DISORDERS
Myasthenia gravis
Lambert-Eaton syndrome
Botulism
Tetanus
Nerve gas poisoning
Black widow spider bite
MUSCLE DISORDERS (MYOPATHIES)
Inherited dystrophies
   Duchenne's muscular dystrophy
   Myotonic dystrophy
Polymyositis (inflammatory, infectious, and toxic)
   Polymyositis
   Eosinophilia-myalgia syndrome
   Trichinosis
   AIDS myopathy
Metabolic
   Steroid myopathy
   Hypokalemic myopathy
   Alcohol myopathy
Mitochondrial myopathies
   Primary mitochondrial myopathies
Progressive ophthalmoplegia
   MELAS and MERRF
NEUROLEPTIC MALIGNANT SYNDROME

AIDS, acquired immunodeficiency syndrome; MELAS, mitochondrial encephalomyelopathy, lactic acidosis, and stroke-like episodes; MERRF, myoclonic epilepsy and ragged-red fibers.

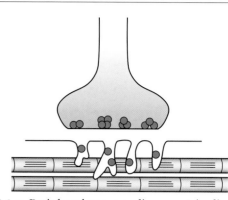

FIGURE 6-1 ■ Peripheral nerve endings contain discrete *packets* or *quanta* of acetylcholine (ACh) that are released in groups of about 200 in response to nerve impulses. The ACh packets cross the synaptic cleft of the neuromuscular junction to reach numerous, deep, and convoluted ACh receptor binding sites. ACh-receptor interactions open cation channels, which induce an *end-plate potential*. If the potential is large enough, it will trigger an *action potential* along the muscle fiber. Action potentials open calcium storage sites, which produce muscle contractions.

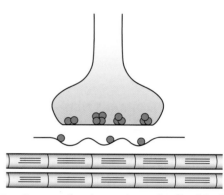

FIGURE 6-2 ■ In myasthenia gravis, antibodies block, destroy, or in other ways inactivate neuromuscular acetylcholine (ACh) receptors. The remaining receptors are abnormally wide and shallow, and present few active binding sites. In addition, the synaptic cleft is widened, which makes neuromuscular transmission inefficient.

associated with myasthenia gravis impair neuromuscular junction but not CNS ACh transmission: One reason is that neuromuscular ACh receptors are nicotinic, but cerebral ACh receptors are mostly muscarinic (see Chapter 21).

Physicians often see a stark contrast between impaired neuromuscular junction activity but preserved CNS ACh activity in myasthenia gravis patients who have almost complete paralysis but normal cognitive status. Similarly, most anticholinesterase medications have no effect on cognitive status or other CNS function because they do not penetrate the blood–brain barrier. One of the few exceptions, physostigmine, penetrates into the CNS, where it can preserve ACh concentrations. Physostigmine had been proposed as a treatment for conditions with low CNS ACh levels, such as Alzheimer's disease. In various experiments with Alzheimer's disease, despite increasing cerebral ACh concentrations, physostigmine produced virtually no clinical benefit (see Chapter 7).

Clinical Features

Myasthenia gravis' characteristic symptoms consist of fluctuating, asymmetric weakness of the extraocular, facial, and bulbar muscles. Repeated activities weaken muscles, and thus symptoms often first develop only in the late afternoon or early evening. Rest temporarily alleviates the weakness whenever it occurs. Almost 90% of patients, who are typically young women or older men, develop diplopia or ptosis as their first symptom. In addition, because patients then develop facial and neck muscle weakness, they begin to grimace when attempting to smile (Fig. 6-3) and have nasal speech. As the disease advances, the neck, shoulder, and swallowing and respiratory muscles become weak (i.e., myasthenia gravis causes bulbar palsy) (see Chapter 4). In severe cases, patients develop respiratory distress, quadriplegia, and an inability to speak (anarthria). Paralysis can spread and worsen so

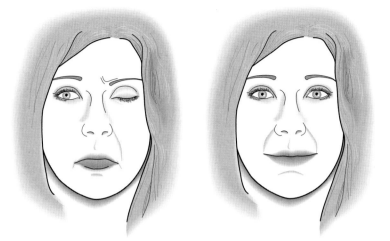

FIGURE 6-3 ■ *Left,* Examination of this young woman, following several weeks of intermittent double vision and nasal speech. Although asymptomatic in the morning, her symptoms tended to develop and worsen in the afternoon and evening. During dinner, her mother feels that the patient is depressed and overtired because of her expressionless face, lack of conversation, and reluctance to eat. The physician found that she had left-sided ptosis and bilateral facial muscle weakness that was especially evident in the loss of the contour of the right nasolabial fold and sagging lower lip. Her weakness was characteristically asymmetric. *Right,* Intravenously administered edrophonium (Tensilon) 10 mg—the Tensilon test—produced a 60-second restoration of eyelid, ocular, and facial strength. This typically brief but dramatic strengthening resulted from edrophonium transiently inhibiting cholinesterase to increase acetylcholine (ACh) activity.

much that patients can reach a "locked-in" state (see Chapter 11).

Absence of certain findings is equally important. Again, in contrast to the physical incapacity, neither the disease nor the medications directly produce mental changes. In addition, although extraocular muscles may be paretic, intraocular muscles are spared. Thus, patients may have complete ptosis and no eyeball movement, but their pupils are normal in size and reactivity to light. Another oddity is that even though patients may be quadriparetic, bladder and bowel sphincter muscle strength will remain normal. Of course, as in muscle disorders, myasthenia does not impair sensation.

Patients with myasthenia gravis can experience exacerbations that occur spontaneously, in conjunction with an intercurrent illness, or following the onset of psychologic stress. In addition, about 40% of pregnant women with myasthenia gravis undergo flare-ups, which occur with equal frequency during each trimester. On the other hand, about 30% of pregnant women with myasthenia gravis enjoy a remission.

The clinical diagnosis of myasthenia can be confirmed by a positive Tensilon (edrophonium) test (see Fig. 6-3), by detecting serum ACh receptor antibodies, or by obtaining certain results on electromyograms (EMGs). About 5% of patients have underlying hyperthyroidism and 10% have a mediastinal thymoma. If these conditions are detected and treated, myasthenia gravis will usually improve.

Differential Diagnosis

Lesions of the oculomotor nerve (cranial nerve III), which result from midbrain infarctions (see Fig. 4-9) or compression by posterior communicating artery aneurysms, can also cause extraocular muscle paresis. In addition to their usually having an abrupt and painful onset, these disorders are identifiable by a subtle finding: The pupil will be widely dilated and unreactive to light because of intraocular (pupillary) muscle paresis (see Fig. 4-6). In addition, many other illnesses cause facial and bulbar palsy: amyotrophic lateral sclerosis (ALS), Guillain-Barré syndrome, Lyme disease, Lambert-Eaton syndrome, and botulism. However, only myasthenia gravis consistently responds to the Tensilon test.

Lambert-Eaton Syndrome and Botulism

Two other illnesses, Lambert-Eaton syndrome and botulism, also stem from impaired ACh neuromuscular transmission and cause weakness. The major physiologic distinction is that myasthenia results from a disorder of *postsynaptic* receptors, but Lambert-Eaton syndrome and botulism result from impaired release of *presynaptic* ACh packets. The presynaptic impairment has different causes. A toxin causes botulism, but an auto-immune disorder—antibodies directed against presynaptic voltage-gated calcium channels—causes Lambert-Eaton syndrome. Whether reduced ACh activity results from impaired presynaptic ACh release or blocked ACh receptors, the ensuing weakness in all these conditions shares some clinical features.

The differences between Lambert-Eaton and myasthenia are numerous. Lambert-Eaton often occurs in conjunction with small-cell carcinoma of the lung. Although it also occasionally occurs with rheumatologic illnesses, Lambert-Eaton is still considered a *paraneoplastic syndrome* (see Chapter 19). It also occurs much less commonly than myasthenia. From a clinical perspective, unlike the weakness in myasthenia, Lambert-Eaton syndrome causes weakness of the limbs. Moreover, repetitive exertion temporarily corrects Lambert-Eaton-induced weakness, presumably by provoking presynaptic ACh release. In addition, Lambert-Eaton syndrome, unlike other neuromuscular junction illnesses, causes autonomic nervous system dysfunction.

In contrast to the cause of Lambert-Eaton, eating contaminated food almost always has been the cause of *botulism*. In this infamous, often fatal disorder, *Clostridium botulinum* spores elaborate a toxin that has a predilection for the presynaptic neuromuscular membrane. (Experts suggest that terrorists might inject these spores into commercial food manufacturing processes, such as milk pasteurizing, to create mass poisonings.)

Botulism victims develop oculomotor, bulbar, and respiratory paralyses that resemble the Guillain-Barré syndrome, as well as myasthenia gravis. In contrast to the symptoms of these illnesses, botulism symptoms arise explosively and include dilated, unreactive pupils. A unique feature, which allows for dramatic life-saving diagnoses, is that often several family members simultaneously develop nausea, vomiting, diarrhea, and fever, and then the distinctive weakness—18 to 36 hours after sharing a meal that subsequently proves to have included a contaminated dish.

Ironically, neurologists now routinely turn botulinum-induced paresis to an advantage. They inject pharmaceutically prepared botulinum toxin to alleviate focal dystonias and dyskinesias, such as blepharospasm, spasmodic torticollis, and writer's cramp (see Chapter 18).

Tetanus

A different *Clostridium* species elaborates the neurotoxin that causes tetanus. In this illness, the toxin from *Clostridium tetani* mostly blocks presynaptic release—not of ACh—but of CNS inhibitory neurotransmitters, particularly gamma-aminobutyric acid (GABA) and glycine. In other words, patients have less inhibitory activity in their brain and spinal cord. The resulting uninhibited muscle contractions cause trismus ("lockjaw"), facial grimacing, an odd but characteristic smile ("risus sardonicus"), and muscle spasms in their limbs. Tetanus most commonly affects drug addicts and workers in farming and scrap metal recovery. When abortions were illegal, they were often complicated by tetanus as well as other infections.

Psychiatrists must not attribute all acutely developing facial or jaw muscle spasmodic contractions to a neuroleptic-induced dystonic reaction. The differential diagnosis includes tetanus and also heat stroke, strychnine poisoning, and rabies.

Nerve Gas and Other Wartime Issues

Most common insecticides are organophosphates that bind and inactivate AChE. With inactivation of its metabolic enzyme, ACh accumulates and irreversibly depolarizes postsynaptic neuromuscular junctions. After insecticides cause initial muscle contractions and fasciculations, they lead to paralysis of respiratory and other muscles. For example, malathion (Ovide), the common shampoo for head lice, is an irreversible AChE inhibitor. It is safe because so little is absorbed through the skin.

On the other hand, people committing suicide, especially in India, often deliberately drink organophosphate pesticides. Similarly, the *nerve gases* that threatened soldiers from World War I through the Persian Gulf Wars bind and inactivate AChE. The common ones—GA, GB, GD, and VX—affect both the CNS and PNS. Some are gaseous, but others, such as sarin (GB), the Tokyo subway poison, are liquid.

Accumulation of ACh causes a *cholinergic crisis*. Its initial features—tearing, pulmonary secretions, and miosis—reflect excessive autonomic cholinergic activity. If the poisons penetrate the CNS, excess ACh causes convulsions, rapidly developing unconsciousness, and respiratory depression.

Ideally, physicians will have a warning and be able to provide pretreatment. They might administer pyridostigmine, which is a reversible AChE inhibitor, as a prophylactic agent because it occupies the vulnerable site on AChE and thereby protects it from irreversible inhibition by the toxin. After nerve gas exposure or liquid ingestion, first aid consists of washing exposed skin with dilute bleach (hypochlorite). Also after exposure, field forces administer *oximes*, because they reactivate AChE and detoxify organophosphates, and atropine, because it is a competitive inhibitor of ACh and blocks the excessive cholinergic activity. In view of a high incidence of seizures, depending on the exposure, field forces also often administer a benzodiazepine. Other antiepileptic drugs are ineffective in this situation.

Survivors of nerve gas poisonings often report developing headaches, personality changes, and cognitive impairment, especially in memory. Their symptoms often mimic those of post-traumatic stress disorder.

Agent Orange, the herbicide sprayed extensively in Southeast Asia during the Vietnam War, allegedly produced peripheral neuropathy, cognitive impairment, psychiatric disturbances, and brain tumors. Although large scientific reviews found no evidence that it actually caused any of those problems, advocacy groups have prodded Congress into accepting a causal relationship.

A recent counterpart, *Persian Gulf War I syndrome*, had similar notoriety. Veterans described varied symptoms, including fatigue, weakness, and myalgias (painful muscle aches). Again, exhaustive studies have found no consistent, significant clinical sign or laboratory evidence of any neurologic disorder. One theory had been that in anticipation of a nerve gas attack, soldiers had been ordered to take a "neurotoxic" antidote (pyridostigmine); however, numerous myasthenia gravis patients had been taking it for decades without adverse effects.

The notion that silicone toxicity from breast implants causes a neuromuscular disorder and other neurologic illness is discussed in the differential diagnosis of multiple sclerosis (see Chapter 15).

Chronic Fatigue Syndrome and Fibromyalgia

Myasthenia gravis and other neurologic disorders are sometimes unconvincingly invoked as an explanation of one of the most puzzling clinical problems: *chronic fatigue syndrome*. Individuals with this condition typically describe not only a generalized sense of weakness, sometimes preceded by myalgias and other flu-like symptoms, but impaired memory and inability to concentrate (i.e., symptoms of cerebral dysfunction).

Unlike myasthenia gravis, chronic fatigue syndrome does not produce weakness in the face or extraocular muscles. Nor does it cause asymmetric weakness. In contrast to most neurologic illnesses, symptoms of different individuals vary greatly. Moreover, their symptoms are unaccompanied by objective findings. Manual muscle testing typically elicits an inconsistent, weak exertion. Blood tests, EMGs, and magnetic resonance imaging (MRI) reveal no significant abnormalities.

Finally, many studies have attributed symptoms, in most cases, to depressive disorders.

Regardless of whether chronic fatigue syndrome is a distinct entity, several well-established illnesses may induce unequivocal fatigue, sometimes as the primary symptom, accompanied by cognitive impairment: Lyme disease, acquired immunodeficiency syndrome (AIDS), mononucleosis, multiple sclerosis, sleep apnea and other sleep disturbances, and eosinophilia-myalgia syndrome. In addition, simple deconditioning from limited physical activity, including weightless space travel and confinement to a hospital bed, frequently causes weakness and loss of muscle bulk.

Fibromyalgia, a cousin of chronic fatigue syndrome, is defined by entirely subjective symptoms of chronic, widespread pain, and multiple tender points. Despite patients' having prominent myalgia, they have no objective clinical, laboratory, or EMG evidence of myositis or any other specific abnormality. Numerous individuals fulfilling the criteria for fibromyalgia also have equally amorphous disorders, such as irritable syndrome, atypical chest pain, and transformed migraine. Also, about 25% of them have concurrent symptoms of depression. As with chronic fatigue syndrome, if fibromyalgia represents a medical entity rather than simply exaggerated pain and weakness, there is no credible evidence that it is a neurologic illness.

MUSCLE DISEASE (MYOPATHY)

Most myopathies have a predilection for the shoulder and hip girdle muscles. They strike these large, "proximal" muscles first, most severely, and often exclusively. Myopathy patients have difficulty performing tasks that require these muscles, such as standing, walking, climbing stairs, combing their hair, and reaching upward. Even with such extensive weakness, patients retain strength in their oculomotor, sphincter, and hand and feet muscles. (Hand and feet muscles are "distal" and are affected more by neuropathies than myopathies.)

Acute inflammatory myopathies lead to myalgias and tenderness. Eventually, both inflammatory and noninflammatory myopathies lead to muscle weakness and atrophy (*dystrophy*). Deep tendon reflexes (DTRs) may be normal but usually hypoactive roughly in proportion to the weakness. Patients do not have Babinski signs or sensory loss because the corticospinal and sensory tracts are not involved. With most myopathies, serum concentrations of muscle-based enzymes, such as creatine phosphokinase (CK) and aldolase, are elevated and EMGs are abnormal. Finally, with a few exceptions (see later), myopathies are free of mental disorders (see later).

Inherited Dystrophies

Duchenne's Muscular Dystrophy

Better known simply as *muscular dystrophy*, Duchenne's muscular dystrophy is the most frequently occurring childhood-onset myopathy. It is a sex-linked genetic illness with expression in childhood. The illness then follows a chronic, progressively incapacitating, and ultimately fatal course. Although women who carry the abnormal gene may have some subtle findings and laboratory abnormalities, for practical purposes this illness is restricted to boys.

Dystrophy typically first affects boys' thighs and shoulders. The first symptom that emerges is a struggle to stand and walk. Subsequently, even though drastically weak, muscles paradoxically increase in size because fat cells and connective tissue infiltrate them (*muscle pseudohypertrophy*, Fig. 6-4, top). Instinctively learning *Gower's maneuver* (see Fig. 6-4, bottom), boys with the illness arise from sitting only by pulling themselves upward or climbing up their own legs. Usually by age 12, when their musculature can no longer support their maturing frame, they become wheelchair-bound and eventually develop respiratory insufficiency.

Psychomotor retardation and an average IQ approximately one standard deviation below normal typically accompany muscular dystrophy. This intellectual impairment is greater than with comparable chronic illnesses and, although stable, often overshadows the weakness. Of course, isolation, lack of education, and being afflicted with a progressively severe handicap account for some psychologic and social, as well as cognitive, impairment. No cure is available, but proposed corrective treatments—transplantation of muscle cells (myoblast transfer) and gene therapy—are on the horizon.

GENETICS

Duchenne's dystrophy results from absence of a crucial muscle-cell membrane protein, *dystrophin*. Thus, Duchenne's dystrophy is one of several myopathies referred to as a *dystrophinopathy*. About 75% of patients carry a mutation in the dystrophin gene—one of the largest genes in the human genome—located on the short arm of the X chromosome. In many cases, the illness arises from a new mutation rather than from an inherited one. Unlike the excessive trinucleotide repeat mutation underlying myotonic dystrophy and several other neurologic disorders (see later), the Duchenne's dystrophy mutation usually consists of a DNA deletion that results in absent or severely dysfunctional dystrophin.

Commercial genetic testing is readily available. Testing blood samples for the DNA deletions or other mutations of the dystrophin gene can diagnose not only individuals with signs of the illness but ones with no signs, such as affected fetuses, females who carry the mutation (carriers), and young boy carriers destined to develop the illness.

A diagnosis of Duchenne's dystrophy can also be based on a muscle biopsy that shows little or no staining for dystrophin (the *dystrophin test*). With modern technology, needle biopsies rather than open surgical procedures provide sufficient tissue.

Becker's Dystrophy

A relatively benign variant of Duchenne's dystrophy, *Becker's dystrophy*, results from a different mutation in the same gene. However, this mutation causes the production of dystrophin that is abnormal but retains some function. Individuals with Becker's dystrophy, which is also a dystrophinopathy, have weakness that begins in their second decade and follows a slowly progressive course that is uncomplicated by cognitive impairment.

Myotonic Dystrophy

The most frequently occurring myopathy of adults is *myotonic dystrophy*. Although also an inherited muscle disorder, it differs in several respects from Duchenne's dystrophy. The symptoms usually appear when individuals are young adults—20 to 25 years—and both sexes are equally affected. Also, rather than having proximal muscle weakness and pseudohypertrophy, patients develop facial and distal limb weakness. Myotonic dystrophy is named after its signature, *myotonia*, which is involuntary prolonged muscle contraction. (The dystrophy, which affects the face and predominantly distal limbs, is also characteristic but not unique.) Myotonia inhibits the release of patients' grip for several seconds after shaking hands or grasping and turning a doorknob. Neurologists elicit this phenomenon by asking patients to make a fist and then rapidly release it. In addition, if the physician lightly taps a patient's thenar (thumb base) muscles with a reflex hammer, myotonia causes a prolonged, visible contraction that moves the thumb medially (Fig. 6-5).

Another characteristic, caused by facial muscle atrophy and balding over the temples, is a sunken and elongated face, ptosis, and a prominent forehead that form a "hatchet face" (see Fig. 6-5). Additional neurologic and non-neurologic manifestations may vary. Patients often develop cataracts, cardiac conduction system disturbances, and endocrine organ failure, such as testicular atrophy, diabetes, and infertility. Treatment is limited to replacement of endocrine deficiencies and, by giving phenytoin quinine, or other medicines, reducing myotonia.

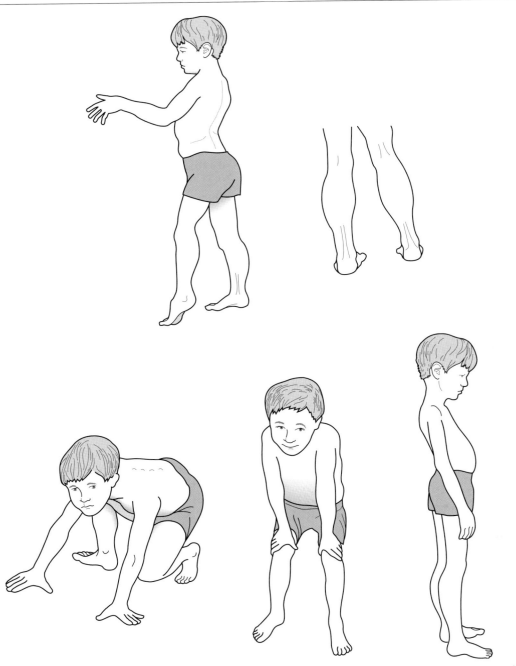

FIGURE 6-4 ■ *Top,* This 10-year-old boy with typical Duchenne's muscular dystrophy has a waddling gait and inability to raise his arms above his head because of weakness of the shoulder and pelvic girdle muscles (i.e., his proximal muscles). His weakened calves are paradoxically enlarged not by exercise but by fat and connective tissue infiltration. This *pseudohypertrophy* of the calf muscles is a classic sign. There is also a typical exaggeration of the normal inward curve of the lumbar spine, *hyperlordosis.* Fund-raising posters frequently feature children with Duchenne's muscular dystrophy. *Bottom, Gower's maneuver,* an early sign of Duchenne's muscular dystrophy, consists of a young victim pushing his hands against his knees then thighs to reach a standing position. He must use his arms and hands because the disease primarily weakens hip and thigh muscles that normally would be sufficient to allow him to stand.

Contrasting somewhat with the nonprogressive cognitive impairment of Duchenne's dystrophy, patients with myotonic dystrophy tend to have not only limited intelligence but also increased cognitive impairment with age. Cognitive impairments correlate with an early age for onset of their dystrophy, which generally reflects more severe disease.

(*Anticipation*, a genetic phenomenon [see later], influences both the age of appearance of symptoms and their severity.) In addition to cognitive impairments, patients' personality tends to be characterized by lack of initiative and progressive blandness. As a group, they are said to have a high incidence of "avoidant personality."

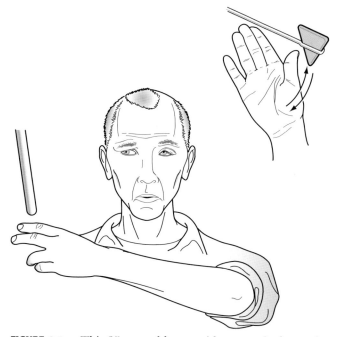

FIGURE 6-5 ■ This 25-year-old man with myotonic dystrophy has the typically elongated, "hatchet" face caused by temporal and facial muscle wasting, frontal baldness, and ptosis. Because of myotonia, a percussion hammer striking his thenar eminence muscles precipitates a forceful, sustained contraction that draws in the thumb for 3 to 10 seconds. Myotonia also prevents him from rapidly releasing his grasp.

GENETICS

Myotonic dystrophy is an autosomal dominant genetic disorder carried on chromosome 19. The mutation in that gene leads to abnormal ion channels in the membranes of muscle and other organ cells. Thus, myotonic dystrophy is an example of a newly described category of illnesses, *channelopathies*.

A crucial aspect of this disease's genetic basis is that it, as well as several other neurologic illnesses, results from excessive repetition of a particular nucleotide base triplet (*trinucleotide repeat*) in the abnormal gene's DNA. In the case of myotonic dystrophy, the trinucleotide base CTG is excessively repeated on chromosome 19.

Other disorders that result from different excessive trinucleotide repeats include ones that are inherited in an autosomal recessive pattern (Friedreich's ataxia), autosomal dominant pattern (spinocerebellar atrophies and Huntington's disease), and sex-linked pattern (fragile X syndrome) (see Chapters 2, 13, and 18, and the Appendix). Whichever the particular trinucleotide base repeat and pattern of inheritance, these illnesses can be easily and reliably diagnosed in symptomatic and asymptomatic individuals by testing white blood cells' DNA.

Illnesses in this group have several features that stem from the expanded trinucleotide repeats. The severity of the symptoms is roughly proportional to the length of the repeats. For example, myotonic dystrophy patients with 50 to 100 trinucleotide repeats have mild and not even all signs, those with 100 to 1000 have all the characteristic signs to a greater or lesser degree, and those with more than 2000 show signs in infancy.

Another characteristic of trinucleotide disorders is that sperm are more likely than eggs to increase their DNA repeats—as if sperm DNA were more genetically unstable than egg DNA. Thus, in these illnesses, children who have inherited the abnormal gene from their father, rather than from their mother, develop symptoms at a younger age and eventually in a more severe form. Similarly, fathers are more apt than mothers to pass along a more severe form of the illness.

In addition, trinucleotide repeat sequences are unstable. When transmitted from parent to child, they tend to expand further rather than self-correcting. The trinucleotide sequences tendency toward greater genetic abnormality and more pronounced symptoms is termed *amplification*.

A clinical counterpart of amplification is *anticipation*: successive generations of individuals who inherit the abnormal gene show signs of the illness at a progressively younger age. For example, a grandfather may not have been diagnosed with myotonic dystrophy until he was 38 years old. At that age, he already had an asymptomatic boy and girl who both carried the gene. The son and daughter typically would not show signs of the illness until they reach 26 years; however, by then, they might each have several children. Anticipation would be further apparent when affected grandchildren show signs in their teenage years. Similarly, in the classic example, Huntington's disease, dementia appears earlier in life and more severely in successive generations, especially when the father has transmitted the abnormal gene (see Chapter 18).

Indications of myotonic dystrophy and other trinucleotide repeat disorders' appearing in progressively younger individuals in a family is due to the earlier emergence of the symptoms in successive generations. Their appearance is not due simply to a heightened vigilance for the condition. In contrast, an apparent increase in incidence resulting from closer scrutiny is an epidemiologic error, called *ascertainment bias*.

Polymyositis

Some infectious and inflammatory illnesses attack only muscles. These illnesses typically cause weakness and myalgias, as in the common "flu," but rarely mental status changes.

Polymyositis is a nonspecific, generalized, inflammatory myopathy characterized by weakness, myalgias, and systemic symptoms, such as fever, and malaise. When these symptoms are accompanied or preceded by a rash—usually on the face and extensor surfaces of the elbows and knees—the diagnosis is usually *dermatomyositis*. In children and many adults, a benign, self-limited systemic viral illness usually causes polymyositis. In other adults, it may be a manifestation of inflammatory diseases, such as polymyalgia rheumatica and polyarteritis nodosa.

Trichinosis, an infectious rather than a purely inflammatory myopathy, is caused by a *Trichinella* infection of muscles. Victims usually develop it from eating undercooked pork or wild game. Thus, in the United States, hunters and recent immigrants from South and Central America are most liable to have ingested *Trichinella* and develop the characteristic muscle pains, fevers, and heliotrope rash.

The *eosinophilia-myalgia syndrome,* more of a toxic than an inflammatory disorder, results from tryptophan or tryptophan-containing products, which are usually taken by insomniacs and health food devotees. The eosinophilia-myalgia syndrome usually consists of several days of severe myalgias and a markedly elevated number and proportion of eosinophils in the blood. Patients often also have fatigue, rash, neuropathy, and cardiopulmonary impairments.

More than half the patients with eosinophilia-myalgia syndrome display mild depressive symptoms that cannot be correlated with their physical impairments, eosinophil counts, or concurrent psychiatric disorders. These patients are in danger of being mislabeled as having chronic fatigue syndrome because of their variable symptoms and, except for the eosinophilia, lack of objective findings.

AIDS myopathy, associated with human immunodeficiency virus (HIV), also causes myalgia, weakness, weight loss, and fatigue. In most patients, the myopathy results from an infection with HIV, but in some, moderate to large doses of zidovudine (popularly known as AZT) seem to be partly or totally responsible. When AZT induces a myopathy, muscle biopsies often show abnormalities in mitochondria and withdrawing the offending medicine usually leads to partial improvement.

Metabolic Myopathies

Muscle metabolism is usually independent of cerebral metabolism, but some disorders induce combinations of muscle and cerebral impairments. For example, prolonged steroid treatment—for organ transplantation, brain tumors, vasculitis, or asthma—frequently produces proximal muscle weakness and wasting (*steroid myopathy*). Steroid treatment also causes a round face, acne, and an obese body with spindly limbs ("cushingoid" appearance). In high doses, steroids can cause mood changes, agitation, and irrational behavior—loosely termed "steroid psychosis." These mental changes are most apt to occur in patients with brain tumors, cerebral vasculitis, and other CNS disorders.

Testosterone and other steroids, when taken in conjunction with exercising, can increase muscle size and strength. Athletes and body-builders use this regimen to enhance their power and appearance. Individuals who abuse steroids also subject themselves to steroid myopathy and steroid psychosis.

An example of the delicate nature of muscle metabolism, sometimes notably independent of cerebral metabolism, is that a low serum potassium concentration (hypokalemia) leads to profound weakness, *hypokalemic myopathy,* and cardiac arrhythmias. Hypokalemic myopathy is often an iatrogenic condition that is caused by administration of diuretics or steroids, which are often surreptitiously self-administered, without potassium supplements. Other causes of hypokalemia that psychiatrists are apt to encounter include laxative abuse and chronic alcoholism when it leads to cirrhosis.

Unlike hypokalemia, which does not alter the mental status, hyponatremia (sodium depletion) causes confusion, agitation, stupor, and seizures. Psychiatrists might encounter patients with hyponatremia and its complications because it results from compulsive water drinking; use of carbamazepine (Tegretol), oxcarbazepine (Trileptal), lithium, and selective serotonin reuptake inhibitors (SSRIs); and numerous medical conditions.

A different disorder involving potassium metabolism is *hypokalemic periodic paralysis,* in which patients have dramatic attacks, lasting several hours to 2 days, of areflexic quadriparesis. During attacks, despite the widespread paralysis, patients remain alert and fully cognizant, breathing normally and purposefully moving their eyes, and their blood tests show serum hypokalemia. Contrary to the illness' name, the attacks' timing is irregular and not "periodic." They tend to occur spontaneously every few weeks, but exercise, sleep, or large carbohydrate meals often precipitate them. The attacks resemble sleep paralysis and cataplexy, but they are differentiated by a longer duration and the hypokalemia. All these conditions differ from psychogenic episodes, including catatonia, by their areflexia as well as hypokalemia.

Usually transmitted in an autosomal dominant pattern, hypokalemic periodic paralysis becomes apparent in adolescent boys. In most cases, it stems from a mutation in the calcium ion channel gene and also represents another channelopathy. An adult-onset variety is associated with hyperthyroidism.

Other common metabolic myopathies sometimes have indirectly related mental status changes. For example, alcoholism leads to limb and cardiac muscle wasting (alcohol cardiomyopathy). In *hyperthyroid myopathy,* weakness develops as part of hyperthyroidism. Although the hyperthyroidism usually causes heat intolerance and hyperactivity, older individuals may have *apathetic hyperthyroidism,* in which signs of overactivity are remarkably absent. As a general rule, metabolic myopathies resolve when normal metabolism is restored.

Some medications, such as clozapine, may cause an elevation of the serum CK concentration but rarely a clinically detectable myopathy. Other medications, such as the lipid-lowering "statins," occasionally cause muscle injury ranging from mild inflammation to life-threatening rhabdomyolysis.

Mitochondrial Myopathies

Mitochondria use cytochrome c oxidase and other enzymes involved in oxidative phosphorylation (respiratory chain system). This metabolic system produces about 90% of the body's energy requirement mostly in the form of adenosine triphosphate (ATP). In turn, the brain is the body's greatest energy consumer. Other high-energy consumers are cardiac, skeletal, and extraocular muscles.

In generating energy, mitochondria must constantly remove *free radicals,* which are highly toxic metabolic by-products. Failure to remove them may lead to Parkinson's disease (see Chapter 18) and other illnesses.

The vital, energy-producing enzymes of mitochondria are delicate and easily poisoned. For example, cyanide rapidly and irreversibly inactivates the mitochondrial respiratory enzymes. With loss of aerobic metabolism in the brain, as well as elsewhere, individuals exposed to cyanide almost immediately lose consciousness. Cyanide has been used for executions in gas chambers and taken by individuals committing suicide, including the several hundred cultists in the murder-suicide massacre in Jonestown, Guyana, in 1978. Also, certain medications might poison mitochondria. For example, nucleoside analogues used to treat HIV infection interfere with the mitochondrial respiratory enzymes and cause weakness and lactic acidosis.

In a newly delineated group of illness, abnormalities in the DNA of mitochondria have been shown to disrupt mitochondrial function. Mitochondrial DNA (mtDNA) differs significantly from chromosomal DNA (nuclear DNA [nDNA]). In contrast to nDNA, which is derived equally from each parent and arranged in familiar pairs, mitochondrial mtDNA is derived entirely from the mother, is double-stranded but ring-shaped, and able to carry only 37 genes. As normal individuals age, they accumulate mutations in mtDNA that are responsible for some age-related changes in the muscles and brain.

Another difference between nDNA and mtDNA is that abnormal mtDNA is passed to daughter cells' mitochondria in random, variable mixtures of normal and abnormal mtDNA. When the proportion of abnormal mtDNA reaches a certain level, the *threshold,* ATP production will be insufficient for cellular function and symptoms will ensue. The daughter cells' mitochondria inherit variable proportions of normal and abnormal mtDNA. The variable proportions, called *heteroplasty,* explain why organs typically have variable proportion of abnormal cells and the illnesses' variable age of onset and clinical features.

Another genetic cause of mitochondrial dysfunction is that nDNA can induce abnormalities in the function of mtDNA. Abnormalities in nDNA that influence mtDNA probably account for many of the problems underlying Wilson's disease (see Chapter 18), Friedreich's ataxia (see Chapter 2), and several other neurologic illnesses. The influence of nDNA on mtDNA can explain why paternally inherited abnormal nDNA can cause malfunction of mtDNA. Moreover, it can explain how a father might transmit a mitochondrial illness to his child.

MtDNA abnormalities typically produce *mitochondrial myopathies,* which are characterized by combinations of impaired muscle metabolism, brain damage, other organ system impairment, and abnormal lipid storage. Muscles, which are almost always included in the multisystem pathology, are filled with a vastly increased number of mitochondria. With special histologic stains, many mitochondrial appear as *ragged-red fibers.* In addition, normal respiratory enzymes, such as cytochrome c oxidase (COX), are absent in many cells—those above the threshold. The inheritance patterns of the mitochondrial myopathies do not follow Mendelian patterns, such as autosomal dominant, but reflect the vagaries of mitochondria's maternal transmission, nDNA influence, heteroplasty, and the threshold effect.

The *primarily mitochondrial myopathies,* which result from mitochondria having deficiencies in cytochrome oxidase or other enzymes, cause weakness and exercise intolerance, short stature, epilepsy, deafness, and episodes of lactic acidosis. Another group of mitochondrial myopathies, *progressive ophthalmoplegia* and its related disorders, cause ptosis and other extraocular muscle palsies along with numerous non-neurologic manifestations, such as retinitis pigmentosa, short stature, cardiomyopathy, and endocrine abnormalities. One mitochondrial DNA disorder, *Leber's optic atrophy,* causes hereditary optic atrophy in young men (see Chapter 12).

The best-known group of mtDNA disorders, *mitochondrial encephalopathies*, is characterized by progressively severe or intermittent mental status abnormalities that usually appear between infancy and 12 years. Children with one of these illnesses typically have mental retardation, progressive cognitive impairment, or episodes of confusion leading to stupor. In other words, mitochondrial disorders cause dementia or intermittent delirium in children. They can also cause paresis of extraocular muscles, psychomotor retardation or regression, migraine-like headaches, and optic atrophy.

The malfunction of mitochondrial respiration characteristically leads to lactic acidosis constantly or only during attacks. (Cyanide poisoning, because it also poisons mitochondria, also leads to lactic acidosis.) In mitochondrial encephalopathies, muscle biopsies show ragged red fibers, which represent accumulation of massive numbers of mitochondria, and a checkerboard pattern of cells that fail to stain for cytochrome c oxidase.

Mitochondrial encephalopathies include two important varieties known best by their colorful acronyms:

- *MELAS*: *m*itochondrial *e*ncephalomyelopathy, *la*ctic *a*cidosis, and *s*troke-like episodes
- *MERRF*: *m*yoclonic *e*pilepsy and *r*agged-*r*ed *f*ibers

Neuroleptic Malignant Syndrome (NMS)

This condition, classically attributed to neuroleptic administration, consists of intense muscle rigidity, fever, and autonomic dysfunction. However, because neuroleptics are not the sole cause, neurologists have sought to change its name to *Parkinson-hyperpyrexia* or *central dopaminergic syndrome.*

Rigidity is so powerful that the muscles crush themselves to the point of causing *rhabdomyolysis* (muscle necrosis). Crushed muscles release their *myoglobin* (muscle protein) into the blood, producing *myoglobinemia* (muscle protein in the blood) and *myoglobinuria* (muscle protein in the urine). At a high enough concentration, especially if a patient is dehydrated, myoglobin precipitates in the renal tubules and impairs renal function.

This series of events is evident in several routine laboratory tests. Rhabdomyolysis causes an elevated concentration of CK. Renal impairment raises the blood urea nitrogen (BUN) and creatinine concentrations. The electroencephalogram (EEG) remains normal or shows only diffuse slowing, which is a mild and nonspecific abnormality indicative either of a toxic disorder or the use of psychotropic medicines (see Chapter 10).

The autonomic dysfunction associated with NMS causes tachycardia and occasionally cardiovascular collapse. Also as a result of intense, generalized muscle contractions, body temperatures rise, sometimes to dangerous levels, and cause cerebral cortex damage. Not surprisingly, the mortality rate has been 15% to 20%.

The *Diagnostic and Statistical Manual, Fourth Edition, Text Revision (DSM-IV-TR)*, which has retained the name NMS, cites severe muscle rigidity and elevated temperature as its primary features. Others features include "changes in level of consciousness ranging from confusion to coma," autonomic dysfunction, leukocytosis, and elevated CK. This description is consistent with the usual clinical criteria of neurologic and internal medical services in acute care hospitals.

NMS has been found most often in agitated, dehydrated men who have received neuroleptics in large doses over a brief period. Medications regularly implicated include the "typical" neuroleptics that primarily block the D_2 receptor. In addition, NMS has been associated in case reports with nonpsychotropic dopamine-blocking medications, such as metoclopramide (Reglan) and "atypical" neuroleptics, such as clozapine. It has also been associated with medications not known primarily as dopamine-blocking agents, such as fluoxetine and lithium. Similarly, abruptly withdrawing dopamine precursors, such as L-dopa (Sinemet), which is comparable to initiating dopamine-blocking neuroleptics, has also precipitated NMS. In cases of phencyclidine (PCP) intoxication, muscle rigidity and high fevers may lead to the NMS.

Although no explanation accounts for all cases, one credible theory is that NMS is an extreme Parkinson-like reaction to sudden dopamine deficiency. Basal ganglia dopamine deficiency could produce intense muscular rigidity, and hypothalamus dopamine deficiency could impair body heat dissipation and other autonomic functions. An alternative theory is that dopamine-blocking psychotropics alter the calcium distribution in muscle cells.

Recommended treatment has included administering L-dopa and the dopamine agonist bromocriptine (Parlodel) in an effort to restore dopamine-like activity. A similar treatment has been proposed: administer apomorphine, which is a dopamine agonist that, unlike other dopamine agonists, is available in an injectable form. (However, its use may be complicated by severe nausea and vomiting.) Another line of treatment has been dantrolene (Dantrium), which was suggested because it restores a normal intracellular calcium distribution. Several studies have advocated ECT, but the rationale and results have been unclear.

Other Causes of Rhabdomyolysis, Hyperthermia, and Altered Mental States

SEROTONIN SYNDROME

This disorder, like NMS, is iatrogenic and marked by muscle hypertonicity. Common features of the serotonin syndrome include tremulousness, myoclonus, clonus (much more striking in the legs than arms), and agitated confusion. Signs of autonomic instability, including mydriasis, diarrhea, tachycardia, hypertension, and fever, characterize severe forms.

The serotonin syndrome has generally been attributed to excessive CNS and PNS serotonin stimulation from individual or combinations of serotoninergic medicines. The medicines most often cited as potential causes of this syndrome include serotonin precursors (such as tryptophan), provokers of serotonin release (amphetamine), serotonin reuptake inhibitors (and tricyclic antidepressants), serotonin metabolism inhibitors (monoamine oxidase inhibitors [MAOIs]), and serotonin agonists (sumatriptan). Even dietary supplements and St. John's wort may cause it. Although in high enough doses, many of these medicines alone might cause illness, the syndrome typically follows administration of a MAOI or SSRI that raised serotonin levels to toxic levels (see Chapter 21). Because serotoninergic medicines are so commonplace, the serotonin syndrome might follow use of antidepressants in a variety of different neurologic illnesses in which depression is commonly comorbid, such as Parkinson's disease, migraines, and chronic pain. In particular, use of the deprenyl, which is a MAOI, should theoretically place a Parkinson's disease patient at risk (see Chapter 18). Despite its proximity to psychiatry, the DSM-IV-TR does not list criteria for the serotonin syndrome.

Unlike NMS, the serotonin syndrome typically causes prominent myoclonus and little or no fever or CK elevation. After removing the responsible medicines, the initial treatment for the serotonin syndrome should attempt to support vital functions, decrease the muscle rigidity, and reduce agitation. Physicians might reverse some of the excessive CNS serotonin activity by using the serotonin 5-HT$_{2A}$ antagonist, cyproheptadine. As a last resort, some authors have recommend chlorpromazine, which is also a serotonin antagonist, or ECT.

MALIGNANT HYPERTHERMIA (MH)

MH, the disorder most often compared and contrasted to NMS, also leads to rhabdomyolysis, hyperthermia, brain damage, and death. In contrast to NMS, MH is precipitated by general anesthesia or by the muscle relaxant succinylcholine. Its underlying cause is excessive calcium release by a calcium channel.

A vulnerability to MH is inherited as an autosomal disorder carried on chromosome 19. Because MH is an inherited condition, physicians should review the family history of patients before they administer succinylcholine prior to ECT or other procedures. If MH were to develop, dantrolene may be an effective treatment.

Additional causes of hyperthermia, altered mental status, and a muscle abnormality other than rigidity include meningitis and other infections, PCP and other hallucinogen ingestion, heat stroke, and delirium tremens (DTs).

Physicians also often include *anticholinergic poisoning*, along with NMS and the serotonin syndrome, in the differential diagnosis of patients with fever and agitated delirium. In addition to those manifestations, anticholinergic poisoning with medications, such as scopolamine, usually produces signs of excessive sympathetic activity, including mydriasis, dry skin, urinary retention, and absent bowel sounds. Physicians faced with a febrile, agitated patient may eliminate anticholinergic poisoning from consideration if the patient has either muscular hypertonicity or bladder and bowel hyperactivity.

LABORATORY TESTS

Nerve Conduction Velocity (NCV) Studies

The NCV studies or simply "nerve conduction studies" can determine the site of nerve damage, confirm a clinical diagnosis of polyneuropathy, and distinguish polyneuropathy from myopathy. In addition, they can help separate neuropathies that have resulted from loss of myelin, such as Guillain-Barré syndrome, in which the conduction velocities slow, from those that have resulted from axon damage, such as with chemotherapy, in which the amplitude is reduced.

NCV is normally 50 to 70 m/second (Fig. 6-6). Nerve damage slows the NCV at the point of injury, which can be located by proper placement of the electrodes (e.g., across the carpal tunnel). With diffuse nerve injury, as in diabetic polyneuropathy, NCVs in all nerves slow to 30 m/second. Myopathies, in contrast, do not slow NCVs.

Electromyography

Neurologists perform EMGs by inserting fine needles into selected muscles. Neurologists record the consequent electrical discharges during complete muscle rest, voluntary contractions, and stimulation of the innervating peripheral nerve. In a myopathy, muscles produce abnormal, *myopathic*, EMG patterns. Several

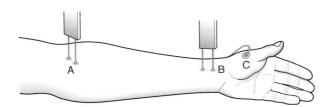

FIGURE 6-6 ■ In determining nerve conduction velocity (NCV), a stimulating electrode that is placed at two points (*A* and *B*) along a nerve excites the appropriate muscle (*C*). The distance between *A* and *B*, divided by the time interval, determines the NCV. In the upper extremities, NCV is normally approximately 50 to 60 m/second and in the lower extremities, approximately 40 to 50 m/second.

diseases—myasthenia gravis, ALS, and myotonic dystrophy—produce distinctive EMG patterns.

Mononeuropathies and peripheral neuropathies also produce abnormal EMG patterns because, in these conditions, improperly innervated muscles malfunction and deteriorate. In other words, the EMG can detect denervated muscles and help determine which peripheral nerve or nerve root is damaged. Neurologists frequently use EMG in cases of lumbar or cervical pain when attempting to document or exclude nerve or nerve root damage.

Serum Enzyme Determinations

Lactic dehydrogenase (LDH), aspartate amino transferase (AST), aldolase, and CK are enzymes concentrated within muscle cells. When illnesses injure muscles, those enzymes escape into the bloodstream. Their serum concentrations rise in rough proportion to the severity of muscle damage. Of the various common conditions, NMS produces the greatest increase in CK. It is also characteristically elevated in Duchenne's dystrophy patients, affected fetuses, and women carriers; metabolic and inflammatory myopathies; and other illnesses affecting muscles. Therefore, for patients with unexplained, ill-defined weakness, as well as those with myopathy or NMS, one of the first laboratory tests should be a determination of the serum CK concentration.

Muscle Biopsy

In expert hands, the microscopic examination of muscle is useful when muscular atrophy might be the result of a neuropathy, ALS, or certain myopathies. The muscle disorders that might be diagnosed in this way include Duchenne's muscular dystrophy, polymyositis, trichinosis, collagen-vascular diseases, mitochondrial myopathies, and several rare glycogen-storage diseases. Electron microscopy as well as routine light microscopy is required to diagnose the mitochondrial myopathies. In many of these disorders, such as MERRF, pathologists stain tissue for the respiratory enzymes and the concentration and morphology of mitochondria. However, although muscle biopsy might be diagnostic in inherited conditions, such as Duchenne's muscular dystrophy and myotonic dystrophy, genetic testing remains easier, more accurate, and more informative in almost all cases.

On the other hand, nerve biopsy remains useful in uncovering only a few rare illnesses. It can add little to the sophistication of clinical evaluations; electrophysiologic studies, such as EMGs; and genetic testing. Also, the biopsy requires removal of a portion of a nerve.

Thermography

Although infrared thermography is frequently performed on the head, neck, lower spine, and limbs, it has little or no value. In particular, thermography is unreliable in the evaluation of herniated disks, headache, or cerebrovascular disease.

REFERENCES

1. Boyer EW, Shannon M: The serotonin syndrome. N Engl J Med 352:1112–1120, 2005.
2. Cummings CJ, Zoghbi HY: Trinucleotide repeats: Mechanisms and pathology. Ann Rev Genomics Hum Genet 1:281–328, 2000.
3. Gervais RO, Russell AS, Green P, et al: Effort testing in patients with fibromyalgia and disability incentives. J Rheumatol 28:1892–1899, 2001.
4. Goetz CG, Bolla KI, Rogers SM: Neurologic health outcomes and Agent Orange: Institute of Medicine report. Neurology 44:801–809, 1994.
5. Hyams KC, Wignall FS, Roswell R: War syndromes and their evaluation: From the U.S. Civil War to the Persian Gulf War. Ann Intern Med 125:398–405, 1996.
6. Kales SN, Christiani DC: Acute chemical emergencies. N Engl J Med 350:800–808, 2004.
7. Krilov LR, Fisher M, Friedman SB, et al: Course and outcome of chronic fatigue in children and adolescents. Pediatrics 102:360–366, 1998.
8. Krup LB, Masur DM, Kaufman LD: Neurocognitive dysfunction in the eosinophilia-myalgia syndrome. Neurology 43:931–936, 1993.
9. Martin CO, Adams HP: Neurologic aspects of biological and chemical terrorism. Arch Neurol 60:21–25, 2003.
10. Meola G, Sansone V, Perani D, et al: Executive dysfunction and avoidant personality trait in myotonic dystrophy type 1 (DM–1) and proximal myotonic myopathy. Neuromusc Dis 13:813–821, 2003.
11. Newmark J: Therapy for nerve agent poisoning. Arch Neurol 61:649–652, 2004.

12. Richmond DP, Agius MA: Treatment of autoimmune myasthenia gravis. Neurology 61:1652–1661, 2003.

13. Said G: Indications and usefulness of nerve biopsy. Arch Neurol 59:1532–1535, 2002.

14. Shapiro RL, Hatheway C, Swerdlow DL: Botulism in the United States: A clinical and epidemiologic review. Ann Intern Med 129:221–228, 1998.

15. Stafford IP, Dildy GA: Myasthenia gravis and pregnancy. Clin Obstet Gynecol 48:48–56, 2005.

16. Wessely S, Hotopf M: Is fibromyalgia a distinct clinical entity? Historic and epidemiological evidence. Baillieres Best Pract Res Clin Rheumatol 13:427–436, 1999.

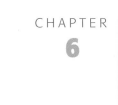

Questions and Answers

1–3. A 17-year-old woman has intermittent double vision when gazing to the left for more than one minute. In each eye alone, her visual acuity is normal. Her examination reveals that she has right-sided ptosis and difficulty keeping her right eye adducted. Her pupils are 4 mm, round, and reactive. Her speech is nasal and her neck flexor muscles are weak. Her strength and deep tendon reflexes (DTRs) are normal.

1. Which disease might explain her intermittent diplopia?
   a. Multiple sclerosis
   b. Psychogenic weakness
   c. Myasthenia gravis
   d. Right posterior communicating artery aneurysm

Answer: c. This is a classic case of myasthenia gravis with ocular, pharyngeal, and neck flexor paresis but no pupil abnormality. She develops diplopia when one or more ocular muscles fatigue. By way of contrast, this pattern of neck flexor paresis, ocular muscle weakness, and ptosis does not occur in multiple sclerosis (MS). Also, although internuclear ophthalmoplegia (INO) frequently occurs in MS, it is causes nystagmus in the abducting eye as well as paresis of the adducting eye (see Chapters 12 and 15). As for psychogenic disturbances, people cannot mimic either paresis of one ocular muscle or ptosis. Compression of the third cranial nerve by an aneurysm produces ptosis and paresis of adduction, but it has a painful onset, and the pupil becomes large and unreactive to light. Furthermore, the bulbar palsy could not be explained by an aneurysm.

2. Which two tests are helpful in confirming the diagnosis?
   a. ACh receptor antibodies
   b. Muscle biopsy
   c. Spine MRI
   d. Tensilon (edrophonium) test
   e. Muscle enzymes: CK, LDH, AST
   f. CSF analysis

Answers: a, d. More than 80% of patients with generalized myasthenia have demonstrable serum antibodies to ACh receptor, but their concentration does not correlate with the severity of the illness. Of myasthenia patients without demonstrable ACh antibodies, about 50% of them will have MuSK antibodies (antibodies to anti*mu*scle-specific *k*inase). The Tensilon test is almost always positive.

3. Which two conditions sometimes underlie the illness?
   a. Hypothyroidism
   b. Hyperthyroidism
   c. Bell's palsy
   d. Thymoma

Answers: b, d. Correction of coexistent hyperthyroidism or thymoma will improve or eliminate myasthenia.

4–5. An 18-year-old dancer develops progressive weakness of her toes and ankles. On examination, she has loss of the ankle reflexes, unresponsive plantar reflexes, and decreased sensation in the toes and feet.

4. Which two diseases are likely causes of her symptoms and signs?
   a. Myasthenia gravis
   b. Toxic polyneuropathy
   c. Polymyositis
   d. Guillain-Barré syndrome
   e. Thoracic spinal cord tumor
   f. Psychogenic mechanisms

Answers: b, d. She has distal lower extremity paresis, areflexia, and hypalgesia, which are signs of a polyneuropathy. Common causes are alcohol, chemicals, and inflammation, such as Guillain-Barré syndrome (acute inflammatory demyelinating polyradiculoneuropathy [AIDP]). Myasthenia rarely affects the legs alone and does not cause a sensory loss. Likewise, the sensory loss and pattern of distal paresis preclude a diagnosis of muscle disease. A spinal cord tumor is unlikely because her ankle reflexes are unreactive, Babinski signs are not present, and she has no "sensory level" or urinary incontinence.

5. Which single test would be most likely to be helpful in making a diagnosis?
   a. EEG
   b. NCV
   c. EMG

d. Tensilon test

e. Muscle enzymes: CK, LDH, AST

f. PET

Answer: b. NCV will probably confirm the presence of a peripheral neuropathy, but it will not suggest a particular cause. CSF analysis in cases of Guillain-Barré syndrome will usually show increased protein and normal or near normal cell count, that is, the "albumino-cytologic disassociation."

6–11. A 5-year-old boy begins to have difficulty standing upright. He has to push himself up on his legs to stand. He cannot run. A cousin of the same age has a similar problem. The patient seems to be unusually muscular and has a normal examination aside from paresis of his upper leg muscles and decreased quadriceps (knee) reflexes.

6. Which single disease is he likely to have?

a. Porphyria

b. Peripheral neuropathy

c. Spinal cord tumor

d. Duchenne's muscular dystrophy

e. A psychogenic disorder

f. Myotonic dystrophy

Answer: d. The boy and his cousin probably have Duchenne's muscular dystrophy because he has the typical findings: Gower's sign (pushing against one's own legs to stand), pseudohypertrophy, and areflexia of weak muscles.

7. Which three tests will help diagnose the case?

a. Muscle dystrophin test

b. NCV

c. EMG

d. Tensilon test

e. Muscle enzymes

f. CSF analysis

Answers: a, c, e. In a definitive finding of Duchenne's muscular dystrophy, muscle dystrophin will be absent on examination of a muscle biopsy. In its variant, Becker's dystrophy, dystrophin will be abnormal. In addition, in Duchenne's muscular dystrophy, EMGs will show abnormal (myopathic potential) patterns and the CK will be markedly elevated. Genetic analysis, the best test for Duchenne's muscular dystrophy, will show mutations on the dystrophin gene, which is located on the X chromosome.

8. What is the sex of the cousin?

a. Male

b. Female

c. Either

Answer: a. Duchenne's muscular dystrophy is a sex-linked trait transmitted by the dystrophin gene. In contrast, myotonic dystrophy is an autosomal dominant trait inherited through the chromosomes in a classic Mendelian pattern of transmission. Several illnesses, such as progressive external ophthalmoplegia, are transmitted by mutations in mitochondrial DNA (mtDNA). mtDNA transmission differs from classic, chromosomal (nDNA) Mendelian transmission. The chief difference is that an individual's mtDNA is derived entirely from the mother. In addition, at a cellular level, mtDNA is *not* equally divided at mitosis between daughter cells, but the mtDNA divides randomly and unequally between them. In cases where the cell contains mutant mtDNA, some daughter cells inherit a large proportion of mutant mtDNA, but others inherit a large proportion of "wild" (normal) mtDNA. The mixture of a cell's mutant and wild mtDNA, "heteroplasty," determines its metabolic status. If the proportion of mutant mtDNA is great enough to interfere with cell function, the "threshold effect" appears and symptoms ensue.

9. Who is the carrier of this condition?

a. Father

b. Mother

c. Either

d. Both

Answer: b.

10. If a sister of the patient is a carrier and the father of all her children does not have the illness, what percent of her female children (girls) will be carriers of Duchenne's dystrophy?

a. 0%

b. 25%

c. 50%

d. 75%

e. 100%

Answer: c.

11. If a sister of the patient is a carrier and the father of all her children does not have the illness what percent of her children will develop Duchenne's dystrophy?

a. 0%

b. 25%

c. 50%

d. 75%

e. 100%

Answer: b. One half of the boys and one half of the girls will inherit the abnormal X chromosome. The boys who inherit it will develop the disease, but the girls who inherit it will only be carriers.

Therefore, 25% of the children (one half of the boys) will have the disease.

12–15. A 68-year-old man has aches and tenderness of the shoulder muscles. He is unable to lift his arms above his head. He has a persistent temperature of 99° to 100.5°F in the afternoons and evenings. A blotchy red rash covers his head, neck, and upper torso.

12. Which three diseases should be considered?
   a. Steroid myopathy
   b. Dermatomyositis
   c. Statin-induced myopathy
   d. Mitochondrial myopathy
   e. Polymyalgia rheumatica
   f. Trichinosis

Answers: b, f. His main symptoms are proximal muscle pain and weakness combined with systemic signs of low-grade fever and a rash. The combination indicates a myopathy that is either inflammatory, such as dermatomyositis, or infectious, such as trichinosis. In each of those cases, the sedimentation rate would be elevated. However, polymyalgia rheumatica does not cause a rash. Similarly, the cholesterol-lowering statin drugs, in 5% to 10% of cases, produce muscle pain and weakness but not a rash. Steroid myopathy and most other metabolic myopathies are painless. Mitochondrial myopathies develop in infants and children.

13. Which two tests are most likely to confirm the diagnosis?
   a. EEG
   b. NCV
   c. EMG
   d. Tensilon test
   e. Muscle enzymes
   f. Skin and muscle biopsy
   g. Nerve biopsy

Answers: e, f. There will be a marked elevation in the CK serum concentration. A biopsy will permit the diagnosis of dermatomyositis, vasculitis, and trichinosis. The best test of polymyalgia rheumatica is a therapeutic trial of small doses of prednisone.

14. Which three conditions are associated with dermatomyositis in the adult?
   a. Dementia
   b. Pulmonary malignancies
   c. Diabetes mellitus
   d. Gastrointestinal malignancies
   e. Delirium
   f. Polyarteritis nodosa

Answers: b, d, f.

15. Which of the above conditions are associated with polymyositis in the child?

Answer: None. In children, polymyositis is associated only with viral illnesses. If an adult develops dermatomyositis, physicians should search for an underlying, occult malignancy because of their close association.

16–24. Which medications are associated with (a) neuropathy, (b) myopathy, (c) both, or (d) neither?

16. Disulfiram
17. Chlorpromazine
18. Nitrofurantoin
19. Isoniazid (INH)
20. Atorvastatin
21. Amitriptyline
22. Nucleoside analogues
23. Lithium carbonate
24. Vitamin B_6

Answers: 16-a, 17-c, 18-a, 19-a, 20-b, 21-d, 22-b, 23-d, 24-a.

25–27. A 50-year-old man has developed low thoracic back pain and difficulty walking. He has mild weakness in both legs, a distended bladder, diminished sensation to pinprick below the umbilicus, and equivocal plantar and DTRs. He has tenderness of the midthoracic spine.

25. Which single condition do his symptoms most clearly indicate?
   a. Polymyositis
   b. Herniated lumbar intervertebral disk
   c. Idiopathic polyneuropathy
   d. Thoracic spinal cord compression

Answer: d. The patient has spinal cord compression at T10 or slightly higher. The reflexes are equivocal because in acute spinal cord compression reflexes are diminished in a phenomenon called "spinal shock." The level is indicated by the sensory changes at the umbilicus. Metastatic tumors are the most frequent cause of spinal cord compression, but herniated intervertebral thoracic disks, multiple sclerosis, tuberculous abscesses, and trauma are sometimes responsible. In contrast, polymyositis affects the arms as well as the legs and does not involve the bladder muscles, produce loss of sensation, or cause spine pain or tenderness.

26. If the routine history, physical examination, and laboratory tests, including a chest x-ray, were normal, which of the following tests should be performed next?

a. CT of the spine
b. X-rays of the lumbosacral spine
c. NCV
d. Tensilon test
e. MRI of the spine
f. PET of the spine

Answer: e. MRI is usually the first test because it is rapid, noninvasive, and readily able to detect soft tissue masses; however, sometimes CT-myelograms are performed.

27. The diagnostic test confirms the clinical impression. If the condition does not receive prompt, effective treatment, which complications might ensue?
   a. Sacral decubitus ulcers
   b. Urinary incontinence
   c. Permanent paraplegia
   d. Hydronephrosis and urosepsis

Answers: a, b, c, d.

28. Which of the following are potential complications of excessive or prolonged use of steroids?
   a. Obesity, especially of the face and trunk
   b. Steroid myopathy
   c. Compression fractures of the lumbar spine
   e. Opportunistic lung and CNS infections
   f. Gastrointestinal bleeding
   g. Opportunistic oral and vaginal infections

Answer: All.

29. Which of the following illnesses that cause weakness can be labeled a (a) dystrophinopathy, (b) channelopathy, (c) both, or (d) neither?
   1. Duchenne's dystrophy
   2. Becker's dystrophy
   3. Myotonic dystrophy
   4. Periodic paralysis
   5. Lambert-Eaton syndrome

Answers: 1-a, 2-a, 3-b, 4-b, 5-b.

30. A 75-year-old woman is hospitalized for congestive heart failure, placed on a low-salt diet, and given a potent diuretic. Although her congestive heart failure resolves, she develops somnolence, disorientation, and generalized weakness. Which of the following is the most likely cause of her mental status change?
   a. Hypokalemia
   b. A cerebrovascular infarction
   c. A subdural hematoma
   d. Cerebral hypoxia from congestive heart failure
   e. Dehydration, hyponatremia, and hypokalemia

Answer: e. Administration of potent diuretics to patients on low-salt diets eventually leads to hypokalemia, hyponatremia, and dehydration. Diuretics are particularly apt to cause obtundation and confusion in the elderly. Hypokalemia alone, however, does not cause mental abnormalities. Physicians should slowly correct the hyponatremia because too rapid correction is associated with the development of a demyelinating injury of the pons, central pontine myelinolysis.

31. Which two myopathies are associated with mental impairment?
   a. Polymyositis
   b. Duchenne's muscular dystrophy
   c. Carpal tunnel syndrome
   d. Myotonic dystrophy
   e. Periodic paralysis
   f. Trichinosis

Answers: b, d. Duchenne's muscular dystrophy and myotonic dystrophy are associated with congenital cognitive impairment. In addition, myotonic dystrophy is associated with personality changes.

32–37. Match the illness with its probable or usual cause.

32. MERRF
33. Myotonic dystrophy
34. Hypokalemic myopathy
35. Cytochrome oxidase deficiency
36. Progressive ophthalmoplegia
37. Periodic paralysis
   a. Autosomal inheritance
   b. Sex-linked inheritance
   c. mtDNA mutation
   d. Viral illness
   e. Underlying malignancy
   f. ACh receptor antibodies
   g. Medications

Answers: 32-c, 33-a, 34-g, 35-c, 36-c, 37- a.

38. Which of the following illnesses is not transmitted by excessive trinucleotide repeats?
   a. Huntington's disease
   b. Myotonic dystrophy
   c. Duchenne's muscular dystrophy
   d. Spinocerebellar ataxia (type 1)
   e. Friedreich's ataxia
   f. Fragile X

Answer: c.

39. Which pattern of inheritance precludes transmission by excessive trinucleotide repeats?

a. Autosomal dominant
b. Autosomal recessive
c. Sex-linked
d. None of the above

Answer: d. Illnesses transmitted by excessive trinucleotide repeats include autosomal dominant (Huntington's disease and most spinocerebellar ataxias), autosomal recessive (Friedreich's ataxia), and sex-linked disorders (fragile X syndrome).

40. What is the role of edrophonium in the Tensilon test?
    a. Edrophonium inhibits cholinesterase to prolong ACh activity.
    b. Edrophonium inhibits cholinesterase to shorten ACh activity.
    c. Edrophonium inhibits choline acetyltransferase to prolong ACh activity.
    d. Edrophonium inhibits choline acetyltransferase to shorten ACh activity.

Answer: a. Edrophonium, which is the generic name for Tensilon, prolongs ACh activity by inhibiting its destructive enzyme, cholinesterase (AChE). Choline acetyltransferase (CAT) is the enzyme that catalyzes the synthesis of ACh.

41. Which type of acetylcholine receptor is damaged in myasthenia gravis?
    a. Muscarinic
    b. Nicotinic
    c. Both
    d. Neither, the problem is in the presynaptic neuron

Answer: b. The number of nicotinic receptors is reduced, and those remaining are rendered less effective.

42. Which two of the following conditions might explain an illness becoming apparent at an earlier age in successive generations?
    a. Ascertainment bias
    b. Age-related vulnerability
    c. Mitochondria DNA inheritance
    d. Anticipation

Answers: a, d. Ascertainment bias is an apparently greater increase in incidence arising from heightened vigilance for a condition. Anticipation is an actual earlier development of an illness' manifestations, usually because of expansion of an abnormal DNA segment in successive generations.

43. For which three of the following conditions is plasmapheresis therapeutic?
    a. Schizophrenia

b. Barbiturate overdose
c. Manic depressive illness
d. Guillain-Barré illness
e. Myasthenia gravis

Answers: b, d, e.

44. Poisoning with which substance causes mental retardation in young children but mononeuropathy in adults?
    a. Copper
    b. Silicone
    c. Lead
    d. Narcotics

Answer: c. Children may develop lead poisoning from eating lead-based paint chips. These children will have cognitive slowing and subsequent school difficulties. Adults may develop lead-induced mononeuropathies, such as a wrist drop, from moonshine or industrial exposure.

45. Which type of ACh receptors predominate in the cerebral cortex?
    a. Nicotinic
    b. Muscarinic
    c. Both
    d. Neither

Answer: b. Muscarinic receptors predominate in the cerebral cortex. They are depleted in Alzheimer's disease. Antibodies directed against nicotinic receptors, which predominate in neuromuscular junctions, characterize myasthenia gravis.

46. Which one of the following is not a characteristic of the Lambert-Eaton syndrome?
    a. Because Lambert-Eaton syndrome is typically found in conjunction with small cell lung carcinoma and other forms of cancer, it is considered a paraneoplastic syndrome.
    b. The syndrome is also associated with rheumatologic diseases.
    c. It results, like myasthenia, from deactivation of ACh at the postsynaptic neuromuscular junction ACh receptor.
    d. The weakness in Lambert-Eaton syndrome primarily involves the limbs. The disorder also causes autonomic nervous system dysfunction.

Answer: c. Although Lambert-Eaton syndrome mimics myasthenia in that it causes weakness and is due to an autoimmune disorder of the neuromuscular junction, Lambert-Eaton syndrome produces primarily limb weakness and dysfunction of the autonomic nervous system. Moreover, its basic abnormality consists of antibodies directed against presynaptic voltage-gated calcium channels that impair ACh release.

47. Which neurotransmitter system does common nerve gases poison?
a. Glycine
b. GABA
c. Serotonin
d. Acetylcholine

Answer: d. Nerve gases, which are typically organophosphorous agents, inactivate acetylcholinesterase (AChE) to produce excessive ACh activity. Tetanus blocks the release of the inhibitory neurotransmitters, particularly glycine and GABA, in the spinal cord and elsewhere in the CNS. Botulinum toxin blocks the release of acetylcholine into neuromuscular junctions.

48. Called to a subway station because of a terrorist attack, a physician is confronted with dozens of passengers in a state of panic who all have abdominal cramps, dyspnea, miosis, weakness, and fasciculations. Many passengers are unconscious and several are having seizures. Which medication should she first administer?
a. Large doses of a minor tranquilizer
b. Small doses of a major tranquilizer
c. Atropine
d. Naloxone

Answer: c. The passengers have been exposed to a terrorist nerve gas poison that has produced PNS dysfunction from excessive ACh activity. In some passengers, the nerve gas has penetrated into the CNS to cause loss of consciousness and seizures. The first antidote to excessive ACh activity is atropine. It penetrates the blood-brain barrier and thus is able to restore CNS as well as PNS ACh activity. Emergency workers also administer an oxime because it restores AChE activity and deactivates the organophosphate poison. In addition, emergency workers often prophylactically administer a benzodiazepine or possibly phenobarbital for their antiepileptic effects. Other antiepileptic drugs are ineffective in this situation.

49. A 52-year-old woman with a history of several episodes of psychosis is brought to the emergency room with agitated confusion, muscle rigidity, and a temperature of 105°F. Her white blood count is 18,000/μL. Although she has marked muscle rigidity and tremulousness, her neck is supple. Her family said that her medications had been changed, but they could provide no other useful information. A head CT and lumbar puncture revealed no abnormalities. Her urine was dark brown. Of the following tests, which one should be performed next?
a. Urine analysis
b. An MRI of the brain
c. An EEG
d. An HIV test

Answer: a. The key to the case is the nature of the urinary pigment. Is it myoglobin or hemoglobin? Are there signs of inflammatory renal damage? The serum chemistry profile might reveal an elevated CK, longstanding renal insufficiency, or other abnormality. In addition to the standard analysis, the urine should be tested for metabolites of cocaine, PCP, and other intoxicants. The other tests are too time-consuming or nonspecific to be helpful for this desperately ill woman. Although meningitis is unlikely in view of the supple neck and normal CSF, many clinicians would administer antibiotics while further evaluation is undertaken. Similarly, whatever the cause, her temperature should be lowered to avoid brain damage.

50. Concerning the preceding question, which two conditions might cause myoglobinuria?
a. Neuroleptic malignant syndrome
b. Porphyria
c. Serotonin syndrome
d. Glomerular nephritis
e. Malaria

Answers: a, c. All these conditions (a–e) can be associated with psychosis and dark urine, but several different pigments may darken urine. Neuroleptic malignant syndrome (NMS) (also known as the hyperpyrexia-rigidity syndrome) and the serotonin syndrome cause myoglobinuria because of muscle breakdown. However, NMS increases CPK and production of myoglobin to a greater degree than the serotonin syndrome. Acute intermittent porphyria produces porphyrins in the urine. Glomerular nephritis and falciparum malaria produce hemoglobinuria.

51–56. Match the disorder with the phenomenon.

51. Unilateral ptosis
52. Facial rash
53. Waddling gait
54. Inability to release a fist
55. Pseudohypertrophy of calf muscles
56. Premature balding and cataracts
a. Myasthenia gravis
b. Duchenne's dystrophy
c. Myotonic dystrophy
d. Polymyositis

Answers: 51-a, 52-d, 53-b, 54-c, 55-b, 56-c.

57. An 8-year-old girl has episodes of confusion and headaches lasting between 1 and 3 days. Between attacks, she has a neurologic examination and all

routine blood tests, head CT, and head MRI. An EEG during attacks showed no epileptiform discharges and between attacks it showed normal alpha rhythm. Eventually, a physician determined that the serum lactic acid concentration rose markedly during every attack but was normal between them. Which should be the next diagnostic test?
a. Lumbar puncture
b. Chromosome analysis for trinucleotide repeats
c. Muscle biopsy
d. Anticardiolipin antibody determination
e. Polysomnography

Answer: c. She probably has a mitochondrial encephalopathy that would be diagnosed with a muscle biopsy's showing proliferation of mitochondria, ragged red fibers, and absence of respiratory enzymes. She most likely has MELAS (*m*itochondrial *e*ncephalopathy, *l*actic *a*cidosis, and *s*troke-like episodes). Other causes of episodic confusion that the Answers suggest—migraines, epilepsy, TIAs, sleep disorders—are reasonable alternatives. However, the repeated elevation of the lactic acid suggests only a mitochondrial encephalopathy.

58. A 50-year-old man has developed erectile dysfunction. As a child, he had poliomyelitis that caused scoliosis and atrophy of his right leg and left arm. DTRs are absent in the affected limbs. What role do the polio-induced physical deficits play in his symptom?

Answer: The polio-induced muscle weakness and atrophy are typically confined to the voluntary muscles of the trunk and limbs. Polio victims have no sensory loss, autonomic dysfunction, or sexual impairment. Although polio survivors sometimes develop a "post-polio" ALS-like syndrome in middle age, it does not cause sensory, autonomic, or sexual dysfunction. This patient's erectile dysfunction must have an explanation other than polio.

59. A corporation's chief executive officer develops ALS. His left arm begins to weaken. Then a multinational conglomerate that claims the executive is losing his mental capabilities initiates a hostile takeover bid. Can this contention be supported by the facts known about ALS?
a. Yes
b. No

Answer: b. Because ALS is strictly a motor neuron disease, no intellectual deterioration can be attributed to it. Although this illness can cause dysarthria and apparent loss of emotional control because of pseudobulbar palsy, ALS does not cause cognitive impairment.

60. A psychiatrist has been called to evaluate a 30-year-old woman for agitation and bizarre behavior. She had been admitted to an intensive care unit for exacerbation of myasthenia gravis and treated with high-dose anticholinesterase medications (e.g., pyridostigmine [Mestinon] and neostigmine). When no substantial improvement occurred, she was given plasmapheresis. The next day she had regained strength, but was confused and agitated. Which is the most likely cause of her mental status change?
a. Anticholinesterase medications
b. Plasmapheresis
c. Cerebral hypoxia
d. Alzheimer-like dementia from CNS depletion of ACh

Answer: c. Mental status abnormalities are a relatively common neurologic problem in severe, poorly controlled myasthenia gravis, Guillain-Barré syndrome, and other neuromuscular diseases—even though the CNS is not directly involved. Mental status abnormalities in myasthenia gravis are not directly attributable to the illness, routine anticholinesterase medications, or plasmapheresis. Instead, generalized weakness, extreme fatigue, or respiratory insufficiency can cause cerebral hypoxia, and high dose steroids can produce psychotic behavior. In addition, being hospitalized in an intensive care unit with a life-threatening illness creates a psychologically stressful situation that, superimposed on medical illnesses and sleep deprivation, can precipitate "ICU psychosis."

61. The family of a 45-year-old man, who had a history of depressive illness, brings him and his girlfriend to the emergency room. Both are comatose and apneic. Their pupils are mid-sized and reactive. Extraocular movements are normal. The CT, illicit drug screening, blood glucose, and other blood tests are all normal except for an anion gap that proves to be due to a markedly elevated lactic acid concentration. Of the following, which is the most likely intoxicant?
a. Botulinum
b. Heroin
c. Cyanide
d. Barbiturates

Answer: c. All of these intoxicants are potential suicide and murder instruments that depress respirations, but only cyanide causes pronounced lactic acidosis. Because cyanide destroys mitochondrial respiratory enzymes, it leads to pronounced lactic acidosis reflected in an anion gap. Botulinum causes dilated pupils and ophthalmoplegia. Routine heroin use causes miosis and overdoses often induce pulmonary edema. Barbiturates overdose also causes miosis.

62. Which one of the following is *not* common to neuroleptic malignant syndrome and malignant hyperthermia?
   a. Fever
   b. Muscle rigidity
   c. Brain damage
   d. Elevated CK
   e. Tachycardia
   f. Familial tendency

Answer: f. Malignant hyperthermia, but not neuroleptic malignant syndrome, has a genetic basis. A vulnerability to the disorder is carried on chromosome 19.

63. Which of the following is a neurotransmitter at the neuromuscular junction as well as CNS?
   a. Dopamine
   b. Serotonin
   c. GABA
   d. Acetylcholine

Answer: d.

64. Which of the following is deactivated more by extracellular metabolism than reuptake?
   a. Dopamine
   b. Serotonin
   c. GABA
   d. Acetylcholine

Answer: d.

65. A 35-year-old woman, who has had myasthenia for 15 years, has been stable on pyridostigmine (Mestinon) 120 mg q.i.d. After a psychologically stressful situation developed, she began to have cramping abdominal pains, diarrhea, rhinorrhea, and excessive pulmonary secretions. Her face, jaw, and neck muscles weakened. Then her limb muscles weakened. Which of the following is most likely to have developed?
   a. Psychogenic fatigue
   b. Cholinergic toxicity
   c. Relapse of her myasthenia
   d. Nerve gas poisoning

Answer: b. Pyridostigmine, which enhances ACh activity at the neuromuscular junction by inactivating cholinesterase, has lead to a cholinergic crisis. Its symptoms mimic those of an organophosphate nerve poison; however, in this case, she probably has developed a medication-induced cholinergic excess. Reducing the pyridostigmine dose will probably reverse the symptoms.

66. Which of the following treatments is not associated with the development of the neuroleptic malignant syndrome?

   a. Metoclopramide
   b. L-dopa withdrawal
   c. Haloperidol
   d. Risperidone
   e. None of the above

Answer: e. This syndrome is generally attributable to sudden deprivation of dopamine activity. Almost all cases are caused by dopamine-blocking antipsychotic medications. However, occasionally nonpsychiatric dopamine-blocking agents, such as metoclopramide, cause it. Similarly, sudden withdrawal of dopamine precursor therapy, such as suddenly stopping L-dopa treatment in Parkinson's disease patients, causes the syndrome.

67. Which are characteristics of myotonic dystrophy but not of Duchenne's dystrophy?
   a. Dystrophy
   b. Cataracts
   c. Baldness
   d. Myotonia
   e. Infertility
   f. Autosomal inheritance
   g. Dementia
   h. Distal muscle weakness
   i. Pseudohypertrophy

Answers: b–f, h.

68. Which conditions are associated with episodic quadriparesis in teenage boys?
   a. Low potassium
   b. REM activity
   c. Hypnopompic hallucinations
   d. Hypnagogic hallucinations
   e. Hyponatremia
   f. 3-Hz spike-and-wave EEG discharges

Answers: a–d. Hypokalemic periodic paralysis and narcolepsy-cataplexy syndrome cause episodic quadriparesis. Hypokalemia causes episodes lasting many hours to days rather than a few minutes. Hyponatremia, when severe, causes stupor and seizures but not quadriparesis. 3-Hz spike-and-wave EEG discharges are associated with absence or petit mal seizures, which do not cause episodic quadriparesis.

69. Which statement concerning mitochondria is not true?
   a. They produce energy mostly in the form of adenosine triphosphate (ATP).
   b. Their DNA is inherited exclusively from the mother.
   c. Their DNA is in a circular pattern.
   d. They generate and must remove toxic free radicals.

e. Compared to the massive energy consumption of the heart and voluntary muscles, the brain's consumption is low.

Answer: e. The brain has the body's greatest energy consumption. The heart and voluntary muscles have the next greatest energy consumption.

70. Which one of the following would not characterize cases of MERRF?
    a. Ragged red fibers in muscle biopsy
    b. Lactic acidosis
    c. Greatly increased numbers of mitochondria in muscle
    d. Uneven staining for cytochrome oxidase enzyme in muscle cells
    e. Absence of dystrophin
    f. Reduced ATP in muscle cells

Answer: e. Absence of dystrophin characterizes Duchenne's muscular dystrophy. The other abnormalities characterizes MERRF and, to a certain extent, other mitochondrial myopathies. Uneven staining for respiratory enzymes reflects the threshold effect and heteroplasty of mtDNA.

71. Which of the following statements regarding dystrophin is false?
    a. Dystrophin is located in the muscle surface membrane.
    b. Dystrophin is absent in muscles affected in Duchenne's dystrophy.
    c. Dystrophin is absent in myotonic dystrophy.
    d. Dystrophin absence in voluntary muscle is a marker of Duchenne's dystrophy.
    e. Dystrophin is present but abnormal in Becker's dystrophy, which results from different mutation of the same gene as Duchenne's dystrophy.

Answer: c.

72. In regard to the genetics of myotonic dystrophy, which are three consequences of its particularly unstable gene?
    a. Males are more likely than females to inherit the illness.
    b. Mitochondrial DNA might be affected.
    c. In successive generations the disease becomes apparent at an earlier age (i.e, genetic anticipation).
    d. In successive generations, the disease is more severe.
    e. When the illness is transmitted by the father rather than the mother, its symptoms are more pronounced.

Answers: c, d, e. The excessive trinucleotide repeats' instability leads to the illness becoming apparent at an earlier age with more severe symptoms (i.e., anticipation) in successive generations. In addition, as in other conditions that result from excessive trinucleotide repeats, when the illness is inherited from the father, its symptoms are more severe because the DNA in sperm is less stable than the DNA in eggs.

73. Which statement concerning mitochondrial abnormalities is not true?
    a. Abnormalities affect the brain, muscles, and retinae in various combinations.
    b. Abnormalities can produce combinations of myopathy, lactic acidosis, and epilepsy.
    c. Mitochondrial myopathies are characterized by ragged red fibers.
    d. Mitochondrial encephalopathies can cause mental retardation or dementia.
    e. The dementia induced by mitochondrial encephalopathies is characterized by certain neuropsychologic deficits.

Answer: e. Although dementia may be superimposed on mental retardation, it is often severe and accompanied by numerous physical deficits but nonspecific in its characteristics.

74. Which of the following may be the result of body-builders taking steroids?
    a. Muscle atrophy
    b. Muscle development
    c. Mood change
    d. Euphoria
    e. Depression
    f. Acne
    g. Compression fractures in the spine
    h. Oral and vaginal infections

Answers: a–h. If taken in excess, steroids produce myopathy, mental changes, infections, and a Cushing's disease appearance.

75–79. Match the condition and its cause.

75. Steroid abuse
76. HIV infection
77. Tryptophan-containing products
78. Alcohol
79. Trichinella
    a. Trichinosis
    b. Eosinophilia-myalgia syndrome
    c. AIDS-associated myopathy
    d. Body building
    e. Cardiac myopathy

Answers: 75-d, 76-c, 77-b, 78-e, 79-a.

80. The serotonin syndrome shares several features with the neuroleptic malignant syndrome. Which one distinguishes the serotonin syndrome?
 a. Results from treatment of nonpsychiatric illnesses
 b. Fever and autonomic nervous system dysfunction
 c. Muscle rigidity and myoglobinuria
 d. Myoclonus
 e. Response to dopaminergic medications
 f. Response to serotonin

Answer: d. Myoclonus is characteristic of the serotonin syndrome, but it is not routinely found in the neuroleptic malignant syndrome (NMS). Both conditions may result from medications used in nonpsychiatric diseases. Both produce fever, autonomic nervous system dysfunction, muscle disorders, and psychosis. The NMS responds to restoration of dopamine activity and the serotonin stimulation responds to serotonin antagonism.

81. An 80-year-old man has had Parkinson's disease for 12 years. For the past several years he has been progressively incapacitated and bed-ridden. His medication regimen includes levodopa-carbidopa and antihypertensive medications. About 1 week before the visit, he began to have weakness and lack of appetite. His neurologist, diagnosing progression of his Parkinson's disease, added deprenyl to the regimen. Over the next several days, he became confused and febrile. His rigidity increased. Which is the most likely cause of his immediate deterioration?

 a. Pneumonia
 b. Neuroleptic malignant syndrome
 c. Serotonin syndrome
 d. Depression

Answer: a. In advanced Parkinson's disease, the most likely cause of physical deterioration, confusion, and fever is pneumonia. In this circumstance, it is often fatal. Depression is also common. Although depression may cause anorexia and increased immobility in advanced Parkinson's disease, it does not cause fever or rigidity. The circumstances of his deterioration and medication regimen would not suggest neuroleptic malignant syndrome. Finally, toxic accumulations of serotonin would be unexpected because serotonin is metabolized by MAO-A and deprenyl is an inhibitor or MAO-B. On the other hand, simultaneously administering a selective serotonin reuptake inhibitor and deprenyl might, at least theoretically, lead to the serotonin syndrome.

82. Which of the following statements regarding mitochondria is false?
 a. They satisfy the entire body's energy requirement.
 b. Oxidative phosphorylation produces most of their energy stores.
 c. Oxidative phosphorylation leads to adenosine triphosphate (ATP).
 d. Most mitochondrial myopathies impair production of ATP.

Answer: a. Mitochondria produce about 90% of the body's energy requirement.

Dementia

Dementia is not an illness but a clinical condition or syndrome of a progressive decline in cognitive function so severe that it impairs daily activities. The neurologic and psychiatric communities both have similar functional or descriptive diagnostic criteria. As stated in the *Diagnostic and Statistical Manual of Mental Disorders, 4th Edition, Text Revision* (DSM-IV-TR), the diagnosis of Dementia of the Alzheimer's Type requires memory impairment plus one or more of the following: aphasia, apraxia, agnosia, or disturbance in executive function (see Chapter 8). Because the diagnosis requires impairments in two domains, it excludes conditions limited to either amnesia (*Greek,* forgetfulness) or aphasia (*Greek,* speechlessness). It also points to different sets of etiologies: in general, conditions that cause either amnesia or aphasia differ from those that cause dementia.

The DSM-IV-TR diagnosis of dementia also requires that the cognitive deficits cause significant impairment in social or occupational function. This requirement defines dementia due to various causes, such as Alzheimer's disease and Huntington's disease. It also helps to differentiate dementia from less pronounced conditions, such as normal aging and *mild cognitive impairment* (see later).

DISORDERS RELATED TO DEMENTIA

Mental Retardation

In contrast to dementia, *mental retardation* consists of *stable* cognitive impairment present since infancy or childhood. Especially when profound, mental retardation is often accompanied by other signs of cerebral injury, such as seizures and "cerebral palsy" (see Chapter 13). In cases of genetic abnormalities, which constitute a small subgroup, mental retardation may be accompanied by distinctive behavioral disturbances and anomalies of non-neurologic organs, such as the face, skin, ocular lenses, kidneys, and skeleton.

The DSM-IV-TR diagnostic criteria for mental retardation are a general intelligence quotient (IQ) of approximately 70 or below; impairment of adaptive functions, such as social skills or personal care; and onset before 18 years of age. In contrast, neurologists

generally limit the age of onset to 5 years, especially because when dementia begins after that time it originates in progressively severe, not congenital, neurologic illness. Whatever the definition, mentally retarded children may, in later life, develop dementia. For example, individuals who have been mentally retarded as a result of trisomy 21 (Down syndrome) almost invariably develop dementia by their fourth or fifth decades (see later).

Amnesia

Memory loss with otherwise preserved intellectual function constitutes *amnesia*. Individuals with amnesia typically can no longer recall events that have recently occurred and cannot remember newly presented information.

DSM-IV-TR criteria for "Amnestic Disorder Due to…" require not only that memory impairment causes inability to learn new information or recall previously learned information but also that it disturbs social or occupational functioning. The criteria exclude episodes that have occurred exclusively during delirium or dementia.

Although related, amnesia and dementia differ. Memory loss alone is not equivalent to dementia. For example, many individuals with amnesia retain sufficient cognitive function to avoid being classified as having dementia. On the other hand, virtually all patients with dementia have memory loss severe enough to be classified as having amnesia.

Neurologists usually attribute amnesia to temporary or permanent dysfunction of the *hippocampus* (*Greek,* seahorse) and other portions of the limbic system, which are based in the temporal and frontal lobes (see Fig. 16-5). Dementia, in contrast, usually results from extensive cerebral cortex dysfunction (see below).

Limbic system dysfunction may be temporary or permanent. *Transient amnesia* is an important, relatively common disturbance consisting of a suddenly occurring period of amnesia lasting only several minutes to several hours. In addition to having several potential medical and neurologic explanations (Table 7-1), transient amnesia might also be mistaken for a psychogenic disorder (see later).

TABLE 7-1 ■ Commonly Cited Causes of Transient Amnesia

TABLE 7-1 ■ Commonly Cited Causes of Transient Amnesia
Alcohol abuse
Wernicke-Korsakoff syndrome
Alcoholic blackouts
Head trauma (e.g., concussion)
Medications
Gamma hydroxybutyrate (GHB)*
Scopolamine
Partial complex seizures
Transient global amnesia

*When used illicitly, GHB is known as the "date-rape drug." GHB is also marketed as oxybate (Xyrem) for treatment of cataplexy (see Chapter 17).

A well-known cause of amnesia lasting several days to several weeks is electroconvulsive therapy (ECT). Although effective for treating mood disorders, ECT almost invariably produces a transient amnesia for events that occurred shortly before or after treatment. ECT-induced amnesia is more pronounced following high electrical dosage and with bilateral rather than unilateral, nondominant hemisphere treatment.

Amnesia from neurologic conditions is often accompanied by other neuropsychologic and physical abnormalities. For example, post-traumatic amnesia, which is due primarily to contusion of the frontal and temporal lobes, is associated with behavioral disturbances, depression, headache, and, depending on the severity of the trauma, physical signs, such as hemiparesis, ataxia, pseudobulbar palsy, and epilepsy (see Chapter 22). Similarly, Wernicke-Korsakoff's syndrome, in addition to its characteristic amnesia, includes ataxia and signs of a peripheral neuropathy (see later).

In another example, *herpes simplex* encephalitis causes long-lasting or permanent amnesia accompanied by other neuropsychologic and physical abnormalities. *H. simplex* is the most common cause of sporadically occurring (nonepidemic) viral encephalitis. (*Human immunodeficiency virus [HIV]* encephalitis is, of course, epidemic.) The virus typically enters the undersurface of the brain through the nasopharynx and invades the frontal and temporal lobes. Destruction of these regions is typically so severe that amnesia, which is inevitable, is accompanied by other manifestations of temporal lobe damage, such as personality changes, partial complex seizures, and the Klüver-Bucy syndrome (see Chapters 12 and 16).

On the other hand, non-neurologic memory impairment may appear as an aspect of several psychiatric illnesses. For example, in a condition that the DSM-IV-TR would label "Dissociative Amnesia," which previous editions labeled "Psychogenic Amnesia," individuals have one or more episodes of amnesia for personal information of a traumatic or stressful nature, such as the circumstances of a family member's death.

The DSM-IV-TR also describes "Dissociative Fugue," which previous editions labeled "Psychogenic Fugue." In this condition, individuals who have some amnesia for past memories, travel away from home. They sometimes assume new identities. Malingerers and fugitives, of course, may adopt symptoms of these disorders. However, DSM-IV-TR criteria for Dissociative Amnesia and Dissociative Fugue exclude amnesia that occurs in the course of any of several other psychiatric disorders, including Posttraumatic Stress Disorder, Acute Stress Disorder, or Somatization Disorder.

Overall, individuals with amnesia from psychiatric illness and malingering lose memory for personal identity or emotionally laden events rather than recently acquired information. Also, such non-neurologic amnesia typically produces inconsistent results on formal memory testing; however, amobarbital (Amytal) infusions may temporarily help restore memories in individuals with non-neurologic amnesia.

Neuropsychologic Conditions

Confabulation is a neuropsychologic condition frequently precipitated by amnesia, in which patients offer implausible explanations in a sincere, forthcoming, typically jovial manner. Although individuals with confabulation disregard the truth, if they are even aware of it, they do not intentionally deceive. Confabulation is a well-known aspect of Wernicke-Korsakoff's syndrome, Anton's syndrome (see cortical blindness, Chapter 12), and anosognosia (see Chapter 8). With these conditions referable to entirely different regions of the brain, confabulation lacks consistent anatomic correlations and physical features.

Aphasia, anosognosia, apraxia, and other neuropsychologic disorders can occur alone, in various combinations, or along with amnesia as components of dementia (see Chapter 8). If a component of dementia, these neuropsychologic disorders indicate that the dementia originates in "cortical" rather than "subcortical" dysfunction (see later). However, each of them is a discrete impairment that alone does not meet the criteria for dementia. Also, these disorders, unlike dementia and amnesia, are attributable to specific, relatively small cerebral lesions. Sometimes only skillful, nonverbal testing can identify these neuropsychologic disorders, tease them apart, and separate them from comorbid dementia.

NORMAL AGING

Beginning at about age 50 years, people are subject to a variety of natural, age-related changes. Many neurologic functions are resistant, but some are especially vulnerable. Those that decline do so at different rates and in uneven trajectories. Up to a point, which has yet to be determined, changes remain within normal limits.

Memory and Other Neuropsychologic Functions

The most common, normal, age-related change is mild, relative memory impairment termed *benign senescence, forgetfulness of old age,* or *age-associated memory impairment.* This impairment is characterized by forgetfulness for people's names. Compared to young adults, older individuals have delayed recall of newly learned lists. However, given enough time, they will be able to retrieve the new material. Although troublesome, their memory problems are not incapacitating.

Other age-related changes include shortened attention span, slowed learning, which leads to slow or imperfect acquisition of new information, and decreased ability to perform complex tasks. A similar but more pronounced and potentially more serious condition, mild cognitive impairment (see later), overlaps these apparently normal, innocuous age-related changes.

On the other hand, several cognitive processes normally resist aging. For example, older people have little or no loss of vocabulary, language ability, reading comprehension, or fund of knowledge. In addition, as determined by the *Wechsler Adult Intelligence Scale-Revised (WAIS-R)*, older individuals' general intelligence declines only slightly. Social deportment and political and religious beliefs continue—stable in the face of a changing society. The elderly remain almost as well-spoken, well-read, and knowledgeable as ever, although possibly becoming set in their ways.

Sleep

Another normal age-related change is that sleep is fragmented, sleep and awakening times are phase-advanced (earlier than usual), and there is less stage 4, non-rapid eye movement (NREM), sleep. Sleep abnormalities that commonly affect the elderly, with or without dementia, are restless leg syndrome and REM behavioral disorder (see Chapter 17).

Motor and Gait

Older people usually lose muscle mass and strength, and develop atrophy of the small muscles of their hands and feet. They lose deep tendon reflex (DTR) activity in their ankles and perception of vibration in their legs. They also have impaired postural reflexes and loss of balance. Most cannot stand on one foot with their eyes closed, which is a standard, simple test.

When combined with age-related skeletal changes, these motor and sensory impairments lead to the common walking pattern of older individuals. This pattern, loosely termed "senile gait," is characterized by increased flexion of the trunk and limbs, diminished arm swing, and shorter steps. Many older individuals instinctively compensate by using a cane.

The neurologic and skeletal changes can lead to incapacitating, potentially fatal falls. Other major risk factors for falls are a previous fall, cognitive impairment, and use of sedatives and antidepressants. Among antidepressants, selective serotonin reuptake inhibitors (SSRIs) carry the same risk as tricyclic antidepressants.

Age-related deterioration of sensory organs impairs hearing and vision. Older individuals typically have small, less reactive pupils and some retinal degeneration. They require greater light, more contrast, and sharper focusing to be able to read and drive. Their hearing tends to be poorer, especially for speech discrimination. Their sense of taste and smell also deteriorate.

Physicians or other professionals must regularly test vision and hearing in elderly patients because loss of these senses accentuates psychologic and physical disabilities and magnifies cognitive impairments. Moreover, many elderly insist on driving, which requires almost full ability in these and other skills. Sensory deprivation, even in mild degrees, can cause or worsen depression, sleep impairment, and perceptual disturbances, including hallucinations.

Electroencephalogram (EEG) and Imaging Changes

As individuals age, the EEG shows slowing of the normal background alpha activity. The dominant frequencies typically slow from 8 to 12 Hz to about 7 to 8 Hz. Computed tomography (CT) and magnetic resonance imaging (MRI) may be normal, but often these studies reveal decreased volume of the frontal and parietal lobes, atrophy of the cerebral cortex, expansion of the Sylvian fissure, and concomitantly increased volume of the lateral and third ventricles (see Figs. 20-2, 20-3, and 20-18). In addition, MRI reveals white matter hyperintensities ("white dots"). Although often striking, these abnormalities are usually innocuous and, by themselves, do not indicate the onset of Alzheimer's disease.

Macroscopic and Microscopic Changes

With advancing age, brain weight decreases to about 85% of normal. Age-associated histologic changes include loss of large cortical neurons and the presence of lipofuscin granules, granulovacuolar degeneration, senile plaques that contain amyloid, and a limited number of neurofibrillary tangles. These changes affect the frontal and temporal lobes more than the parietal lobe. In addition, advancing age leads to loss of neurons in many important brainstem and other deeply situated structures, including the locus ceruleus, suprachiasmatic nucleus, substantia nigra, and nucleus basalis of Meynert; however, the mamillary bodies remain unaffected (see later).

MILD COGNITIVE IMPAIRMENT

Mild cognitive impairment (MCI) straddles age-associated memory impairment and dementia. Although the DSM-IV-TR does not define it, most neurologists and psychiatrists consider that MCI consists of memory impairments accompanied by abnormal memory test scores, but normal cognitive function and preserved activities of daily living. One measure the physician might apply is to compare patients' cognitive capacity and functioning to their peers. Unlike individuals with dementia, those with MCI continue to socialize, work, and maintain their hobbies.

Most important, MCI also represents a precursor to dementia for many individuals. Compared to individuals of the same age with normal cognitive function, who develop dementia at a rate of 1% to 2% yearly, those with MCI progress to dementia at a rate of 10% to 20% yearly. Risk factors for MCI progressing to dementia are the degree of cognitive impairment as well as the usual risk factors for Alzheimer's disease (see later). Many MCI individuals already have Alzheimer-like pathologic changes at autopsy. Because correctable causes of dementia might present with MCI, physicians should evaluate MCI patients with the same testing as they would dementia patients.

DEMENTIA

Causes and Classifications

Because seemingly innumerable illnesses can cause dementia, a traditional classification by etiology is only slightly more enlightening than an alphabetical list. Although quality and depth of the cognitive deficits are interesting, such information is not distinctive enough for a diagnosis. In other words, neuropsychologic tests alone cannot diagnose a particular dementia-causing illness with sufficient reliability to forego imaging studies and other testing that might exclude other illnesses and particularly reversible

causes of dementia. The following classifications based on salient clinical features, although overlapping, are practical and easy to learn:

- *Prevalence:* The most common causes of dementia are Alzheimer's disease; dementia with Lewy bodies (DLB); frontotemporal dementia; and vascular dementia. All together they account for 95% of cases of dementia.
- *Patient's age at the onset of dementia:* Beginning at age 65 years, those same illnesses cause almost all cases of dementia; however, between 21 and 65 years, HIV disease, substance abuse, severe head trauma, end-stage multiple sclerosis, and vascular disease cause dementia. In adolescence (Table 7-2) and in childhood, the causes are different.
- *Accompanying physical manifestations:* Dementia can be associated with gait apraxia (see later), myoclonus (see later), peripheral neuropathy (see Table 5-2), chorea and other involuntary movement disorders (see Table 18-4), and, in numerous structural lesions, lateralized signs.
- *Genetics:* Among frequently occurring illnesses, dementia is transmitted in an autosomal dominant pattern in Huntington's disease and in a percentage of families with Alzheimer's disease, Creutzfeldt-Jakob disease, and frontotemporal dementia, but in an autosomal recessive pattern in Wilson's disease.
- *Reversibility:* The most common conditions that physicians usually list as "reversible causes of dementia" are depression, overmedication, hypothyroidism, B_{12} deficiency, and other metabolic abnormalities. Dementia due to many conditions, including subdural hematomas and normal pressure hydrocephalus, is theoretically

TABLE 7-2 ■ Causes of Dementia in Adolescents

Cerebral neoplasms
  Chemotherapy (intrathecal)
  Radiotherapy treatment
Degenerative illnesses
  Huntington's disease
  Metachromatic leukodystrophy
  Other rare, usually genetically transmitted, illnesses
Drug, inhalant, and alcohol abuse, including overdose
Head trauma, including abuse
Infections
  Acquired immunodeficiency syndrome (AIDS) dementia
  Variant Creutzfeldt-Jakob disease (vCJD)
  Subacute sclerosing panencephalitis (SSPE)
Metabolic abnormalities
  Adrenoleukodystrophy
  Wilson's disease

reversible, but substantial, sustained improvement is unusual. Overall, reversible dementias are rightfully sought, but the results are discouraging. Using current, relatively strict criteria, only about 9% of dementia cases are potentially reversible and less than 1% have been partially or fully reversed. Also, most reversible cases consist of only MCI of less than 2 years' duration.

- *"Cortical" and "subcortical dementias"*: In this controversial distinction, cortical dementias consist of illness in which dementia is accompanied by other neuropsychologic signs of cortical injury, typically aphasia, agnosia, and apraxia. Because the brain's deeper areas are relatively untouched, patients remain alert, attentive, and ambulatory. Alzheimer's disease serves as the prime example.

In contrast, subcortical dementias are typified by only mild to moderately severe intellectual and memory dysfunction, but by pronounced apathy, affective changes, slowed mental processing, and gait abnormalities. Examples include DLB, vascular dementia, normal pressure hydrocephalus, HIV-associated dementia (HAD), multiple sclerosis, and Huntington's and Parkinson's diseases.

Although the cortical-subcortical classification persists, it has been slipping into disuse because of several problems. The presence or absence of aphasia, agnosia, and apraxia does not reliably predict the category of dementia. In addition, because the DSM-IV-TR requires these neuropsychologic deficits for the diagnosis of dementia, whatever the etiology, it would classify virtually all patients with dementia as being "cortical." Moreover, this system cannot account for the prominent exceptions inherent in several illnesses, including the mixed picture in frontotemporal dementia and other illnesses, subcortical pathology in Alzheimer's disease, motor problems in DLB, and cortical abnormalities in Huntington's disease.

Of these dementia-producing illnesses, this chapter discusses Alzheimer's disease, other commonly occurring ones, and those that are otherwise important. Under separate headings, it adds discussions of the companion topics of pseudodementia and toxic-metabolic encephalopathy. Subsequent chapters discuss other dementia-producing illnesses, which are typically characterized by their physical manifestations, such as several childhood illnesses; Huntington's, Parkinson's, and Wilson's diseases; brain tumors; and head trauma.

Mental Status Testing

Screening Tests

Neurologists and psychiatrists often use screening tests—ones easily administered in 1 hour or less—to detect, estimate the severity, and follow the course of cognitive deficits. Several screening tests are widely used, standardized, and have foreign language versions. However, they also carry several caveats. Unless these tests are carefully corrected, they tend to overestimate cognitive impairment in elderly people, those who have been poorly educated (8 years or less of school), and ethnic minorities. Moreover, they cannot reliably distinguish between dementia produced by Alzheimer's disease from dementia produced by other illnesses, depression-induced cognitive impairment, or delirium. Finally, in evaluating a highly educated person, screening tests may not detect cognitive impairment.

MINI-MENTAL STATE EXAMINATION (MMSE) (FIG. 7-1)

Physicians so regularly administer the MMSE that it has risen to the level of the standard screening test. Moreover, its results correlate with histologic changes.

In addition to detecting current cognitive impairment, the MMSE has predictive value. For example, when well-educated individuals' scores are borderline, as many as 10% to 25% may develop dementia in the next 2 years. The MMSE can also cast doubt on a diagnosis of Alzheimer's disease as the cause of dementia under certain circumstances: (1) If scores on successive tests remain stable for 2 years, the diagnosis should be reconsidered because Alzheimer's disease almost always causes a progressive decline; and (2) If scores decline precipitously, illnesses that cause a rapidly advancing dementia, such as a glioblastoma or Creutzfeldt-Jakob disease, become the more likely diagnosis.

However, critics describe the test as "too easy" because it permits MCI and even early dementia to escape detection. It may also fail to test adequately for executive function and may miss cases of frontotemporal dementia. Also, because the MMSE depends so heavily on language function, it may be inadequate in measuring conditions, such as multiple sclerosis and toluene abuse, in which the subcortical white matter receives the brunt of the damage.

ALZHEIMER'S DISEASE ASSESSMENT SCALE (ADAS)

The ADAS consists of cognitive and noncognitive sections. Its cognitive section (*ADAS-Cog*) (Fig. 7-2) includes not only standard tests of language, comprehension, memory, and orientation but also tests of visual-spatial ability, such as drawing geometric figures, and physical tasks that reflect ideational praxis, such as folding a paper into an envelope. Patients obtain scores of 0 to 70 points in proportion to worsening performance.

MINI-MENTAL STATE
EXAMINATION (MMSE)

Maximum score	Patient's score	Ask the patient, "Please ... (tell me) ..."
		Orientation
5	_____	What is the day, date, month, year, and season?
5	_____	Where are we: city, county, state; floor of hospital/clinic?
		Registration
3	_____	Repeat the names of 3 common objects that I say.
		Attention and Calculation
5	_____	Either subtract serial 7's from 100 or spell backwards the word "World."
		Recall
3	_____	Repeat the 3 names learned in "registration."
		Language
2	_____	Name a pencil and a watch.
1	_____	Repeat "No and's, if's, or but's."
3	_____	Follow this 3 step request: "Take a paper in your right hand, fold it in half, and put it on the floor."
1	_____	Read and follow this request: "Close your eyes."
1	_____	Write any sentence.
1	_____	Copy this figure:
_____30_____	_____	**Patient's total score**

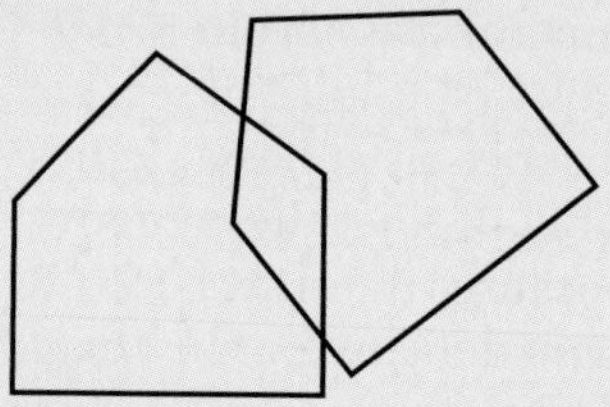

FIGURE 7-1 ■ Mini-Mental State Examination (MMSE). Points are assigned for correct answers. Scores of 20 points or less indicate dementia, delirium, schizophrenia, or affective disorders alone or in combination. These low scores are not found in normal elderly people or in those with neuroses or personality disorders. In addition, MMSE scores fall in proportion of impairments in daily living. For example, scores of 20 correlate with inability to keep appointments and use a telephone. Scores of 15 correlate with inability to dress and groom. (Adapted from Folstein MF, Folstein SE, McHugh PR: "Mini-mental state": A practical method for grading the cognitive state of patients for the clinician. J Psychiatr Res 12:189–198, 1975. © 1975, 1998 MiniMental LLC.)

Compared to the MMSE, the ADAS-Cog is more sensitive, reliable, and less influenced by educational level. However, it is more complex and subjective. Test-givers, who need not be physicians, must undergo special training, and the testing usually requires 45 to 60 minutes. Alzheimer's disease researchers, especially those involved in pharmaceutical trials, routinely use the ADAS-Cog to monitor the course of Alzheimer's disease and measure the effect of medication.

Further Testing

If the results of a screening test yields borderline or otherwise inadequate results, a battery of neuropsychologic tests may clarify the situation. These tests, which usually require at least 3 hours, assess the major realms of cognitive function, such as language (which should be tested first to ensure the validity of the entire test), memory, calculations, judgment, perception, and construction. Neuropsychologic tests are not required for a diagnosis of dementia and are not part of a standard evaluation, but they can help in several situations:

- For extremely intelligent, well-educated, or highly functional individuals with symptoms of dementia whose screening tests fail to show a cognitive impairment
- For individuals whose ability to execute critical occupational or personal decisions, including legal competency, must be ensured

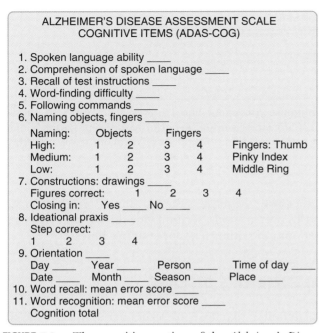

ALZHEIMER'S DISEASE ASSESSMENT SCALE
COGNITIVE ITEMS (ADAS-COG)

1. Spoken language ability ____
2. Comprehension of spoken language ____
3. Recall of test instructions ____
4. Word-finding difficulty ____
5. Following commands ____
6. Naming objects, fingers ____

Naming:	Objects		Fingers		
High:	1	2	3	4	Fingers: Thumb
Medium:	1	2	3	4	Pinky Index
Low:	1	2	3	4	Middle Ring

7. Constructions: drawings ____
   Figures correct: 1   2   3   4
   Closing in: Yes ____ No ____
8. Ideational praxis ____
   Step correct:
   1   2   3   4
9. Orientation ____
   Day ____   Year ____   Person ____   Time of day ____
   Date ____   Month ____   Season ____   Place ____
10. Word recall: mean error score ____
11. Word recognition: mean error score ____
    Cognition total

FIGURE 7-2 ■ The cognitive section of the *Alzheimer's Disease Assessment Scale* (*ADAS-Cog*), the standard test for assessing pharmacologic intervention, has been designed to measure many important aspects of cognitive function that are apt to deteriorate in Alzheimer's disease. The noncognitive section measures mood, attention, delusions, and motor activity, such as pacing and tremors. As dementia begins or worsens, patients' responses change from no impairment (where the patient receives 0 points) to severe cognitive impairment (5 points). In other words, as dementia worsens, patients accumulate points. ADAS-Cog scores for patients with mild to moderate Alzheimer's disease range from 15 to 25 and, as cognitive function declines, scores increase by 6 to 12 points yearly. This scoring system has a greater magnitude and is inverse the one used in the MMSE. (From Rosen WG, Mohs RC, Davis KL: A new rating scale for Alzheimer's disease. Am J Psychiatry 141:1356–1364, 1984. Reprinted with permission from the American Journal of Psychiatry, Copyright 1984. American Psychiatric Association.)

■ For individuals with confounding problems, such as mental retardation, learning disabilities, minimal education, deafness, or aphasia
■ In distinguishing dementia from depression, other psychiatric disturbances, and malingering
■ In distinguishing Alzheimer's disease from frontotemporal dementia

Numerous neuropsychologic tests, often administered in various combinations, have well-substantiated findings. For example, in the case of well-educated individuals with suspected dementia, neuropsychologists might administer the *Graduate Record Examination* (*GRE*) and compare the results to prior performances, which are often available.

A helpful format that complements neuropsychologic tests measures patients' functional status and the impact of cognitive impairment on their daily activities. For example, using the *Functional Capacity Assessment* (Fig. 7-3), the physician, with the help of family members, measures the patient's performance on daily activities that require judgment, memory, and attentiveness. Another test, the *Clinical Dementia Rating* (*CDR*), which nonmedical as well as medical personal can administer, assesses function in memory, orientation, problem solving, judgment, community affairs, home and hobbies, and personal care.

Laboratory Evaluation

Depending on the clinical evaluation, neurologists generally request a series of laboratory tests (Table 7-3). Although testing is expensive (Appendix 2), it may allow a firm diagnosis, disclose a correctable cause of dementia, or reveal an underlying medical disorder.

Because CT can detect most structural abnormalities, including brain tumors, subdural hematomas, and normal pressure hydrocephalus, it is usually sufficient as a screening test in cases of dementia. The MRI is superior because it is better able to diagnose multiple infarctions, demyelinating diseases, and small lesions. However, neither CT nor MRI can firmly diagnose Alzheimer's disease because cerebral atrophy and an enlarged third ventricle, which are virtually the only abnormalities usually evident on imaging studies, are also present in people with normal age-related changes and numerous illnesses, such as trisomy 21, alcoholic dementia, HAD, and some varieties of schizophrenia.

The EEG is not indicated for routine evaluation of dementia because in Alzheimer's disease, its variants, and vascular dementia—the common dementia-producing illnesses—it shows only minor, nonspecific abnormalities. Moreover, those abnormalities are often indistinguishable from normal age-related changes. On the other hand, an EEG may help if patients have shown certain unusual clinical features, such as seizures or myoclonus; a rapid decline in cognitive function; or stupor. An EEG is specifically indicated in suspected cases of Creutzfeldt-Jakob disease or subacute sclerosing panencephalitis (SSPE) (see later), where patients have myoclonus and the EEG shows relatively specific "periodic sharp-wave complexes" or "burst-suppression patterns" (see Fig. 10-6).

The EEG can also contribute to a diagnosis of depression-induced dementia, when a patient's poor performance on mental status tests contrasts with an EEG's normal or only mildly slowed background activity. It should also help in diagnosing metabolic encephalopathy.

FUNCTIONAL CAPACITY ASSESSMENT
Fulfills professional/occupational responsibilities
Maintains financial records: checkbook, credit accounts, etc.
Continues hobbies
Shops, keeps house, cooks
Travels independently to work, friends, or relatives

FIGURE 7-3 ■ The Functional Capacity Assessment is not a quantitative assessment but a survey. The physician should determine whether the patient performs these common activities. If an activity cannot be performed, the physician should determine if the reason is impaired intellectual ability, emotional disturbance, social isolation, or physical incapacity, including impaired special senses.

TABLE 7-3 ■ Screening Laboratory Tests for Dementia
Routine tests
Chemistry profile of electrolytes, glucose, liver function, renal function
Complete blood count
Specific blood tests
B$_{12}$ level^
Human immunodeficiency virus (HIV) antibodies[+]
Lyme titers[+]
Syphilis test*[+]
Thyroid function (e.g., thyroxine [T4])
Neurologic tests
Electroencephalogram (EEG)[+]
Computed tomography (CT)[#]

*In testing for neurosyphilis, either the fluorescent treponemal antibody absorption (FTA-ABS) or treponemal microhemagglutination assay (MHA-TP) test is preferred to the Venereal Disease Research Laboratory (VDRL) or rapid plasma reagin (RPR) (see text).

^Serum folate level determinations, previously a routine test, are indicated only if patients have anemia or suspected nutritional impairments.

[+] For individuals in risk groups (see text).

[#] The MRI is not standard because the CT is usually sufficient.

A lumbar puncture (LP) is also not a routine test because it cannot add direct support to the diagnosis of Alzheimer's disease or vascular dementia. However, neurologists perform an LP to test the cerebrospinal fluid (CSF) when patients with dementia have indications of certain infections, such as neurosyphilis, SSPE, or Creutzfeldt-Jakob disease. They also perform it to measure the pressure and withdraw fluid in cases of suspected normal pressure hydrocephalus. Although CSF analysis may reveal altered concentrations of amyloid and tau proteins—markers of Alzheimer's disease—the sensitivity and specificity of such testing remain too low to allow it to be routine.

Physicians should also reserve other tests for particular indications. For instance, if adolescents or young adults develop dementia, an evaluation might include blood tests for HIV; serum ceruloplasmin determination and slit-lamp examination for Wilson's disease; urine toxicology screens for drug abuse; and, rarely, urine analysis for metachromatic granules and arylsulfatase-A activity for metachromatic leukodystrophy (see Chapter 5). Likewise, physicians should judiciously request systemic lupus erythematosus (SLE) preparations, serum Lyme disease titer determinations, and other tests for systemic illnesses.

ALZHEIMER'S DISEASE

A "definite" diagnosis of Alzheimer's disease, the illness that most commonly causes dementia, requires histologic examination of brain tissue. However, a "probable" diagnosis, which is accepted for clinical purposes and is consistent with psychiatric criteria, is acceptable if adults have (1) the insidious onset of a progressively worsening dementia and (2) clinical and laboratory evaluations (see Table 7-3) that exclude alternative neurologic and systemic illnesses. These criteria yield an antemortem diagnostic accuracy of almost 90%. They would even be more reliable if they excluded patients with signs of either extrapyramidal system or frontal lobe dysfunction.

Clinical Features

Cognitive Decline

Alzheimer's disease typically causes a progressive loss of cognitive function, but its rate of progression can differ among individuals. Also, in many patients the decline is uneven, with about 10% experiencing several years of a plateau.

In the early stage, patients may remain conversant, sociable, able to perform routine work-related tasks, and physically intact. Nevertheless, the spouse or caregiver will probably report that they suffer from memory impairment for facts, words, and ideas; a tendency to lose their bearings at night and in new surroundings; and slowness in coping with new situations. Mental status testing will probably disclose impairments in judgment or other cognitive functions, as well as memory disturbances.

As Alzheimer's disease progresses, it causes further memory loss, unequivocal impairment in other cognitive functions, and often psychopathology. Language impairment includes a decrease in spontaneous verbal output, an inability to find words (*anomia*), and the use of incorrect words (*paraphasic errors*)—elements of aphasia. When patients try to circumvent forgotten words, they may veer into tangentialities. Eventually, patients' verbal output declines until they become mute.

Several Alzheimer's disease symptoms stem from deterioration in visual-spatial abilities. This impairment, which develops early in the illness, causes patients to lose their way in familiar surroundings or while following well-known routes. It also explains *constructional apraxia*, the inability to translate an idea or mental picture into a physical object, organize visual information, or integrate visual and motor functions. The MMSE and other tests can reveal constructional apraxia when they ask patients to draw a clock or figures such as the intersecting pentagons. Asking patients to manipulate small objects, such as matchsticks, often also elicits constructional apraxia. Signs of deterioration in visual-spatial abilities include—in addition to inability to copy a drawing or reproduce matchstick figures—simplification, impaired perspective, perseverations, and sloppiness.

Neuropsychiatric Manifestations

As the *Neuropsychiatric Inventory (NPI)* has shown, the majority of Alzheimer's disease patients demonstrate apathy or agitation. In addition, many demonstrate dysphoria and abnormal behavior. Delusions, which emerge in about 20% to 40% of Alzheimer's disease patients, are usually relatively simple but often incorporate paranoid ideation.

Occurring about half as frequently as delusions, hallucinations are usually visual but sometimes auditory or even olfactory. Whatever their form, hallucinations portend behavioral disturbances, rapid decline of cognitive function, markedly abnormal EEGs, and an overall poor prognosis. Hallucinations are also associated with a slow, shuffling (parkinsonian) gait, as well as pronounced cognitive impairment.

Their development, however, carries several clinical caveats. Often a superimposed toxic-metabolic condition, such as pneumonia, rather than progression of dementia, causes or precipitates hallucination. More important, visual hallucinations early in the course of dementia, particularly if the patient has a shuffling gait, suggests a different illness—DLB (see later). In cases of Alzheimer's disease, low doses of antipsychotic agents will suppress hallucinations and thereby reduce agitation—allowing patients a measure of calm and comfort. On the other hand, if the patient actually suffers from DLB, antipsychotic agents will readily cause disabling extrapyramidal symptoms. Moreover, both typical and atypical agents place elderly patients with dementia at a slightly increased but probably equal risk of stroke (see Chapter 11).

A particularly troublesome behavioral manifestation of Alzheimer's disease is wandering. Although not peculiar to Alzheimer's disease, wandering probably originates in a combination of various disturbances: memory impairment, visual-spatial perceptual difficulties, delusions, and hallucinations; akathisia; side effects from other medicines; sleep disturbances; and mundane activities, such as looking for food or seeking old friends. Whatever its etiology, wandering is dangerous to the patient.

Alzheimer's patients also lose their normal circadian sleep-wake pattern to a greater degree than cognitively intact elderly people. Their sleep becomes fragmented throughout the day and night. Most important, the breakdown in their sleep parallels the severity of their dementia.

Disturbingly, Alzheimer's patients' motor vehicle accident rate is greater than comparably aged individuals, and it increases with the duration of their illness. Clues to unsafe driving include missing exits, under- or over-turning, inability to parallel park, and delayed braking. Accidents are more apt to occur on local streets than on the highway.

(Yet, 16- to 24-year-old men have an even higher rate of motor vehicle accidents than Alzheimer's patients!) Several states require that physicians report patients with medical impairments, presumably including Alzheimer's disease, that would interfere with safe driving. Another potentially disruptive activity of patients with Alzheimer's disease dementia is that approximately 60% of them vote.

Physical Signs

Patients with Alzheimer's disease characteristically have little physical impairment until the illness is advanced. Until then, for example, they are ambulatory and coordinated enough to feed themselves. The common sight of an Alzheimer's disease patient walking steadily but aimlessly through a neighborhood characterizes the disparity between intellectual and motor deficits. Physicians can typically elicit only frontal release signs (Fig. 7-4), increased jaw-jerk reflex (see Fig. 4-13), and Babinski signs. Unlike patients with vascular dementia, those with Alzheimer's disease do not have grossly apparent lateralized signs, such as hemiparesis or homonymous hemianopsia.

When patients reach the end stage, their physical as well as cognitive deficits become profound. They then become mute, fail to respond to verbal requests, remain confined to bed, and assume a decorticate (fetal) posture. They frequently slip into a persistent vegetative state (see Chapter 11).

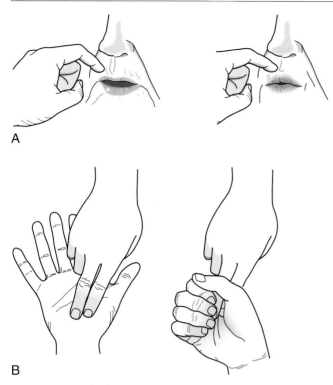

FIGURE 7-4 ■ The frontal lobe release reflexes that are found frequently in elderly individuals with severe dementia are the snout and grasp reflexes. *A*, The snout reflex is elicited by tapping the patient's upper lip with a finger or a percussion hammer. This reflex causes the patient's lips to purse and the mouth to pout. *B*, The grasp reflex is elicited by stroking the patient's palm crosswise or the fingers lengthwise. The reflex causes the patient to grasp the examiner's fingers and fail to let go despite requests.

Tests

"Testing" for Alzheimer's disease is a misnomer because no test possesses the requisite diagnostic sensitivity and specificity (nor can testing diagnose two frequently occurring related diseases: DLB and frontotemporal dementia). When neurologists suspect Alzheimer's disease in a patient with dementia, they perform tests primarily to exclude other causes.

The first EEG change in Alzheimer's disease, slowing of background activity, is not universal and is difficult to distinguish from expected age-related slowing. In advanced disease, the EEG usually shows slow, disorganized background activity, which is also nonspecific.

CT shows nonspecific cerebral atrophy and a widened third ventricle. Serial studies typically show a rapidly progressive, yet still nonspecific, atrophy.

MRI similarly shows a sequential, progressive atrophy: first the hippocampus, then the temporal and parietal lobes, and eventually the frontal lobes. As with CT, MRI shows widening of the third ventricle

as well as the atrophy. However, not only is the cerebral atrophy nonspecific, but even in established cases of Alzheimer's disease, it has no predictive value. In fact, MRIs of patients with schizophrenia also reveal enlarged ventricles and atrophy of the anterior hippocampus.

In about one half of Alzheimer's patients, positron emission tomography (PET) shows areas of decreased cerebral oxygen and glucose metabolism in the bilateral parietal and temporal cortical association cortex. These areas of hypometabolism are vague at first, but as the disease progresses, they become more distinct and spread to the frontal lobe cortex. Nevertheless, PET remains unsuitable for routine use mostly because of poor sensitivity and specificity, and its exorbitant cost.

Single photon emission computed tomography (SPECT) is a less expensive and less cumbersome version of PET. However, it produces nonspecific results.

Cerebral cortex biopsies for diagnostic purposes are virtually never indicated—mostly because routine evaluation is about 90% reliable. In addition, histologic findings of Alzheimer's disease differ only quantitatively, rather than qualitatively, from age-related changes. As a rare last resort, cerebral cortex biopsies can provide a diagnosis of Creutzfeldt-Jakob disease or its variant and, mostly by excluding other illnesses, they may help establish cases of familial Alzheimer's disease.

Various other less invasive tests—psychologic, serologic, and radiographic—are constantly proposed to diagnose Alzheimer's disease. However, they lack the specificity or sensitivity to surpass the current reliability of about 90%.

$$\text{Sensitivity} = \frac{\text{true-positives}}{(\text{true-positives} + \text{false-negatives})}$$

$$\text{Specificity} = \frac{\text{true-negatives}}{(\text{true-negatives} + \text{false-positives})}$$

Pathology

Compared to age-matched controls, brains of Alzheimer's disease patients are more atrophic. The cerebral atrophy in Alzheimer's disease, although generalized, primarily affects the cortical association areas, such as the parietal-temporal junction, and the limbic system. It particularly strikes the hippocampus and prominently involves the locus ceruleus and entire olfactory nerve. In contrast, reflecting the disease's absence of paresis, sensory loss, and blindness, the atrophy spares the cerebral regions governing motor, sensory, and visual functions.

The atrophy leads to compensatory dilation of the lateral and third ventricles. Of these, the temporal horns of the lateral ventricles expand disproportionately. Nevertheless, in Alzheimer's disease and most other illnesses that cause dementia, the anterior horns of the lateral ventricles maintain their concave (bowed inward) shape because of the indentation on their lateral border by the head of the preserved caudate nucleus (see Figs. 20-2 and 20-18). The exception is Huntington's disease, in which atrophy of the head of the caudate nucleus allows the ventricle to expand laterally and assume a convex shape (bowed outward) (see Fig. 20-5).

"Plaques and tangles" remain the most conspicuous histologic feature of Alzheimer's disease. Although present in normal aging and other illnesses, in Alzheimer's disease, the plaques and tangles are more plentiful and tend to cluster, like the atrophy, in the cortex association areas, limbic system, and hippocampus.

The *neurofibrillary tangles,* which also characterize dementia pugilistica, SSPE, and other neurologic illnesses, are composed of paired, periodic helical filaments within neurons. Their concentration parallels the dementia's duration and severity. Neurofibrillary tangles cluster within hippocampus neurons and disrupt the normal cytoskeletal architecture. The clusters are composed largely of a hyperphosphorylated form of *tau protein,* which is a microtubule binding protein. In other words, an intraneuronal protein—tau—aggregates in Alzheimer's disease and contributes to the death of neurons.

The *neuritic plaques,* a form of *senile plaques,* are extracellular aggregates composed of an amyloid core surrounded by abnormal axons and dendrites (*neurites*). Up to 50% of the amyloid core contains an insoluble 42 amino acid peptide, *amyloid β-peptide (Aβ)* (see later). Plaques follow a completely different geographic distribution than tangles. Although amyloid-containing plaques correlate with dementia, the association of neurofibrillary tangles and dementia is stronger.

Another histologic feature of Alzheimer's disease is the *loss of neurons* in the frontal and temporal lobes. More striking, the loss of neurons in the *nucleus basalis of Meynert* (also known as the *substantia innominata*), which is a group of large neurons located near the septal region beneath the globus pallidus (see Fig. 21-4), is distinctive and has important neurotransmitter ramifications. Of all these histologic features, loss of synapses correlates most closely with dementia.

Amyloid Deposits

Returning to the formation of Aβ, enzymes encoded on chromosome 21 cleave *amyloid precursor protein (APP)* to precipitate Aβ in the plaques (Fig. 7-5). Aβ differs from the amyloid deposited in viscera as the

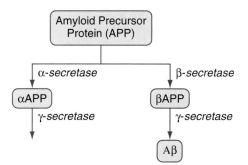

FIGURE 7-5 ■ The amyloid precursor protein (APP) is a 770 amino acid protein. Three secretase enzymes (α-, β-, and γ-) cleave APP into polypeptide fragments. α-secretase creates a polypeptide (αAPP) that is further cleaved by γ-secretase into a soluble and therefore nontoxic polypeptide. However, β-secretase creates a polypeptide (βAPP) that when cleaved by γ-secretase creates Aβ, which is an insoluble, toxic, 42 amino acid polypeptide.

result of various systemic illnesses, such as multiple myeloma and amyloidosis. In Alzheimer's disease, insoluble Aβ accumulates early, uniformly, and permanently in the cerebral cortex and vital subcortical regions.

Several lines of evidence have given rise to the theory that the conversion of APP to Aβ and its accumulation serves as the critical mechanism in producing Alzheimer's disease, which is known as the *amyloid cascade hypothesis.* The evidence includes several powerful observations.

- All known genetic mutations associated with Alzheimer's disease increase Aβ production (chromosomes 1, 14, 21) or aggregation (chromosome 19) (see later).
- The clearest established genetic risk factor, which involves *apolipoprotein E (Apo-E)* (see later), promotes Aβ deposition. Aβ is toxic in vitro.
- In several experiments, Aβ helped precipitate tau aggregates.
- Antibodies to Aβ reduce clinical and pathologic aspects of Alzheimer's disease.

Biochemical Abnormalities

Under normal circumstances, neurons in the basal nucleus of Meynert synthesize *acetylcholine (ACh).* Using the enzyme *choline acetyltransferase (ChAT),* these neurons convert acetylcoenzyme-A (acetyl-CoA) and choline to ACh:

$$\text{Acetyl-CoA} + \text{Choline} \xrightarrow{\textit{ChAT}} \text{ACh}$$

Normally, the neurons emanating from the basal nucleus of Meynert project upward to virtually the entire cerebral cortex and the limbic system to provide cholinergic (i.e., acetylcholine [ACh]) innervation. Alzheimer's disease is characterized—virtually identified—by a loss of the neurons in the basal nucleus of Meynert. Their loss leads to a marked reduction in cerebral cortex ACh concentrations, ChAT activity, and cerebral cholinergic activity. As with the distribution of the macroscopic and microscopic changes in Alzheimer's disease, ACh activity is particularly depressed in the cortical association areas and limbic system. Curiously, ChAT is depleted only in advanced Alzheimer's disease but not in earlier stages or MCI.

Alzheimer's disease is also associated with reduced concentrations of other established or putative neurotransmitters: somatostatin, substance P, norepinephrine, vasopressin, and several other polypeptides. However, compared to the ACh loss, their concentrations are not decreased profoundly or consistently, and do not correlate with dementia.

The *cholinergic hypothesis*, drawn from these biochemical observations, postulates that reduced cholinergic activity causes the dementia of Alzheimer's disease. The primary evidence supporting this hypothesis is the finding that even in normal individuals, blocking cerebral ACh receptors causes profound memory impairments. For example, an injection of scopolamine, which has central anticholinergic activity, induces a several-minute episode of Alzheimer-like cognitive impairment that can be reversed with physostigmine (Fig. 7-6). The cholinergic hypothesis led to the therapeutic approach of attempting to preserve ACh activity by inactivating its metabolic enzyme, cholinesterase (see Fig. 7-6).

Although the ChAT deficiency in Alzheimer's disease is striking, it is not unique. Pronounced ChAT deficiencies are also found in the cortex of brains in trisomy 21, Parkinson's disease, and DLB but not in those of Huntington's disease.

Risk Factors and Genetic Causes

Researchers have established several risk factors for Alzheimer's disease. Age older than 65 years is the most statistically powerful risk factor for Alzheimer's disease because, after that point, the incidence doubles every 5 years. Thus, the prevalence rises from 10% among individuals aged 65 years, to almost 40% among individuals older than 85 years.

Other well-established risk factors include trisomy 21 and several other mutations, having a twin or a first-degree relative with Alzheimer's disease, and Apo-E 3/4 or 4/4 (see later). Researchers have proposed other associations, most of which remain generally weak, inconsistent, or as yet unproven, including

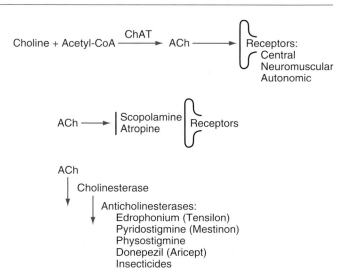

FIGURE 7-6 ■ *Top*, The enzyme choline acetyltransferase (ChAT) catalyzes the synthesis of choline and acetyl-coenzyme-A (ACoA) to form acetylcholine (ACh) in central, peripheral, and autonomic nervous system neurons. When released from its presynaptic neurons, ACh interacts with postsynaptic ACh receptors. *Middle*, However, ACh may be blocked from interacting with the receptors by various substances. For example, scopolamine, which readily crosses the blood–brain barrier, blocks ACh-receptor interaction in the central nervous system (CNS). Atropine blocks ACh receptors but predominantly those in the autonomic nervous system. Unless large quantities are administered, atropine does not cross the blood–brain barrier. *Bottom*, ACh is metabolized by cholinesterase. Thus, its action is terminated under normal conditions by enzyme degradation rather than, as with dopamine and serotonin, being terminated by reuptake. However, if cholinesterase is inhibited or blocked, ACh will be preserved. Various substances—anticholinesterases or cholinesterase inhibitors—block the enzyme and preserve ACh concentrations. For example, edrophonium (Tensilon) and pyridostigmine (Mestinon) are anticholinesterase medicines used to treat myasthenia gravis by preserving neuromuscular junction ACh (see Fig. 6-2). Anticholinesterases are also widely used in insecticides that cause paralysis by creating excessive ACh activity at neuromuscular junctions. Physostigmine, a powerful anticholinesterase medicine that can cross the blood–brain barrier, is administered to correct ACh deficits in Alzheimer's disease and purported in tardive dyskinesia (see Chapter 18). It might also be administered to counteract excessive anticholinergic activity in tricyclic antidepressant overdose or the effects of scopolamine or atropine.

impaired olfactory acuity, myocardial infarction, elevated homocysteine levels, moderate to severe head trauma, hypertension, hyperthyroidism, exposure to aluminum, and a history of psychologic distress.

Family history of Alzheimer's disease is clearly a risk factor. Although most cases of Alzheimer's disease occur sporadically, it develops in about 20% of patients' offspring, 10% of second-degree relatives, and 5% of age-matched controls.

Apo-E, a cholesterol-carrying serum protein produced in the liver and brain, confers a substantial risk. Circulating Apo-E binds to Aβ. Neuritic plaques accumulate the mixture.

Chromosome 19 encodes the gene for Apo-E in three alleles: Apo-E2, Apo-E3, and Apo-E4. Everyone inherits one of three alleles (E2, E3, E4) from each parent, giving each person an allele pair (E2-E2, E2-E3, E2-E4, E3-E4, etc.). Approximately 10% to 20% of the population inherits E3-E4 or E4-E4, which are the pairs most closely associated with Alzheimer's disease.

Having two alleles (being homozygous) for E4—and to a lesser degree having one allele (being heterozygous) for E4—is unequivocally associated with an increased risk of developing or earlier appearance of Alzheimer's disease. More than 50% of Alzheimer's disease patients carry one E4 allele. Of individuals carrying no E4 alleles, only about 20% develop Alzheimer's disease; of those carrying one E4 allele, 50% develop the disease; and of those carrying two E4 alleles, 90% develop it. Not only does the E4 allele put the individual at risk for developing the disease, it also hastens development of the disease. For example, compared to individuals carrying no E4 alleles, those carrying one E4 allele develop Alzheimer's disease 5 to 10 years earlier, and those with two E4 alleles develop the disease 10 to 20 years earlier.

On the other hand, having one or even two E4 alleles is neither necessary nor sufficient for development of Alzheimer's disease. The association of E4 with Alzheimer's disease, although very close, is not close enough to be etiologic. In other words, E4 remains a powerful risk factor, but not a cause, of Alzheimer's disease. Thus, researchers refer to the Apo gene as a "susceptibility" gene.

Because the Apo-E determinations lack the specificity and sensitivity required for a reliable diagnostic test, current recommendations limit its use. According to current neurologic standards, physicians should not test for E4 alleles either in individuals who have developed dementia or in asymptomatic individuals as a predictive test for Alzheimer's disease.

In Parkinson's disease, as with Alzheimer's disease, Apo-E4 is associated with an increased risk and decreased age of onset of the illness. Several, but not all, studies have associated Apo-E4 with an increased risk of permanent cognitive impairment following traumatic brain injury.

In contrast to these risk factors for Alzheimer's disease, several factors are associated with a decreased incidence or postponed onset of the symptoms. For example, formal education seems to offer a measurable degree of protection against dementia in general and Alzheimer's disease in particular. A formal education presumably forms an underlying complex neuronal network that provides a framework for a cognitive reserve. Also, if to prove the old saying that "fish is brain food," studies have shown that eating fish with a high omega-3 fatty acid content, such as herring, mackerel, and salmon, once a week may substantially reduce the incidence of Alzheimer's disease. In addition, some studies have shown that certain diets, folic acid, tocopherol (vitamin E), other vitamins, antioxidants, *Ginkgo biloba*, and dietary supplements also reduce the risk of developing Alzheimer's disease.

Other studies have shown that certain leisure activities—playing board games, reading, playing musical instruments, and ballroom dancing—provide measurable protection against dementia. Use of nonsteroidal anti-inflammatory drugs (NSAIDs) may serve as a protective factor; however, once the disease has developed, they do not alter the decline. Surprisingly, smoking is associated with a reduced incidence of Alzheimer's disease, even after adjusting for premature death.

Genetic Causes

Unlike the gene on chromosome 19, which determines apolipoprotein alleles and thus confers varying degrees of risk, genes on at least three other chromosomes—1, 14, and 21—unequivocally cause Alzheimer's disease, presumably through increased Aβ production (Table 7-4). In other words, although the Apo-E gene confers susceptibility, these genes—"obligate" or "causative" genes—actually produce the illness. All of them transmit Alzheimer's disease in a familial pattern that is usually autosomal dominant, produce symptoms at a relatively young age (30 to 60 years), promote Aβ production, and lead to its deposition in plaques. Nevertheless, although these genetic abnormalities determine the fate of many individuals and provide a window into the pathogenesis of Alzheimer's disease, they account for less than 5% of all cases.

Treatment

Dementia

In light of the plausibility of the cholinergic hypothesis and the finding that postsynaptic cholinergic receptors remain relatively intact, several treatments aim at restoring ACh activity. In attempting to copy the successful strategy of administering a dopamine precursor, levodopa (L-dopa), to Parkinson's disease patients, Alzheimer's disease researchers administered ACh precursors, such as choline and lecithin (phosphatidyl choline). Similarly, they tried ACh agonists, such as arecoline, oxotremorine, acetyl-L-carnitine, and bethanechol. Whether administered by intraventricular or traditional

TABLE 7-4 ■ Genetic Abnormalities Associated with Alzheimer's Disease

Chromosome	Gene	Percent of Cases	Age of Onset (years)
1	Presenilin 2	<1%	50–65
14	Presenilin 1	1%–5%	30–60
19	Apolipoprotein-E (Apo-E)	50%–60%	>60
21	Amyloid precursor protein (APP)	<1%	45–60

routes, none of these strategies produced a consistent, significant benefit.

A complementary strategy, similar to maintaining ACh neuromuscular junction activity in myasthenia (see Chapter 6), attempts to maintain cerebral ACh concentration by reducing its metabolism by cholinesterases. Cholinesterase inhibitors that penetrate the blood–brain barrier, such as physostigmine, increase cerebral ACh concentrations. In Alzheimer's disease treatment, several commercially available cholinesterase inhibitors—donepezil, rivastigmine, and galantamine—produce modest, temporary (approximately 9–12 month) improvement in cognitive tests, "global evaluations," and measurements of quality of life. They also either reduce certain neuropsychologic symptoms, such as depression, psychosis, and anxiety, or the need for psychotropics to suppress them. In addition, cholinesterase inhibitors help in DLB, which is also characterized by an ACh deficit (see later). As an expectable side effect of cholinesterase inhibitors because they increase cholinergic (parasympathetic) intestinal activity, they frequently trigger abdominal cramps.

Some therapeutic trials were based on replenishing other deficient presynaptic neurotransmitters, such as somatostatin, vasopressin, and other polypeptides. Despite their promise, all were unsuccessful.

Another theory postulated that cholesterol-lowering medicines, common known as "statins," would leach cholesterol from neuritic plaques and thereby prevent or improve Alzheimer's disease. Rigorous analysis, however, showed that whatever the coronary artery benefits, statin treatment failed to protect against or correct Alzheimer's disease. Moreover, studies showed that statin treatment failed to protect against stroke and vascular dementia.

Researchers initially expected that estrogen replacement therapy (ERT), which suppresses menopausal symptoms, would also delay the onset of Alzheimer's disease or slow its progression. However, women taking ERT developed the disease at the same rate and followed the same or a more accelerated course as did a control group.

Although reduced cerebral blood flow is a result, not a cause, of Alzheimer's disease, researchers attempted to improve blood flow with cyclospasmol and an ergot alkaloid. A minimal improvement that followed such treatment was attributed to its antidepressant properties.

In an attempt to protect neurons, researchers administered an N-methyl-D-aspartate (NMDA) receptor antagonist, memantine (Namenda), with the expectation that it would block toxic glutamine excitatory neurotransmission. When given with donepezil, memantine produced some improvement in memory and learning in patients with moderate to severe Alzheimer's disease for several months.

One of the most novel approaches consisted of immunizations against amyloid. The expectation was that antibodies would attack and destroy amyloid plaques. Researchers first administered an anti-amyloid vaccine to mice with an inherited Alzheimer-like illness and then to patients with Alzheimer's disease. Although the vaccination program was successful in the mice, humans developed inflammatory encephalitis. Researchers are also attempting to interrupt the synthesis of Aβ by inhibiting β-*secretase* and γ-*secretase* (see Fig. 7-5).

As for preventing progression of MCI to dementia, although donepezil reduces the risk of progression for as long as 1 year, neither it nor vitamin E has an effect at 36 months. However, it may be more helpful in MCI patients homozygous for Apo-E4.

Other Symptoms

Because depression may complicate Alzheimer's disease and even cause or worsen cognitive impairment, neurologists often prescribe therapeutic trials of antidepressants. However, in view of the ACh deficiency in Alzheimer's disease, physicians should avoid psychotropics with anticholinergic activity. In particular, they should avoid prescribing tricyclic antidepressants because they tend to cause confusion and orthostatic hypotension. Instead, serotonin and possibly norepinephrine reuptake inhibitors may alleviate depression, as much or more than tricyclic antidepressants, and produce fewer side effects.

Anxiety and agitation also complicate Alzheimer's disease. Neurologists usually prescribe a benzodiazepine or other anxiolytic. They often prescribe a typical or atypical antipsychotic agent for agitation, especially if it exhausts the patient; however, psychopharmacology provides only a modest relief.

Similarly, psychotropics offer little benefit for wandering and other dangerous behavior. "Behavior management techniques" (BMT), which are nonpharmacologic alternatives, such as removing doorknobs and constructing large indoor and outdoor "safe zones," will painlessly confine the patient. Also, frequently scheduled snacks and trips to the toilet may reduce wandering.

Alzheimer's disease patients' sleep disruptions often represent the family's most burdensome problem. When mild, sleep disturbances may be reduced by providing daytime exercise, exposure to sunlight, and restricted naps. Otherwise, for everybody's benefit, sleep disruptions usually require preemptive, early evening administration of hypnotic, anxiolytic, or antipsychotic agents.

In the absence of definitive studies comparing one psychotropic to another, neurologists have only a few general rules. For example, they target one symptom and begin treatment with small doses of a single medicine and then proceed to an effective dose. They try to avoid confusing medication side effects, especially sedation, with disease progression. Before adding new medicines or increasing the dose of current ones, they assess the patient's entire medication regimen. Because many elderly patients are overmedicated rather than undermedicated, their first strategy is often to subtract rather than add a medicine. They periodically reassess need for psychotropics because, as the disease progresses, symptoms change or even disappear. Although the patient should conventionally remain the focus of attention, physicians caring for Alzheimer's disease patients must consider the spouse, who is often old and infirm, or other persons who act as caregivers. Physicians often prescribe medicines to ease a caregiver's duties, physical limitations, sleep requirements, and mental well-being.

As the burdens of care threaten the family, physicians might advise the relatives that care at home is not in either the patient's or their best interest. Inability to walk, incontinence, highly demanding nursing requirements, and, mostly, night-time outbursts and other disruptive behavior—not cognitive decline—eventually compel families to place these patients in nursing homes. Physicians can help families by keeping their expectations realistic, preserving their financial and emotional resources, securing help from social service agencies, and preventing a hopeless situation from dominating family life.

RELATED DISORDERS

Trisomy 21

Almost all individuals with trisomy 21, if they live to 40 years, develop an Alzheimer-like dementia superimposed on their mental retardation. Moreover, their brains show Alzheimer-like changes: atrophy, cholinergic depletion, amyloid plaques, neurofibrillary tangles, and loss of neurons in the nucleus basalis. Likewise, CT, MRI, and PET studies show Alzheimer-like changes. Even women who give birth to a child with trisomy 21 have a five-fold increase in Alzheimer's disease. These striking similarities between trisomy 21 and Alzheimer's disease led to an early suggestion that in certain families Alzheimer's disease resulted from an abnormality inherited on chromosome 21. (Subsequent research not only showed that chromosome 21 was responsible in those families, but also implicated other chromosomes—1, 14, and 19—in other families [see previous].)

Dementia with Lewy Bodies (DLB)

Another illness that typically causes dementia in individuals older than 65 years is *dementia with Lewy bodies (DLB)*, which has also been called *Lewy body variant, Lewy body disease,* or *diffuse Lewy body disease.* Possibly accounting for up to 30% of cases initially diagnosed as Alzheimer's disease, DLB may be merely a variant of Alzheimer's disease rather than a distinct illness. Perhaps because of its recent separation from Alzheimer's disease, the DSM-IV-TR does not specifically include DLB among "other general medical conditions," such as head trauma and Huntington's disease, that cause dementia.

Researchers named DLB for its microscopic pathology: an abundance of intracytoplasmic inclusions (Lewy bodies) in cerebral cortex neurons that stain with α-*synuclein antibodies.* Therefore, while tau aggregates in neurons in Alzheimer's disease, α-synuclein aggregates in neurons in DLB.

In DLB, the concentration of Lewy bodies in the cerebral cortex correlates with dementia. Until DLB's description, Lewy bodies had been reported almost exclusively in relationship to the substantia nigra in Parkinson's disease. (α-synuclein, as well as Lewy bodies, also aggregates in neurons in Parkinson's disease.)

To a certain extent, DLB mimics Alzheimer's disease. Both illnesses arise in older individuals and cause similar nonspecific cognitive deficits. Also, as in Alzheimer's disease, in DLB the brain concentrations of ChAT and acetylcholine are diminished and their loss correlates with the degree of cognitive impairment. In fact, the loss of ChAT is greater in DLB than Alzheimer's disease.

However, DLB and Alzheimer's disease differ in their noncognitive clinical features. DLB is characterized by mild extrapyramidal (Parkinson-like) features, particularly a masked face, bradykinesia, and gait impairment. These akinetic-rigid features, more so than tremor, accompany the onset of dementia or arise within 1 year. Also, DLB patients experience sudden, unexpected changes in cognition, attentiveness, and alertness. Their fluctuations in mental status, which are characteristic, mimic episodes of delirium or toxic-metabolic encephalopathy. Visual hallucinations, another characteristic feature, also plague patients at the onset of DLB and throughout its course. The hallucinations, which include visions of people and animals, are typically so detailed and vivid that they provoke fear and precipitate confusion. They are associated with Lewy bodies in the temporal lobes. (Visual hallucinations also frequently develop in patients with advanced Alzheimer's and Parkinson's diseases—but usually not at the onset of these illnesses.)

Another disturbing symptom typical of DLB, which often begins before the dementia and ultimately occurs in about 50% of patients, is *rapid eye movement (REM) sleep behavior disorder* (see Chapter 17). (Just as with the accumulations of Lewy bodies and α-synuclein, this characteristic sleep disorder also occurs in Parkinson's disease.) Normal individuals, during REM sleep, are rendered quadriparetic except for respiratory and ocular movement. However, individuals with REM sleep behavior disorder, whether from DLB or Parkinson's disease, are immune to the usual REM-induced paralysis and behave as though they are acting out their dreams. They make running, punching, and similar motions while fast asleep.

Physicians should be aware of several caveats related to medicines in DLB. Although the illness' extrapyramidal signs seem typical of Parkinson's disease, L-dopa or other Parkinson's disease medicines provide little benefit and often create unpleasant side effects, including visual hallucinations. A related caveat is that although visual hallucinations, whether illness-related or iatrogenic, might prompt the administration of antipsychotic agents, dopamine-blockers readily produce pronounced extrapyramidal signs. Because of DLB patients' unusual sensitivity, even small amounts of antipsychotic agents cause akinesia and board-like rigidity.

Cholinesterase inhibitors stabilize or improve cognitive function and reduce visual hallucinations for several months. Long-acting benzodiazepines, such as clonazepam, suppresses the REM sleep behavior disturbance.

Frontal Lobe Disorders

Injuries

The frontal lobes contain the main centers for personality, emotions, and executive decisions. Executive function—itself a higher cortical function—includes integrating various conventional cognitive functions, considering potential solutions, weighing probable outcomes, and initiating a response.

Equally important to centers that initiate responses, the frontal lobes also contain centers that inhibit instinctive behaviors in mature adults. Patients with frontal lobe damage—from physical injury or disease—show characteristic, uninhibited physical, emotional, and behavioral changes.

Patients with extensive frontal lobe damage are generally apathetic: indifferent or unresponsive to their surroundings, ongoing events, and underlying illness. They also have comparable mental slowness. During neuropsychologic testing, these impairments prevent patients from making transitions, changing sets, and adopting alternative strategies.

These patients, who have slowed thoughts and lack of emotions, reduce their verbal output. If an illness or injury damages the dominant frontal lobe's language center, patients will also have impaired verbal output as a manifestation of aphasia. In general, frontal lobe damage leads to a paucity of speech that can range from reticence to silence (*abulia*).

Their movements tend to be slow (*bradykinetic*), repetitive (*perseverated*), or absent (*akinetic*). Walking becomes awkward and uncertain (*apraxic*). Absence of voluntary movement can accompany an absence of speaking and expression (*akinetic mutism*). Patients' viscous thinking and bradykinesia combine to cause *psychomotor retardation*.

Their impaired inhibitory systems tend to promote flighty and inappropriate thoughts and comments, bladder or bowel incontinence, and unrestrained expression of sexual urges. Because patients cannot inhibit a natural tendency to attend to new stimuli, they are easily distracted from their tasks. They may be so incapable of disregarding new stimuli that they become "stimulus bound." Also, uninhibited patients characteristically display a superficial, odd jocularity with uncontrollable, facetious laughter (*witzelsucht*). On a different, somber note regarding uninhibited behavior, neurologic evaluations have revealed that the majority of murderers have frontal lobe dysfunction.

Despite all its attendant neuropsychologic deficits, frontal lobe damage does not necessarily cause dementia. Patients with frontal lobe damage typically retain memory, simple calculation ability, and visual-spatial perception because these cognitive domains are based largely in the parietal and temporal lobes or distributed throughout the cerebral cortex. Indeed, patients' IQ tests often yield normal results.

Physical signs of frontal lobe injury often accompany these neuropsychologic abnormalities. For example, examination of these patients may reveal pseudobulbar palsy (see Chapter 4), nonfluent aphasia, and frontal release reflexes (see later). Also, because of the olfactory nerves' location on the undersurface of the frontal lobes, patients with frontal lobe injuries often have anosmia.

Commonly cited causes of bilateral frontal lobe damage include traumatic brain injury, invasive glioblastoma multiforme, metastatic tumors, metachromatic leukodystrophy, multiple sclerosis plaques, ruptured anterior cerebral artery, and infarction of both anterior cerebral arteries. In the abandoned *frontal lobotomy*, neurosurgeons injected the cortex with sclerosing agents or severed the large white matter tracts underlying the frontal lobes' cortex (see Fig. 20-23). Patients who underwent a frontal lobotomy had less agitation but usually at the expense of developing apathy, restricted spontaneous verbal output, indifference to social conventions, and impaired abstract reasoning.

In contrast to bilateral frontal lobe injury producing extensive neuropsychologic impairments, careful surgical removal of the anterior, nondominant frontal lobe causes little if any impairment. Neurosurgeons routinely perform this procedure on this "silent area" of the brain to remove cerebral malignancies, arteriovenous malformations, or a seizure focus refractory to antiepileptic drugs. Epilepsy patients, who preoperatively had required treatment with several antiepileptic drugs in substantial doses, are often clearer and more cognizant in the postoperative period if only because the surgery allowed a reduction in their antiepileptic drug regimen.

Frontotemporal Dementia

Frontotemporal dementia is a heterogeneous, degenerative syndrome that encompasses *Pick's disease* and several related illnesses. Its course consists of an insidious onset of dementia at an average age of approximately 53 years, followed by a fatal progression usually lasting less than 4 years. Thus, compared to Alzheimer's disease, frontotemporal dementia has a younger age of onset and a considerably shorter course.

The characteristic symptoms of frontotemporal dementia reflect loss of frontal and, to a less extent, the temporal lobe function. Patients show a broad decline in insight, social skills, interpersonal conduct, and executive function. They display combinations of mental rigidity, impersistence, and easy distractibility; labile affect; and speech and language impairments, such as echolalia and perseveration. In addition, probably as a result of their temporal lobe damage, patients have prominent memory problems and elements of the Klüver-Bucy syndrome, such as "hyperorality" and disinhibition (see Chapter 16).

Symptoms, which are often apparent only in retrospect, usually emerge in patients' sixth and seventh decades. Their onset precedes those of Alzheimer's disease by one to two decades and leads to a fatal conclusion within 4 years.

If the disease encompasses the frontal and temporal lobe portion of the perisylvian language arc, patients' speech may contain paraphasias or anomias. As the disease progresses, patients display muscle rigidity, slow gait, re-emergence of frontal release reflexes, and then urinary incontinence. In contrast to symptoms of early Alzheimer's disease, frontotemporal dementia's early features do not include impairments in visual-spatial ability—a function governed largely by the parietal lobes. For example, frontotemporal dementia patients maintain their ability to copy a picture but not to draw one from their memory. Also, they do not lose their sense of direction, even in new surroundings, and they do not manifest constructional apraxia.

Because of the prominent personality and behavioral disturbances accompanied by only relatively mild memory impairment, some physicians place frontotemporal dementia in the category of neurobehavioral illnesses rather than dementia-producing illnesses. Moreover, physicians have been more prone to misdiagnose frontotemporal dementia patients, compared to patients with other common forms of dementia, as having depression, manic-depressive illness, chronic fatigue syndrome, or other psychiatric illness. In particular, patients' paucity of language, affect, and movement potentially leads to an erroneous diagnosis of depression.

The DSM-IV-TR terms the disorder "Dementia Due to Pick's Disease"; however, that designation fails to acknowledge that, in frontotemporal dementia, behavioral disturbances outweigh cognitive impairments and that individuals with true Pick's disease comprise only a minority of cases of frontotemporal dementia. Astute clinicians will not confuse frontotemporal dementia with Alzheimer's disease (Table 7-5).

As the researchers named DLB for its microscopic appearance, researchers named frontotemporal dementia for its gross appearance, which correlates with its clinical features: the frontal and anterior temporal lobes are atrophic, leaving the parietal and occipital lobes apparently intact. Plaques and tangles are either uncommon or absent.

Cases with neurons containing argentophilic (silver-staining) inclusions (*Pick bodies*), which are a minority, are designated Pick's disease. In other words, Pick's disease is now considered a histologic variant of frontotemporal dementia rather than a distinct illness.

TABLE 7-5 ■ Features Distinguishing Alzheimer's Disease and Frontotemporal Dementia

Feature	Alzheimer's Disease	Frontotemporal Dementia
Age at onset (years)	>65	53 years (mean age)
Memory impairments	Early and most pronounced	Subtle, at least initially
Language impairment	Except for anomias, none until late stage	Reticence, paraphasias, anomic aphasia
Behavior abnormalities	None until middle or late stage	Early and prominent disinhibition, but often apathy
CT/MRI appearance	General atrophy, but especially parietal and temporal lobes	Frontal and temporal lobe atrophy

CT = computed tomography; MRI = magnetic resonance imaging.

Moreover, because antibodies to tau stain Pick bodies, many researchers attribute Pick's disease, if not most cases of frontotemporal dementia, to an abnormality in tau metabolism. (Thus, some neurologists, coining new terms, group Alzheimer's and frontotemporal dementia into tauopathies, and DLB and Parkinson's disease into *synucleinopathies*.)

Frontotemporal dementia may account for about 15% of all cases of dementia and a much higher proportion in individuals younger than 65 years. It tends to occur in multiple family members because many cases seem to have been inherited in an autosomal dominant pattern. About 10% of cases have been linked to a mutant gene on chromosome 17, which codes for tau. Also, approximately 10% of frontotemporal dementia patients have comorbid ALS-like physical abnormalities (see Chapter 5).

CT and MRI changes, which are predictable in view of the gross pathology, consist of frontal and anterior temporal lobe atrophy with normal-sized parietal lobes (see Fig. 20-6). By contrast, CT and MRI changes in Alzheimer's disease affect the entire cortex, but primarily affect the parietal and temporal lobes, which host most association areas. Despite an overall poor sensitivity and specificity, PET and SPECT often show hypometabolism in frontal lobes but relatively normal metabolism in parietal and occipital lobes.

OTHER DEMENTIAS

Vascular Dementia

Vascular dementia, resulting from multiple cerebral infarctions, is the most frequent cause of dementia after Alzheimer's disease and DLB. Testing reveals dementia in approximately 20% of patients following an ischemic stroke. Although previous editions and many neurologists previously have referred to the condition as "multiinfarct dementia," the DSM-IV-TR describes similar criteria for Vascular Dementia and Dementia of the Alzheimer's Type.

Infarctions that cause dementia usually take the form of critically situated infarctions, multiple large or small (lacunar) infarctions, or infarctions almost exclusively in the white matter (Binswanger's disease). Any of these insults can be superimposed on either clinically silent or overt Alzheimer's disease.

In vascular dementia—unlike in Alzheimer's disease, DLB, and frontotemporal dementia—focal or lateralized physical signs equal or dominate cognitive impairments. The physical signs that may appear alone or in various combinations during the course of vascular dementia include dysarthria, hemiparesis, hemianopsia, and ataxia. In addition, pseudobulbar palsy and aphasia often complicate the dementia and alter its expression. Compared to Alzheimer's disease patients, vascular disease patients tend to have more symptoms of depression and anxiety. Patients with either illness are equally at risk for psychosis.

Another characteristic of vascular dementia is its course. Unlike the other illnesses, vascular dementia tends to present with both physical and cognitive impairments, and then progress through a *stepwise* parallel accumulation of additional cognitive and physical deficits. A clinical history and CT or MRI evidence of two or more ischemic strokes support the clinical diagnosis.

Hypertension, probably because it is a powerful risk factor for strokes, is a powerful risk factor for vascular dementia. Even a suggestion of cerebrovascular disease, such as a gait abnormality in an elderly person without dementia, is a risk factor. Similarly, vascular disease in other organs, such as coronary artery disease, poses a risk for vascular dementia. Coronary artery bypass surgery can also cause immediate and delayed postoperative cognitive decline. However, vascular dementia is not associated with isolated hypercholesterolemia.

Frequently coexisting aphasia, other neuropsychologic deficits, and critical physical impairments, particularly dysarthria and pseudobulbar palsy, potentially confound vascular dementia's neuropsychologic picture. In addition, frequently associated illnesses, such as renal and cardiac disease, and the medicines used to treat them can exacerbate its cognitive and physical impairments. Perhaps only because of the frequent comorbidity of Alzheimer's disease, cholinesterase inhibitors provide symptomatic benefit in vascular dementia. Thus, with multiple underlying mechanisms, neuropsychologic manifestations and associated physical deficits, and comorbidity with Alzheimer's disease, vascular dementia is a heterogeneous condition.

Wernicke-Korsakoff Syndrome

Chronic, excessive alcohol consumption leads to cognitive impairment and other signs of central nervous system (CNS) and peripheral nervous system (PNS) damage. Although any particular neurologic complication may predominate, *Wernicke-Korsakoff syndrome* encompasses most of them.

Alcohol-induced cognitive impairment is proportional to the lifetime consumption of alcohol and develops in about 50% of all chronic alcoholics. It typically begins with a *global confusional state.* Perhaps on account of denial and inability to appreciate their impairments, chronic alcoholics are oblivious to their disabilities. Contrary to traditional descriptions, confabulation is usually absent or inconspicuous.

The signature of Wernicke-Korsakoff syndrome is amnesia that includes impaired memory for previously known facts (*retrograde amnesia*) coupled with an inability to remember new ones (*anterograde amnesia*). By itself, this amnesia—like aphasia and the frontal lobe syndrome—does not constitute dementia. If the amnesia worsens, however, it interferes with various memory-based cognitive functions, especially learning, and eventually evolves into an Alzheimer-like dementia.

In acute stages of Wernicke-Korsakoff syndrome, patients also display combinations of ataxia and ocular motility abnormalities that include conjugate gaze paresis, abducens nerve paresis, and nystagmus. However, only a minority has all these abnormalities. With chronic alcoholism, with or without Wernicke-Korsakoff syndrome, patients develop a peripheral neuropathy and cerebellar atrophy. Because the cerebellar atrophy particularly affects the vermis (see Chapter 2), chronic alcoholism leads to the distinctive gait ataxia (see Fig. 2-13).

CTs and MRIs may be normal or show only cerebral and cerebellar atrophy. The EEG is usually normal or near normal. Characteristic petechial hemorrhages develop in the mamillary bodies and structures surrounding the third ventricle and aqueduct of Sylvius (see *periaqueductal gray matter*, Fig. 18-2). Because the mamillary bodies are an important element of the limbic system, a basic component of the memory circuit, Wernicke-Korsakoff syndrome produces the amnesia (see Fig. 16-5). Also, because the periaqueductal gray matter contains the nuclei of cranial nerves three and six and is adjacent to the medial longitudinal fasciculus (see Chapters 4 and 12), Wernicke-Korsakoff syndrome produces ocular motility abnormalities.

Wernicke-Korsakoff syndrome is not restricted to alcoholics. Similar clinical and pathologic changes have developed in nonalcoholic individuals who have undergone starvation, dialysis, chemotherapy, or gastric or bariatric surgery. It has also developed on rare occasion in individuals with eating disorders—anorexia nervosa, prolonged vomiting, and self-induced fasting.

Therefore, Wernicke-Korsakoff syndrome is not merely the result of alcohol toxicity. In fact, it probably results primarily from a profound nutritional deficiency of thiamine (vitamin B_1), an essential coenzyme in carbohydrate metabolism. Thiamine administration preventing or even partially reversing Wernicke-Korsakoff syndrome confirms this probability. Most neurologists immediately inject thiamine in both equivocal and clear-cut cases. Although thiamine treatment may reverse many manifestations of acute Wernicke-Korsakoff syndrome, only 25% of patients recover from chronic alcohol-induced dementia.

The DSM-IV-TR, no longer requiring a thiamine deficiency, applies the term "Alcohol-Induced Persisting Amnestic Disorder" to Wernicke-Korsakoff syndrome. It does not address the ocular motility disturbances and other physical neurologic abnormalities. When alcoholism leads to dementia, the DSM-IV-TR applies the term "Alcohol-Induced Persisting Dementia."

Other Causes of Dementia in Alcoholics

Alcoholics are prone to motor vehicle accidents because of impaired judgment, slowed physical responses, and a tendency to fall asleep while driving. Because of motor vehicle accidents, as well as simple falls, they develop head trauma that causes contusions and subdural hematomas, which lead to permanent cognitive impairment and other neurologic sequelae. Those with Laënnec's cirrhosis, especially following gastrointestinal bleeding, develop hepatic encephalopathy. Even low-grade or subtle hepatic encephalopathy may continually or intermittently cause cognitive or personality change.

Rarely, but interestingly, alcoholics can develop degeneration of the corpus callosum that causes a "split brain syndrome" (see Marchiafava-Bignami syndrome, Chapter 8). They are also susceptible to seizures from either excessive alcohol use or alcohol withdrawal. In either case, because the seizures result from metabolic aberrations, they are more likely to be generalized, tonic-clonic seizures rather than partial complex seizures. Infants of severely alcoholic mothers are often born with the *fetal alcohol syndrome,* which includes facial anomalies, low birth weight, microcephaly, and tremors. Most important, fetal alcohol syndrome can lead to mental retardation.

Medication-Induced Dementia

Medication-induced cognitive impairment remains one of the few correctable causes of dementia or delirium. In fact, neurologists prescribe many medicines—opioids, antiepileptic drugs, antiparkinson agents, steroids, and psychotropics—that routinely produce cognitive impairment and other neuropsychologic abnormalities. Some medicines, such as cimetidine, do so infrequently but unpredictably. Even medicines instilled into the eye may be absorbed into the systemic circulation and cause mental changes. Also, seemingly innocuous over-the-counter medicines, such as St. John's wort, may directly produce a mental aberration or cause an adverse interaction that produces one.

Normal Pressure Hydrocephalus

Neurologists commonly refer to normal pressure hydrocephalus (NPH) as a cause of dementia identifiable by its physical manifestations and a correctable cause of dementia. Despite it promise, the condition is fraught with problems. Neurologists are able to identify and then successfully treat few patients. Clinical and laboratory diagnostic tests lack sensitivity and specificity. Treatment, which consists of neurosurgical placement of a shunt, is hazardous and inconsistently effective.

Most cases of NPH are idiopathic, but meningitis or subarachnoid hemorrhage often precedes NPH. In those cases, blood or inflammatory material probably clog the arachnoid villi overlying the brain and impair reabsorption of CSF. As CSF production continues despite inadequate reabsorption, excessive CSF accumulates in the ventricles and distends them to the point of producing hydrocephalus (Fig. 7-7).

NPH is a clinical syndrome—not an illness itself—comprising three elements: dementia, urinary incontinence, and gait apraxia. Neurologists consider the dementia "subcortical" because it entails slowing of thought and gait (psychomotor retardation), but sparing of cortical features, such as naming and language skills. Whatever its features, the dementia is less impressive than the physical features.

Gait apraxia is usually the first and most prominent physical feature of NPH (Fig. 7-8). Although gait apraxia is also a manifestation of frontal lobe disorders, it represents the single most consistent manifestation of NPH. Moreover, it is the first symptom to improve with treatment (see later). Urinary incontinence, which also improves with treatment, initially consists of urgency and frequency that progress to

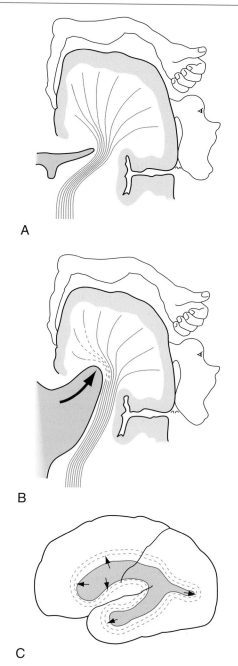

A

B

C

FIGURE 7-7 ■ *A* and *B*, Ventricular expansion, as in normal pressure hydrocephalus, results in compression of brain parenchyma and stretching of the myelinated tracts of the internal capsule (see Fig. 18-1). Gait impairment (apraxia) and urinary incontinence are prominent normal pressure hydrocephalus (NPH) symptoms because the tracts that govern the legs and the voluntary muscles of the bladder are the most stretched. *C*, Also, because the cerebrospinal fluid (CSF) exerts force equally in all directions, pressure on the frontal lobes leads to dementia and psychomotor retardation.

incontinence. These physical features separate NPH from Alzheimer's disease and make it the quintessential subcortical dementia.

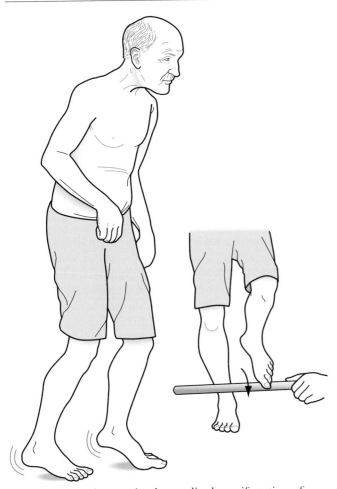

FIGURE 7-8 ■ Gait apraxia, the cardinal manifestation of normal pressure hydrocephalus (NPH), can be seen in several aspects of gait testing. Patients with gait apraxia fail to alternate their leg movements and do not shift their weight to the forward foot. They tend to pick up the same leg twice in a row or elevate the weight-bearing foot. When their weight remains on the foot that they attempt to raise, that foot appears to be stuck or "magnetized" to the floor. Gait apraxia is most pronounced when patients start to walk or begin a turn. However, because their stepping reflex is relatively preserved, they can sometimes step over a stick or other obstacle.

In NPH, CTs and MRIs show ventricular dilation, particularly of the temporal horns (see Figs. 20-7 and 20-19), and sometimes signs of CSF reabsorption across ventricular surfaces. The imaging studies show minimal or no cerebral atrophy. Nevertheless, identification of NPH by CTs and MRIs is unreliable. The findings are nonspecific, particularly because they resemble cerebral atrophy with resultant hydrocephalus, *hydrocephalus ex vacuo* (see Fig. 20-3). Isotopic cisternography, a technique that outlines the ventricles and the cisterns, provides a profile of CSF absorption; however, it too is not reliable enough for therapeutic

decisions. The CSF pressure and its protein and glucose concentrations are normal. The EEG and neuropsychologic tests are also not helpful for a diagnosis.

Common, helpful tests are simply to withdraw 30 mL of CSF by LP or to perform a series of three LPs. Each maneuver presumably transiently reduces hydrocephalus. Following CSF removal, improvement in the patient's gait—not necessarily the dementia—indicates NPH and predicts a benefit from permanent CSF drainage.

NPH can be relieved, at least theoretically, by placement of a shunt into a lateral ventricle to drain CSF into the chest or abdominal cavity where it can be absorbed. However, a clinically beneficial response to shunt installation occurs in as few as 50% of cases in which a cause of NPH, such as a subarachnoid hemorrhage, is established, and only 15% of idiopathic cases. Moreover, despite the apparent simplicity of shunting, neurosurgical complications, which can be devastating, occur in 13% to 28% of patients.

INFECTIONS

Neurosyphilis

Caused by persistent *Treponema pallidum* infection, neurosyphilis had been largely of historic interest until the late 1980s, when it afflicted many acquired immunodeficiency syndrome (AIDS) patients. Secondary syphilis causes *acute syphilitic meningitis*. Only a small fraction of patients eventually develop tertiary neurologic complications, such as dementia or stroke-like insults in the spinal cord or brain.

If dementia does develop, it initially causes only mild, nonspecific personality changes and amnesia. Delusions of grandeur, despite their notoriety, occur rarely. However, a wide variety of physical abnormalities—dysarthria, tremors, Argyll-Robertson pupils (see Chapter 12), tabes dorsalis, steppage gait, and optic atrophy—may accompany syphilis-induced dementia.

When AIDS patients contract syphilis, compared to others who contract the disorder, neurologic complications are more likely to ensue and follow a more aggressive course. AIDS impairs syphilis patients' ability to suppress the illness at its secondary stage and its emergence from a latent stage. AIDS patients with syphilis require intravenous rather than intramuscular penicillin. Although complete clinical recovery is rare, vigorous penicillin treatment may improve cognitive impairment and reverse CSF abnormalities.

Diagnosis of neurosyphilis in AIDS patients is difficult in part because they cannot mobilize the immunologic responses that produce positive results on serologic tests. Also, imaging studies in neurosyphilis typically reveal cerebral atrophy but rarely the diagnostic gummas.

Standard serologic tests for syphilis are the *Venereal Disease Research Laboratory (VDRL)* and the newer *rapid plasma reagin (RPR)* tests. However, neither is sufficiently sensitive and specific for neurologic purposes. Only about 85% of neurosyphilis patients have a positive blood test result. False-negative findings may result from the naturally occurring resolution of serologic abnormalities; prior, sometimes inadequate, treatment; or AIDS-induced immunologic impairment. False-positive results, also common, are usually attributable to old age, addiction, the antiphospholipid syndrome, and other autoimmune diseases (the "4 As").

Refinements of the standard tests are the treponemal or confirmatory serologic tests, the *fluorescent treponemal antibody absorption (FTA-ABS)* and the *treponemal microhemagglutination assay (MHA-TP)*. Both are more sensitive and more specific. They yield positive results in more than 95% of neurosyphilis cases. Moreover, although false-positive FTA-ABS and MHA-TP test results may occur with other spirochete infections, misleading results are otherwise exceedingly rare. In fact, when evaluating a patient for neurosyphilis, rather than first ordering a VDRL or RPR test, the physician might simply order a FTA-ABS or MHA-TP test.

Physicians should order CSF testing when individuals who have developed dementia have either clinical evidence of neurosyphilis, positive FTA-ABS or MHA-TP tests, or have AIDS. The VDRL test remains the only currently available one for the CSF. In about 60% of neurosyphilis cases, the CSF contains an elevated protein concentration (45 to 100 mg/dL) and a lymphocytic pleocytosis (5 to 200 cells/mL).

CSF test results in AIDS patients sometimes pose two potentially confusing situations. In AIDS patients *without* syphilis, the CSF often contains an elevated protein concentration and a lymphocytic pleocytosis—abnormalities that might lead to a misdiagnosis of syphilis. On the other hand, in AIDS patients *with* neurosyphilis, the CSF, as well as routine serologic tests, may be false-negative because of the paralysis of the immune system.

One guideline is that a positive CSF VDRL test result provides an unequivocal diagnosis of neurosyphilis. On the other hand, in as many as 40% of cases, the CSF VDRL test is false-negative. Neurosyphilis can nevertheless usually be diagnosed by the clinical situation and the CSF profile. Another guideline is that penicillin remains the best treatment for neurosyphilis. Even in equivocal situations, physicians should consider administering it.

Subacute Sclerosing Panencephalitis (SSPE)

SSPE is a rare infectious illness that develops predominantly in children or adolescents. Its earliest manifestations consist of poor schoolwork, behavioral disturbances, restlessness, and personality changes. As the illness progresses, victims develop dementia and characteristic myoclonus. When SSPE develops in adults, which is rare, its manifestations consist of visual impairment and various motor deficits (spastic hemiparesis, bradykinesia, and rigidity) as well as myoclonus. In most cases, SSPE is fatal in 1 to 2 years. Although currently available antiviral medicines may arrest its course, victims who survive usually remain in a vegetative state.

A clinical diagnosis of SSPE may be confirmed by finding an elevated CSF measles antibody titer and, during the initial phase of the illness, periodic sharp-wave complexes or a burst-suppression pattern on the EEG (see Fig. 10-6). (The EEG pattern in Creutzfeldt-Jakob disease and SSPE is similar, but the clinical picture and histology are entirely different.) Histologic sections in SSPE reveal intranuclear eosinophilic inclusions (Cowdry bodies). By way of contrast, Lewy bodies are intracytoplasmic eosinophilic inclusions.

Several observations implicate a defective measles (rubeola) virus as the cause. Before the introduction of a vaccine, SSPE complicated approximately 1 in 40 cases of measles, but today almost no vaccinated children develop measles or SSPE. Also, about 50% of SSPE patients contracted measles before 2 years of age. Most important, CSF measles antibody titers are very high in SSPE patients. Finally, SSPE persists in countries without measles immunization programs and when defective vaccines were administered.

Creutzfeldt-Jakob and Related Diseases

In most cases, Creutzfeldt-Jakob disease, like SSPE, causes a triad of dementia, myoclonus, and distinctive EEG patterns. Compared to Alzheimer's disease, Creutzfeldt-Jakob disease appears at a younger age (50 to 64 years) and causes death more rapidly (in about 6 months). Neurologists cannot offer effective treatment.

Although the dementia of Creutzfeldt-Jakob disease lacks specific qualities, it is typically accompanied by myoclonus. In addition, pyramidal, extrapyramidal, or cerebellar signs sometimes develop. The illness' distinctive laboratory tests and cerebral histology can confirm a clinical diagnosis. The DSM-IV-TR cites Creutzfeldt-Jakob disease, along with only several other neurologic illnesses, as a specific cause of dementia.

Although researchers cannot transmit Alzheimer's disease, DLB, or vascular dementia from patients to animals, they routinely transmit Creutzfeldt-Jakob disease to primates by inoculating their brains with tissue from Creutzfeldt-Jakob patients. Transmitting the illness to laboratory animals demonstrates that the illness is infectious, as well as transmissible, and that *inter*species transmission can occur. In addition, accidents have transmitted it between humans—*intra*species transmission—by corneal transplantation, intracerebral EEG electrodes, and neurosurgery specimens. In a well-known iatrogenic tragedy, growth hormone extracted from human cadaver pituitary glands transmitted the illness to a group of children undergoing treatment for pituitary insufficiency.

Most cases of Creutzfeldt-Jakob disease are sporadic and rare ones are iatrogenic. Individuals with this disorder on a familial basis (*Gerstmann-Sträussler-Scheinker* [*GSS*]) disease, who comprise about 15% of the total, follow an autosomal dominant pattern and have an earlier age of onset. GSS patients presumably have a genetic susceptibility due to a mutation on the PrP gene (see later) situated on chromosome 20.

Prions

In work for which he was honored with the Nobel Prize in 1997, Dr. Stanley B. Prusiner showed that a novel group of pathogens, labeled *prions* (*pro*teina-ceous *in*fective agents), composed entirely or almost entirely of protein and completely lacking DNA and RNA, caused Creutzfeldt-Jakob disease and related illnesses. Prions remain the only known example of infectious agents lacking nucleic acid. Also unlike conventional infectious agents, prions resist routine sterilization, heat, formaldehyde, and treatments that hydrolyze nucleic acids. However, because they are protein-based, prions are susceptible to procedures that denature proteins, such as exposure to proteases.

Prion protein (*PrP*), an amyloid protein encoded on chromosome 20, is the predominant or sole constituent of prions. It probably has a role in the formation of synapses, signaling between cells, and copper transportation. Normally, PrP exists in a PrP^c isoform, which is folded in a certain configuration, soluble, and easily digested by proteases. In Creutzfeldt-Jakob disease and related illnesses, PrP^c is transformed to the PrP^{Sc} isoform, which is folded differently, insoluble in most detergents, protease resistant, and probably toxic. Although PrP^{Sc} does not reproduce itself in the conventional sense, it continuously reconfigures PrP^c into aggregates of intraneuronal PrP^{Sc}.

As PrP^{Sc}-induced changes accumulate, the cerebral cortex takes on a distinctive microscopic, vacuolar (sponge-like) appearance (*spongiform encephalopathy*). Special histologic stains can detect PrP^{Sc}. Surprisingly, histologic specimens lack the inflammatory cells normally seen in infections. Overall, Creutzfeldt-Jakob disease serves as the primary example of a *transmissible spongiform encephalopathy* induced by a *prion infection*.

Testing

During the course of Creutzfeldt-Jakob disease, the EEG usually shows periodic sharp-wave complexes or a burst-suppression pattern that can confirm a clinical impression. In almost 90% of cases, CSF contains a protein marker, the "14–3-3 protein." Although valuable, finding this protein in the CSF is not peculiar to Creutzfeldt-Jakob disease because it is also present in other illnesses characterized by sudden neuron death, such as encephalitis, hypoxia, and tumors. The CSF in Creutzfeldt-Jakob disease, as in Alzheimer's disease, usually contains an elevated concentration of tau protein. MRIs might suggest Creutzfeldt-Jakob disease as well as exclude mass lesions for consideration. Some studies have tentatively diagnosed Creutzfeldt-Jakob disease by locating PrP^{Sc} deposits in olfactory nerves and even in extraneural tissue, such as the spleen and muscle.

If all else fails, neurologists consider a brain biopsy. If the diagnosis is correct, cerebral tissue shows spongiform changes. However, because of the dangers in obtaining and processing the tissue, and the absence of effective treatment, neurologists and neurosurgeons usually perform cerebral biopsies only to resolve diagnostic dilemmas or when reasonable alternative diagnoses might be amenable to treatment.

Other Spongiform Encephalopathies

Several spongiform encephalopathies, in addition to Creutzfeldt-Jakob disease, affect humans or animals. In general, their symptoms typically do not appear until after an incubation period of many years and reflect only CNS involvement. As with Creutzfeldt-Jakob disease, the symptoms consist primarily of mental deterioration accompanied by myoclonus and ataxia, and their course is relentlessly progressive and ultimately fatal.

Interspecies transmission of prion infections occurs naturally as well as during laboratory experiments. When it does, incubation time is long. In contrast, intraspecies transfer is relatively easy and incubation time is short.

Several spongiform encephalopathies have remained confined to animals. For example, *scrapie* causes sheep and goats to scrape against walls to denude themselves. (PrP^{Sc} is named after the "scrapie prion.") In *transmissible mink encephalopathy*, affected mink develop more vicious, antisocial behavior than normal, followed by progressive deterioration of motor function.

Some spongiform encephalopathies are restricted to humans, although possibly only those with a genetic susceptibility. *Fatal familial insomnia* is a recently described sleep disorder that clearly depends on a genetic vulnerability. *Kuru,* characterized by dementia, tremulousness, dysarthria, and ataxia, developed in members of the Fore Tribe of New Guinea. Until United States health officials stopped the practice, tribe members, usually women and their children preparing for cannibalism rituals, evidently infected themselves with brain tissue. The incubation was 4 years to 30 years, but once symptoms were apparent, death ensued within the year.

Bovine spongiform encephalopathy (BSE), commonly known as "mad cow disease," is the notorious veterinarian spongiform encephalopathy that struck 180,000 British cattle. BSE caused belligerence and apprehension in normally docile cows. They developed tremulousness and then ataxia before collapsing. Although its origin remains a mystery, the subsequent intraspecies transmission of BSE probably resulted from slaughterhouses' incorporating scraps of infected brain and spinal cord into animal feed (offal). The wholesale slaughter of almost 4 million cattle eradicated the epidemic in Britain; however, isolated animals with the disease, many exported from Britain, have been found in the United States, Japan, and Western Europe.

In an American counterpart of BSE, which has also been brought under control through draconian methods, *chronic wasting disease (CWD) of deer and elk* developed in animals of those species living in the Rocky Mountain states, western provinces of Canada, and as far east as Wisconsin. Affected animals lost muscle, strength, and vitality before succumbing. Because elk and deer are not carnivorous, this illness is probably transmitted by exchange of bodily fluids.

Variant Creutzfeldt-Jakob Disease

The alarm over BSE arose when several British citizens succumbed to *variant Creutzfeldt-Jakob disease* (the human counterpart of BSE). In this probable interspecies transfer of BSE, victims developed striking psychiatric disturbances, painful peripheral sensory disturbances, and ataxia that progressed to death in about one year. The psychiatric symptoms—usually

appearing first, most prominently, and progressively—consisted of dysphoria, withdrawal, and anxiety during the first 4 months; memory impairment, inattention, and aggression during the fourth through sixth months; and, before death, agitation, dementia, and psychosis with hallucinations. Aside from a minority of victims having painful paresthesias in their limbs, neurologic symptoms did not develop until the middle stage of the illness. Then they would also develop gait impairment and dysarthria. Toward the end, they would develop limb and truck ataxia, myoclonus, and finally decorticate posture. Ultimately almost 150 individuals—almost all of them British citizens or visitors—fell victim to variant Creutzfeldt-Jakob disease.

Variant Creutzfeldt-Jakob disease differs from common Creutzfeldt-Jakob disease in that its victims are younger (mean age 26 years); its course, although also fatal, is longer (average 1 year); its primary symptoms are psychiatric and sensory disturbances; EEG reveals nonspecific slowing rather than the characteristic periodic pattern; and MRI diffusion weight images usually show abnormalities in the pulvinar (a posterior portion of the thalamus). Several conditions mimic variant and common Creutzfeldt-Jakob diseases. Lithium or bismuth intoxication or thyroid (Hashimoto) encephalopathy may produce myoclonus with dementia; however, these conditions usually cause more of a delirium than dementia, and all are readily detectable with specific blood tests. Remote effects of carcinoma might also produce wasting, myoclonus, and dementia (Chapter 19). Also, physicians might consider variant Creutzfeldt-Jakob disease as one of the causes of dementia in adolescents or young adults (see Table 7-2).

Lyme Disease

Acute Lyme disease (*neuroborreliosis*), when it involves the nervous system, can cause facial palsy, headache, peripheral neuropathy, meningitis, or encephalitis. With CNS infection, patients can be delirious. In this stage, serum and CSF tests for Lyme disease are usually positive and CSF will almost always be abnormal: its typical profile consists of pleocytosis, elevated protein concentration, reduced glucose concentration, and Lyme antibodies. With antibiotic treatment, the clinical manifestations and abnormal CSF tests promptly resolve.

After antibiotic treatment of the acute illness, approximately 15% of patients remain with numerous and variable physical symptoms, such as headache, muscle and joint pain, sleep disturbances, and fatigue. These patients, who physicians label as having "chronic Lyme disease," also describe cognitive and mood disturbances, including irritability, depressed mood, inattention, and memory impairment.

Chronic Lyme symptoms remain enigmatic. Not even all patients with chronic symptoms have a persistently positive serum Lyme titer. Even so, the persistence would be analogous to life-long abnormal serologies after successful syphilis treatment. When Lyme tests are positive, titers do not correlate with memory impairments. At the same time, routine tests for systemic illnesses, such as the sedimentation rate and white cell count, are generally normal. An infectious etiology is doubtful given that several studies have shown that these patients' symptoms do not improve with repeated courses of antibiotics.

Some symptoms mimic multiple sclerosis, but the most prominent ones fall into the category of chronic fatigue syndrome (Chapter 6) or depression. Confusing matters somewhat, because the infectious agent, *Borrelia burgdorferi*, is a spirochete as in syphilis, serum FTA-ABS and VDRL tests may be positive in Lyme disease.

HIV-Associated Dementia (HAD)

The nomenclature of HAD has evolved. Previously called *AIDS dementia, AIDS dementia complex, HIV dementia*, or, according to the DSM-IV-TR, *Dementia Due to HIV Disease*, this disorder remains one of the most important complications of AIDS and a relatively frequent cause of dementia in young and middle-aged adults.

HIV infection of the brain (*encephalitis*) causes HAD. Although virologists classify HIV as "neurotropic," it primarily infects macrophages and microglia rather than neurons. In some patients, cytomegalovirus (CMV) or toxoplasmosis encephalitis or other AIDS-related condition may contribute to the cognitive impairment.

Risk factors for HAD include duration of AIDS, low CD_4 counts, and high viral loads. Ironically, because HAD develops in proportion to the duration of the illness, its prevalence has increased as treatment has improved longevity. Also, treatment has allowed HAD to develop in AIDS patients with relatively high CD_4 counts.

Manifestations

HAD causes rapid decline, over weeks to a few months, in three domains: cognition, behavior, and motor ability. In contrast, language function, at least initially, is preserved, and patients remain articulate. Patients typically develop impaired memory and shortened concentration that are soon accompanied by

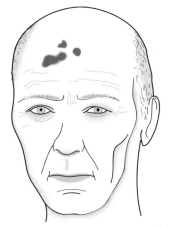

FIGURE 7-9 ■ Kaposi's sarcoma lesions, which appear as small, slightly raised, dry, and purple or red-brown patches, suggest acquired immunodeficiency syndrome (AIDS). They are most often found in homosexual male AIDS patients.

psychomotor retardation, apathy, and withdrawal from social interactions. A clinical caveat is that HAD-induced blunted affect, social withdrawal, and vegetative symptoms, such as anorexia and sleeplessness, can mimic depression.

Slowness and clumsiness impair patients' walking. They also lose dexterity and their large limb movements slow. The development of psychomotor retardation and gait impairment is so consistent that neurologists consider HAD a prime example of subcortical dementia.

HAD can cause or worsen depression, mania, and psychosis. Although AIDS patients' suicide rate is 17 to 36 times greater than in a healthy population, some of these suicides are attributable, as in Huntington's disease, to impetuous behavior and impaired judgment rather than depression or despair.

Patients often decline into a persistent vegetative state, in which they are akinetic, severely demented, incontinent, paraplegic, and mute. Seizures, myoclonus, slowed ocular saccades and pursuits, and extrapyramidal signs may complicate this portion of their downhill course. In addition, patients' systemic symptoms, such as weight loss and fever, further burden their already impaired cognitive and emotional status. Although the purple plaques of Kaposi's sarcoma (Fig. 7-9) are characteristic of AIDS, they are not a marker for dementia.

Treatment

Highly active antiretroviral therapy (HAART), a combination of several antiviral medicines administered on a complex schedule, actually improves cognitive function in HAD patients and prolongs their lives.

Despite its benefits, HAART requires a complicated, arduous regimen that many patients with HAD, especially if they also have depression, cannot follow. Several of the components of the regimen, such as efavirenz and zidovudine, can cause psychosis. Those metabolized by the cytochrome P450 enzyme system potentially create adverse drug-drug interactions. Furthermore, although some interfere with methadone and can precipitate opiate withdrawal symptoms, others produce neuropathy or, because they interfere with mitochondria metabolism, myopathy (see Chapters 5 and 6).

As for treatment of the neurobehavioral symptoms, stimulants, such as dextroamphetamine and methylphenidate, may ameliorate psychomotor retardation and fatigue. Stimulants may also reverse social withdrawal and improve patients' mood. Physicians can administer antidepressants and antipsychotics for the usual indications even though the underlying problem is HAD.

Testing

In HAD, both CTs and MRIs show cerebral atrophy with enlarged ventricles and basal ganglia abnormalities. In addition, MRIs may also show nonspecific scattered white matter abnormalities.

CSF typically reveals a mild lymphocytic pleocytosis, normal or slightly elevated protein concentration, and, as a reflection of inflammation, oligoclonal bands. If tested, CSF shows HIV. Physicians measure the CD_4 count and viral load in the blood. Depending on the circumstance, they might perform blood tests for illnesses, in addition to AIDS, that are associated with drug abuse or unsafe sex, such as hepatitis, bacterial endocarditis, and syphilis.

At autopsy, the brain is atrophic and pale. Changes are most apparent in the frontal lobes and basal ganglia. Microscopic examination shows perivascular infiltrates, gliosis of the cerebral cortex, demyelination, microglial nodules, and multinucleated giant cells. HIV can be isolated from the brains and CSF of virtually all patients with HAD. Overall, clinical changes outweigh histologic abnormalities.

AIDS-Induced Cerebral Lesions

Infectious or neoplastic AIDS-induced cerebral lesions, like other cerebral lesions, cause headache, focal seizures, lateralized signs, and increased intracranial pressure. Moreover, they can exacerbate HAD.

Another caveat is that physicians are liable to misdiagnose headaches as a manifestation of depression or "tension." In fact, headaches are a particularly ominous symptom in AIDS patients. The majority of AIDS patients who develop them harbor serious underlying pathology, such as cryptococcal meningitis and cerebral toxoplasmosis.

Second to HIV, *Toxoplasma gondii* causes the most common AIDS-related CNS infections, *cerebral toxoplasmosis*. This protozoon typically produces multiple ring-shaped enhancing lesions that are readily detectable by CT or MRI (see Fig. 20-11). Because toxoplasmosis is so common in AIDS, imaging studies can be almost diagnostic, and antibiotics are highly effective, neurologists usually prescribe an antibiotic trial and reserve a cerebral biopsy for patients who do not respond.

Other opportunistic organisms that cause cerebral lesions in AIDS patients include fungi, such as *Candida* and *Aspergillus*, and viruses, such as CMV and polyoma virus. In addition, a DNA *JC virus* causes *progressive multifocal leukoencephalopathy (PML)*. As its name suggests, PML produces multiple widespread, but sometimes confluent, lesions in the white (*leuko*) matter, which is the myelin, of the brain and spinal cord. PML typically produces combinations of cognitive impairment, hemiparesis, spasticity, blindness, and ataxia. In AIDS patients, the development of PML is near terminal complication. After the diagnosis, their mean life expectancy is 4 months.

Although the neurologic findings and MRI appearance of PML mimic multiple sclerosis (see Chapter 15), which is another demyelinating illness of young adults, the vastly different clinical situations, course of the illnesses, and HIV testing readily eliminate confusion. Although most opportunistic infections develop in AIDS patients only once their CD_4 count decreases to below 200 cells/mm^3, PML frequently develops in AIDS patients who have more than 400 cells/mm^3. PML also develops in patients with immunosuppression from leukemia, lymphoma, chemotherapy, and organ transplant regimens. In PML, whatever the underlying condition, the CSF usually contains JC virus nuclei acid, which reflects the etiology and serves as a diagnostic marker.

HIV disease patients who also contract syphilis tend to develop virulent acute syphilitic meningitis and meningovascular complications. However, because antibiotics are so effective for these patients, syphilis' primary or secondary stages rarely progress to a tertiary stage, such as tabes dorsalis.

The most common cerebral neoplasm-complicating HIV disease is *primary cerebral lymphoma*. Although this tumor's clinical and CT features mimic toxoplasmosis, it occurs less frequently and usually presents as a solitary lesion. Compared to common systemic lymphomas, primary cerebral lymphomas respond poorly to radiotherapy, steroids, and other treatment. In HIV disease, lymphomas also develop in the spinal canal and compress the spinal cord. Less frequently, gliomas, metastatic Kaposi's sarcoma, and other malignancies complicate HIV disease.

Other AIDS-Related Conditions

Depending on which portion of the nervous system is primarily infected, patients can develop HIV encephalitis, myelitis, or meningitis. Similarly, all CNS tissue, especially CSF, is infectious.

The spinal cord is subject to HIV infection, as well as the development of lymphomas. Spinal cord infection (*myelitis*) with HIV, *vacuolar myelopathy*, produces paraparesis, the Romberg sign, and other indications of spinal cord injury. The damage in vacuolar myelopathy is located predominantly in the posterior columns (the fasciculus gracilis and f. cuneatus [see Chapter 2]). Although this pattern resembles combined system disease, vitamin B_{12} treatment does not relieve HIV myelitis.

A virus related to HIV, the *human T-cell lymphotrophic virus type 1* (*HTLV-1*), similarly infects the spinal cord and causes paraparesis; however, it does not lead to cognitive impairment. As with HIV, HTLV-1 is transmitted sexually and by blood transfusion. Because HTLV-1 myelopathy is endemic in the Caribbean region and Africa, it had previously been known as "tropical spastic paraparesis."

AIDS patients with or without dementia may develop *meningitis* from HIV infection, tuberculosis (TB), syphilis, or, most commonly, cryptococcosis. In addition to causing headache, fever, and malaise, meningitis in AIDS patients brings on delirium.

The PNS is also frequently involved. HIV or CMV infections lead to polyneuropathy, a Guillain-Barré syndrome, mononeuropathies, and myopathies. In AIDS patients, many of these conditions, unlike their usual presentation, are extraordinarily painful. In addition, some painful neuropathies are medication-induced.

PSEUDODEMENTIA

When a psychiatric disturbance produces, mimics, exacerbates, or merely coexists with cognitive impairment, the condition is termed *pseudodementia*. Depression most often mimics cognitive impairment, but other psychiatric illnesses, such as anxiety or schizophrenia, may produce the same effect.

However, when diagnosing and treating Alzheimer's disease patients, physicians should separate dementia from depression. Depression should not significantly impair performance on cognitive testing if testers provide enough time and encouragement.

Also, when depression seems to accompany dementia, its symptoms rarely reach the level of a major mood disorder.

On the other hand, a potential pitfall for the physician evaluating a patient with cognitive impairment is to disregard affective and vegetative disturbances. Another pitfall is overestimating the significance of age-related neurologic test results, such as mild EEG slowing and cerebral atrophy on CTs or MRIs. The physician making these errors might miss the opportunity to treat the patient for depression.

Perhaps the most important aspect of patients' seeming to have depression-induced cognitive impairments is that they develop dementia from Alzheimer's disease almost six times as frequently as their age-adjusted counterparts. Furthermore, the risk of eventually developing dementia rises with increasing numbers of depression and bipolar episodes. Thus, contrary to older medical literature citing pseudodementia as the most frequent "correctable cause of dementia," both pseudodementia and depression often act as harbingers of Alzheimer's disease.

TOXIC-METABOLIC ENCEPHALOPATHY

Characteristics

Toxic-metabolic encephalopathy, a term commonly applied by neurologists, consists of a fluctuating state of consciousness, confusion, and other mental disturbances induced by an exogenous or endogenous *chemical* imbalance. When an evaluation identifies the cause, neurologists specify the condition, such as uremic or hepatic encephalopathy. They usually call similar disturbances caused by infectious agents "encephalitis," and those without an identifiable cause, "acute confusional state."

In DSM-IV-TR, the criteria for *Delirium* due to specific medical conditions require primarily a disturbance of the level of consciousness (usually reduced awareness and attention span), and either change in cognition (such as disorientation) or development of perceptual deficits. These symptoms, which neurologists also accept, must have developed over hours to days and subsequently fluctuate. Although the two labels—delirium and toxic-metabolic encephalopathy—refer to almost identical conditions, this text uses the latter term because it conforms to most neurologists' practice.

Toxic-metabolic encephalopathy can be distinguished from dementia primarily by the patient's level of consciousness acutely deteriorating and subsequently fluctuating. For example, dementia takes at least 6 months or longer to appear in the most rapidly developing illnesses, such as Creutzfeldt-Jakob disease. Once individuals develop dementia, the cognitive impairment remains on a stable, although deteriorating, course that may be exacerbated by a toxic-metabolic encephalopathy. In contrast, those with toxic-metabolic encephalopathy develop confusion and obtundation over several hours to days. Their sensorium fluctuates with the vicissitudes of the underlying illness and its response to treatment. Also, the underlying illness may first cause seizures or coma. Partial spontaneous improvements allow patients to regain their awareness; however, even when alert, they are apt to be inattentive, disoriented, and disorganized. Also, they are apt to misinterpret stimuli and develop delusions and hallucinations. Although most patients are at least sleepy and oblivious to their surroundings, sometimes patients' awareness is abnormally heightened, and they are hypervigilant.

Physical features associated with toxic-metabolic encephalopathy also distinguish it from dementia. Toxic-metabolic encephalopathy typically causes signs of autonomic system hyperactivity, such as tachycardia, sweating, and fever. Like the depressed sensorium, autonomic system hyperactivity develops suddenly and then fluctuates. Depending on the etiology,

specific physical findings, routine laboratory tests, and EEG may reveal characteristic abnormalities.

Young children, individuals older than 65 years, and those with pre-existing dementia or brain injury are particularly susceptible to toxic-metabolic encephalopathy. In addition, immobility, hearing impairment, and visual impairment intensify the symptoms. Whether or not dementia pre-exists, manifestations of toxic-metabolic encephalopathy are similar.

Despite successful treatment of the underlying medical problem, the encephalopathy can lag in its improvement or occasionally deteriorate (Fig. 7-10). If undetected, chronic encephalopathy can cause low-grade cognitive impairment and mimic dementia or even depression. Renal, hepatic, or pulmonary insufficiency often leads to such cognitive impairment.

Most physical abnormalities accompanying a toxic-metabolic encephalopathy are nonspecific, but some point to a specific diagnosis and allow an astute bedside diagnosis. For example, in Wernicke-Korsakoff syndrome, patients have oculomotor palsies, nystagmus, ataxia, and polyneuropathy. Patients with hepatic or uremic encephalopathy have *asterixis* (Fig. 7-11). Those with uremia, penicillin intoxication, meperidine (Demerol) treatment, and other metabolic encephalopathies have myoclonus. Narcotic and barbiturate

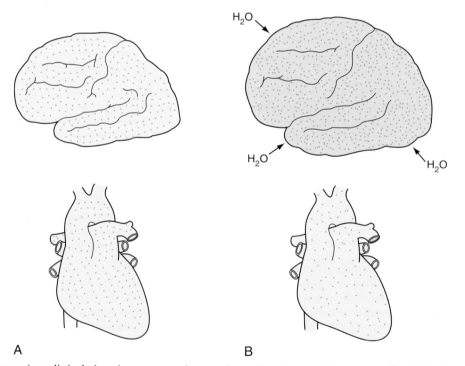

A   B

FIGURE 7-10 ■ A distressing clinical situation occurs when patients deteriorate—become confused, lethargic, and agitated—after apparent correction of certain metabolic abnormalities. *A*, As portrayed in the sketches on the left, in cases of uremia or hyperglycemia, the brain and blood contain an approximately equal concentration of solute (dots). *B*, Overly vigorous dialysis or insulin administration clears solute more rapidly from the blood than the brain, leaving solute concentration in the brain much greater than in the blood. The concentration gradient causes free water to move into the brain, which produces cerebral edema.

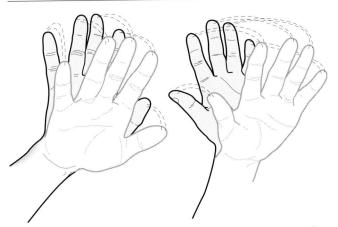

FIGURE 7-11 ■ Asterixis, a sign of a toxic-metabolic encephalopathy, is elicited by having patients extend their arms and hands, as though they were stopping traffic. Their hands intermittently quickly move downward and slowly return, as though waving good-bye.

intoxication causes miosis (contracted pupils), and amphetamines, atropine, and other sympathomimetic drugs dilate pupils.

In almost all cases of toxic-metabolic encephalopathy, EEGs show pronounced slowing and other nonspecific abnormalities. These changes begin at the onset of mental aberrations and continue throughout the course of the illness. One EEG finding suggestive of a specific etiology is that triphasic waves suggest a hepatic, uremic, or other metabolic encephalopathy. CTs and MRIs are normal unless they show atrophy or a coexisting structural lesion, such as a subdural hematoma. CSF is abnormal in meningitis, encephalitis, subarachnoid hemorrhage, and severe hepatic encephalopathy; however, it is normal in most toxic-metabolic encephalopathies.

Causes

Of numerous potential causes of toxic-metabolic encephalopathy, a limited number explain the majority of cases in acute care hospitals (Table 7-6). Reading the chart will usually reveal the diagnosis. Many cases result from readily apparent organ failure; iatrogenic causes; or are self-induced, occasionally as a suicide attempt. Especially in older patients, some may be the first manifestation of a fatal illness.

Medicines and illicit drugs are outstanding offenders. The offending medicine might even have been administered in a small dose, but in a previously unexposed patient. Medicine-related problems also include interference by a drug with hepatic metabolism, other drug-drug interactions, or absorption of ocular or topical medicines. In particular, medicines for CNS disorders—anticholinergic, antiepileptic, antiparkinson,

TABLE 7-6 ■ **Commonly Cited Frequent Causes of Toxic-Metabolic Encephalopathy**

Narcotics and alcohol
Medications
Major surgery
Hepatic or uremic encephalopathy
Fluid or electrolyte imbalance, especially dehydration
Pneumonia or other non-neurologic infection

hypnotic, narcotics, and psychotropics—are the ones most likely to produce an encephalopathy. Antihypertensives represent another dangerous group because, through orthostatic hypotension and sometimes dehydration, they can produce mental status changes.

Another category is withdrawal of medicines or other substances. Unlike the depressed sensorium associated with typical toxic-metabolic encephalopathy, withdrawal from alcohol, benzodiazepines, narcotics, or nicotine causes agitation, confusion, hallucinations, and hypervigilance. Also, withdrawal from alcohol, barbiturates, and benzodiazepines causes seizures. Physicians can reverse these disturbances, at least temporarily, by restoring the missing substance or providing a reasonable facsimile, such as methadone to a narcotic addict or a nicotine patch to an inveterate cigarette smoker.

Hepatic Encephalopathy

A particularly interesting and relatively common variety of toxic-metabolic encephalopathy is *hepatic encephalopathy*. If a liver fails, mental function and consciousness steadily decline. Mild confusion with either lethargy or, less frequently, agitation may precede coma and overtly abnormal liver function tests. Asterixis and EEG changes characteristically develop.

Hepatic encephalopathy has traditionally been attributed to an elevated concentration of ammonia (NH_3). This theory is consistent with the common situation of patients with cirrhosis developing hepatic encephalopathy following gastrointestinal bleeding or after meals with a high protein content, such as red meat. In both these situations, because of cirrhosis-induced portal hypertension, NH_3 released by protein in food or blood is shunted into the systemic circulation. Being small and nonionic (uncharged), NH_3 readily penetrates the blood–brain barrier. Treatment has been directed at converting ammonia (NH_3) to ammonium (NH_4^+), which is ionic and unable to penetrate the blood–brain barrier.

Alternative explanations for hepatic encephalopathy include the following: production of false neurotransmitters, substances that bind to benzodiazepine-gamma aminobutyric acid (GABA) receptors and increase GABA activity, and disturbances in cellular energy generating systems. Clinicians sometimes reduce hepatic encephalopathy when they give flumazenil, a benzodiazepine antagonist that interferes with benzodiazepine-GABA receptors.

REFERENCES

Age-Related Changes and Mild Cognitive Impairment

1. Clarfield AM: The decreasing prevalence of reversible dementias. Arch Intern Med 163:2219–2229, 2003.
2. Grigoletto F, Zappala G, Anderson DW, et al: Norms for the Mini-Mental State Examination in a healthy population. Neurology 53:315–320, 1999.
3. Knopman DS, Boeve BF, Petersen RC: Essentials of the proper diagnoses of mild cognitive impairment, dementia, and major subtypes of dementia. Mayo Clin Proc 78:1290–1308, 2003.
4. Knopman DS, DeKosky ST, Cummings JL, et al: Practice parameter: Diagnosis of dementia (an evidence-based review). Neurology 56:1143–1153, 2001.
5. Morris JC, Storandt M, Miller JP, et al: Mild cognitive impairment represents early-stage Alzheimer's disease. Arch Neurol 58:397–405, 2001.
6. Mungas D, Marshall SC, Weldon M, et al: Age and education correction of Mini-Mental State Examination for English- and Spanish-speaking elderly. Neurology 46:700–706, 1996.
7. Petersen RC, Stevens JC, Ganguli, et al: Practice parameter: Early detection of dementia: Mild cognitive impairment (an evidence-based review). Report of the Quality Standards Subcommittee of the American Academy of Neurology. Neurology 56:1133–1142, 2001.
8. Petersen RC, Thomas RG, Grundman M, et al: Vitamin E and donepezil for the treatment of mild cognitive impairment. N Engl J Med 352:2379–2388, 2005.

Alzheimer's Disease

9. Cummings JL: Alzheimer's disease. N Engl J Med 351:56–67, 2004.
10. Doody RS, Stevens JC, Beck C, et al: Practice parameter: Management of dementia (an evidence-based review). Report of the Quality Standards Subcommittee of the American Academy of Neurology. Neurology 56:1154–1166, 2001.
11. Dubinsky RM, Stein AC, Lyons K: Practice parameter: Risk of driving and Alzheimer's disease. Report of the Quality Standards Subcommittee of the American Academy of Neurology. Neurology 54:2205–2211, 2000.
12. Folstein MR, Folstein SE, McHugh PR: "Mini-Mental State": A practical method for grading the cognitive state of patients for the clinician. J Psychiatr Res 12:189–198, 1975.
13. Fleminger S, Oliver DL, Lovestone S, et al: Head injury as a risk factor for Alzheimer's disease. J Neurol Neurosurg Psychiatry 74:857–862, 2003.
14. Galvin JE, Lee VMY, Trojanowski JQ: Synucleinopathies: Clinical and pathological implications. Arch Neurol 58:186–190, 2001.
15. Holmes C, Wilkinson D, Dean C, et al: The efficacy of donepezil in the treatment of neuropsychiatric symptoms of Alzheimer's disease. Neurology 63:213–219, 2004.
16. Kawas CH: Early Alzheimer's disease. N Engl J Med 349:1056–1063, 2003.
17. Marson DC, Chatterjee A, Ingram KK, et al: Toward a neurologic model of competency: Cognitive predictors of capacity to consent in Alzheimer's disease using three different legal standards. Neurology 46:666–672, 1996.
18. Morris MC, Evans DA, Bienias JL, et al: Consumption of fish and n-3 fatty acids and risk of incident Alzheimer disease. Arch Neurol 60:940–946, 2003.
19. Ott BR, Heindel WC, Papandonatos GD: A survey of voter participation by cognitively impaired elderly patients. Neurology 60:1546–1548, 2003.
20. Paulsen JS, Salmon DP, Thal LJ, et al: Incidence of and risk factors for hallucinations and delusions in patients with probable AD. Neurology 54:1965–1971, 2000.
21. Reisberg B, Doody R, Stoffler A, et al: Memantine in moderate-to-severe Alzheimer's disease. N Engl J Med 348:1333–1341, 2003.
22. Rocchi A, Pellegrini S, Siciliano G, et al: Causative and susceptibility genes for Alzheimer's disease: A review. Brain Res Bull 61:1–24, 2003.
23. Rosen WG, Mohs RC, Davis KL: A new rating scale for Alzheimer's disease. Am J Psychiatry 141:1356–1364, 1984.
24. Schupf N, Kapell D, Nightingale B, et al: Specificity of the fivefold increase in AD in mothers of adults with Down syndrome. Neurology 57:979–984, 2001.
25. Teri L, Logsdon RG, Peskin E, et al: Treatment of agitation in AD: A randomized, placebo-controlled clinical trial. Neurology 55:1271–1278, 2000.
26. Verghese J, Lipton RB, Katz MJ, et al: Leisure activities and the risk of dementia in the elderly. N Engl J Med 348:2508–2516, 2003.
27. Wilson RS, Evans DA, Bienias JL, et al: Proneness to psychological distress is associated with risk of Alzheimer's disease. Neurology 61:1479–1485, 2003.

HIV-Associated Dementia

28. Geraci AP, Simpson DM: Neurological manifestations of HIV-1 infection in the HAART era. Compr Ther 27:232–241, 2001.
29. Shor-Posner G: Cognitive function in HIV-1-infected drug users. J Acquir Immune Defic Syndr 25(Suppl 1): S70–73, 2000.
30. Treisman GJ, Kaplin AL: Neurologic and psychiatric complications of antiretroviral agents. AIDS 16:1201–1215, 2002.

Dementia with Lewy Bodies

31. Fernandez HH, Trieschmann ME, Burke MA, et al: Quetiapine for psychosis in Parkinson's disease versus dementia with Lewy bodies. J Clin Psychiatry 63:513–515, 2002.
32. Geser F, Wenning GK, Poewe W, et al: How to diagnose dementia with Lewy bodies: State of the art. Mov Disord 12(Suppl 12):S11–S20, 2005.
33. Harding AJ, Broe GA, Halliday GM: Visual hallucinations in Lewy body disease relate to Lewy bodies in the temporal lobe. Brain 125:391–403, 2002.
34. McKeith IG, Dicjson DW, Lowe J, et al: Diagnosis and management of dementia with Lewy bodies: Third report of the DLB consortium. Neurology 65:1863–1872, 2005.
35. Simard M, Reekum RV, Cohen T: A review of the cognitive and behavioral symptoms in dementia with Lewy bodies. J Neuropsychiatry Clin Neurosci 12:425–450, 2000.

Depression and Pseudodementia

36. Kessing LV, Andersen PK: Does the risk of developing dementia increase with the number of episodes in patients with depressive disorder and in patients with bipolar disorders? J Neurol Neurosurg Psychiatry 75:1662–1666, 2004.
37. Powlishta KK, Storandt M, Mandernach TA, et al: Absence of effect of depression on cognitive performance in early-stage Alzheimer's disease 61:1265–1268, 2004.
38. Visser PJ, Verhey FRJ, Ponds RWHM, et al: Distinction between preclinical Alzheimer's disease and depression. J Am Geriatr Soc 48:479–484, 2000.

Frontotemporal Dementia

39. Hodges JR, Davies RR, Xuereb JH, et al: Clinicopathological correlates in frontotemporal dementia. Ann Neurol 56:399–406, 2004.
40. Kucharski A: History of frontal lobotomy in the United States, 1935–1955. Neurosurgery 14:762–772, 1984.

Lyme Disease

41. Kaplan RF, Trevino RP, Johnson GM, et al: Cognitive function in post-treatment Lyme disease. Do additional antibiotics help? Neurology 60:1916–1922, 2003.
42. Klempner MS, Hu LT, Evans J, et al: Two controlled trials of antibiotic treatment in patients with persistent symptoms and a history of Lyme disease. N Engl J Med 345:85–92, 2001.

Prion Illnesses and Related Disorders

43. Chong JY, Rowland LP, Utiger RD: Hashimoto encephalopathy. Arch Neurol 60:164–171, 2003.
44. Henry C, Knight R: Clinical features of variant Creutzfeldt-Jakob disease. Rev Med Virol 12:143–150, 2002.
45. Prusiner SB: Neurodegenerative diseases and prions. N Engl J Med 344:1516–1526, 2001.
46. Rabinovici GD, Wang PN, Levin J, et al: First symptom in sporadic Creutzfeldt-Jakob disease. Neurology 66:286–287, 2006.

47. Snowden JS, Mann DMA, Neary D: Distinct neuropsychological characteristics in Creutzfeldt-Jakob disease. J Neurol Neurosurg Psychiatry 73:686–694, 2002.
48. Spencer DM, Knight RSG, Will RG: First hundred cases of variant Creutzfeldt-Jakob disease: Retrospective case note review of early psychiatric and neurologic features. BMJ 324:1479–1482, 2002.
49. Williams ES, Miller MW: Chronic wasting disease in deer and elk. Rev Sci Tech Off 1:305–316, 2002.

Toxic-Metabolic Encephalopathy

50. Abramowicz M (ed): Drugs that may cause cognitive disorders in the elderly. Med Lett 42:111–112, 2000.
51. Inouye SK, Bogardua ST, Charpentier PA, et al: A multicomponent intervention to prevent delirium in hospitalized older patients. N Engl J Med 340:669–676, 1999.
52. Mayer SA, Chong JY, Ridgway E, et al: Delirium from nicotine withdrawal in neuro-ICU patients. Neurology 57:551–553, 2001.
53. Riordan SM, Williams R: Treatment of hepatic encephalopathy. N Engl J Med 337:473–479, 1997.
54. Trzepacz PT, Mulsant BH, Dew MA, et al: Is delirium different when it occurs in dementia? J Neuropsychiatry Clin Neurosci 10:199–204, 1998.

Vascular Dementia

55. Ballard C, Neill D, O'Brien J, et al: Anxiety, depression and psychosis in vascular dementia: prevalence and associations. J Affect Disord 59:97–106, 2000.
56. Groves WC, Brandt J, Steinberg M, et al: Vascular dementia and Alzheimer's disease: Is there a difference? J Neuropsychiatry Clin Neurosci 12:305–315, 2000.

Miscellaneous

57. Black DW: Pathologic laughter: A review of the literature. J Nerv Ment Dis 170:67–71, 1982.
58. Blake PY, Pincus JH, Buckner C: Neurologic abnormalities in murderers. Neurology 45:1641–1647, 1995.
59. Lair L, Naidech AM: Modern neuropsychiatric presentation of neurosyphilis. Neurology 63:1331–1333, 2004.
60. Newman MF, Kirchner JL, Phillips-Bute B, et al: Longitudinal assessment of neurocognitive function after coronary-artery bypass surgery. N Engl J Med 344:395–402, 2001.
61. Singer C, Lang AE, Suchowersky O: Adult-onset subacute sclerosing panencephalitis. Mov Disord 12:342–353, 1997.
62. Verghese J, Lipton RB, Hall CB, et al: Abnormality of gait as a predictor of non-Alzheimer's dementia. N Engl J Med 347:1761–1768, 2002.
63. Savolainen S, Hurskainen H, Paljarvi L et al: Five-year outcome of normal pressure hydrocephalus with or without a shunt: Predictive value of the clinical signs, neuropsychological evaluation and infusion test. Acta Neurochir (Wien) 144:515–523, 2002.

Questions and Answers

1. Which of the following statements is true regarding individuals with mild cognitive impairment (MCI)?
   a. They have impairment of their social or occupational activities.
   b. They are at risk for Alzheimer's disease, but not illnesses, such as combined system disease, that cause dementia.
   c. Approximately 10% to 20% progress to Alzheimer's disease each year.
   d. The risk factors associated with their progressing to dementia are different than those for developing Alzheimer's disease.

   Answer: c. Each year, approximately 10% to 20% of MCI individuals progress to dementia—almost always from Alzheimer's disease. While they maintain their social and occupational activities, MCI individuals cannot be diagnosed as having dementia. The risk factors associated with MCI individuals progressing to dementia are similar to those for all individuals developing Alzheimer's disease. For example, individuals carrying the Apo E4-E4 are likely to progress to dementia. Even though the cognitive changes are mild, physicians should have MCI patients undergo tests for correctable causes of dementia.

2. Advancing age leads to loss of neurons in the cerebral cortex and many deep structures. Which of the following structures is not subject to age-related neuron loss?
   a. Locus ceruleus
   b. Suprachiasmatic nucleus
   c. Substantia nigra
   d. Nucleus basalis of Meynert
   e. Mamillary bodies

   Answer: e. Despite advancing age, the mamillary bodies remain largely unscathed. Changes in the other structures contribute to age-related disturbances in affect (locus ceruleus), sleep (locus ceruleus and suprachiasmatic nucleus), and locomotion (substantia nigra).

3. In a 70-year-old man who has normal cognitive and physical function, which sensation is most likely to be lost?
   a. Joint position
   b. Vibration
   c. Pain
   d. Temperature

   Answer: b. In normal individuals older than 65 years, vibration sensation is lost to a greater degree than other sensations. Although loss of position sense is less pronounced, that loss is more troublesome because it leads to gait impairment and falls. In contrast, pain and temperature sensations are relatively well preserved.

4. The diagnosis of normal pressure hydrocephalus (NPH) has received much attention in the literature because installation of a ventricular-peritoneal shunt may correct the dementia. Which statement is the most correct regarding conditions that predispose a patient to NPH?
   a. Hypothyroidism causes dementia, gait apraxia, and incontinence.
   b. Meningitis causes obstructive hydrocephalus that mimics NPH.
   c. Subarachnoid hemorrhage, like meningitis, causes obstructive hydrocephalus that mimics NPH.
   d. No particular illness seems to be the cause in the majority of NPH cases.

   Answer: d. Both meningitis and subarachnoid hemorrhage can cause communicating hydrocephalus and sometimes NPH. However, most cases of NPH are idiopathic. Unless patients have had preceding meningitis or subarachnoid hemorrhage, only 25%, at most, benefit from placement of a shunt.

5. True or False: A cerebral cortex biopsy assists in the routine diagnosis of Alzheimer's disease.

   Answer: False. Although a diagnosis is often highly desirable, a cerebral cortex biopsy cannot provide a diagnosis in Alzheimer's disease because its changes are quantitative rather than qualitative. For example, normal aged brains contain the characteristic plaques and tangles—although in lesser concentrations and different distributions.

6. With which feature is Alzheimer's disease dementia most closely associated?
   a. Large ventricles
   b. Increased concentration of plaques
   c. Increased concentration of tangles
   d. Degree of synapse loss

   Answer: d. Although neurofibrillary tangles and, to a lesser extent, plaques are associated with dementia, loss of synapses is most closely correlated with dementia. On a macroscopic level, atrophy of the hippocampus is most closely associated with Alzheimer's disease.

7. A 75-year-old man who had played professional football stated that over the past 3 to 5 years he has become generally weaker and has lost muscle bulk, particularly in his hands. He has also lost the ability to ride a bicycle. Nevertheless, he is still able to play golf, walk a mile, and perform his activities of daily living. A routine medical evaluation reveals no particular abnormality. Which is the most likely explanation for his symptoms?
   a. He merely has normal, age-related muscle and coordination changes.
   b. Professional football has led to neurologic complications.
   c. The problem is not trauma itself, but CNS trauma that led to an ALS-like condition.
   d. He has an undetected neuropathy.

Answer: a. His loss of muscle bulk, particularly in the intrinsic hand muscles, generalized decrease in strength, and mild incoordination all represent normal age-related changes. Advanced age, certain occupations (such as carpentry), and injuries from many sports (such as boxing) lead to cervical spondylosis. Whatever its cause, cervical spondylosis produces weakness and atrophy of hand muscles and gait impairment. ALS has not been associated with such injuries.

8. What is the pattern of inheritance (a–d) of the following diseases (1–4)?
   1. Wilson's
   2. Huntington's
   3. Familial Creutzfeldt-Jakob
   4. Familial Alzheimer's
   a. Sex-linked recessive
   b. Autosomal recessive
   c. Autosomal dominant
   d. None of the above

Answers: 1-b, 2-c, 3-c, 4-c.

9. Which feature is *not* common to the dementia of Alzheimer's disease and trisomy syndrome?
   a. An abnormal gene carried on chromosome 21
   b. Low concentrations of cerebral choline acetyltransferase
   c. Amyloid precursor protein (APP) abnormalities
   d. Low concentrations of cerebral acetylcholine
   e. Abnormalities in the nucleus basalis of Meynert
   f. Heritability
   g. Abundant plaques and tangles

Answer: f. Alzheimer's disease often develops in families. In 5% or fewer cases, Alzheimer's disease is associated with the presenilin genes 1 and 2 (transmitted by chromosomes 14 and 1, respectively) or the APP gene (transmitted by chromosome 21); it follows an autosomal dominant pattern; and symptoms appear in relatively young patients (e.g., 40 to 65 years old). Although trisomy 21, Down's syndrome, conveys an almost certain risk of all features of Alzheimer's disease, it is virtually never inherited from a parent.

10. Which enzyme converts amyloid precursor protein (APP) to αAPP and βAPP?
   a. Monamine oxidase
   b. Tyrosine hydroxylase
   c. Secretase
   d. Catecholamine transferase

Answer: c. α-secretase converts APP to αAPP and β-secretase converts APP to βAPP.

11. Which enzyme converts βAPP to amyloid β-peptide (Aβ)?
   a. Monamine oxidase
   b. Tyrosine hydroxylase
   c. Secretase
   d. Catecholamine transferase

Answer: c. A series of secretase enzymes cleaves APP into a soluble and insoluble amyloid. γ-secretase converts βAPP to Aβ, which is the insoluble, major constituent of amyloid plaques.

12. Match the histologic finding in Alzheimer's disease with its description.
   1. Paired, hyperphosphorylated helical filaments
   2. Cluster of degenerating nerve terminals with an amyloid core
   3. Group of neurons beneath the globus pallidus
   a. Neurofibrillary tangles
   b. Neuritic plaque
   c. Substantia innominata or nucleus basalis of Meynert

Answers: 1-a, 2-b, 3-c.

13. Which variety of amnesia is typically accompanied by a peripheral neuropathy?
   a. Alcohol-related neurologic changes
   b. Alzheimer's disease
   c. Vascular dementia
   d. Traumatic brain injury

Answer: a. Wernicke-Korsakoff syndrome is probably the result of alcohol-related nutritional deprivation. At its onset, Wernicke-Korsakoff syndrome consists of amnesia, rather than dementia, accompanied by oculomotor gaze palsy, nystagmus, ataxia, and neuropathy. In time, alcoholism leads to dementia.

14. Which is the most common EEG finding in patients with early Alzheimer's disease?
    a. Theta and delta activity
    b. Periodic sharp-wave complexes
    c. High-voltage fast activity
    d. Normal or slight slowing of the background activity
    e. K complexes
    f. Rapid eye movement (REM) activity

Answer: d. Early Alzheimer's disease creates little or no change in the EEG. Moreover, its changes overlap those attributable to older age or minimal cognitive impairment. Thus, the EEG is not a good diagnostic test for Alzheimer's disease. Theta and delta activity and, particularly, K complexes are associated most often with sleep; however, theta and delta activity can indicate structural lesions or metabolic aberrations. Periodic sharp-wave complexes are a hallmark of Creutzfeldt-Jakob disease.

15. With which condition is cerebral atrophy, as detected by CT or MRI, most closely associated?
    a. Alzheimer's disease
    b. Intellectual impairment
    c. Old age

Answer: c. Although cerebral atrophy is closely correlated with advanced age and numerous neurologic illnesses, it has a poor correlation with Alzheimer's disease or minimal cognitive impairment. Alzheimer's disease is most closely associated with an enlarged third ventricle and atrophy of the hippocampus.

16. Which two conditions feature α-synuclein?
    a. Alzheimer's disease
    b. Parkinson's disease
    c. Dementia with Lewy bodies
    d. Frontotemporal dementia
    e. Huntington's disease

Answers: b, c. Lewy bodies characterize the histology of both Parkinson's disease and dementia with Lewy bodies. These round, eosinophilic, intracytoplasmic inclusions stain for α-synuclein whether they are located in the basal ganglia in Parkinson's disease or the cerebral cortex in dementia with Lewy bodies. In other words, α-synuclein is the intraneuronal protein aggregate in Parkinson's disease and dementia with Lewy bodies.

17. Which two conditions feature intraneuronal tau proteins?
    a. Alzheimer's disease
    b. Parkinson's disease
    c. Dementia with Lewy bodies
    d. Frontotemporal dementia
    e. Huntington's disease

Answers: a, d. Tau acts as a microtubule binding protein. In contrast to the preceding question about α-synuclein, tau is the intraneuronal protein aggregate in Alzheimer's disease and frontotemporal dementia.

18. From which area of the brain do the majority of cerebral cortex cholinergic fibers originate?
    a. Hippocampus
    b. Basal ganglia
    c. Frontal lobe
    d. Nucleus basalis of Meynert

Answer: d

19–22. What is the effect of the following substances on cerebral acetylcholine (ACh) activity?

19. Cholinesterase inhibitors that penetrate the blood–brain barrier
20. Scopolamine
21. Organic phosphate insecticides
22. Physostigmine
    a. Increases ACh activity
    b. Decreases ACh activity
    c. Does not change ACh activity

Answers: 19-a. Centrally acting cholinesterase inhibitors, such as donepezil (Aricept), which are often prescribed as treatment for Alzheimer's disease, increase cerebral ACh activity. In contrast, peripherally acting anticholinesterases, such as pyridostigmine (Mestinon), correct the neuromuscular junction ACh activity deficit in myasthenia, but they have no effect on cognition or other cerebral function.

20-b. Scopolamine is a centrally acting anticholinergic medication similar to atropine. In routine pharmacologic doses, neither scopolamine nor atropine crosses the blood–brain barrier; however, in high doses both penetrate the blood–brain barrier and cause a toxic psychosis

21-a. Organic phosphate insecticides usually contain anticholinesterases that overwhelm the neuromuscular junction with an overabundance of ACh.

22-a. Physostigmine is also a centrally acting anticholinesterase, but it has a short half-life.

23. Which of the following features does not characterize the Alzheimer's disease Assessment Scale (ADAS-Cog)?
    a. The testing requires about 45 minutes.
    b. The testing, including scoring, must be performed by a trained individual.
    c. Patients with Alzheimer's disease typically increase their scores by 9 points yearly.
    d. Despite the advantages of the ADAS-Cog, the Mini-Mental State Examination (MMSE) is

the standard test in assessing pharmacologic treatment in Alzheimer's disease.

Answer: d. The ADAS, which has cognitive and noncognitive sections, measures mood and behavior, and is the standard test in assessing pharmacologic treatment in Alzheimer's disease.

24. Which is not a feature of Wernicke-Korsakoff syndrome?
    a. Petechial hemorrhages into the periaqueductal gray matter
    b. Petechial hemorrhages into the mamillary bodies
    c. Hemorrhage into portions of the limbic system
    d. Dementia

Answer: d. Wernicke-Korsakoff syndrome is characterized by amnesia, not dementia. Hemorrhages into the mamillary bodies, which are part of the limbic system, probably explain the amnesia.

25. Which one of the following histologic features of Alzheimer's disease is an intraneuronal abnormality?
    a. Neurofibrillary tangles
    b. Neuritic plaques
    c. Senile plaques
    d. β-amyloid deposits

Answer: a. Neurofibrillary tangles are composed of intraneuronal, paired helical filaments of hyperphosphorylated tau proteins. Plaques, whose main constituent is β-amyloid, are extraneuronal.

26. A test for Alzheimer's disease purportedly has a high sensitivity but a low specificity. In a revision of the test, what would be the most likely effect of reducing the proportion of false-positive results?
    a. The sensitivity would increase.
    b. The specificity would increase.
    c. Both the sensitivity and specificity would increase.
    d. Neither the sensitivity nor specificity would increase.

Answer: b. Specificity would increase because it is calculated by dividing the true negatives by the sum of true negatives and false positives. In simple terms, with fewer false positives the results would be more specific because a positive result is more likely to be reliable. With Alzheimer's disease, diagnoses based on neurologic examination and routine testing are approximately 90% accurate. Any new test must have a high sensitivity and specificity to add value to current diagnostic criteria.

27. Which of the following is the most specific blood test for syphilis?
    a. VDRL
    b. Microhemagglutination assay (MHA-TP)
    c. Wassermann
    d. Colloidal gold curve
    e. RPR

Answer: b. The MHA-TP and FTA-ABS are specific for syphilis and other spirochete infections, including Lyme disease. The Wassermann and colloidal gold curve tests for syphilis are outdated. The VDRL and RPR tests, which are termed reagin tests, are nonspecific and carry a high false-positive rate.

28. Which is not a potential early clinical feature of frontotemporal dementia?
    a. Dementia with prominent memory impairment
    b. Familial tendency
    c. Loss of inhibition (disinhibition)
    d. Anomic aphasia
    e. Aggressive personality changes, including features of the Klüver-Bucy syndrome

Answer: a. In frontotemporal dementia, which includes Pick's disease, patients typically present with prominent personality changes, behavioral disturbances, and limited language abnormality, such as anomic aphasia. Those neurobehavioral changes dwarf the cognitive impairment, which consists more of impaired judgment than memory impairment (amnesia).

29. Which one of the following conditions is not a complication of professional boxing?
    a. Dementia pugilistica
    b. Intracranial hemorrhage
    c. Parkinsonism
    d. Slowed reaction times
    e. Progression of dementia, even after retirement
    f. Peripheral neuropathy

Answer: f. Unless trauma injures particular nerves, boxers do not develop a peripheral neuropathy. However, they are subject to repeated blows to the head, which can cause an acute intracranial hemorrhage or chronic, progressive cognitive and motor skills deterioration (dementia pugilistica).

30. During an experiment to reproduce Alzheimer's-like cognitive deficits, a subject is administered excessive scopolamine. Of the following, which would be the best antidote?
    a. Atropine
    b. Edrophonium
    c. Neostigmine
    d. Physostigmine

Answer: d. Scopolamine and atropine block acetylcholine receptors. Reducing cerebral cholinergic activity is a *forme fruste* of CNS anticholinergic poisoning that mimics the cognitive changes of Alzheimer's disease. The antidote is cholinergic-enhancing medications that cross the blood–brain barrier. Although edrophonium, neostigmine, and physostigmine each inhibit cholinesterase and thus enhance cholinergic activity, only physostigmine readily crosses the blood–brain barrier. As a general rule, scopolamine and atropine are anticholinergic and counterbalance the cholinesterase inhibitor physostigmine.

31. Which movement disorders are associated with cognitive impairment?
    a. Choreoathetosis
    b. Parkinson's disease
    c. Dystonia musculorum deformans (torsion dystonia)
    d. Tourette's syndrome
    e. Essential tremor
    f. Rigid form of Huntington's disease
    g. Wilson's disease
    h. Spasmodic torticollis

Answers: a (associated with mental retardation in many but not all cases), b (in the middle to late stages), f, g.

32. A woman brought her husband to the emergency room because he suddenly became "confused" during sexual intercourse. On examination, the 65-year-old patient was fully alert and attentive but distraught. He was unable to recall recent events, the date, or any of three objects after a 3-minute delay; however, he recalled his social security number, home address, and other detailed personal information. Also, his language function and judgment seemed normal to the doctors and his wife. His symptoms resolved after 2 hours. Which of the following conditions is most likely?
    a. Dissociative state
    b. Dementia
    c. Fugue state
    d. Transient global amnesia
    e. Transient ischemic attack (TIA)

Answer: d. The patient had a 2-hour episode of memory impairment with preservation of consciousness, perception, and judgment. Amnesia is usually caused by temporal lobe dysfunction from ischemia, infarction, partial complex seizures, Wernicke-Korsakoff syndrome, or certain medications, such as scopolamine. In this case, the problem was *transient global amnesia (TGA)*. The term is somewhat of a misnomer because the amnesia was not truly global: as in most cases of TGA, he could recall deeply ingrained personal information. This amnesia differs from the amnesia in psychogenic disorders, in which all memories or only repugnant ones are lost.

TGA is probably attributable to ischemia of the posterior cerebral arteries, which supply the temporal lobe; however, some neurologists believe that it is a manifestation of seizure. It is most common in individuals older than 65 years and may be precipitated by sexual intercourse, physical stress, or strong emotions.

33–35. Match the following conditions, which produce confabulation, with the location of the underlying brain damage.

33. Wernicke-Korsakoff syndrome
34. Anton's syndrome
35. Nondominant hemisphere syndrome
    a. Right parietal lobe
    b. Periventricular gray matter, mamillary bodies
    c. Occipital lobes, bilaterally
    d. Dominant parietal lobe

Answers: 33-b, 34-c, 35-a.

36. According to his coworkers, a 60-year-old male bank manager has lost his ability to complete financing arrangements. Although he seemed to know the individual facts of each deal, he failed to go through the sequence of the established procedures. In addition, his wife reported that, in a change of character, he had begun to tell off-color jokes. At home he tended to speak little and often only when prodded for a response. His MMSE score was 25. A general neurologic examination revealed no myoclonus, hemiparesis, or ataxia. Which is the most likely cause of his impairment at work?
    a. Alzheimer's disease
    b. Depression
    c. Frontotemporal dementia
    d. Diffuse Lewy body disease

Answer. c. The problem at work consists of a failure to complete the proper sequence of steps in financing a deal rather than memory impairment or general cognitive ability. His problem is executive impairment that might be termed "ideational apraxia" (see Chapter 8). In combination with his reduced inhibition, seen in his joke-telling and reticence at home, his executive impairment probably is a manifestation of frontotemporal dementia. As in this case, frontotemporal dementia often primarily causes neurobehavioral changes rather than dementia. Moreover, the changes consist more of violating sexual conventions, misjudgments, poor planning, and language problems than of memory impairment.

37. A 35-year-old man with HIV disease for 17 years and a CD_4 count of 190 cells/mm^3 presents with an evolution over several weeks of left hemiparesis

and bilateral ataxia. His cognitive function is within normal limits. His MRI shows several large areas of demyelination, without mass effect, in various areas of the cerebrum and brain. Which test would most likely indicate the diagnosis?
a. CSF titers for JC virus nucleic acid
b. CSF test for oligoclonal bands
c. Brain biopsy for toxoplasmosis
d. Brain biopsy for lymphoma

Answer: a. He probably has developed PML, in which case CSF would contain JC virus nucleic acid. PML tends to develop only in patients with CD_4 counts below 200 cells/mm^3, but several patients undergoing highly active retroviral therapy have develop PML despite CD_4 counts substantially higher than 200 cells/mm^3. A variety of inflammatory neurologic illnesses, particularly MS, result in oligoclonal bands in CSF. Both toxoplasmosis and lymphoma are mass lesions that would have caused headaches from increased intracranial pressure and changes reflecting mass effects on imaging studies. Also, lymphomas are usually solitary lesions in HIV patients.

38. Match the histologic finding (a–h) with the disease (1–7).
    a. Argentophilic intraneuronal inclusions
    b. Cowdry bodies
    c. Lewy bodies
    d. Neurofibrillary tangles
    e. Spongiform encephalopathy
    f. Kayser-Fleischer rings
    g. Staining with α-synuclein antibodies
    h. Accumulation of tau
    1. Creutzfeldt-Jakob disease
    2. Wilson's disease
    3. Frontotemporal dementia
    4. Dementia with Lewy bodies
    5. Parkinson's disease
    6. Alzheimer's disease
    7. Subacute sclerosing panencephalitis (SSPE)

    Answers:
    a. 3 (in cases of Pick's disease)
    b. 7
    c. 4 and 5
    d. 6 and dementia pugilistica and SSPE
    e. 1 and variant Creutzfeldt-Jakob disease, kuru, fatal familial insomnia, scrapie, and other animal spongiform encephalopathies
    f. 2
    g. 4, 5
    h. 3 and, less so, 6

39. Which skin lesion is most closely associated with AIDS?

a. Lymphoma
b. Herpes simplex
c. Kaposi's sarcoma
d. Chancre
e. Herpes zoster

Answer: c. Kaposi's sarcoma is so closely linked to AIDS that it is an AIDS-defining illness. Herpes zoster is an infection of the dorsal root ganglia, which is common in AIDS patients and occurs in all stages of the illness. It leads to zoster of the skin ("shingles") and often postherpetic neuralgia.

40. Which of the following descriptions may be applied to patients in the end-stages of Alzheimer's disease?
    a. Locked-in syndrome
    b. Persistent vegetative state
    c. Electrocerebral silence
    d. Slow wave sleep

Answer: b. The persistent vegetative state results from extensive cerebral cortex damage. End stage Alzheimer's and Parkinson's diseases, cerebral anoxia, and severe traumatic brain injury are the most common causes of the persistent vegetative state. In contrast, the locked-in syndrome usually results from a massive but incomplete lower brainstem injury. Occlusions of the basilar artery and amyotrophic lateral sclerosis are frequently occurring causes. Electrocerebral silence (the absence of EEG activity) characterizes brain death, barbiturate overdose, or deep anesthesia. Slow wave sleep is normal stage 3 and 4 NREM sleep.

41. Which of the following diseases will be supported by finding the 14-3-3 protein in the CSF?
    a. Alzheimer's
    b. Parkinson's
    c. Dementia with Lewy bodies
    d. Creutzfeldt-Jakob

Answer: d. The CSF in Creutzfeldt-Jakob disease usually contains 14-3-3 protein; however, CSF in encephalitis and tumors may also contain this marker. Although not completely specific, in the setting of compatible clinical and EEG findings, it has a strong enough association to obviate a neurosurgical biopsy. The CSF in Creutzfeldt-Jakob disease also usually contains elevated levels of tau protein, but that finding is even more nonspecific.

42. What is the most common cause of multiple, discrete cerebral lesions in AIDS patients?
    a. Lymphoma
    b. Kaposi's sarcoma
    c. Cryptococcus
    d. Toxoplasmosis

e. Tuberculosis

Answer: d. Of all potential cerebral mass lesions that can complicate AIDS, toxoplasmosis is the most common. It characteristically produces multiple ring-enhancing masses. Lymphomas, the second most common lesions, are usually single.

43. Which is the most frequently occurring, nonepidemic form of encephalitis?
   a. HIV encephalitis
   b. *Herpes simplex* encephalitis
   c. *Herpes zoster* encephalitis
   d. Meningococcal encephalitis

Answer: b. *Herpes simplex* is the most common non-epidemic infectious agent that causes encephalitis. This virus typically invades the temporal lobes and, because it devastates the limbic system, causes partial complex seizures, amnesia, and the Klüver-Bucy syndrome. HIV and meningococcus are epidemic infections. Meningococcus causes meningitis much more often than encephalitis. *Herpes zoster* only rarely invades the brain or spinal cord.

44. In Alzheimer's disease, into which substance is amyloid precursor protein (APP) converted?
   a. Amyloid β-peptide (Aβ)
   b. Neurofibrillary tangles
   c. αAPP
   d. Tau

Answer: a. APP is converted to Aβ, which is insoluble, accumulates, and appears to form the nidus of plaques.

45. Which of the following illnesses is most closely associated with suicide?
   a. Alzheimer's disease
   b. Dementia with Lewy body disease
   c. Huntington's disease
   d. Creutzfeldt-Jakob disease
   e. Parkinson's disease

Answer: c. In Huntington's disease, suicide neither stems from depression nor deliberate, well-planned actions. Rather, it usually stems from an impetuous action.

46. Amnesia in Alzheimer's disease may be most closely associated with deficiency of which of the following substances?
   a. Dopamine
   b. Scopolamine
   c. Somatostatin
   d. Acetylcholine
   e. Serotonin

Answer: d. Although studies have shown that each of these transmitters, to a greater or lesser extent, is deficient in Alzheimer's disease, the acetylcholine deficit is greatest and most closely associated with amnesia.

47. Which group of drivers has the highest rate of motor vehicle accidents (MVAs)?
   a. Healthy individuals older than 65 years
   b. Alzheimer's disease patients older than 65 years
   c. Teenage drivers
   d. Men younger than 25 years

Answer: d. Individuals older than 65 years have a higher rate of MVAs than the average driver's rate. Those with Alzheimer's disease have a greater rate than same-aged drivers, and their rate increases with the duration and severity of their illness. Factors that explain the increased MVA rate include poor judgment, impaired eye-hand-foot coordination, slowed reaction time, diminished vision and hearing, and excessive day-time sleepiness. Teenagers have a high rate, with young adult men having the highest rate. Often, in addition to lacking judgment and experience, they use alcohol.

48. Of the following, which is the greatest reason that Alzheimer's patients are placed in nursing homes?
   a. Dementia
   b. Incontinence
   c. Hallucinations
   d. Sundowning
   e. Disruptive behavior

Answer: e. Disruptive behaviors—agitation, the interruption of the family's sleep, dangerous activities, and wandering—are the most likely precipitants of placing Alzheimer's patients in a nursing home. Other important causes are incontinence, requiring help with bathing and toileting, and the development of a medical illness that alone would not be sufficient. All these problems place tremendous stress on the spouse or other caregiver. Frequently, the loss through death or disability of the caregiver is the precipitating factor in placing the patient.

49. Which of the following statements regarding dementia with Lewy bodies is false?
   a. It is, at most, 15% as common as Alzheimer's disease.
   b. The microscopic feature consists of Lewy bodies concentrated in the substantia nigra.
   c. The disease typically produces symptoms in the fifth and sixth decades.
   e. Lewy bodies are eosinophilic intracytoplasmic inclusions that stain for tau.
   f. The ChAT loss in dementia with Lewy bodies is greater than in Alzheimer's disease.

Answer: b. Lewy bodies dispersed throughout the cerebral cortex are the signature of dementia with Lewy bodies. In Parkinson's disease, Lewy bodies are confined to the substantia nigra. In both illnesses, the Lewy bodies are eosinophilic intracytoplasmic inclusions that stain for α-synuclein. Dementia with Lewy bodies probably occurs 30% as frequently as Alzheimer's disease.

50. Which chromosome codes for the amyloid precursor protein (APP)?
    a. 14
    b. 19
    c. 21
    d. All of the above

Answer: c. Chromosome 21 codes for APP. Mutations on the gene lead to an excess production of amyloid and deposition of Aβ amyloid. Not surprisingly, individuals with three copies of that chromosome, particularly in trisomy 21 (Down's syndrome), almost invariably develop all the features of Alzheimer's disease.

51. Infections, trauma, infarctions, and possibly febrile convulsions may damage the mesial portion of both temporal lobes. Which neuropsychologic deficit will such damage produce?
    a. Amnesia
    b. Anosognosia
    c. Apraxia, ideational
    d. Apraxia, ideomotor
    e. Abulia

Answer: a. Bilateral mesial temporal injury characteristically produces amnesia that is usually most pronounced in an anterograde pattern, that is, patients will have impairment in memorizing new information, but have a relatively preserved ability to recall previously learned information. Anosognosia is the inability to appreciate an illness or deficit, typically a left hemiparesis. Ideomotor apraxia, essentially impaired conversion of an idea into an action, is usually a left-sided frontal or parietal lobe infarction (see Chapter 8). Ideational apraxia is impairment of an individual's ability to perform a sequence of steps requiring a simple plan and continual monitoring. It usually reflects either frontal lobe injuries or diffuse cerebral disease (see Chapter 8). Abulia, complete or nearly complete loss of spontaneous speech and other expression, results from lateral frontal lobe injury (see Chapter 8). In addition to causing retrograde amnesia, mesial temporal lobe injuries characteristically lead to partial complex seizures.

52. Regarding the association between apolipoprotein-E (Apo-E) and Alzheimer's disease, which one of the following statements is false?

a. Because people inherit 1 of 3 alleles (E2, E3, E4) from each parent, everyone has 2 alleles, forming one pair, such as E2-E3, E2-E4, E2-E2, etc.
b. Apolipoprotein binds to β-amyloid and forms neuritic plaques.
c. Inheriting the E4-E4 pair causes Alzheimer's disease.
d. Approximately 10% to 20% of the population has the pair E3-E4 or E4-E4, which are closely associated with Alzheimer's disease.

Answer: c. Even inheriting the E4-E4 pair does not necessarily lead to Alzheimer's disease. Although the Apo-E gene, which is carried on chromosome 19, is a powerful risk factor, the gene is neither a causative nor an obligate factor. Apo-E4 alleles increase the risk of Alzheimer's disease. Moreover, they advance, by as much as 20 years, the appearance of the first symptoms. In contrast, the presenilin and APP genes are causative genes.

53. Through which structure is CSF normally absorbed?
    a. Cerebral ventricles
    b. The brain parenchyma
    c. Choroid plexus
    d. Arachnoid villi

Answer: d. CSF is secreted through the choroid plexus, which is located mostly in the lateral ventricles. CSF circulates through all the ventricles and then over and around the brain and spinal cord. CSF is absorbed through the arachnoid villi to enter the venous circulation. Sometimes following subarachnoid hemorrhage or meningitis, blocked arachnoid villi lead to communicating hydrocephalus.

54. Which is a cause of obstructive hydrocephalus?
    a. Aqueductal stenosis
    b. Chronic meningitis
    c. Subarachnoid hemorrhage
    d. Hydrocephalus ex vacuo

Answer: a. Stenosis or obstruction of the aqueduct of Sylvius, which allows CSF to pass from the third to the fourth ventricle, causes obstructive hydrocephalus. The ventricular expansion that results from cerebral atrophy is termed hydrocephalus ex vacuo. As noted in the previous question, subarachnoid hemorrhage and meningitis block arachnoid villi and lead to communicating hydrocephalus.

55. Which statement is false regarding the gait of the normal elderly?
    a. It is characterized by a short stride.
    b. It frequently causes falls.
    c. Orthopedic changes are as important as most neurologic illness.

d. It is characterized by apraxia.

e. Peripheral nerve changes are an important component.

Answer: d.

56. Of the following risk factors for falls in the elderly, which is most common?
    a. Use of sedatives
    b. Transient ischemic attacks
    c. Neuropathy
    d. History of a stroke

Answer: a. Additional risk factors are cognitive impairment, musculoskeletal changes, and a history of a fall.

57. Which feature is usually absent in Creutzfeldt-Jakob disease?
    a. Inflammatory cells in cerebral cortex biopsies
    b. Dementia
    c. Burst suppression pattern or periodic sharp-wave EEG changes
    d. Survival less than 1 year
    e. Spongiform changes in cerebral cortex biopsies
    f. PrP^{Sc}
    g. Myoclonus

Answer: a. Even though Creutzfeldt-Jakob disease is an infectious illness, transmitted by prions, brain biopsies fail to reveal inflammatory cells, which would be a typical response. Biopsies show spongiform changes and, with special stains, PrP^{Sc} (scrapie protein).

58. Which statement is *false* regarding the infective agent in spongiform encephalopathies?
    a. It is largely, if not totally, composed of protein.
    b. It is resistant to formalin fixation and conventional sterilization techniques.
    c. Interspecies transfer is possible but requires a large inocula and a long incubation time.
    d. Similar agents cause SSPE.

Answer: d. Prions cause spongiform encephalopathies: Creutzfeldt-Jakob disease, variant Creutzfeldt-Jakob disease, its familial variant, Gerstmann-Sträussler disease, and fatal familial insomnia; however, a mutation of the measles virus probably causes SSPE. Prions also cause spongiform diseases in animals, including bovine encephalopathy ("mad cow disease"), wasting disease of elk and deer, scrapie, and mink encephalopathy.

59. What is the effect of highly active antiretroviral therapy (HAART) on HIV-associated dementia?
    a. HAART improves cognitive function in patients with HAD.
    b. Although HAART improves life-expectancy, it has no demonstrable effect of HAD.

c. HAART both improves life expectancy and, in AIDS patients living longer, reduces HAD.

d. HAART has no interaction with other medications that AIDS patients are likely to take.

Answer: a. HAART improves cognitive function in patients with HAD. Although it increases their longevity, AIDS patients are apt, even with relatively high CD$_4$ counts, to develop HAD. Because HAART medications are metabolized by the cytochrome P450 system, drug-drug interactions may occur. HAART medications may compete with methadone and, when added to a methadone regimen, precipitate opiate-withdrawal symptoms.

60. In which condition are the anterior horns of the lateral ventricles convex (bowed outward)?
    a. Alzheimer's disease
    b. Parkinson's disease
    c. Dementia with Lewy bodies
    d. Frontotemporal dementia
    e. Huntington's disease

Answer: e. Atrophy of the head of the caudate nucleus allows the anterior horns of the lateral ventricles to bow outward. Although the ventricles expand in the other conditions, their configuration is preserved.

61. Which of the following are risk factors for HAD in AIDS patients?
    a. Anemia
    b. Weight loss
    c. Late stages of AIDS
    d. High viral load
    e. All of the above

Answer: e. Before the introduction of HAART, HAD would develop only if CD$_4$ counts fell below 200 cells/mm^3. Subsequently, AIDS patients with CD$_4$ counts of 200–400 cells/mm^3 have been developing HAD.

62. With which illness are visual hallucinations most closely associated?
    a. Alzheimer's disease
    b. Dementia with Lewy bodies
    c. Vascular dementia
    d. Frontotemporal dementia

Answer: b. Visual hallucinations are characteristic of dementia with Lewy bodies. However, they are also associated with Parkinson's disease dementia and use of dopaminergic medications. In contrast, visual hallucinations are relatively infrequent in Alzheimer's disease during its early stages. When they do occur in Alzheimer's disease, visual hallucinations may develop in the context of delirium.

63. After being given a medication, a 66-year-old man developed forgetfulness, dry mouth, blurred vision, and urinary retention. Which was the most likely type of medication?
   a. Anticholinergic
   b. β-blocker
   c. Cholinesterase inhibitor
   d. Dopamine agonist

Answer: a. He has developed classic anticholinergic side effects. Patients older than 65 years and those with dementia are particularly vulnerable to anticholinergic side effects.

64. According to the cortical-subcortical classification of dementia, which of the following illnesses would lead to cortical dementia (c) or subcortical dementia (sc)?
   a. Frontotemporal dementia
   b. Parkinson's disease
   c. Huntington's disease
   d. Normal pressure hydrocephalus
   e. Alzheimer's disease
   f. HAD (AIDS dementia)

Answers: Frontotemporal dementia—cortical; Parkinson's disease—subcortical; Huntington's disease—subcortical; normal pressure hydrocephalus—subcortical; Alzheimer's disease—cortical; HAD—subcortical.

65. Which statement is false concerning hepatic encephalopathy?
   a. Ammonia (NH_3) crosses the blood–brain barrier more readily than ammonium (NH_4^+).
   b. Toxins bind to benzodiazepine-GABA and increase GABA activity.
   c. Ammonia (NH_3) is the primary cause of hepatic encephalopathy, and concentrations of NH_3 directly correlate with its severity.
   d. Benzodiazepine receptor antagonists, such as flumazenil, can briefly reverse hepatic encephalopathy.

Answer: c. Although therapy usually aims at reducing NH_3, its concentration correlates poorly with the severity of hepatic encephalopathy.

66. A variety of tests are administered to a 50-year-old man with the onset of personality changes but no significant cognitive impairment. In the Wisconsin Card Sorting Test, the tester deals him 4 playing cards: 3 of clubs, 7 of clubs, 9 of clubs, and 7 of hearts. The tester asks the patient to point to the card that does not belong. He picks the 7 of hearts after explaining that it is the only red card. The

tester then deals another 4 cards: the 5 of clubs, 6 of hearts, 5 of spades, 5 of diamonds, and 6 of clubs. When again asked to pick the one that does not belong, the patient without hesitancy picks the 5 of diamonds. Which disorder does his choice indicate?
   a. Frontal lobe dysfunction
   b. Visual-spatial impairment
   c. Dementia
   d. Occipital cortex impairment
   e. Color blindness

Answer: a. In this element of the Wisconsin Card Sorting Test, the patient cannot change from sorting by color to sorting by number. His inability to "switch sets" is indicative of frontal lobe dysfunction.

67. A 76-year-old right-handed man who had developed confusion was asked to draw a clock. What problem does his drawing most likely represent?
   a. Alzheimer's disease
   b. Normal aging
   c. A dominant frontal lobe infarction
   d. A nondominant frontal lobe infarction
   e. A dominant parietal lobe infarction
   f. A nondominant parietal lobe infarction

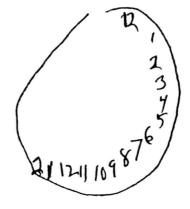

Answer: f. The drawing shows a neglect of the left field and constructional apraxia. The clock is an incomplete, poorly drawn circle with uneven spacing between the digits and the circle. There is also perseveration of the digits. Constructional apraxia can be a manifestation of dementia, mental retardation, and both frontal and parietal lobe injuries, on either side; however, it is most closely associated with nondominant parietal lobe lesions. The left-sided neglect is also referable to a nondominant parietal lobe lesion.

68. Which DSM-IV criteria distinguish Alzheimer's disease dementia from vascular dementia?
   a. Alzheimer's disease, but not vascular dementia, must include memory impairment.

b. Alzheimer's disease, but not vascular dementia, must include at least one of the following: aphasia, apraxia, agnosia, or disturbance in executive functioning.

c. Alzheimer's disease, but not vascular dementia, must impair social or occupational functioning.

d. Alzheimer's disease, but not vascular dementia, need not be accompanied by focal neurologic symptoms and signs.

e. None of the above.

Answer: e. Both Alzheimer's and vascular dementia must include memory impairment and at least one of the following: aphasia, apraxia, agnosia, or disturbance in executive functioning. In addition, both must impair social or occupational functioning. Focal neurologic symptoms and signs must accompany vascular dementia but not Alzheimer's disease.

69. Which of the following statements concerning the MMSE is false?
   a. It is sensitive.
   b. Unlike the ADAS-Cog, the MMSE can be administered without special training.
   c. It reliably distinguishes Alzheimer's dementia from vascular dementia.
   d. Educational levels influence the MMSE more than the ADAS-Cog.
   e. Low scores can reflect metabolic aberrations, thought disorders, or mood disorders, as well as dementia.

Answer: c. Although the MMSE will identify most cases of dementia, it cannot determine the cause. Although the MMSE is helpful in the diagnosis of dementia, it is nonspecific in terms of the dementia's etiology. Moreover, some false-positive results occur. ADAS-Cog testing is more involved than the MMSE. The test takes about one hour to complete. A skilled person is required to administer and score it. Nevertheless, despite its complexity, the ADAS-Cog is the standard test in Alzheimer's disease pharmaceutical trials.

70. Which of the following is least likely to reduce an individual's score on the MMSE?
   a. Gender
   b. Less than an eighth grade education
   c. Being an ethnic minority
   d. Being older than 75 years

Answer: a. Although an individual's gender has almost no effect on the MMSE score, limited education, being a member of a minority group, and advancing age all reduce the score. Correction factors can reduce the adverse effects of age and limited education. Spanish versions of the test are available.

71. A 45-year-old man with AIDS and a CD_4 count of 50 cells/mm^3 reports slowly developing a generalized, dull headache and inability to concentrate. The neurologic examination reveals no focal findings or indication of increased intracranial pressure. An MRI shows no intracranial pathology. Which of the following would be the best diagnostic test?
   a. A lumbar puncture
   b. Determining serum toxoplasmosis titers
   c. A therapeutic trial of an antidepressant
   d. A therapeutic trial of a serotonin agonist

Answer: a. About 85% of AIDS patients with headaches have serious intracranial pathology rather than a tension-type headache, migraine, or depression. Almost one half of them have *Cryptococcus* meningitis or cerebral toxoplasmosis. In this case, the normal neurologic examination and head MRI in almost all cases excludes toxoplasmosis and other mass lesions.

72. A family brought a 45-year-old man to the emergency room because he had been confused and behaving strangely during the past day. The patient, they state, has not experienced any unusual event, stress, or trauma. A neurologist found no physical abnormalities and extensive testing, including toxicology, EEG, MRI, and LP, showed no abnormality. The patient cannot state his name, birthday, or address. He cannot recall any personal events of the previous 6 months or any current political events. His affect is appropriate and language function is normal. Which of the following is the most likely diagnosis?
   a. Transient global amnesia
   b. Dissociative amnesia
   c. Wernicke-Korsakoff syndrome
   d. Frontal lobe dysfunction

Answer: b. Personal identification—name, birthday, address, and telephone number—is deeply embedded information that is actually "overlearned." Only an extensive, devastating brain injury, such as advanced Alzheimer's disease or major head trauma, would dislodge this information. (Those conditions would also impair his affect, language function, and motor function.) This patient's amnesia most likely does not have an organic basis. However the information at hand is insufficient to make a firm diagnosis of Dissociative Amnesia, formerly known as "Psychogenic Amnesia," or distinguish it from Dissociative Identity Disorder, Somatization Disorders, or malingering.

73. Which of the following is usually not considered a domain of cognitive function?
   a. Language
   b. Mood

c. Praxis

d. Visual-spatial conceptualization

Answer: b. The traditional domains of cognitive function are memory, calculation, and judgment. Other domains are visual-spatial conceptualization, performance skills, and learned motor actions (praxis). Mood, affect, and emotions, although they originate in cerebral function, are not domains of cognitive function.

74. What percent of Alzheimer's disease cases are attributable to the causative genes: amyloid precursor protein (APP) (chromosome 21), presenilin 1 (chromosome 14), and presenilin 2 (chromosome 1)?

a. 5%

b. 10%

c. 25%

d. 50%

Answer: a. Despite their importance, this group of genes determines less than 5% of Alzheimer's disease cases. When these genes cause Alzheimer's disease, the illness usually follows an autosomal dominant pattern and victims develop symptoms at a relatively young age (30 to 60 years).

75. A 77-year-old man was asked, as part of an evaluation for dementia, to copy a sequence of four sets of three squares followed by a circle. Almost immediately after beginning the task, he began to tell the physician a nonsensical joke with sexual innuendo. After briefly returning to the task, he was distracted first by a small defect in the paper and then by soft noise outside the room. Finally, he excused himself to go the men's room, but only after he let some urine escape and wet his pants. On returning, he recounted a similar joke and said he could not concentrate because of all the distractions. He scored 22 on the MMSE and had no lateralized neurologic findings. Which area of the brain does this man's behavior reflect?

a. The cortical association areas, as in Alzheimer's disease

b. The parietal lobes, as in hemi-inattention disorders

c. The frontal lobes, as in frontal lobe dysfunction

d. The limbic system, as in Klüver-Bucy syndrome

Answer: c. This man has easy distractibility, marked disinhibition, inappropriate jocularity, and a suggestion of urinary incontinence, in the absence of frank dementia. The distractibility is a manifestation of inability to suppress attentiveness to new stimuli, another form of disinhibition. He was unable to inhibit shifting his attention to new stimuli as they appeared: He was "stimulus bound." All these phenomena reflect frontal lobe damage. They are complementary to the patient's difficulties in Question 66. Some elements of frontal lobe damage are similar to limbic system damage largely because the limbic system is partly based in the frontal lobes. Moreover, as is probably the diagnosis is this case, frontotemporal dementia causes all these symptoms.

In contrast, Alzheimer's disease particularly strikes cerebral cortical association areas. Although causing dementia, it usually produces apathy. Its behavioral abnormalities are less severe and less predictable than those of frontotemporal dementia. Damage to the non-dominant parietal lobe typically causes hemi-inattention and related symptoms. Damage to the limbic system, which may be a component of frontotemporal dementia, typically causes amnesia and Klüver-Bucy syndrome.

76. In an attempt to commit suicide, an elderly person swallows an entire bottle of donepezil. He becomes unconscious, hypotensive, and markedly bradycardic. Which medication should be administered?

a. A different anticholinesterase inhibitor PO

b. Pyridostigmine IV

c. Atropine IV

d. Edrophonium (Tensilon) IV

Answer: c. The overdose of donepezil, which is an anticholinesterase inhibitor, created excessive ACh concentration. The excessive cholinergic activity led to the bradycardia. Atropine, an anticholinergic agent, must be given IV to counteract the cholinergic-induced bradycardia. Pyridostigmine and edrophonium, like donepezil, increase ACh activity and would exacerbate the bradycardia.

77. A 19-year-old exchange student from Britain began to have deterioration in her personality, cognitive impairment, painful burning sensations in her feet, and myoclonic jerks. There was no family history of neurologic or psychiatric illness. Results of the following tests were normal: CT, MRI, CSF, B_{12}, T_4, RPR, CSF measles antibodies, serum ceruloplasmin, urine for metachromatic granules, heavy metal screening, toxicology, porphyrin screening, HIV, Lyme titer, and chromosome studies for excessive trinucleotide repeats. The EEG had disorganization and a slow background, but it lacked distinctive abnormal features. After exhaustive noninvasive testing, a cerebral biopsy was performed. It showed microscopic vacuoles. She died after a 1-year course. Which is the most likely etiology of her neurologic illness?

a. A retrovirus

b. A prion

c. Drug or alcohol abuse

d. A psychiatric illness

Answer: b. The clinical presentation of progressive, fatal mental deterioration with burning paresthesias and myoclonus is consistent with several illnesses, but the biopsy showing spongiform changes (microscopic vacuoles) indicates that the diagnosis in this case is the *variant Creutzfeldt-Jakob disease (vCJD)*. This illness represents an interspecies transmission of bovine spongiform encephalopathy (BSE). Unlike classic Creutzfeldt-Jakob disease, vCJD occurs in teenagers and young adults, has prominent psychiatric symptoms, leads to sensory disturbances, and lacks the characteristic EEG changes (periodic sharp-wave complexes). Almost all victims have been young adults who have lived in Britain, and the majority of them consulted a psychiatrist when their symptoms first developed.

78. An 80-year-old retired janitor, who has developed mild forgetfulness, scores 19 on the MMSE. The physical portion of the neurologic examination discloses no abnormalities. The standard blood tests and head CT are unremarkable; however, the apolipoprotein E (Apo-E) test shows an E4 allele. Which statement is the most valid in this case?
   a. Neurologists routinely recommend Apo-E screening of individuals at risk for dementia, as well as those already afflicted with dementia.
   b. A single Apo-E4 determination, with dementia, is diagnostic of Alzheimer's disease.
   c. Little or no education and Apo-E4 alleles are associated with Alzheimer's disease.
   d. Determining Apo-E4 alleles never has a role in cases of Alzheimer's disease.

Answer: c. Being uneducated and having one or both Apo-E4 alleles are risk factors for Alzheimer's disease; however, neither causes the disease. Apo-E determinations have a role in investigations of multiple family members with early onset Alzheimer's disease; however, neurologists do not use this test as a screening procedure for individuals with or without dementia.

79. What do the following conditions have in common: toluene abuse, multiple sclerosis (MS), progressive multifocal leukoencephalopathy (PML), metachromatic leukodystrophy, and adrenoleukodystrophy?
   a. All are commonly associated with seizures.
   b. All are infectious illnesses.
   c. All are leukoencephalopathies.
   d. All cause dementia early in their course

Answer: c. All these conditions primarily injure CNS white matter, that is, they all cause leukoencephalopathy. Because these illnesses spare cerebral cortex gray matter, they rarely cause seizures or dementia until

the late stages of the illness. PML is an opportunistic infection. MS is suspected of being infectious. Metachromatic leukodystrophy and adrenoleukodystrophy are inherited illnesses.

80. In Alzheimer's disease, which region of the brain contains the greatest concentration of β-amyloid plaques?
   a. Frontal lobe
   b. Parietal lobe
   c. Hippocampus
   d. Nucleus basalis
   e. Caudate nuclei

Answer: c. The concentration of β-amyloid plaques and neurofibrillary tangles is greatest in the hippocampus. Other sites of high concentrations are the cerebral cortex association areas.

81–84. At the risk of oversimplification, match each dementia-producing illness with its characteristic presenting feature(s).

81. Alzheimer's disease
82. Dementia with Lewy bodies
83. Frontotemporal dementia
84. Vascular dementia
   a. Aggressiveness and other behavioral disturbances
   b. Memory impairment
   c. Akinetic-rigid parkinsonism
   d. Stepwise motor and cognitive deterioration
   e. REM sleep behavior disorder

Answers: 81-b, 82-c and e, 83-a, 84-d.

85. A hospital review board refers a 60-year-old well-respected male psychiatrist to a psychiatrist in a neighboring county for evaluation because he has been accused of improper sexual advances toward several female patients. Two independent sources have substantiated the accusations. During the examination, the psychiatrist has good cognitive function, although he does not seem as thoughtful or verbal as the examining psychiatrist had expected. He also seems reticent, but impetuous, when he speaks. When commenting on the accusations, he dismisses their seriousness and their validity. He also relates several episodes of his recent uncharacteristic, public verbal attacks on junior colleagues. He has continued to work, maintain family life, and pursue his hobbies. A neurologist, who previously examined the psychiatrist, has already reported that his MMSE score was 27, physical neurologic testing showed no abnormalities, and MRI of the brain and an EEG were within normal limits. Which of the following conditions has most likely developed?

a. Mild cognitive impairment
b. Dementia from Alzheimer's disease
c. Dementia from diffuse Lewy body disease
d. Dementia from another illness

Answer: d. The psychiatrist-patient has shown uninhibited behavior and impaired judgment in the inappropriate sexual advances and impetuousness. In addition, some of his behavior might have been aggressive, such as the attacks on colleagues. His reticence contrasts to his overactivity in other areas. He does not fulfill criteria for dementia because he can still function at work and at home, and his MMSE score, although lower than expected, is normal. Although he does not have dementia, he is not normal. Because his abnormal behavior dwarfs his cognitive impairment, he most likely has developed frontotemporal dementia. (In a slightly different scenario, hypomania or bipolar disorder might have been a better a diagnosis.)

86. In the previous case, which abnormality would probably be found on immunologic staining?
    a. Argentophilic inclusions
    b. Tau deposits
    c. Alpha-synuclein inclusions
    d. Lewy bodies in the cortex

Answer: b. In about 50% of frontotemporal dementia cases, standard histologic staining shows argentophilic inclusions (Pick bodies). Immunologic staining consistently shows tau deposits in frontotemporal dementia and several other neurodegenerative illnesses. Frontotemporal dementia is associated with mutations in the tau gene. Alpha-synuclein inclusions and Lewy bodies in the cortex characterize dementia with Lewy bodies.

87. A wife brought her 70-year-old husband to a psychiatrist because for the last 3 to 6 months he was having increasingly severe hallucinations, especially at night, and memory problems. During the initial evaluation, he was alert and oriented. His MMSE score was 25/30. He had reduced spontaneous movements and increased tone in his wrist and elbow muscles. His gait was shuffling, and he had a positive "pull test." A CT and routine blood tests, including those for dementia, revealed no abnormalities. During the follow-up evaluation, he was lethargic and scored only 20/30 on the MMSE. However, still untreated, he was alert during the next examination. The wife confirmed that he had a fluctuating sensorium. Which is the most likely disorder?
    a. Parkinson's disease
    b. Side effect from a medication

c. Alzheimer's disease
d. Dementia with Lewy bodies

Answer: d. Dementia with Lewy bodies presents with features of both Alzheimer's and Parkinson's diseases. In addition, with its characteristic fluctuating level of consciousness, this illness mimics a toxic-metabolic encephalopathy. Of course, physicians should exclude toxic-metabolic encephalopathy before making a diagnosis of dementia with Lewy bodies. An interesting harbinger of dementia with Lewy bodies is the development of REM sleep behavior disorder. In addition to sharing clinical features with Alzheimer's disease and toxic-metabolic encephalopathy, dementia with Lewy bodies is similar to long-standing Parkinson's disease, except that rigidity and akinesia predominate tremor. The important distinction is that, at its onset, Parkinson's disease causes neither cognitive impairment nor visual hallucinations, but dementia with Lewy bodies typically presents with such changes.

88. Which of the following structures are intranuclear inclusion bodies?
    a. Cowdry bodies
    b. Lewy bodies
    c. Pick bodies
    d. Neurofibrillary tangles

Answer: a. All of these intraneuronal abnormalities are seen with illnesses that cause dementia. Cowdry bodies are intranuclear inclusion bodies, typically found in SSPE, that are probably residue of measles or another virus infection. Lewy bodies, Pick bodies, and neurofibrillary tangles are all intracytoplasmic inclusions.

89. A 68-year-old man, who had recently sustained a right cerebral infarction, was asked to reproduce the physician's 10-block pyramid (left). He attempted 4 times (right), but it always fell before completion. What is the implication of his inability to reproduce the pyramid?

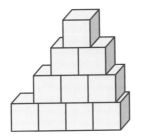 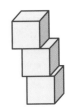

a. Dementia
b. Executive impairment
c. Left hemi-inattention
d. Left homonymous hemianopsia

Answer: c. He has left hemi-inattention—not a hemianopsia—in failing to appreciate both sides of the pyramid. He probably also has an element of constructional apraxia in failing to instinctively know that his unbalanced structure would topple.

90. A 40-year-old woman developed sudden paresis of her left upper and lower face. Her blood test for Lyme disease was positive, and physicians treated her with intravenous antibiotics for 2 weeks. During the treatment she began to describe fatigue, irritability, memory impairment, and depression. After these symptoms persisted for 6 months and her Lyme titer remained reactive, her physician prescribed a second course of antibiotics. Nevertheless, her chronic fatigue and memory impairment remained so disabling that she could not work. Which statement is true?
   a. An additional course of antibiotics would not relieve the symptoms more than a placebo.
   b. An additional course of antibiotics is indicated because her Lyme serology remains positive.
   c. An additional course of antibiotics is warranted whether or not her Lyme serology remains positive.
   d. Her chronic symptoms are attributable to the antibiotics.

Answer: a. Several studies have shown that additional courses of antibiotics for "chronic Lyme disease" do not reverse the neurocognitive symptoms or the chronic fatigue in either seropositive or seronegative patients. The antibiotics themselves do not cause these symptoms.

91. A 16-year-old girl loses interest in school and then in her friends. When she becomes apathetic, her parents bring her for a full evaluation. The neurologist detects mild dementia and subtle myoclonus. An extensive evaluation, including an MRI, is normal except that the EEG shows periodic sharp-wave complexes. The CSF shows a markedly elevated level of antibodies to measles but no cells and no 14-3-3 protein. Which illness does the evaluation indicate?
   a. Variant Creutzfeldt-Jakob
   b. SSPE
   c. Schizophrenia
   d. Metachromatic leukodystrophy

Answer: b. Antibodies to measles in CSF indicate SSPE. Unlike the conventional disease, variant Creutzfeldt-Jakob disease typically affects teens and young adults, and the EEG does not contain periodic complexes. In schizophrenia, the EEG is normal and the CSF does not contain any consistently reliable marker. Metachromatic leukodystrophy, which usually develops in children, reveals its demyelinating nature on the MRI.

92. In assessing for dementia, in which condition would the MMSE be most valuable?
   a. Alzheimer's disease
   b. Parkinson's disease
   c. Frontotemporal dementia
   d. Toluene abuse

Answer: a. The MMSE is a standard tool in assessing the presence and progression of dementia in Alzheimer's disease. The other conditions, in contrast, produce subcortical dementia. Their manifestations cannot readily be measured by a test, such as the MMSE, that relies primarily on language.

93. The family of a 70-year-old man brings him to a psychiatrist because he has developed visual hallucinations during the previous 3 weeks. Only 2 months before the consultation, a neurologist, who performed an extensive evaluation, had diagnosed minimal cognitive impairment. An internist found no particular abnormality. The patient takes no medicines except aspirin. The psychiatrist finds that the man does not have a mood or thought disorder, and that his MMSE score is 24. The hallucinations, which are often vivid, occur during the daytime as well as during sleep and last many minutes. They vary in content and emotion but are often threatening or otherwise disturbing. The psychiatrist also notes that the patient has a paucity of speech and voluntary movement. He has reduced arm swing when walking and turns *en bloc*. When shaking his hand, the psychiatrist noted that his muscle tone is mildly increased. Which is the best treatment for the hallucinations?
   a. Antipsychotic agents
   b. Antidepressants
   c. Levodopa (L-dopa)
   d. Dopamine agonists
   e. Cholinesterase inhibitor
   f. None of the above

Answer: a. In view of his parkinsonism and mild cognitive impairment, the patient probably has dementia with Lewy body disease, an illness where visual hallucinations are an early, characteristic feature. Although Alzheimer's and Parkinson's diseases—and the medicines used to treat them—may also cause visual hallucinations, that manifestation usually occurs relatively late in the course and only when patients have unequivocal dementia. In this case, antipsychotic agents, but only in small doses, are indicated to suppress the hallucinations. Routine doses of antipsychotic agents will convert his bradykinesia and increased muscle tone to akinesia and immobility. Atypical rather than typical dopamine-blocking agents are preferable because they are less likely to aggravate the parkinsonism. Many neurologists would also add a cholinesterase inhibitor.

Aphasia and Related Disorders

Neurologists utilize the anatomic and physiologic correlates of language, language impairment (*aphasia*), and related disorders to deduce how the normal brain functions and to advance linguistics studies. They test for language-related disorders, often quite striking in their presentation, to help localize and diagnose neurologic disease.

Aphasia, the flagship of neuropsychologic disturbances, can disrupt cognition, halt certain functions, and produce mental aberrations. Aphasia and its related disorders appear prominently in many psychiatric conditions. The *Diagnostic and Statistical Manual of Mental Disorders, 4th Edition, Text Revision* (*DSM-IV-TR*) omits a definition of common adult-onset aphasia.

LANGUAGE AND DOMINANCE

The *dominant hemisphere*, by definition, governs language function and houses the brain's language centers. In its *association areas*, the dominant hemisphere also integrates language with intellect and emotion as well as tactile, auditory, and visual sensations. Because of its crucial role, the dominant hemisphere serves as the brain's main portal for expression of thoughts, emotions, and many facets of cognitive activity.

Language development begins in infancy, which is also the period of greatest brain *plasticity* (ability to be remodeled). By the age of 5 years, the brain establishes dominance for language. Then, as vocabulary, verbal nuance, and language complexity increase throughout life, plasticity declines. For example, after puberty, children usually cannot learn new (second) languages without preserving traces of their native (primary) language. Also after puberty, the nondominant hemisphere can no longer assume a meaningful role in language following injury of dominant hemisphere.

Language includes more than speaking, listening, reading, and writing. It also includes sign language and tone-dependent languages, such as Chinese. The dominant hemisphere's *perisylvian language arc* (see later) processes all forms of languages. Thus, lesions in this region impair all language forms, to a greater or lesser extent. Thus, with dominant hemisphere strokes, for example, deficits in reading parallel deficits in writing. (One notable exception is alexia without agraphia [see later].)

However, the dominant hemisphere does not necessarily govern languages learned as adults, including a second language, or use of obscenities, which is usually an expression of strong emotions. The *nondominant* hemisphere bestows on speech its *prosody*, which consists of the mixture of inflection, rhythm, and manner, that determines its affect and shades of meaning.

Cerebral hemisphere dominance includes more than governance of language. It also regulates certain motor and sensory functions. The dominant hemisphere controls fine, rapid hand movements (handedness) and, to a lesser degree, reception of vision and hearing. For example, right-handed people, who have left cerebral hemisphere dominance, not only rely on their right hand for writing and throwing a ball but they also use their right foot for kicking, right eye when peering through a telescope, and right ear for listening to words spoken simultaneously in both ears (*dichotic listening*).

Anatomically, the dominant hemisphere is distinctive in being virtually the only exception to the left-right symmetry of the brain. The dominant temporal lobe's superior surface—the *planum temporale*—has a much greater cortical area than its nondominant counterpart because it has more gyri and deeper sulci. Not only does the relatively large cortical area of the dominant planum temporale allow for greater language development but it probably also allows for greater musical ability because it is larger in musicians than nonmusicians and largest in musicians with perfect pitch. However, this normal asymmetry is lacking or even reversed in many individuals with dyslexia, autism, and chronic schizophrenia—conditions with prominent language abnormalities.

HANDEDNESS

About 90% of all people are right-handed and correspondingly left hemisphere dominant. In addition, most left-handed people are also left hemisphere dominant.

Most left-handed people have naturally occurring right hemisphere dominance, but in others, congenital injury to their left hemisphere forced their right hemisphere to assume dominance. Left-handedness is over-represented among individuals with an overt neurologic impairment, such as mental retardation or epilepsy, and certain major psychiatric disorders, such as schizophrenia and autism. Moreover, it is over-represented among children with subtle neurologic abnormalities, such as dyslexia, other learning disabilities, stuttering, and general clumsiness.

Left-handed people are also disproportionately represented among musicians, artists, mathematicians, athletes, and recent U.S. presidents. (In the last 30 years, left-handed presidents have included Gerald Ford, George H. Bush, Bill Clinton, and, for the most part, Ronald Reagan. Right-handed presidents numbered only two: Jimmy Carter and George W. Bush.)

Athletes who are left-handed tend to be more successful than right-handed ones, but only in sports involving direct confrontation, such as baseball, tennis, fencing, and boxing, because they benefit from certain tactical advantages, such as a left-handed batter being closer to first base. They have no greater success in sports without direct confrontation, such as swimming, running, pole-vaulting, and other track and field events.

Unlike right-handed individuals, left-handed ones become aphasic after injury to either cerebral hemisphere. In addition, if left-handed individuals develop aphasia, its variety relates less closely to the specific injury site (see later) and their prognosis is relatively good.

Many individuals are ambidextrous probably because they have mixed dominance. Seemingly endowed with language, music, and motor skill function in both hemispheres, they tend to excel in sports and performing on musical instruments.

Although the left hemisphere is dominant in approximately 95% of all people (and the rest of this chapter assumes it always is), sometimes dominance must be established with certainty. For example, when the temporal lobe must be partially resected because of a tumor or intractable partial complex epilepsy (see Chapter 10), only a limited resection of the dominant temporal lobe would be feasible. Too large a resection might create aphasia or memory impairment.

The *Wada test*—direct injection of sodium amobarbital into a carotid artery—can establish cerebral dominance. When the amobarbital perfuses the dominant hemisphere, it renders the patient temporarily aphasic. Similarly, infusion of amobarbital into a temporal lobe may cause temporary amnesia if the other temporal lobe is already damaged. Another diagnostic test, functional magnetic resonance imaging (fMRI), in which subjects essentially undergo language evaluation during an MRI, is potentially better.

MUSIC

In general, musically gifted people tend to process music, as language, in their dominant hemisphere. Those with *perfect pitch*—the ability to identify a tone in the absence of a reference tone—have distinctive fMRI patterns when listening to music. Also, their dominant hemisphere planum temporale is relatively enlarged. If these musically gifted people develop aphasia, they also lose a great deal of their musical ability.

In contrast, individuals without any particular musical ability rely on their nondominant hemisphere to carry a tune. For them, perhaps the proximity of their musical and emotional systems, both in the nondominant hemisphere, explains the emotional effects of music. The primary location of music in the nondominant hemisphere for most people may also explain why many aphasic individuals, handicapped in language, often retain their ability to recognize music and to sing.

APHASIA

The Perisylvian Language Arc

Impulses conveying speech, music, and simple sounds travel from the ears along the acoustic (eighth cranial) nerves into the brainstem, where they synapse in the *medial geniculate body*. Then postsynaptic, crossed and uncrossed brainstem tracts bring the impulses to the primary auditory cortex, *Heschl's gyri*, in each temporal lobe (see Fig. 4-16). Most music and some other sounds remain based in the nondominant hemisphere. However, the brain transmits language impulses to *Wernicke's* area, which is situated in the dominant temporal lobe. From there, they travel in the *arcuate fasciculus*, coursing posteriorly through the temporal and parietal lobes, and then circling anteriorly to the frontal lobe's *Broca's area*. This vital language center—located immediately anterior to the motor center for the right face, larynx, pharynx, and arm (Fig. 8-1)—receives processed, integrated language and converts it to speech. A horseshoe-shaped region of cerebral cortex, which surrounds the sylvian fissure, the *perisylvian language arc*, contains Wernicke's area, the arcuate fasciculus, and Broca's area.

Using the perisylvian language arc model, researchers have established normal and abnormal language patterns. For example, when normal people repeat aloud what they hear, auditory impulses go first to

FIGURE 8-1 ■ The left cerebral hemisphere contains *Wernicke's area* in the temporal lobe and *Broca's area* in the frontal lobe, where it sits between Heschl's gyrus (see Fig. 4-16) and the cerebral cortex motor area for the right hand, face, and language. The *arcuate fasciculus,* the "language superhighway," connects Wernicke's and Broca's areas. It curves rearward from the temporal lobe to the parietal lobe. It then passes through the angular gyrus and forward to the frontal lobe. These structures surrounding the sylvian fissure, which comprise the *perisylvian language arc,* form the central processing unit of the language system.

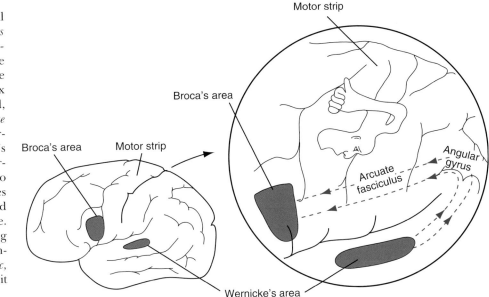

Wernicke's area, then pass around the arcuate fasciculus, and finally arrive in Broca's area for speech production (Fig. 8-2, *A*). Reading aloud is a complicated variation of repeating aloud because reading requires both hemispheres and a learned system of decoding symbols, that is, having been taught to read. As people read, their geniculocalcarine pathway transmits visual impulses from the lateral geniculate bodies to the calcarine (visual) cortex in both the left and right occipital lobes (see Fig. 4-1). Impulses from the left visual field go to the right occipital cortex. Then those impulses must travel through the posterior corpus callosum to reach the left (dominant) cerebral hemisphere. The impulses that have crossed from the right visual cortex merge with those already in the left hemisphere in its parietal lobe. Decoded, coherent language information then travels from the left parietal lobe via the arcuate fasciculus to Broca's area for articulation (see Fig. 8-2, *B*).

Clinical Evaluation

Before diagnosing aphasia, the clinician must keep in mind normal language variations. Normal people may struggle and stammer when confronted with a novel experience, such as a neurologic examination. Individuals have their own style and rhythm. Some may be reticent, uneducated, intimidated, or hostile. Some, before speaking, consider each word and formulate every phrase as though carefully considering which item to chose from a menu, but others just impulsively blurt out the first thing on their mind.

In diagnosing aphasia, the clinician can use various classifications. A favorite distinguishes *receptive (sensory)*

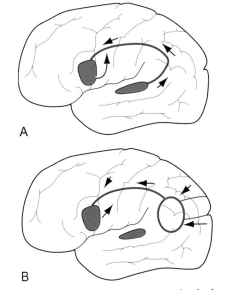

FIGURE 8-2 ■ *A,* When people *repeat aloud,* language is received in Wernicke's area and then transmitted through the parietal lobe by the arcuate fasciculus to Broca's area. This area innervates the adjacent cerebral cortex for the tongue, lips, larynx, and pharynx. *B.* When people *read aloud,* visual impulses are received by the left and right occipital visual cortex regions. Both regions send impulses to a left parietal lobe association region (the oval), which converts text to language. Impulses from the left visual field, which are initially received in the right cortex, must first pass through the posterior corpus callosum to reach the language centers (see Fig. 8-4).

from *expressive (motor)* aphasia based on relative impairment of verbal reception versus expression. However, a major drawback of that classification is that most aphasic patients have a mixture of impairments that do not allow specific diagnosis.

TABLE 8-1 ■ Salient Features of Major Aphasias

Feature	Nonfluent	Fluent
Previous descriptions	Expressive	Receptive
	Motor	Sensory
	Broca's	Wernicke's
Spontaneous speech	Nonverbal	Verbal
Content	Paucity of words, mostly nouns and verbs	Complete sentences with normal syntax
Articulation	Dysarthric, slow, stuttering	Good
Errors	Telegraphic speech	Paraphasic errors, nonspecific phrases, circumlocutions
Response on testing		
Comprehension	Preserved	Impaired
Repetition	Impaired	Impaired
Naming	Impaired	Impaired
Associated deficits	Right hemiparesis (arm, face > leg)	Hemianopsia, hemisensory loss
Localization of lesion frontal lobe	Temporal or parietal lobe	Occasionally diffuse

The most clinically useful and perhaps most widely used classification, *nonfluent-fluent*, derives from the patient's verbal output (Table 8-1). Fluent and nonfluent aphasias are usually evident during conversation, history taking, or mental status examination.

A standard series of simple verbal tests identify and further classify these aphasias. This entire test sequence can be repeated with written requests and responses; however, with one notable exception (described later), written deficits parallel verbal ones. The standard aphasia tests evaluate *three basic language functions*: *comprehension*, *naming*, and *repetition* (Table 8-2).

- Comprehension is tested by asking the patient to follow simple requests, such as picking up one hand, opening and closing eyes, and protruding the tongue.
- Naming is tested by asking the patient to say the name of common objects, such as a pen or key.
- Repetition is tested by asking the patient to recite several short phrases, such as, "The boy went to the store."

Nonfluent Aphasia

Characteristics

Paucity of speech characterizes nonfluent aphasia. Patients are nonverbal. Whatever speech they produce consists almost exclusively of single words and short phrases, with preferential use of basic words, particularly nouns and verbs. Their speech lacks modifiers, such as adjectives, adverbs, and conjunctions. Longer phrases typically consist entirely of stock phrases or sound bites, such as, "Not so bad" or "Get out of here."

TABLE 8-2 ■ Clinical Evaluation for Aphasia

Spontaneous speech: fluent versus nonfluent
Verbalization tests
  Comprehension
    Ability to follow simple requests, "Please, pick up your hand."
    Ability to follow complex requests, "Please, show me your left ring finger, and stick out your tongue."
  Naming
    Common objects: tie, keys, pen
    Uncommon objects: watchband, belt buckle
  Repetition
    Simple phrases: "The boy went to the store."
    Complex phrases: "No ands, ifs, or buts."
Reading and writing (repeat above tests)

Nonfluent speech is also slow. Its rate is typically less than 50 words per minute, which is much slower than normal (100 to 150 words per minute). Another hallmark is that the flow of speech is so interrupted by excessive pauses that its pattern is sometimes termed "telegraphic." For example, in response to a question about food, a patient might stammer "fork...steak...eat...no."

Patients with nonfluent aphasia may be unable to say either their own name or the names of common objects. They cannot repeat simple phrases. At the same time, they have relatively normal comprehension that can be illustrated by their ability to follow verbal requests, such as "Please, close your eyes" or "Raise your left hand, please."

Localization and Etiology

Lesions responsible for nonfluent aphasia are usually situated in or near Broca's area (Fig. 8-3, *A*). Their

FIGURE 8-3 ■ *A*, Lesions that cause *nonfluent aphasia* are typically located in the frontal lobe and encompass Broca's area and the adjacent cortex motor strip. *B*, Those causing *fluent aphasia* are in the temporoparietal region, may even consist of diffuse injury, such as from Alzheimer's disease, and encompass Wernicke's areas and the posterior regions. They usually spare the motor strip. *C*, Those causing *conduction aphasia*, which are relatively small, interrupt the arcuate fasciculus in the parietal or posterior temporal lobe. *D*, Those causing isolation aphasia are circumferential injuries of the watershed region that spare the perisylvian language arc.

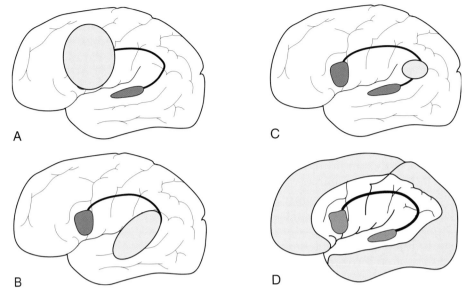

etiology is usually a middle cerebral artery stroke or other discrete structural lesion; however, their location, not their nature, produces the aphasia. Whatever their etiology, these lesions tend to be so extensive that they damage neighboring structures, such as the motor cortex and the posterior sensory cortex. Moreover, because they are usually spherical or conical, they damage underlying white matter tracts, including the visual pathway. Diffuse cerebral injuries, such as metabolic disturbances or Alzheimer's disease, practically never cause nonfluent aphasia.

Neurologists originally termed nonfluent aphasia "expressive" or "motor" because of the prominent speech impairment or "Broca's" because of the responsible lesion's location.

Associated Deficits

Because the lesion usually damages the motor cortex and other adjacent and underlying regions, nonfluent aphasia characteristically occurs in association with a right hemiparesis, with particular weakness of the arm and lower face, and with poor articulation (dysarthria). Lesions with any depth also cause a right homonymous hemianopsia (visual field cut). One of the most common syndromes in neurology is an occlusion of the left middle cerebral artery that produces the combination of nonfluent aphasia and right-sided hemiparesis with the arm much more involved than the leg, right-sided homonymous hemianopsia, and right-sided hemisensory impairment.

Lesions causing nonfluent aphasia often simultaneously produce *buccofacial apraxia*, also called "oral apraxia." This apraxia, like others, is not paresis or any kind of involuntary movement disorder, but the inability to execute normal voluntary movements of the face, lip, and tongue. When buccofacial apraxia occurs in conjunction with nonfluent aphasia, it adds to the dysarthria.

To demonstrate buccofacial apraxia, the examiner must ask the patient to say "La . . Pa . . La . . Pa . . La . . Pa"; protrude the tongue in different directions; and pretend to blow out a match and suck through a straw. Patients with buccofacial apraxia will be unable to comply, although they may be able to use the same muscles reflexively or when provided with cues. For example, patients who cannot speak might sing, and those who cannot pretend to use a straw might be able to suck water through an actual one.

Regarding another aspect of aphasia, lesions obliterating Broca's area often render patients mute (*aphemic*). Nevertheless, they can often express themselves with left hand gestures and shoulder shrugs, and they can also comprehend verbal requests. Their communication, albeit limited, distinguishes them from patients with psychogenic mutism.

Lesions completely damaging both frontal lobes reduce patients to a paucity or absence of speech (*abulia*) with little emotion, responsiveness, or voluntary movement (akinesia). This extensive damage, which constitutes a loss far more profound than nonfluent aphasia, invariably produces a neurologic-based depression.

Even without such extensive loss, patients with nonfluent aphasia, who typically remain aware of and frustrated by their impairments, often develop comorbid depression. An admittedly simple psychologic explanation proposes that patients with aphasia have suffered a major loss and naturally feel sad, hopeless, and frustrated. A neurologic explanation is that because aphasia-producing lesions are generally located in the frontal lobe, they produce concomitant apathy and abulia (see Frontal Lobe Disorders, Chapter 7). Psychiatrists face obstacles when assessing mood in aphasic patients because they often appear apathetic, cannot communicate, and offer potentially misleading facial expressions. In these patients, physicians might utilize a visual analog mood scale similar to those used to measure pain (see Chapter 14).

Alternatively, signs of depression in aphasic patients, particularly those who have had several strokes, may actually be manifestations of dementia or pseudobulbar palsy. The situation is complicated because nonfluent aphasia, dementia, pseudobulbar palsy, and depression share several aspects. Moreover, all four neuropsychologic conditions are manifestations of frontal lobe injury and they often occur together in various combinations. For example, frontotemporal dementia and multiple strokes routinely produce dementia and aphasia, and sometimes the other symptoms.

When strokes or head trauma cause aphasia, patients improve to a greater or lesser extent because ischemic areas of the brain recover and surviving neurons form new connections. Little or no documentation supports the usefulness of speech therapy or medication.

Global Aphasia

Extensive dominant hemisphere damage abolishes so much language function that it results in an extreme form of nonfluent aphasia, *global aphasia*. Aside from uttering some unintelligible sounds, patients with global aphasia are mute. Although they can follow some gestured requests, which bypass the language arc, they cannot comply with verbal ones.

Moreover, patients with global aphasia tend to be uncommunicative in any way and emotionally unresponsive. They also usually have comparably severe physical deficits, including right hemiplegia, right homonymous hemianopsia, and conjugate deviation of the eyes toward the left. Frequent causes are dominant hemisphere tumors, internal carotid or middle cerebral artery occlusions causing extensive cerebral ischemia, cerebral hemorrhages, and penetrating wounds.

Fluent Aphasia

Paraphasias and Other Characteristics

Fluent aphasia is characterized by the inability to comprehend language along with incessant use of *paraphasic errors* or *paraphasias*, which are incorrect or even nonsensical words. Patients insert paraphasias within relatively complete, well-articulated, grammatically correct sentences that are spoken at a normal rate. Enough paraphasias can render conversation unintelligible.

Paraphasias most often consist of a word substitution, such as "clock" for "watch" or "spoon" for "fork" (*related paraphasias*), in which the substitute word arises from the same category. Less commonly, the words involved have little relation, such as "glove" for "knife" (*unrelated paraphasia*), or a nonspecific relation, such as "that" for any object (a *generic substitution*). Paraphasias may also consist of altered words, such as "breat" for "bread" (*literal paraphasia*).

Fluent aphasia patients also insert strings of nonsensical coinages (*neologisms*), such as "I want to fin gunt in the fark." They can bounce several times from one word to another with a close sound but little or no shared meaning (*clang associations*, from the German *klang*, sound). For example, a patient making a clang association might ask, "What's for dinner, diner, slimmer, greaser, bouncer . . ."

As if to circumvent their word-finding difficulty, patients often speak in *circumlocutions*. They may also tend toward *tangential diversions*, as though once having spoken the wrong word, they pursue the idea triggered by their error. They string together meaningfully related words until they reach an absurd point. For example, when attempting to name a pencil, the patient said, "pen, paper, tree, forest . . ."

Nevertheless, because nondominant hemisphere functions remain unaffected, nonverbal expressions are preserved (see later). For example, prosody remains consistent with patients' mood. Patients continue to express their feelings through facial gestures, body movements, and cursing. Similarly, most patients retain their ability to produce a melody even though they may be unable to repeat the lyrics. For example, patients can hum a tune, such as "Jingle Bells," but if they attempt to sing it, their lyrics are strewn with paraphasias.

Associated Deficits

Unlike nonfluent aphasia, fluent aphasia is not associated with significant hemiparesis because the responsible lesion is distant from the cerebral cortex motor strip. Signs of corticospinal tract injury are minimal. Physicians typically elicit only right-sided hyperactive deep tendon reflexes (DTRs) and a Babinski sign. However, they may detect a right-sided sensory impairment and visual field cut because the underlying lesions often interrupt sensory and visual cerebral pathways.

Strikingly, patients are often strangely unaware of their paraphasias, unable to edit them, and often oblivious to their listener's consternation. Sometimes patients must sense their inability to communicate and develop anxiety, agitation, or paranoia. Clinicians not seeing any hemiparesis and unable to capture the patient's attention for detailed testing often do not appreciate the neurologic basis of the abnormal language, thought, or behavior. For many psychiatry liaison consultations, the sudden onset of fluent aphasia often turns out to be the explanation for an "acute psychosis," marked change in behavior, or management problem.

Localization and Etiology

Usually, discrete structural lesions, such as small strokes, in the temporoparietal region are the cause of fluent aphasia (see Figs. 8-3, *B* and 20-16). Although these lesions do not necessarily damage Wernicke's area, the arcuate fasciculus, or the sensory cortex, neurologists have often labeled fluent aphasia "Wernicke's" or "sensory" aphasia. Unlike nonfluent aphasia, it is sometimes caused by diffuse cerebral injury, including Alzheimer's disease.

Varieties of Fluent Aphasia

Differences in the varieties of fluent aphasia tend to be subtle largely because their identity turns on fine points. Moreover, clinical-pathologic correlations are subject to great individual variations in anatomy, language production, and cognitive capacity.

Anomia

A common variety of aphasia, *anomic aphasia* or *anomia*, is simply inability to name objects. Small strokes most often produce this aphasia. Less commonly, anomia results from a neurodegenerative illness, such as Alzheimer's disease or, more likely, frontotemporal dementia. For patients with these illnesses, anomia rather than memory impairment might explain their inability to state the names of familiar places, objects, and people.

Transcortical or Isolation Aphasia

Some lesions damage only the cerebral cortex surrounding the language arc. By sparing the language pathway, these lesions leave basic language function intact but isolated from other functions. *Transcortical* or *isolation aphasia*, another aphasia variety, stems from cerebral injuries that, while sparing the perisylvian arc, damage the entire surrounding cerebral cortex. Because the language system remains intact, patients with isolation aphasia retain their ability to repeat whatever they hear, but they cannot interact in a conversation, follow requests, or name objects. Moreover,

because of damage to the entire remaining cortex, patients have severe cognitive impairment. Depending on the injury, patients may also tend to assume a decorticate posture (see Fig. 11-5).

The salient feature of isolation aphasia is the disparity between seeming muteness but preserved ability to repeat long, complex sentences readily, involuntarily, and sometimes compulsively. This parrot-like echoing of others' words is called *echolalia*. A cursory evaluation could understandably confuse this speech pattern with irrational jargon.

The etiology of isolation aphasia lies in the precarious blood supply of the cerebral cortex. Although major branches of left middle cerebral artery perfuse the perisylvian arc, only thin, fragile, distal branches of middle, anterior, and posterior cerebral arteries perfuse its border with the surrounding cortex (the *watershed area*). When these vessels deliver insufficient cerebral blood flow to this portion of the cortex, it suffers a *watershed infarction*, which, in turn, leads to isolation aphasia (see Fig. 8-3, *D*). Thus, cardiac or respiratory arrest, suicide attempts using carbon monoxide, and other hypotensive or hypoxic episodes cause isolation aphasia. When Alzheimer's disease strikes cerebral areas except the language and motor regions, which is uncommon, it too can cause isolation aphasia.

If desired, clinicians can further divide transcortical aphasia into sensory and motor varieties. Both are characterized by preserved ability to repeat. Transcortical *sensory* aphasia is essentially a fluent aphasia with preserved ability to repeat. Transcortical *motor* aphasia is essentially a nonfluent aphasia that also preserves, despite paucity of verbal output, ability to repeat.

Conduction Aphasia

In contrast to lesions that damage the cortex surrounding the perisylvian language arc and spare the language pathway, some lesions damage only the arcuate fasciculus and thereby interrupt the language arc. Damage to the arcuate fasciculus—the tract connecting Broca's and Wernicke's areas—produces another, unique variety of aphasia. In *conduction aphasia*, a small, discrete arcuate fasciculus lesion, usually in the parietal or posterior temporal lobe (see Fig. 8-3, *C*), interrupts or *disconnects* Wernicke's and Broca's areas. (It therefore may be seen as one of the *disconnection syndromes* [see later].) Conduction aphasia patients are fluent and retain good comprehension, but they cannot repeat phrases or short sentences. In contrast to patients with isolation aphasia, they are particularly maladept at repeating strings of syllables.

The most frequent cause of conduction aphasia is a small, embolic stroke in the posterior temporal branch of the left middle cerebral artery. The infarctions are usually so small that they cause little or no physical deficit. At worst, patients have right lower facial weakness.

MENTAL ABNORMALITIES WITH LANGUAGE IMPAIRMENT

Dementia

Although aphasia by itself is not equivalent to dementia, it can be a component of dementia or it can mimic dementia. For example, when aphasia impairs routine communications, such as saying the date and place, repeating a series of numbers, and following requests, it mimics dementia. At times, patients with severe aphasia seem so bizarre that they appear incoherent. Because people think in words, aphasia also clouds thinking and memory.

The two conditions also differ in their time course. Dementia develops slowly, but aphasia begins abruptly, except in the unusual case when it heralds a neurodegenerative illness. Nonfluent aphasia further differs from dementia in its accompanying physical aspects: dysarthria and obvious lateralized signs, such as a right-sided hemiparesis and homonymous hemianopsia. Paraphasias readily characterize fluent aphasia.

Occasionally patients have both aphasia and dementia. This combination often occurs with one or more strokes superimposed on Alzheimer's disease and with frontotemporal dementia. These situations notoriously defy classification because aphasia so often invalidates standard cognitive tests.

Distinguishing aphasia from dementia and recognizing when the two conditions coexist are more than an academic exercise. A diagnosis of aphasia almost always suggests that a patient has had a discrete dominant cerebral hemisphere injury. Because a stroke or other structural lesion would be the most likely cause, the appropriate evaluation would include a computed tomography (CT) or magnetic resonance imaging (MRI). In contrast, a diagnosis of dementia suggests that the most likely cause would be Alzheimer's disease, frontotemporal dementia, or another diffuse process, and the evaluation might include various blood tests as well as a CT or MRI.

Schizophrenia

Distinguishing fluent aphasia from *schizophrenic speech* can, theoretically at least, prove even more troublesome. Circumlocutions, tangential diversions, and neologisms are common manifestations. As the thought disorder of schizophrenia develops, its language abnormalities increase in frequency and

similarity to aphasia. In a different situation, previously healthy people suddenly developing aphasia can be so frightened and confused that they become agitated and irrational.

However, many differences can be discerned. Schizophrenic speech usually develops gradually in patients who are relatively young (in their third decade) and have had long-standing psychiatric illness. Their neologisms and other paraphasias occur relatively infrequently and tend toward the inconspicuous. Unlike most patients with fluent aphasia, those with schizophrenia can repeat polysyllabic words and complex phrases.

In contrast, aphasia usually appears suddenly in the seventh or eighth decade. Except for some patients with fluent aphasia, most retain awareness that they cannot communicate and very often request help in this regard. Also, possibly because of self-monitoring, they keep their responses short and pointed. Any right-sided hemiparesis or hemianopsia clinches the diagnosis.

Other Disorders

Language abnormalities appear early and prominently as in the DSM-IV-TR criteria of many of the *Pervasive Developmental Disorders*, including *Autistic Disorder*, *Rett's Disorder*, and *Childhood Disintegrative Disorder*. In addition, although Asperger's disorder children have no significant delay in language and remain fluent, they fail to appreciate the nuances and affective components of language. Likewise, a generalized language regression appears after several years of normal development in Rett's syndrome (see Chapter 13). Overall, when language regression strikes children, particularly boys and those younger than 3 years, they face a high likelihood of developing an autistic disorder.

Autistic children typically begin to speak later than normal and ultimately demonstrate impairments in all aspects of language: articulation (phonology), prosody, grammar, reception and especially expression, conversation, and facial and bodily communication. In addition, their speech in many cases features a myriad of nonsensical repetitions (stereotypies), idiosyncrasies, and echolalia.

Mutism and apparent language abnormalities can also be manifestations of psychogenic disturbances (see Chapter 3). In these cases, apparent language impairment is usually inconsistent and amenable to suggestion. Acquired stuttering also often indicates a psychogenic language impairment. For example, a patient with psychogenic aphasia might stutter and seem to be at a loss for words but communicate normally by writing. Sometimes, amobarbital infusion during an interview might be appropriate.

A common psychogenic, aphasia-like condition is the sudden, unexpected difficulty in remembering someone's name (blocking). The classic example remains the Freudian slip. (Freud's work on aphasia presaged his exploration of analysands' unconscious, in part, through words spoken in "error.") Depending on one's viewpoint, everyday word substitutions may be termed either paraphasias or insights into the unconscious. For example, when a physician's former secretary, being evaluated for a neurologic disorder, says that she has been Dr. So-and-So's "medical cemetery," a clinician could interpret the comment as either her feelings about the competence of the doctor, an indication of the patient's own fears of death, or a paraphasia that is referable to a dominant hemisphere lesion.

DISORDERS RELATED TO APHASIA

Dyslexia

In most cases, reading impairment despite normal or near normal intelligence and education represents a developmental disorder, *developmental dyslexia* (Greek, *lexis*, word or phrase). If observed closely, approximately 10% of all school children display some degree of developmental dyslexia. Moreover, alone or comorbid with related problems, developmental dyslexia occurs in 80% of all children with learning disabilities. Teachers usually detect it when children first try to read, but occasionally, mild forms escape detection until older children confront the complicated reading tasks of high school or college. In about 25% of children and, to a lesser extent, in some adults, dyslexia is comorbid with attention deficit hyperactivity disorder (ADHD). Regardless of when it first appears and acknowledging that some educational strategies ameliorate the problem, developmental dyslexia persists throughout life. For dyslexic students who are otherwise bright, studying mathematics and science helps circumvent the disability.

Dyslexia affects boys with disproportionate severity and frequency, such that the boy-to-girl ratio lies between 2:1 and 5:1. Many children come from families in which several other members also have dyslexia. Studies have implicated several autosomal dominant and sex-linked genes. Imaging and pathologic studies reveal that the brains of dyslexic individuals lack the normal planum temporale asymmetry. In other words, their brains are symmetric, which is abnormal.

In older children and adults, strokes, trauma, or other lesions can produce dyslexia or completely impair reading ability (*acquired alexia*). In those cases, acquired alexia is usually a component of aphasia and accompanied by right-sided motor deficits. More important, with one famous exception, *agraphia* (inability to write) invariably accompanies the alexia.

Alexia and Agraphia

In the notable exception, *alexia without agraphia* (Fig. 8-4), patients demonstrate little or no impairment in comprehending speech or expressing themselves verbally or by writing; however, they simply cannot read. For example, such patients can transcribe another person's dictation and write their own thoughts but then are unable to read their own handwriting. Alexia without agraphia, which should really be called "alexia with graphia," results from a destructive lesion encompassing the dominant (left) occipital lobe and adjacent posterior corpus callosum (see Fig. 20-24). Aside from having a right homonymous hemianopsia, patients lack physical deficits.

Gerstmann's Syndrome

Gerstmann's syndrome, a classic disorder, consists of four neuropsychologic disturbances: *acalculia* (impaired arithmetic skills), *finger agnosia* (inability to identify fingers), *left/right confusion*, and agraphia. When all four elements occur, which is exceedingly rare, neurologists usually attribute the syndrome to a lesion in the *angular gyrus* of the dominant parietal lobe (see Fig. 8-1).

One the other hand, neurologists question the existence of this syndrome as a distinct clinical entity.

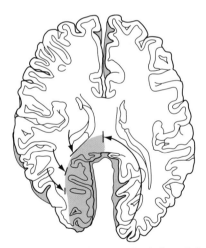

FIGURE 8-4 ■ Lesions that damage the left occipital lobe and the posterior corpus callosum cause *alexia without agraphia* (see Fig. 20-24). Patients are unable to see anything in their right visual field because of the left occipital cortex damage. Left visual images still reach the right cortex, but they cannot be transmitted to the left cerebral language centers because the critical posterior corpus callosum is damaged. Thus, patients cannot comprehend written material presented to either visual field. In contrast, they can still write full sentences from memory, imagination, or dictation because these forms of information still reach the language centers.

Patients rarely display all the components and those with three or four usually also have aphasia or dementia. Nevertheless, the constellation, even if it does not constitute a syndrome, is useful. Clinicians can seek these neuropsychologic disturbances in both adults with strokes and children with learning disabilities. For example, children with dyscalculia also frequently display poor handwriting (agraphia) and clumsiness from left/right confusion. Those impairments are accompanied by subtle physical signs of dominant hemisphere injury, such as right-sided hyperactive DTRs and a Babinski sign without hemiparesis.

Apraxia

Roughly the motor system's equivalent of nonfluent aphasia, *apraxia* is inability to execute learned actions despite normal strength, sensation, and coordination. Neurologists attribute apraxia to disruption of links between motor centers and the perisylvian language arc, frontal lobe executive centers, and other vital neuropsychologic regions.

Although apraxia can be readily differentiated from simple paresis, it is often inseparable from aphasia or dementia. In fact, apraxia often appears as a symptom of Alzheimer's disease and other cortical dementias (see Chapter 7).

In demonstrating apraxia, the examiner generally first tests the patient's buccofacial (lips, face, tongue) and limb movements in making gestures or "symbolic acts" (Table 8-3). Next, the examiner asks the patient to perform imagined actions, first on pretend objects and then on actual ones. After seeing the examiner perform an action, patients with apraxia typically can copy it. Similarly, when patients with apraxia are given an actual object, which gives them a cue, they can often perform the object's intended action. For example, a patient with apraxia might not be able to mimic using a comb, but when presented with one he or she would use it appropriately.

Overall, their inability to use a common tool, such as a comb or spoon, most reliably demonstrates their apraxia. Further testing, depending on circumstances, includes performing a series of steps, copying figures, arranging matchsticks, walking, or dressing.

Patients typically remain unaware of their apraxia because they usually do not spontaneously attempt the various tests, such as saluting an unseen officer or using an imaginary screwdriver. Moreover, an unsophisticated clinician might incorrectly attribute a motor impairment due to apraxia to paresis or incoordination.

Despite its complexity, neurologists designate several clinically useful categories of apraxia. *Ideomotor apraxia*, the most common category, consists basically of the inability to convert an idea into an action. For example, patients with ideomotor apraxia cannot pretend to perform an action (pantomime) at an examiner's request despite possessing a clear understanding and retaining the physical ability to comply. Clinicians might envision ideomotor apraxia as the result of a disconnection between cognitive or language regions and motor regions (Fig. 8-5). Almost invariably, a left-sided frontal or parietal lobe lesion gives rise to the apraxia. Thus, ideomotor apraxia often coexists with aphasia, particularly nonfluent aphasia, and inability of the right hand to pantomime.

One of its two varieties, *buccofacial apraxia*, as previously discussed, is a feature of nonfluent aphasia. In the other variety, *limb apraxia*, patients cannot execute simple requests involving their right arm or leg. They cannot salute or move their hand in certain abstract patterns. They cannot pretend to brush their teeth, turn a key, comb their hair, or kick a ball. When asked to pretend to *use* an object, these patients characteristically use their hand as though it *were* the actual object. For example, they will brush their teeth with their forefinger instead of pretending to hold a toothbrush.

In *ideational apraxia*, patients cannot conceive and then perform a sequence of steps. For example, they cannot pretend to fold a letter, place it into an envelope, address the envelope, and then affix a stamp. In contrast to ideomotor apraxia, which is associated with nonfluent aphasia, ideational apraxia is almost inseparable from dementia. In particular, ideational apraxia is a hallmark of frontotemporal dementia, where it reflects executive dysfunction. In addition,

		Action	
	Gesture*	**Imagined**	**Real**
Buccofacial	Kiss the air	Pretend to blow out a match	Blow out a match
	Repeat "Pa"	Pretend to suck on a straw	Drink water through a straw
Limb	Salute	Pretend to use a comb	Comb the hair
	Stop traffic	Pretend to write	Write with a pencil or pen

TABLE 8-3 ■ Testing for Ideomotor Apraxia

*Symbolic acts.

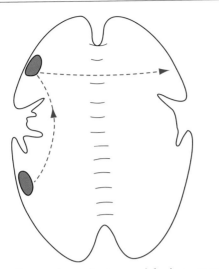

FIGURE 8-5 ■ In a schematic transaxial view, requests for *normal movements* travel to Wernicke's area in the dominant (left) posterior temporal lobe. They are transmitted anteriorly to the motor regions and, through the anterior corpus callosum, to the contralateral motor strip. Interruptions of the path within the left cerebral hemisphere result in ideomotor apraxia of both arms, causing bilateral limb apraxia. Lesions in the anterior corpus callosum interrupt only those impulses destined to control the left arm and leg, which causes unilateral left arm and leg ideomotor apraxia.

Alzheimer's disease and multiple strokes, because they lead to dementia and impaired planning and execution, often cause ideational apraxia.

This book covers several other apraxias in more detail elsewhere. *Construction* and *dressing apraxias* are typically manifestations of nondominant hemisphere lesions (see later). *Gait apraxia* is a hallmark of normal pressure hydrocephalus (see Fig. 7-8).

NONDOMINANT HEMISPHERE SYMPTOMS

Neuropsychologic symptoms arising from nondominant hemispheres injury tend to be short-lived and subtle. Their expression often depends on the patient's premorbid intelligence, personality, and defense mechanisms. Moreover, the symptoms occur not only individually but also in various combinations and in interrelated fashions. Neither a nondominant syndrome nor its components are defined in the DSM-IV-TR. Detecting them requires considerable clinical acumen.

Their cause is almost always a structural lesion that has rapidly developed, such as trauma, a stroke, or malignant tumor. Neurodegenerative illnesses rarely cause such symptoms. Thus, "nondominant symptoms" appear abruptly and unexpectedly. Their development often leaves patients perplexed and dumbfounded.

Hemi-Inattention

Patients with nondominant hemisphere injury typically display *hemi-inattention (hemispatial neglect)* as their most prominent symptom. These injuries usually originate in a stroke or other structural lesion of the nondominant parietal lobe cortex and the underlying thalamus and reticular activating system. Damage to these regions causes hemi-inattention and related symptoms by impairing arousal and distribution of spatial attention.

Patients with hemi-inattention ignore visual, tactile, and other sensory stimuli that originate from their left side (Fig. 8-6). For example, they disregard, fail to perceive, or misinterpret objects in their left visual field (Fig. 8-7). Sometimes men with this condition leave the left side of their face unshaven. In contrast to patients with homonymous hemianopsia, who usually develop some awareness and thus make compensatory movements to keep objects in the preserved visual field, those with hemi-inattention remain oblivious to their situation and make no normal exploratory eye or limb movements.

Another manifestation of hemi-inattention—*extinction on double simultaneous stimulation (DSS)*—occurs when an examiner stimulates both sides of a patient's body, but the patient neglects the left-sided stimulation. For example, when the examiner touches both arms, the patient reports that only the right one was touched, but when the examiner touches only the left arm, the patient correctly reports that it was touched. Another example of DSS can occur with visual stimulation. A patient might correctly perceive a flash of light in the left visual field, but when the examiner simultaneously flashes light in both visual fields, the patient would report seeing only the one in the right-sided visual field.

In a related symptom, *dressing apraxia* (impaired ability to dress), patients with a nondominant hemisphere lesion may leave their left side partly undressed or they may completely fail to dress. Patients with dressing apraxia may not merely leave their left limbs out of their clothing, they may put both hands into one sleeve, misalign buttons, and become befuddled when presented with their clothing turned inside out. Moreover, patients generally remain unaware that their clothing is disheveled. Even though their dressing apraxia may require hemi-inattention and other perceptual problems, neurologists label it an apraxia because of the initial, obvious problem with skilled movements.

An extreme form of hemi-inattention occurs in the *alien hand syndrome*. In this disorder, a patient's left hand retains some rudimentary motor and sensory functions, but the patient cannot control the movements or appreciate the sensations. Without the

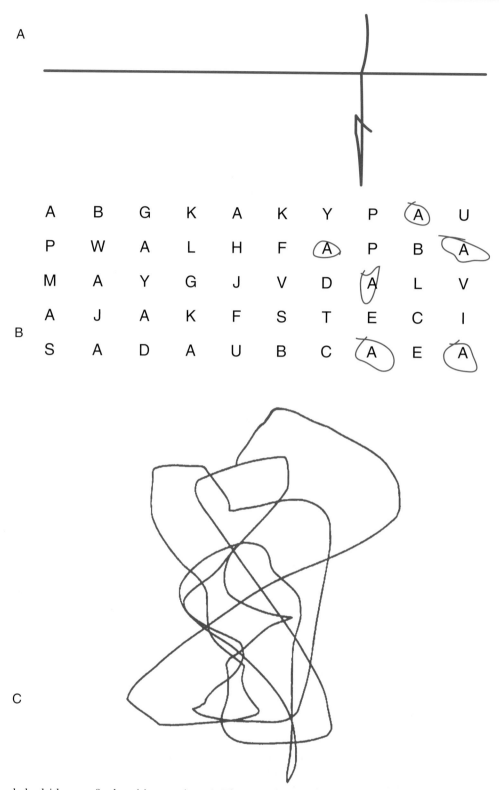

FIGURE 8-6 ■ Simple bedside tests for hemi-inattention. *A,* The examiner has asked the patient, who has just sustained a right middle cerebral infarction, to bisect a horizontal line. The patient, neglecting a portion of the line's left side, draws the vertical line off-center to the right, bisecting only the portion of the line's perceived segment. *B,* Then the examiner asks the patient to circle all the "A"s on the page. Again neglecting the left side of the page, the patient circles only those on the right. *C,* An examiner has asked a 4-year-old boy, recovering from right parietal trauma, to draw a man. Because of a combination of hemi-inattention and constructional apraxia (see later), he merely scribbles on the right side of the paper.

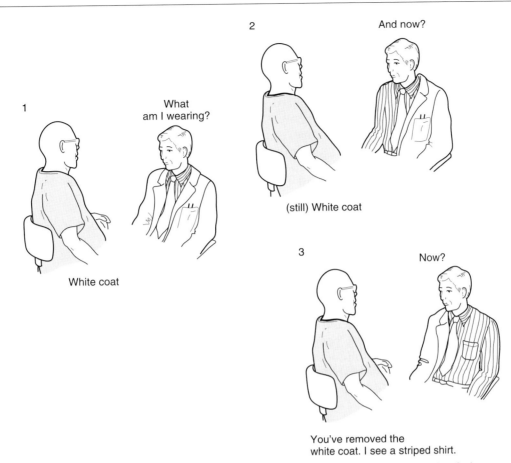

FIGURE 8-7 ■ In a classic demonstration of left *hemi-inattention*, the patient, neglecting left-sided stimulation, perceives only what the examiner is wearing in his right visual field. Even if the patient's problem were simply a left homonymous hemianopsia, he still would have explored and discovered, with his intact right visual field, that the examiner was half-dressed.

patient's awareness, the hand moves semipurposefully, making its own explorations and performing simple tasks, such as scratching or moving bedclothes. In an often-quoted example, a patient reported that her hand intermittently attempted to choke her.

The alien hand syndrome rests on the patient having at least two misperceptions: (1) the patient does not possess the hand and (2) because the hand's movements take place independent of the patient's knowledge and control, another person (the alien) governs them. Most patients feel divorced from the hand or, at least, accept only a tenuous relationship to it. Several cases have occurred in the context of corpus callosum injury, suggesting that the alien hand syndrome is another disconnection syndrome (see later).

Anosognosia, inability to acknowledge a physical deficit (usually a left hemiparesis), is an aspect of hemi-inattention of profound clinical importance. Patients typically cannot identify the affected part of their body (*somatotopagnosia* or *autotopagnosia*). For example, they might claim that the examiner's limb is really theirs; deny ownership of their own paretic limb; or refuse to accept that the obviously paralyzed limb is even weak.

Sometimes they attribute the weakened limb to a third person, such as their roommate. That ploy holds instant appeal if the roommate has an immobilized limb from a stroke or fracture. Alternatively, even while accepting their hand weakness, patients might offer an improbable explanation, such as that they merely fell asleep on it and its strength will return in a few hours. In other words, patients with anosognosia notoriously employ denial, projection, and rationalization, and other defense mechanisms.

The origin of anosognosia, as with other nondominant symptoms, remains unknown. Some researchers attribute it to a loss of afferent sensory input. Clinical experience, however, shows that although loss of sensation may be a prerequisite, it alone is insufficient. For example, patients with a thoracic spinal cord transection lose feeling in their lower trunk and legs, but they remain acutely aware of their paraparesis and incontinence as well as anesthesia. Another theory, better supported by evidence, suggests that disordered attentiveness and arousal, arising from damage of the underlying thalamus and reticular activating system, produce inattention and anosognosia.

Patients with anosognosia, especially if they adhere to denial, often refuse to accept physical therapy and other hospital routines. They can become belligerent and insist on leaving the hospital. On the other hand, they may seem so oblivious to their deficit that they appear to display *la belle indifférence*. Many of them are likely to have comorbid depression. Therefore, from the perspective of a consultation-liaison psychiatrist asked to evaluate behavioral disturbances, unrealistic plans, or mood changes in a patient with left hemiparesis, the psychiatrist should evaluate the patient for anosognosia as well as its frequent companion, depression. While examining the patient, all clinicians should also refrain from confronting the patient with the physical and neuropsychologic deficits. Crude attempts at educating such a patient might produce a catastrophic reaction. Fortunately, anosognosia clears in most cases within 10 days and in almost all by 3 months.

Denial and confabulation are not restricted to nondominant hemisphere injury. Both are prominent signs in suddenly occurring cortical blindness (see Anton's syndrome, Chapter 12). Confabulation is also found in Wernicke-Korsakoff syndrome (see Chapter 7).

Another manifestation of nondominant hemisphere injury is *constructional apraxia*, which is a *visual-spatial* perceptual impairment. Patients with this disorder cannot organize visual information or integrate it with fine motor skills. For example, they cannot copy simple figures or arrange matchsticks in patterns (Fig. 8-8). More so than other nondominant symptoms, constructional apraxia cannot be reliably ascribed to a nondominant lesion. It can also be found in patients with mental retardation, diffuse cerebral dysfunction, and executive dysfunction from frontal lobe disease.

Aprosody

Aprosody constitutes the inability to recognize emotional or affective qualities of other individuals' speech. Thus, nondominant hemisphere lesions interfere with patients' innate capacity to discern emotions from others' tone of voice. For example, a patient with aprosody would be unable to appreciate the contrasting feelings in the question "Are you going home?" asked first by a jealous hospital roommate and then by a gleeful spouse. On a more subtle level, patients also might not perceive the emotions conveyed by a spouse.

In addition, aprosody restricts the ability to impart emotional qualities to speech. With no inflection or style, patients' speech sounds bland and unfeeling.

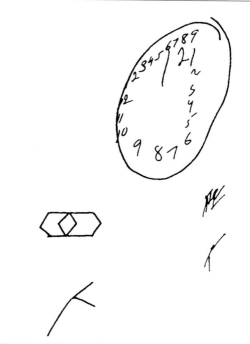

FIGURE 8-8 ■ When asked to draw a clock, a patient with *constructional apraxia* drew an incomplete circle, repeated (perseverated) the numerals, and placed them asymmetrically. When attempting to copy the top left figure, the patient repeated several lines, failing to draw any figure. The patient also misplaced and rotated the position of the bottom left figure (see also Fig. 2-8). Such abnormalities are not peculiar to nondominant hemisphere injuries, and they often appear in Bender-Gestalt and WAIS testing.

To assess prosody, the examiner re-creates a short version of the aphasia examination. During spontaneous speech, the examiner notes the patient's variations in volume, pitch, and emphasis. The examiner might have the patient ask a question, such as "May I have the ball?" in the manner of a friend and then a stern schoolteacher using appropriate vocal and facial expressions. The examiner then asks a similar question, impersonating the various characters while the patient tries to identify them. As an alternative, the examiner might ask the patient to describe pictures of people obviously displaying emotions.

Loss of nonverbal communication tends to accompany aprosody. In particular, patients lose meaningful face and limb expressions, popularly called "body language" or technically called speech's *paralinguistic component*. These physical aspects of communication lend conviction, emphasis, and affect to spoken words. Indeed, such gestures seem independent and sometimes more credible than speech. Well-known examples are children crossing their fingers when promising, adults who wink while telling a joke, and people who smile while relating sad events.

Extending the concept that the nondominant hemisphere confers affect on language, several authors have suggested that the nondominant hemisphere governs perception and expression of emotion and other complex nonverbal processes. The dominant hemisphere, they suggest, is responsible for verbal, sequential, analytic cognitive processes and reflection.

DISCONNECTION SYNDROMES

Almost all mental processes require communication pathways between two or more cerebral cortical areas located within one cerebral hemisphere, and many require communication between areas in opposite hemispheres. The arcuate fasciculus, for example, provides intrahemispheric communication between Wernicke's and Broca's areas. For interhemispheric communication, myelin-coated axonal (white matter) bundles, often called *commissures*, provide the pathway. The most conspicuous interhemispheric commissure is the *corpus callosum.*

Injuries that sever communication pathways, but spare the actual area, cause uncommon but interesting phenomena, the *disconnection syndromes.* Neurologists predicted their existence before verifying them in actual patients, much as physicists have predicted certain subatomic particles before discovering them. This chapter has previously discussed several disconnection syndromes: (1) alexia without agraphia, (2) conduction aphasia, and (3) ideomotor apraxia with its varieties, buccofacial and limb apraxia. Subsequent chapters will present other disconnection syndromes, including the medial longitudinal fasciculus (MLF) syndrome, also known as intranuclear ophthalmoplegia (INO) (see Chapters 12 and 15).

In the *anterior cerebral artery syndrome,* in which an occlusion of both anterior cerebral arteries leads to an infarction of the frontal lobes and anterior corpus callosum, information cannot pass between the left hemisphere language centers and the right hemisphere motor centers. Although the patient's left arm and leg will have normal spontaneous movement, those limbs fail to follow an examiner's verbal or written requests to move them. In other words, the patient will have unilateral (left-sided) limb apraxia (see Fig. 8-5).

Surprisingly, other injuries of the corpus callosum may not produce disconnection syndromes. For example, the corpus callosum occasionally fails to develop in utero (*congenital absence*), but unless other anomalies are present, patients may have no overt impairment. In *Marchiafava-Bignami syndrome* or *disease,* which has been attributed to excessive consumption of Italian red wine in a minority of cases, patients may show disconnection signs, but only as part of extensive cerebral dysfunction.

Split-Brain Syndrome

The most important disconnection syndrome referable to the corpus callosum is the *split-brain syndrome.* Now rare, this disorder previously resulted from a longitudinal surgical division of the corpus callosum (commissurotomy) performed in an effort to control intractable epilepsy (see Chapter 10). The commissurotomy almost completely isolated each cerebral hemisphere.

In cases of the split-brain syndrome, examiners may present certain information to only a single, isolated hemisphere. For example, examiners can show pictures, writing, and other visual information within one visual field to present information to only the patient's contralateral hemisphere (Fig. 8-9). Likewise, examiners can present tactile information to only the contralateral hemisphere by having a blindfolded patient touch objects with the one hand. However, auditory information cannot be presented exclusively—only predominantly—to one hemisphere. (Because pathways are duplicated in the brainstem [see Fig. 4-16], sounds detected in one ear are transmitted, after the medial geniculate synapse, to both hemispheres, but predominantly to the contralateral hemisphere.)

The interruption of the corpus callosum prevents the right hemisphere from sharing information with the entire brain, particularly the left hemisphere's language centers. As could be anticipated, the right hemisphere's information, experience, and emotion cannot reach the patient's consciousness, at least to the level of verbal expression. For example, if an object is placed in a blindfolded patient's left hand, the patient cannot name or describe it, and the right hand cannot choose an identical object. Similarly, if one hand learns to follow a maze, the other hand will have to be taught separately.

Not only can each hemisphere separately perceive visual and tactile information, but also each can separately perceive emotions. For example, if a humorous picture were shown to the right visual field, a patient might laugh and be able to describe the picture's humorous content; however, if the same picture were shown to the patient's left visual field, it might provoke an amused sensation but one that the patient could not verbalize or even fully comprehend. If a sad picture were shown in the left visual field and a humorous one in the right, the patient's amused response would be distorted because of the conflict.

Split-brain studies have suggested that normal people have, in their two hemispheres, neuropsychologic

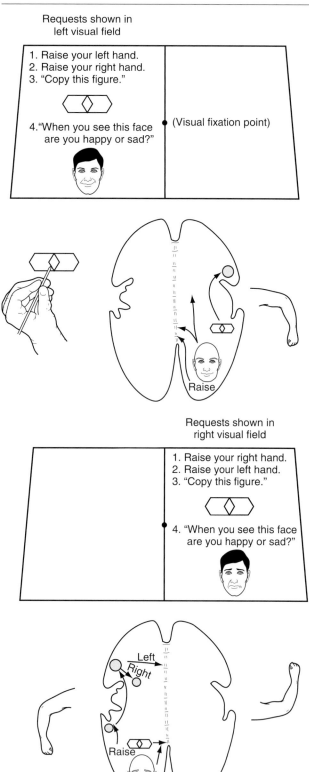

Requests shown in
left visual field

1. Raise your left hand.
2. Raise your right hand.
3. "Copy this figure."

4. "When you see this face
are you happy or sad?"

(Visual fixation point)

Raise

Requests shown in
right visual field

1. Raise your right hand.
2. Raise your left hand.
3. "Copy this figure."

4. "When you see this face
are you happy or sad?"

Left
Right

Raise

FIGURE 8-9 ■ After a *commissurotomy*, patients typically have the *split-brain syndrome*. Each hemisphere can be tested individually by showing requests, objects, and pictures in the contralateral visual field. *Upper,* Objects and written requests shown in the left visual field are perceived by the right visual field. Because connections to the ipsilateral motor area are intact, the *left* hand can copy figures. However, because the right hemisphere is unable to transmit information through the corpus callosum to the dominant left cerebral hemisphere, which governs language function, patients cannot read the requests or describe the objects. Although patients cannot speak of the feelings evoked by emotionally laden pictures shown in their left visual field, they have sympathetic, nonverbal responses. *Lower,* Written requests and objects shown in the right visual field are perceived by the left hemisphere. Patients can read those written requests, copy those objects with the right hand, and comply with the requests; however, because the language areas cannot send information through the corpus callosum, the left hand cannot comply. When patients describe emotions portrayed in a picture, their language lacks affect, derived from the nondominant hemisphere.

systems that are independent, parallel, and capable of simultaneous reasoning. Also, in normal people, the systems usually complement each other, but they potentially conflict.

REFERENCES

1. Absher JR, Benson DF: Disconnection syndromes: An overview of Geschwind's contributions. Neurology 43:862–867, 1993.
2. Basso A, Scarpa MT: Traumatic aphasia in children and adults: A comparison of clinical features and evolution. Cortex 26:501–514, 1990.
3. Basso A, Farabola M, Grassi MP, et al: Aphasia in left-handers. Comparison of aphasia profiles and language recovery in non-right-handed and matched right-handed patients. Brain Lang 38:233–252, 1990.
4. Benton AL: Gerstmann's syndrome. Arch Neurol 49:445–447, 1992.
5. Besson M, Schon D: Comparison between language and music. Ann NY Acad Sci 930:232–258, 2001.
6. Brust JC: Music and the neurologist. Ann NY Acad Sci 930:143–152, 2001.
7. Buxbaum LJ, Ferraro MK, Veramonti T, et al: Hemispatial neglect. Neurology 62:749–756, 2004.
8. Faber R, Abrams R, Taylor MA, et al: Comparison of schizophrenic patients with formal thought disorder and neurologically impaired patients with aphasia. Am J Psychiatry 140:1348–1351, 1983.
9. Feinberg TE, Schindler RJ, Flanagan NG, et al: Two alien hand syndromes. Neurology 42:19–24, 1992.
10. Greener J, Enderby P, Whurr R: Speech and language therapy for aphasia following stroke. Cochrane Database Syst Rev 2:CD000425, 2000.
11. Gazzaniga MS: The split brain revisited. Sci Am 51–55, July 1998.
12. Hemenway D: Bimanual dexterity in baseball players. N Engl J Med 309:1587, 1983.
13. Hickok G, Bellugi U, Klima ES: Sign language in the brain. Sci Am 59–65, June 2001.

14. Klein SK, Masur D, Farber K, et al: Fluent aphasia in children: Definition and natural history. J Child Neurol 7:50–59, 1992.

15. Laurent-Vannier A, Pradat-Diehl P, Chevignard M, et al: Spatial and motor neglect in children. Neurology 60:202–207, 2003.

16. Motley MT: Slips of the tongue. Sci Am 253:116–125, 1985.

17. Mesulam MM: Primary progressive aphasia—a language-based dementia. N Engl J Med 349:1535–1542, 2003.

18. Portal JM, Romano PE: Patterns of eye-hand dominance in baseball players. N Engl J Med 319:655, 1988.

19. Shinnar S, Rapin I, Arnold S, et al: Language regression in childhood. Pediatr Neurol 24:183–189, 2001.

20. Stern RA: Assessment of mood states in aphasia. Semin Speech Lang 20:3–49, 1999.

1–5. Formulate the following cases.

CASE 1

A 68-year-old man suddenly develops right hemiparesis. He only utters "Oh, Oh!" when stimulated. He makes no response to questions or requests. His right lower face is paretic, and the right arm and leg are flaccid and immobile. He is inattentive to objects in his right visual field.

CASE 2

A 70-year-old man, since suffering a stroke the previous year, can only say "weak, arm," "go away," and "give...supper me." His speech is slurred. He can raise his left arm, protrude his tongue, and close his eyes. He can name several objects, but he cannot repeat phrases. His right arm is paretic, but he can walk.

CASE 3

Over a period of 6 weeks, a previously healthy 64-year-old woman has developed headaches, progressively severe difficulty in finding words, and apparent confusion. She speaks continuously and incoherently: "Go to the warb," "I can't hear," "My heat hurts." She is unable to follow requests, name objects, or repeat phrases. On examination, there is pronation of the outstretched right arm, a right Babinski sign, and papilledema. Visual fields cannot be tested.

CASE 4

A 34-year-old man with mitral stenosis has the sudden onset of aphasia after a transient left-sided headache. Although articulate and able to follow requests and repeat phrases, he has difficulty in naming objects. For example, when a pen, pin, and penny are held up in succession, which serves as a frequently used test, he substitutes the name of one for the other and repeats the name of the preceding object; however, he can point to the "money," "sharp object," and "writing instrument" when these objects are placed in front of him. No abnormal physical signs are present.

CASE 5

A 54-year-old man, over several months, has developed difficulty in thinking and the inability to remember the word he desires. Although his voice quivers, he is fully conversant and articulate. He is able to write the correct responses to questions; however, he has slow and poor penmanship. He is able to name six objects, follow double requests, and repeat complex phrases. On further testing, he has difficulty recalling six digits, three objects after 3 minutes, and both recent and past events. Judgment seems intact. The remainder of the neurologic examination is normal.

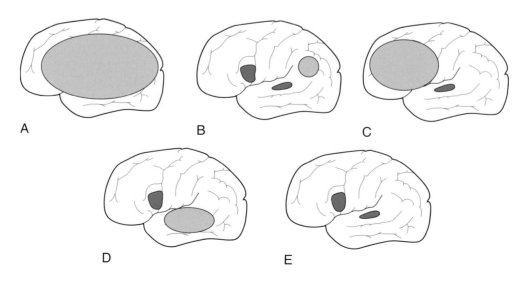

A   B   C

D   E

Answers: 1–5

Case 1. He has complete loss of language function, *global aphasia,* accompanied by right hemiplegia and homonymous hemianopsia. The cause is probably an occlusion of the left internal carotid artery creating an infarction of the entire left hemisphere. However, the lesion's particular etiology is much less important than its location in determining the presence and variety of aphasia.

Case 2. Because he can manage only a few phrases or words in a telegraphic pattern, this man has nonfluent aphasia. Although only about one third of cases of aphasia can be neatly characterized, this man has a "textbook case." As with other textbook cases, his nonfluent aphasia is accompanied by right hemiparesis, in which the arm is more paretic than the leg. Nonfluent aphasia is usually caused by an occlusion of the left middle cerebral artery. An underlying infarction would encompass Broca's area and the adjacent cortical motor region but spare the cortical fibers for the leg, which are supplied by the anterior cerebral artery. However, trauma, tumors, and other injuries in this location may produce the same picture.

Case 3. The patient has fluent aphasia characterized by a normal quantity of speech interspersed with paraphasic errors, but only subtle right-sided corticospinal tract abnormalities. She probably has a lesion in the left parietal or posterior temporal lobe. The headaches and papilledema, given her age and the course of the illness, suggest that it is a mass lesion, such as a glioblastoma multiforme, rather than a CVA.

Case 4. He has anomic aphasia, which is a variety of fluent aphasia in which language impairment is restricted to the improper identification of objects (a naming impairment). Its origin may be Alzheimer's disease or other neurodegenerative illness, but in view of the history of mitral stenosis and headache, the origin was probably a small embolic CVA (see Chapter 11).

Case 5. The patient does not have aphasia. His difficulty with memory could be either an early dementia or psychogenic inattention. Further evaluations might include neuropsychologic studies and evaluation for dementia.

6–10. Match the lesions that are pictured schematically with those expected in cases 1–5.

Answers: *Case 1,* drawing A; *Case 2,* drawing C; *Case 3,* drawing D; *Case 4,* drawing B or D; *Case 5,* drawing E.

11–26. Match the lesion with the expected associated finding(s).

11. Paresis of one recurrent laryngeal nerve
12. Pseudobulbar palsy
13. Bulbar palsy
14. Dominant hemisphere temporal lobe lesion
15. Lateral medullary syndrome
16. Laryngitis
17. Dominant hemisphere angular gyrus lesion
18. Dominant hemisphere parietal lobe lesion
19. Nondominant hemisphere parietal lobe lesion
20. Bilateral frontal lobe tumor
21. Bilateral anterior cerebral artery infarction
22. Streptomycin toxicity
23. Alcohol intoxication
24. Periaqueductal hemorrhagic necrosis (Wernicke's encephalopathy)
25. Phenytoin (Dilantin) toxicity
26. Infarction of left posterior cerebral artery

    a. Dysarthria, including hoarseness
    b. Dysphagia
    c. Dementia
    d. Dyscalculia
    e. Fluent aphasia
    f. Constructional apraxia
    g. Dyslexia
    h. Deafness
    i. Mutism
    j. Left-right disorientation
    k. Finger agnosia
    l. Hyperactive reflexes
    m. Sixth cranial nerve palsy
    n. Alexia
    o. Ataxia
    p. Dressing apraxia
    q. Anosognosia
    r. Hemi-inattention
    s. Left limb apraxia
    t. Delirium

Answers: 11-a; 12-a, b, l; 13-a, b; 14-e; 15-a, b, o; 16-a; 17-d, j, k (Gerstmann's syndrome); 18-d, e, g, j, k; 19-f, p, q, r; 20-c, possibly also a, b, and i; 21-s and possibly c and i; 22-h, o; 23-a, d, o, t; 24-m, o, t; 25-o, t; 26-n.

27. EMS workers revived a 34-year-old man after he attempted suicide by sitting in a garaged car with the motor running. During the next week he only sat in bed and looked out the window. He displayed no emotion and did not respond to requests. Although he was otherwise mute, he seemed to repeat in intricate detail whatever he was asked and occasionally whatever was spoken on television. Physicians found brisk deep tendon reflexes and bilateral palmomental reflexes, but only equivocal plantar reflexes. The examiner was uncertain whether the patient had depression, dementia, or other neuropsychologic abnormality. Please discuss the case and suggest further evaluation.

Answer: The patient was probably exposed to excessive carbon monoxide. As in many cases of survival following cardiac arrest or strangulation, cerebral anoxia creates cerebral cortex damage. When patients permanently lose all intellectual and voluntary motor function, they are said to be in the *persistent vegetative state* (see Chapter 11).

In this case, the cerebral damage was incomplete. It probably isolated the perisylvian language arc of the cerebral cortex comprising Wernicke's area, the arcuate fasciculus, and Broca's area. Isolation of this crucial region from the rest of the cerebral cortex caused *transcortical* or *isolation aphasia*, which permits repetition of words and phrases, no matter how complex. In this disorder, language formation does not interact with the rest of the brain's language system, and patients cannot name objects or follow requests. Because a large portion of the cerebral cortex is damaged, patients usually have dementia, paresis, frontal release signs, and cortical blindness.

In cases in which cerebral cortex damage is superimposed on depressive illness or other psychologic aberrations, the clinical picture is unpredictable. In these patients, detailed testing of language function must be part of the mental status examination.

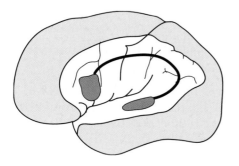

In isolation aphasia, which is usually caused by cerebral hypoperfusion, the most vulnerable portions of the cerebral cortex are damaged. Because the perisylvian language arc is well-perfused, it escapes damage. Language processes may continue within this region, but they receive no input from other regions of the cerebral cortex.

28. A left-handed 64-year-old male schoolteacher sustained a thrombosis of the right middle cerebral artery. What might be predicted regarding language function?
    a. He will certainly develop aphasia.
    b. He will have left hemiparesis if he has aphasia.
    c. If he develops aphasia, his prognosis is relatively good.
    d. If he has aphasia, he will have a homonymous hemianopsia.

Answer: c. Left-handed individuals who have normal intelligence remain either predominantly left-hemisphere dominant or mixed cerebral dominant. Also, their language centers in the right hemisphere are not arranged analogously to either those of a person with left hemisphere dominance or their own right hemisphere motor and visual tracts. If left-handed individuals suffer an infarction of the right cerebral hemisphere, they do not necessarily develop aphasia or the usual associated deficits. In fact, they may develop aphasia if they have an infarction in the left cerebral hemisphere. Also, left-handed individuals, compared to right-handed ones, have a better prognosis for the resolution of aphasia.

29. If the patient in the previous question were discovered to have a resectable tumor in the right temporal lobe, how could language function of the right cerebral hemisphere be established before surgery?
    a. An MRI could be performed.
    b. A CT could show differences in the *planum temporale*.
    c. Barbiturates infused into the carotid artery of the dominant hemisphere would cause aphasia.
    d. A PET study would indicate cerebral dominance for language.

Answer: c. Infusion of barbiturates directly into the dominant carotid artery produces aphasia (the *Wada test*). This test can determine if a cerebral hemisphere is dominant before removal of cerebral neoplasms or an epilepsy scar focus. PET scans are difficult to perform because they require short-lived cyclotron generated substrates. The scan shows relatively poor resolution of metabolic function. Although the *planum temporale* (the superior surface of the temporal lobe cortex) has a greater area in the dominant than nondominant temporal lobe, the difference is not always present. Even when present, the difference cannot be reliably visualized with a CT or MRI. Functional MRI (fMRI), which is under development, may replace the

Wada test in locating the language regions and determining other functional areas of the brain.

30. In which conditions are confabulations *not* found?
    a. Anton's syndrome
    b. Gerstmann's syndrome
    c. Anosognosia
    d. Wernicke-Korsakoff syndrome

Answer: b. Gerstmann's syndrome is a controversial entity that consists of the combination of right and left confusion, dyslexia, dyscalculia, and finger agnosia. It is usually attributed to lesions in the angular gyrus of the parietal lobe of the dominant hemisphere. In denial of blindness (Anton's syndrome), blind patients typically confabulate or fantasize about the appearance of objects presented to them. Although bilateral strokes, simultaneously or in succession, often cause Anton's syndrome, it occurs most often in elderly people who undergo ophthalmologic surgical procedures and cannot temporarily see out of either eye. Failure to acknowledge a left hemiparesis or similar deficit (anosognosia) is often accompanied by confabulation, denial, and other defense mechanisms. Although confabulations are described in the Wernicke-Korsakoff's syndrome, they are actually an uncommon symptom. When they do occur, the patients usually also have marked memory impairment.

31. Match the speech abnormality (dysarthria) (a–d) with the illness (1–4).
    a. Hypophonia
    b. Scanning speech
    c. Nasal speech
    d. Strained and strangled speech
    1. Myasthenia gravis
    2. Parkinsonism
    3. Multiple sclerosis
    4. Spasmodic dysphonia

Answer: a-2, b-3, c-1, d-4.

32. Which conditions *usually* cause aphasia?
    a. Chronic subdural hematomas
    b. Myasthenia gravis
    c. Multiple sclerosis
    d. Parkinsonism
    e. None of the above

Answer: e. Subdural hematomas are located in the extra-axial space. Although chronic subdural hematomas typically cause headaches and dementia, they usually do not cause aphasia or other localized neurologic symptoms. Myasthenia gravis is a disorder of the neuromuscular junction and therefore does not cause

dementia, aphasia, or other signs of CNS dysfunction. Multiple sclerosis (MS) affects the cerebral white matter to a large extent only late in its course. Although MS may then cause dementia, it rarely causes aphasia. Parkinsonism may cause dysarthria (hypophonia and tremor) and, late in the illness, dementia; however, it rarely if ever causes aphasia.

33. A 45-year-old airplane pilot reported that when she awoke earlier in the morning, for approximately 5 minutes she had "expressive aphasia," by which she meant that she was unable to speak or gesture, but she understood most of the news on the radio. During that time, she had no other symptoms. Which of the following conditions are reasonable explanations for her episode?
    a. Seizure
    b. TIA
    c. Migraine
    d. Sleep disorder
    e. All of the above

Answer: e. All of those conditions are reasonable explanations. She might have had a partial seizure originating in the left frontal lobe that led to postictal aphasia and a right hemiparesis. A TIA in the distribution of the left carotid artery might also have caused aphasia with or without right hemiparesis. Hemiplegic migraines, which can cause speech or language impairment, can occasionally affect adults. An episode of sleep paralysis, such as hypnopompic cataplexy, may cause brief quadriparesis and mutism. The possible etiologies of transient aphasia and transient hemiparesis are similar (see Hemiplegic Migraines, Chapter 9, and Carotid Artery TIAs, Chapter 11).

34. A 70-year-old man suddenly developed inability to read. Although he can write his name and most sentences that are dictated to him, he cannot read aloud or copy written material. His speech is fluent and contains no paraphasic errors. He can see objects only in his left visual field. What is this man's difficulty, and where is the responsible lesion(s)?
    a. Alexia without agraphia
    b. Cortical blindness
    c. Psychogenic impairments
    d. Fluent aphasia
    e. Nonfluent aphasia

Answer: a. He clearly has alexia, as demonstrated by his inability to read, and also a right homonymous hemianopsia. He does not have agraphia because he can transcribe dictation and write words from memory. Nor does he have aphasia. Thus, he has the syndrome of alexia without agraphia. A lesion in the left occipital lobe and posterior corpus callosum causes this syndrome. The left occipital lesion would explain the failure of visual information to pass from the intact right visual cortex through the corpus callosum to the left (dominant) hemisphere for integration (see Fig. 8-4). Because memory and auditory circuits, as well as the corticospinal system, are intact, he can write words that he hears or remembers. Such lesions are usually caused by infarctions of the left posterior cerebral artery or by infiltrating brain tumors, such as a glioblastoma multiforme.

35. A 68-year-old man had a car accident because he drifted into oncoming traffic. He has a left homonymous hemianopsia and a mild left hemiparesis, which he fails to appreciate. Which neuropsychologic problem describes his denying his left arm weakness?
    a. Anosognosia
    b. Aphasia
    c. Anton's syndrome
    d. Alexia

Answer: a. After having the accident because a left homonymous hemianopsia prevented him from seeing oncoming traffic, he fails to recognize his deficits, which is anosognosia. This perceptual distortion is a characteristic manifestation of a parietal lobe lesion.

36. Which one of the following statements concerning Heschl's gyrus is false?
    a. Heschl's gyrus is bilateral and located adjacent to the planum temporale.
    b. Words and sound heard in the right ear are transmitted to the right cerebral cortex.
    c. Each Heschl's gyrus reflects auditory stimulation predominantly from the contralateral ear.
    d. Heschl's gyrus appears to sort auditory stimuli for direction, pitch, loudness, and other acoustic properties rather than words for their linguistic properties.

Answer: b. Words and sound heard in the right ear are transmitted to the both the right and, more so, left cerebral cortex The dominant hemisphere planum temporale, which is integral to language function, has greater surface area than its counterpart. Each hemisphere's Heschl's gyrus, which processes the auditory qualities of sound, is symmetric (see Figs. 4-16 and 8-1).

37. Patients with nondominant hemisphere lesions are reported to have loss of the normal inflections of speech and diminished associated facial and limb gestures. What are the technical terms used to describe these findings?
    a. Limb apraxia
    b. Buccolingual apraxia
    c. Hypophonia
    d. Aprosody and loss of paralinguistic components of speech

Answer: d. Aprosody is the loss of the normal inflections of speech and emotional content. Diminished facial and limb gestures constitute loss of paralinguistic components of speech.

38. Physicians show a man who has undergone a commissurotomy for intractable seizures a written request to raise both arms. What will be his response when the request is shown in his left visual field?
    a. He will raise only his left arm.
    b. He will raise only his right arm.
    c. He will raise both arms.
    d. He will raise neither arm.

Answer: d. When the request is shown in his left visual field, he will not raise either arm because the request, which he must read, does not reach the left hemisphere language centers. In contrast, when the request is shown in his right visual field, the request reaches the language centers and he will raise his right hand, but the request to move his left hand may not reach the right hemisphere's motor center.

39–44. With which conditions are the various forms of apraxia (a-h) associated?
39. Gait
40. Constructional
41. Ideational
42. Limb
43. Buccofacial
44. Ideomotor
    a. Aphasia
    b. Hemi-inattention
    c. Dementia
    d. Dysarthria
    e. Incontinence
    f. Left homonymous hemianopsia
    g. Right homonymous hemianopsia
    h. Aprosody

Answers: 39-c, e (in normal pressure hydrocephalus); 40-b, f, h (in nondominant parietal lobe syndromes); 41-c; 42-a, g; 43-a, d, g; 44-a, g.

45. In asking, "How does aphasia in left-handed people differ from aphasia in right-handed people?" which potential response is incorrect?
    a. Aphasia can result from lesions in either hemisphere.
    b. The variety of aphasia is less clearly related to the site of cerebral injury.
    c. The prognosis is better.
    d. The etiologies are different.

    Answer: d.

46. Which of the following is not a disconnection syndrome?
    a. Internuclear ophthalmoplegia
    b. Conduction aphasia
    c. Split-brain syndrome
    d. Isolation aphasia
    e. Alexia without agraphia

    Answer: d. Disconnection syndromes refer to disorders in which lesions sever connections between primary neuropsychologic centers. Although not generally considered a disconnection syndrome, internuclear ophthalmoplegia results form damage of interconnecting fasciculi. In contrast, isolation aphasia results from extensive cerebral cortex injury that preserves the language arc, and its elements remain connected. Extensive destruction of the entire language arc leads to global aphasia.

47. Which artery supplies most of the perisylvian language arc?
    a. Anterior cerebral artery
    b. Middle cerebral artery
    c. Posterior cerebral artery
    d. Vertebrobasilar artery system

    Answer: b.

48. What is the term applied to the area of the cerebral cortex between branches of the major cerebral arteries?
    a. Watershed area
    b. Limbic system
    c. Cornea
    d. Arcuate fasciculus

    Answer: a. A geographic region or divide drained by a river or stream was originally called "watershed." To neurologists, the term means areas of the cerebral cortex that are perfused by the terminal branches of arteries. During hypotension or anoxia, the already tenuous blood supply falls to an insufficient level in watershed cerebral regions.

49. Which is true regarding sign language?
    a. Sign language, like spoken language, is based in the dominant hemisphere in congenitally deaf individuals.
    b. Middle cerebral artery occlusions in deaf people typically cause aphasia in sign language.
    c. Sign language relies on visual rather than auditory input.
    d. American Sign Language (ASL) is the proper name for the common, gesture-based sign language in the United States.
    e. All of the above.

    Answer: e.

50. In nonfluent aphasia, why is the arm typically more paretic than the leg?
    a. The motor cortex for the arm is supplied by the middle cerebral artery, which is usually occluded. The motor cortex for the leg is supplied by the anterior cerebral artery, which is usually spared.
    b. The arm has a larger cortical representation.
    c. The infarct occurs in the internal capsule.
    d. The motor cortex for the arm is supplied by the anterior cerebral artery, which is usually occluded. The motor cortex for the leg is supplied by the middle cerebral artery, which is usually spared.

    Answer: a.

51. After a right parietal infarction, patients may develop an alien hand syndrome. Which two of the following characteristics describe this phenomenon?
    a. Persistent burning pain in the hand of someone with hemiparesis
    b. The misperception that a paralyzed hand is normal
    c. Attraction to another person's hand
    d. A perception that the paralyzed hand is not the patient's
    e. A perception that the paralyzed hand acts independently or under another person's control

    Answers: d, e. The perception of one's hand seems to be particularly vulnerable. Persistent burning pain in a paretic hand may be a manifestation of the thalamic pain syndrome (see Chapter 14). The misperception that a paralyzed hand is normal constitutes anosognosia. Attraction to another person's hand is not a neurologic condition.

52. Which variety of apraxia is most closely associated with normal pressure hydrocephalus?
    a. Ideational
    b. Dressing
    c. Ideomotor
    d. Buccofacial
    e. Oral
    f. Gait

Answer: f. Gait apraxia, incontinence, and dementia are the primary manifestations of normal pressure hydrocephalus. Gait apraxia is usually the first and most prominent symptom. It is also the first symptom to resolve following successful treatment.

53. In which disorders is echolalia a symptom?
    a. Autism
    b. Isolation aphasia
    c. Dementia
    d. Tourette's syndrome
    e. All of the above

Answer: e. Echolalia, an involuntary repetition of visitors' or examiners' words, is a manifestation of diverse neurologic conditions.

54. Which disconnection syndrome stems from corpus callosum damage?
    a. Split-brain syndrome
    b. Internuclear ophthalmoplegia (INO)
    c. Conduction aphasia

Answer: a. Although all the conditions are disconnection syndromes, only corpus callosum damage, which causes an interhemispheric disconnection, produces the split-brain syndrome.

55. Which conclusion has stemmed from studies of patients who have undergone a commissurotomy?
    a. The corpus callosum is vital to the auditory system.
    b. Patients with the split-brain syndrome have gross, readily identifiable physical and cognitive abnormalities.
    c. Emotions generated in the right hemisphere are not as readily described as those generated in the left hemisphere.
    d. Emotions generated in the left hemisphere are not as readily described as those in the right hemisphere.

Answer: c.

56. A 60-year-old man who has undergone a commissurotomy has his hands placed in a closed box containing many objects. A set of keys is placed in his left hand. By voice and gesture, he is asked to identify them. Which would be his most accurate response?
    a. He would say, "A set of keys."
    b. With his right hand, he would write, "A set of keys."
    c. Although unable to say, "A set of keys," he would be able to pick another set of keys from the various objects.
    d. He would be unable to comply with the request under any circumstance.

Answer: c. The commissurotomy isolates the language center from his right hemisphere, but he is still capable of comprehending the request, especially if it is gestured.

57. A psychiatrist sees a 74-year-old woman in the nursing home because she constantly reports intruders in her nursing home room. On multiple occasions, security guards found no evidence of an intrusion. Her family had placed her in the nursing home following partial recovery from a right-sided parietal stroke. Its residual deficits were a mild left hemiparesis and hemisensory impairment but no dementia. The psychiatrist finds that the woman has a tenuous relationship to her hand, which moves freely and, without her knowledge, pulls at her clothing. The woman does not deny that she had a stroke, but disclaims the hand at the end of her arm. "I am not moving it. Who is?" she finally asks the psychiatrist. Which is the most likely description for her perception?
    a. Delusions or hallucinations associated with a nondominant hemisphere infarction
    b. The alien hand syndrome
    c. Anosognosia
    d. Dementia

Answer: b. She has the alien hand syndrome because of a nondominant stroke. She typically proposes the following: The independently moving hand, which she does not fully feel or control, belongs to someone else, such as an intruder.

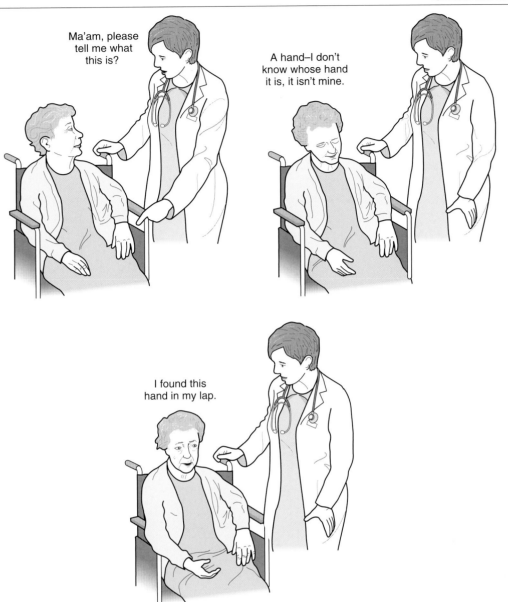

58. Which structure relays visual information from the brainstem to the visual cortex?
    a. The medial geniculate body
    b. The lateral geniculate body
    c. The optic chiasm
    d. The Edinger-Westphal nucleus

    Answer: b. The optic tract transmits visual information to the lateral geniculate body. After the synapse, it sends the information through the geniculocalcarine tract to the occipital lobe's visual cortex. The Edinger-Westphal nucleus relays information regarding light intensity to adjust pupil size.

59. Which structure relays auditory information from the brainstem to the auditory cortex?

    a. The medial geniculate body
    b. The lateral geniculate body
    c. The optic chiasm
    d. The Edinger-Westphal nucleus

    Answer: a. The medial geniculate body receives auditory information from ipsilateral and contralateral brainstem auditory tracts. After the synapse, the medial geniculate sends the information to the temporal lobe's auditory cortex. Unlike transmission of visual information only to the contralateral visual cortex, both ears transmit information to each auditory cortex, but each ear's signals go predominantly to the contralateral cortex. Auditory signals regarding language go predominantly to the dominant hemisphere cortex.

60. When asked to identify a tie, an aphasic patient said, "Fly, sigh, my, my, my, bye..." Which term best describes the response?
   a. Paraphasias
   b. Tangentialities
   c. Clang associations
   d. Jargon speech

Answer: c. The string of words is associated by sound rather than meaning, which constitutes clang associations. If their meaning had associated the words, the string would have best been described as a tangentiality.

Headaches

In the most widely accepted categorization, the International Headache Society (IHS) recognizes three major categories: Primary Headaches, Secondary Headaches, and Cranial Neuralgias. Primary headaches include *tension-type, migraine,* and *cluster headaches.* Although not life-threatening, primary headaches may create severe pain, incapacitate patients, and, with frequent attacks, reduce their quality of life. Neurologists diagnose headaches, not by physical examination or laboratory tests, which are characteristically normal, but by their distinctive symptoms. Despite several credible theories, their etiologies remain unknown.

Secondary headaches are often manifestations of an underlying serious, sometimes life-threatening, illness. This category includes *temporal arteritis, intracranial mass lesions, idiopathic intracranial hypertension (pseudotumor cerebri), meningitis, subarachnoid hemorrhage,* and *postconcussion headaches* (see Chapter 22, Head Trauma). This category also includes *Headache Attributed to Psychiatric Disorder.* Unlike the diagnosis of primary headaches, the diagnosis of secondary headaches usually rests on physical or laboratory abnormalities.

PRIMARY HEADACHES

Tension-Type Headache

Tension-type headache (TTH), previously called "tension headache," is a common headache disorder characterized by intermittent dull pain usually located bilaterally in the frontal or cervical regions. The manifestations are restricted to pain. Patients have little or no associated symptoms, such as photophobia, hyperacusis, phonophobia, nausea, or other autonomic disturbance. This headache plagues women more than men and often affects multiple family members. Patients with TTH complain, but they usually go about their business. (In contrast, patients who are unable to function during headaches probably have migraine.)

TTH has traditionally been attributed to contraction of the scalp, neck, and face muscles (Fig. 9-1), as well as emotional "tension." Fatigue, cervical spondylosis, bright light, loud noise, and, at some level, emotional factors were said to produce or precipitate them.

However, because studies have demonstrated that this headache results from neither muscle contractions nor psychological tension, the designation "muscle contraction" or "tension" probably represents a misnomer. The term "tension-type" headache is, at least, more appropriate. In fact, many neurologists place this headache at the opposite end of a headache spectrum from migraine, where both result from a common, but unknown, physiologic disorder.

Treatment

Neurologists generally first assure patients that their headache does not represent a brain tumor or other potentially fatal illness, which are frequently unspoken fears. On the other hand, their headaches are liable to become a chronic condition. Risk factors for a poor outcome include comorbid migraine, being unmarried, and sleep disorders.

For headaches that occur less than twice a week, neurologists usually suggest "acute therapy"—medicines taken at the headache's onset to abort an

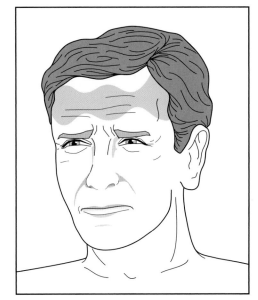

FIGURE 9-1 ■ Tension-type headaches produce a band-like, squeezing, symmetric pressure at the neck, temples, or forehead.

incipient attack or reverse a full-blown one. Over-the-counter medicines, such as aspirin, aspirin-caffeine compounds, acetaminophen, and nonsteroidal anti-inflammatory drugs (NSAIDs), usually suffice. Patients keep these medicines readily available in the car, at work, and in pocketbooks to take at any inkling of a headache. However, physicians should be mindful that their daily use often leads to "chronic daily headaches" or "medication overuse headaches," previously termed "rebound headaches" (see later).

Neurologists recommend "preventive therapy"—medicines taken daily—under several circumstances: if headaches occur more frequently than two or three times per week, acute therapy is ineffective, or analgesic consumption is excessive. For example, even if patients have no history of depression, neurologists often prescribe small night-time doses of a tricyclic antidepressant (TCA). Similarly, even if patients have no history of epilepsy, neurologists often prescribe certain antiepileptic drugs (AEDs), such as valproate/divalproex (Depakote) and topiramate (Topamax). However, they usually avoid prescribing benzodiazepines. Although the muscle contraction explanation for this headache has been all but discredited, several studies have found that botulinum toxin injections into scalp and cervical muscles, which prevents muscle spasms, helped some patients.

Rigorous scientific studies have yet to substantiate the numerous, popular suggestions that alternative treatments, such as acupuncture and biofeedback, alleviate headaches. In adults, insight-oriented psychotherapy and psychoanalysis, when directed toward headaches, do not reduce them; however, they may provide insight, reduce anxiety, treat depression, and offer other benefits. Stress management therapy, especially when combined with a TCA, is modestly effective. In children and adolescents, relaxation and cognitive-behavioral therapy (CBT) reduce the frequency and severity of chronic headache.

Migraine

In clinical practice, the essential diagnostic criteria for migraine consist of episodic, disabling headaches associated with nausea and photophobia. The nonheadache symptoms, in fact, often overshadow or replace the headache. The headaches' qualities—throbbing and unilateral—are typical but not essential even though they are included in the HIS criteria (Table 9-1).

Neurologists grossly divide migraine into two subtypes—defined primarily by the presence or absence of an *aura*. Although migraine symptoms are complex and variable, they are usually consistent from headache to headache for the individual patient.

Approximately 12% of all Americans suffer from migraine, with women predominating by a 3:1 ratio. Migraine may first appear in childhood, but most often not until adolescence. The prevalence increases until age 40 years.

Migraine with Aura

Previously labeled *classic migraine, migraine with aura* affects only about 10% of migraine patients. The aura, which can be almost any symptom of cortex or brain dysfunction, typically precedes or accompanies the headache (Table 9-2). The headache itself is similar to the headache in *migraine without an aura* (see later).

Auras usually appear and then evolve over 4 to 10 minutes, persist for less than 1 hour, and evaporate with the headache's onset. They typically consist of a transient visual phenomenon, but sometimes a simple olfactory or auditory hallucination. Instead of a disturbance in one of the special senses, aura occasionally consists of language impairment similar to aphasia, sensory misperception, or personality change. In children, but not adults, recurrent colic or "cyclic abdominal pain" with nausea and vomiting can constitute an aura.

TABLE 9-1 ■ Criteria for Migraine*

Recurrent (≥5) attacks of headache each with a duration of 4–72 hours (untreated or unsuccessfully treated)

At least 2 of the following characteristics

a. Unilateral location

b. Pulsating quality (throbbing pain)

c. Moderate or severe in intensity

d. Aggravation by routine physical activity

The headache is accompanied by at least 1 of the following symptoms:

a. Nausea and/or vomiting

b. Photophobia and phonophobia

*Essential features of the HIS classification.

TABLE 9-2 ■ Auras of Migraine

Sensory phenomena

  Special senses

    Visual, olfactory, auditory, gustatory

  Paresthesias, especially lips and hand

Motor deficits

  Hemiparesis, hemiplegia

Neuropsychologic changes

  Aphasia

  Perceptual impairment, especially for size, shape, and time

Emotional and behavioral

  Anxiety, depression, irritability, (rarely) hyperactivity

When not followed by a headache, auras may represent recurrent hallucinations. Moreover, visual auras can be a manifestation of several other neurologic disorders (see Table 12-1).

The most common migraine auras are visual hallucinations (see Chapter 12). They usually consist of a graying of a region of the visual field (*scotoma*) (Fig. 9-2, *A*), flashing zigzag lines (*scintillating* or *fortification scotomata*) (see Fig. 9-2, *B*), crescents of brilliant colors (see Fig. 9-2, *C*), tubular vision, or distortion of objects (*metamorphopsia*). Unlike visual auras attributable to other neurologic conditions, these typically involve the simultaneous appearance of positive phenomena, such as scintillations, and negative ones, such as opaque areas.

Migraine without Aura

Previously labeled *common migraine, migraine without aura* affects about 75% of migraine patients. Migraine, which is devoid of an aura, typically lasts 4 to 24 hours and occurs episodically. In about 60% of cases, migraine is throbbing and located on one side of the head (hemicranial). The pain is located predominantly behind a temple (temporal), around one eye (periorbital), or behind one eye (retro-orbital). Of those attacks that begin unilaterally, about 50% move to the opposite side or become generalized (Fig. 9-3). Frequent attacks can evolve into a dull, symmetric, and continual pain that mimics TTH.

Although the throbbing quality and initial unilateral location of migraine headaches are typical, those features are not essential for diagnosis and do not distinguish them from TTH. What distinguishes migraine from TTH are its nonheadache symptoms, including sensory hypersensitivity (photophobia and phonophobia), autonomic dysfunction (nausea and vomiting), and disability. In common terms, people with migraine have episodes of moderately severe headaches accompanied by nausea, and during a painful attack, they usually go to a dark, quiet room.

In conjunction with their tendency to seek seclusion, migraine patients often have changes in their mood and attentiveness that can mimic depression, partial complex seizures, and other neurologic disturbances (Table 9-3). Although some patients with migraine become feverishly active, most become despondent or distraught. Partly because of autonomic dysfunction, migraine sufferers tend to drink large quantities of water or crave certain foods or sweets, particularly chocolate. Children often become confused and overactive. After an attack clears, especially when it ends with sleep, migraine sufferers may experience a sense of tranquility or even euphoria.

Also in contrast to TTH, migraine attacks typically begin in the early morning rather than the afternoon.

In fact, they often have their onset during early morning rapid eye movement (REM) periods (see Chapter 17). Sometimes they begin exclusively during sleep (*nocturnal migraine*). In women, migraine often first develops at menarche, recurs premenstrually, and is aggravated by some oral contraceptives. During pregnancy, about 70% of women with migraine experience dramatic relief, but usually only during their second or third trimesters. However, pregnancy can also have adverse effects. About 10% of women with migraine go through their first attack during pregnancy. Furthermore, 10% to 20% of pregnant women with migraine have more frequent or more severe attacks than usual. Nevertheless, pregnancies beset by migraine are no more likely than ones free of migraine to suffer miscarriage, eclampsia, or fetal malformations. Although postpartum headaches may represent a recurrence of migraine, they may instead represent more serious conditions, such as cortical vein thrombosis, complication of epidural anesthesia, or pituitary infarction.

Another important characteristic of migraine is that it can be precipitated—especially in susceptible individuals—by certain factors called "triggers," such as skipping meals or fasting on religious holidays, too little or excessive sleep, menses, psychologic or occupational stress, overexertion, head trauma, and alcoholic drinks. (Alcohol can also provoke attacks of cluster headaches [see later].) Red wine and brandy are the alcoholic drinks most likely to trigger an attack, with vodka and white wine the least likely. Additionally, cheap wine may be more likely than fine wine to cause headaches. In contrast, alcoholic beverages tend to ameliorate TTH.

To the chagrin of many patients, migraine attacks often coincide with weekends and the start of a vacation. Many of the factors associated with these periods likely contribute to this paradox: withdrawal from work-related stress, anxieties associated with leisure periods, too little sleep, sleeping later than usual (which extends REM periods and does not allow the customary morning cup of coffee [see later]), and holiday meals, which typically include foods spiced with monosodium glutamate (MSG) accompanied by alcoholic beverages.

Psychiatric Comorbidity

Contrary to old views, migraine is not restricted to individuals in upper-income brackets or among those who are rigid, perfectionist, and competitive. The "migraine personality" is now considered an outmoded concept.

Anxiety, panic attacks, major depression, and, less so, bipolar disorder are comorbid with migraine. However, despite migraine's chronicity and widespread neurophysiologic changes, it has no long-term effect on cognitive function.

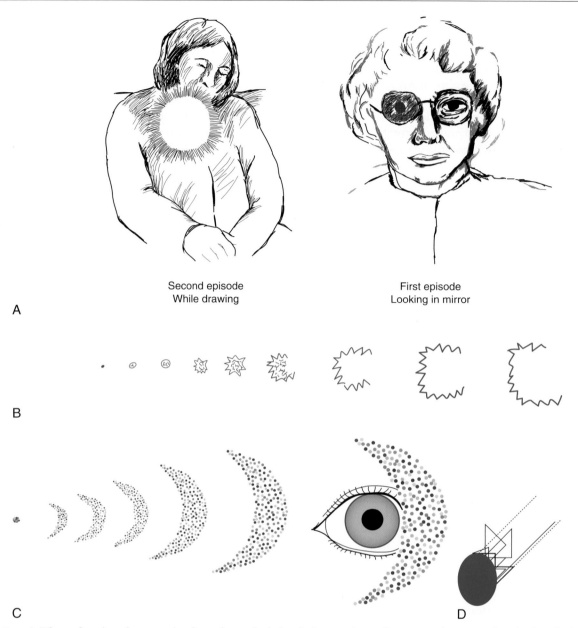

FIGURE 9-2 ■ *A,* These drawings by an artist show the typical visual obscurations of a *scotoma* that precedes the headache phase of her migraine attacks. In both cases, a small circular area near the center of vision is lost entirely or reduced in clarity. Even though the aura is gray and has a relatively simple shape, she is captivated by it. Despite the impending headache they signal, migraine-induced visual hallucinations mesmerize patients. *B,* The patient who drew this aura, a *scintillating scotoma,* wrote, "In the early stages, the area within the lights is somewhat shaded. Later, as the figure widens, you can sort of peer right through the area. Eventually, it gets so wide that it disappears." This scotoma, which is typical, consists of an angular, brightly lit margin and an opaque interior that begins as a star and expands into a crescent. It scintillates at 8 to 12 Hz. Angular auras are sometimes called *fortification scotomas* because of their similarity to ancient military fortresses. *C,* A 30-year-old woman artist in her first trimester of pregnancy had several migraine headaches that were heralded by this scotoma. It began as a blue dot and, over 20 minutes, enlarged to a crescent of brightly shimmering, multicolored dots. When the crescent's intensity was at its peak, she was so dazzled that she lost her ability to see and think clearly. *D,* Having patients draw visual hallucinations has great diagnostic value. One patient, who had no artistic talent, reconstructed this "visual hallucination" using a computer drawing program. Children might provide similar valuable diagnostic information if they are asked to draw what they "see" before a headache.

When depression is comorbid with migraine, the conditions seem reciprocal. Major depression increases the risk of migraine but not of other severe headaches. Similarly, unlike other headache disorders, migraine increases the risk of major depression. Studies differ as to the effect of comorbid depression on the

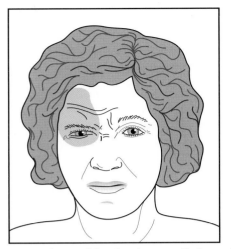

FIGURE 9-3 ■ Patients with migraine usually have throbbing, hemicranial headaches that, in about 50% of cases, either move to the other side of the head or become generalized. However, the headache's severity, quality, and geography, although characteristic and sometimes agonizing, are not as indicative of migraine as their nonheadache features—prostration, nausea, photophobia, and tendency to seek seclusion.

TABLE 9-3 ■ Common Neurologic Causes of Transient Mood Disturbance or Altered Mental Status

Drugs
    Illicit
    Medicinal
Metabolic aberrations
    Hypoglycemia
    Hepatic encephalopathy
Migraine
Mitochondrial encephalopathy
Seizures (see Chapter 10)
    Absence
    Partial complex
    Frontal lobe
Sleep attacks (e.g., narcolepsy, sleep apnea naps [see Chapter 17])
Transient global amnesia (see Chapter 11)
Transient ischemic attacks (see Chapter 11)

frequency or disability of migraine. In an effect that seems to be restricted to women, adverse life events increase headache frequency.

Therapy for patients with migraine and comorbid depression should start with simple behavioral advice, such as get sufficient sleep on a regular schedule, exercise moderately, avoid alcohol and drugs, and keep a "headache diary" (see later). CBT, as an adjunct to medication, may be helpful.

TCAs are not only effective for treating migraine comorbid with depression, they are more effective than selective serotonin reuptake inhibitors (SSRIs)

in treating migraine with or without depression. Also, SSRIs, when administered concurrently with one of the commonly used antimigraine serotonin (5-hydroxytryptamine) agonists, such as a "triptan" (see later) or dihydroergotamine (DHE), carry a low but definite risk of producing the serotonin syndrome (see Chapter 6).

Recognizing the neurologic basis of migraine, the *Diagnostic and Statistical Manual of Mental Disorders, 4th Edition, Text Revision (DSM-IV-TR)* requires including headaches on Axis III. Comorbid psychiatric disorders, such as depression and anxiety, would remain on Axis I (i.e., migraine with comorbid depression would not be considered a single condition but two separate disorders). Alternatively, if depression played an important role in an individual's migraine, the diagnosis might change to a *Pain Disorder Associated with Both Psychologic Factors and a General Medical Condition.* In the rare situation where patients fabricate reports of severe, intractable migraine to sustain a narcotic addiction, the diagnosis would be *Malingering.*

Other Subtypes of Migraine

Childhood migraine is not simply migraine in "short adults." Compared to migraine in adults, the headache component of childhood migraine is briefer (frequently less than 2 hours), more severe, and less likely to be unilateral (only one third of cases). As with migraine in adults, the nonheadache components may overshadow the headache. Childhood migraine can produce episodes of confusion, incoherence, or agitation. In addition, it often leaves children incapacitated by nausea and vomiting. (Physicians caring for children with such episodes should also consider mitochondrial encephalopathy as an alternative, although rare, diagnosis [see Chapter 6].)

Children are particularly susceptible to migraine variants, such as basilar-type and hemiplegic migraine. In *basilar-type migraine,* the headache is accompanied or even overshadowed by ataxia, vertigo, dysarthria, or diplopia—symptoms that reflect brain dysfunction in the basilar artery distribution (the cerebellum, brainstem, and posterior cerebrum [see Fig. 11-2]). In addition, when basilar migraine impairs the temporal lobes, located in the posterior cerebrum, patients may experience temporary generalized memory impairment, for example, transient global amnesia (see Chapter 11).

Hemiplegic migraine is defined by various grades of hemiparesis often combined with hemiparesthesia, aphasia, or other cortical symptoms. These symptoms usually precede or accompany an otherwise typical migraine headache, but they may also develop without any other migraine symptom. In evaluating a patient who has had transient hemiparesis, the physician might consider hemiplegic migraine along with transient ischemic attacks (TIAs), stroke, postictal (Todd's) hemiparesis, and conversion disorder.

In *familial hemiplegic migraine,* patients develop transient hemiparesis before or during the headache. This rare variety of migraine is transmitted in an autosomal dominant pattern by a genetic abnormality on chromosome 19. The basic mechanism is a calcium channel abnormality—a "channelopathy." Other channelopathies include myotonic dystrophy, also transmitted by an abnormal gene on chromosome 19; varieties of episodic ataxias; and varieties of epilepsy.

Occasionally the hemiparesis persists indefinitely. In this stroke-like situation, the migraine is termed *complicated.* Only migraine with aura serves as a risk factor for stroke. For practical purposes, the risk may be restricted to women migraineurs who both smoke cigarettes and use oral contraceptives. The risk is so pronounced that oral contraceptives are counterindicated in women with migraine who smoke.

Migraine-Like Conditions: Food-Induced Headaches

Certain foods and medications can cause nonspecific headaches. Moreover, in susceptible individuals, they can even trigger migraine. However, other than alcohol, the role of foods and chocolate is overemphasized: food precipitates migraine in only about 15% of patients.

The two clearest examples of foods precipitating headaches occur in the *Chinese restaurant syndrome,* in which the offending agent is MSG, and the *hot dog headache,* in which it is the nitrite in processed meats. A different situation is the *ice cream headache,* in which any very cold food that overstimulates the pharynx acts as the trigger. Some people—but fewer than generally assumed—develop migraine-like headaches after eating foods containing tyramine, such as ripened cheese, or ones containing phenylethylamine, such as chocolate. In view of its tendency in some individuals to precipitate attacks, migraine sufferers' frequent chocolate craving before an attack seems ironic. Nevertheless, migraine sufferers should probably avoid the "Four 'C's:" chocolate, cheese, Chinese food, and alcohol [C_3H_5OH].

On the other hand, people who miss their customary morning coffee typically develop the *caffeine-withdrawal syndrome* consisting of moderate to severe headache often accompanied by anxiety and depression. Although this syndrome is almost synonymous with coffee deprivation, withdrawal of other caffeine-containing beverages or medications can precipitate it (Chapter 17). Herein lies a dilemma: sudden withdrawal of caffeine can cause the withdrawal syndrome, but excessive caffeine leads to irritability, palpitations, and gastric acidity.

Medication-Induced Headaches

Antianginal medicines, such as nitroglycerin or isosorbide (Isordil), perhaps because they contain nitrites or dilate cerebral as well as cardiac arteries, cause headaches. Elderly patients who have cerebrovascular atherosclerosis are particularly vulnerable. Curiously, whereas some calcium channel blockers, such as nifedipine (Procardia), trigger headaches, others, such as verapamil (Calan), may prevent them. For the psychiatrist, the most notorious iatrogenic headache, which is often complicated by cerebral hemorrhage, is produced by the interaction of monoamine oxidase inhibitor (MAOI) antidepressants with other medications or foods (see later).

Sex-Related Headaches

Sexual intercourse or masturbation, with or without orgasm, may trigger a migraine-like headache. Currently termed *primary headache associated with sexual activity,* these headaches were previously termed *coital cephalgia* or *orgasmic headache,* depending on the circumstances. Sex-related headaches, which are especially common in individuals with migraine, typically last for several minutes to several hours. The pain may be severe and incapacitating, but the neurologic problem is almost always benign. Nevertheless, before dismissing severe headaches occurring during sexual activity or any vigorous activity, physicians might consider intracerebral or subarachnoid hemorrhage (see later). When the diagnosis of sex-related headaches is secure, taking propranolol or indomethacin before sex can usually prevent the ensuing headache.

Proposed Causes of Migraine

A once popular theory postulated that constriction of cerebral arteries caused a migraine aura and then, when constriction fatigued, arteries dilated and allowed unsuppressed pulsations to pound the arterial walls, which produced the headache. A current, more credible theory attributes migraine to "spreading neuronal depression," which postulates that impaired metabolism of cerebral neurons spreads—first as increased neuronal activity and then as inhibited neuronal activity—from the posterior to anterior cerebral cortex. This theory suggests that the trigeminal nucleus in the pons triggers the release of serotonin, substance P, neurokinin, various neuropeptides, and other vasoactive neurotransmitters. These neurotransmitters incite painful vasodilation and perivascular inflammation.

Other theories postulate faulty serotonin (5-hydroxytryptamine [5-HT]) neurotransmission. Although studies have established no single serotonin mechanism, several observations are important. Most serotonin-producing neurons are in the brainstem's dorsal raphe nuclei. The triptans act primarily as serotonin receptor agonists in the cerebral vessels' trigeminal nerve endings.

Whatever the biochemical mechanism, a genetic abnormality predisposes certain individuals to migraine. About 70% of migraine patients have a close relative with the disorder, and studies of twins show a high concordance. The risk of migraine is 50% or greater in relatives of an individual with migraine, and this risk increases with the severity of attacks. In the case of hemiplegic migraine, the genetic basis is well established.

Acute Treatment

In attempting to identify migraine triggers, neurologists usually suggest that patients create a headache diary to record headache days, medications, diet, menses, school examinations, and other potential precipitants. If patients cannot avoid triggers, they should at least anticipate them. For some individuals, relaxation techniques or other forms of CBT may be helpful. In contrast, scientific studies have not yet documented the purported benefits of hypnosis, acupuncture, transcutaneous electrical stimulation, or spinal manipulation.

Successful treatment of migraine usually requires medications to dampen the headache and ameliorate the accompanying nausea and vomiting. Treatment regimens for children and adolescents differ slightly from those for adults. As with TTH, patients take medications on an acute basis to abort an incipient migraine or reverse a full-blown one. For acute treatment of occasional, mild attacks, simple analgesics, NSAIDs, and other oral, over-the-counter medicines may arrest the headache and produce minimal side effects.

Although opioids may suppress headaches, neurologists have remained wary of initiating or rewarding drug-seeking behavior (see Chapter 14). In the majority of patients undergoing opioid treatment, their emergency room visits and hospitalizations decrease, but their headaches and disability persist. Moreover, they commonly misuse opioids. Nevertheless, neurologists prescribe them in limited, controlled doses when vasoactive or serotoninergic medications carry too many risks, such as for pregnant or elderly patients. For pregnant women, neurologists may first prescribe acetaminophen, caffeine, or, only during the first two trimesters, ibuprofen. If these provide inadequate relief, rather than expose the mother and fetus to potentially harmful serotonin agonists or ergotamines, neurologists often prescribe morphine, meperidine, or other opioid. The data concerning triptan treatment of pregnant women are inadequate. To reduce the chance of their patients' abusing opioids, physicians often have them sign contracts with rules regarding doses, lost medicines, monitoring requirements, and not obtaining opioids from other physicians.

Triptans, which are $5HT_{1B/1D}$ serotonin receptor agonists, include eletriptan (Relpax), rizatriptan (Maxalt), sumatriptan (Imitrex), and zolmitriptan (Zomig). They are rapidly effective for moderate to severe migraine. These medications are all available as pills and some as injections, sublingual wafers, and nasal sprays. The variety of forms allows patients to administer their medicines without any delay, even when in public or suffering from nausea. For menstrually related migraine, women might suppress attacks by taking a triptan during the several days before menses. Their use during pregnancy, however, remains controversial.

Ergotamine and dihydroergotamine, which are primarily vasoconstrictors, are also rapidly effectively. Their excessive use may lead to persistent, excessive vasoconstriction (*ergotism*) in the digits, coronary arteries, and elsewhere. Because they might precipitate a miscarriage or cause fetal malformations, they are counterindicated in pregnant women.

Many of these migraine medications have worrisome side effects. Similar to the analgesics used to treat TTH, frequent use of these medicines—as little as two to three times a week—may lead to "chronic daily headache" or "medication overuse headache" (see later). Excessive ergotamine use can lead to chronic daily headache as well as ergotism. As previously mentioned, administering a SSRI concurrently with a triptan or other serotonin agonist may lead to the serotonin syndrome.

Migraine often leads to nausea and vomiting. Paradoxically, these problems may also represent a side effect of DHE or another medicine. Even when minor, these symptoms preclude orally administered medication. Rectal or intravenous antiemetics sometimes can serve as the primary medicine or act synergistically with the migraine medicine. One caveat remains: Dopamine-blocking antiemetics may cause acute and permanent dystonic reactions similar to those of antipsychotic medicines (see Chapter 18).

Under certain circumstances, neurologists hospitalize patients with severe, uninterrupted migraine refractory to outpatient treatment. Migraine lasting more than 3 days (*status migrainosus*) usually leads to prostration, prolonged painful distress, and dehydration. Affected patients benefit substantially from parenteral medication, intravenous fluids, antiemetics, and a quiet, dark refuge. Medically supervised withdrawal from over-the-counter medications or narcotics may also require hospitalization.

Preventative Treatment

Neurologists prescribe preventative treatment under several circumstances: migraine occurring more than four times a month; migraine causing 3 to 4 days of disability per month; acute medicines losing their effectiveness; or patients' taking excessive medicine. Preventative medicines fall into four categories: β-blockers, TCAs, calcium channel blockers, and AEDs.

Neurologists often prescribe β-blockers for migraine prophylaxis, as well as for treatment of essential tremor (see Chapter 18). However, they avoid prescribing them to patients with comorbid depression because they may precipitate or exacerbate mood disorder.

TCAs, particularly amitriptyline and nortriptyline, prevent or reduce the severity, frequency, and duration of migraine. Apart from their mood-elevating effect, these antidepressants may be useful in migraine treatment because they decrease or alter REM sleep, when many migraine attacks begin. In addition, because they enhance serotonin, they are analgesic (see Chapter 14). As most migraine patients are young and require only small doses, compared to those used to treat depression, the side effects of TCAs are rarely a problem. SSRIs are less effective than TCAs in preventing migraine.

Calcium channel blockers, such as verapamil (Calan), may also be effective and have a relatively low incidence of side effects. However, neurologists cannot reliably predict their benefit.

Certain AEDs, such as topiramate and valproate/divalproex, offer preventative treatment for migraine, as well as for neuropathic pain and epilepsy. Valproate/divalproex is suitable for migraine sufferers with or without affective disorders. It may suppress migraine by reducing 5-HT neurons firing in the dorsal raphe nucleus or by altering trigeminal $GABA_A$ receptors in the meningeal blood vessels.

Chronic Daily Headaches

After many years, headaches often increase in frequency to a daily or near daily basis. Practicing neurologists label these *chronic daily headaches* (CDH), although the IHS terms them "Daily Persistent Headache." Most cases of CDH follow chronic TTH or migraines where medication overuse complicated their treatment. However, CDH in adolescents is an exception: in them, CDH often develops in the absence of medication overuse.

TABLE 9-4 ■ Comparison of Tension-type and Migraine Headaches		
	Tension-type	**Migraine**
Location	Bilateral	Hemicranial*
Nature	Dull ache	Throbbing*
Severity	Slight–moderate	Moderate–severe
Associated symptoms	None	Nausea, hyperacusis, photophobia
Behavior	Continues working	Seeks seclusion
Effect of alcohol	Reduces headache	Worsens headache

*In approximately half of patients, at least at onset.

CDH patients typically have a continual discomfort or dull pain. They seem to suffer from a combination of migraine and TTH—to the extent that they can be differentiated (Table 9-4)—that blend, vary, and recur. However, their headaches typically lack further defining characteristics, such as an aura, throbbing sensation, nausea, photophobia, or even a discrete onset.

As with migraine, major depression and panic disorders are comorbid with CDH. In addition, CDH is comorbid with various somatic illnesses, particularly chronic pain, fibromyalgia, sleep disturbances, and chemical dependancy (medication abuse). Risk factors for CDH include frequent use of medications, female gender, limited education, head trauma, and obesity.

Many cases of CDH are clearly attributable to daily or near daily use of medications for either TTH or migraine. On the other hand, abrupt withdrawal of these medicines ironically leads to *withdrawal* or *rebound headaches.*

Although chronic overuse of almost any headache medication may lead to CDH, those most closely associated with withdrawal headaches are ergotamine, aspirin-butalbital-caffeine compounds (e.g., Fiorinal), benzodiazepines, sedatives, and opioids. Even overuse of triptans and NSAIDs can lead to CDH. Moreover, triptans lead to CDH in less than 2 years, but analgesics take almost 5 years.

Treatment of CHD may first require addressing comorbid psychiatric and medical conditions. Antidepressants and mood-modulating medications, such as valproic acid, would be particularly suitable for depression comorbid with CDH. Withdrawal symptoms from headache medications can be as worrisome as ones from opioids. Neurologists often recommend hospitalization for CDH patients with severe depression as well as those attempting to withdraw from barbiturates and opioids.

Cluster Headaches

Cluster headaches usually occur in groups (clusters). Each headache lasts 45 minutes to 1.5 hours (if untreated), and attacks occur from one to eight times daily for a period of several weeks to months. The demography of this disorder is unique. It affects men six to eight times more commonly than women and has little familial tendency. It typically develops in men between ages 20 and 40 years. More than 80% of those affected smoke and about 50% drink alcohol excessively.

Most cluster attacks have a predictable, cyclic pattern. For example, some develop every spring or fall. During a cluster period, headaches occur randomly throughout the day; however, alcoholic drinks and REM sleep can readily precipitate them. Cluster-free intervals range from a few months to several years.

An individual headache consists of severe, sharp, nonthrobbing pain that most often bores into one eye and the adjacent region. Ipsilateral eye tearing, conjunctival injection, nasal congestion, and a partial Horner's syndrome (Figs. 9-4 and 12-16)—ipsilateral autonomic symptoms—typically accompany the headache. Unlike migraine, attacks of cluster headaches are brief, but their pain is extraordinarily intense and always unilateral. The pain is so severe that it drives patients to agitation and restlessness. Also unlike migraine, cluster headache is not preceded by an aura, accompanied by nausea, or alleviated by bedrest or seclusion.

Cause and Treatment

A different but unknown form of cerebrovascular dysfunction than occurs in migraine causes cluster

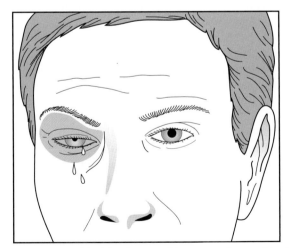

FIGURE 9-4 ■ As with this 43-year-old man, patients with cluster headaches usually experience unilateral periorbital pain accompanied by ipsilateral tearing and nasal discharge, along with ptosis and miosis (a partial Horner's syndrome). He has a right-sided partial Horner's syndrome, tearing, and a typical instinctual compensatory elevation of the right eyebrow to uncover the right eye.

headaches. Nevertheless, because the two probably result from cerebrovascular dysfunction, share several features, and respond to many of the same medications, both are called "vascular headaches."

Orally administered acute migraine medications are ineffective mostly because each cluster headache's abrupt, unexpected onset and relatively short duration does not allow enough time for the patient to take the medicine and absorb it. However, sumatriptan or dihydroergotamine injections and, in a unique treatment, oxygen inhalation at 8 to 10 L/minute may abort them. Preventative medicines include lithium, steroids, and valproic acid. (Neurologists introduced lithium because cluster headaches, like bipolar episodes, follow a cyclic pattern and affect middle-aged individuals.)

SECONDARY HEADACHES

Temporal Arteritis/Giant Cell Arteritis

Temporal arteritis (giant cell arteritis) is a disease of unknown etiology in which the temporal, other cranial arteries, and often also medium-sized arteries throughout the body develop overt inflammation. Because histologic examination of affected arteries reveals giant cells and the disease is systemic, this condition is more properly called giant cell arteritis than the more restrictive term temporal arteritis.

Patients are almost always older than 55 years, making temporal arteritis one of the several headache conditions that predominantly affect the elderly (Table 9-5). The pain is usually dull, continual, and located in one or both temples. Jaw pain on chewing ("jaw claudication") is unusual but almost pathognomic. In advanced cases, the temporal arteries are tender and red from induration. Signs of systemic illness, such as malaise, low-grade fever, and weight loss, often accompany the headache. In about 25% of cases, polymyalgia rheumatica or another rheumatologic disorder accompanies giant cell arteritis.

Because untreated arterial inflammation leads to arterial occlusion, serious complications may develop

---

TABLE 9-5 ■ Causes of Headaches Predominantly in the Elderly

Brain tumors: glioblastoma, metastases
Cervical spondylosis
Vasodilators and other medications
Postherpetic neuralgia
Subdural hematomas after little or no trauma
Temporal arteritis (giant cell arteritis)
Trigeminal neuralgia

when the diagnosis is delayed. Two dreaded complications, which stem from occlusions of the ophthalmic, ciliary, and cerebral arteries, are blindness and strokes. In more than 90% of cases, the erythrocyte sedimentation rate (ESR) rises above 40 mm. A temporal artery biopsy remains the definitive test, but it is sometimes unnecessary, hazardous, or impractical. Timely treatment with high-dose steroids will relieve the headaches and prevent complications.

Intracranial Mass Lesions

The first symptom of brain tumors and chronic subdural hematomas—common mass lesions (see Chapter 19 and Fig. 20-9)—is most often headaches. However, brain tumor headache qualities are nonspecific or even misleading. For example, brain tumor headaches usually mimic TTH because they are bilateral and dull. When headaches are unilateral, they are on the side opposite the tumor in 20% of cases. Although brain tumor headaches notoriously begin during early morning REM sleep and awaken patients, that pattern develops in less than half the patients. Moreover, numerous other headaches display the same early morning onset: migraine, cluster headaches, carbon dioxide retention, sleep apnea, and caffeine withdrawal.

Characteristically, at least subtle cognitive and personality changes accompany headaches attributable to mass lesions. In addition, even if not present initially, lateralized signs usually develop within 8 weeks. However, overt signs of increased intracranial pressure—papilledema and stupor—may not develop until late in the course, if at all.

To avoid missing mass lesions and to calm the fears of patients, their families, and medical colleagues, neurologists readily order computed tomography (CT) or magnetic resonance imaging (MRI) for almost all patients with unexplained progressive headaches. In addition, for patients with headaches beginning after 55 years, they order an ESR.

Chronic Meningitis

Chronic meningitis, like mass lesions, produces weeks of a dull, continual headache accompanied by progressive cognitive impairment and personality changes. However, with chronic meningitis, symptoms and signs of a systemic infectious illness, such as tuberculosis, may predominate. Meningeal inflammation at the base of the brain causes other distinguishing features. The inflammation chokes various cranial nerves, leading to facial palsy (from seventh cranial nerve injury), hearing impairment (eighth nerve), or extraocular muscle palsy (third, fourth, or sixth nerves). It

also impairs the reabsorption of cerebrospinal fluid (CSF) through the arachnoid villa, which leads to hydrocephalus.

A variety of infectious agents can cause chronic meningitis, but generally only in susceptible individuals. For example, *Cryptococcus* commonly causes it almost only in patients who have impaired immune systems, particularly those taking long-term steroids, chemotherapy, or other immunosuppressants and those with AIDS. With almost any variety of chronic meningitis, CT or MRI typically shows hydrocephalus, reflected in elevated CSF pressure. CSF analysis, which is critical, typically shows a lymphocytic pleocytosis, low glucose concentration, elevated protein concentration, and often specific antigens.

Idiopathic Intracranial Hypertension (Pseudotumor Cerebri)

Scientific groups have changed the popular terms "pseudotumor cerebri" and "benign intracranial hypertension" to *idiopathic intracranial hypertension.* This term reflects the potentially serious nature of this condition.

Idiopathic intracranial hypertension, which originates in cerebral edema, develops predominantly in young, obese women who have menstrual irregularity. Excessive vitamin A and outdated tetracycline use preceded several cases. Recent studies suggest that the cause in many cases is elevated intracranial venous sinus pressure.

Whatever the underlying cause, intracranial hypertension gives rise to papilledema and, as in so many other conditions, a dull, generalized headache. When intracranial pressure markedly rises, patients develop florid papilledema. If untreated, the papilledema leads to expanded visual fields and eventually optic atrophy and blindness (see Chapter 12). Increased intracranial pressure also sometimes stretches and then damages one or both of the abducens (sixth) cranial nerves. Abducens nerve palsy leads to unilateral or bilateral inward eye deviation because of the unopposed, intact third cranial nerves (see Fig. 4-8).

Surprisingly, many intracranial hypertension patients suffer from severe headaches and have florid papilledema, but their neurologic examination is otherwise normal. Moreover, they usually have no depression of their intellect or mood.

Neurologists, cognizant that the differential diagnosis of pseudotumor is tumor, routinely order a CT or MRI. In pseudotumor cerebri, these studies typically reveal cerebral swelling and compressed, small ventricles, but no mass lesions.

CSF pressure is typically greater than 300 mm H_2O, but often reaches levels greater than 400 mm.

11. Holroyd KA, O'Donnell FJ, Stensland M, et al: Management of chronic tension-type headache with tricyclic antidepressant medication, stress management therapy, and their combination. A randomized controlled trial. JAMA 285:2208–2215, 2001.
12. Headache Classification Committee of the International Headache Society: The International Classification of Headache Disorders (2nd ed). Cephalalgia 24:1–160, 2004.
13. Juang KD, Wang SJ, Fuh JL, et al: Comorbidity of depressive and anxiety disorders in chronic daily headache and its subtypes. Headache 40:818–823, 2000.
14. Kaufman DM, Solomon S: Migraine visual auras: A medical update for the psychiatrist. Gen Hosp Psychiatry 14:162–170, 1992.
15. Lewis D, Ashwal S, Hershey A, et al: Practice parameter: Pharmacological treatment of migraine headache in children and adolescents. Report of the American Academy of Neurology Quality Standards Subcommittee and the Practice Committee of the Child Neurology Society. Neurology 63:2215–2224, 2004.
16. Linde K, Rossnagel K: Propranolol for migraine prophylaxis. Cochrane Database Syst Rev 2: CD003225, 2004.
17. Lipton RB, Stewart WF: Migraine headaches: Epidemiology and comorbidity. Clin Neurosci 5:2–9, 1998.
18. Littlewood JT, Glover V, Davies PTG, et al: Red wine as a cause of migraine. Lancet 1:558–559, 1988.
19. Loder E: Prophylaxis of menstrual migraine with triptans: Problems and possibilities. Neurology 59:1677–1681, 2002.
20. Lyngberg AC, Rasmussen BK, Jørgensen T, et al: Prognosis of migraine and tension-type headache: A population-based follow-up study. Neurology 65:580–585, 2005.
21. Mathew NT: Antiepileptic drugs in migraine prevention. Headache 41(Suppl 1):S18–S24, 2001.
22. Rasmussen BK: Migraine and tension-type headache in a general population: Precipitating factors, female hormones, sleep pattern and relation to lifestyle. Pain 53:65–72, 1993.
23. Reynolds DJ, Hovanitz CA: Life event stress and headache frequency revisited. Headache 40:111–118, 2000.
24. Rozen TD: Antiepileptic drugs in the management of cluster headache and trigeminal neuralgia. Headache 41(Suppl 1):S25–S32, 2001.
25. Sacks OW: Migraine: Revised and Expanded. Berkeley, University of California Press, 1992.
26. Saper JR, Lake AE, Hamel RL, et al: Daily scheduled opioids for intractable head pain. Long-term observations of treatment program. Neurology 62:1687–1694, 2004.
27. Silberstein SD: Comprehensive management of headache and depression. Cephalalgia 21:50–55, 1998.
28. Silberstein SD: Practice parameter: Evidence-based guidelines for migraine headache. Report of the Quality Standards Subcommittee of the American Academy of Neurology. Neurology 55:754–762, 2000.
29. Silberstein SD, Welch KMA: Painkiller headache. Neurology 59:972–974, 2002.
30. Silverman K, Evans SM, Strain EC, et al: Withdrawal syndrome after the double-blind cessation of caffeine consumption. N Engl J Med 327:1109–1114, 1992.
31. Wang AJ, Fuh JL, Lu SR, et al: Chronic daily headache in adolescents: Prevalence, impact, and medication overuse. Neurology 66:193–197, 2006.
32. Zwart JA, Dyb G, Hagen K, et al: Depression and anxiety disorders associated with headache frequency. Eur J Neurol 10:147–152, 2003.

Questions and Answers

1. Over the previous 6 hours, a 17-year-old Marine recruit has developed a severe generalized headache, lethargy, nuchal rigidity, and fever. Which should be considered first?
   a. Acute bacterial meningitis
   b. A subarachnoid hemorrhage
   c. Migraine headache
   d. Encephalitis

   Answer: a. Acute bacterial meningitis, particularly meningococcal meningitis, is a common, often fatal disease in military recruits, schoolchildren, and other young people brought into confined areas from diverse backgrounds. Subarachnoid hemorrhages, which can cause lethargy and nuchal rigidity, usually have a cataclysmic onset. Migraine causes prostration and a tendency for sufferers to seek seclusion, but this patient has nuchal lethargy, rigidity, and a fever. Encephalitis usually develops in an epidemic fashion and does not cause nuchal rigidity.

   The possibility of bacterial meningitis merits immediate investigation with a lumbar puncture (LP) for cerebrospinal fluid (CSF) analysis. With bacterial meningitis, the CSF reveals a low glucose concentration (0–40 mg/100 mL), high protein concentration (greater than 100 mg/100 mL), and a polymorphonuclear pleocytosis (greater than 100/mL). Although alternatives have been suggested, penicillin (20 million U/day intravenously) remains the standard antibiotic regimen.

2. Following 5 days of moderate bitemporal headaches, a woman brought her 45-year-old husband for psychiatric evaluation because he began to develop episodes of purposeless, repetitive behavior. On examination, he was febrile, disoriented, inattentive, and unable to recall any recent or past events. Computed tomography (CT) revealed no abnormalities in the brain or sinuses. His CSF contained 89 white blood cells (WBCs), of which 90% were lymphocytes; 45 mg% glucose; and 80 mg% protein. An electroencephalogram (EEG) showed spikes overlying both temporal lobes. Which is the most likely diagnosis?
   a. Acute bacterial meningitis
   b. Subarachnoid hemorrhage
   c. Migraine headache
   d. Encephalitis

   Answer: d. His partial complex seizures and amnesia reflect temporal lobe dysfunction. Small infarctions

and infections are not visible on CT, but physicians can see them on magnetic resonance imaging (MRI). In view of the delirium, fever, and the CSF profile, the underling illness is most likely an infectious process. Herpes simplex encephalitis, the most common non-epidemic encephalitis, has a predilection for the temporal lobes, which house major portions of the limbic system. It produces this picture of fever, delirium, partial complex seizures, and amnesia. Severe cases of herpes simplex encephalitis cause temporal lobe hemorrhagic infarctions, which allows some blood to seep into the CSF. Survivors of severe cases may exhibit a human form of the Klüver-Bucy syndrome (see Chapter 16).

3. Which symptoms most accurately differentiate migraine from other forms of headache?
   a. Headaches that are unilateral and throbbing
   b. Headaches that are exacerbated by physical activity
   c. Headaches that respond only to opioids for relief
   d. Headaches that are disabling and accompanied by nausea and photophobia

   Answer: d. Autonomic symptoms distinguish migraine from other primary headache disorders. The quality and location of the headache, although important, are not critical.

4. In which age group does migraine most often first develop?
   a. Childhood
   b. Adolescence
   c. Young adult years
   d. Middle age

   Answer: b. The peak incidence of the first migraine attack is in mid to late adolescence. The prevalence continues to rise until approximately age 40 years. Women are affected more than men (almost 3:1).

5. Which of the following statements about migraine during pregnancy is true?
   a. Pregnancy usually increases the frequency and severity of attacks.
   b. Migraine during pregnancy is associated with complications.
   c. In almost 10% of cases, women with migraine had their first attack during pregnancy.
   d. In women who have migraine, postpartum headaches usually represent depression.

Answer: c. Although almost 10% of women with migraine had their first attack during pregnancy, pregnancy reduces the frequency and intensity of migraine attacks in women who suffered from migraine before conceiving. Even if migraine persists throughout pregnancy, it does not lead to miscarriage, eclampsia, or fetal malformations. Although postpartum depression may intensify postpartum headaches, the headaches themselves in migraine patients usually represent a recurrence of migraine. Depending on the particular case, physicians might evaluate the patient for other postpartum neurologic complications, such as cortical vein thrombosis, headaches from epidural anesthesia, and pituitary necrosis.

6. A 4-year-old boy has headaches with incapacitating nausea and vomiting complicated by confusion, incoherence, and agitation. However, he has no paresis or nuchal rigidity. His mother has a history of migraine. Between attacks, he appears normal. Serum lactate and pyruvate levels are elevated. Which of the following is the most likely explanation for the child's attacks?
    a. Tension-type headache
    b. Brain tumor
    c. Diabetes
    d. Mitochondrial encephalopathy

Answer: d. The elevated serum lactate and pyruvate levels indicate a mitochondrial encephalopathy.

7. Which of the following is the least significant risk factor for chronic daily headache (CDH)?
    a. Frequent if not daily use of headache medicines
    b. History of tension-type headache
    c. History of migraine
    d. History of cluster headache
    e. Head trauma

Answer: d. Tension-type and migraine headaches, but not cluster headaches, are significant risk factors for CDH. In adolescents compared to adults, medication overuse is less of a risk factor for developing CDH.

8. If a patient with major depression were treated with a SSRI, what would be the risk of administering a triptan for migraine?
    a. Eruptions at the mucocutaneous border
    b. Hypertension leading to a cerebral hemorrhage
    c. Delirium, fever, myoclonus
    d. Muscle rigidity, rhabdomyolysis, fever, and renal failure

Answer: c. If triptans, which are serotonin agonists, are administered in conjunction with an SSRI, patients may develop the serotonin syndrome. Eruptions at the mucocutaneous border are a manifestation of an allergic reaction, for example, the Steven-Johnson syndrome. Hypertension leading to a cerebral hemorrhage can complicate treatment with a monamine oxidase inhibitor (MAOI). Muscle rigidity, rhabdomyolysis, fever, and renal failure are manifestations of the neuroleptic malignant syndrome.

9. Which is the cause of hemiplegic migraine?
    a. Mitochondrial DNA abnormality
    b. Excessive use of headache medications
    c. Calcium channel abnormality, carried on chromosome 19
    d. Excessive trinucleotide repeats on chromosome 4

Answer c. A calcium channel abnormality, carried on chromosome 19, causes hemiplegic migraine. Other disorders attributable to calcium channel abnormalities are myotonic dystrophy, which is also attributable to an abnormal gene on chromosome 19, and several other episodic disorders, such as varieties of ataxia and epilepsy. Excessive CAG trinucleotide repeats on chromosome 4 causes Huntington's disease.

10. A young hypertensive woman suddenly develops severe right periorbital pain, prostration, a right third cranial nerve palsy, and nuchal rigidity. What is the most likely explanation?
    a. A ruptured aneurysm in the circle of Willis
    b. An ocular migraine
    c. Myasthenia gravis
    d. None of the above

Answer: a. Although several illnesses may cause a severe periorbital pain, the third nerve palsy indicates that her right posterior communicating artery aneurysm ruptured and caused a subarachnoid hemorrhage. Myasthenia gravis may cause extraocular muscle weakness that can mimic a third nerve palsy; however, because myasthenia gravis spares the pupillary muscles, pupils remain round, equal, and reactive to light. Also, it does not cause either pain or nuchal rigidity. More important, neither myasthenia gravis nor medications that treat it cause cognitive impairment.

11. While watching television, a middle-aged hypertensive man had the sudden onset of the worst headache of his life. On examination, he is able to speak coherently, but has nausea and vomiting. Of the following, which is the most likely cause?
    a. An intracranial hemorrhage
    b. Migraine
    c. Seizure
    d. Brain tumor

Answer: a. The symptom, "the worst headache of my life," indicates a cerebral or subarachnoid hemorrhage. Migraine or cluster headaches, which may appear in middle age, might be considered; however, those diagnoses should be entertained only when headaches have become a chronic illness (often requiring months of observation) and when potentially fatal conditions have been excluded.

12. An elderly, depressed man developed a continual, moderately severe, generalized headache. He has a decreased attention span and a short-stepped gait. Which illness is least likely to be present?
    a. Giant cell arteritis
    b. Subdural hematoma
    c. Brain tumor
    d. Dementia with Lewy bodies
    e. Depression

Answer: d. Dementia with Lewy bodies does not cause headache. To a certain extent, a short-stepped gait and decreased attention span normally develop as individuals age. The elderly are particularly vulnerable to giant cell arteritis, trigeminal neuralgia, subdural hematomas that develop either spontaneously or following trivial injuries, primary or metastatic brain tumors, depression, and side effects of medications.

13. Which two of the following headaches is always unilateral and on the same side?
    a. Migraine
    b. Trigeminal neuralgia
    c. Cluster
    d. Idiopathic intracranial hypertension

Answer: b, c. Migraine headaches are frequently but not exclusively unilateral, and they often switch sides or generalize. Idiopathic intracranial hypertension causes a generalized headache.

14–25. Match the disease (Questions 14–25) with the characteristic symptoms (a–m). Some questions may have more than one answer.
14. Tic douloureux
15. Bell's palsy
16. Idiopathic intracranial hypertension
17. Basilar migraine
18. Subarachnoid hemorrhage
19. Temporal arteritis
20. Angle-closure glaucoma
21. Subdural hematoma
22. Postconcussion headache
23. Medulloblastoma
24. Viral meningitis
25. Hemiplegic migraine
    a. Severe ocular pain, "red eye," markedly decreased vision
    b. Papilledema, generalized headache, obesity, and menstrual irregularity
    c. Mastoid pain followed by facial palsy

    d. Lancinating pain on one side of the jaw
    e. Moderate headache, focal seizures, and fever
    f. Mild headache and hemiparesis after a fortification scotoma
    g. Chronic pain, depressed sensorium
    h. Unilateral forehead pain, malaise, jaw claudication, high sedimentation rate
    i. Daily dull headaches, inattention, insomnia, depression, and anxiety
    j. Apoplectic headache, nuchal rigidity
    k. Horner's syndrome
    l. Headache, nausea, vomiting, diplopia, and ataxia
    m. Several days of headache, fever, and photophobia, with lymphocytic pleocytosis in the CSF

Answers: 14-d, 15-c, 16-b, 17-l, 18-j, 19-h, 20-a, 21-g, i, or l, 22-i, 23-l, 24-m, 25-f.

26. Which of the following is not an indication for changing from acute to preventative therapy for migraine?
    a. More than four migraine headaches monthly
    b. Tinnitus from aspirin-containing medications
    c. Ergotism
    d. Habitual narcotic use
    e. Once monthly migraine with aura

Answer: e.

27. What are common triggers of migraine headaches?

Answer: Menses, glare, alcohol, missing meals, too much or too little sleep, and relief from stress may precipitate migraine attacks. REM sleep is also a trigger, but it is more closely associated with the development of cluster headaches.

28. How do migraine headaches in children differ from those in adults?

Answer: Although migraine patients of all ages may have autonomic dysfunction, these symptoms may be the primary or exclusive manifestation in children. Children are also more prone to develop basilar artery migraine. They are also more likely to have behavioral disturbances, such as agitation or withdrawal, and are particularly prone to cyclic vomiting and abdominal pain as the primary or sole manifestation of migraine.

29. Which neurologic disorders cause visual hallucinations?

Answer: Visual hallucinations may be a manifestation of migraine, seizures originating in the temporal or occipital lobes, narcolepsy (hypnopompic or hypnagogic hallucinations), hallucinogens (such as LSD), or alcohol withdrawal (DTs).

30. In which part of the brain are serotonin-containing neurons concentrated?
a. Limbic system
b. Frontal lobes
c. Dorsal raphe nucleus
d. Cerebellum

Answer: c.

31. Concerning migraine, to which process does "spreading neuronal depression" refer?
a. The organically based changes in affect that accompany migraine
b. The wave of neuron hypometabolism that precedes and may cause the migraine
c. The inability of the cortex to respond to the migraine
d. The comorbid depressive disorder

Answer: b. Spreading neuronal depression refers to cerebral neuron hypometabolism that spreads—first as increased neuronal activity and then as inhibited neuronal activity—posteriorly to anteriorly over the cerebral cortex. It precedes and may cause the migraine.

32. Which of the following does "xanthochromic CSF" not imply?
a. The CSF is yellow.
b. Subarachnoid bleeding probably occurred within the previous several days.
c. The serum bilirubin concentration or CSF protein concentration may be highly elevated.
d. The CSF is opaque.

Answer: d.

33. Which type of headache do brain tumors most often mimic?
a. Tension-type
b. Migraine
c. Cluster
d. Subarachnoid hemorrhage
e. Trigeminal neuralgia

Answer: a.

34–37. Which of the following headache types is ameliorated by sleep? (Yes/No)
34. Migraine with aura
35. Trigeminal neuralgia
36. Cluster
37. Temporal arteritis

Answers: 34-Yes. Sleep typically relieves migraine attacks, although REM sleep may actually trigger them. 35-No. Sleep has no effect on trigeminal neuralgia and, conversely, trigeminal neuralgia has no effect on sleep. 36-No. REM sleep typically precipitates cluster headaches. 37-No. Temporal arteritis is independent of sleep.

38–44. Which of these conditions often awaken patients from sleep? (Yes/No)
38. Migraine
39. Sleep apnea
40. Brain tumor
41. Subdural hematoma
42. Tension-type headaches
43. Cluster headaches
44. Chronic obstructive pulmonary disease

Answers: 38-Yes, 39-Yes, 40-Yes, 41-Yes, 42-No, 43-Yes, 44-Yes.

45. During which stage of sleep do migraine and cluster headaches begin?
a. REM
b. NREM
c. Slow-wave
d. None of the above

Answer: a.

46. Which common laboratory tests yield abnormal results in patients with migraine?
a. CT
b. MRI
c. EEG
d. None of the above

Answer: d. None of the above. Although the EEG is often abnormal, the abnormalities are not sufficiently frequent or characteristic to help in the diagnosis.

47. A graduate student develops severe periorbital headaches every winter when he goes to Miami. Which form of headache does this pattern indicate?
a. Depression-induced
b. Tension-type
c. Migraine
d. Cluster
e. Trigeminal neuralgia
f. Giant cell arteritis

Answer: c or d. Going on vacation, especially when it entails psychologic stress, disrupted sleep, or excessive alcohol consumption, may precipitate migraines. Alternatively, cluster headaches are characterized by, and named for, their temporal grouping, which usually occurs around predictable events.

48. Which of the following two conditions cost industry the largest number of lost work-hours?
a. Low back pain
b. Epilepsy
c. Headache

d. Cerebrovascular disease
e. Brain tumors
f. Neck pain

Answers: a and c.

49–51. Which of the following headaches follow family patterns? (Yes/No)
49. Migraine
50. Cluster
51. Tension-type

Answers: 49-Yes, 50-No, 51-Yes.

52. A 35-year-old man who suffers several migraine attacks a year developed a uniquely severe headache during sexual intercourse. He described it as "the worst headache" of his life. Two evenings later, this headache recurred during masturbation. Which variety of headache is he most likely experiencing?
a. Psychogenic
b. Cluster
c. Coital
d. Tension-type

Answer: c. Most likely, he has sex-induced benign headaches. These are common and fall under the rubric of "coital migraine" or "headache associated with sexual activity." On the other hand, the development of a severe headache, especially during vigorous activity, usually requires further evaluation. In particular, the physician might consider a subarachnoid or intracerebral hemorrhage and order a CT, MRI, or lumbar puncture because of the possibility of a potentially fatal subarachnoid hemorrhage.

53. When are women's migraine attacks often more severe or frequent?
a. Premenstrual days
b. Menopause
c. When taking oral contraceptives
d. Menarche
e. All of the above

Answer: e.

54. What is the minimum frequency of headaches required for a diagnosis of "chronic daily headache" (CDH)?
a. Once or more daily
b. Half the days of each month
c. Once a week
d. Clusters, during which 2 or more occur daily
e. None of the above

Answer: b. CDH, also called "persistent daily headache," occurs at least 15 times per month. Cluster

headache occurs daily in clusters, but usually only for periods of a few weeks.

55. Which cranial nerve innervates the meninges?
a. Olfactory
b. Oculomotor
c. Trigeminal
d. Facial
e. None of the above

Answer: c.

56. Which of the following statements concerning serotonin (5HT) is false?
a. Serotonin is metabolized to 5-hydroxyindolacetic acid (5HIAA).
b. Platelet serotonin concentration falls at the onset of migraine attacks.
c. Sumatriptan, dihydroergotamine, and ergotamine all act on serotonin receptors.
d. Serotonin containing neurons are concentrated in the dorsal raphe.
e. During a migraine, urinary serotonin and 5-HIAA concentrations fall.

Answer: e.

57–60. Match each medication with its common adverse effect.
57. SSRI and a triptan
58. Propranolol
59. Cafergot
60. Aspirin
a. Vascular spasm, claudication, muscle cramps (with prolonged use)
b. Myoclonus, fever
c. Gastric distress and bleeding, easy bruisability
d. Bradycardia, asthma, fatigue
e. None of the above

Answers: 57-b (serotonin syndrome), 58-d, 59-a (ergotism), 60-c.

61. Which condition is usually cyclic or periodic, develops predominately in men, and responds to lithium?
a. Migraine
b. Cluster headaches
c. Trigeminal neuralgia
d. Giant cell arteritis

Answer: b.

62. A 40-year-old woman has had migraine since adolescence and depression for 10 years. Her psychiatrist changed her antidepressant to a SSRI. The medicine initially seemed to reduce her headaches and improve her mood. However, after 1 month her headaches returned with even greater severity. Her family brought her to the emergency room when she developed agitated confusion and tremulousness. Her blood pressure is 110/70 mmHg and her temperature, 100°F. Her urine contains a small quantity of myoglobin. Which of the following is the most likely cause of her condition?

a. Neuroleptic malignant syndrome
b. SSRI overdose
c. Serotonin syndrome
d. A MAOI crisis

Answer: c. She has the serotonin syndrome because she apparently took an antimigraine serotonin agonist, such as a triptan, in addition to the SSRI. She lacks the muscle rigidity and high temperature of neuroleptic malignant syndrome. A MAOI crisis would almost invariably cause hypertension.

63. Which of the following headache varieties is most often associated with a mood change?

a. Cluster
b. Trigeminal neuralgia
c. Giant cell arteritis
d. Migraine
e. Idiopathic intracranial hypertension

Answer: d.

64. Which of the following headache varieties occurs more often in men than women?

a. Migraine with aura
b. Migraine without aura
c. Idiopathic intracranial hypertension
d. Trigeminal neuralgia
e. Tension-type
f. Cluster

Answer: f.

65. Which two CNS structures are pain-sensitive?

a. Optic nerves
b. Meninges
c. Cerebral neurons
d. Ventricles

Answers: a, b.

66–73. Match the headache with its most likely cause.

66. Tic douloureux
67. Hot-dog headache
68. Sinusitis with seizures
69. Idiopathic intracranial hypertension
70. Temporal arteritis
71. Chinese restaurant syndrome
72. Nocturnal migraine
73. Antianginal medication-induced headaches

a. Inflammation of extracranial and intracranial arteries
b. Autonomic nervous system dysfunction
c. Vascular compression of the trigeminal nerve
d. Nitrites
e. Monosodium glutamate (MSG)
f. Cerebral edema
g. Nightmares
h. REM sleep
i. NREM sleep
j. Infection causing meningitis or a brain abscess
k. Cerebral artery as well as coronary artery dilation

Answers: 66-c, 67-d or e, 68-j, 69-f, 70-a, 71-e, 72-h, 73-k.

74. Which of the following is an invalid reason for why tricyclic antidepressants (TCAs) help migraine sufferers who do not have overt depression?

a. TCAs improve sleep patterns.
b. TCAs increase the concentration of serotonin, which is analgesic.
c. TCAs themselves are analgesic.
d. TCAs are endorphins.
e. Depression is often comorbid with migraine.

Answer: d.

75. Which of the following complications are more likely to develop in pregnant women with migraine than in pregnant women without migraine?

a. Miscarriage
b. Eclampsia
c. Fetal malformations
d. All of the above
e. None of the above

Answer: e. Pregnant women beset by migraine are not at increased risk of miscarriage, eclampsia, or fetal malformations.

CHAPTER 10

Epilepsy

Epilepsy, a tendency to have recurrent seizures, affects about 6 of every 1000 people. It embodies several important neurologic problems facing psychiatrists. Seizures can mimic psychiatric disturbances, and vice versa. Epilepsy is often comorbid with cognitive impairment, depression, and other psychiatric illnesses. Moreover, many antiepileptic drugs (AEDs), which also alleviate pain, headache, other neurologic conditions, and several psychiatric illnesses, tend to induce cognitive impairment and mood changes.

ELECTROENCEPHALOGRAM (EEG)

Normal and Abnormal

Invented in the first half of the 20th century and improved by upgrades, such as computerization, the EEG remains the most specific laboratory test for seizures. In addition, it still helps in the diagnosis of several other neurologic conditions.

The routine EEG records cerebral electrical activity detected by "surface" or "scalp" electrodes (Fig. 10-1). Four frequency bands of cerebral activity, represented by Greek letters, emanate from the brain (Table 10-1).

EEG readers first determine the display of the electrodes (the *montage*). They also note the time scale, which is determined by vertical lines on the EEG paper or displayed as 1-second horizontal bars. Although approaches vary, most readers then determine the EEG's *dominant* or *background rhythm* (see later), organization, and symmetry. EEG readers accord special attention to abnormal patterns, especially if they occur in paroxysms. They judge all these features in relation to whether the patient is awake, asleep, unresponsive, or having observable seizure activity.

The normal dominant EEG activity is in the *alpha* range of 8 to 13 cycles-per-second, or Hertz (Hz), and detectable mostly over the occipital region (Fig. 10-2). Alpha activity is prominent when individuals are relaxed with their eyes closed, but disappears if they open their eyes, concentrate, or become anxious. Because alpha activity reflects an anxiety-free state, it represents the goal in "alpha training," biofeedback, and other behavior modification techniques. Alpha

activity also disappears when people fall asleep or take medicines that affect mental function. In the elderly, the background rhythm typically slows but remains within the alpha range. In many illnesses that affect the brain, background EEG activity not only slows but also becomes disorganized. However, in the early stages of Alzheimer's disease, the background activity, although slower than normal, often remains organized and in the alpha range.

Beta activity consists of high (> 13 Hz) frequency activity, usually with low voltage overlying the frontal lobes. Beta activity replaces alpha activity when people concentrate, become anxious, or take medications,

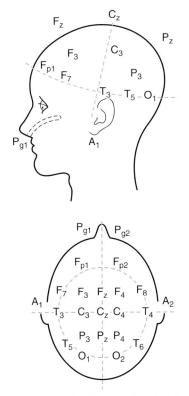

FIGURE 10-1 ■ In the standard array of scalp electrodes, most are named for the underlying cerebral region (e.g., frontal, temporal central, parietal, and occipital). Odd-numbered ones are on the left, and even-numbered ones on the right. The P_g electrodes attach to nasopharyngeal leads and the A electrodes, the ears (aural leads).

such as benzodiazepines. The usual background EEG activity in adults consists mostly of alpha and beta activity.

Theta (4 to 7 Hz) and *delta* (< 4 Hz) activities occur normally in children and everyone during deep sleep but are usually absent in healthy alert adults. When present over the entire brain, theta or delta activity often indicates a degenerative illness or metabolic derangement. In a different situation, continuous focal slow activity with *phase reversal* in bipolar montages (Fig. 10-3) indicates an underlying cerebral lesion; however, its absence certainly does not exclude one.

Pointed waves—"spikes" or "sharp waves"—and slow waves occur in about 3% of the general population; however, they may signal a cerebral lesion or a predisposition to seizures. When sharp waves or spikes are phase-reversed in bipolar montages, they are an even stronger indication of an irritative focus with potential to produce a seizure. Although isolated spikes or sharp or slow waves do not allow a diagnosis of epilepsy, paroxysms of them suggest the diagnosis.

Seizures

During a seizure (*ictus*), the EEG reveals paroxysmal activity usually consisting of bursts of spikes, slow waves, or complexes of spike-and-waves or polyspike-and-waves. However, muscle or movement artifacts may obscure the ictal EEG abnormalities. After the seizure, in the *postictal period*, EEGs commonly show only slow low voltage activity, *postictal depression*, often followed by diffuse high voltage slowing.

EEGs obtained between seizures, in the *interictal period*, contain abnormalities that support—but do not prove—a diagnosis of epilepsy in most patients. On the other hand, because many epilepsy patients have normal interictal EEGs, a normal interictal EEG cannot exclude a diagnosis. Furthermore, about 15% of the general population demonstrates nonspecific EEG changes, such as an isolated slow wave, sharp wave, or spike—a finding that further confuses the EEG's value. These same nonspecific EEG changes also confound studies of patients with various neurologic, psychiatric, or medication-induced disorders.

EEG technicians employ certain maneuvers to provoke EEG abnormalities in patients suspected of having primary generalized epilepsy (see later). For example, they ask these patients to hyperventilate for 3 minutes or look toward a stroboscopic light during the test. If these strategies fail to yield diagnostic EEG patterns and a strong suspicion of seizures persists, physicians might repeat an EEG following sleep deprivation. In about 30% of epileptic patients, a *sleep-deprived EEG* reveals abnormalities not apparent in routine studies.

In some epilepsy patients, specially placed electrodes reveal abnormalities undetectable by ordinary

TABLE 10-1 ■ Common EEG Rhythms		
Activity	**Hz (cycles/sec)**	**Usual Location**
Alpha	8–13	Posterior
Beta	> 13	Anterior
Theta	4–7	Generalized*
Delta	< 4	Generalized*

EEG, electroencephalogram.
*May be focal.

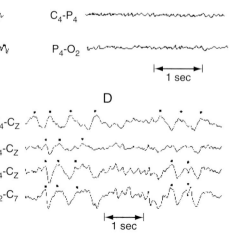

FIGURE 10-2 ■ *A, Alpha* rhythm consists of regular 11-Hz activity overlying the occipital lobe. *B, Beta* rhythm consists of low voltage, irregular 17-Hz activity overlying the frontal lobe. *C, Theta* rhythm consists of 5-Hz activity overlying the right frontal lobe. *D, Delta* activity consists of high voltage 2- to 3-Hz activity present over the entire hemisphere.

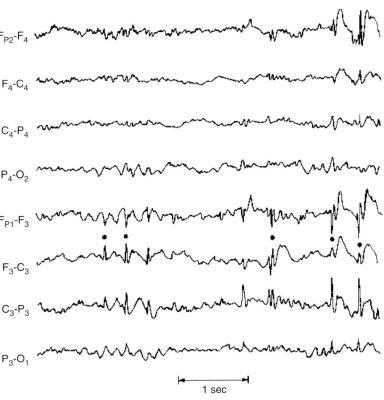

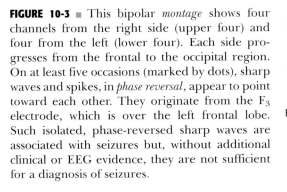

FIGURE 10-3 ∎ This bipolar *montage* shows four channels from the right side (upper four) and four from the left (lower four). Each side progresses from the frontal to the occipital region. On at least five occasions (marked by dots), sharp waves and spikes, in *phase reversal*, appear to point toward each other. They originate from the F₃ electrode, which is over the left frontal lobe. Such isolated, phase-reversed sharp waves are associated with seizures but, without additional clinical or EEG evidence, they are not sufficient for a diagnosis of seizures.

scalp electrodes. For example, anterior temporal scalp, nasopharyngeal, or sphenoidal electrodes can detect discharges from the temporal lobe's inferior-medial (mesial or medial) surface (Fig. 10-4). Electrodes surgically implanted in the dura, subdural space, or cerebral cortex can pinpoint an epileptic focus and also show that a seizure focus seen on scalp electrodes may only be a reflection ("mirror") of the actual focus.

Another diagnostic strategy, *continuous EEG-video monitoring*, consists of several days of split-screen videotaped clinical and EEG recordings usually undertaken in hospital epilepsy units. The monitoring system should record any seizures, changes in behavior, and effects of sleep. At the same time, physicians might check serum AED concentrations and various physiologic data. Continuous EEG-video monitoring has become the gold standard for many epilepsy studies, including diagnosing, classifying, and determining the frequency of seizures; evaluating patients for epilepsy surgery; treating patients who seem to suffer from *refractory seizures* (frequent seizures that do not respond to AEDs); and identifying disorders that mimic seizures, particularly psychogenic seizures (see later).

Quantitative EEG analysis (QEEG) or *EEG brain mapping* involves topographic displays and comparisons of a patient's EEG to standard results. This technique, used mostly in research, remains too unreliable for clinical evaluation of patients with epilepsy, minor and moderate head injury, postconcussive syndrome,

learning disabilities, attention deficit-hyperactivity disorder, and psychiatric illnesses. QEEG's fledging status should preclude its introduction in litigation.

With children, an evaluation could actually begin with parents' videotaping episodes of suspected seizures or other intermittent disturbances, including temper tantrums, breath-holding spells, night terrors or other parasomnias (see Chapter 17), and dopamine responsive dystonia and certain other abnormal movements (see Chapter 18), for review with the physician.

Toxic-Metabolic Encephalopathy

During the initial phase of toxic-metabolic encephalopathy (delirium), when patients have only subtle behavioral or cognitive disturbances, the EEG almost always loses alpha activity and develops generalized theta and delta activity. Its organization deteriorates as the patient's sensorium disintegrates. In addition to causing EEG slowing and disorganization, some forms of metabolic encephalopathy, notably hepatic and uremic encephalopathy, characteristically produce *triphasic waves* (Fig. 10-5). In fact, with hepatic failure, triphasic waves often appear before bilirubin levels rise.

Just like a toxic-metabolic encephalopathy almost always produces EEG abnormalities, the converse holds equal weight. A normal EEG reliably precludes a toxic-metabolic encephalopathy.

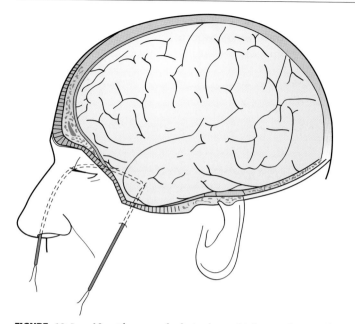

FIGURE 10-4 ■ *Nasopharyngeal electrodes,* which are inserted through the nostrils, reach the posterior pharynx. There, separated by the thin sphenoid bone, they are adjacent to the temporal lobe's medial surface, which is the focus, or origin, of about 80% of partial complex seizures. (Figures in Chapter 20 show the relatively large distance between the temporal lobe's medial surface and the scalp, and the close relationship between the temporal lobe and the sphenoid bone.) *Sphenoidal* electrodes are inserted through the skin to reach the lateral surface of the sphenoid wing. Electrodes in this location are near the temporal lobe's inferior surface. (However, specially placed scalp electrodes, new arrays, electronic filters, and critical reading of the EEG may be just as accurate.) To pinpoint a seizure focus in anticipation of its surgical removal, neurosurgeons may place a grid of electrodes in the subdural space.

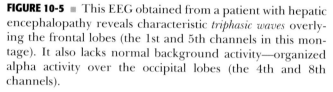

100µv L___
1 sec

FIGURE 10-5 ■ This EEG obtained from a patient with hepatic encephalopathy reveals characteristic *triphasic waves* overlying the frontal lobes (the 1st and 5th channels in this montage). It also lacks normal background activity—organized alpha activity over the occipital lobes (the 4th and 8th channels).

Dementia

In early Alzheimer's disease, the background alpha activity usually slows from about 10 to 12 Hz down to 8 Hz. This decrease is subtle and, especially for people older than 65 years, remains within the normal range. In moderately advanced Alzheimer's disease, however, the background EEG is unequivocally slow and often disorganized.

Vascular dementia also induces EEG abnormalities. However, these changes cannot reliably differentiate vascular dementia from Alzheimer's disease dementia (see Chapters 7 and 11).

In contrast, the EEG is almost definitive in diagnosing subacute sclerosing panencephalitis (SSPE) and Creutzfeldt-Jakob disease (see Chapter 7). In these conditions—characterized clinically by dementia and myoclonic jerks—the EEG shows *periodic sharp-wave complexes* (Fig. 10-6). However, *variant*

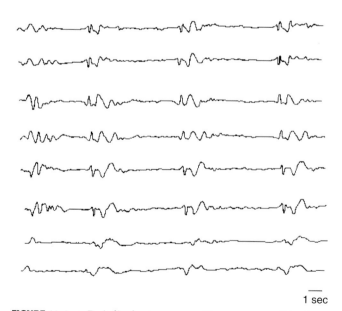

___
1 sec

FIGURE 10-6 ■ *Periodic sharp-wave complexes* appear all in channels as four fairly regular bursts of electrical activity followed by minimal activity. This alternating pattern is termed "burst-suppression." Periodic complexes' clinical counterpart may be myoclonic jerks. Together they are cardinal features of two illnesses characterized by dementia: subacute sclerosing panencephalitis (SSPE) and Creutzfeldt-Jakob disease (see Chapter 7).

Creutzfeldt-Jakob disease fails to produce these EEG changes (see Chapter 7).

The EEG can also help distinguish between *pseudodementia* and dementia—to the extent that they constitute separate entities (see Chapter 7). In pseudodementia the EEG ideally would remain normal, but in dementia from almost any cause, it would show slowing. However, in the many patients with a mixture of depression and mild dementia, the EEG cannot measure each condition's relative contribution to cognitive impairment.

Even though EEGs are relatively inexpensive and carry no risk, neurologists do not routinely order them in the evaluation of a patient with dementia except under certain circumstances: when dementia develops in less than 3 to 6 months; myoclonus accompanies dementia, which suggests Creutzfeldt-Jakob disease or a related illness; fluctuations in the patient's behavior or level of consciousness indicate a toxic-metabolic encephalopathy; or the diagnosis of dementia is equivocal.

Structural Lesions

The EEG does not reliably detect or exclude structural lesions, even those that cause seizures, such as brain tumors, cysticercosis, bacterial abscesses, strokes, or subdural hematomas. In fact, the EEG is normal in many of these conditions, and even when abnormal, it does not distinguish among them. Computed tomography (CT) and especially magnetic resonance imaging (MRI) are standard and, despite their expense, cost-effective tests for detecting structural lesions (see Chapter 20). Although CT generally suffices, MRI better detects small structural lesions. MRI is especially effective in detecting mesial temporal sclerosis, which underlies many partial complex seizures (see later).

Altered States of Awareness

The EEG shows distinctive changes during normal progressively deeper stages of sleep and during dreaming. Coupled with monitors of ocular movement and muscle activity in the polysomnogram (PSG), the EEG is critical in diagnosing sleep disturbances (see Chapter 17).

The EEG is also useful in diagnosing the *locked-in syndrome*, a condition in which patients cannot speak or move their trunk or limbs. Although they appear comatose or demented, they remain fully alert and in possession of their cognitive capacity (see Chapter 11). The locked-in syndrome commonly results from either an infarction in the lower brainstem or

extensive cranial and peripheral nerve damage. With their cerebral hemispheres and upper brainstem intact, patients retain normal cerebral activity and normal EEG activity.

The locked-in syndrome must be differentiated from the *persistent vegetative state* (PVS), which is also characterized by patients' inability to speak. PVS typically follows cerebral cortex anoxia from cardiac arrest, drug overdose, or carbon monoxide poisoning. Most important, because these patients have sustained extensive cerebral cortex injury, they have profound dementia. Nevertheless, their vegetative functions, such as breathing and digesting food, continue. Also, their eyes continue to open and close, but mostly randomly or in response to light. As would be predicted, the extensive cerebral cortical damage leads to slow and disorganized EEG activity.

Finally, absence of EEG activity (*electrocerebral silence*), in most circumstances, indicates "brain death." Making that determination before the heart stops beating permits harvesting organs for transplantation. The exceptions—hypothermia or drug overdose—preclude a diagnosis of brain death based on the EEG. For example, people may fully recover from either barbiturate overdose or drowning in icy water that initially left them with no obvious signs of life and a "flat" EEG.

Psychiatric Disturbances and Psychotropics

Although a psychiatrist (Hans Berger) developed the EEG in 1929 to aid in diagnosing psychiatric illness, it never filled that role. Obtaining EEGs on a routine basis for psychiatric patients is not warranted. Most EEGs would show normal patterns or only minor, nonspecific abnormalities, such as excessive beta or theta activity, or a few sharp waves or spikes. Moreover, there is simply no consensus as to the nature or frequency of various EEG patterns in psychiatric illnesses.

Further confounding any potential diagnostic value, psychotropic medications induce EEG changes. Although these changes are usually minor and nonspecific, some are prominent and persist for up to 2 months after medications are withdrawn. In fact, the EEG changes may simply reflect a medication's intended effect on the brain.

There are few guidelines for assessing psychotropics' EEG effects. Most produce intermittent or continuous background slowing with theta or even delta activity. Benzodiazepines and barbiturates typically produce beta activity, which is sometimes a telltale sign of surreptitious drug use. Phencyclidine (PCP) and other excitatory drugs cause generalized, paroxysmal discharges. Phenothiazines also produce sharp waves, even at therapeutic serum concentrations. Lithium at toxic levels, clozapine, and tricyclic antidepressants (TCAs) cause spikes and sharp waves. Of the antipsychotics, clozapine, olanzapine, and trifluoperazine generally produce the most EEG changes, and quetiapine, loxapine, and haloperidol, the least.

Electroconvulsive therapy (ECT) also induces EEG changes. During and immediately after ECT, EEG changes resemble those of a generalized tonic-clonic seizure and its aftermath. Subsequently, EEG slow-wave activity develops over the frontal lobes or the entire cerebrum and persists for up to 3 months. When ECT is unilateral, EEG slowing is less pronounced and more restricted to the treated side. Although ECT-induced EEG slowing is associated with memory impairment, it is also associated with more effective treatment of depression.

SEIZURE VARIETIES

The two major seizure categories are *partial seizures* and *primary generalized (generalized) seizures*. Although most partial seizures are classified either as *partial with elementary symptoms* or *partial with complex symptoms*, most generalized seizures are classified as either *absence seizures (absences)* or *tonic-clonic seizures* (Table 10-2).

Partial seizures are said to have *elementary* symptoms when their clinical manifestations consist of only a particular movement or sensation without alteration in consciousness. Impaired consciousness, with or without psychologic abnormalities, constitutes a *complex* symptom. Both varieties of partial seizures originate from paroxysmal electrical discharges in a discrete region of the cerebral cortex—the *focus*. For example, partial seizures with motor symptoms are attributable to a focus in the contralateral frontal lobe. These and other seizures consist of similar, stereotyped symptoms for a given patient in almost every episode. Thus, variable symptoms suggest a nonepileptic disorder.

TABLE 10-2 ■ International Classification of Epilepsies by Seizure Type (Modified Version)

Partial (or focal) epilepsies
    Partial seizures with elementary symptomatology:
        Without impairment of consciousness
    Partial seizures with complex symptomatology:
        With impairment of consciousness
    Partial seizures with secondary generalization
Generalized epilepsies
    Absences
    Tonic-clonic (grand mal)

Most partial seizures last between several seconds and several minutes. However, in a condition known as *epilepsia partialis continua* or *partial (focal) status epilepticus*, seizures continue for 30 minutes to many hours. As long as the discharge remains confined to its focus, the original symptoms persist. Continual seizures interfere with complex mental and physical activity and render patients dull and immobile. Nevertheless, they can continue to perform routine activities. For example, despite the seizure, patients may continue to drive familiar routes, dress in their usual clothing, and continue eating.

However, the cerebral cortex discharges tend to spread in a slow, brush-fire-like manner to adjacent cortical areas, which produces additional symptoms. Discharges may eventually spread over the entire cortex or travel directly through the corpus callosum to the contralateral cerebral hemisphere. If the discharges engulf the entire cerebral cortex (*secondary generalization*), patients lose consciousness, develop bilateral motor activity, and show generalized EEG abnormalities. Despite the seizure's final, all-encompassing nature, it would still be called a "partial seizure with secondary generalization" because the nomenclature is based on initial manifestations.

In primary generalized seizures, the thalamus or other subcortical structure presumably generates discharges. These immediately spread upward, exciting the entire cerebral cortex. Primary generalized seizures are bilateral, symmetric, and without focal clinical or EEG findings.

Usually caused by a genetic propensity (from one or more genes) or a metabolic aberration, primary generalized seizures are characterized by unconsciousness and generalized EEG abnormalities; however, they do not necessarily generate gross motor activity. Generalized tonic-clonic seizures may persist for many hours, in which case they become a life-threatening condition, *generalized status epilepticus*.

PARTIAL ELEMENTARY SEIZURES

Partial seizures with elementary *motor* symptoms, formerly called focal motor seizures, most often consist of rhythmic jerking (clonic movement) of a body region that may be limited to one finger or extend to an entire side of the body (Fig. 10-7). These seizures may evolve into partial status epilepticus or undergo secondary generalization. Sometimes, in a "Jacksonian march," a seizure discharge spreads along the motor cortex, and movements that began in one finger extend to the entire arm and then the face.

After a partial motor seizure, affected muscles may remain temporarily weak. Such postictal (*Todd's*) monoparesis or hemiparesis may persist for up to 24 hours.

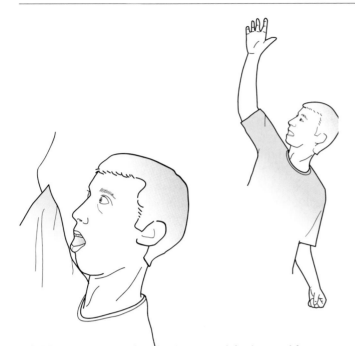

FIGURE 10-7 ■ In a patient having a partial seizure with motor symptoms, his head, neck, and eyes deviate toward the right; his right arm extends; and his left arm flexes. In this case, a focal epileptic discharge in the contralateral left frontal lobe produces this "adversive posture."

Thus, the differential diagnosis of transient hemiparesis includes transient ischemic attacks (TIAs), hemiplegic migraines, conversion disorder, and Todd's hemiparesis.

Seizures with elementary *sensory* symptoms, which usually are attributed to a focus in the parietal lobe's sensory cortex, most frequently consist of tingling or burning paresthesias in body regions with extensive cortical representation, such as the face. Sometimes sensory loss, a "negative symptom," might be a seizure's only manifestation.

Partial elementary seizures with "special sensory" symptoms consist of specific simple auditory, visual, or olfactory sensations. Although these symptoms are so vivid that they can be described as "hallucinations," patients readily recognize them as manifestations of cerebral dysfunction rather than actual events.

Patients with auditory symptoms, which are attributable to temporal lobe lesions, frequently report hearing repetitive noises, musical notes, or single meaningless words. Visual symptoms, which are attributable to occipital lesions, usually consist of relatively simple or elementary bright lights. Sometimes though, they may form lines, spots, or splotches of color that move slowly across the visual field or, like a view through a kaleidoscope, rotate around the center of vision. Physicians must distinguish between elaborate visual seizure phenomena and visual hallucinations due to other causes (see Table 12-1).

Olfactory symptoms classically consist of perceiving vaguely recognizable odors, such as the frequently cited one of burning rubber. However, contrary to popular belief, these odors are not necessarily repugnant. Because olfactory hallucinations usually result from discharges in the amygdala or the *uncus* (the anterior inferior tip of the temporal lobe), partial seizures with olfactory symptoms are often called *uncinate seizures* or *fits*. As with other sensory symptoms, olfactory hallucinations represent the initial phase of the seizure rather than merely the warning of one. If discharges spread from sensory regions to engulf a larger area of the temporal lobe, they trigger partial simple or complex seizures.

EEG and Etiology

During partial elementary seizures, EEGs show spikes, sharp or slow waves, or spike-wave complexes overlying the seizure focus. For example, during seizures with motor symptoms, EEG abnormalities may be prominent in channels over the frontal lobe (Fig. 10-8), and, during the interictal period, EEGs may still show occasional spikes in the same channels.

Depending mostly on the patient's age when seizures begin, particular lesions may be suspected. When young children develop partial seizures, typical causes are congenital cerebral injuries (see later), neonatal meningitis, and neurocutaneous disorders (see Chapter 13).

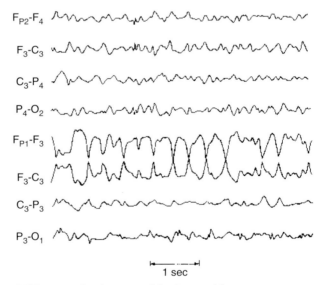

FIGURE 10-8 ■ During a partial seizure with motor symptoms, this EEG contains a paroxysm of 4-Hz sharp wave activity with phase reversals referable to the F_3 electrode. Because the F_3 electrode overlies the left frontal region, the seizure probably consists of right face or arm motor activity and, in some of the cases, a deviation of the head and eyes to the right.

In young adults, common causes of partial elementary seizures are head trauma, arteriovenous malformations (AVMs), and previously asymptomatic congenital injuries, such as cortical dysgenesis. Posttraumatic seizures are not associated with trivial head injuries but with serious trauma, such as injuries causing more than 30 minutes of unconsciousness, depressed (not just linear) skull fractures, intracranial hematomas, or penetrating wounds. Young adults with major psychiatric disturbances are prone to seizures. For example, about 30% of autistic individuals develop epilepsy by the time they are adults. Also, genetic abnormalities in sodium or calcium channels or the gamma-aminobutyric acid (GABA)$_A$-receptor subunit can cause both partial and generalized seizures.

Because drug and alcohol abuse carries multiple neurologic ramifications, neurologists often consider these etiologies in young adults presenting with seizures. Especially when seizures are accompanied by psychotic or otherwise abnormal behavior, physicians should suspect cocaine, PCP, and amphetamine intoxication. Cocaine reduces seizure threshold, causes strokes, leads to noncompliance with AED regimens, and disrupts sleep. However, although neonates may develop seizures during opiate withdrawal, adult opiate addicts generally do not develop seizures during heroin use, withdrawal, or detoxification. Also, marijuana does not lead to seizures and actually has a slight antiepileptic effect.

In contrast, withdrawal from daily use of benzodiazepines (especially alprazolam) or substantial amounts of alcohol also produces seizures within several days to a week. These seizures often evolve into status epilepticus. Most cases of benzodiazepine-withdrawal seizures are associated with prescription medicines rather than "street" drugs.

Although a seizure associated with drug or alcohol abuse can reveal dependency or addiction, it does not necessarily constitute epilepsy. Moreover, a life-threatening neurologic complication of substance abuse, rather than of withdrawal, may produce seizures. For example, cocaine routinely causes cerebral hemorrhages that in turn cause seizures. Similarly, although heroin may not directly produce seizures, its intravenous use can lead to bacterial endocarditis, episodes of cerebral anoxia, acquired immunodeficiency syndrome (AIDS), hepatitis, and vasculitis, which all can cause seizures.

Adults aged 40 to 60 years most often develop seizures because of a structural lesion, such as a primary or metastatic brain tumor. By contrast, older people are more likely to have a stroke rather than a tumor. In young adults with AIDS, the cause is most likely cerebral toxoplasmosis. The patient's geography also suggests the cause. For example, in South and Central America, cerebral cysticercosis is the most common cause of

seizures. In the Indian subcontinent, tuberculomas are one of the most common causes.

PARTIAL COMPLEX SEIZURES

Partial complex seizures most often begin in late childhood or early adulthood. Affecting about 65% of epilepsy patients, they are the most common seizure variety. Psychiatry consultations are often solicited for epilepsy patients because of partial complex seizures' variable and often ambiguous ictal manifestations, postictal and interictal symptoms, and frequent comorbid conditions, including depression, cognitive impairment, and psychogenic seizures. Psychiatrists may also be asked about appropriate psychotropics for the psychiatric comorbidities because antidepressants and antipsychotics have potential adverse reactions in epilepsy patients.

Continuous EEG-video monitoring studies have defined ictal and postictal manifestations and separated them from psychogenic seizures and other nonepileptic disturbances. Epidemiologic studies indicate that, within broad ranges, cognitive impairment, depression, and other psychiatric conditions are routinely comorbid with epilepsy.

Before discussing partial complex seizures, a preliminary note on nomenclature will clarify the topic. Older literature applied less accurate titles, such as *psychomotor seizures* and *temporal lobe seizures* or *temporal lobe epilepsy* (*TLE*). However, the term "psychomotor seizures" is properly applied only to rare partial complex seizures with exclusively behavioral abnormalities. Likewise, the term TLE is not entirely appropriate because the seizure focus in about 10% of cases is not located in the temporal lobe but in the frontal lobe or other extratemporal region (see later, Frontal Lobe Seizures). Finally, TLE is inconsistent with the current classification of seizures according to symptoms rather than anatomic origin.

Etiology

Mesial temporal sclerosis, probably the most common cause of partial complex seizures, is characterized by sclerosis of the hippocampus and atrophy of the temporal lobe. Although anoxia, other perinatal insult, and prolonged febrile seizures—but not occasional febrile seizures—might lead to most cases of mesial temporal sclerosis, recent research suggests that trauma and infections with herpesvirus or prions may have caused some cases. Other lesions that cause partial complex seizures include temporal lobe hamartomas, astrocytomas, and those that cause partial elementary seizures (see above).

Except in about 10% of cases (see later, Frontal Lobe Seizures), the responsible lesion is within the temporal lobe. Menses, intercurrent illness, or low AED serum concentration may precipitate partial complex as well as other varieties of seizures. For example, up to 80% of women with epilepsy report an increase in seizure frequency around their menses.

Ictal Symptoms

Symptoms of partial complex seizures in 20% to 80% of patients include a characteristic premonitory sensation, called an *aura*. Not merely a warning, it constitutes the first portion of the seizure.

During most of a partial complex seizure, patients usually display a blank stare and are inattentive and uncommunicative. They always—by definition—have impaired consciousness. In most cases, they also have partial or complete memory loss, called *amnesia*, presumably because the limbic system in the temporal lobe is beset with seizure discharges. The amnesia is so striking that it may seem to be a patient's only symptom. (Partial complex seizures, therefore, must be strongly considered among the neurologic causes of the *acute amnestic syndrome* [see Table 7-1].)

Physical manifestations of partial complex seizures consist of only simple, repetitive, purposeless movements (*automatisms*) of the face and hands. Present in about 80% of partial complex seizures originating in the temporal lobe, common automatisms include repetitive swallowing, kissing, lip smacking, fumbling with clothing, scratching, and rubbing the abdomen (Fig. 10-9). Other physical manifestations are simple actions, such as standing, walking, pacing, or even driving; however, sometimes these actions are simply ingrained tasks that continue despite the seizure. In

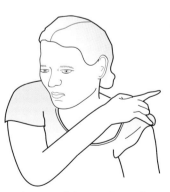

FIGURE 10-9 ■ During partial complex seizures, patients are typically dazed. They perform rudimentary, purposeless actions, such as pulling on their clothing, paying little or no attention. Their hands and fingers move in clumsy and misdirected patterns. Repetitive, simple body movements, *automatisms*, such as lip smacking, occur in approximately 80% of cases with a temporal lobe focus.

addition, more than 25% of patients utter brief phrases or unintelligible sounds.

Many times the environment triggers actions and words. For example, a child may clutch and continually stroke a nearby stuffed animal while repeating an endearing phrase. Impaired consciousness, apparent self-absorption, and subsequent failure to recall the event would distinguish this activity from normal behavior.

Partial complex seizures occasionally cause elaborate visual or auditory hallucinations accompanied by appropriate emotions. Although often dramatic, these symptoms are rare.

Physicians should maintain skepticism regarding nonspecific "experiential phenomena"—*déjà vu* (French, previously seen or experienced), *jamais vu* (French, never seen or experienced), dream-like states, mind-body dissociations, and floating feelings. Having crept into the popular vocabulary, these terms have lost most of their diagnostic value. Moreover, reliable symptoms and signs and EEG findings rarely corroborate their relationship to seizures.

Another frequently encountered symptom with a dubious association with partial complex seizures is the *rising epigastric sensation*. It consists of a sensation of swelling in the abdomen that, as if progressing upward within the chest, turns into tightness of the throat and then a sensation of suffocation. Although it could be an aura, the rising epigastric sensation may also represent a panic attack or *globus hystericus*, a common psychogenic disturbance in which people feel a similar tightening of the throat and an inability to breathe. Likewise, when seizures originate in the amygdala, they are said to cause overwhelming fear as the primary or only symptom. However, the medical literature does not support the notion that pronounced fear, as an isolated sensation, is a seizure manifestation. More likely, it would represent a panic attack.

Many partial complex seizures, like simple partial seizures, intermittently undergo secondary generalization. In *partial status epilepticus*, seizures are prolonged or recur in quick succession. In *nonconvulsive status epilepticus*, patients demonstrate hours of neuropsychologic aberrations, such as thought disorder, language impairment, or change in sensorium, accompanied only by automatisms. Their behavior may be so bizarre that the condition merits the label *ictal psychosis*.

Sex, Violence, and Aggression

During seizures, patients sometimes fumble with buttons, tug at their clothing, scratch their perineum, or make rudimentary masturbatory movements. They may even seem to undress partially. However, these patients are not exposing themselves or attempting to engage in sex. Except for very rare instances, seizures are unaccompanied by erotic or interactive sexual behavior. On the other hand, most seizure-like symptoms that develop during sexual activity, such as hyperventilation, are simply manifestations of anxiety.

Continuous EEG-video monitoring has demonstrated that *ictal* violence, allowing for rare exceptions, consists only of random shoving, pushing, kicking, or verbal abuse, such as screaming. This behavior is fragmented, unsustained, and, most important, unaccompanied by rage or anger. Moreover, violence, which occurs in less than 0.1% of cases, is virtually never the sole manifestation of a partial complex or any other type of seizure.

A different form of violence associated with seizures, belligerence or *resistive violence,* occurs when patients fight restraints during their ictal or postictal period. Much more frequently occurring than ictal violence, it stems largely from patients' fighting off health care workers or family members who attempt to restrain them or give them injections.

Physicians must distinguish ictal violence, with its lack of aggression, from both criminal violence, which is characterized by aggression, and episodic dyscontrol syndrome (see later). To be considered aggression, behavior must be directed, have a conscious or unconscious rationale, and be accompanied by a consistent affect. Although aggression may consist only of threats or taking control, it often leads to deliberate personal and property damage.

During seizures, patients cannot engage in sequential activities, premeditated actions, or meaningful interactions with other people—the critical elements of criminal activity. They also lack the cognitive ability to operate mechanical devices. These limitations preclude violent crimes either in the midst of a seizure or as a manifestation of a seizure. Overall, most neurologists accept violence, but neither aggression nor criminal acts, as a rare manifestation of seizures.

Postictal Symptoms

Following an actual partial complex seizure, with an average duration of 2 to 3 minutes, patients characteristically experience confusion, clouding of the sensorium, disorientation, flat affect, and sleepiness; however, some patients experience postictal agitation leading to violence. Postictal confusion may be intensified in seizures involving the brain's language region that cause transient aphasia (see Chapter 8). Similarly, if the seizure focus includes the cortical areas involved with motor function, patients may have a Todd's hemiparesis. For 15 to 30 minutes after the seizure, approximately 40% of patients have an elevated serum prolactin concentration and some may also have focal postictal EEG depression.

Astute physicians are unlikely to mistake partial complex seizures for psychotic episodes. Partial complex seizures last only a few minutes, consist of stereotyped symptoms, necessarily include impaired consciousness, and have postictal manifestations characterized by sleepiness, amnesia, behavioral withdrawal, and dulled thinking. After a seizure, patients gradually return to their interictal personality, which admittedly might be abnormal. In contrast, psychotic episodes, which are frequently triggered by factors in the environment, typically last at least several days. Their manifestations vary greatly and often include hypervigilance. Finally, neither sleepiness nor amnesia follows the episode.

Frontal Lobe Seizures

Frontal lobe seizures, named for the region of the brain where they originate, constitute a distinct, important variety of partial complex seizures. Compared to typical partial complex seizures, their manifestations more often consist of abrupt, aura-less onset of vocalizations, bilateral complex movements, relatively short duration (less than 1 minute), and little or no postictal confusion. In addition, frontal lobe seizures tend to begin in the adult years, occur relatively frequently (several times a month), develop predominantly during sleep, and produce discharges difficult to detect by conventional EEG.

With their manifestations so bizarre and paroxysmal changes so rarely detectable on a routine EEG, frontal lobe seizures mimic psychogenic seizures. Also, when they begin exclusively during sleep, frontal lobe seizures mimic sleep disorders (see Chapter 17).

Comorbid Conditions and Their Treatment

Depression

Depression is the most common comorbid condition in epilepsy. It is even more common in epilepsy than in other chronic illnesses, including asthma and diabetes. Its prevalence in epilepsy patients ranges between approximately 7.5% and, in intractable seizure patients, 55%. Given those prevalence rates, many authors assert that physicians underdiagnose and undertreat depression in epilepsy patients.

Risk factors for depression include partial complex seizures, onset of epilepsy in late adult years, and, in most studies, frequent seizures. Also, some studies associate depression with a failure of partial seizures to undergo secondary generalization—as though experiencing a generalized seizure ameliorates underlying depression. Once depression complicates epilepsy, seizure frequency increases. For example, depression-associated behavior, such as sleep deprivation, noncompliance with an AED regimen, or substance abuse, precipitates seizures. Depressed patients may also consciously or unconsciously superimpose psychogenic seizures on epileptic ones. Additionally, depressed epilepsy patients are more likely to require hospitalization than patients suffering from depression alone. Moreover, depression worsens patients' quality of life and acts as one of several risk factors for suicide (see later). On the other hand, current studies no longer find that a long history of epilepsy or the laterality of the seizure focus to be powerful risk factors for depression in epilepsy.

Physicians should direct initial therapy of depression comorbid with epilepsy not toward depression but toward better seizure control. Seizure control will probably improve patients' mood, reduce behavioral disturbances, and restore some cognitive function. Fortunately, certain AEDs, such as carbamazepine (which bears a structural similarity to TCAs), lamotrigine, and valproate, raise serotonin levels and possess both anticonvulsant and mood-stabilizing properties.

Physicians should add antidepressants as standard practices indicate; however, their use carries several caveats. Although antidepressants improve patients' mood, they may not reduce the frequency of their seizures. Another potential problem is that many AEDs and other psychotropic medicines act as substrates, inhibitors, or inducers of cytochrome P450. The addition of a psychotropic drug renders certain AEDs ineffective or toxic. For example, adding an enzyme-inhibiting antidepressant, such as fluoxetine, to carbamazepine or phenytoin, leads to toxic levels of the AED. Even some apparently benign, readily available substances may alter AED serum concentrations. For example, grapefruit juice can increase concentrations of carbamazepine and zonisamide, and St. John's wort can decrease their concentrations.

Most important, antidepressants, perhaps more than any other class of medication, tend to cause seizures. They even cause seizures in patients with no history of epilepsy. In general, risk factors for psychotropic-induced seizures include a history of epilepsy; other neurologic disorders, including Alzheimer's disease and traumatic brain injury; prior ECT; and drug or alcohol abuse.

The most common situation in which psychotropic-induced seizures occur is with overdose. TCAs lead to seizures in approximately 5% to 25% of overdose cases, and the incidence following overdose of amoxapine and maprotiline is even greater. Overdose-induced seizures most often appear within 3 to 6 hours, but almost never after 24 hours.

With routine antidepressant treatment, the risk of seizures is dose-dependent. Seizures most often occur during the first week of treatment, following sudden large elevations in dose, or with regimens involving multiple medicines. Still, the incidence of seizures with TCAs at a dose of 200 mg daily or with bupropion at up to 400 mg daily is less than 1%; however, with higher doses, the incidence rises to unacceptable levels. In an exception, clomipramine led to seizures in 1.5% of patients taking 300 mg or less per day. This relatively high rate represents clomipramine's most significant adverse reaction. Moreover, this risk does not diminish over time, as is the case with most other antidepressants.

In contrast to the relatively high rates of seizures associated with tricyclic and heterocyclic antidepressants, monamine oxidase inhibitors, selective serotonin reuptake inhibitors (SSRIs), and other serotonin-nor-epinephrine reuptake inhibitors produce seizures in less than 0.3% of cases.

As an alternative to antidepressant medicines, ECT can help alleviate depression in epilepsy patients. Although prolonged seizures may unexpectedly follow ECT, that complication is rare and readily responds to AEDs. (On an historical note, ECT originated in neuropsychiatrists' observation that depressed epileptic patients' mood improved after a seizure. The first treatments consisted of inducing hypoglycemic seizures by injections of large amounts of insulin. Only later attempts used electricity.)

Even though most psychotropic medicines in epileptic patients are safe, some words of warning are necessary. Despite all precautions, adding a psychotropic medication will often cause an increased frequency of seizures. Physicians can reduce the risk by introducing psychotropics slowly, attempting to use low doses of a single medicine, checking potential drug-drug interactions, and monitoring serum concentrations of medicine.

If a patient taking a psychotropic medication were to develop a seizure, physicians must guard against reflexively blaming the psychotropic medicine. For example, a structural lesion, such as a brain tumor or subdural hematoma, or other neurologic condition might be the cause of both the seizure and symptoms of depression. Similarly, a seizure in depressed patients may result from a deliberate medicine overdose or failure to take prescribed AEDs. Finally, some seizure-like episodes may represent psychogenic disturbances.

Bipolar Disorder

Bipolar symptoms comorbid with epilepsy are uncommon, but more frequently occurring than in either the general population or individuals with other medical disorders. When developing in epilepsy patients, dependent childish behavior, fluctuating moods, and rapid cycling characterize mania. Also, patients postoperative for temporal lobectomy, particularly right-sided procedures, and those with preoperative bilateral EEG abnormalities may develop mania.

Anxiety

Various studies suggest that anxiety is comorbid with epilepsy in 20% to more than 60% of cases. Patients' reports and physicians' interpretation of the symptom may help explain the variations in frequency. For example, in the face of an impending seizure, many patients are reasonably fearful and may panic. Additionally, a seizure's aura may have anxiety-like components. In other cases, anxiety may be a manifestation of a generalized anxiety or panic disorder. Physicians may freely treat anxiety comorbid with epilepsy with benzodiazepines, as well as with antidepressants. Benzodiazepines have antiepileptic effects; however, their abrupt withdrawal may precipitate seizures that even lead to status epilepticus.

Psychosis

Periods of psychosis may appear during the postictal period, which encompasses the several days immediately after a seizure. In fact, psychosis follows as many as 7% of refractory partial complex seizures. A flurry of seizures—several in quick succession—is the greatest risk factor. Other risk factors include low intelligence and bilateral seizure foci. During episodes of psychosis, patients may become violent and suicidal. Recurrent episodes may lead to interictal psychosis and cognitive decline.

Unlike risk factors for depression, risk factors for psychosis—and several other interictal psychiatric disorders comorbid with epilepsy—are signs of brain damage, such as low intelligence; childhood onset of epilepsy; frequent seizures; multiple seizure types; seizures that require multiple AEDs; physical neurologic abnormalities; and anatomic abnormalities visualized by CT or MRI.

Interictal psychosis is akin, but not identical, to "schizophreniform psychosis," which is also known as "schizophrenia-like psychosis of epilepsy." This disorder generally arises when patients are about 30 years old and their epilepsy began in childhood, especially between 5 and 10 years of age. Its symptoms include hallucinations, paranoia, and social isolation. Unlike typical schizophrenic patients, seizure patients with schizophreniform psychosis retain a relatively normal affect, do not deteriorate, and do not have an increased incidence of schizophrenia in their families.

Epilepsy patients with psychosis also have neuropathologic, as well as clinical, signs of brain damage.

Their brains have large cerebral ventricles, periventricular gliosis, and focal damage. In an interesting comparison, multiple sclerosis (MS) patients, despite having equally extensive cerebral damage, rarely have schizophrenic symptoms.

Whether the thought disorder is termed interictal psychosis, schizophreniform psychosis, or schizophrenia-like psychosis of epilepsy, its clinical features are inconsistent and do not constitute a distinct psychiatric entity. In *Diagnostic and Statistical Manual of Mental Disorders, 4th Edition, Text Revision* (*DSM-IV-TR*), the psychosis associated with epilepsy—whether it occurs during, immediately afterward, or between seizures—might have to be included in the category of *Psychosis Due to a Medical Condition* (*Epilepsy*). In other words, the DSM-IV-TR does not specifically define intraictal, postictal, and interictal psychoses despite their frequency and psychiatric features.

A different condition, which neurologists sometimes call *forced normalization* ("alternative psychosis"), occurs when AEDs have suddenly controlled long-standing seizures and "forced" the EEG to be normal. Subjected to forced normalization, patients may develop either psychosis or depression. Some researchers propose that the seizures, although troublesome, had suppressed a thought or mood disorder. Although the details surrounding forced normalization remain controversial, physicians might closely monitor patients who rapidly achieve complete seizure control.

In the opposite scenario, *withdrawal-emergent psychopathology,* physicians who suddenly discontinue AEDs may produce or unmask psychiatric disorders—particularly anxiety or depression. In these patients the AEDs apparently suppressed a psychiatric disorder along with the epilepsy. Withdrawal-emergent psychopathology may also come into effect after neurosurgery has greatly reduced patients' seizure frequency and allows them to curtail their AED regimen, after which psychiatric disturbances emerge (see later).

In treating comorbid psychoses, many of the same rules apply as when prescribing antidepressants for comorbid depression. Most important, AEDs should remain the mainstay of treatment.

An overdose of an antipsychotic, just like an overdose of antidepressant, can lead to seizures. Among antipsychotics, an overdose of chlorpromazine is more likely than one of haloperidol, thioridazine, fluphenazine, or the newer atypical agents to cause seizures.

In therapeutic doses, antipsychotic-induced seizures are dose-dependent, occur with large increases in the dose, and develop more frequently in patients with epilepsy or underlying brain damage. In the therapeutic as well as the overdose range, chlorpromazine again remains most apt to provoke seizures. Except for clozapine, which leads to seizures in 4% of patients taking more than 600 mg daily, atypical antipsychotics carry a seizure risk of less than 1%. Physicians forced to restart an antipsychotic following a medication-induced seizure should, while excluding other causes of psychosis and seizures (previously discussed), reintroduce the same or different antipsychotic slowly and, after checking for potential adverse interactions, consider adding an AED.

Cognitive Impairment

Of individuals with either mental retardation or cerebral palsy, 10% to 20% have epilepsy (see Chapter 13). In them, epilepsy usually appears before age 5 years and its incidence increases in proportion to their physical and intellectual impairments, number of seizure types, and frequency of seizures. Of individuals institutionalized because of mental retardation, 40% have epilepsy.

When brain damage underlying seizures is progressive—as in tuberous sclerosis, storage diseases, and mitochondrial encephalopathies—seizure control, cognitive capacity, and motor function all decline. Conversely, progressive cognitive decline or increasingly refractory seizures suggest a progressive, rather than a congenital, static neurologic disorder. As with interictal psychosis, many risk factors for cognitive decline reflect underlying brain damage.

Partial complex seizures are closely associated with increasingly severe cognitive impairment in many patients. If epilepsy surgery or adjustment of AEDs in these patients prevents seizures, their cognitive decline may cease and partly reverse. However, if surgery does not arrest the seizures, the cognitive impairment may worsen at an increased rate. Moreover, unsuccessful surgery may lead to depression.

According to one explanation for the progressive cognitive impairment associated with partial complex seizures, the underlying mesial temporal sclerosis leads to damage of the surrounding limbic system. Another explanation, which pertains to all seizure types, and to children as well as adults, proposes that AEDs burden cognitive function. AED-induced cognitive impairment develops most often following rapid introduction, high doses, and an AED regimen with more than one medicine. Some AEDs, such as topiramate (in moderate to high doses), levetiracetam, and phenobarbital, can produce various neuropsychologic and behavioral disturbances, as well as cognitive dysfunction. When physicians prescribe AEDs for conditions other than epilepsy, such as migraines, neuropathic pain, or psychiatric disorders, neuropsychologic side effects develop less frequently because the AED dose is smaller, it is often the only psychoactive medicine, and patients do not have underlying cerebral disease. However, with rapid introduction, high dose, and polypharmacy, these side effects frequently develop.

Destructive Behavior

SUICIDE

Suicide occurs four to five times more frequently in epilepsy patients than in the general population. Among epilepsy patients, suicide occurs most frequently among those with partial complex seizures. Risk factors for suicide in epilepsy are psychotic disturbances, borderline personality disorder, and other interictal psychopathology, as well as risk factors present in the general population, such as depression, poor physical health, life stress, previous suicide attempts, and access to firearms. As in other neurologic illnesses, such as Huntington's disease, impaired judgment and poor impulse control, rather than deliberate planning, may prompt the suicide.

CRIME AND INTERICTAL VIOLENCE

The consensus among neurologists is that criminal violence cannot be a manifestation of a seizure. However, epilepsy, head trauma, and congenital or acquired brain injury lead to poor impulse control, lower socioeconomic status, and other conditions that steer people toward crime. Although the incidence of epilepsy is at least four times greater among men in prison than in the general population, crimes of epileptic prisoners are no more violent than those of nonepileptic ones. Moreover, the prevalence of epilepsy is the same in nonviolent criminals as violent ones. Also, EEG abnormalities do not correlate with violent offenses.

Interictal violence rather than ictal violence, which was discussed previously, usually consists of only verbal and minor physical acts. It tends to occur in epilepsy patients who are antisocial, schizophrenic, or mentally retarded. These patients show no differences, compared to nonviolent epilepsy patients, in the variety or frequency of seizures, EEG abnormalities, or AED treatment.

Personality Traits

Classic studies described "temporal lobe epilepsy" patients as distinctively circumstantial in thinking, hyposexual, humorless, "sticky" in interpersonal relations, and overly concerned with general philosophic and religious questions. These patients often wrote excessively and compulsively (hypergraphia). Supporting studies suggested that the presence of these abnormal traits depended on whether the seizure focus was in the right or left temporal lobe. Right-sided foci supposedly predisposed patients to anger, sadness, and elation, but left-sided ones to ruminative and intellectual tendencies.

Recent studies, based on continuous EEG-video monitoring and strict methodology, have either not corroborated the presence of those personality traits or found them in as few as 7% partial complex seizure patients. In fact, the same traits were found in patients without epilepsy. For example, hypergraphia can be a symptom of schizophrenia or bipolar disorder. The studies also found no difference in personality traits when foci are in different temporal lobes or even other brain areas and no difference in personality traits among patients with different varieties of epilepsy. As a general rule, personality changes and cognitive impairment in epilepsy patients may serve as clinical markers of brain damage.

In view of the underlying brain damage, previous editions of the *Diagnostic and Statistical Manual of Mental Disorders* classified personality changes associated with epilepsy under the rubric "organic personality disorder." The current edition, DSM-IV-TR, classifies them—in equally broad terms—as *Personality Disorder NOS* or a *Personality Change Due to a General Medical Condition.*

Delirium

Epilepsy patients may present with disorientation, amnesia, and possibly aphasia. Occasionally they act in an irrational, agitated, and belligerent manner. Most often such patients are simply in a delirium from a prolonged postictal period.

Another common cause of delirium in epilepsy patients is AED intoxication. In particular, the addition of a psychotropic, a second AED, or any other medication that alters the metabolism often leads to toxic increases in serum AED concentrations. For example, adding lamotrigine to valproate (valproic acid/divalproex) increases valproate concentrations, possibly to toxic levels. The addition of a psychotropic to an AED regimen, depending on the particular combination, might create the same adverse effect. Occasionally patients deliberately or inadvertently cause AED intoxication by self-administering excessive quantities of their medicines or mixing them with alcohol.

Partial complex or absence status epilepticus, especially nonconvulsive status epilepticus, may present with delirium. Because those seizure varieties may cause mental changes without overt physical abnormalities, a diagnosis based solely on clinical grounds without a corroborating EEG is unreliable.

When seizures lead to head trauma, patients may sustain traumatic brain injury, including intracranial bleeding and subdural hematomas, that lead to acutely or permanently altered mental states. Even without serious injury, repeated minor head injuries cause memory impairment, other symptoms of the postconcussion syndrome (see Chapter 22), and behavioral disturbances.

Testing During and After Partial Complex Seizures

EEG

During a partial complex seizure, the EEG most often shows paroxysms of spikes, slow waves, or other abnormalities in channels overlying the temporal or frontotemporal region. Even though a seizure focus may be unilateral, bilateral EEG abnormalities may appear because of additional foci, interhemispheric projections, or "reflections." Nasopharyngeal and other specially placed leads may capture temporal lobe discharges that routine scalp electrodes fail to detect (Fig. 10-10).

In the interictal period, the routine EEG contains spikes or spike-and-wave complexes over the temporal lobes in about 40% of cases. When accompanied by an appropriate history, these EEG abnormalities are specific enough to corroborate the diagnosis. Looking at the situation in reverse, about 90% of persons with anterior temporal spikes on the EEG will have partial complex seizures. Nevertheless, diagnosis of seizures should not be based only on EEG spikes. Diagnosis of partial complex or other seizures requires correlation of EEG abnormalities with symptoms and signs.

If diagnosis remains a problem, especially where episodic behavioral abnormalities are believed to result from seizures, physicians should arrange for continuous EEG-video monitoring. EEG corroboration of partial complex seizures might begin with a routine EEG, but it has only a 40% yield. Although EEGs performed during sleep and wakefulness or following sleep deprivation might offer a greater yield, EEG-video monitoring offers virtually a 100% yield.

Other Tests

Because partial elementary and partial complex seizures usually originate from structural lesions, neurologists routinely order MRIs unless patients have a

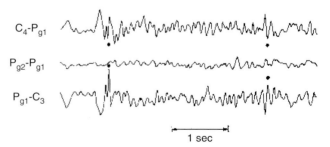

FIGURE 10-10 ■ An interictal EEG with nasopharyngeal electrodes (P_{g1} and P_{g2}) shows phase-reversed spikes that routine scalp electrodes may not detect.

contraindication (see Chapter 20). With even greater resolution than CT and freedom from artifacts produced by the bones surrounding the middle fossa, MRI reveals mesial temporal lobe sclerosis, tuberous sclerosis nodules, small strokes, and cryptic AVMs, as well as overt lesions (see Fig. 20-26). (MRI with thin cuts through the temporal lobes is often required to detect mesial temporal lobe sclerosis.) Neurologists also order MRI for tonic-clonic seizures because clinical and EEG data may not distinguish primary generalized seizures from partial seizures with secondary generalization. With drug- or alcohol-withdrawal seizures and absences (see later), these scans may add little or no information.

Positron emission tomography (PET), which illustrates cerebral metabolism, facilitates surgery in epilepsy patients with partial complex seizures. During the interictal period, PET shows hypometabolism in a region far larger than the focus indicated by MRI. Because of technical requirements, obtaining PET during the seizure remains difficult. Moreover, its relatively low resolution does not permit a precise localization.

Magnetoencephalography (MEG) diagrams magnetic fields of the brain. Coupled with the EEG, MEG can merge electrophysiologic data and magnetic images. MEG by itself does not yet substantially assist in the diagnosis of epilepsy or other illness.

TREATMENT

AEDs

Neurologists routinely prescribe AEDs—rather than hypnosis, nutrition therapy, or lifestyle changes, for example—as the primary treatment for epilepsy (Table 10-3). With numerous medicines and relatively few direct comparison studies, clinical experience provides only several reliable guidelines. Treatment with AED monotherapy is preferable to AED polypharmacy. Monotherapy minimizes side effects, noncompliance, and cost. Although neurologists occasionally attempt AED polypharmacy, only a minority of patients benefits from the addition of a second AED, and less than 5% benefit from the addition of a third. Neurologists refrain from routinely instituting AED therapy following a first idiopathic seizure, which itself does not constitute epilepsy. Except for status epilepticus or other emergency situation, neurologists slowly initiate AED therapy. Finally, AEDs within a category appropriate for the seizure variety often have similar effectiveness but differ substantially in their potential side effects.

Because the liver metabolizes many AEDs, these drugs may alter the metabolism of various psychotropics and each other. For example, many AEDs may reduce the serum concentration and thus lower the effectiveness of haloperidol, clozapine, methadone, and oral contraceptives. Similarly, beginning phenytoin or carbamazepine—either as an AED or mood stabilizer—in a patient enrolled in a methadone program may bring on narcotic withdrawal. In this case, physicians might first increase the daily methadone dose. Moreover, several AEDs, including phenytoin, carbamazepine, and phenobarbital, induce enzymes that may so greatly increase metabolism of contraceptives that even women conscientiously taking them may conceive. As an added danger, the fetus will then be exposed to their potential teratogenic effects.

Paradoxically, even AEDs can cause seizures. For example, carbamazepine and oxcarbazepine may induce hyponatremia severe enough to cause seizures.

TABLE 10-3 ■ Commonly Used AEDs		
AED	**Usual Daily Dose (mg)**	**Therapeutic Serum Concentration (μ/mL)***
Carbamazepine (Tegretol) ^	600–1200	5–12
Divalproex (Depakote)	1500–2000	50–100
Ethosuximide (Zarontin)	2000	40–100
Gabapentin (Neurontin)	900–1800	
Lamotrigine (Lamictal)	100–500	
Phenytoin (Dilantin)	300–400	10–20
Topiramate (Topamax)	400	

AEDs, antiepileptic drugs.

*Recommended concentrations vary and should be altered depending on the clinical situation. Often a "subtherapeutic level" is sufficient, and increasing the dose will create side effects without improving seizure control.

^To reach a steady state, five "half-lives" are required (e.g., carbamazepine 4–6 days, phenytoin 5–10 days, and valproate 3–6 days).

These AEDs have mostly replaced phenobarbital and its closely related AED, primidone (Mysoline), which both cause sedation, cognitive impairment, and depression. Also, barbiturates, particularly when used in children and adults with brain damage, may produce a "paradoxical reaction" of excitement and hyperactivity rather than sedation. On the other hand, most children with epilepsy and comorbid hyperactivity may safely use stimulants.

Mental Side Effects

In general, excessive concentrations of AEDs cause cognitive impairment, confusion, lethargy, and, at very high serum concentrations, stupor. Cognitive impairment typically consists of memory difficulties, intellectual dulling, and inattention. AEDs can have this effect both on individuals coping with neurologic deficits as well as on psychiatric patients.

Cognitive impairment from AEDs may result from polypharmacy, excessive medication concentration, rapid introduction of the medication, or use of phenobarbital or primidone. Impairment from phenytoin is partly attributable to slowed motor activity that impairs performance on timed psychologic tests. Phenytoin, carbamazepine, and valproate—the older AEDs—do not otherwise differ in the incidence or type of cognitive impairment they cause. Preliminary information on the newer AEDs indicates that gabapentin and lamotrigine produce only minimal impairments, but that topiramate may initially impair attention and word fluency.

AEDs may also produce severely disordered thinking and personality changes that may rise to the level of psychosis. The primary example, although rare, is forced normalization (see previous). AED-induced behavioral changes are most apt to develop in individuals with a history of epilepsy that had an early onset, secondarily generalized seizures, and EEGs showing bilateral changes and those with a history of psychosis or affective disorder.

Physical Side Effects

As with other classes of medications, AEDs generally tend to cause a group of side effects and individual ones potentially cause additional ones. For example, even at therapeutic levels, most AEDs can cause liver abnormalities and bone marrow suppression.

Recent work has discovered that several AEDs enhance age-related osteoporosis and leave epilepsy patients with increased vulnerability to hip fractures from falls. Women older than 65 years, individuals confined to wheelchairs or bed, and those receiving little sunlight are particularly susceptible. AEDs associated with decreased bone density include carbamazepine, phenytoin, phenobarbital, which all induce cytochrome P450 enzymes, and valproate, which does not. Prescribing many AEDs often involves checking patients' bone density scans, as well as their white blood count, liver function tests, and serum AED concentration.

As mentioned previously, individual AEDs may have drug-specific side effects. For example, valproate increases patients' weight, lamotrigine and levetiracetam are weight-neutral, and topiramate and zonisamide reduce weight—although not to the degree and safety to be considered part of a weight loss program.

Phenytoin intoxication causes a well-known constellation of nystagmus, ataxia, and dysarthria. Many times AEDs induce a benign rash, but occasionally and unpredictably they may cause a fulminant, potentially fatal mucocutaneous allergic reaction, the *Stevens-Johnson syndrome* (erythema multiforme). This condition, which begins as a rash, consists of blisters on the mouth, eyes, and skin that are often weeping and confluent. The disrupted skin and mucus membranes leak serum, fluid, and electrolytes and allow bacteria to invade the blood stream.

AEDs and Pregnancy

Apart from the possibility of fetal exposure to AEDs, epilepsy itself carries a considerable teratogenic risk. For mothers with epilepsy, the rate of fetal malformations—exclusive of AED-induced malformations—is 4% to 8%. In comparison, the rate for nonepileptic mothers is lower—2% to 4%—but still substantial. If only the father has epilepsy, there remains an increased but lesser teratogenic risk.

Fetal exposure to AEDs increases the rate of malformations, some of which are devastating. Most AEDs cross the placenta. The malformation rate is increased if the mother takes an AED during the first trimester, requires AED polypharmacy, or has a low serum folate level. No AED is risk-free, and none exclusively induces a particular malformation. The Food and Drug Administration (FDA) has classified carbamazepine and valproate as Category D ("dangerous") and lamotrigine, levetiracetam, oxcarbazepine, and topiramate as a somewhat safer Category C ("caution").

Malformations associated with AEDs are probably induced during the first trimester when organs, particularly the central nervous system (CNS), are forming. The most serious—*meningomyelocele* and other *neural tube defects* (see Chapter 13)—have been closely, but not exclusively, associated with both carbamazepine (0.5%) and valproate (1%). In addition, AEDs increase the rate of cleft lip, cleft palate, and ventricular septal defect.

Less severe fetal malformations are likewise not exclusively associated with any specific AED. In particular, the *fetal hydantoin* (phenytoin) *syndrome*, which includes craniofacial abnormalities and limb defects, is not peculiar to prenatal phenytoin therapy.

Notwithstanding the risks associated with taking AEDs during pregnancy, having generalized tonic-clonic seizures from undertreatment also poses a substantial threat to the mother and fetus. For example, seizures increase the risks of obstetric complications.

Several strategies may reduce AEDs' teratogenic potential. Physicians should review both prospective parents' family histories for congenital malformations, epilepsy, and other neurologic problems. In addition, physicians ideally should taper if not discontinue AEDs from before conception through at least the first trimester. If patients must continue an AED, they should take just one (achieve monotherapy) and that one should not be valproate, carbamazepine, or phenobarbital. Because serum AED concentrations tend to fall during pregnancy, physicians should frequently check blood levels.

Neonatologists, neurologists, and psychiatrists should be mindful that many AEDs cross into breast milk. Ethosuximide, lamotrigine, phenobarbital, and topiramate concentrations may reach therapeutic levels in breast-feeding neonates. However, aside from sleepiness, symptoms of toxicity rarely develop. In contrast, carbamazepine, phenytoin, and valproate are relatively safe in the postpartum period. An important consequence of transplacental transfer of medications occurs when pregnant women taking phenobarbital or opioids, including methadone, induce dependance in the fetus. During the first several postpartum days, unless neonatologists replace these medicines, the fetus may experience withdrawal symptoms including seizures.

In addition, women—whether or not they are taking AEDs—should take folic acid or folate before conception and throughout the pregnancy, particularly to reduce the risk of neural tube defects. Physicians should avoid prescribing carbamazepine and valproate during this period because of their association with neural tube defects. Once pregnant, women should undergo a serum α-fetoprotein determination, an ultrasound examination, and possibly other obstetrical tests to detect fetal neural tube defects.

Another potential problem is that some AEDs (including phenobarbital, primidone, phenytoin, and carbamazepine) produce a deficiency in vitamin K-dependent clotting factors. Because the resulting anticoagulant effect may lead to intracerebral hemorrhage, obstetricians administer vitamin K.

AEDs may also induce CNS abnormalities later in life. For example, phenytoin therapy initiated before puberty may retard normal cerebellar growth. Through their effect on the hepatic cytochrome P450 oxidases, AEDs may also increase or decrease serum concentration of other medications with wide-ranging unintended consequences. For example, carbamazepine, phenytoin, and phenobarbital induce P450 enzymes, valproate inhibits them, and gabapentin and several other newer AEDs have little or no effect. Finally, carbamazepine, phenytoin, topiramate, and oxcarbazepine elevate the serum homocysteine level, which is a risk factor for strokes and heart attacks.

Vagus Nerve Stimulation

Vagus nerve stimulation (VNS), a new technique for reducing refractory seizures, consists of an implanted pacemaker-like device that stimulates the segment of the vagus nerve (cranial nerve X) in the neck. The vagus nerve seems the most appropriate conduit to the brain because it is readily accessible in its cervical portion, contains almost entirely afferent fibers but few pain-conveying ones, and has, on the left side, few efferent cardiac fibers.

The VNS device sends electric impulses regularly, such as for 30 seconds every 5 minutes, and also when the patient senses an aura and activates it. The impulses ascend along the vagus nerve's afferent fibers to synapse in the medulla's nucleus solitarius, which projects to the cortex, hypothalamus, and limbic system (see Chapter 4).

VNS helps suppress generalized and partial seizures in children and adults. Over 5 years, it reduces the mean seizure frequency by about 30%. In addition, it decreases AED requirements. For seizures with bilateral foci, VNS has almost completely replaced commissurotomy (see later); however, for seizures emanating from a single focus, surgical resection remains more effective.

In addition to suppressing seizures, VNS reduces depression and anxiety comorbid with epilepsy. It even improves the mood of depressed patients without epilepsy. Despite its benefits, VNS causes an expectable side effect: Its electrical stimulation briefly impairs the vagus nerve's function causing hoarseness and dyspnea.

Surgery

Under the appropriate circumstances, surgical removal of a seizure focus, with or without a surrounding portion of the brain, has risen to the level of a standard treatment. Although many patients who undergo temporal lobectomy must continue taking an AED, approximately two thirds enjoy almost a complete cessation of seizures and many of the others enjoy a significant reduction.

If only by reducing the need for multiple or high doses of AEDs, surgery also often improves cognitive function. Furthermore, most depressed patients experience an improvement in their mood. Even those who have suffered from refractory epilepsy enjoy a lessening, if not almost a complete resolution, of depression and anxiety. Overall, most patients eventually enjoy a general improvement in quality of life.

With proper preoperative planning, surgeons can remove large areas of the temporal lobe without producing either language or memory impairment. Even with extensive resections, the surgical morbidity and mortality remain very low.

If three trials of appropriate AEDs at therapeutic doses fail to suppress seizures, neurologists consider epilepsy to be "refractory." Children, adolescents, and adults who suffer from refractory epilepsy become candidates for surgery. For many epilepsy patients with partial complex seizures, surgery holds many advantages over prolonged AED therapy even if it suppresses seizures.

In addition to refractory seizures or AED intolerance, surgical candidates should have a single frontal or temporal lobe lesion that is clearly identifiable on clinical, EEG, and radiographic testing. They often must also undergo a Wada test, functional MRI, or similar testing (see Chapter 8) to determine if surgery, which entails removal of a portion of the temporal lobe, would lead to aphasia, amnesia, or other neuropsychologic problems. If both temporal lobes were injured from birth or during surgery, patients may suffer permanent amnesia or the Klüver-Bucy syndrome (see Chapters 12 and 16).

Despite the substantial benefits of epilepsy surgery, patients and physicians should anticipate several potential postoperative issues. Improvements may require many years to become evident. Additionally, surgery provides little benefit for psychosis. In fact, many patients experience postoperative psychiatric complications, including personality changes, depression, and mania during the first two postoperative months. In addition, psychosis sometimes emerges, but usually only if seizures recur. The depression is long-lasting in about 10% of patients. Also, if surgery fails to control seizures, behavioral and cognitive capacity may actually deteriorate more rapidly than if patients had not undergone surgery.

Even if surgery eliminates seizures, postoperative psychiatric disorders may prevent patients from returning to their preoperative life. These disorders may originate in the surgery unmasking a psychiatric disorder, reduction in AEDs that had been suppressing psychiatric symptoms as well as seizures, or, akin to AED-induced forced normalization, sudden surgery-induced complete seizure control.

A different and more invasive procedure may rarely be indicated in individuals with intractable bilateral frontal seizures or infants with atonic seizures ("drop attacks"). In a *commissurotomy* or *corpus callosotomy,* a neurosurgeon longitudinally severs the anterior two-thirds or entire corpus callosum, interrupting the spread of discharges between cerebral hemispheres. Because the procedure "splits" apart the cerebral hemispheres, it may cause the *split-brain syndrome* (see Fig. 8-9).

Rolandic Epilepsy

Rolandic epilepsy (childhood epilepsy with centrotemporal spikes), the most common form of partial epilepsy in childhood, almost always begins between ages 5 and 9 years, occurs predominantly in boys, and remits by puberty. The seizures consist of unilateral paresthesias, movements of the face, and speech arrest. They tend to undergo secondary generalization during sleep. Interictal EEG changes consist of high voltage spikes in the central temporal region (Rolandic spikes) during sleep. AEDs readily suppress the seizures.

Unlike other partial epilepsies, Rolandic seizures are restricted to childhood, not associated with an underlying structural lesion, and inherited (in an autosomal dominant pattern). In contrast to children with absences (see later), those with Rolandic epilepsy are not at risk of eventually developing other varieties of epilepsy.

GENERALIZED SEIZURES

Immediate loss of consciousness accompanied by bilateral, symmetric, synchronous, paroxysmal EEG discharges characterizes generalized seizures. These seizures may result from either an autosomal dominant genetic disorder, a physiologic disturbance, or a metabolic aberration, including drug and alcohol withdrawal. In contrast to partial seizures, generalized seizures lack an aura, lateralized motor or sensory disturbances, and focal EEG abnormalities. Also, generalized seizures, as opposed to secondary generalized seizures, almost never result from brain tumors, cerebral infarctions, or other structural lesions. Most generalized seizures are of either the absence (previously called *petit mal*) or tonic-clonic (*grand mal*) variety.

Absences

Absences usually begin between ages 4 and 10 years and disappear in early adulthood. The seizures, which may occur many times daily, consist of 2- to 10-second lapses in attention accompanied by automatisms, subtle clonic limb movements, or blinking (Fig. 10-11). The blinking sometimes occurs rhythmically at 3 Hz, which is the frequency of the associated EEG abnormality. During the seizure, children maintain muscle tone and bladder control. However, they cannot carry on mental and physical activities. With frequent seizures, they may appear inattentive, dull, or even mentally retarded. After a seizure, as though it had never occurred, children have no retrograde amnesia, confusion, agitation, or sleepiness.

Absence status epilepticus can sometimes lead to a several-hour episode of apathy, psychomotor retardation, and confusion. Such an attack usually develops in children or young adults with a history of absences or other seizures who suddenly stopped taking their AEDs. Absence status epilepticus in any age group mimics acute psychosis. If an EEG confirms a clinical diagnosis of absence status epilepticus, intravenous benzodiazepine will abort an attack.

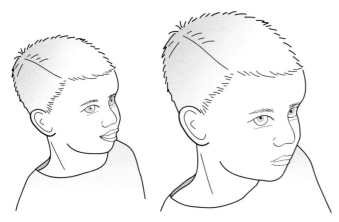

FIGURE 10-11 ■ In the midst of an absence, which lasts for only 2 to 10 seconds, this 8-year-old boy has a staring spell that suddenly and unexpectedly interrupts his discussion with a friend. He becomes glassy-eyed and mute, his eyes roll upward, and he blinks at 3 Hz. Although he loses consciousness, he maintains bodily tone and does not become incontinent. At the end of his seizure, he resumes talking and is unaware that he sustained one.

EEG, Etiology, and Treatment

During an absence, the EEG shows synchronous 3-Hz spike-and-wave complexes in all channels (Fig. 10-12). Even in the interictal period, an EEG reveals occasional asymptomatic bursts of 3 Hz spike-and-wave complexes lasting 1 to 1.5 seconds. This pattern reflects an underlying abnormality in the reciprocal circuits between the thalamus and the cerebral cortex.

In patients with absences, either hyperventilation or photic stimulation can precipitate the characteristic clinical and EEG abnormalities. Just as the EEG abnormality reflects generalized cerebral dysfunction, PET scans performed during absences show increased metabolism in the thalamus and the entire cortex.

Patients' relatives often also have absences or 3-Hz spike-and-wave complexes that can be precipitated by hyperventilation. This finding supports the hypothesis that patients inherit a predisposition in an autosomal dominant pattern. In contrast to tonic-clonic seizures, absences are not associated with drug withdrawal, metabolic aberrations, or structural lesions. Therefore, as a general rule, CTs and MRIs are not indicated.

Neurologists treat absences with ethosuximide, valproate, or occasionally clonazepam, but most children readily respond to ethosuximide. About two thirds of children enjoy a permanent remission during adolescence. In them, AEDs can be discontinued. In other children, tonic-clonic or other generalized seizures develop as a replacement for or in conjunction with the absences.

FIGURE 10-12 ■ Absences are often so brief and liable to be confused with either inattention or partial complex seizures that neurologists often attempt to precipitate them for diagnostic purposes in an EEG laboratory. One common practice consists of asking a child suspected of having absences to count numbers slowly while hyperventilating. An absence would be evident when the counting pauses and the EEG shows regular, symmetric, and synchronous 3-Hz spike-and-wave complexes arising from and returning to a normal EEG background—as in this reproduction.

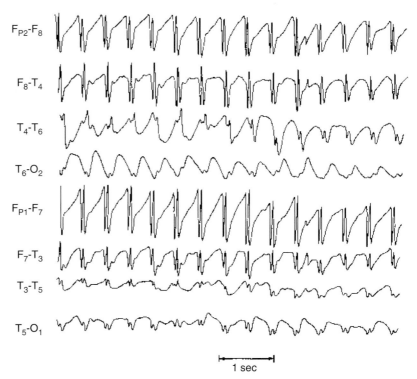

1 sec

TABLE 10-4 ■ Comparison of Partial Complex and Absence Seizures

Feature	Partial Complex	Absence
Aura	Often	Never
Consciousness	Impaired	Lost at onset
Movements	Usually simple, repetitive but may include complex activity	Blinking and facial and finger automatisms
Postictal behavior	Amnesia, confusion, and tendency to sleep	No abnormality, except amnesia for ictus
Frequency	1 to 2 per week	Several daily
Duration	2 to 3 minutes	1 to 10 seconds
Precipitants		Hyperventilation, photic stimulation
EEG	Spikes and polyspike and waves, usually over both temporal regions	Generalized 3-Hz spike-and-wave complexes
AEDs	Carbamazepine, phenytoin	Ethosuximide, valproate

EEG, electroencephalogram; AEDs, antiepileptic drugs.

Although absences bear a superficial resemblance to partial complex seizures, physicians should distinguish the two conditions. They have different manifestations, EEG abnormalities, and treatment (Table 10-4).

Tonic-Clonic Seizures

Unlike absences, tonic-clonic seizures begin at any age after infancy, persist into adulthood, and cause massive motor activity and profound postictal residua. Although patients may have a prodrome of malaise or a depressed mood, tonic-clonic seizures are usually an unheralded explosion. In the initial tonic phase, patients lose consciousness, roll their eyes upward, and extend their neck, trunk, and limbs, as if to form an arch. Immediately afterward, in the dramatic clonic phase, patients violently and symmetrically jerk their limbs, neck, and trunk (Fig. 10-13).

A potential diagnostic problem is that during this terrible episode of tonic-clonic movement, a primary generalized seizure resembles a partial seizure that has undergone secondary generalization. Often only a detailed history, a trained observer, or an intraictal EEG can distinguish between them.

If electronic filters can eliminate the superimposed muscle EEG artifact during the tonic phase, the EEG shows repetitive, increasingly higher amplitude spikes occurring with increasing frequency in all channels. In the clonic phase, slow waves interrupt the spikes, which become less frequent (Fig. 10-14).

After the clonic phase, the EEG shows postictal depression. The postictal EEG is often the only one available, but it can confirm the diagnosis. Similarly, after ECT, the EEG is slow. After most tonic-clonic or ECT-induced seizures, as well as after approximately 40% of partial complex seizures, the serum prolactin level rises for 10 to 20 minutes. About 50% of patients with tonic-clonic seizures have interictal asymptomatic, brief bursts of spikes, polyspikes, or slow waves on the EEG. Photic stimulation or hyperventilation may precipitate seizures and accompanying EEG abnormalities.

Etiology

Many cases of tonic-clonic epilepsy result from an autosomal dominant trait expressed between the ages of 5 and 30 years. Patients often have a history of childhood absences. Various factors, such as sleep deprivation, can precipitate these seizures in susceptible individuals. Medical house officers who have worked all night are susceptible to tonic-clonic seizures during the next day.

Most seizures arising in sleep emerge during stage 2 of nonrapid eye movement (NREM) sleep (see Chapter 17). Rapid eye movement (REM) sleep, in contrast, remains relatively seizure-free. Some epileptic patients have seizures predominantly or exclusively during sleep, and many others experience them only on awakening. To avoid committing a diagnostic error, physicians should evaluate patients with exclusively sleep-related episodes for a sleep disorder masquerading as epilepsy (see later and Chapter 17).

Alcohol can precipitate seizures in cases of profound intoxication or alcohol-induced hypoglycemia. Abrupt withdrawal from chronic, excessive alcohol consumption produces alcohol-withdrawal seizures after about 1 to 3 days of abstinence. Although the clinical and EEG manifestations of these seizures resemble those of genetically determined seizures, their interictal EEG is normal.

A small group of children, adolescents, and some adults have *reflex epilepsy*—absences or tonic-clonic seizures in response to particular sensory stimulation. In its most common variety, *photosensitive* or *photoconvulsive epilepsy*, seizures are triggered by specific visual stimuli, such as discotheque strobe lights, television pictures that have lost their vertical stability, televised cartoons, or video games. Even stationary patterns of certain letters, words, or figures may trigger seizures. Likewise, particular musical passages may trigger seizures.

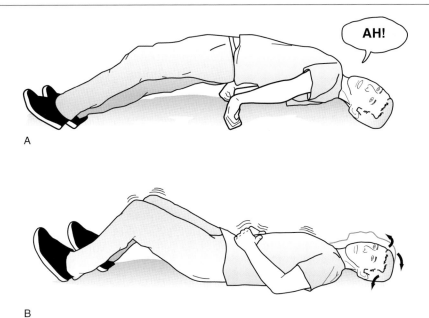

A

B

FIGURE 10-13 ■ *A,* This man in the tonic phase of a tonic-clonic seizure arches his torso and extends his arms and legs. He assumes this position because of the relatively greater strength of the extensor muscles compared to the flexor muscles. Simultaneous diaphragm, chest wall, and laryngeal muscle contractions force air through his tightened larynx to produce the shrill "epileptic cry." During this phase, he may also bite his tongue and lose control of his urine. *B,* In the clonic phase, the patient's head, neck, and legs contract symmetrically and forcefully for about 10 to 20 seconds. Saliva, which becomes aerated and often blood-tinged from tongue lacerations, froths from his mouth. His pupils dilate and he sweats profusely. Finally, his muscular contractions become progressively less frequent and weaker. The seizure usually ends with a sigh, followed by stertorous breathing. In the immediate postictal period, he remains unresponsive. Before regaining consciousness, he often passes through a state of confusion and agitation, loosely termed "postictal psychosis."

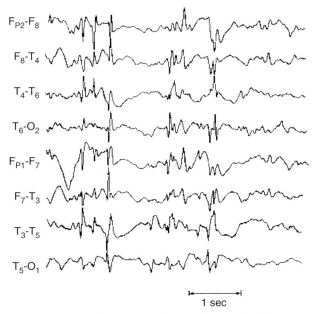

FIGURE 10-14 ■ During a tonic-clonic seizure, the EEG ideally shows paroxysms of spikes, polyspikes, and occasional slow waves in all channels; however, muscle artifact can obscure this pattern. Even during interictal periods, the EEG contains multiple bursts of generalized spikes in the background. In contrast to occasional temporal lobe spikes, this pattern confirms a diagnosis of epilepsy in patients with seizures.

Treatment

As in their initial treatment of partial seizures, neurologists attempt to suppress seizures with monotherapy. They commonly prescribe valproate, phenytoin, carbamazepine, or another AED for tonic-clonic seizures.

Febrile Seizures

Febrile seizures, occurring at least once in 2% to 4% of all children, are the most common variety of childhood seizure. These seizures usually last less than 30 seconds and lack focal findings. Older literature suggested that febrile seizures often cause mesial temporal sclerosis, which in turn would lead to partial complex epilepsy. However, recent studies demonstrate that children experiencing febrile seizures have little or no increased risk of partial complex seizures.

Pediatricians and neurologists, in the past, would routinely prescribe prophylactic phenobarbital or valproic acid. However, those and other AEDs not only provide little protection, they impair cognitive function and produce hyperactivity. Today, pediatricians and neurologists usually recommend oral or rectal diazepam only when fevers develop to prevent febrile seizures.

NONEPILEPTIC CONDITIONS

Psychogenic Seizures

Psychogenic seizures and physiologic seizure-like events, such as breath-holding spells, fall within the category of *nonepileptic seizures*. Psychogenic seizures, which occur 5% to 10% as frequently as epileptic seizures, usually develop in females aged 19 to 35 years, relatives of patients with psychogenic seizures, and individuals reporting a history of abuse.

Psychiatrists originally classified all psychogenic seizures as symptom of a conversion disorder. Those using the DSM-IV-TR label individual cases of psychogenic seizures as a Conversion Disorder or a pseudoneurologic symptom of a Somatization Disorder. However, psychiatrists rarely attribute psychogenic seizures to psychosis or eating disorders. Although the literature is scant in the following regard, physicians might sometimes find that psychogenic seizures are a manifestation of factitious illness or malingering.

On several occasions, a group of people—particularly female adolescents—has simultaneously or in succession succumbed to seizure-like episodes during a period of weeks to months. When multiple individuals are affected by seizure-like episodes or similar disturbances, the neurologic literature terms the small epidemic "mass hysteria."

As with epileptic seizures, psychogenic seizures tend to be stereotyped for the individual. The most important difference is that, despite the apparent generalized nature of some psychogenic seizures, consciousness is preserved. Also, patients with psychogenic seizures often demonstrate slow development of flailing, struggling, agitation, and alternating limb movements that are asymmetric (out-of-phase) and lack a tonic period. Additionally, the head often moves rhythmically and side-to-side and the trunk moves with suggestive pelvic thrusts.

Sometimes, as in epileptic seizures, psychogenic seizure patients bite their lip or tip (but not the side) of their tongue and urinate on themselves. Even if patients speak, they often stutter or stammer. When turned from side-to-side, they consistently direct their gaze toward the floor. As fatigue ensues, the movements decline in intensity and regularity, but often resume after rest. The duration of psychogenic seizures—typically 2 to 5 minutes—exceeds that of the average epileptic seizure.

Unless they deliberately mimic an epileptic seizure, psychogenic seizure patients recover immediately. They have no postictal symptoms, such as confusion, headache, retrograde amnesia, or hemiparesis.

EEGs obtained during a psychogenic seizure would ideally be normal, but muscle movement artifact obscures the tracing. An EEG performed after the episode, which is more feasible, would lack the usual postictal depression. Also, the serum prolactin concentration would not rise.

If routine testing fails to provide a diagnosis, continuous EEG-video monitoring would probably differentiate psychogenic seizures from epileptic seizures. The portion of the EEG monitoring obtained during sleep is especially important because epileptic seizures—not psychogenic seizures—may arise from genuine sleep.

The extremes are readily identifiable, but several subtle diagnostic pitfalls remain. Psychogenic seizures can be quite convincing. They can include urination and, in as many as 20% of cases, deliberate or inadvertent self-injury. Applying only clinical criteria, the distinction between psychogenic and epileptic seizures in most studies is no more accurate than 80% to 90%.

Another pitfall remains as to whether patients with psychogenic seizures also have epileptic ones. Recent studies have shown an unexpectedly low comorbidity: Only 5% to 10% of patients with psychogenic seizures have comorbid epileptic seizures. In cases when they are comorbid, epilepsy patients' psychogenic seizures so closely mimic their epileptic seizures that physicians must perform continuous EEG-video monitoring to distinguish them. The combination of psychogenic and epileptic seizures may occasionally explain "refractory epilepsy." Still another pitfall is that some frontal lobe and partial complex seizures produce such bizarre behavior that neurologists might summarily dismiss the patient.

Even compared to patients with epileptic seizures, patients with psychogenic seizures, whether or not they also have epileptic ones, often fare poorly. In the majority of patients with both types of seizures, AEDs and psychotropics are unsuccessful, patients remain at least partially dependent on caregivers, and their quality of life ratings are especially low.

Episodic Dyscontrol Syndrome/ Intermittent Explosive Disorder

The episodic dyscontrol syndrome—roughly equivalent to the DSM-IV-TR condition, *Intermittent Explosive Disorder*—usually consists of violently aggressive, primitive outbursts, including screaming, punching, wrestling, and throwing objects that injure people or destroy property. Minor external stimuli, such as verbal threats, anger, or frustration, especially after consuming even small amounts of alcohol, usually provoke the episodes. (If alcohol actually causes the episodes, the DSM-IV-TR does not classify them as Intermittent Explosive Disorder.) A highly charged affect often precedes and then accompanies the outburst. After it, patients claim justification, repentance, or amnesia.

In contrast to violent partial complex seizures (see previous), which are rare, episodic dyscontrol episodes are nonstereotyped, at least momentarily purposeful, and highly emotional. Furthermore, these violent attacks have a clear aggressive intent. They occur predominantly in young men who have congenital or traumatic brain injury, borderline intelligence, and minor physical neurosis abnormalities. Many have interictal EEG abnormalities. Although the neurologic community does not accept episodes of episodic dyscontrol syndrome (Intermittent Explosive Disorder) as seizures, neurologists suggest AEDs, mood stabilizers, and abstinence from alcohol.

RELATED ISSUES

Driving

Patients with epilepsy have a motor vehicle accident rate seven-fold greater than the general population. Not only might they have seizures while driving, AEDs can make them sleepy enough to cause traffic accidents. Epilepsy patients also have increased rates of traffic violations, including driving under the influence of alcohol or drugs. As in the general population, automobile accidents are most closely associated with male drivers younger than 25 years.

Almost all states require a waiting period for a driving license or renewals after having a seizure, but modifications are sometimes allowed for seizures arising from an isolated medical illness, such as hypoglycemia, and for those with a prolonged aura. Most states set a waiting period of 3 to 12 months, but several, including New York and California, allow some flexibility for noncommercial driving. They also require applicants to reveal any history of seizures or loss of consciousness (for any reason). In addition, several states require physicians to report drivers with seizures ("mandatory physician reporting").

Although many patients with epilepsy die suddenly and unexpectedly, certain activities represent known hazards. Drowning is probably the most common cause of accidental death. In addition, patients sometimes sustain head trauma, dislocations, lacerations, and ocular injuries during seizures.

Alcohol

Drinking alcoholic beverages in moderation should not give rise to seizures in epileptic patients. On the other hand, AEDs will not prevent seizures that arise from alcohol abuse or withdrawal mostly because when people drink, they usually neglect to take their medicines. Even if they do, AEDs will not prevent such seizures. Thus, neurologists do not prescribe AEDs to alcoholics who develop alcohol-withdrawal seizures. If one were to occur, benzodiazepines, probably because of their similarity to alcohol, act as an effective AED.

Cerebrovascular Disturbances

TIAs resemble partial seizures because both may involve momentarily impaired consciousness and physical deficits (see Chapter 11). In general, however, TIAs have slower onset and rarely cause loss of consciousness.

Of the various cerebrovascular disturbances, *transient global amnesia (TGA)* most closely resembles partial complex seizures (see Chapter 11). During a TGA episode, a frequent cause of transient amnesia (see Table 7-1), patients cannot remember new information, such as the date, location, and examining physicians; however, they retain basic memories, such as their name, address, and telephone number. This discrepancy separates TGA from psychogenic amnesia, in which basic as well as new information is lost.

During TGA, the EEG shows spikes but not paroxysmal bursts. MRIs show bilateral temporal lobe abnormalities indicative of ischemia. In the absence of reliable laboratory data, neurologists diagnose TGA, although with some uncertainty, by its clinical features.

Migraines, which also have an element of vascular disturbance, may induce episodes of confusion and personality change followed by a tendency to sleep (see Chapter 9). Migraines particularly mimic seizures when they lead to transient hemiparesis and abnormal EEGs. In fact, migraine patients have a greater than usual incidence of seizures, making migraines a risk factor for epilepsy. The correct diagnosis of migraines relies on the patient's history and response to medications.

Sleep Disorders

Bizarre behavior during the night might not be a nocturnal seizure but a sleep disorder (see Chapter 17). Some sleep disorders so closely mimic seizures that only polysomnography or continuous EEG-video monitoring can distinguish them. For example, children might have a *night terror* or another *parasomnia*, and older adults are liable to develop *REM behavior disorder*. In patients who experience repeated bouts of unresponsiveness, the *narcolepsy-cataplexy syndrome*, which includes several seizure-like symptoms, such as momentary loss of body tone (cataplexy) and dream-like hallucinations, represents a diagnostic alternative to seizure disorder. Unlike seizures, the narcolepsy-cataplexy syndrome has no aura, motor activity, incontinence, or subsequent symptoms. Moreover, during attacks of narcolepsy, an EEG or polysomnography shows REM activity.

Metabolic Aberrations

Of the various metabolic aberrations that can mimic seizures, reactions to medicines are probably the most common. Many medicines, including some administered as eyedrops, produce transient mental and physical alterations; however, they almost never induce stereotyped movements or thoughts.

Hyperventilation commonly induces giddiness, confusion, and other psychologic symptoms that can be confused with seizures (see Chapter 3). When prolonged and deep, hyperventilation may precipitate seizures, but probably only in epileptic individuals.

Hypoglycemia, which can result from excessive insulin, alcohol intoxication, skipping meals, and prediabetic states, can induce anxiety attacks and seizure-like symptoms. Similar symptoms occur with excessive coffee intake. Although the severity and frequency of these symptoms are probably overestimated, small frequent meals and reduction of caffeine consumption should remedy most cases.

REFERENCES

AEDs, Surgery, and Other Treatments

AEDs

1. Bourgeois BF: Determining the effects of antiepileptic drugs on cognitive function in pediatric patients with epilepsy. J Child Neurol 19(Suppl 1):S15–S24, 2004.
2. Ensrud KE, Walczak TS, Blackwell T, et al: Antiepileptic drug use increases rates of bone loss in older women: A prospective study. Neurology 62:2051–2057, 2004.
3. Farhat G, Yamout B, Mikati MA, et al: Effect of antiepileptic drugs on bone density in ambulatory patients. Neurology 58:1348–1353, 2002.
4. French JA, Kanner AM, Bautista J, et al: Efficacy and tolerability of the new antiepileptic drugs I: Treatment of new onset epilepsy. Report of the Therapeutics and Technology Assessment Subcommittee of the American Academy of Neurology and the American Epilepsy Society. Neurology 62:1252–1260, 2004.
5. French JA, Kanner AM, Bautista J, et al: Efficacy and tolerability of the new antiepileptic drugs II: Treatment of refractory epilepsy. Report of the Therapeutics and Technology Assessment Subcommittee of the American Academy of Neurology and the American Epilepsy Society. Neurology 62:1261–1273, 2004.
6. Hagg S, Spigset O: Anticonvulsant use during lactation. Drug Saf 22:425–440, 2000.
7. Hirz D, Berg A, Bettis D, et al: Practice parameter: Treatment of the child with a first unprovoked seizure: Report of the Quality Standards Subcommittee of the American Academy of Neurology and the Practice Committee of the Child Neurology Society. Neurology 60:166–175, 2003.
8. Holmes LB, Harvey EA, Coull BA, et al: The teratogenicity of anticonvulsant drugs. N Engl J Med 344:1132–1138, 2001.
9. Kaaja E, Kaaja R, Hiilesmaa V: Major malformations in offspring of women with epilepsy. Neurology 60:575–579, 2003.
10. Ketter TA, Malow BA, Flamini R, et al: Anticonvulsant withdrawal-emergent psychopathology. Neurology 44:55–61, 1994.
11. Lee S, Sziklas V, Andermann F, et al: The effects of adjunctive topiramate on cognitive function in patients with epilepsy. Epilepsy 44:339–347, 2003.
12. Loring DW, Meador KJ: Cognitive side-effects of antiepileptic drugs in children. Neurology 62:872–877, 2004.
13. Martin R, Kuzniecky R, Ho S, et al: Cognitive effects of topiramate, gabapentin, and lamotrigine in healthy young adults. Neurology 52:321–327, 1999.
14. Meador KJ, Lorning DW, Hulihan JF, et al: Differential cognitive and behavioral effects of topiramate and valproate. Neurology 60:1483–1488, 2003.
15. Olafsson E, Hallgrimsson JT, Hauser WA, et al: Pregnancies of women with epilepsy. Epilepsia 39:887–892, 1998.
16. Pacia SV, Devinsky O: Clozapine-related seizures: Experience with 5,629 patients. Neurology 44:2247–2249, 1994.
17. Penovich P, Gaily E: What can we say to women of reproductive age with epilepsy? Neurology 64:938–939, 2005.
18. Petty SJ, Paton LM, O'Brien TJ, et al: Effect of antiepileptic medication on bone mineral measures. Neurology 65:1358–1363, 2005.
19. Quality Standards Subcommittee of the American Academy of Neurology: Practice parameter: Management issues for women with epilepsy. Neurology 51:944–948, 1998.
20. Salinsky MC, Storzbach D, Spencer DC, et al: Effects of topiramate and gabapentin on cognitive abilities in healthy volunteers. Neurology 64:792–798, 2005.
21. White JR, Walczak TS, Leppik IE, et al: Discontinuation of levetiracetam because of behavioral side-effects: A case-control study. Neurology 61:1218–1221, 2003.

Surgery

22. Altshuler L, Rausch R, Delrahim S, et al: Temporal lobe epilepsy, temporal lobectomy, and major depression. J Neuropsychiatry Clin Neurosci 11:436–443, 1999.
23. Carran MA, Kohler CG, O'Connor MJ, et al: Mania following temporal lobectomy. Neurology 61:770–774, 2003.
24. Devinsky O, Barr WB, Vickrey BG, et al: Changes in depression and anxiety after resective surgery for epilepsy. Neurology 65:1744–1749, 2005.

25. Spencer SS, Berg AT, Vickrey BG, et al: Initial outcomes in the Multicenter Study of Epilepsy Surgery. Neurology 61:1680–1685, 2003.
26. Wiebe S, Blume WT, Girvin JP, et al: A randomized, controlled trial of surgery for temporal-lobe epilepsy. N Engl J Med 345:311–318, 2001.

Vagus Nerve Stimulation

27. Chavel SM, Westerveld M, Spencer S: Long-term outcome of vagus nerve stimulation for refractory partial epilepsy. Epilepsy Behav 4:302–309, 2003.
28. Privitera MD, Welty TE, Ficker DM: Vagus nerve stimulation for partial seizures. Cochrane Database Syst Rev 1: CD002896, 2002.
29. Schachter SC: Vagus nerve stimulation therapy summary: Five years after FDA approval. Neurology 59(Suppl 4):S15–S20, 2002.
30. Uthman B, Reichl AM, Dean JC, et al: Effectiveness of vagus nerve stimulation in epilepsy patients: A 12-year observation. Neurology 63:1124–1126, 2004.

Other Treatments

31. Krystal AD, Coffey CE: Neuropsychiatric considerations in the use of electroconvulsive therapy. J Neuropsychiatry 9:283–292, 1998.
32. Sackheim HA, Prudic J, Devanand DP, et al: Effects of stimulus intensity and electrode placement on the efficacy and cognitive effects of electroconvulsive therapy. N Engl J Med 328:839–846, 1993.

Interictal Comorbidities and Their Treatment

33. Adachi N, Matsuura M, Okubo Y, et al: Predictive variables of interictal psychosis in epilepsy. Neurology 55:1310–1314, 2000.
34. Alldredge BK: Seizure risk associated with psychotropic drugs: Clinical and pharmacokinetic considerations. Neurology 53(Suppl 2):S68–S75, 1999.
35. Attarian H, Vahle V, Carter J, et al: Relationship between depression and intractability of seizures. Epilepsy Behav 4:298–301, 2003.
36. Bear DM, Fedio P: Quantitative analysis of interictal behavior in temporal lobe epilepsy. Arch Neurol 34:454–467, 1977.
37. Blum D, Metz A: Prevalence of major affective disorders and manic/hypomanic symptoms in persons with epilepsy: A community survey. Neurology 58(Suppl 3):A175, 2003.
38. Blumer D, Montouris G, Davies K, et al: Suicide in epilepsy: Psychopathology, pathogenesis, and prevention. Epilepsy Behav 3:232–241, 2002.
39. Blumer D, Wakhlu S, Montouris G, et al: Treatment of the interictal psychoses. J Clin Psychiatry 61:110–122, 2000.
40. Boylan LS, Flint LA, Labovitz DL, et al: Depression but not seizure frequency predicts quality of life in treatment-resistant epilepsy. Neurology 62:258–261, 2004.
41. Bruton CJ, Stevens JR, Frith CD: Epilepsy, psychosis, and schizophrenia. Neurology 44:34–42, 1994.
42. Cramer JA, Blum D, Reed M, et al: The influence of comorbid depression on seizure severity. Epilepsia 44:1578–1584, 2003.
43. Ettinger AB, Kanner AM (eds): *Psychiatric Issues in Epilepsy.* Philadelphia, Lippincott, Williams & Wilkins, 2001.
44. Ettinger AB, Reed ML, Goldberg JF, et al: Prevalence of bipolar symptoms in epilepsy vs other chronic health disorders. Neurology 65:535–540, 2005.
45. Flor-Henry P: Psychosis and temporal lobe epilepsy. Epilepsia 10:363–395, 1969.
46. Gross A, Devinsky O, Westbrook LE, et al: Psychotropic medication use in patients with epilepsy: Effect on seizure frequency. J Neuropsychiatry Clin Neurosci 12:4, 2000.
47. Hansotia P, Broste SK: The effect of epilepsy or diabetes mellitus on the risk of automobile accidents. N Engl J Med 324:22–26, 1991.
48. Harden CL: The co-morbidity of depression and epilepsy: Epidemiology, etiology, and treatment. Neurology 59(Suppl 4):S48–S55, 2002.
49. Helmstaedter C, Kurthen M, Lux S, et al: Chronic epilepsy and cognition: A longitudinal study in temporal lobe epilepsy. Ann Neurol 54:425–432, 2003.
50. Jones JE, Hermann BP, Barry JJ, et al: Rates and risk factors for suicide, suicidal ideation, and suicide attempts in chronic epilepsy. Epilepsy Behav 4(Suppl 3):S31–S38, 2003.
51. Kanemoto K, Kawasaki J, Mori E: Violence and epilepsy: A close relation between violence and postictal psychosis. Epilepsia 40:107–109, 1999.
52. Kanner AM: The complex epilepsy patient: Intricacies of assessment and treatment. Epilepsia 44(Suppl 5):3–8, 2003.
53. Krauss GL, Ampaw L, Krumholz A: Individual state driving restrictions for people with epilepsy in the US. Neurology 57:1780–1785, 2001.
54. Kudo T, Ishida S, Kubota H, et al: Manic episode in epilepsy and bipolar I disorder: A comparative analysis of 13 patients. Epilepsia 42:1036–1042, 2001.
55. Lee KC, Finley PR, Alldredge BK: Risk of seizures associated with psychotropic medications: Emphasis on new drugs and new findings. Expert Opin Drug Saf 2:233–247, 2003.
56. Meador KJ: Newer anticonvulsants: Dosing strategies and cognition in treating patients with mood disorders and epilepsy. J Clin Psychiatry 64(Suppl 8):30–34, 2003.
57. Mendez MF, Doss RC, Taylor JL: Interictal violence in epilepsy: Relationship to behavior and seizure variables. J Nerv Ment Dis 181:566–569, 1993.
58. Mendez MF, Doss RC, Taylor JL, et al: Depression in epilepsy: Relationship to lesion laterality. J Neurol Neurosurg Psychiatry 57:232–233, 1994.
59. Mendez MF, Doss RC, Taylor JL, et al: Depression in epilepsy: Relationship to seizures and anticonvulsant therapy. J Nerv Ment Dis 181:444–447, 1993.
60. Mendez MF, Grau R, Doss RC, et al: Schizophrenia in epilepsy: Seizure and psychosis variables. Neurology 43:1073–1077, 1993.

61. Mendez MF, Lanska DJ, Manon-Espaillat R, et al: Causative factors for suicide attempts by overdose in epileptics. Arch Neurol 46:1065–1068, 1989.
62. Morrell MJ, Sperling MR, Stecker M, et al: Sexual dysfunction in partial epilepsy: A deficit in physiologic arousal. Neurology 44:243–247, 1994.
63. Nathaniel-James DA, Brown RG, Maier M, et al: Cognitive abnormalities in schizophrenia and schizophrenia-like psychosis of epilepsy. J Neuropsychiatry Clin Neurosci 16:472–479, 2004.
64. Pillmann F, Rohde A, Ullrich A, et al: Violence, criminal behavior, and the EEG. J Neuropsychiatry Clin Neurosci 11:454–457, 1999.
65. Pincus JH: Violence: The neurologic contribution. Arch Neurol 49:595–603, 1992.
66. Pisani F, Oteri G, Costa C, et al: Effects of psychotropic drugs on seizure threshold. Drug Saf 25:91–110, 2002.
67. Roach ES, Langley RL: Episodic neurological dysfunction due to mass hysteria. Arch Neurol 61:1269–1272, 2004.
68. Rodin E, Schmaltz S: The Bear-Fedio personality inventory and temporal lobe epilepsy. Neurology 34:591–596, 1984.
69. Sachdev P: Schizophrenia-like psychosis and epilepsy: The status of the association. Am J Psychiatry 155:325–336, 1998.
70. Schachter SC (ed): *Visions: Artists Living With Epilepsy.* Elsevier, 2003.
71. Slater E, Beard AW: The schizophrenic-like psychosis of epilepsy. Br J Psychiatry 109:95–150, 1963.
72. Trimble M, Schmitz B (eds): *The Neuropsychiatry of Epilepsy.* New York, Cambridge University Press, 2002.
73. Whitman S, Coleman TE, Patmon C, et al: Epilepsy in prison: Elevated prevalence and no relationship to violence. Neurology 34:775–782, 1984.

Psychogenic Seizures

74. Alper K, Devinsky O, Perrine K: Nonepileptic seizures and childhood sexual and physical abuse. Neurology 43:1950–1953, 1993.
75. Benbadis S, Agrawal V, Tatum WO: How many patients with psychogenic nonepileptic seizures also have epilepsy. Neurology 57:915–917, 2001.
76. Martin R, Burneo JG, Prasad A, et al: Frequency of epilepsy in patients with psychogenic seizures monitored by video-EEG. Neurology 61:1791–1792, 2003.
77. Reuber M, Pukrop R, Bauer J, et al: Prognostic factors in psychogenic nonepileptic seizures. Ann Neurol 53:305–311, 2003.
78. Roach ES, Langley RL: Episodic neurological dysfunction due to mass hysteria. Arch Neurol 61:1269–1272, 2004.
79. Sigurdardottir KR, Olafsson E: Incidence of psychogenic seizures in adults: A population-based study in Iceland. Epilepsia 39:749–752, 1998.

80. Szaflarski JP, Hughes C, Szaflarski M, et al: Quality of life in psychogenic nonepileptic seizures. Epilepsia 44:236–242, 2003.

Seizures and Epilepsy

81. Boro A, Haut S: Medical comorbidities in the treatment of epilepsy. Epilepsy Behav 4:S2–S12, 2003.
82. Chang BS, Lowenstein DH: Epilepsy. N Engl J Med 349:1257–1266, 2003.
83. Devinsky O, Westbrook L, Cramer J, et al: Risk factors for poor health-related quality of life in adolescents with epilepsy. Epilepsia 40:1715–1720, 1999.
84. Flicker DM: Sudden unexplained death and injury in epilepsy. Epilepsia 41(Suppl 2):S7–S12, 2000.
85. Goossens LAZ, Andermann F, Andermann E, et al: Reflex seizures induced by calculation, card or board games, and spatial tasks: A review of 25 patients and delineation of the epileptic syndrome. Neurology 40:1171–1176, 1990.
86. Greenlee BA, Ferrell RB, Kauffman CI, et al: Complex partial seizures and depression. Curr Psychiatry Rep 5:410–416, 2003.
87. Laskowitz DT, Sperling MR, French JA, et al: The syndrome of frontal lobe epilepsy: Characteristics and surgical management. Neurology 45:780–787, 1995.
88. Lings S: Increased driving accident frequency in Danish patients with epilepsy. Neurology 57:435–439, 2001.
89. Manford M, Fish DR, Shorvon SD: An analysis of clinical seizure patterns and their localizing value in frontal and temporal lobe epilepsies. Brain 119:17–40, 1996.
90. Saygi S, Katz A, Marks DA, et al: Frontal lobe partial seizures and psychogenic seizures. Neurology 42:1274–1277, 1992.
91. Tarkka R, Pääkkö E, Pyhtinenj J, et al: Febrile seizures and mesial temporal sclerosis: No association in a long-term follow-up study. Neurology 60:215–218, 2003.
92. Yerby MS, Kaplan P, Tran T: Risks and management of pregnancy in women with epilepsy. Cleve Clin J Med 71(Suppl 2):S25–37, 2004.

Testing

93. Centorrino F, Price BH, Tuttle M, et al: EEG abnormalities during treatment with typical and atypical antipsychotics. Am J Psychiatry 159:109–115, 2002.
94. Hughes JR: A review of the usefulness of the standard EEG in psychiatry. Clin Electroencephalogr 27:35–39, 1996.
95. Therapeutics and Technology Assessment Subcommittee of the American Academy of Neurology: Assessment: Magnetoencephalography (MEG). Neurology 42:1–4, 1992.
96. Therapeutics and Technology Assessment Subcommittee of the American Academy of Neurology: Assessment of digital EEG, quantitative EEG, and EEG brain mapping. Neurology 49:277–292, 1997.

Questions and Answers

1–4. Match each EEG with the appropriate interpretation (see pages 230–231).
1. Fig. EEG-A
2. Fig. EEG-B
3. Fig. EEG-C
4. Fig. EEG-D
   a. Spike and polyspike-and-wave
   b. 3-Hz spike-and-wave
   c. Normal
   d. Temporal spike focus

Answers: 1-c, 2-d, 3-b, 4-a.

5–8. Match the EEG abnormality with its associated seizure.
5. Interictal temporal lobe spikes
6. Generalized 3-Hz spike-and-wave
7. Generalized spike and polyspike-and-wave
8. Occipital spike-and-wave
   a. Tonic-clonic (grand mal)
   b. Partial elementary
   c. Partial complex
   d. Absence (petit mal)

Answers: 5-c, 6-d, 7-a, 8-b.

9–16. Match the EEG pattern with its most likely cause.
9. Delta activity, phase reversed over left posterior cerebrum
10. Bifrontal beta activity
11. Alpha rhythm
12. Triphasic waves
13. Rapid extraocular movement artifact
14. Periodic complexes
15. Unilateral cerebral theta and delta activity
16. Electrocerebral silence
   a. Normal resting state
   b. Hepatic encephalopathy
   c. Benzodiazepine use
   d. Occipital lobe tumor
   e. Cerebral death
   f. Dream-filled sleep
   g. Unilateral ECT
   h. Psychosis
   i. Creutzfeldt-Jakob disease
   j. Barbiturate overdose

Answers: 9-d, 10-c, 11-a, 12-b, 13-f (REM sleep), 14-i, 15-g, 16-e and j.

17. In which four conditions will an EEG be helpful in suggesting a specific diagnosis?
   a. Cerebral tumor
   b. Hepatic encephalopathy
   c. Neurosis
   d. Huntington's disease
   e. Cerebral abscess
   f. Creutzfeldt-Jakob disease
   g. Psychogenic seizures
   h. Bipolar illness
   i. Cerebellar tumor
   j. SSPE
   k. Psychosis
   l. Multiple sclerosis
   m. Early Alzheimer's disease

Answers: b, f, g, j.

18–20. Match each AED complication with its definition.
18. Stevens-Johnson syndrome
19. Forced normalization
20. Paradoxical hyperactivity
   a. Suppression of seizure activity and conversion to a normal EEG that may trigger a psychosis
   b. Sometimes fatal allergic reaction primarily involving the gastrointestinal mucosa
   c. Psychosis as an allergic reaction
   d. Excitement instead of sedation, especially with phenobarbital treatment of children and adults with brain damage

Answers: 18-b, 19-a, 20-d.

21–24. Identify the following statements as true or false.
21. Use of EEG in diagnosing psychiatric illness is complicated by psychotropic-induced EEG changes.
22. Benzodiazepines and barbiturates induce beta EEG activity.
23. Lithium at toxic levels, clozapine, and tricyclic antidepressants cause spikes and sharp waves.
24. Clozapine, olanzapine, and trifluoperazine produce the most EEG changes, and quetiapine, loxapine, and haloperidol the least.

Answers: 21-True, 22-True, 23-True, 24-True.

25. Carbamazepine is often used in the treatment of epilepsy patients with comorbid depression.

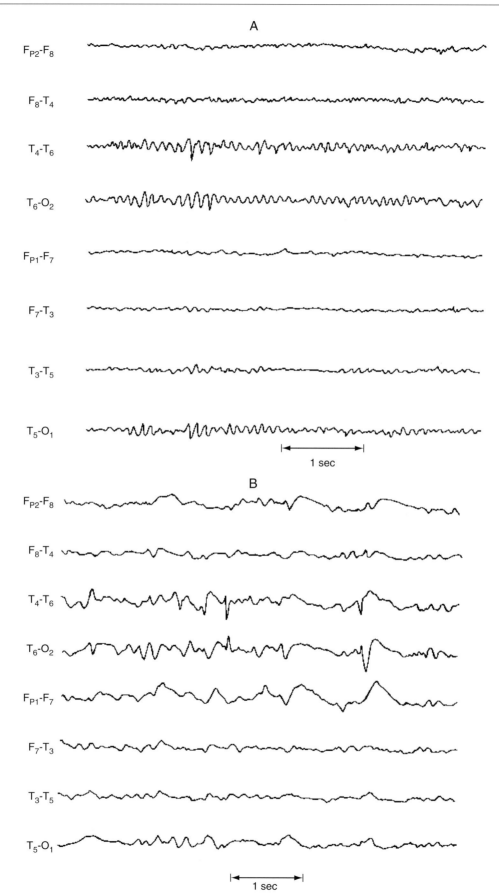

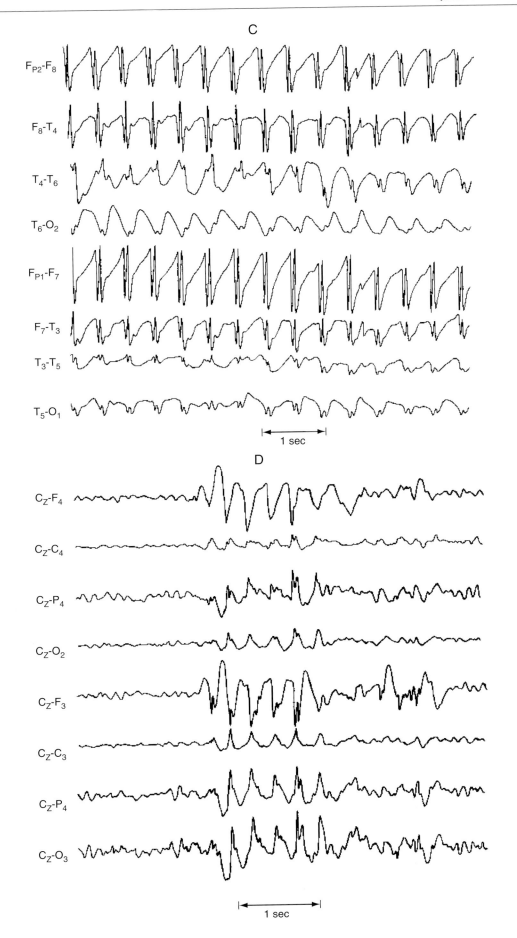

C

1 sec

D

1 sec

Which of the following medications has a chemical structure most similar to carbamazepine?
a. Lithium
b. Phenytoin
c. Imipramine
d. Haloperidol
e. Phenelzine
f. Tranylcypromine

Answer: c. Imipramine has a chemical structure most like carbamazepine.

26. For which condition is QEEG accepted as a clinical test?
    a. Attention deficit hyperactivity disorder
    b. Postconcussive syndrome
    c. Head trauma
    d. Depression
    e. Epilepsy
    f. Learning disabilities

Answer: e. QEEG remains an investigational diagnostic technique for almost all conditions. Even in epilepsy, QEEG still requires sophisticated data analysis.

27. Which application of ECT is least likely to produce amnesia?
    a. Unilateral, nondominant hemisphere
    b. Unilateral, dominant hemisphere
    c. Bilateral
    d. Each pattern will produce similar incidence and severity of amnesia.

Answer: a. Although ECT in a unilateral pattern over the nondominant hemisphere may be least effective in reversing depression, it will produce the least amnesia.

28. Which feature indicates a frontal lobe seizure rather than another form of partial complex seizure?
    a. Childhood onset
    b. Olfactory auras
    c. Absence of an aura, duration of less than 1 minute, and little postictal symptomatology
    d. The ability of sleep to suppress these seizures

Answer: c. Frontal lobe seizures, unlike other partial complex seizures, usually develop in adults and consist of numerous, relatively brief episodes of bizarre activity devoid of aura, automatisms, and postictal confusion. On the basis of their clinical manifestations alone, physicians are especially apt to misdiagnose them as psychogenic episodes. Frontal lobe seizures develop predominantly during sleep. A routine EEG is often unable to assist in the diagnosis.

29. A 28-year-old man was admitted to the hospital following several seizures. He denied prior seizures,

head trauma, and systemic symptoms. He had been maintained in a methadone program for narcotic addiction. His seizures were finally attributed to a congenital cerebral injury. His physicians gave him phenytoin and renewed his methadone prescription. Several days later developed agitation, anxiety to the point of incoherence, diaphoresis, and tachycardia. Which should be the consulting psychiatrist's first step?
a. Administer a tranquilizer
b. Administer an SSRI
c. Administer an atypical neuroleptic
d. Increase the daily methadone dose
e. Increase the phenytoin dose
f. Change the AED

Answer: d. Because phenytoin decreases methadone activity, it precipitates narcotic withdrawal. To avoid this problem, physicians should increase the dose of methadone. The alternative—stopping the phenytoin—may precipitate additional seizures or even cause status epilepticus. Changing phenytoin to another AED would require 5 to 10 days.

30. How do carbamazepine and phenytoin interact with oral contraceptives?
    a. These AEDs increase the contraceptive's effectiveness, permitting lower estrogen preparations to be effective.
    b. These AEDs decrease the contraceptive's effectiveness, risking conception.
    c. These AEDs have no effect on a contraceptive's effectiveness.
    d. In contrast to these AEDs having a teratogenic effect, other AEDs have been shown to be risk-free.

Answer: b. Several AEDs that induce enzymes, including carbamazepine, phenobarbital, phenytoin, and topiramate, greatly increase the metabolism of oral contraceptives, possibly inactivating them.

31. In which phase of sleep is a seizure least likely to occur?
    a. Stage 2 NREM
    b. REM
    c. Sleep following sleep deprivation
    d. Awakening from sleep

Answer: b. Seizures are most likely to emerge during stage 2 NREM sleep and least likely during REM sleep.

32. Which statement regarding the incidence of depression in epilepsy patients is true?
    a. Studies show that seizure frequency is proportionate to the incidence of depression.

b. The frequency of secondary generalized partial complex seizures is inversely proportionate to the incidence of depression.

c. Compared to depression without comorbid epilepsy, depression comorbid with epilepsy is more often bipolar.

d. ECT is contraindicated in epilepsy.

Answer: b. Most studies find that seizure frequency is a risk factor for depression. Several studies conclude that epilepsy patients suffer more depressive episodes when partial complex seizures fail to undergo secondary generalization. The incidence of bipolar disorder in epilepsy patients is near or only slightly higher than that of the general population. ECT treatment is an acceptable option for depression comorbid with epilepsy.

33. Which statement regarding the schizophreniform psychosis that develops in epilepsy is false?

a. Schizophreniform psychosis is associated with intractable epilepsy.

b. Epileptic patients who develop schizophreniform psychosis have larger cerebral ventricles and more cerebral damage than those who do not.

c. The incidence of schizophrenia in first-degree relatives of epileptic schizophreniform psychosis patients is similar to the incidence of schizophrenia in first-degree relatives of nonepileptic schizophrenia patients.

d. Butyrophenones are preferred over chlorpromazine as treatment for acute psychosis in epilepsy patients.

Answer: c. In contrast to first-degree relatives of nonepileptic schizophrenic patients, who have an increased incidence of schizophrenia, first-degree relatives of epileptic patients with schizophreniform psychosis show no increased incidence of schizophrenia. Chlorpromazine, more often than butyrophenones, precipitates seizures in epileptic patients.

34–43. The patient's age when partial (elementary or complex) seizures begin suggests the cause. Match the cause with the age(s) when associated seizures are likely to appear (the same answer may be applicable to different questions).

34. Head injury
35. Congenital cerebral malformation
36. Arteriovenous malformation
37. Glioblastoma multiforme
38. Metastatic brain tumor
39. Cocaine use
40. Cerebrovascular accident
41. Pseudoseizure
42. Medial temporal sclerosis

43. Perinatal cerebral hypoxia

a. Childhood
b. Adolescence
c. Middle age

Answers: 34-b, 35-a, 36-a and b, 37-c, 38-c, 39-b, 40-c, 41-b, 42-a and b, 43-a.

44–46. The family of a previously healthy 60-year-old man brings him to the emergency room in a state of confusion and excitement. A neurologist finds that he has poor memory for recent and past events, but he can recall his own and his wife's name and their address. His judgment, language, and other cognitive processes are slow but intact. The examination shows no physical abnormalities. He gradually improves over a period of 2 hours.

44. What is the best diagnosis for his condition?

a. Delirium
b. Dissociative fugue (formerly called psychogenic fugue)
c. Acute amnestic syndrome
d. Dissociative amnesia (formerly called psychogenic amnesia)

45. Which one of the following is *not* an acceptable explanation for his condition?

a. Partial complex seizures
b. Wernicke-Korsakoff syndrome
c. Psychogenic disturbances
d. Medication side effects
e. Transient global amnesia
f. AED intoxication

46. Dysfunction of which area of the brain is most likely responsible for his condition?

a. Temporal lobe
b. Entire cerebrum
c. Thalamus
d. Frontal lobe

Answers: 44-c. Preserved recollection of personal information distinguishes acute amnestic syndrome from dissociative (psychogenic) states. In this case, amnesia is a better diagnosis than delirium because of the circumscribed neuropsychologic problem, the stable, rather than fluctuating, level of consciousness, and the more specific terminology. His lack of traveling also distinguishes an amnestic syndrome from dissociative (psychogenic) fugue. 45-f. AED intoxication can cause delirium and cognitive impairment but not so limited an impairment as amnesia. By contrast, the other conditions are capable of impairing memory without damaging other cognitive functions. 46-a.

47. A 6-year-old boy has absence seizures with paroxysms of 3-Hz spike-and-wave EEG activity. He was unable to tolerate ethosuximide (Zarontin). Which AED should be tried next?
    a. Phenytoin
    b. Carbamazepine
    c. Valproic acid
    d. Phenobarbital

Answer: c. Absences with 3-Hz spike-and-wave activity are usually first treated with ethosuximide, but valproic acid is appropriate if ethosuximide is unacceptable or if grand mal seizures accompany the absence seizure.

48. A 23-year-old medical student was experimenting with smoking marijuana. Its effect, completely different than he anticipated, was anxiety and fear. The student was brought to the emergency room with hallucinations, agitation, fever, and nystagmus. Increasing mental and physical agitation soon developed, culminating in a seizure. Of the following, which is the most likely culprit?
    a. Marijuana
    b. Phencyclidine (PCP)
    c. Cocaine
    d. Demerol

Answer: b. PCP, even in minute amounts, can cause hallucinations, nystagmus, and seizures. Drug users sometimes mix it with marijuana. Cocaine not only produces hallucinations and seizures, it may cause cerebral hemorrhage, stroke, or vasculitis. When health care personnel develop seizures, treating physicians should consider drug abuse.

49. After developing lethargy and confusion, a 30-year-old woman with a history of partial complex seizures is brought to the emergency room. Which of the following conditions is the most likely cause?
    a. Expansion of a temporal lobe tumor
    b. Development of a subdural hematoma from head trauma
    c. Partial complex status epilepticus
    d. AED intoxication
    e. Development of a systemic disorder, such as renal failure

Answer: d. Although all these problems must be considered, the usual cause in such cases is AED intoxication or prolonged postictal confusion. If AED intoxication is profound or recurs, physicians should consider the possibility that the episode was a deliberate overdose or an adverse interaction of her AED with a psychotropic.

50. Which six of the following signs may indicate AED intoxication?
    a. Hemiparesis
    b. Ataxia of gait
    c. Nystagmus
    d. Aphasia
    e. Dysarthria
    f. Lethargy or stupor
    g. Dysmetria on heel-shin testing
    h. Tremor on finger-nose testing
    i. Papilledema

Answers: b, c, e, f, g, h.

51. In which part of the skull are the temporal lobes located?
    a. Sella
    b. Anterior fossa
    c. Posterior fossa
    d. Middle fossa

Answer: d. The temporal lobes occupy the entire middle fossae. The posterior fossa holds the cerebellum, medulla, fourth ventricle, and vertebral and basilar arteries.

52. What is the duration of the serum prolactin level elevation after a generalized tonic-clonic or partial complex seizure?
    a. 24 hours
    b. 12 hours
    c. 2 hours
    d. Less than 1 hour

Answer: d. Following a majority of tonic-clonic and ECT-induced seizures and a minority of partial complex ones, the serum prolactin level briefly rises for approximately 10 to 20 minutes. It does not rise following a psychogenic seizure.

53. Which of the following statements are true?
    a. Epileptic individuals are more likely than others to be convicted of a crime and sent to prison.
    b. Epileptic criminals are no more likely than other criminals to commit violent crimes.

Answers: a-True, b-True.

54. Which one of the following statements concerning neural tube defects is false?
    a. Meningomyeloceles may be induced by AED treatment of pregnant women.
    b. The incidence of neural tube defects is reduced by folic acid diet supplements.
    c. The neural tube is derived from the endoderm.

d. The neural tube forms the brain and the spinal cord.

Answer: c. Soon after conception the ectodermal layer of the embryo invaginates to form the neural tube.

55. Which of the following antiepileptic drugs lead to weight loss?
    a. Valproate
    b. Levetiracetam
    c. Topiramate
    d. Phenytoin
    e. Gabapentin

Answer: c. Valproate often causes weight gain. Topiramate often leads to a small weight loss. The others have little effect on weight.

56. If a medication that inhibited CYP 3A4 metabolic enzymes were administered to an individual taking carbamazepine, what would happen to the carbamazepine plasma concentration?
    a. The plasma concentration of carbamazepine would increase.
    b. The plasma concentration of carbamazepine would decrease.
    c. The plasma concentration of carbamazepine would remain unchanged.
    d. None of the above.

Answer: a. Medications that inhibit CYP 3A4 enzymes, including erythromycin and fluoxetine, raise the plasma concentration of carbamazepine, possibly to toxic levels.

57. If a medication that induced CYP 3A4 metabolic enzymes were administered to an individual taking carbamazepine, what would happen to the carbamazepine plasma concentration?
    a. The plasma concentration of carbamazepine would increase.
    b. The plasma concentration of carbamazepine would decrease.
    c. The plasma concentration of carbamazepine would remain unchanged.
    d. None of the above.

Answer: b. Medications that induce CYP 3A4 enzymes, including phenobarbital, phenytoin, and carbamazepine itself, decrease the plasma concentration of carbamazepine, possibly to subtherapeutic levels. In the case of carbamazepine therapy, increasing doses are often required to maintain a therapeutic concentration. Moreover, carbamazepine-induced enzymes decrease plasma concentrations of alprazolam, clozapine, haloperidol, oral contraceptives, and valproate.

58. Which of the following AEDs is an inhibitor of cytochrome P450 enzymes?
    a. Phenytoin
    b. Phenobarbital
    c. Carbamazepine
    d. Valproate

Answer: d. Valproate is an inhibitor of P450 enzymes, but the others induce the enzyme.

59. Although electrocerebral silence on an EEG often indicates brain death, other conditions may produce the same finding. Of the following, which two other conditions also produce electrocerebral silence?
    a. Psychogenic unresponsiveness
    b. Depression
    c. Severe Alzheimer's disease
    d. Barbiturate overdose
    e. Hypothermia
    f. Locked-in syndrome

Answers: d, e. Before declaring brain death on the basis of an EEG, the physician must be certain that the patient's body temperature is near normal and that blood tests do not detect barbiturates.

60. Which is the best test for demonstrating mesial temporal sclerosis?
    a. MRI of the brain
    b. SPECT of the brain
    c. CT of the brain
    d. CT with contrast of the brain
    e. EEG
    f. EEG with nasopharyngeal leads

Answer: a.

61. Which one of these statements regarding epilepsy, the EEG, and ECT treatment is false?
    a. When unilateral right-sided ECT is administered, the EEG changes are found predominantly over the right hemisphere.
    b. Generalized EEG changes after ECT are associated with more successful treatment of depression.
    c. Generalized EEG changes after ECT are associated with greater amnesia.
    d. ECT may precipitate status epilepticus in patients with epilepsy or a structural lesion.
    e. ECT is contraindicated when epilepsy is comorbid with depression

Answer: e. ECT is an acceptable strategy when epilepsy is comorbid with depression.

62. Which statement regarding the normal EEG is false?

a. Anxiety or concentrating on a simple problem will abolish alpha activity.
b. Hyperventilation will produce slow waves or slow the background activity.
c. The normal background rhythm is low voltage and "fast."
d. Drowsiness, as well as sleep, will slow the background activity.
e. Stroboscopic lights may capture cerebral activity.

Answer: c. The normal background rhythm is alpha activity, which is 8–12 Hz and medium in voltage. By contrast, beta activity, which is faster and lower in voltage, replaces alpha when the EEG subject experiences anxiety or concentrates on mental activities. It also replaces alpha activity if the subject takes sedatives or minor tranquilizers, including benzodiazepines.

63. A man with alcoholism and epilepsy is taking phenytoin. He presents with confusion, nystagmus, and ataxia. A routine medical and neurologic evaluation reveals no abnormal findings, except that he has alcohol on his breath. What should be the two first steps?
    a. Determine the blood alcohol and glucose concentrations
    b. Obtain an EEG
    c. Administer more phenytoin
    d. Administer thiamine

Answers: a, d. Many alcoholic individuals have epilepsy. When inebriated, they pose several dilemmas. Wernicke-Korsakoff syndrome, hypoglycemia from liver disease, or head trauma could each cause confusion and obtundation. Although the confusion, nystagmus, and ataxia suggest phenytoin intoxication, that condition is unlikely because during binges alcoholics usually do not take their AEDs. In addition, they may omit their insulin and antihypertensives.

64–65. A 32-year-old left-handed woman has suffered partial complex seizures since age 14 years. Her seizures have not responded to monotherapy. When taking two or three AEDs, which were only slightly more effective in suppressing seizures than taking one, she usually developed AED intoxication. EEG-video monitoring documented partial complex seizures despite therapeutic AED concentrations. EEGs also showed a left anterior temporal lobe seizure focus.
64. In contemplating surgery, what test should be performed next?
    a. Amobarbital interview
    b. Withdrawal of AEDs
    c. PET scan
    d. Wada test

Answer: d. The patient, who may be right-hemisphere dominant for language, might benefit from a partial or complete left temporal lobectomy. However, if her left temporal lobe were dominant, which is usually the case, she would be able to withstand only a limited resection. Functional MRI may, in the future, provide results as reliable as the Wada test.

65. Assuming a temporal lobectomy is safely performed, what is the likelihood of complete or near-complete remission of her seizures?
    a. 25%
    b. 50%
    c. 75%
    d. Almost 100%

Answer: c. In approximately 75% of cases, epilepsy surgery completely eliminates seizures or allows their control with fewer AEDs and lower doses.

66. Which of the following statements regarding Rolandic epilepsy is true?
    a. It is also called childhood epilepsy with centrotemporal spikes.
    b. The most common cause is mesial temporal sclerosis.
    c. When children with the condition become adults, they are prone to develop other varieties of seizures.
    d. The diagnosis often requires EEG-video monitoring, and if a single focus is identified, a partial lobectomy is indicated.

Answer: a. Rolandic epilepsy, an inherited condition, is restricted to the childhood years. EEGs performed during sleep may be necessary for diagnosis, but elaborate monitoring is rarely necessary. Once diagnosed, Rolandic epilepsy is readily responsive to AEDs. Unlike generalized absences, which lead to later development of tonic-clonic or other seizures in one third of cases, Rolandic epilepsy usually remits in adolescence.

67–71. Match the condition with its closest description (the same answer may be applicable to different questions).
67. Nonconvulsive status epilepticus
68. Seizure-like activity under conscious control
69. Activity not under conscious control that mimics seizures
70. Withdrawal emergent psychopathology
71. Forced normalization
    a. Psychiatric disturbances, including psychotic behavior, arising after AEDs rapidly and completely suppress frequent seizures
    b. Psychiatric disturbances, especially anxiety and depression, developing after withdrawal of AEDs
    c. Psychogenic seizures

d. Repetitive or prolonged seizures with mental impairment as the primary or exclusive symptom

Answers: 67-d, 68-c, 69-c, 70-b, 71-a.

72. Which two statements regarding the relationship of interictal violence to epilepsy are true?
   a. Violence is associated with epilepsy patients taking two or more AEDs.
   b. Violence tends to occur in schizophrenic or mentally retarded epilepsy patients but rarely in other epilepsy patients.
   c. Crimes of adult epileptic incarcerated criminals are no more violent than those of non-epileptic ones.
   d. The prevalence of epilepsy is no greater in prisoners than in the general population.

Answers: b, c.

73. Which variety of seizure do physicians most often misdiagnose as a psychogenic seizure?
   a. Partial complex seizure that originates in the temporal lobe
   b. Partial complex seizure that originates in the frontal lobe
   c. Febrile seizure
   d. Absence
   e. Drug withdrawal seizure

Answer: b. Physicians are most likely to misdiagnose frontal lobe seizures because they often induce bizarre behavior, such as pelvic thrusting, flailing limb movements, and alternating head movements.

74. Which of the following is associated with postictal EEG depression?
   a. Vegetative symptoms
   b. Tendency toward suicide
   c. Sleep-wake disturbances
   d. Slow, low voltage EEG activity

Answer: d. Postictal EEG depression refers not to a mood disorder but to the slow, low voltage EEG patterns that follow seizures, including those induced by ECT. However, postictal EEG depression is not detectable following psychogenic seizures or certain partial (focal) seizures.

75. A commercial airliner from South America to New York crashed after exhausting its fuel supply. A young man who had been one of the passengers was brought to the hospital with blunt abdominal trauma. Shortly after arriving in the emergency room, he became agitated, incoherent, diaphoretic, and hypertensive. Although physicians found no sign of head injuries, he developed status epilepticus and unstable vital signs. During one seizure,

several ruptured condoms passed through his rectum. Other condoms, still intact and containing a white powder, subsequently passed out of his rectum. What is the most likely cause of his seizures and unstable vital signs?
   a. Epidural hematoma
   b. Cysticercosis
   c. Subdural hematoma
   d. Cocaine overdose
   e. Hypoxia

Answer: d. Swallowing condoms filled with contraband is a common method of smuggling cocaine into the United States. If a condom breaks, cocaine spills into the intestine, and toxic quantities are absorbed into the systemic circulation. The resulting cocaine overdose causes psychosis, cardiac instability, and seizures. Although irrelevant in this case, the most common cause of seizures in South and Central America is cysticercosis.

76. Which AED is associated with polycystic ovaries and hyperandrogenism?
   a. Carbamazepine
   b. Valproate
   c. Phenytoin
   d. Topiramate
   e. a and b
   f. b and c

Answer: f. Older AEDs adversely affect many endocrine-based functions in women. Carbamazepine and valproate increase the risk of neural tube defects. Valproate treatment is also associated with transient thinning of hair and obesity, as well as with polycystic ovaries and hyperandrogenism. Both phenytoin and carbamazepine reduce the effectiveness of oral contraceptives, and phenytoin usually also causes increased facial hair.

77. Which one of the following statements does not describe Todd's paralysis?
   a. Todd's paralysis is apparent only during the first 24 hours following a seizure.
   b. Todd's hemiparesis may follow any seizure.
   c. Todd's hemiparesis may be accompanied by other lateralized deficits, such as aphasia.
   d. Todd's paralysis suggests a partial, rather than a generalized, seizure disorder.

Answer: b. Todd's paralysis, typically a transient postictal hemiparesis, rather than a quadriparesis or paraparesis, usually follows partial motor seizures. It does not follow absences and several other seizure varieties.

78. Valproate and carbamazepine induce neural tube closure defects. Which of the following is not a neural tube closure defect?

a. Meningomyelocele
b. Meningocele
c. Spina bifida
d. Encephalocele
e. Tetralogy of Fallot

Answer: e. Meningomyelocele, meningocele, and spina bifida—in decreasing severity of malformation—are neural tube closure deficits of the lumbar spine and spinal cord. An encephalocele is the cerebral counterpart.

79. Which of the following is an untrue statement regarding EEG changes associated with bilateral ECT?
    a. During and immediately after ECT, EEG changes resemble those of a generalized tonic-clonic seizure.
    b. EEG slow-wave activity persists for up to 3 months after bilateral ECT.
    c. ECT-induced EEG slowing is associated with memory impairment.
    d. ECT-induced EEG slowing is associated with ineffective treatment of depression.

Answer: d. ECT-induced EEG slowing is associated with more effective treatment of depression. However, it is also associated with prolonged amnesia.

80. Which is the least significant risk factor for seizures in patients receiving therapeutic doses of antidepressants?
    a. A seizure focus in the left temporal lobe
    b. A history of epilepsy
    c. Abnormalities on a pretreatment EEG
    d. Underlying brain damage

Answer: a. The effect of the laterality of the seizure focus remains controversial. Seizures induced by antidepressants are related to excessive or sudden elevations in serum antidepressant concentration, use of multiple medications, and various indications of brain damage, such as a history of epilepsy, abnormal physical findings, and an abnormal EEG. The seizures usually occur in the first week of treatment.

81. Which of the following psychotropics is most likely to cause a seizure?
    a. Clozapine
    b. Aripiprazole
    c. Olanzapine
    d. Risperidone
    e. Quetiapine
    f. Ziprasidone

Answer: a. Clozapine carries a seizure risk of approximately 4% when administered in high doses,

that is, more than 600 mg daily. In therapeutic doses, the other antipsychotics carry a risk of less than 1%.

82. Which of the following is the greatest risk factor for depression complicating epilepsy?
    a. Duration of epilepsy
    b. Partial complex epilepsy
    c. Family history of epilepsy
    d. Frequent seizures

Answer: b. Among epilepsy patients, depression occurs particularly in those who have partial complex seizures or require multiple AEDs. The duration of epilepsy, seizure frequency, and family history of depression are less significant. Epilepsy-associated depression is rarely bipolar. When it is comorbid with epilepsy, depression reduces patients' quality of life—even more than seizure frequency or severity.

83. In rating the potential teratogenic risks of AEDs, which group carries the FDA label of Category D (dangerous)?
    a. Carbamazepine and valproate
    b. Lamotrigine, levetiracetam, oxcarbazepine, and topiramate
    c. Phenobarbital and phenytoin
    d. Ethosuximide

Answer: a. The FDA has labeled carbamazepine and valproate, which are both associated with neural tube defects, as Category D. The FDA has labeled lamotrigine, levetiracetam, oxcarbazepine, and topiramate as Category C (caution).

84. What proportion of individuals with well-documented psychogenic seizures also has epileptic seizures?
    a. <10%
    b. 25%
    c. 50%
    d. 66%

Answer: a. Although early reports indicated that approximately 50% of patients with psychogenic seizures also have epilepsy, recent studies suggest that psychogenic seizures are comorbid with epilepsy in only 5% to 10% of cases.

85. What is the effect of drinking large quantities of grapefruit juice on the serum concentration of carbamazepine?
    a. Increased concentrations
    b. Decreased concentrations
    c. No effect

Answer: a. Grapefruit juice by inducing enzymes increases concentrations of carbamazepine, zonisamide, and several psychotropic medications.

86. What is the effect of pregnancy on seizure frequency?
  a. Seizures tend to decrease in frequency.
  b. Seizures tend to increase in frequency.
  c. Pregnancy has no effect on seizure frequency.

Answer: b. During pregnancy seizure frequency increases because serum AED levels drift downward as their clearance increases, and women's body mass increase dilutes AED concentration.

87. If two AEDs fail to suppress seizures, what is the likelihood that the addition of a third will be successful?
  a. <5%
  b. 25%
  c. 75%
  d. 100%

Answer a. If two AEDs do not suppress seizures, the likelihood of success with the addition of a third is <5%. Moreover, such polypharmacy often creates unbearable side effects. If AEDs cannot suppress seizures, physicians should reassess the diagnosis of epilepsy, variety of seizure(s), appropriate AED, and the patient's compliance (by measuring blood levels). If optimal medical management remains ineffective, neurologists often consider vagus nerve stimulation or neurosurgery.

88. Which of the following AEDs often causes paradoxical hyperactivity in young children and adults with traumatic brain injury?
  a. Clonazepam
  b. Phenobarbital
  c. Valproate
  d. Carbamazepine
  e. Lamotrigine

Answer: b. Phenobarbital and sometimes other sedating medicines may cause paradoxical hyperactivity in individuals with an immature or damaged brain.

89. Which of the following is the least significant risk factor for interictal psychosis?
  a. Early age of onset of epilepsy
  b. Low intelligence
  c. Certain EEG patterns
  d. Family history of psychosis

Answer: c. Although no specific EEG abnormality predicts interictal psychosis, signs of brain damage and a family history of psychosis are risk factors for interictal psychosis.

90. Which of the following AEDs crosses the placenta?
  a. Phenobarbital
  b. Methadone

  c. Carbamazepine
  d. Topiramate
  e. All of the above

Answer: e. AEDs and many other medications and substances pass through the placenta into the fetal circulation. For example, opioids pass through and, with continued use, may lead to fetal dependancy. Unless neonatologists provide a substitute at delivery, the neonate may undergo opioid withdrawal and experience a seizure.

91. Which of the following are readily transferred through breast milk?
  a. Topiramate
  b. Lamotrigine
  c. Phenobarbital
  d. Ethosuximide
  e. Zonisamide
  f. All of the above

Answer: f. Most AEDs pass into breast milk and, in breast-feeding neonates, some reach substantial serum concentrations. Although usually their only effect is sleepiness, more serious reactions may occur.

92. Which group of antidepressants has the greatest likelihood of inducing seizures?
  a. Bupropion, clomipramine
  b. Nefazodone
  c. Fluoxetine, paroxetine, sertraline

Answer: a.

93. Which group of antipsychotics has the greatest likelihood of inducing seizures?
  a. Chlorpromazine, clozapine
  b. Haloperidol
  c. Risperidone

Answer: a.

94. Which of the following AEDs is least likely to cause bone loss?
  a. Carbamazepine
  b. Phenytoin
  c. Levetiracetam
  d. Valproate
  e. Phenobarbital

Answer: c. Carbamazepine, phenytoin, phenobarbital, and valproate cause bone reabsorption, which enhances age-related osteoporosis. Bone density scans in patients taking these AEDs show decreased mineralization. The AEDs implicated in bone loss, with the exception of valproate, all induce cytochrome P450 enzymes. Neurologists often follow women taking these AEDs with bone scans and switch them to another AED if the scans detect osteoporosis.

95. A 32-year-old woman suffered from partial complex seizures that began when she was 18 years old. Multiple AED regimens had produced mental dulling and other side effects and still allowed one or two seizures each week. One year before a psychiatric consultation underwent partial left temporal lobectomy for seizure control. Subsequently she remained seizure-free even without any AEDs. However, she developed postoperative anxiety, fearfulness, dysphoria, and "moodiness." CCTV-EEG monitoring during this time showed no epileptic activity. Which would be the best strategy to restore her preoperative mental status?

a. Prescribe an antidepressant
b. Prescribe an anxiolytic
c. Reinstitute an AED, such as valproate
d. Install a vagus nerve stimulator

Answer: c. Following neurosurgical removal of a seizure focus in the temporal lobe, many patients experience postoperative psychiatric complications, particularly personality changes and depression. Psychosis sometimes emerges, but usually only if seizures recur. Although this patient probably is not experiencing seizures, a mood-stabilizing AED would probably re-establish her equilibrium.

TIAs and Strokes

Transient ischemic attacks (TIAs) and *strokes* (or *cerebrovascular accidents [CVAs]*) cause readily recognizable constellations of transient or permanent neurologic deficits. Well-informed psychiatrists should be able to recognize their physical manifestations and anticipate their most common accompanying neuropsychologic manifestations, including amnesia, dementia, depression, and altered levels of consciousness. Psychiatrists should also be able to distinguish TIAs and strokes from related conditions, such as brain tumors, that produce similar clinical manifestations.

TRANSIENT ISCHEMIC ATTACKS

As the name suggests, TIAs are temporary interruptions in cerebral circulation that give rise to neurologic deficits. TIAs typically last from 30 to 60 minutes. Although about 10% of TIAs last up to 4 hours, many that last longer than 1 hour represent the onset of a stroke. Most result from platelet emboli arising from the inner surface of atherosclerotic, stenotic, and ulcerated plaques in the *extracranial arteries* that comprise the cerebral blood supply: the carotid and vertebral arteries and the aorta. When an embolus courses through a cerebral artery, it interrupts circulation and induces ischemia. Cardiac arrhythmias and other causes of hypotension also produce TIAs.

Not only do TIAs cause neurologic deficits, they also herald underlying atherosclerotic cerebrovascular disease and increased risk of sustaining stroke (see later). TIAs lead to strokes when either an atherosclerotic plaque throws off a large embolus that permanently blocks a "downstream" cerebral artery or a plaque grows large enough to occlude an extracerebral vessel.

TIAs mimic other transient neurologic conditions, particularly partial seizures, postictal confusion and (Todd's) hemiparesis, migraine, and metabolic aberrations. In addition, when they produce aphasia or another neuropsychologic deficit but no physical deficit, TIAs mimic psychogenic episodes.

Carotid Artery TIAs

Platelet emboli that form on plaques at the common carotid artery bifurcation (Fig. 11-1) lead to cerebral hemisphere TIAs. These TIAs are characterized by (contralateral) hemiparesis, hemisensory loss, paresthesias, or hemianopsia. In addition, because the ophthalmic artery is the first branch of the internal carotid artery, emboli that flow into the ophthalmic artery can cause several minutes of visual obscuration or blindness in that eye. Patients with this distinctive symptom—*amaurosis fugax* (Greek, fleeting darkness) or transient blindness—typically describe a "blanket of gray" descending slowly in front of one eye (Table 11-1). However, TIAs rarely cause headache.

Between TIAs, patients typically appear to be normal. However, occasionally auscultation over the carotid artery bifurcation reveals a harsh systolic sound (*bruit*) that suggests carotid artery stenosis or at least atherosclerotic cerebrovascular disease. Retinal emboli (Hollenhorst plaques) of atheromatous material, which are observable on funduscopy, strongly suggest carotid artery stenosis.

Carotid artery TIAs often induce neuropsychologic aberrations that may be unaccompanied by hemiparesis or other physical impairments. For example, dominant hemisphere TIAs may suddenly, but briefly, cause aphasia. Similarly, nondominant hemisphere TIAs may cause brief hemi-inattention (see Chapter 8).

TIAs in patients with pre-existing early stage Alzheimer's disease may convert a mild, compensated intellectual impairment into a brief but marked confusional state. A similar episode may occur after atherosclerosis slowly occludes one carotid artery forcing the other carotid artery to supply both cerebral hemispheres through the circle of Willis (Fig. 11-2, top right). In this case, emboli from the patent artery produce bilateral cerebral ischemia.

Laboratory Tests

Because TIAs are a precursor for strokes, neurologists test patients for highly stenotic atherosclerotic plaques that might be amenable to correction (see later).

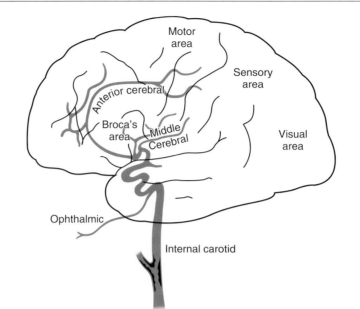

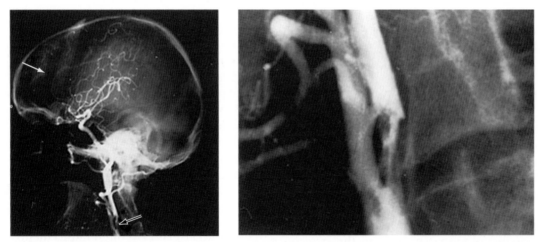

FIGURE 11-1 *Top,* At its bifurcation in the neck, the common carotid artery divides to form the external and internal carotid arteries. Within the skull, the internal carotid artery gives rise to the ophthalmic artery, and then it branches into the anterior and middle cerebral arteries. It also gives rise to the posterior communicating artery—not the posterior cerebral artery. Thus, each internal carotid artery perfuses the ipsilateral eye and most of the ipsilateral cerebral hemisphere. Each *middle cerebral artery* supplies the deep and midsection of the hemisphere that contains most of the motor cortex, sensory cortex, and, in the dominant hemisphere, the language arc (see Fig. 8-1). Each *anterior cerebral artery* supplies the frontal lobe, including the medial surface of the motor cortex, which contains the motor innervation for the leg (see Fig. 7-6). The *posterior cerebral arteries* (not pictured) originate from the basilar artery and supply the occipital and most of the temporal lobes. *Bottom left,* An arteriogram of the carotid artery and its branches prominently displays the bifurcation (*closed arrowhead*), the typical "candelabra" of branches of the middle cerebral artery rather than a single vessel, and a faint anterior cerebral artery that sweeps from anterior to posterior (*open arrowhead*). *Bottom right,* A magnification of the bifurcation shows that an extensive circumferential plaque constricts the internal carotid artery. The remaining blood flow appears as an "apple core." The rough interior surface of the artery gives rise to retinal and cerebral emboli.

Ultrasound (Doppler and duplex) studies, which can measure blood flow and show artery structure, are a generally reliable technique for detecting carotid artery stenosis. The traditional, definitive diagnostic procedure has been arteriography (angiography). However, because it requires catheterization of an artery followed by injection of iodinated contrast material this procedure may cause a stroke or other serious complications. Magnetic resonance imaging angiography (MRA), which has been supplanting traditional arteriography, readily permits noninvasive observation of extra- and intracerebral vessels (see Chapter 20).

Computed tomography (CT) is often an acceptable test; however, magnetic resonance imaging (MRI)

TABLE 11-1 ■ Carotid Artery TIAs

Symptoms
  Contralateral hemiparesis, hemianopsia, hemisensory loss
  Aphasia
  Ipsilateral amaurosis fugax
Associated findings
  Carotid bruit
  Retinal artery emboli
Tests
  Ultrasonography (carotid Doppler and duplex studies)
  Magnetic resonance imaging angiography (MRA)
  Cerebral arteriography
Therapy
  Medical: platelet inhibitors (e.g., aspirin)
  Surgical: carotid endarterectomy, if stenosis >70% and symptomatic

TIAs, transient ischemic attacks.

offers greater resolution and better visualization of posterior fossa structures. Unlike routine MRI sequences, diffusion-weighted MRI sequences can identify ischemic strokes within their initial 48 hours. Depending on the symptoms, a routine evaluation for transient neurologic deficits sometimes includes an electrocardiogram (ECG), a 24-hour study of the cardiac rhythm (Holter monitor), electroencephalogram (EEG), blood glucose determinations, and an evaluation for systemic illness.

Preventative Measures

TIAs not only create troublesome neurologic problems, but they are also one of many risk factors for stroke (see later). In addition, because TIAs and strokes are both manifestations of cerebrovascular disease, they have the same set of risk factors and preventative measures.

One common preventative measure for TIAs is inhibiting platelet aggregation. This strategy reduces the incidence of TIAs by approximately 30%. Common aspirin (one 81-mg tablet daily), on balance, remains the most effective platelet aggregation inhibitor; however, it may induce gastrointestinal bleeding. Other platelet inhibitors, such as clopidogrel (Plavix) or dipyridamole in combination with aspirin (Aggrenox), may hold an advantage for individual patients. Anticoagulation with warfarin (Coumadin) is suitable for patients with atrial fibrillation, mitral stenosis, and certain other cardiac conditions, but rarely for TIAs in the absence of such conditions.

Carotid endarterectomy is an invasive, delicate procedure in which surgeons briefly open the carotid artery to remove atherosclerotic plaque. Although effective, it is dangerous because the cerebral blood supply may be briefly interrupted or pieces of the plaque may fly into the cerebral circulation and cause a stroke. Nevertheless, carotid endarterectomy or another corrective procedure, such as a stent (see later), is indicated for patients with carotid artery TIA symptoms whose arteriography, MRA, or ultrasound study shows at least 70% carotid artery stenosis. A corrective procedure for asymptomatic individuals with comparably severe carotid stenosis may also be indicated, but the criteria remain uncertain. No procedure is feasible for complete occlusion of the artery.

An alternative to endarterectomy is intravascular insertion of perforated tubes (stents) that are expanded at atherosclerotic obstructions (see Fig. 20-28). Stents are suitable for correcting stenosis of vertebral and, in experimental circumstances, intracerebral arteries, as well as stenosis of the carotid arteries. They serve as permanently implanted tubular scaffolding that preserves arterial blood flow. Also, by securing underlying atheromatous debris against the inner surface of arterial walls, they reduce the likelihood of emboli flying from a large to small artery and causing a stroke. Placing a stent, which is performed under local anesthesia, carries less risk than an endarterectomy. Already widely used, stents have an established safety record in correcting coronary artery disease and abdominal aneurysms.

Basilar Artery TIAs

The two vertebral arteries join to form the basilar artery at the undersurface of the brain. This group of vessels, which is usually called the *vertebrobasilar system*, *basilar artery system*, or simply the *posterior circulation*, supplies the brainstem, cerebellum, and the posterior-inferior portion of the cerebrum (the occipital and medial-inferior portion of the temporal lobes [see Fig. 11-2]). Emboli-generating plaques tend to develop at both the origin of the vertebral arteries (in the chest) and their junction.

Symptoms and signs of basilar artery TIAs, which usually result from patchy brainstem ischemia, are distinctly different from those of carotid artery TIAs (Table 11-2). Typical basilar artery TIA symptoms include tingling around the mouth (circumoral paresthesias), dysarthria, nystagmus, ataxia, and vertigo. On rare occasions, when all blood flow through the basilar artery momentarily stops, the entire brainstem becomes ischemic. The brainstem ischemia interrupts consciousness and body tone, which causes patients to collapse. This TIA, termed a *drop attack*, strikes suddenly and unexpectedly. (It appears similar to cataplexy [see Chapter 17].)

Vertigo represents one of the most characteristic symptoms of basilar artery TIAs. As a medical

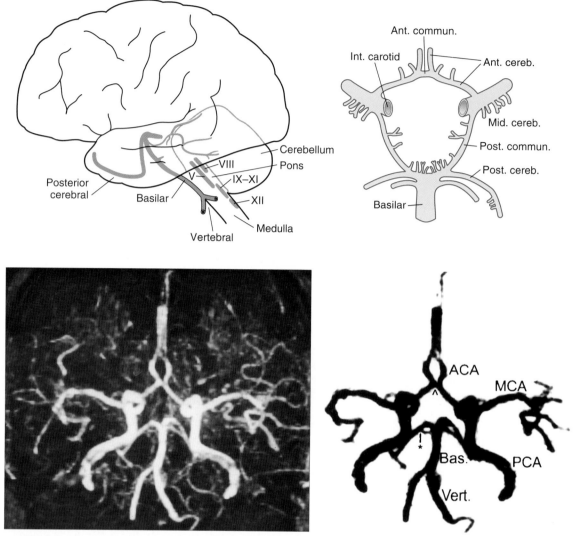

FIGURE 11-2 *Top left,* After ascending encased in the cervical vertebrae, the two vertebral arteries enter the skull. They join to form the basilar artery at the base of the brain. Small, delicate branches from the basilar artery supply the brainstem. (The Roman numerals refer to cranial nerve nuclei.) Large branches, as if wrapping their arms around the brainstem, supply the cerebellum and posterior portion of the cerebrum (i.e., the occipital lobes and inferomedial portions of the temporal lobes). The posterior cerebral arteries are, for practical purposes, the terminal branches of the basilar artery. They supply the occipital cortex and the posterior, inferior aspect of the temporal lobes. *Top right,* The circle of Willis, the "great anastomoses," is completely patent only in only about 20% of people. It is formed by connections between the basilar and internal carotid arteries, and gives off the anterior, middle, and posterior cerebral arteries. The circle also potentially provides anastomoses between anterior-posterior and right-left cerebral circulations. Although the circle confers advantages, junctions of the arteries are weak spots. Defects may balloon outward, form berry aneurysms, rupture, and produce subarachnoid hemorrhages. *Bottom left,* This axial MRA shows the major cerebral arteries that form the circle of Willis and anterior and posterior circulations. *Bottom right,* This rendition of the MRA image highlights the major cerebral arteries. The anterior circulation consists primarily of the middle cerebral (MCA), and anterior cerebral (ACA) arteries. The anterior communicating artery (^) joins the ACAs. The posterior circulation consists primarily of the two vertebral (Vert.), basilar (Bas.), posterior communicating (*), and the posterior cerebral arteries (PCA).

symptom, vertigo means a sensation of the patient or the surroundings revolving or otherwise moving. The thoughtful physician should accept no other descriptions. In particular, the common complaint of "dizziness" has no clinical value because it can also mean imbalance, lightheadedness, anxiety, confusion, impending trouble, or psychologic decompensation.

The evaluation of basilar artery symptoms typically includes—as with carotid artery symptoms evaluation—ultrasound evaluation, MRA, and evaluation for cardiac and systemic illness. In addition, a transcranial Doppler examination, which harmlessly penetrates the skull, may portray the vertebrobasilar system's architecture. Neurologists rely on the same

TABLE 11-2 ■ Vertebrobasilar Artery TIAs

Symptoms
   Vertigo, vomiting, tinnitus
   Circumoral paresthesias or numbness
   Dysarthria, dysphagia
   Transient global amnesia
   Drop attacks
Associated findings
   Nystagmus
   Ataxia
   Cranial nerve abnormalities
Tests
   Ultrasonography (transcranial Doppler studies)
   Magnetic resonance imaging angiography (MRA)
   Cerebral arteriography
Therapy
   Medical: platelet inhibitors (aspirin)
   Surgical: none

TIAs, transient ischemic attacks.

medications used for carotid artery TIAs. Because the usual sites of vertebrobasilar stenosis remain shielded by the chest, vertebrae, and skull, an endarterectomy would not be feasible. However, stents can be inserted through critical stenoses to restore normal blood flow and reduce the chance of a stroke.

Transient Global Amnesia

TIAs sometimes impair the circulation of the basilar artery's terminal branches, the posterior cerebral arteries, that supply the temporal lobes (see Fig. 11-2). Because the temporal lobes contain portions of the limbic system (see Fig. 16-5), these TIAs cause episodes of temporal lobe ischemia that induce temporary amnesia and personality change—called *transient global amnesia* (*TGA*). Although, migraine, partial complex seizures, metabolic aberrations, and drug intoxications have been suggested as alternative etiologies for TGA, the most likely remains a basilar artery TIA.

A suddenly developing period of amnesia is the cardinal feature of TGA. During an attack, patients cannot memorize or learn new information, such as a sequence of digits, that is, they have *anterograde amnesia*. In addition, they cannot recall recently acquired information, such as the events of the last several hours or days, that is, they also have *retrograde amnesia*. Patients typically do not know how they came to the physician's office or the emergency room. Their recall of other recent events is also filled with gaps. They lose track of their responses during an interview by a physician, who may have to be reintroduced several times during the examination.

As a secondary aspect, some patients understandably become perplexed, distraught, or even agitated.

Unable to comprehend their situation, they may panic. Some patients, as if recoiling, appear apathetic and immobile.

TGAs typically occur in middle aged and older individuals who are apt to have cerebrovascular disease. They typically develop in the midst of frightening events or physical exertion, particularly sexual activity—coincidences that might erroneously lead to various psychologic interpretations. After its abrupt onset, TGA lasts for 3 to 24 hours, with its intensity most pronounced during the initial 1 to 2 hours. By definition, the total duration must not exceed 24 hours. The recurrence rate is about 10%.

In contrast to their amnesia for recently learned facts, TGA patients characteristically retain their general knowledge and fundamental personal information. For example, they are typically able to recite their name, address, telephone number, and occupation. TGA patients may also be able to perform complex tasks that were learned before the TGA. (All this preserved memory contradicts the term *global* in TGA.)

Even without a confirmatory laboratory test for TGA, its clinical features differentiate it from other conditions. Although physicians might be tempted to label a distraught patient with no recall of recent, sometimes distressing events, as having a psychiatric disturbance, TGA patients' retention of fundamental personal information distinguishes them from individuals with dissociative amnesia and other psychiatric disturbances (see later). In addition, their preserved intellect and general knowledge, as well as their remaining fully conscious, distinguishes them from individuals with delirium. TGA patients, despite their amnesia, also do not confabulate in the manner of Wernicke-Korsakoff patients. Because their motor system is completely spared, they walk and talk normally—making TGA a prime example of a transient mental disturbance unaccompanied by physical deficits. Of the conditions that most closely mimic a TGA, partial complex seizures differ by producing dulling of the sensorium, simple repetitive actions, paroxysmal or other epileptiform EEG changes, and a high rate of recurrence (see Chapter 10).

In contrast, *Dissociative Amnesia*, as described in the *Diagnostic and Statistical Manual of Mental Disorders, 4th Edition, Text Revision (DSM-IV-TR)*, consists of one or more episodes of amnesia for fundamental personal information "usually of a traumatic or stressful nature." The amnesia might be highly selective regarding prior events and not include an anterograde component. For example, individuals who just survived a devastating earthquake might develop dissociative amnesia. Thus, dissociative amnesia may partly overlap acute and post-traumatic stress disorders.

In a related DSM-IV-TR disorder, *Dissociative Fugue*, previously called *Psychogenic Fugue*, individuals travel away from home or work. Sometimes they assume a new identity. As a secondary aspect of this disorder, they seem to be amnestic for personal information concerning their past life. Although having retrograde amnesia, they have no anterograde amnesia. In other words, once their new location or personality is established, they are able to recall the new relevant information, but have forgotten their history. They may not recall, for example, previous spouses, debts, or crimes.

STROKES (CEREBROVASCULAR ACCIDENTS)

Strokes cause permanent physical and neuropsychologic deficits. Most result from an arterial thrombosis, embolus, or hemorrhage that disrupt cerebral blood flow.

Risk Factors

Reflecting the necessity of preventing strokes, innumerable studies have investigated risk factors for stroke. They are numerous, replicate to a certain extent those for myocardial infarction, have different statistical strength in their association with each other as well as with stroke, and, in some cases, are modifiable.

The most powerful risk factor for stroke is age older than 65 years, after which the incidence of strokes rises almost exponentially. Yet, about 25% of stroke victims are younger than 65 years and some are children and young adults (Table 11-3).

Hypertension, the other, frequently occurring major risk factor, leads to strokes in the victims younger than 65 years, as well as in those older than 65

TABLE 11-3 ■ Risk Factors for Strokes in Children and Young Adults

Antiphospholipid syndrome
Cardiac disease*
Drug abuse
Homocystinuria
Migraine^
Mitochondrial disorders+
Sickle cell disease and other blood dyscrasias
Vasculitis and congenital vascular malformations

*Mitral stenosis and other valvular abnormalities, congenital defects, and arrhythmias predispose to strokes.
^The incidence of strokes is increased only in migraine with aura and hemiplegic migraine.
+Strokes are an integral part of mitochondrial encephalopathy, lactic acidosis, and stroke-like episodes (MELAS) and other mitochondrial disorders (see Chapter 6).

years. It is also probably the cause of most cases of stroke-induced dementia (see vascular dementia later). Hypertension—both systolic and diastolic—is associated with both thrombotic and hemorrhagic strokes. Increasingly widespread treatment of hypertension has led to a steady decline, since 1915, in stroke-related deaths in the United States. (On the other hand, antihypertensive medications may have bothersome side effects [see later].)

As previously mentioned, TIAs are a risk factor for stroke. Within the first year following a TIA, approximately 12% of patients develop a stroke. Each year thereafter, an additional 5% develop a stroke.

Various cardiac conditions—valvular disease, prosthetic valves, acute myocardial infarction, and atrial fibrillation—comprise another risk factor because they tend to produce thromboses on valves and endocardial surfaces that embolize to the brain and elsewhere. Treatment with an anticoagulant, such as warfarin (Coumadin), in patients with any of these risk factors greatly reduces the incidence of embolic stroke.

Diabetes mellitus and elevated total cholesterol are powerful risk factors for myocardial infarction but less so for stroke. For individuals younger than 45 years, elevated cholesterol has no association with stroke, and for all individuals, only cholesterol levels greater than 300 mg/mL are a risk for stroke. Nevertheless, cholesterol-lowering statins, but not dietary interventions, reduce the incidence of strokes and TIAs in individuals with elevated cholesterol.

Cigarette smoking conveys a grave risk for stroke that has been overshadowed by its other hazards. Compared to nonsmokers, former cigarette smokers retain an almost two-fold greater risk of stroke, and active cigarette smokers have a four-fold greater risk. More striking, smokers who are hypertensive have a 20-fold greater risk. Although judicious alcohol drinking (one drink daily to weekly) provides a slight protective effect, heavy alcohol intake poses a risk.

Migraine—in general—represents a risk factor of minor influence. Moreover, any increased risk is probably restricted to migraineurs who smoke, use oral contraceptives, or have headaches with aura. Drug abuse frequently causes strokes through intravenous injection of particulate material, episodes of anoxia and hypotension, cerebral vasculitis, hypertension, and vasospasm. For example, amphetamines, cocaine, ecstasy, and pseudoephedrine are sympathomimetic stimulants that induce bursts of hypertension and prolonged arterial vasospasm that lead to stroke or myocardial infarction (see Chapter 21). In particular, cocaine alkaloid ("crack cocaine") notoriously leads to cerebral hemorrhage; however, marijuana intoxication or chronic use is not associated with strokes. Studies have also implicated over-the-counter medicines, including weight-loss pills, cough suppressants, and sympathomimetic stimulants, such as phenylpropanolamine and ephedra. Because of their association with strokes, the Food and Drug Administration (FDA) has banned many of them.

Estrogen, when used alone as hormone replacement, slightly increases the stroke risk for postmenopausal women. In contrast, the danger from oral contraceptives is probably restricted to the original, high-dose estrogen preparations. Currently available low-dose estrogen preparations confer only a negligible risk for stroke.

Recent studies have revealed that elevated concentration of homocysteine, which is an amino acid that normally circulates in the blood, either increases the risk of stroke or serves as marker for an increased risk. In the autosomal recessive genetically determined condition, *homocystinuria,* children develop with a Marfan-like habitus, ocular lens displacement, and other anatomic abnormalities. More important, they routinely suffer strokes in childhood (see Table 11-3). Elevated homocysteine levels in adults are associated with use of antiepileptic drugs and coronary artery and peripheral vascular disease, as well as stroke. Elevated levels increase the risk of stroke as much as cigarette smoking. Although folic acid supplements reduce elevated serum homocysteine concentrations (see Fig. 5-8) and probably reduce the incidence of neural tube defects, studies so far do not show that they reduce the incidence of strokes.

Most risk factors discussed so far relate to atherosclerosis as the major underlying etiology for stroke. However, some data suggest that vascular inflammation or infection gives rise to strokes. For example, C-reactive protein (CRP), which serves as a serum protein marker for inflammation, roughly parallels the cholesterol concentration; however, the two markers are not identical and CRP has the stronger association with strokes. In addition, antiphospholipid and anticardiolipin antibodies predispose patients to various complications of a hypercoagulable state, including venous thrombosis, miscarriage, and migraine, as well as stroke, in the *antiphospholipid syndrome.* Other, compelling data that link stroke with vascular inflammation, independent of other risk factors, shows that severe periodontal disease presages stroke, at least in men and those younger than 60 years. Not only does this association point to a nonatherosclerotic etiology of stroke but it also illustrates a treatable risk factor.

Pregnancy itself is not associated with a significantly increased incidence of common, ischemic strokes. However, several pregnancy- or delivery-related problems, such as eclampsia, cortical vein thrombosis, and ruptured aneurysms, may lead to stroke-like brain damage. During the first six postpartum weeks, however, the risk of thrombotic and hemorrhagic strokes rises multiple times.

Among elderly patients with dementia, atypical and typical antipsychotic agents carry the same, slightly increased, stroke risk compared to a placebo. The risk prompted a "black box warning" on the package insert.

Some studies have also proposed psychologic distress, depressive symptoms, anger, and negative emotions as stroke risk factors. Also, some life-styles known to carry an increased stroke and myocardial infarction risk—cigarette smoking, heavy alcohol drinking, and lack of exercise—may reflect underlying psychiatric disturbances. On the other hand, some data suggest that psychologic distress predicts only fatal—not nonfatal—ischemic strokes and that "Type A" personality does not convey a risk factor for strokes. In any case, studies have failed to prove that altering these psychologic factors reduces the risk of stroke.

With these factors in mind, individuals could optimize their chance of avoiding a stroke (and myocardial infarction) simply by first controlling their blood pressure, stopping tobacco and excessive alcohol use, and exercising. Most individuals would probably also profit by taking low-dose aspirin or another antiplatelet agent. If their cholesterol were elevated, they should take a statin in addition to modifying their diet, and, if their homocysteine were elevated, folic acid. They may also be able to modify other risk factors.

Thrombosis and Embolus

Thrombosis, a clot that propagates within an atherosclerotic extracranial or intracerebral artery and simply occludes it, causes the majority of strokes. Because it interrupts the blood supply and deprives the "downstream" brain of oxygen, a thrombosis leads to *ischemic stroke.*

Another cause of an ischemic stroke is an embolus from the heart, extracranial artery, or intracranial artery that lodges in a cerebral artery. When the source of the embolus is an artery, this stroke is termed an *arterial-arterial embolus.* Other causes of thrombosis and embolism include vasculitis, drug abuse, sickle-cell disease, and other blood dyscrasias. In short, the most frequent causes of strokes consist of abnormalities of the heart, blood vessels, or blood.

On a cellular level, ischemic strokes lead to cell death by *necrosis.* Although this process requires no cellular energy, the necrotic debris elicits a cellular inflammatory response. Necrosis also takes place in brain injury, brain tumors, and many other insults. In contrast, cell death by *apoptosis,* which requires cellular energy and does not evoke an inflammatory response, takes place in amyotrophic lateral sclerosis (ALS), Huntington's disease, and many other neuro-degenerative diseases. Also unlike necrosis, apoptosis is a stage of normal development for some organs, such as the thymus.

Infarctions in the Carotid Artery Distribution

Cerebral artery thrombosis and embolism produce cerebral infarction in the distribution of the artery that creates well-known patterns of clinical deficits (see Fig. 11-1 and Table 11-4).

- *Anterior* cerebral artery infarction damages the anterior and medial aspects of the frontal lobe. It typically causes paresis and apraxia of the con-tralateral leg. With bilateral anterior cerebral ar-tery infarctions, the resulting extensive frontal lobe damage causes pseudobulbar palsy, apathy, mutism, urinary incontinence, and the other signs of frontal lobe dysfunction (see Chapter 7), along with motor impairment of both legs.
- *Middle* cerebral artery infarction, which is the most common, results in contralateral hemipar-esis, hemisensory loss, aphasia with dominant hemisphere lesions, and hemi-inattention with nondominant hemisphere strokes.

TABLE 11-4 ■ Common Manifestations of Strokes

Carotid artery
  Anterior cerebral
    Contralateral lower extremity paresis
    Mutism, apathy, pseudobulbar palsy*
  Middle cerebral
    Contralateral hemiparesis
    Hemisensory loss
    Aphasia
    Hemi-inattention
  Posterior cerebral
    Contralateral homonymous hemianopsia
    Alexia without agraphia
Vertebrobasilar system
  Basilar artery
    Total occlusion
      Coma
      Locked-in syndrome^
    Occlusion of branch
      Cranial nerve palsy with contralateral hemiparesis^
      Internuclear ophthalmoplegia^
  Vertebral artery
    Lateral medullary (Wallenberg's) syndrome^

---

*With bilateral infarctions.
^No cognitive impairment.

Although the geography of the lesions determines their neurologic deficits, the time course suggests whether they have originated in an embolus or a thrombosis. Cerebral emboli-induced infarctions de-velop suddenly as the embolus lodges in a cerebral vessel. Usually deficits are maximal at the onset of the stroke and resolve over the next several days. Cerebral thromboses, in contrast, generally develop slowly or intermittently, begin during sleep, and are relatively painless. The majority of the deficits are permanent. With both embolic and thrombotic strokes, the region surrounding the infarction becomes edematous. During the third to fifth days, when edema is most severe, neurologic deficits are most pronounced. Some clinical recovery occurs as the edema resolves; however, the infarction remains a functionless scar.

Moreover, CVA scars are potentially epileptogenic. Approximately 50% of seizures that develop in adults older than 65 years originate from strokes (see Chapter 10). Thus, in patients with cerebrovascular disease, a brief episode of confusion or unresponsive-ness may result from a TIA, TGA, or partial complex seizure.

Infarctions in the Basilar Artery Distribution

Infarctions in the basilar artery distribution cause brainstem, cerebellar, or posterior cerebral injuries. In contrast to cerebral hemisphere infarctions, brain-stem infarctions generally do not cause language or intellectual impairment (see Table 11-4). Small brain-stem infarctions usually cause constellations of cranial nerve injuries and hemiparesis. Large ones usually cause coma, if not immediate death.

The posterior cerebral arteries, as previously noted, are really branches of the basilar artery. Infarction of a posterior cerebral artery causes a contralateral homonymous hemianopsia and occasionally alexia without agraphia (see Chapter 8). Bilateral posterior cerebral artery strokes can cause (cortical) blindness (see Chapter 12).

Precise localization of small brainstem infarctions is often desirable for both clinical and academic reasons. Lesions of the midbrain cause ipsilateral oculomotor nerve and contralateral paresis (see Fig. 4-9). Pontine lesions cause ipsilateral abducens nerve and contralat-eral paresis (see Fig. 4-11). Midline pons or midbrain infarctions cause the medial longitudinal syndrome (MLF) syndrome (see Chapters 12 and 15). Finally, lateral medullary infarctions, which are the most com-mon brainstem infarction, cause ipsilateral limb ataxia, palatal paresis, Horner's syndrome, and alternating hypalgesia (see Wallenberg's syndrome, Fig. 2-10).

The clinical implication of localization indicates that if the lesion is situated in the brainstem, the patient's mental function will remain intact. For example, a patient with right hemiparesis and a left sixth cranial nerve palsy is unlikely to have aphasia.

Hemorrhages

Cerebral or cerebellar hemorrhages typically occur abruptly and, because of increased intracranial pressure, produce headaches, nausea, and vomiting. Patients usually lose consciousness and have profound neurologic deficits determined by the hemorrhage's location. One special example is the *cerebellar hemorrhage* because it rapidly leads to compression of the fourth ventricle, which causes obstructive hydrocephalus, and then compression of the brainstem, which leads to depressed respiratory drive and coma. Physicians can diagnose cerebellar hemorrhage by its clinical characteristics—occipital headache, gait ataxia, dysarthria, and lethargy. Once the diagnosis is confirmed, neurosurgeons usually should immediately evacuate it.

Hemorrhages, which are most often the result of hypertension, usually erupt in the basal ganglia, thalamus, and pons, as well as the cerebellum (see Figs. 20-13 and 20-14). Sympathomimetic drugs, such as crack cocaine, also cause hemorrhages, but their location is not as predictable as with hypertension. Another example closely related to sympathomimetic drugs causing cerebral hemorrhage is the patient who takes an antidepressant monamine oxidase inhibitor and then inadvertently receives certain foodstuffs, such as aged cheese, meperidine (Demerol), or red wine (see Chapter 9).

Treatment options, other than supportive care, are limited. However, neurologists and neurosurgeons have recently introduced coagulant factors and stereotactic drainage to halt bleeding and evacuate hematomas.

When not caused by trauma, *subarachnoid hemorrhage (SAH)* usually results from a ruptured berry aneurysm (a balloon-like dilation of an artery). It most often causes a prostrating headache and nuchal rigidity, but not necessarily any physical deficits. Sexual activity, straining at stool, and other usually benign exertion can rupture an aneurysm and precipitate a SAH. Sometimes a SAH mimics coital cephalalgia or a migraine (see Chapter 9). However, when an aneurysm ruptures, CT, even more reliably than MRI, usually reveals blood in the subarachnoid space at the base of the brain or within the ventricles. Also, a lumbar puncture yields bloody or xanthochromic (yellow) cerebrospinal fluid (CSF).

The traditional treatment has consisted of a craniotomy to clamp the neck of the aneurysm. Even for aneurysms located in accessible positions, surgery was fraught with complications, including rupture of an aneurysm that had only been leaking and inadvertent occlusion of the parent vessel. Current treatment options now include intravascular insertion of coils and "glues" that trigger clotting within the aneurysm and other minimally invasive procedures.

NEUROPSYCHOLOGIC SEQUELAE

Vascular dementia, often labeled *multi-infarct dementia*, represents a moderate but unknown proportion of cases of dementia. However, not only do Alzheimer's disease and its relative, dementia with Lewy bodies (see Chapter 7), represent a much greater proportion of cases of dementia, but the majority of individuals with vascular dementia have comorbid Alzheimer's disease.

Among risk factors for vascular dementia, pre-existing cognitive impairment—from Alzheimer's disease or other dementia-producing illness—is foremost. Similarly, depression, whether it preceded the stroke or developed only after it struck, is another powerful risk factor for vascular dementia.

In addition, several stroke-related mechanisms may lead to vascular dementia. In the most common one, strokes simply obliterate large areas of brain tissue. In this situation, dementia develops without regard to the extent or location of the strokes. Sometimes, in another mechanism, several small strokes strike strategic regions of the brain. Another common mechanism consists of hypertension-induced multiple small subcortical strokes or *lacunes*. In this condition, numerous 0.5- to 1.5-cm scars in the white matter and other regions of the brain produce the *état lacunaire*, also labeled *Binswanger's disease*.

Vascular dementia is typically accompanied by focal neurologic deficits, such as hemiparesis, dysarthria, clumsiness, and gait impairment. Sometimes signs of frontal lobe injury—apathy, emotional instability, impaired executive ability, incontinence, and pseudobulbar palsy—often overshadow the intellectual impairment. Gait impairment is so prominent that it places most cases of vascular dementia in the subcortical dementia category (see Chapter 7). If a clinician were asked to distinguish between Alzheimer's disease and vascular dementia, the diagnostic value of focal neurologic deficits would far outweigh the nature and severity of cognitive deficits. Also, although delusions and, less frequently, hallucinations complicate both conditions, depression is more common in vascular dementia.

Another important, although not pathognomonic, feature of vascular dementia is that neurologic function deteriorates in a stepwise pattern. Presumably, an irregular succession of strokes progressively adds physical and cognitive impairments.

In evaluating a patient for vascular dementia, CT and MRI can reveal cerebral infarcts and other signs of cerebrovascular disease. Although rarely necessary, positron emission tomography (PET) and single positron emission computed tomography (SPECT) show multiple, almost random hypometabolic regions in vascular dementia. In contrast, hypometabolism in Alzheimer's disease involves the temporal and parietal association cortex regions and eventually the frontal lobes.

Cholinesterase inhibitors (see Chapter 7) seem to retard the progression or actually reduce the severity of vascular dementia. Their benefit, however, might be attributable to their effect on the portion of the dementia that represents comorbid Alzheimer's disease.

The *DSM-IV-TR* criteria for Vascular Dementia, previously called Multi-Infarct Dementia, reproduce those for Alzheimer's disease dementia, but also require either focal neurologic signs or laboratory evidence, presumably by CT or MRI, of cerebrovascular disease that can explain the dementia. Unlike the criteria in previous editions, vascular dementia's characteristic stepwise, often abrupt, course is no longer required.

Other Neuropsychologic Sequelae

Well-known, stroke-induced specific neuropsychologic disturbances are manifestations of strokes in critical areas of the cerebral cortex. As previously discussed, dominant hemisphere lesions may, for example, cause aphasia, Gerstmann syndrome, or apraxia. Nondominant ones may cause hemi-inattention and forms of apraxia (see Chapter 8). Bilateral frontal lobe lesions may cause pseudobulbar palsy and frontal lobe dysfunction.

Infarctions of the large areas of the cerebral cortex tenuously perfused at the periphery of the cerebrovascular perfusion network, the *watershed areas*, produce other, more extensive or more variable neuropsychologic deficits. Watershed areas are vulnerable because delicate terminal branches of the cerebral arteries provide a tenuous blood supply. Episodes of severe anoxia, hypotension, carbon monoxide poisoning, or similar insult often reduce the blood supply and produce a *watershed infarction*. Depending on the infarction's extent and severity, patients are often left with dementia, a persistent vegetative state (PVS), cortical blindness, or, sparing the perisylvian language arc because it is relatively well-perfused, isolation aphasia (see Chapter 8).

Depression

Most studies find that between 30% and 50% of stroke patients display symptoms of depression, ranging from minor disturbances in mood to those of a major depression. In all its varieties, depressive symptoms follow stroke more frequently than they follow either a medical illness or orthopedic injury that produces similar disabilities. Neurologists loosely diagnose all depression symptoms following a stroke as *poststroke depression*. Psychiatrists may use the roughly comparable DSM-IV-TR term, Mood Disorder due to a General Medical Condition.

In its mildest form, depressive symptoms—sadness, psychic slowness, lack of energy, and impaired concentration—affect about 40% of patients at 6 months after their stroke. Compared to nondepressed patients, these patients have greater neurologic deficits and more frequently a prehospitalization history of dementia or depression. Once 3 years have elapsed, these symptoms have remitted on about 80% of patients. However, about one third of patients with minor poststroke depression go on to develop major depression.

With or without preceding minor depression, the incidence of major depression peaks at 3 to 6 months after a stroke and has a mean duration of 6 to 9 months. Although the majority of depressed patients enjoy a remission within the year, 30% remain depressed at 1 year and 20% at 3 years.

Risk factors for poststroke depression begin with the usual risk factors for depression, such as a history of depression, close family member with depression, and ill health. In addition, several risk factors reflect the severity of stroke-induced deficits, particularly the degree of paresis, functional impairment, curtailed activities of daily living (ADLs), and neuropsychologic deficits, such as cognitive impairment and aphasia. Poststroke depression also correlates with crying, more so than apathy, immediately after the stroke and young age of onset.

On the other hand, physicians might confuse some stroke-induced symptoms with depression. For example, patients with a nondominant hemisphere stroke may deny having a hemiparesis because of anosognosia and lose their ability to express or comprehend emotions because of aprosody (see Chapter 8). Strokes—individually or in succession—that damage both frontal lobes frequently result in apathy, pathologic crying and emotional incontinence because of pseudobulbar palsy (see Chapter 4), and a paucity of verbal output (abulia, see Chapter 7). Following several strokes, patients often develop sleep disturbances and vegetative symptoms.

Similarly, medical care may produce complications that mimic depression. For example, some medications—beta-blockers, diuretics, and antiepileptic drugs—routinely administered to stroke patients may induce mood changes or cognitive impairment. Also, sleep deprivation, uncomfortable or painful procedures, and psychologic factors, such as disorientation, fear, and isolation, may express themselves as changes in mood.

Patients with these neurologic or iatrogenic conditions that mimic depression might have coexisting, but hidden, poststroke depression. An astute physician can discern the various components of the patient's illness and then treat them.

Several recent studies have challenged the classic notion that strokes in the left frontal lobe most often cause depression. These studies report equally strong correlations between depression and lesions in the right as well as the left cerebral hemisphere, and in the basal ganglia, thalamus, and other subcortical structures. Overall, they show little or no relationship between poststroke depression and lesion localization or even laterality.

Whatever its associations or underlying cause, poststroke depression carries several serious consequences. Depressed stroke patients do not fully participate in their rehabilitation programs. They fail to optimize their remaining motor, cognitive, and language functions. They preserve fewer ADLs. Conversely, physicians might investigate patients for depression if they "underachieve" in rehabilitation programs.

Despite the rationale and some studies that support treatment of depressed stroke patients with antidepressants, psychotherapy, or electroconvulsive therapy (ECT), rigorously derived evidence is lacking. Although few or imperfect, studies have described successful treatment of poststroke depression with tricyclic antidepressants, selective serotonin reuptake inhibitors, psychostimulants (especially in the elderly), and ECT. In addition, some studies have reported improved cognitive function accompanying resolution of poststroke depression. Although ECT may cause more confusion than usual in stroke victims, it is safe in poststroke depression.

Other Psychiatric Complications

In contrast to the frequent occurrence of poststroke depression, mania following a stroke rarely occurs. Moreover, when mania follows a stroke, its characteristics and underlying pathology are poorly understood.

Approximately 25% of stroke patients, particularly women and younger patients, have anxiety. Of them, the majority has comorbid depression. Even without comorbid depression, poststroke anxiety impairs function and rehabilitation, persists for years, and diminishes long-term outcome. As with the other poststroke psychiatric comorbidities, the anxiety has no consistent clinical-anatomic correlation.

Delusions, hallucinations, and other symptoms of psychosis also rarely develop after a stroke. When such symptoms develop, they typically reflect pre-existing dementia. However, patients with anosognosia following a nondominant hemisphere stroke constitute a potential exception. Sometimes, unconsciously going to extraordinary lengths to deny their deficits, they employ confabulation, delusions, and irrational explanations. Moreover, if physicians confront them with their disability, patients may have a catastrophic psychologic reaction.

ALTERED LEVELS OF CONSCIOUSNESS

Strokes and many other conditions frequently depress the patient's level of consciousness. Neurologists usually describe the levels of consciousness, in descending order, as *alert, lethargic, stuporous,* or *comatose.* Not to belabor the obvious, but alert patients are characteristically awake and have their eyes open. Being alert is a prerequisite—but not a guarantee—for the essential human qualities of awareness, cognitive status, and emotional capability. Moreover, being alert reflects an underlying, well-functioning cerebral cortex, brainstem, and reticular activating system.

Patients who appear alert have not necessarily retained consciousness or their essential human qualities. For example, advanced Alzheimer's disease patients who seem awake and have open eyes may have severe, incapacitating cognitive impairment. Similarly, patients who seem awake and have open eyes may have been reduced by cerebral anoxia or other insult to the PVS and have lost all of their human qualities (see later). In the opposite situation, some patients deprived of all their motor function, such as those in the locked-in syndrome, retain all their human qualities (see later).

In a deeper level of unconsciousness, lethargic patients remain with their eyes closed and appear asleep; however, with stimulation, they open their eyes and temporarily assume an alert state. Even when aroused, these patients are typically inattentive, disoriented, and cognitively impaired.

Although lethargy is a variation of normal, such as when individuals are sleep-deprived, it can also represent the first symptom of diffuse cerebral cortical dysfunction. The most common conditions that cause lethargy and more depressed levels of consciousness include toxic-metabolic aberrations, large destructive lesions, and increased intracranial pressure. These conditions usually damage both cerebral hemispheres; the brainstem, particularly its reticular activating system; or the entire brain.

Whatever its etiology, lethargy may be an aspect of delirium, which neurologists call "toxic-metabolic encephalopathy." In this widespread condition, lethargic patients may have hallucinations, hypervigilance rather than somnolence, and physical agitation.

Compared to lethargy, stupor connotes a more depressed level of consciousness. Stuporous patients remain unarousable with their eyes closed. They respond with only rudimentary motor or verbal responses to verbal or tactile stimuli. Although metabolic aberrations, structural lesions, and increased intracranial pressure can all cause stupor, structural lesions usually also produce lateralized signs, such as hemiparesis.

Coma, which can be graded by the Glasgow Coma Scale (see Chapter 22), is the most profound depression of consciousness. Comatose patients always have closed eyes, make little or no verbal responses, and move their limbs just reflexively. This profound depth of unconsciousness reflects profound disturbance of both cerebral hemispheres or the brainstem.

In practice, these states of depressed levels of consciousness last from several hours, several days, or, at most, several weeks. If the underlying illness spares vital structures, it usually either leaves the patient unscathed or beset by permanent neurologic deficits. Nevertheless, even those patients with widespread neurologic deficits, if they survive, eventually resume the appearance of an alert repose with open eyes. Sometimes the patient returns from coma to the locked-in syndrome, PVS, or minimally responsive state.

Locked-In Syndrome

Among the innumerable patients who have sustained strokes or other structural lesions and appear completely incapacitated, physicians should search for the patient in the *locked-in syndrome*. This rare but important condition describes patients who are mute, quadriplegic, bedridden, and totally dependent on caregivers; however, these patients remain alert, have *intact cognitive capacity*, and can communicate by moving their eyes. In other words, their completely disabled body encases (locks-in) an intact mind.

The locked-in syndrome usually results from an infarction of the base or ventral surface of the pons (basis pontis, see Fig. 2-9) or medulla (bulb), usually because a thrombosis or embolus has occluded a branch of the basilar artery (see Fig. 11-2). Bulbar palsy and bilateral interruption of the corticospinal tracts render patients mute and quadriplegic. They almost always require tracheostomy, ventilator support, and feeding tubes.

Several peripheral nervous system (PNS) diseases, as well as bulbar lesions, may cause the locked-in

syndrome. For example, myasthenia gravis, ALS, Guillain-Barré syndrome, and other PNS illnesses (see Chapters 5 and 6) may cause severe and extensive enough paresis of cranial and limb muscles to cause the locked-in syndrome.

Despite the devastating neurologic damage, the upper brainstem, bulb's dorsal surface (including the reticular activating system), and cerebral cortex remain intact. Moreover, the physiologic circuits between the cerebral cortex and upper brainstem, including the thalamus, continue to reverberate (Fig. 11-3). Thus, locked-in patients retain normal cognition, affective capacity, and, given sufficient clues, a sleep-wake cycle. Although otherwise almost totally paralyzed, patients can still purposefully move their eyes and eyelids. By closing their eyelids in a "yes" or "no" pattern, patients can communicate by answering questions. The preserved circuits between the thalamus and cerebral cortex allow for a relatively normal EEG.

The medical, social, and legal management of locked-in syndrome patients should be based on their being cognizant. They can remain alert and

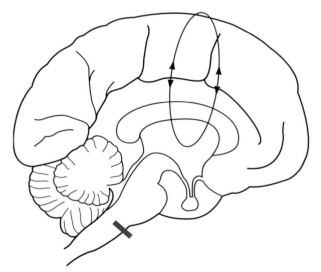

FIGURE 11-3 The locked-in syndrome usually results from an infarction of the ventral or basilar portion of the lower brainstem, typically at the basis pontis (see Fig. 2-9). A lesion in this area (indicated by the bar) would sever the corticospinal tracts and directly injure cranial nerves IX through XII. However, it would not damage several vital systems: (1) the reticular activating system of the brainstem; (2) the cerebral hemispheres, particularly the cerebral cortex; and (3) the cerebral and brainstem system that governs ocular movement (see Fig. 12-12). This lesion, which is nowhere near the cortex, would not affect the brain's cognitive, language, or visual centers. The EEG is relatively normal because the reverberating circuits between the thalamus and the cerebral cortex (indicated by the loop), which generate the organized, relatively regular background EEG activity, are also unharmed.

comprehend people talking and reading to them. They can convey their wishes, including decisions regarding their care. Although locked-in syndrome patients who have suffered a brainstem infarction partially recover, their overall prognosis is poor. In contrast, patients debilitated from a PNS illnesses often fully recover.

Physicians might examine stroke victims (and those with severe, extensive PNS disease) for the locked-in syndrome if they are unable to speak or move their limbs but have their eyelids open and can voluntarily look from side to side. The physician should ask these patients to blink a certain number of times. If they respond, a system of communication can be developed. (One patient communicated freely using eyelid blinks in Morse code.) If patients can blink meaningfully, the physician should test their ability to see and calculate. Afterward, physicians can undertake detailed mental status testing.

Persistent Vegetative State

Extensive cerebral damage, in either children or adults, may cause the *persistent vegetative state* (PVS), which is much more common than the locked-in syndrome. PVS patients, unlike those in a locked-in syndrome, lack self-awareness and cognizance of their surroundings, have lost all cognitive capacity, and cannot communicate in any manner (Fig. 11-4). Moreover, they are bedridden with quadriparesis and incontinence (Fig. 11-5). In what might constitute a misleading appearance, these patients seem alert with open eyes, retain sleep-wake periods, breathe without respirators, withdraw a limb from noxious stimulation, and maintain hypothalamic and brainstem reflexes (vegetative functions). Their eyes, moving spontaneously and randomly, may momentarily fix on a face or reflexively turn toward voices or other sounds. The vegetative activity and seeming wakefulness are rudimentary. With their lack of consciousness, patients in the PVS can neither perceive pain nor suffer.

Unfortunately, relatives may misinterpret patients' appearance, eye movements, and other activities as appreciating their presence or understanding their words. Relatives often not only overestimate the patient's cognitive capacity, they may treat the patients as if they are suffering, in a state of suspended animation, or temporary unconsciousness.

Acute, massive cerebral insults, including major traumatic brain injury, cerebral anoxia from cardiac arrest or drug overdose, profound hypoglycemia, and massive strokes, or progression of neurodegenerative illnesses, such as Alzheimer's disease and childhood-onset metabolic disorders, may lead to a vegetative state. After 1 month of existing in a vegetative state, patients fall into the category of *persistent* vegetative

state. Following acute insults, most patients are typically comatose for days to weeks before entering a vegetative state. Patients with neurodegenerative illnesses usually slip into a PVS without first entering coma. Once patients have been in PVS from head trauma for 1 year or from degenerative illness for 3 months, they have no realistic chance of recovery.

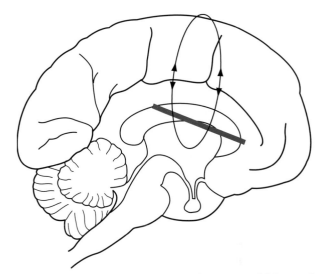

FIGURE 11-4 The persistent vegetative state, which can be caused by cerebral anoxia or numerous other conditions, results from extensive damage to the cerebral cortex or the tissue immediately underlying it (indicated by the bar). These injuries impair all cerebral functions, including cognitive ability, purposeful motor activity, vision, and speech. The brainstem, being relatively unaffected by these conditions, becomes independent of cerebral control. It then operates by reflex to regulate the body's vegetative functions: swallowing, digestion, breathing, metabolism, and temperature regulation. The EEG is abnormal because the cerebrum and its interactions with the brainstem (indicated by the loop) are damaged.

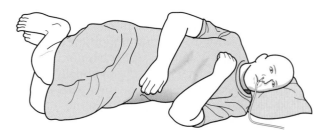

FIGURE 11-5 Patients in the persistent vegetative state tend to assume a decorticate (flexed or fetal) posture because of extensive cerebral damage. Although they are awake, have roving eye movements, retain a sleep-wake cycle, and usually do not require a respirator, they are mute, virtually motionless, and unable to respond to visitors or examiners. Patients are almost always dependent on combinations of nasogastric tubes, intravenous lines, urinary catheters, tracheostomies, and other mechanical devices. Being immobile, they are vulnerable to aspiration pneumonia, urinary tract infections, and pressure sores.

Beyond its heart-wrenching neurologic aspects, PVS raises important ethical and legal considerations. Acting on patients' living wills or other directions that they "not live like a vegetable," their relatives have sought to discontinue nutrition and artificial supports. Several well-known legal cases have explored the limits of maintaining PVS patients in accordance with their wishes or in the absence of any known wish. In general, the courts have allowed the health care proxy or closest relative to make decisions regarding the patient in the vegetative state, including removing food and nutrition.

Minimally Responsive State

Several authors have recently described a related condition, the *minimally responsive state,* in which patients have lost almost their entire cognitive capacity and voluntary movements. They require complete bodily care. The salient feature of the minimally responsive state is that patients retain a fragment of mental function. Unlike patients in the PVS, ones in the minimally responsive state are conscious and interactive—albeit in the smallest ways—with their environment, visitors, or family members. Nevertheless, their reactions are only miniscule, inconsistent, and liable to be "seen" only by wishful relatives. To distinguish this condition from the PVS, patients must at least follow simple requests, gesture in a "yes" or "no" manner, or demonstrate vocal, facial, motor, or emotional purposeful behavior. Also, unlike the EEG and PET in the PVS, which fail to show meaningful cerebral cortical activity, these studies in the minimally responsive state may reflect some organized cerebral cortical activity.

The causes of the minimally responsive state are similar to those for the PVS. However, the prognoses of these conditions differ. Although the vegetative state is almost always permanent, the minimally responsive state may be transient. Another important difference rests with the legal system because it has not yet determined the status of patients in the minimally responsive state, especially regarding their capacity for medical decision making. Because some of these patients improve and some have a modicum of comprehension, medical and legal authorities will have to judge each patient on a case-by-case basis.

MANAGING STROKE

Laboratory Tests

In most cases, CT or MRI confirms a diagnosis of a stroke or reveals common alternatives, such as a brain tumor, abscess, or subdural hematoma (see Figs. 20-8, 20-9, 20-15). CT indicates the presence and location of most strokes, except those that are acute, small, or located in the brainstem or posterior fossa (where bone artifacts may obscure them). As diagnostic tests in this situation, skull x-rays and EEGs are superfluous. MRA can visualize the extra- and intracranial cerebral arteries.

Examination of the CSF through a lumbar puncture (LP) may reveal signs of a SAH or infection, such as meningitis and encephalitis, that might mimic a stroke. However, an LP is unnecessary for a routine stroke and should be avoided in the presence of an intracranial mass lesion (see Transtentorial Herniation, Fig. 19-3).

Therapy

For ischemic strokes, neurologists may administer thrombolytic agents, such as tissue plasminogen activator (tPA), that ideally will dissolve cerebral arterial occlusions and restore cerebral blood flow. As could be anticipated, tPA carries the potential complication of cerebral hemorrhage. Because of its dangers, neurologists must administer tPA according to a demanding set of guidelines, including giving it within 3 hours after stroke onset and only after CT shows no blood. Other thrombolytic agents, which are administered by angiography directly to an occlusion, and "neuroprotective agents" (medications that preserve ischemic brain tissue) are in development. Steroids, oxygen, and vasoactive medicines have no proven benefit.

Medical and nursing care is directed at preventing complications: aspiration pneumonia, decubitus ulcers, deep vein thromboses, and urinary tract infections. If the patient is not alert or the gag reflex is diminished, medications and nutrition must be given intravenously or by a nasogastric tube. To prevent decubiti, which are unsightly, malodorous, and liable to lead to sepsis, physicians usually order air mattresses, sweat-absorbent bed surfaces (e.g., artificial sheepskins), and elbow and heel cushions for paretic limbs. Because urinary incontinence adds to the likelihood of developing decubitus ulcers, leaves patients cold and wet, and creates repugnant odors, physicians generally order catheters.

The patient's bed should be placed against the wall so that visitors and staff approach the patient from the side without perceptual impairment. For example, the staff should place the bed of a patient with a left hemiparesis and a left homonymous hemianopsia with the wall to the left. That placement will allow visitors to approach from the right side, patients to see them with their right visual field, and the patients' right hand to grasp important objects from a bedside table (e.g., call-buttons, television controls, and telephone).

In the initial phase, caregivers of stroke patients can be helpful by orienting the patient and bringing a luminous dial clock, a calendar, and pictures; repositioning the patient and moving paretic limbs to avoid contractures; and locating appropriate rehabilitation facilities.

Eventually many caregivers have difficulty in coping with the patients' disabilities. Whatever the patients' symptoms, their caregivers develop depression at about three times the usual rate.

Physical therapy will often maintain the patient's muscle tone, forestall decubitus ulcers, and prevent contractures. It will usually help patients with simple hemiparesis to regain the ability to walk, circumvent some impediments, and avoid maladaptive but expeditious physical compensations. Speech therapy may help with dysarthria and offer patients encouragement; however, it probably does not restore language function in aphasia. "Cognitive and perceptual skill training" for impaired mentation, sensory impairment, and visual loss remains without proven value.

Hemi-inattention and anosognosia usually resolve spontaneously within the first month. However, aphasia usually improves to almost its fullest extent by 4 to 6 weeks. Deficits present after that time usually do not resolve. Poor prognostic factors for recovery—as any physician might sense—are advanced age, dementia, persistent hemi-inattention, incontinence, bilateral brain damage, and prior strokes.

REFERENCES

1. Aben I, Denollet J, Lousberg R, et al: Personality and vulnerability to depression in stroke patients. Stroke 33:2391–2395, 2002.
2. Abramowicz M (ed): Atypical antipsychotics in the elderly. Med Lett 47:61–62, 2005.
3. Carota A, Berney A, Aybek S, et al: A prospective study of poststroke depression. Neurology 64:428–433, 2005.
4. Carson AJ, MacHale S, Allen K, et al: Depression after stroke and lesion location: A systematic review. Lancet 356:122–126, 2000.
5. Chemeriniski E, Robinson RG: The neuropsychiatry of stroke. Psychosomatics 41:5–14, 2000.
6. Chen C, Biller J, Willing SJ, et al: Ischemic stroke after using over the counter products containing ephedra. J Neurol Sci 217:55–60, 2004.
7. Giacino JT, Ashwal S, Childs N, et al: The minimally conscious state: Definition and diagnostic criteria. Neurology 58:349–353, 2002.
8. Gill SS, Rochon PA, Herrmann N, et al: Atypical antipsychotic drugs and risk of ischemic stroke: Population based retrospective study. BMJ 330:445, 2005.
9. Grau AJ, Becher H, Ziegler CM, et al: Periodontal disease as a risk factor for ischemic stroke. Stroke 35:496–501, 2004.
10. Hackett ML, Anderson CS, House AO: Interventions for treating depression after stroke. Cochrane Database Syst Rev 3:CD003437, 2004.
11. House A: Depression associated with stroke. J Neuropsychiatry 8:453–457, 1997.
12. Inzitari D, Pantoni L, Lamassa M, et al: Emotional arousal and phobia in transient global amnesia. Arch Neurol 54:866–873, 1997.
13. Kaufman D, Lipton R: The persistent vegetative state: An analysis of clinical correlates and costs. NY State J Med 92:381–387, 1992.
14. Kim JS, Choi-Kwon S: Poststroke depression and emotional incontinence. Neurology 54:1805–1810, 2000.
15. Kimura M, Robinson RG, Kosier JT: Treatment of cognitive impairment after poststroke depression: A double-blind treatment trial. Stroke 31:1482–1486, 2000.
16. Koton S, Tanne D, Bornstein NM, et al: Triggering risk factors of ischemic stroke. A case-crossover study. Neurology 63:2006–2010, 2004.
17. Kurth T, Slomke MA, Kase CS, et al: Migraine, headache, and the risk of stroke in women: A prospective study. Neurology 64:1020–1026, 2005.
18. Levine JS, Branch W, Rauch J: The antiphospholipid syndrome. N Engl J Med 346:752–763, 2002.
19. Malouf R, Birks J: Donepezil for vascular cognitive impairment. Cochrane Database Syst Rev 1:CD004395, 2004.
20. May M, McCarron P, Stansfield S, et al: Does psychologic distress predict the risk of ischemic stroke and transient ischemic attack? The Caerphilly study. Stroke 33:7–12, 2002.
21. Multi-Society Task Force on PVS: Medical aspects of the persistent vegetative state. N Engl J Med 330:1499–1508, 1572–1579, 1994.
22. Ohira T, Iso H, Satoh S, et al: Prospective study of depressive symptoms and risk of stroke among Japanese. Stroke 32:903–908, 2001.
23. Penovich P, Gaily E: What can we say to women of reproductive age with epilepsy? Neurology 64:938–939, 2005.
24. Petiti DB, Sidney S, Bernstein A, et al: Stroke in users of low-dose oral contraceptives. N Engl J Med 335:8–15, 1996.
25. Quality Standards Subcommittee of the American Academy of Neurology: Practice parameters: Assessment and management of patients in the persistent vegetative state. Neurology 45:1015–1018, 1995.
26. Qureshi AI, Tuhrim S, Broderick JP, et al: Spontaneous intracerebral hemorrhage. N Engl J Med 344:1450–1460, 2001.
27. Sachdev PS, Brodaty H, Valenzuela MJ, et al: The neuropsychological profile of vascular cognitive impairment in stroke and TIA patients. Neurology 62:912–919, 2004.
28. Savitz SI, Caplan LR: Vertebrobasilar disease. N Engl J Med 352:2618–2626, 2005.

29. Tatemichi TK, Desmond DW, Paik M, et al: Clinical determinants of dementia related to stroke. Ann Neurol 33:568–575, 1993.

30. Verdelho A, Hénon H, Lebert F, et al: Depressive symptoms after stroke and relationship with dementia: A three-year follow-up study. Neurology 62:905–911, 2004.

31. Williams JE, Nieto FJ, Stanford CP, et al: The association between trait anger and incident stroke risk. Stroke 33:13–20, 2002.

32. Whyte EM, Mulsant BH, Vanderbilt J, et al: Depression after stroke: A prospective epidemiological study. J Am Geriatr Soc 52:774–778, 2004.

Questions and Answers

1-10. Match the neurologic deficit (1-10) with the most likely artery of infarction (a-k).

DEFICIT

1. Left hemiparesis with relative sparing of the leg
2. Left lower extremity monoparesis
3. Monocular blindness from optic nerve ischemia
4. Left homonymous hemianopsia
5. Left palate paresis, left limb ataxia
6. Right third cranial nerve palsy with left hemiparesis
7. Right hemiparesis with aphasia
8. Quadriplegia and mutism with intact mentation
9. Left sixth and seventh cranial nerve palsy with right hemiparesis
10. Coma, quadriparesis

ARTERY

a. Right posterior cerebral
b. Left posterior cerebral
c. Right anterior cerebral
d. Right middle cerebral
e. Left anterior cerebral
f. Left middle cerebral
g. Ophthalmic
h. Vertebral or posterior inferior cerebellar
i. Perforating branch of basilar
j. Anterior spinal
k. Basilar

Answers: 1-d, 2-c, 3-g, 4-a, 5-h, 6-i, 7-f, 8-i and k, 9-i, 10-k.

11-20. Match the type of transient neurologic deficit with the artery involved.

DEFICIT

11. Transient global amnesia
12. Monocular amaurosis fugax
13. Paresthesias of right arm and aphasia
14. Vertigo, nausea, nystagmus, and ataxia
15. Migraine
16. Locked-in syndrome
17. Diplopia
18. Cortical blindness
19. Transient hemiparesis
20. Paraparesis and anesthesia below the chest, but preserved position and vibration sensation

ARTERY

a. Carotid
b. Basilar
c. Both
d. Neither

Answers: 11-b, 12-a (ophthalmic artery), 13-a, 14-b, 15-a usually but sometimes b, 16-b, 17-b, 18-b, 19-c, 20-d. Occlusions of the anterior spinal artery, which is an occasional complication of surgery involving the aorta, injure the spinal cord except for its posterior columns.

21-30. After having a steadily worsening left-sided headache for one week, a 74-year-old man seeks a neurologic evaluation. The examination reveals a nonfluent aphasia and right-sided hemiparesis, hyperreflexia, a Babinski sign, and homonymous hemianopsia. Which of the following should be considered as likely possibilities (Yes/No)?

21. Cerebral hemorrhage
22. Subarachnoid hemorrhage
23. Brain tumor
24. Subdural hematoma
25. Basilar artery occlusion
26. Carotid artery occlusion
27. Brain abscess
28. Toxoplasmosis
29. Cerebral embolus
30. Multiple sclerosis

Answers

21. No. Cerebral hemorrhages are usually catastrophic processes that develop during several hours.
22. No. The headaches of a subarachnoid hemorrhage would also be sudden and incapacitating. The examination would show nuchal rigidity.
23. Yes. A brain tumor is a likely cause and a good choice in the differential diagnosis. However, several clinical features distinguish a tumor from

a stroke. Tumors produce increasingly greater symptoms over a period of weeks—even in the fastest growing varieties, such as metastasis or glioblastoma. Also, the first indication of a tumor is frequently a seizure or newly developing, intractable headache.

24. Unlikely. Although the headache and hemiparesis are consistent, masses outside the brain substance (i.e., extra-axial lesions) rarely cause aphasia or hemianopsia.

25. No. A basilar artery occlusion would interrupt the reticular activating system causing coma and quadriplegia.

26. Yes. During a week, carotid artery stenosis can lead to complete occlusion and infarction of an entire cerebral hemisphere.

27. Yes. As with a brain tumor, an abscess and its surrounding edema can grow rapidly enough to impair an entire cerebral hemisphere.

28. No. Cerebral toxoplasmosis develops almost only as a complication of AIDS. Moreover, because toxoplasmosis typically produces multiple infections, it usually does not cause such a localized, unilateral constellation of symptoms.

29. No. Although the deficits are compatible, emboli occur acutely.

30. No. The headache, extent of the lesion, single focus, and his age are inconsistent.

31-36. After a stroke, a 65-year-old man is alert, but he is mute and unable to move his palate, arms, or legs. He has bilateral hyperreflexia and Babinski signs. He responds appropriately to verbal and written questions by blinking his eyelids.

31. Does this man have a fluent, nonfluent, or global aphasia?
32. Is his vision impaired?
33. Has he sustained cerebral damage?
34. How would the EEG appear?
35. What is this syndrome called?
36. Where is the lesion?

Answers

31. No. Because he can understand spoken language and respond appropriately, he does not have aphasia.
32. No. He can read written questions.
33. No. The palate weakness and other motor pareses may be the result of brainstem damage. Cortical functions seem to be intact.
34. The EEG should appear normal because cortical functions are intact.
35. His being fully alert, cognizant, and communicative, but almost completely paralyzed, indicate that he suffers from the locked-in syndrome.

36. The lesion is in the ventral surface of the lower brainstem (i.e., the base of the pons or basis pontis).

37-41. A 64-year-old man had sustained a right cerebral infarction the previous year from which he has a residual left-sided hemiparesis. His family has just brought him to the emergency room after he developed the sudden, painless onset of right hemiparesis and mutism. On examination, he has bilateral paresis and no verbal output. Although his eyes are frequently open, he fails to respond to either voice or gesture. He has no papilledema. He seems to have normal sleep-wake cycles.

37. Where is the probable site of the recent injury?
38. What is the probable cause?
39. Would the EEG be normal?
40. If he were not paralyzed, would he be able to write?
41. Would he have bulbar or pseudobulbar palsy?

Answers

37. The new lesion is in the left (dominant) hemisphere. With the history of a prior right cerebral infarction, he now has bilateral cerebral infarctions.
38. The sudden, painless onset suggests a thrombotic or embolic stroke. The rapid onset and lack of indication of increased intracranial pressure exclude a mass lesion, such as a tumor or abscess.
39. The EEG will be abnormal because of extensive cerebral damage.
40. No. Aphasic patients generally have impairment in all modes of communication. Moreover, as the result of extensive cerebral cortex damage, he probably has dementia (i.e., vascular dementia).
41. He would probably have pseudobulbar palsy because, in the setting of bilateral cerebral infarctions, he is mute, bilaterally weak, and unresponsive to voice. Moreover, because he has evidence of no cognitive function and the EEG is abnormal, he is vegetative. His ability to open his eyes and achieve a discernible sleep-wake cycle is consistent with the vegetative state. If he makes no improvement in 1 month, he will probably evolve into a persistent vegetative state.

42-52. A 20-year-old woman awakens from sleep and finds that she has a mild left hemiparesis. Which are the possible causes of her deficit (Yes/No)?

42. Cerebral thrombosis associated with high-dose estrogen oral contraceptives
43. Cerebral vasculitis from lupus or drug abuse
44. Cerebral embolus from mitral stenosis
45. Cerebral embolus from drug abuse

46. Septic cerebral embolus from bacterial endocarditis
47. Cerebral embolus from an atrial myxoma
48. Cocaine-induced stroke
49. Infarction from sickle cell disease
50. Migraine-induced transient paresis (i.e., hemiplegic migraine)
51. A prolonged postictal (Todd's) paresis
52. Multiple sclerosis

Answers: 42-49. All yes. Strokes in young people are the result of diseases of the heart, blood, or blood vessels. The other processes (50-52), although not strictly strokes, may mimic strokes.

53-56. A 20-year-old woman is brought to the emergency room by her family because she suddenly lost her ability to speak or move her right arm or leg. The patient looks directly forward, but does not follow verbal requests. On inspection of her fundi, her eyes constantly evert. She seems to respond to visual images in all fields. The right arm and leg are flaccid and immobile, but her face is symmetric. The neurologist finds symmetric deep tendon reflexes (DTRs) and no pathologic reflexes. She does not react to noxious stimuli on the right side of her face or body.

53. Where does the lesion appear to be located?
54. (a) What pathologic features usually found with such a lesion are not present in the patient?
(b) What non-neurologic features are present?
55. What is the most likely origin?
56. What readily available laboratory tests would lend great support to the diagnosis?

Answers

53. A patient who seems to have global aphasia and a right hemiparesis would usually have a left cerebral hemisphere lesion.
54. (a) She does not have the usual paresis of the lower (right) face, asymmetrical DTRs, Babinski signs, or a right homonymous hemianopsia. (b) Eversion of the eyes during inspection is almost always a voluntary act. Inability to perceive noxious stimuli is rare in cerebral lesions. Likewise, a sharply demarcated sensory loss (splitting the midline) is not neurologic.
55. A psychogenic disturbance is the most likely cause.
56. A normal EEG, CT, or MRI would support the diagnosis of a psychogenic disturbance.

57-60. A 70-year-old man has the sudden onset of a severe occipital headache, nausea, vomiting, and an inability to walk. He has no paresis but a downward drift of the right arm and symmetrically hyperactive DTRs with equivocal plantar response. He has dysmetria on right finger-nose and heel-shin movements. His gait is so ataxic that he must be supported when he attempts to walk.

57. Where is the lesion?
58. Which side?
59. What is its origin?
60. What is the consequence of the increased size of the lesion?

Answers

57. The lesion is in the cerebellum.
58. Abnormal cerebellar findings are referable to the ipsilateral hemisphere, which, in this case, is the right side.
59. In view of the patient's age and the sudden onset of the cerebellar deficits, a stroke is the most likely cause. Because he has a severe headache, physicians must give cerebellar hemorrhage first consideration.
60. If the hemorrhage were to expand, it would compress the fourth ventricle and cause obstructive hydrocephalus. With further expansion, the hemorrhage would compress the brainstem. Unless neurosurgeons were to evacuate the cerebellar hematoma, coma and death would soon follow.

61. Which one of the following is a typical finding in a 65-year-old man with transient global amnesia (TGA)?
a. Retaining ability to recall his name and address
b. Having underlying psychopathology
c. Having several prior episodes
d. Ability to perform mathematics

Answer: a. Patients with TGA, despite gross amnesia otherwise, can typically state their personal identifying facts. The primary deficit consists of inability to recall recently acquired information. Preservation of their identity characteristically sets TGA patients apart from those with a psychogenic disturbance. In addition, unlike partial complex seizures, TGA episodes rarely recur.

62. Elevated serum concentration of homocysteine is a risk factor for stroke and myocardial infarction. Which is the best method to reduce an elevated serum homocysteine concentration?
a. High protein diet
b. Statin medication
c. Folic acid
d. None of the above

Answer: c. Folic acid (folate) will reduce homocysteine concentration. However, that strategy, although innocuous, inexpensive, and easy to enact, has not yet actually been shown to reduce the risk of stroke or myocardial infarction.

63. In B_{12} deficiency, which two serum constituents rise?

a. Homocysteine
b. Methylmalonic acid
c. Folate
d. Cystathionine

Answers: a and b. Homocysteine and methylmalonic acid will accumulate in the absence of B_{12}, which acts as a coenzyme in the metabolic process. Administration of folate, which acts as a coenzyme along with B_{12}, will alleviate some features of B_{12} deficiency, such as megaloblastic anemia. However, without concomitant administration of B_{12}, folate will not prevent combined system disease (see Fig. 5-8).

64. A 35-year-old woman sought chiropractic treatment of her neck. In the middle of vigorous manipulation, she suddenly developed vertigo, nausea, and vomiting. On examination, she had dysarthria; nystagmus; right-sided ptosis and miosis; numbness of the left arm, leg, and trunk; and ataxia on right finger-to-nose movements. What is the most likely etiology of her condition?

a. Basilar artery occlusion
b. Drug-induced brainstem injury
c. Food poisoning
d. A torsion-induced dissection of the right vertebral artery

Answer: d. Traumatic vertebral artery dissections occasionally follow forceful, twisting neck movements, such as occurs in wrestling, whiplash neck injuries, and chiropractic manipulation. As in this case, vertebral artery dissections, like atherosclerotic occlusions, typically cause the lateral medullary syndrome.

65. Which medication category will reduce the incidence of vascular dementia?

a. Cholesterol-lowering medications, such as the "statins"
b. Antioxidants, such as deprenyl and alpha-tocopherol
c. Antihypertensives
d. Nonsteroidal anti-inflammatory drugs

Answer: c. Because antihypertensive medications unarguably reduce the incidence of strokes, their use is associated with a lower incidence of strokes' consequences, including dementia. The benefit on Alzheimer's disease of the other medications is suggestive but remains unproven.

66-67. Found wandering about in a confused manner, a 45-year-old woman is brought to the emergency room. She is lethargic, inattentive, and confused. Although she has word-finding difficulties, she is able to follow requests and repeat. Her pupils are equal and reactive, and her fundi are normal. Extraocular movements are full. All her extremities move well. She has hyperactive DTRs and bilateral Babinski signs.

66. Where is the lesion?

67. What is the most likely cause?

Answers

66. Because the woman has no lateralizing signs or indications of increased intracranial pressure, a physician cannot say that she has a "lesion." She is more likely to have a toxic-metabolic encephalopathy (delirium).

67. Causes of delirium are most often metabolic alterations (uremia, hypoglycemia), postictal confusion, infectious processes (encephalitis), intoxications (medications, alcohol, drugs, barbiturates), and head trauma.

68. Which of the following varieties of stroke most often appears as patients awaken in the morning?

a. Cerebral hemorrhage
b. Cerebral thrombosis
c. Cerebral embolus
d. Subarachnoid hemorrhage

Answer: b.

69. Which of the varieties of stroke described in Question 68 most often develops during sexual intercourse?

Answer: d.

70. Of the following, which is the most important stroke risk factor?

a. "Type A" personality
b. High cholesterol diet
c. Obesity
d. Cigarette smoking
e. Hypertension
f. Lack of exercise

Answer: e.

71. Which of the following is the standard therapy for vertebrobasilar artery TIAs?

a. Endarterectomy
b. Surgical anastomosis
c. Coumadin
d. Aspirin

Answer: d.

72. Which of the following is the most important cause of vascular dementia?
   a. Carotid bifurcation atherosclerosis
   b. Cerebral emboli
   c. Generalized atherosclerosis
   d. Hypertension with small vessel disease

Answer: d.

73. Which is aspirin's mechanism of action in reducing TIAs?
   a. It interferes with platelet adhesion.
   b. It retards prostaglandins production.
   c. It inactivates the NMDA receptor.
   d. It is a vasodilator.

Answer: a.

74. A 28-year-old man with mild generalized headache has had a 3-day history of increasing left arm weakness and clumsiness. Examination reveals only mild left arm weakness and hyperactive DTRs in that arm. Routine medical evaluation reveals no abnormalities. Both CTs and MRIs show five large ring-enhancing cerebral lesions. Of the following, which is the most likely cause of his neurologic difficulties?
   a. Cerebral infarction
   b. Cerebral hemorrhage
   c. Toxoplasmosis
   d. Glioblastoma
   e. Meningioma

Answer: c. The most common cause of multiple ring-enhancing cerebral lesions in young adults is toxoplasmosis, which is a typical manifestation of AIDS. Cerebral lymphoma is another complication, but it usually causes only a single lesion. Cerebral cysticercosis (not offered as a choice) remains endemic in South and Central America. It develops insidiously and usually presents with a seizure. Cerebral infarctions in a 28-year-old man are rare; however, cocaine use, sickle cell disease, trauma, and cardiac diseases that lead to emboli can cause them. With cerebral infarctions, the scans usually show a "pie-shaped" pattern. Cerebral hemorrhage is typically a sudden event, associated with blood-density on scans. A glioblastoma would also be rare in a 28-year-old individual, and the scans would have indicated an infiltrating tumor. A meningioma is likewise rare in young adults. When it does occur, a meningioma is extra-axial and slowly growing.

75-86. Match the sign (75-86) with the locked-in syndrome (a), persistent vegetative state (b), both (c), or neither (d).
75. Mutism
76. Quadriparesis

77. Voluntary eye movement
78. Reflexive movement to light and sound
79. Sleep-wake cycles may be preserved
80. Capacity to suffer
81. Cognitive capacity intact
82. Cognitive capacity lost
83. Due to lesion in base of pons that spares reticular activating system
84. Due to lesions that damage virtually all of cerebral cortex
85. May be caused by Guillain-Barré syndrome or myasthenia gravis
86. May be caused by anoxia or insulin injections, as in attempted murder

Answers: 75-c, 76-c, 77-a, 78-c, 79-c, 80-a, 81-a, 82-b, 83-a, 84-b, 85-a, 86-b.

87. Which of the following characteristics most reliably distinguishes vascular dementia from Alzheimer's dementia?
   a. Stepwise development
   b. MRIs that show atrophy
   c. Aphasia
   d. Focal physical findings
   e. Greatest cognitive deficit is loss of memory
   f. Absence of plaques and tangles

Answer: d. Focal physical findings, such as hemiparesis, homonymous hemianopsia, and pseudobulbar palsy, which are manifestations of infarctions of the cerebrum, cerebellum, or brainstem, characterize vascular dementia. A stepwise development of vascular dementia is frequent but it is not the most characteristic aspect and no longer a requirement in DSM-IV-TR for the diagnosis. Both vascular dementia and Alzheimer's disease dementia follow progressive as well as stepwise patterns. Atrophy is seen in both conditions. However, in underlying vascular dementia, infarctions are often visible on an MRI or CT. Aphasia is a characteristic finding of vascular dementia, but anomic aphasia is also sometimes found in Alzheimer's disease. Loss of memory is a common feature and diagnostic criteria for both conditions. Alzheimer's-like pathology is present in many cases of vascular dementia.

88. In patients with symptomatic carotid stenosis, what degree of stenosis justifies a carotid endarterectomy?
   a. 50%
   b. 60%
   c. 70%
   d. 80%
   e. 90%
   f. 100%

Answer: c. A 70% or greater stenosis of the suspected carotid artery in a symptomatic individual justifies a carotid endarterectomy, provided that it can be performed with little risk (i.e., 3% or less). Arteries with 100% stenosis (total occlusion) are inoperable. The data are less clear on the severity of carotid stenosis in an asymptomatic individual. Once enough data are available on the use of stents for carotid stenosis, different criteria may probably be applied.

89. Which pattern is most likely found on positron emission tomography (PET) and single positron tomography (SPECT) in an individual with multi-infarct (vascular) dementia?
    a. Multiple, scattered hypometabolic regions
    b. Hypometabolism in the temporal and parietal association cortex
    c. Hypometabolism in the frontal lobes
    d. None of the above

Answer: a. The multiple discrete areas probably reflect the underlying strokes. Alzheimer's disease scans show hypometabolism in the temporal and parietal association cortex and eventually hypometabolism in the frontal lobes.

90. Which are the following characteristics of the N-methyl-D-aspartate receptor?
    a. It is usually called the NMDA receptor.
    b. It regulates calcium channels.
    c. Excitatory neurotransmitters, such as glutamate, bind onto this receptor.
    d. Overstimulation of the receptor leads to cell death by calcium flooding.
    e. All of the above.

Answer: e.

91. A 73-year-old woman arises from a vigorous hair washing at her local beauty parlor and finds that she is vertiginous and nauseated. A physician detects nystagmus and ataxia of her limbs and trunk. Her symptoms and signs resolve over 1 hour. Which is the most likely cause of her disturbance?
    a. Carotid artery TIA
    b. Vertebrobasilar artery TIA
    c. A chemical in the hair wash
    d. Ordinary lightheadedness

Answer: b. She probably has had hyperextension (excessive backward bending) of her neck that crimped her vertebral arteries and caused a vertebrobasilar artery TIA. This condition is most common in elderly people who have narrowed, atherosclerotic vertebral arteries and spinal osteophytes that press against the vertebral arteries as they pass upward through the cervical spine. This disorder is sometimes called the *vanity syndrome* because it was first described in patrons of beauty parlors who had their hair washed in basins (vanities).

92. Which condition involving neuron death is characterized by cellular infiltrates but does not require cellular energy?
    a. Stroke
    b. Amyotrophic lateral sclerosis (ALS)
    c. Involution of the ductus arteriosus
    d. Involution of the thymus

Answer: a. Cellular infiltrates characterize necrosis, which is the histology of stroke, trauma, and most infections. In contrast, ALS, many other degenerative illnesses, and normal age-related changes lead to cell death by apoptosis, which is programmed, energy-requiring, and free of cellular infiltrates.

93. With which disability is poststroke depression least associated?
    a. Functional disability, particularly hemiplegia
    b. Aphasia
    c. Cognitive impairment
    d. Bulbar palsy

Answer: d. Poststroke depression is associated with physical, language, and cognitive deficits, and pseudobulbar palsy. In other words, when asked to evaluate a stroke victim for depression, the conscientious psychiatrist should watch for neurologic disorders that can mimic, precipitate, or co-exist with a stroke.

94. Studies consistently correlate poststroke depression with strokes of the left frontal lobe. (True/False)

Answer: False. Although classic studies reported an association of poststroke depression with stroke of the left frontal lobe, newer studies have implicated the right cerebral hemisphere, other lobes, and subcortical structures, such as the basal ganglia and thalamus.

95. Which of the following would be the least statistically significant risk factor for stroke?
    a. Periodontal disease
    b. Marijuana use
    c. Cocaine use
    d. Elevated C-reactive protein (CRP)
    e. Elevated homocysteine levels

Answer: b. Although cocaine and other sympathomimetic stimulants lead to stroke by causing hypertension and vasoconstriction, marijuana has little or no relationship to stroke. Newly elucidated risk factors, which are related to vascular inflammation and atherosclerosis, include periodontal disease, elevated homocysteine levels, and elevated CRP. CRP is complementary to cholesterol and perhaps more powerful. Although the risk associated with CRP and cholesterol overlap, they are not identical.

96. The parents of a 9-year-old boy bring him to the emergency room after he suddenly developed aphasia and right-sided hemiparesis. There is no indication of trauma. CT confirms the clinical impression of a left middle cerebral artery stroke. Routine blood tests are normal except for an elevated CPK concentration and indications of lactic acidosis. Sickle cell testing and determination of homocysteine levels are normal. Which of the following would be the most appropriate diagnostic test?
    a. Cerebral arteriography
    b. Temporal artery biopsy
    c. Muscle biopsy
    d. Chromosome analysis

Answer: c. Lactic acidosis in a child who has suffered a stroke indicates a mitochondrial myopathy, such as MELAS (*m*itochondrial *e*ncephalomyelopathy, *l*actic *a*cidosis, and *s*troke-like episodes). A muscle biopsy in MELAS and other mitochondrial disorders will reveal abnormal numbers, distribution, and enzyme content of mitochondria.

97. Which of the following statements most closely describes the course of poststroke depression in the majority of cases?
    a. The incidence of major depression peaks 3 to 6 months after a stroke and has a mean duration of 6 to 9 months.
    b. The incidence of major depression peaks within the first month after a stroke and has a mean duration of 1 to 2 months.
    c. Major depression begins almost immediately after a stroke and its incidence progresses steadily upward during the following 1 to 2 years.
    d. Major depression begins soon after the onset of the stroke, but its symptoms change during the next 6 months to a year.

Answer: a. Depression often begins soon after a stroke, but usually subsides by the end of the first year. Although the majority of depressed patients enjoy a remission within the year, 30% remain depressed at 1 year and 20% at 3 years.

98. Which of the following groups is least closely associated with poststroke depression?
    a. History of depression or poor physical health before the stroke
    b. Severity of the physical deficits
    c. Curtailed activities of daily living
    d. Poststroke psychosis

Answer: d. Delusions, hallucinations, and other forms of psychosis rarely develop after a stroke and they have little relationship to depression. Moreover, when poststroke psychosis occurs, it is associated with pre-existing dementia.

99. Which of the following statements concerning patients with poststroke depression is untrue?
    a. They tend to perform poorly in physical rehabilitation programs.
    b. They fail to optimize their remaining motor, cognitive, and language abilities.
    c. If ECT is indicated, it can be given with impunity.
    d. Some studies reported that successful treatment of depression improved cognitive function.

Answer: c. Although it is effective, ECT may cause more confusion than usual in stroke victims.

100-101. When asked to evaluate a 79-year-old man 6 months after two strokes and a cardiac arrest, a psychiatrist finds that the patient remains alert throughout a long evaluation but confined to bed, quadriplegic, mute, and dependent on health care workers for all activities of daily living, including feeding. The patient can establish eye contact with the psychiatrist and begin to follow several simple requests, such as "Please, show me your hand," but not more complicated ones, such as "Please, close your eyes and pick up your thumb." The patient can also indicate when a stimulus is painful and if he is thirsty. He seems to take no pleasure in food, television, or family members' visits.

100. Which of the following terms best describes the patient's condition?
    a. Locked-in syndrome
    b. Persistent vegetative state
    c. Minimally responsive state
    d. Delirium
    e. Coma

Answer: c. Because the patient remains alert and attentive to the psychiatrist, he is neither in coma nor delirium. His attentiveness, responses to requests, and appreciation of pain and thirst exclude the persistent vegetative state. In view of his having only those rudimentary neurologic functions and inability to appreciate any pleasure, his condition would best be described as either severe dementia or the minimally responsive state.

101. In this patient, what would an EEG most likely show?

a. Alpha activity over the occipital lobes
b. Slow and disorganized background activity
c. Triphasic waves
d. Electrocerebral silence

Answer: b. The patient probably has extensive, severe cerebral injury, which would cause slow and disorganized background activity. Alpha activity over the occipital lobes is the normal pattern of alert individuals with their eyes closed who are neither concentrating nor anxious. Triphasic waves are associated with hepatic encephalopathy and other disorders that cause delirium. In the locked-in syndrome, the EEG might show either normal or slow and disorganized activity. PET, another ancillary test, in the persistent vegetative state shows no cerebral cortical activity; however, in the minimally responsive state, PET shows small areas of cerebral cortex activity.

102. A 40-year-old man reported suddenly developing weakness in his left arm and leg after slipping on ice and striking his neck and back. When the neurologist examined him, she found that the degree of weakness was inconsistent, the DTRs were normal, and plantar reflexes were flexion. CTs of his head, neck, and lower back showed no abnormalities. When he still seemed to have left hemiplegia, she re-examined him. When asked to raise his right leg, he pushed down (extended) his left. His strength was so great in left leg extension that, using it as a level, she raised his lower trunk from the bed. Similarly, when asked to push downward with the right leg, he reflexively raised his left leg. What is the best description of his left leg movements?
a. She elicited a Hoover's sign.
b. The patient demonstrated left-sided hemi-in-attention.
c. He has anosognosia.
d. He has a spinal cord stroke.

Answer a. The neurologist has demonstrated the Hoover's sign, which is an indication of psychogenic hemiparesis. Another sign of psychogenic hemiparesis is the abductor sign (see Fig. 3-3). Other suggestions of psychogenic hemiparesis included the intermittent nature of his weakness, normal DTRs, and absence of Babinski signs.

103. In the recovery room following coronary artery bypass surgery, an 85-year-old man complained that he was unable to move his legs. Neurologists found that he had a clear sensorium, good memory and judgment, intact cranial nerves, and, in his arm and hands, good strength and normal DTRs. They also found that he had flaccid areflexic paraplegia, hypalgesia to pin below the umbilicus, and urinary retention that he did not appreciate. In contrast, position and vibration sensations were preserved in his legs and feet. Where is the lesion?
a. Bilateral anterior cerebral arteries
b. Cervical spinal cord
c. Thoracic spinal cord
d. Peripheral nervous system
e. Cauda equina

Answer: c. The patient sustained an infarction of the anterior spinal artery where it perfuses the thoracic spinal cord, that is, a stroke of the spinal cord. The anterior spinal artery is thin and delicate. It and its parent artery, which feeds from the aorta, are vulnerable to trauma and atheromatous debris dislodged during any surgery involving the aorta. The anterior spinal artery supplies the anterior two thirds of the spinal cord (see Figure below and Chapter 2). Infarctions of this artery cause paraplegia and anesthesia because of damage to the corticospinal and lateral spinothalamic tracts. Immediately after acute spinal cord injuries, patients lose DTRs and muscle tone because of "spinal shock," but several days to weeks later they develop hyperactive DTRs, Babinski signs, and spasticity. Because multiple, small intercostal arteries supply the posterior portion of the spinal cord, infarction of the anterior spinal artery spares the posterior columns. In this infarction, position and vibration sensations are spared.

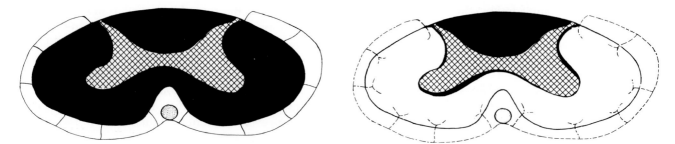

Left, A cross section of a myelin stain of the normal thoracic spinal cord shows that the anterior spinal artery perfuses the anterior two thirds of the cord. This region contains the corticospinal and lateral spinothalamic tracts (see Fig. 2-15). *Right,* If atheromatous material were to occlude the anterior spinal artery, this region of the spinal cord would undergo infarction. The patient would lose strength in the legs and sensation below the site of the infarction. However, because this infarction spares the posterior columns, the patient would still perceive position and vibration sensation.

Bilateral anterior cerebral artery infarctions can cause paraplegia, but cognitive and personality changes are more prominent. Also, DTRs become hyperactive and Babinski signs are often present.

104-106. A 75-year-old man came to the emergency room because he suddenly developed right hemiparesis. One year before he had sustained a right middle cerebral artery occlusion that resulted in a left hemiparesis. Neurologists had diagnosed him many years before with Alzheimer's disease. CT showed an acute left middle cerebral artery distribution infarction and the old right middle cerebral artery infarction. Although the patient was breathing satisfactorily, he was unresponsive to verbal and tactile stimulation. He was quadriplegic. His eyes were closed and he moaned but did not speak.

104. Which of the following terms best describes his level of consciousness?
 a. Lethargic
 b. Stuporous
 c. Comatose
 d. Locked-in state
 e. Persistent vegetative state

Answer: c. Assessing the three main clinical parameters—eye opening, verbal response, and motor response—shows that this patient is comatose.

105. If he survives the acute stroke superimposed on his pre-existing stroke and Alzheimer's disease, which will most likely be his status?
 a. He will remain permanently comatose.
 b. Within several weeks, his eyes will open and he will resume periods of sleep and wakefulness, but he will never regain cognitive or emotional capacity.
 c. Within the year, he will eventually regain his cognitive and emotional capacity but remain quadriplegic and mute.
 d. The strokes will have devastating psychologic effects and he will go into deep depression.

Answer: b. Each of the two strokes and the Alzheimer's disease irreparably damage the cerebral cortex. Although his brainstem will continue to function and govern eating, sleeping, and reflex activity, he will not regain cognitive and emotional capacity.

106. Which of the following terms will least likely describe his condition at the end of 1 year?
 a. Locked-in syndrome
 b. Persistent vegetative state
 c. Minimally responsive state

Answer: a. The locked-in syndrome describes patients who retain cerebral function and their cognitive and emotional capacity but have quadriplegia and anarthria. This patient has had devastating cerebral insults and undoubtedly has lost all or almost all cerebral function.

Visual Disturbances

Visual disturbances are frequent and complex. This chapter describes several common neuro-ophthalmologic problems likely to occur in psychiatric patients, including decreased visual acuity, glaucoma, visual field loss, and visual hallucinations (Table 12-1). It also describes several ophthalmologic causes of visual impairment in the elderly (Table 12-2).

EVALUATING VISUAL DISTURBANCES

After determining the patient's specific visual symptom, the physician's initial examination typically includes inspecting the globe or "eyeball" (Fig. 12-1) and eyelids; assessing visual acuity, visual fields, and optic fundi; and testing pupil reflexes and ocular movement. Physicians must perform additional examinations for psychogenic blindness, visual agnosia, and other perceptual disturbances (see later).

Physicians routinely measure visual acuity by having the patient read from either a Snellen wall chart or a handheld card (Fig. 12-2). A person with "normal" visual acuity can read $\frac{3}{8}$-inch letters at a distance of 20 feet. This acuity, which is the reference point of the system, is designated 20/20. People with 20/40 acuity must be as close as 20 feet to see what a person with normal vision can see at a distance of 40 feet.

Optical Disturbances

In *myopia,* due to a lens that is too "thick," a globe that is too "long," or other optical abnormality, people have increasingly blurred vision at increasingly greater distances (Fig. 12-3). Myopia first becomes troublesome during adolescence when it causes difficulty with seeing blackboards, watching movies, and driving. Because reading and other close-up activities are unimpaired, people with myopia are labeled "nearsighted." Occasionally medicines cause myopia. For example, topiramate (Topamax), a widely prescribed medication for migraine and epilepsy, may produce an acutely occurring but transient myopia. (It can also cause angle-closure glaucoma [see later].)

In its counterpart, *hyperopia* or hypermetropia, the lens is usually too "thin" rendering its refractive strength insufficient, although the globe may be too "short." People with hyperopia have increasing visual difficulty at increasingly shorter distances. They are often labeled "farsighted."

In *presbyopia,* older individuals cannot focus on closely held objects because their relatively inelastic and dehydrated lenses are unable to change shape. With their impaired near vision, people with

---

TABLE 12-1 ■ Common Neurologic Causes of Visual Hallucinations

Blindness
  Blindness, especially with hearing impairment (e.g., sensory deprivation)–Charles Bonnet syndrome
  Palinopsia
Delirium tremens (DTs)
Dementia-producing diseases
  Alzheimer's
  Dementia with Lewy bodies*
  Parkinson's^
Intoxications
  Alcoholic hallucinosis
  Hallucinogens
    Amphetamines
    Cocaine
    Lysergic acid diethylamide (LSD), mescaline
    Phencyclidine (PCP, angel dust)
  Medicines
    Atropine
    L-dopa
    Penicillin
    Scopolamine
    Steroids
Migraine with aura (classic migraine)
Narcolepsy: Hypnopompic (awakening) and hypnagogic (falling asleep) hallucinations (see Chapter 17)
Seizures (see Chapter 10)
  Frontal lobe
  Elementary (visual)
  Complex partial

---

*Although visual hallucinations are likely to complicate almost any form of dementia, they are characteristic of dementia with Lewy body disease.

^Antiparkinson medications, such as levodopa-carbidopa (Sinemet) are more likely than Parkinson's disease itself to produce hallucinations.

TABLE 12-2 ■ Common Causes of Visual Impairments in Individuals Older than 65 Years
Cataracts
Diabetic retinopathy
Macular degeneration
Glaucoma
Presbyopia and other accommodation problems
Temporal (giant cell) arteritis
Visual agnosia and cortical blindness from multiple strokes or Alzheimer's disease

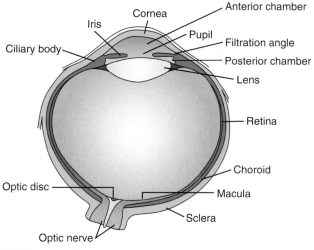

FIGURE 12-1 ■ The eye.

4 7 9 3 $\frac{20}{200}$

5 3 2   **X O O**   **ɯ ɯ Ǝ** $\frac{20}{100}$

7 9 0 2 5   **X O X**   **E E Ǝ** $\frac{20}{50}$

852437   OXX   E ɯ $\frac{20}{30}$

739426   OOX   ɯ E Ǝ $\frac{20}{20}$

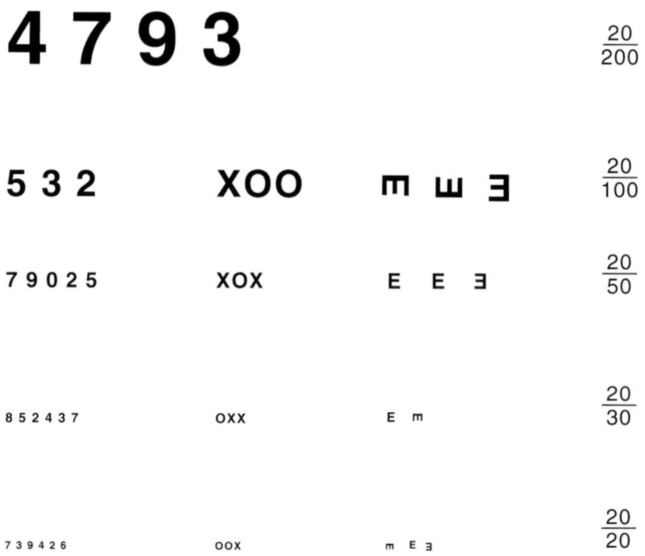

FIGURE 12-2 ■ This hand-held visual acuity chart should be held 14 inches from the patient. The acuity is the smallest line that can be read without a mistake. Each eye should be tested individually. For neurologic evaluations, patients should wear their glasses or contact lenses.

hyperopia and those with presbyopia tend to hold newspapers and sew with needles at arms' length. Reading glasses usually can compensate for the problem by bringing the focal point into the proper working distance. Older individuals also tend to have small pupils, which should not be mistaken for Argyll-Robinson pupils (see later).

Disruption of the *accommodation reflex* is another common cause of optical disturbance. Normally, when a person looks at a closely held object, this reflex contracts the ciliary body muscles to thicken the lens so that it focuses the image on the retina. It also causes miosis and increases convergence muscle tone. For example, when a person begins to read a newspaper, the eyes slightly converge, the pupils constrict, and the lens thickens to provide greater refraction of the closely held newsprint onto the retina.

Because the parasympathetic nervous system mediates the accommodation reflex, medications with anticholinergic side effects impair visual acuity for closely held objects. In *drug-induced accommodation paresis*, patients have visual acuity impairment for closely held objects (Fig. 12-4). For example, selective serotonin reuptake inhibitors (SSRIs), tricyclic

antidepressants, and clozapine, which have well-known anticholinergic properties, produce blurred vision mostly because they impair the accommodation reflex. In addition, venlafaxine (Effexor) causes paresis of accommodation in 9% of patients taking 75 mg daily, and sertraline (Zoloft) and paroxetine (Paxil) cause blurred vision in approximately 4% of patients. This side effect may be unsuspected because these medicines can impair accommodation without producing other anticholinergic effects, such as dry mouth, constipation, and urinary hesitancy.

Abnormalities of the Lens, Retina, and Optic Nerve

Cataracts (loss of lens transparency) result from complications of old age (senile cataract), trauma, diabetes, myotonic dystrophy (see Chapter 6), and chronic use of certain medicines, such as steroids. In prolonged, high doses, phenothiazines and atypical neuroleptics produce minute lens opacities but they are rarely sufficiently dense to impair vision.

Pigmentary changes in the retina can be a manifestation of congenital injuries, degenerative diseases, diabetes, or the use of massive doses of phenothiazines (Fig. 12-5). In addition, acquired immunodeficiency syndrome (AIDS) often leads to serious opportunistic retinal infection with unusual pathogens, such as cytomegalovirus. Current anti-AIDS medical regimens have greatly reduced the visual morbidity.

FIGURE 12-3 ■ Image focusing in hyperopic and myopic eyes. *A,* In normal eyes, the lens focuses the image on to the retina. *B,* In hyperopic eyes, the shorter globe or improperly focusing lens causes the image to fall behind the retina. *C,* In myopic eyes, the longer globe or improperly focusing lens causes the image to fall in front of the retina. Lenses can compensate for the refractive errors of hyperopia and myopia. Alternatively, laser or surgical "flattening" of the lens corrects myopia in many individuals.

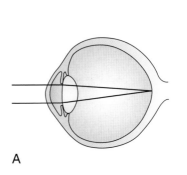
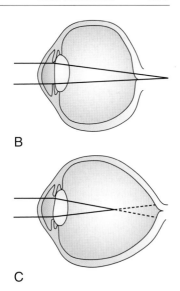

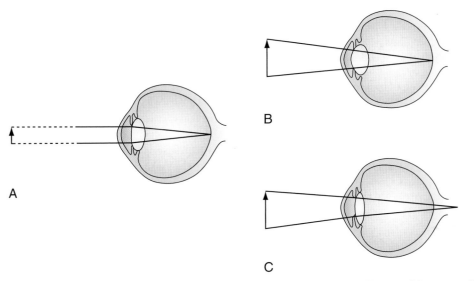

FIGURE 12-4 ■ Accommodation and accommodation paresis. *A,* When looking at a distant object, parallel light rays are refracted little by a relatively flat lens onto the retina. *B,* Accommodation: when looking at a closely held object, ciliary muscle contraction increases the curvature of the lens, greatly refracting the light rays. *C,* Accommodation paresis: if the ciliary muscles are paretic, the lens cannot form a rounded shape. Its weakened refractive power focuses light rays from closely held objects behind the retina; however, parallel light rays from distant objects still focus on the retina. Therefore, accommodation paralysis blurs closely held objects but leaves distant ones distinct.

In 25% or more of Americans older than 65 years, the cells of the retina's pigment epithelium, mostly in the macula, degenerate through a variety of mechanisms, including proliferation of the underlying blood vessels. When degeneration involves cells in the macula, a condition known as *macular degeneration,* it impairs patients' fine, critical central vision. Patients characteristically lose their reading ability and have distorted images of faces of friends and relatives. Despite devastating losses in central vision, some peripheral vision remains, permitting patients to negotiate around their living areas. Following a course of slow, progressive deterioration, patients typically lose all their vision. As with individuals who develop blindness from any cause, patients with macular degeneration risk losing their self-sufficiency, developing visual hallucinations (especially if they have hearing or cognitive impairments [see Table 12-1]), and appearing to have more severe cognitive dysfunction.

The extreme forces on the eyes brought about by child abuse (nonaccidental head injury), other causes of violent head shaking, or direct trauma often result

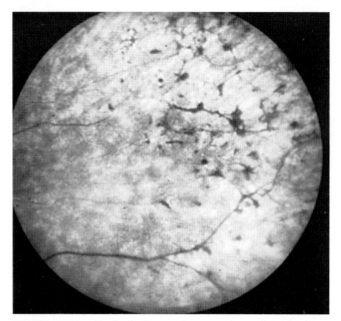

FIGURE 12-5 ■ Retinal hyperpigmentation—described as "black bone spicules" or "salt and pepper"—can be induced by massive doses of thioridazine (Mellaril). Before these retinal pigmentary changes are visible on funduscopic examination, patients may complain of blurred vision or impaired night-time vision.

in retinal hemorrhages. When due to child abuse, other stigmata of repeated trauma—fractures of the long bones, multiple skull fractures, and burns (see Chapter 22)—frequently accompany retinal hemorrhages.

Optic Nerve

Injuries of the optic nerve generally produce sudden and marked visual loss and impairment of the afferent limb of the light reflex (see Fig. 4-2). With time, the optic nerve undergoes atrophy. Unless a "common denominator" has also affected the cerebrum, illnesses that injure the optic nerves do not produce mental aberrations. Conditions injuring both areas include lysosomal storage diseases, multiple sclerosis (MS), methanol (methyl alcohol) and other intoxications, and chronically increased intracranial pressure, as with pseudotumor cerebri (idiopathic intracranial hypertension, see Chapter 9).

A classic example of simultaneous injury of both the optic nerve and cerebrum is an olfactory groove or sphenoid wing *meningioma*. This tumor compresses the nearby optic nerve (see Chapter 19 and 20) and burrows into the overlying frontal or temporal lobe. The cerebral damage can cause intellectual and personality changes and trigger partial complex seizures. At the same time the optic nerve damage causes blindness in one eye.

Tumors of the pituitary region, such as *adenomas* or *craniopharyngiomas*, can produce visual loss accompanied by psychologic changes. Unless detected and removed early, these tumors grow slowly upward to compress the optic chiasm and hypothalamus and downward to infiltrate the pituitary (see Fig. 19-4). Long-standing compression of the optic chiasm causes optic atrophy and bitemporal hemianopsia. Compression of the hypothalamus and pituitary causes headache, decreased libido, diabetes insipidus, and loss of secondary sexual characteristics.

Inflammation of the optic nerve, called *optic* or *retrobulbar neuritis*, causes sudden, painful visual loss in one eye (Fig. 12-6). One aspect of the loss is that patients perceive the color red as less intense or "desaturated." For example, they "see" red in the American flag in less vivid hues than normal and they cannot easily distinguish red from green. Because the optic nerve serves as the afferent limb of the light reflex, a classic feature of optic neuritis consists of the *afferent pupillary defect*: When the examiner shines light into the eye with optic neuritis, both pupils fail to constrict; however, when the same light shines into the unaffected eye, both pupils normally constrict (see Fig. 4-2).

When optic neuritis affects the optic disk, which is the most anterior segment of the optic nerve, physicians will often see inflammation of the disk (papillitis) on funduscopic examination. If, as in retrobulbar neuritis, the neuritis affects only a segment of the optic nerve posterior to the disk, physicians will be unable to see any abnormality on funduscopic examination during the acute phase.

Although many illnesses can cause optic neuritis, MS is one of the most common causes. In other words, patients who develop optic neuritis are at risk for developing MS (see Chapter 15). For example, if an optic neuritis patient's MRI shows lesions in the brain and the CSF contains oligoclonal bands, that patient has greater than 50% risk of developing MS. On the other hand, an optic neuritis patient without either MRI lesions or CSF oligoclonal bands has a less than 15% risk of developing MS.

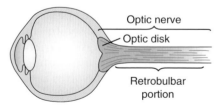

FIGURE 12-6 ■ Physicians consider the long segment of the optic nerve behind the eye its *retrobulbar* portion. If multiple sclerosis or inflammatory conditions attack it, patients develop *optic* or *retrobulbar neuritis*, which is characterized by pain and loss of vision (see Fig. 15-2).

With recurrent optic neuritis attacks, whatever their origin or location within the nerve, the optic nerve becomes atrophic, the disk white, the pupil unreactive, and the eye blind. A course of high-dose, intravenous steroids may shorten the attack but probably not alter the ultimate outcome. Physicians must use this treatment cautiously because it can produce mental aberrations, including euphoria, agitation, and, in the extreme, psychosis.

Toxins can also damage the optic nerves. For example, if alcoholics inadvertently drink methanol, an adulterant of everyday ethyl alcohol (ethanol) beverages, they develop a combination of gastroenteritis, delirium, and diffuse neurologic dysfunction. Moreover, the methanol damages the optic nerves so severely that it causes atrophy and blindness.

An inflammatory condition of the arteries that supply the optic nerve, *temporal* or *giant cell arteritis*, often leads to ischemia of the optic nerves. Moreover, the arteritis tends to spread to the cerebral arteries (see Chapter 9). Typically affecting only people older than 65 years, temporal arteritis often first causes a mild to moderate subacute headache and systemic symptoms, such as malaise, prolonged aches, and pains. The number and variety of these initial nonspecific symptoms understandably give the appearance of depression or the beginning of a somatoform disorder. However, physicians should avoid missing the diagnosis of temporal arteritis because, unless they promptly treated the patient with steroids, it can cause blindness and strokes. Finding giant cells and other signs of inflammation on a temporal artery biopsy will confirm the diagnosis.

Leber's hereditary optic atrophy, an illness attributable to a point mutation in mitochondrial DNA, also involves the optic nerves. Most commonly affecting young males, it causes visual loss culminating in blindness in one and then, within months, the other eye. As with mitochondrial disorders of muscle (see Chapter 6) and possibly Parkinson's disease, Leber's atrophy serves as a prime example of an abnormality in mitochondrial DNA-determined energy production causing serious neurologic illness.

GLAUCOMA

In most cases, glaucoma is elevated intraocular pressure resulting from obstructed outflow of aqueous humor through the *filtration angle* of the anterior chamber of the eye (Fig. 12-7). Two common varieties—*open-angle* and *angle-closure*—are recognized, and the angle-closure variety occasionally results from psychotropic medications. If glaucoma remains untreated, it damages the optic nerve, causes visual field impairments, and eventually leads to blindness.

Open-Angle Glaucoma

Open-angle or *wide-angle glaucoma* occurs seven times more frequently than closed-angle glaucoma. People at greatest risk are older than 65 years, diabetic, myopic, and relatives of glaucoma patients. Because symptoms are usually absent at the onset, glaucoma might be diagnosed only when an ophthalmologist detects elevated intraocular pressure, certain visual field losses, or changes in the optic nerve. Later, when central vision or acuity is impaired, the optic cup is abnormally deep and permanently damaged. Lack of symptoms in the initial phase of open-angle glaucoma is one of the most compelling reasons for routine ophthalmologic examinations.

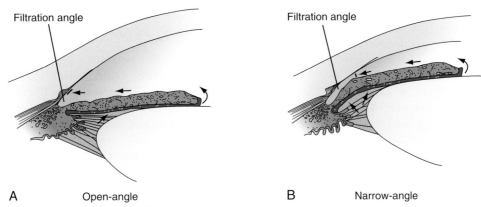

A   Open-angle   B   Narrow-angle

FIGURE 12-7 ■ *A,* Open-angle glaucoma: the aqueous humor does not drain despite access to the absorptive surface of the angle. Impaired flow from the eye leads to gradually increased intraocular pressure (glaucoma). *B,* Narrow-angle glaucoma: when the iris is pushed forward, as may occur during pupil dilation, the angle is narrowed or even closed. Obstruction of aqueous humor flow, which usually occurs suddenly, leads to angle-closure glaucoma.

Open-angle glaucoma usually responds to topical medications (eye drops) or laser surgery. Psychotropic medications do not precipitate open-angle glaucoma. In general, patients with open-angle glaucoma may be given antidepressants and other psychotropic medications provided that their glaucoma treatment is continued.

Angle-Closure Glaucoma

In *angle-closure glaucoma*, which is also called *closed-angle* or *narrow-angle glaucoma,* intraocular pressure is usually elevated by impaired aqueous humor outflow at the filtration angle (see Fig. 12-7). In one variety, the fluid becomes trapped behind the iris. Patients with narrow-angle glaucoma, like those with open-angle glaucoma, usually are older than 40 years and often have a family history of the disorder, but they also have had a history of hyperopia and long-standing narrow angles. Few have had symptoms, such as seeing halos around lights, preceding an attack of angle-closure glaucoma. In contrast to the relatively normal appearance of the eye in open-angle glaucoma, in acute angle-closure glaucoma the eye is red, the pupil dilated and unreactive, and the cornea hazy. Moreover, the eye and forehead are painful, and vision is impaired.

Angle-closure glaucoma is sometimes iatrogenic. For example, when pupils are dilated for ocular examinations, the "bunched-up" iris can block the angle (see Fig. 12-7B). Likewise, medicines with anticholinergic properties, probably because they dilate the pupil, can precipitate angle-closure glaucoma.

Despite the attention to the potential problem, the complication rate of glaucoma with tricyclic antidepressant use is low and, with SSRIs, almost nonexistent. With the shift to SSRIs, psychiatrists are able to avoid the potential problem of tricyclic antidepressant-induced glaucoma. However, as physicians prescribe tricyclics for increasingly numerous, mostly neurologic conditions—chronic pain, urinary incontinence, headache, and diabetic neuropathy—many patients remain vulnerable. In addition, other medications for neurologic diseases, such as the antiepileptic drug, topiramate, can cause angle-closure glaucoma.

Whatever the cause of angle-closure glaucoma, prompt treatment can preserve vision. Topical and systemic medications open the angle (by constricting the pupil) and reduce aqueous humor production. Laser iridectomy immediately and painlessly creates a passage directly through the iris that drains aqueous humor.

Because glaucoma poses such a threat, individuals older than 40 years should have intraocular pressure measured every 2 years and those older than 65 years, every year. Most patients who are under treatment

for either form of glaucoma may safely receive psychotropic medications. Glaucoma medications, such as pilocarpine (a cholinergic medicine that constricts the pupils), and ophthalmic beta-blockers, such as timolol (Timoptic), may be absorbed into the systemic circulation and create cardiovascular and psychologic side effects. Their absorption can also cause orthostatic lightheadedness, bradycardia, and even heart block. Not surprisingly, elderly patients who use beta-blocker eyedrops sometimes experience brief periods of confusion.

Children are also susceptible to systemic absorption. For example, when given scopolamine or other atropine-like eye drops for ocular examination, they often develop agitation. On the other hand, marijuana, despite claims of its proponents, is no more effective than standard medications for treating glaucoma.

CORTICAL BLINDNESS

Bilateral occipital cortex injuries can produce severe visual impairment, called *cortical blindness.* The underlying cause may be damage limited to the posterior cerebrum from bilateral posterior cerebral artery occlusions or traumatic occipital lobe injury. Alternatively, extensive brain injury from anoxia, multiple strokes, or MS may cause cortical blindness along with other impairments. Reflecting occipital lobe damage, electroencephalograms (EEGs) characteristically lose their normal, posterior 8- to 12-Hz (alpha) rhythm. Whether the cortical blindness results from limited or generalized cortex injury, the pupils are normal in size and reactivity to light because all elements of the pupillary light reflex remain intact: the midbrain and optic and oculomotor nerves (see Fig. 4-2).

Anton's Syndrome

The dramatic neuropsychologic phenomenon of *Anton's syndrome*—blind patients insisting that their vision is intact—characteristically complicates cortical blindness. The syndrome consists of an irrational response to the sudden onset of blindness rather than the blindness itself. As with patients displaying anosognosia (see Chapter 8), those with Anton's syndrome respond to their visual loss primarily with the defense mechanism of denial. They also confabulate by "describing" their room, clothing, and various other objects. In addition, they often behave as though they had normal vision and proceed to stumble about their room.

For example, a 76-year-old man sustained a right-sided posterior cerebral artery stroke that was superimposed on a left-sided posterior cerebral stroke from the previous year. He first blamed his inability to see the examiner's blouse on poor lighting and then claimed to be disinterested in it. When pressed, still denying his blindness, he confabulated by calmly describing the blouse as "lovely" and "becoming," at times elaborating that it was "obviously made from fine material."

Signs of generalized cerebral cortex injury, especially delirium and dementia, accompany many cases of Anton's syndrome. If an underlying stroke or other lesion extends beyond the occipital lobes, amnesia (from bilateral temporal lobe injury) or anosognosia for other deficits (from right-sided parietal lobe injury) may accompany Anton's syndrome.

VISUAL PERCEPTUAL DISTURBANCES

Visual perceptual disturbances usually consist of impaired processing of visual information or inability to integrate visual information with other neuropsychologic information at the cerebral cortical level. Beware that although these fascinating disturbances seem to be neatly defined, patients usually have incomplete forms. Moreover, illnesses often superimpose visual perceptual disturbances on other neuropsychologic disorders, such as dementia, aphasia, and apraxia. In these cases, patients' problems more than coexist: they multiply.

Palinopsia

Palinopsia (Greek, *palin,* again; *opsis,* vision), which may be likened to "visual perseveration," consists of recurrent or persistent images following removal of the visual stimulus. Technically a form of hallucinations, the visions usually appear to the patient within an area of incomplete visual loss in the left lateral field. Patients with palinopsia can have recurrent images of objects, scenes, or family members. Frequently, several afterimages reappear as "visual echoes" in rapid succession, but sometimes only after hours or days. Because palinopsia duplicates images of actual common inanimate objects, it usually does not elicit an emotional response.

Both the left lateral visual impairment and superimposed hallucinations stem from right-sided occipital and parietal lobe lesions, such as stroke, tumor, or trauma. In some cases, palinopsia has coincided with focal EEG seizure activity, in which case it may represent a failure of the cortex to capture only a single image. When images recur following a long interval, seizures may be the underlying cause of the palinopsia.

Agnosia

Another visual perceptual disturbance, *visual agnosia,* consists of inability to appreciate the meaning of an object by sight, despite an intact visual system and the absence of aphasia and dementia. Patients with visual agnosia simply cannot comprehend what they see. For example, a man shown a stop sign might recognize and describe it but fail to comprehend what action he must take.

With visual agnosia, language function is normal when vision is bypassed (as when patients touch objects). In contrast, bypassing language by relying on hearing does not alter the language deficits in aphasia.

Visual agnosia develops most often in the setting of cerebral strokes or Alzheimer's disease. Although physicians can think of it as representing a disconnection of the occipital visual cortex from cognitive centers, research has not yet defined its underlying pathophysiology—certainly not as well as it has with aphasia (see Chapter 8).

Visual agnosia is also a major aspect of the infamous, although relatively rare, *Klüver-Bucy syndrome.* Neurosurgeons have produced this behavioral disorder in monkeys by resection of both anterior temporal lobes, which contain the amygdalae and components of the limbic system. The resulting limbic system damage produces visual agnosia so severe that the monkeys not only touch all objects, but they compulsively identify all objects by putting them into their mouth ("psychic blindness"). Their behavior can be repetitive, compulsive, and indiscriminate.

When the Klüver-Bucy syndrome occurs in humans (see Chapter 16), it includes a muted version of psychic blindness, *oral exploration.* This component of the syndrome consists of patients' placing inedible objects in their mouth but only intermittently, briefly, partly, and absent-mindedly.

Color agnosia is a particular inability to identify colors by sight. The affected individual's problem is neither common color blindness, which is a sex-linked inherited retinal abnormality, nor aphasia. The real problem is that patients cannot specify (by speech or writing) the name of colors. When shown painted cards, for example, they cannot say or write the name of the colors. In striking contrast, they behave as though they appreciate colors. Patients can typically match pairs of cards of the same color, read Ishihara plates (pseudoisochromatic numbered cards), and recite the colors of well-known objects, such as the American flag.

In a related impairment, *prosopagnosia,* patients cannot recognize *familiar faces* (Greek, *prosōpon,* face, person; *agnosia,* lack of knowledge). However, they can identify the same people by their voice, dress, and mannerisms. Prosopagnosia is often accompanied by an inability to identify objects out of their usual (visual) context, such as a shirt pocket cut from a shirt. Neurologists usually attribute it to either bilateral occipitotemporal or right-sided temporal lesions. Alternatively, they attribute it to neurodegenerative illnesses, such as Alzheimer's disease or, more often, frontotemporal dementia. In a variation of prosopagnosia, patients with right cerebral lesions cannot match pairs of pictures of *unfamiliar* faces. This condition probably represents a visual perceptual impairment induced by a nondominant parietal lobe lesion.

Balint's Syndrome

Balint's syndrome, which has been attributed to bilateral parietal-occipital region damage from strokes or Alzheimer's disease, consists of three related, admittedly overlapping elements concerned with visual attention: *ocular apraxia* (sometimes called "*psychic paralysis of fixation*"), *optic ataxia,* and *simultanagnosia.* Ocular apraxia is the neuropsychologic inability of a patient to shift attention by looking away from an object to one located in the periphery of vision. Patients behave as though they were mesmerized by the original object or as a radar system that has locked onto an approaching hostile aircraft. By briefly closing their eyes, which momentarily interrupts attention, patients can shift their gaze.

Optic ataxia, another element of Balint's syndrome, is the inability to look or search in a deliberate pattern. A common manifestation consists of inability to read in methodical visual sweeps.

The third element, simultanagnosia consists of being able to attend only to objects immediately in the center of vision. When simultaneously confronted with objects in the center and in the periphery of vision, patients will invariably ignore the one in the periphery even though it might be important or attractive. Because of simultanagnosia, patients cannot comprehend complicated scenes or objects. For example, they would be unable to recognize a baseball game, but instead able to see only an individual player, a base, or the distant expanse of grass.

Psychogenic Blindness

Cases of *psychogenic blindness* that convincingly mimic true blindness are rare. Because people lack an

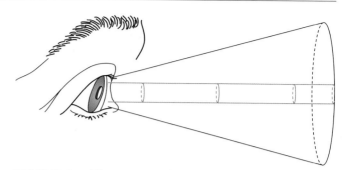

FIGURE 12-8 ■ The area seen by a person normally increases conically in proportion to the distance from the object. In *tubular* or *tunnel vision,* which defies the laws of optics, the visual area is constant despite increasing distance.

intuitive knowledge of visual pathways, neurologists can readily discover nonanatomic patterns of psychogenic blindness. Even bedside testing can easily reveal its spurious nature. Also, patients cannot easily maintain psychogenic blindness because it is burdensome and incapacitating.

Psychogenic blindness occurs in malingering and various psychiatric disorders, most notably conversion disorder. Its most common patterns are complete visual loss (or generalized impairment), blindness in the eye ipsilateral to a psychogenic hemiparesis, and *tubular* or *tunnel vision* (Fig. 12-8). The combination of monocular visual loss and hemiparesis defies the laws of neuroanatomy: the division of optic pathways at the optic chiasm provides that a cerebral lesion causing hemiparesis may also cause hemianopsia—not monocular blindness. (Brainstem lesions may cause hemiparesis and diplopia, but neither hemianopsia nor monocular blindness.)

Similarly, loss of vision in a tubular pattern defies the laws of optics: the visual area should expand with increasing distance. (An important exception to this law, however, sometimes occurs in migraine with aura [see Chapter 9], in which patients may have the perception of peripheral vision constriction.) Uncommon, but relatively sophisticated patterns of psychogenic blindness are homonymous hemianopsia and combinations of monocular loss and a contralateral hemianopsia.

To unmask most varieties of psychogenic blindness, an uninhibited examiner simply might make childlike facial contortions or ask the patient to read some four-letter words. The patient's reaction to these provocations would reveal the ability to see. When only one eye is affected by psychogenic blindness, fogged, colored, or polarized lenses in front of the unaffected eye will often confuse (or fatigue) a patient into revealing that vision is present. Visual field testing in cases of psychogenic visual loss often reveals a spiral or other physiologically nonsensical pattern.

Another technique that reveals intact vision is to spin a vertically striped cylinder (drum) in front of a person. The drum will elicit *optokinetic* nystagmus in individuals with normal vision, even those too young to speak. Likewise, having patients look at a large, moving mirror irresistibly compels everyone with intact vision to follow their own image.

Another, easy test is to offer patients lenses with negligible optical value. A pair of glasses with these lenses allows patients to extract themselves from psychogenic blindness without embarrassment.

If clinical tests are inconclusive, EEG and other electrophysiologic testing may help. Alpha rhythm overlying the occipital lobes of patients at rest with their eyes closed, and loss of that activity when they open their eyes, indicates an intact visual system. However, because patients' anxiety or concentration suppresses alpha activity, its absence is not as significant as its presence. In visual evoked response (VER) testing, another noninvasive electrophysiologic test, visual system injuries produce abnormal potentials (see Chapter 15).

Visual Hallucinations

Unlike auditory hallucinations, which typically result from psychiatric disorders, visual hallucinations in adults usually result from neurologic disorders. In children, however, they may be a symptom of schizophrenia. Qualities of visual hallucinations that should prompt a neurologic evaluation include development of stereotyped visions, alteration in the patient's level of consciousness, and concurrent behavioral abnormalities. Although patients may require an imaging study, at least routine blood tests, urinary toxicology studies, and an EEG, the clinical setting and character of the images often suggest the correct diagnosis.

Visual hallucinations can originate in dysfunction of the frontal or temporal, as well as the occipital, cortex. Problems as diverse as toxic-metabolic encephalopathy, dementia-producing diseases, medication side effects, and structural lesions can produce them (see Table 12-1).

Tumors, strokes, and other structural lesions can cause partial elementary, frontal lobe, or complex seizures (see Chapter 10)—all of which can produce visual symptoms. These hallucinations, which tend to be stereotyped and brief, can be "seen" in both eyes and may even appear in a hemianopic area. They range from simple geometric forms in partial elementary seizures to detailed visions accompanied by sounds, thoughts,

emotions, smells, and, characteristically, impairment of consciousness, in partial complex seizures.

The "aura" in migraine with aura (previous termed "classic migraine") consists of sensory disturbances—olfactory, sensory, or visual. In almost all cases, the aura includes stereotyped visual hallucinations (Fig. 9-2). The most common migraine-induced visual hallucinations consist of distinctive crescent scotomata or scintillating, patterned zigzag lines (fortification spectra) that move slowly across the visual field for 1 to 20 minutes before yielding to a hemicranial headache. In a potentially confusing situation, visual auras sometimes represent the sole manifestation of migraine. In rare individuals, migraine aura consists of elaborate visual distortions, such as *metamorphopsia*, in which individuals and objects appear, to the patient, to change size or shape, as in the celebrated Alice in Wonderland syndrome.

As an element of narcolepsy (see Chapter 17), visual hallucinations intrude into a patient's partial consciousness. Similar to dreams but unlike migraine aura, these visual hallucinations are composed of variable, unpredictable—not stereotyped—intricate visions accompanied by rich thoughts and strong emotions. They tend to occur while patients fall asleep (hypnagogic hallucinations) or awaken (hypnopompic hallucinations). As with normal dreams, these hallucinations are associated with flaccid, areflexic paresis and rapid eye movements (REMs).

Visual hallucinations are also a hallmark of neurodegenerative diseases that cause dementia, particularly Alzheimer's, Lewy body, and Parkinson's diseases (see Chapters 7 and 18). When manifestations of these disorders, hallucinations tend to be visually complex, have a paranoid aspect, and occur predominantly at night. As a clue to dementia with Lewy body disease, visual hallucinations occur frequently and begin early in its course. When visual hallucinations develop in Alzheimer's disease, they occur in its late stages. Hallucinations in Parkinson's disease are usually partly medication-induced.

Many classes of medicines, in addition to anticholinergics or dopamine enhancers, may cause hallucinations. Similarly, illicit stimulants, by design, may cause hallucinations.

In general, but not always, medicine- or drug-induced hallucinations develop in the context of delirium. Even withdrawal from certain substances can also cause visual hallucinations. The best known example is alcohol-withdrawal causing *delirium tremens* (*DTs*). In most patients with DTs, varied, sometimes frightening hallucinations stem from the environment and are accompanied by agitation, confusion, sweating, and tachycardia. Alternatively, some patients, petrified by the hallucinations, become reticent and immobile.

Finally, acute visual loss routinely produces "release" visual hallucinations. In the most common example, cortical blindness induces hallucinations. Similarly, sudden blindness from ocular injury induces hallucinations.

Examples of blindness causing or releasing visual hallucinations include soldiers with extensive eye wounds who have periods of "seeing" brightly colored forms and even entire scenes. Similarly, visual hallucinations along with disorientation and agitation often complicate eye surgery in elderly patients. Thus, elderly patients and others who may have cognitive impairment should not undergo simultaneous bilateral ophthalmologic surgical procedures.

Whether acute or chronic, visual loss represents sensory deprivation. In situations involving acute blindness, the brain acts as though it has lost the normal visual input required to suppress spontaneous, unregulated visual cortex activity. Especially when superimposed on hearing and cognitive impairments, visual loss also precipitates other mental aberrations. Many elderly patients with visual impairment from any cause have frequently occurring, varied, picturesque colored or black-and-white hallucinations of benign, familiar objects that last minutes to several hours. In this condition, the *Charles Bonnet syndrome,* elderly, visually handicapped patients sit and have quiet, harmless hallucinations that they disclose only reluctantly. However, the hallucinations occasionally upset the patients and precipitate restlessness, insomnia, and delusions. Physicians may calm the situation by reassuring these patients that their visual loss commonly leads to their hallucinations.

With seizures, migraine, or narcolepsy, appropriate treatment of the underlying condition will usually eliminate visual hallucinations. Antipsychotic agents easily suppress hallucinations that complicate neurodegenerative illnesses, intoxications, and visual loss; however, physicians should avoid administering dopamine-blocking ones to patients with dementia with Lewy bodies (see Chapter 7).

VISUAL FIELD LOSS

The patterns of visual loss (Fig. 12-9) serve as a time-honored and reliable guide to localization and diagnosis. As in so much of neurology, anatomy determines destiny. The following guidelines apply to visual field loss:

Optic nerve lesions, such optic neuritis or trauma, lead to loss of an area of the visual field, *scotoma,* of the ipsilateral eye. This area is usually oval or kidney-shaped and, unlike most other visual field defects, crosses the midline. If a lesion damages the entire optic nerve, that eye will lose all vision and the patient will have *monocular blindness.* In striking contrast to the marked visual loss, the optic disk appears normal on funduscopy during the acute phase of optic neuritis and many other nerve injuries. After several weeks, however, optic atrophy develops and the disk loses its pink-orange color and appears pale.

Pituitary adenoma, the lesion that most often compresses the optic chiasm, usually rises upward and disrupts the inferior nasal crossing fibers. The damage to these fibers causes *bitemporal superior quadrantanopsia.* If the adenoma continues to expand and grow upward, it disrupts the superior as well as the inferior crossing fibers. The increased damage to the nasal crossing fibers expands the visual field deficit to a *bitemporal hemianopsia.* To the extent that the optic nerves are compressed, they develop optic atrophy. By that time, patients have hypopituitarism and an elevated serum prolactin level.

Injuries of the optic tract between the optic chiasm, the synapse in the lateral geniculate bodies, and the occipital cortex cause contralateral homonymous quadrantanopsias or hemianopsias. For example, strokes in the distribution of the left posterior cerebral artery cause infarctions of the left occipital cortex that result in a right homonymous hemianopsia. Similarly, strokes in the distribution of the left middle cerebral artery cause infarctions of a segment of the optic tract anterior to the occipital lobe but still cause a right homonymous hemianopsia.

Moreover, strokes in the frontal or parietal lobes usually cause physical and neuropsychologic deficits in addition to a homonymous hemianopsia. In those strokes, ocular deviation, hemiparesis, hemisensory loss, and certain neuropsychologic deficits typically accompany homonymous hemianopsia. For example, right-sided homonymous hemianopsia is often associated with conjugate ocular deviation to the left, right-sided hemiparesis and hemisensory loss, and nonfluent aphasia. Similarly, left-sided homonymous hemianopsia is often associated with conjugate ocular deviation to the right, left-sided hemiparesis and hemisensory loss, and left-sided anosognosia and hemi-inattention (see Chapter 8).

Unlike scotoma from optic nerve lesions and many cases of psychogenic visual loss, homonymous and bitemporal hemianopsias respect the midline. Although occipital lesions sometimes do not involve the center of vision (see later), hemianopsias never drift over the center vertical line to affect portions of the other visual field.

Another feature of those strokes is that because the injury affects the optic *tract* rather than optic *nerve,* the optic disks do not undergo atrophy.

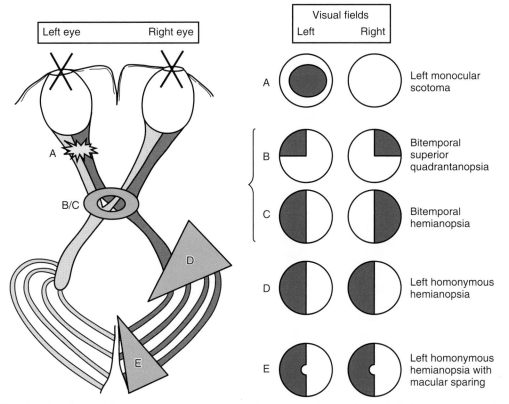

FIGURE 12-9 ■ The visual pathway (also see Fig. 4-1), extending from the retina to the occipital cortex, is exquisitely vulnerable throughout its entire course. Lesions produce characteristic visual field defects. The defects, in turn, indicate the lesion's location, etiology, and associated findings. *A*, Optic nerve lesions typically produce ipsilateral scotoma. *B*, Optic chiasm lesions, from below, when small (smaller ring), produce superior bitemporal quadrantanopsia. *C*, Optic chiasm lesions when large (larger ring) produce bitemporal hemianopsia. *D*, Cerebral lesions that interfere with the anterior optic tract result in contralateral homonymous hemianopsia. *E*, Lesions that interfere with the occipital cortex result in contralateral homonymous hemianopsia, sometimes with macular sparing. Although the determination of visual fields serves as a highly reliable sign of localized neurologic disease, their display is one of clinical neurology's most confusing aspects. In the standard manner, these sketches portray visual field defects as crosshatched areas from the *patient's perspective*. For example, the sketch of the left homonymous hemianopsia *(D)* portrays the abnormal areas on the left side of each circle—as when the patient looks at the paper. The sketch of cerebral optic tract pathways portrays the tracts as though a picture had been taken from above the patient's brain (e.g., see Fig. 8-4). However, CTs and MRIs traditionally show the brain in right-to-left reversal. A CT, for example, will show a left cerebral lesion on the right side of the study. Medical illustrations should include a notation to orient the reader.

A rare but important variation is the *homonymous superior quadrantanopia* (Fig. 12-10). This visual field deficit may be the only physical manifestation of a contralateral temporal lobe lesion. Thus, it may represent the only interictal physical finding in patients who have partial complex seizures. Another clinically important association is that a temporal lobectomy for trauma or intractable epilepsy may leave this visual defect.

When lesions damage only the occipital portion of the optic tract, patients develop a contralateral homonymous hemianopsia. Unlike with damage of the anterior portion, precise determinations of the visual fields in occipital lobe lesions may demonstrate that the center of vision is preserved within the hemianopsia. As though the macula, which transmits the center of vision, were represented bilaterally in the occipital cortex, the preservation of this visual area is termed, *macular sparing*. With or without macular sparing, homonymous hemianopsia from lesions confined to the occipital lobe is typically unaccompanied by physical defects. Also, as with anterior cerebral lesions, the optic nerves do not undergo atrophy.

CONJUGATE OCULAR MOVEMENT

Both eyes normally move together in a paired, coordinated (*conjugate*) manner that allows people to look (*gaze*) laterally and follow (*pursue*) moving objects.

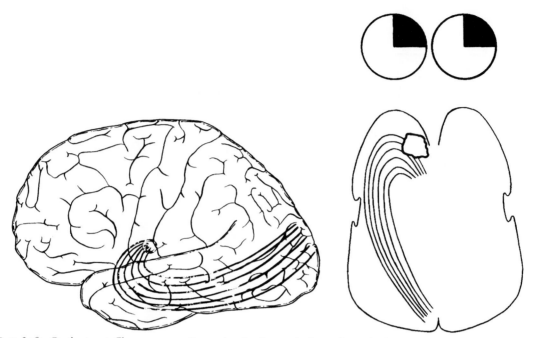

FIGURE 12-10 ■ *Left,* Optic tract fibers sweep from the brainstem's lateral geniculate body to the occipital lobe's visual cortex. The tract's inferior fibers first sweep anteriorly—through the temporal lobe's anterior tip—before heading posteriorly. These fibers convey visual information from the contralateral superior temporal quadrant. *Right,* A large lesion or a surgical resection of the left temporal lobe has damaged the inferior optic tracts to produce a contralateral (right) superior quadrantanopsia.

A succession of cerebral then brainstem *gaze centers,* modulated by cerebellar and visual input, generates conjugate eye movement. Conjugate movements are considered to be under *supranuclear* control because cerebral cortical centers, through corticobulbar tracts, drive and coordinate the activity of the oculomotor, trochlear, and abducens cranial nerve nuclei.

Conjugate eye movement originates in each frontal lobe's *cerebral conjugate gaze center.* When a person is at rest, each cerebral center continuously emits impulses that go through a complicated pathway to "push" the eyes contralaterally. With the counterbalancing activity of each cerebral gaze center, the eyes remain midline (Fig. 12-11). When a person wants to look to one side, the contralateral cerebral gaze center increases activity. For example, when someone wants to look toward a water glass on the right, the left cerebral gaze center activity increases, and, as if pushing the eyes away, the eyes turn to the right. If this person wished to reach for the glass, the left cerebral motor strip, which is situated adjacent to the gaze center, would mobilize the right arm.

Partial seizures also increase activity of the conjugate gaze center. They push the eyes contralaterally and, because the seizures usually encompass the adjacent corticospinal tract, they push the head and neck contralaterally and produce tonic-clonic activity of the contralateral arm and leg.

In contrast, when patients have unilateral destructive cerebral injuries, such as large strokes, the activity of the gaze center on that side is abolished. The activity of the other center, being unopposed, pushes the eyes toward the injured side. ("The eyes look toward the [cerebral] stroke.") For example, with a left cerebral stroke, the eyes deviate toward the left. Also, because the corticospinal tract is usually damaged, the right side of the body is paralyzed. (Here the saying is "When the eyes look away from the paralysis, the stroke is cerebral.")

When intact, each cerebral gaze center produces conjugate eye movements by stimulating a contralateral *pontine gaze center,* which is also called the *pontine paramedian reticular formation (PPRF).* In contrast to the movement generated by the cerebral center, each pontine center *pulls* the eyes toward its own side (Fig. 12-12). A stroke on one side of the pons thus allows the eyes to be pulled toward the opposite side. For example, if the right pontine gaze center were damaged, the eyes would deviate to the left. Also, because the right pontine corticospinal tract would be damaged, the left arm and leg would be paralyzed. With a pontine lesion, in short, the eyes "look toward the paralysis."

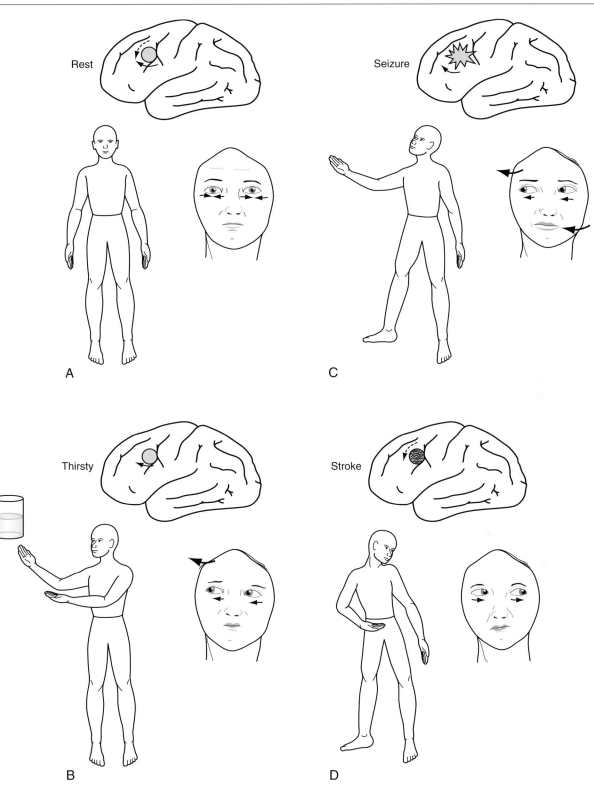

FIGURE 12-11 ■ *A,* At rest, the eyes are midline because the impulses of each frontal lobe conjugate gaze center are balanced, each "pushing" the eyes contralateral. Maintaining eyes in one position is an active process. *B,* Voluntarily increased activity of the left cerebral gaze center drives the eyes to the right (contralateral). *C,* Involuntarily increased cerebral activity also drives the eyes contralateral. Also, seizure activity in the left cerebral hemisphere causes right arm and leg tonic-clonic activity. *D,* A stroke destroys the left cerebral gaze center, permitting the right center to push the eyes toward the lesion. It also destroys the cerebral motor strip, causing contralateral paresis. The eyes "looking" away from the hemiparesis characterize this common stroke.

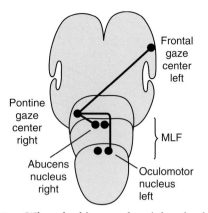

FIGURE 12-12 ■ When looking to the right, the left frontal conjugate gaze center stimulates the right (contralateral) pontine gaze center, which is also called the *pontine paramedian reticular formation (PPRF)*. The pontine center, in turn, stimulates the right (adjacent) abducens nerve nucleus and, upward through the left medial longitudinal fasciculus (MLF), the left (contralateral) oculomotor nerve nucleus, which is in the midbrain.

When the pontine gaze center receives impulses from the contralateral cerebral conjugate gaze center, it activates one abducens nucleus and the contralateral oculomotor nucleus to produce conjugate lateral eye movement: the adjacent abducens (sixth cranial nerve) nucleus and, through the *medial longitudinal fasciculus (MLF)*, the contralateral oculomotor (third cranial nerve) nucleus (see Figs. 15-3 and 15-4). If the brain were to simultaneously activate both abducens nuclei, both eyes would turn outward. On the other hand, if it were to simultaneously stimulate both oculomotor nuclei, both eyes would turn inward.

MLF injury, as often occurs in MS and brainstem strokes, produces the *MLF syndrome* or *internuclear ophthalmoplegia (INO)*. This condition, which spares the cranial nuclei and nerves, causes a classic pattern of ocular movement impairment identifiable primarily by inability of the eye ipsilateral to the lesion to adduct past the midline (see Chapter 15).

Another important ocular movement abnormality is *nystagmus* (rhythmic horizontal, vertical, or rotatory eyeball oscillation). Several central nervous system (CNS) injuries, including MS and brainstem strokes, cause nystagmus. In addition, it may be the most prominent physical finding in use of diazepam, barbiturates, alcohol, antipsychotics, or antidepressants. Nystagmus in a delirious patient suggests drug or alcohol use or intoxication. In this situation, physicians should consider Wernicke-Korsakoff syndrome and phencyclidine (PCP) intoxication.

Neurologists routinely find nystagmus in epilepsy patients taking therapeutic doses of phenytoin (Dilantin) or phenobarbital. Likewise, its absence may suggest noncompliance with their anticonvulsant regimen.

Although typically a sign of CNS dysfunction, nystagmus may be a normal variant. For example, many normal individuals have horizontal nystagmus (end point nystagmus) when looking far laterally. Some people have congenital nystagmus, which may be disconcerting to people looking at them, but it does not interfere with their vision. Congenital nystagmus is usually pendular (no alternation of fast and slow phases), direction-changing, and absent when they look toward a particular point (the null point). Although vertical nystagmus suggests a CNS lesion, predominantly horizontal nystagmus is often caused by labyrinthitis, in which case it is associated with vertigo, nausea, and vomiting.

Saccades and Pursuit Movement

Under ordinary circumstances, when an object enters the periphery of the visual field, the eyes dart toward it to redirect the line of sight and refocus attention. The eyes rotate conjugately, smoothly, and rapidly. Their movement does not disturb the eyelids or head. These ocular movements, *saccades*, are characterized by their rapidity, which may exceed 700 degrees per second.

Neurologists examine saccades by asking patients to stare at an object 45 degrees to one side and then suddenly shift their gaze to an object 45 degrees to the other side. At the bedside, the primary abnormality is slowness. Other abnormalities are overshooting or undershooting (hypermetria and hypometria), irregular or jerky movements, and—a subtle one—initiating the saccade by blinking or a head jerk (Fig. 12-13).

Many conditions, including strokes, MS, tumors, neurodegenerative illnesses, and schizophrenia, can damage the intricate mechanisms that generate saccades. The responsible lesions may be located in the cerebral cortex, cerebellum, pons, or occasionally elsewhere in the CNS. Abnormal saccades are a signature of Huntington's disease (see Chapter 18). Depending on the task used to demonstrate saccades, schizophrenics and their first-degree relatives may have abnormal saccades.

Although saccades are responsible for rapid shift of gaze from one object to another, *pursuit* or *smooth pursuit* is the slow continual ocular tracking of a moving object, such as a bird in flight. The bedside test consists of asking the patient to follow the examiner's finger as it moves horizontally at about 30 degrees per second. The eyes should remain on the target and smoothly track the finger through its 6-second path from one side to the other. The primary abnormality would be an irregular path instead of a smooth curve.

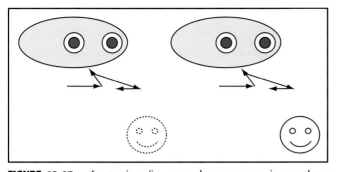

FIGURE 12-13 ■ In testing for saccades, an examiner asks a patient with Huntington's disease to shift his gaze from the examiner's nose to an object 3 feet to the left; however, after the patient's eyes shift conjugately to the left, they jerk momentarily to the right, then resume their leftward movement, but overshoot the target. They finally come to rest on the object. This path, made jerky by "intrusions," characterizes the abnormal saccades of Huntington's disease and possibly many cases of schizophrenia. Another characteristic of abnormal saccades is that they provoke patients to initiate them by tossing their head in the direction of the desired gaze, blinking, or widely opening their eyelids.

Numerous lesions and illnesses—even fatigue and inattention—impair smooth pursuit (Table 12-3). For example, parietal, temporal, or occipital cortex lesions; brainstem lesions; numerous medications; advanced age; and several neurologic and psychiatric illnesses cause irregular, rapid ocular movement.

In addition, although not specific enough to be diagnostic of schizophrenia, abnormalities in smooth pursuit serve as a neurophysiologic marker. Schizophrenia is more closely linked to abnormalities in smooth pursuit than to abnormalities in saccades. Schizophrenia patients' smooth pursuit eye movements are characteristically jerky and interrupted. Not only are these intrusions detectable early in schizophrenic patients, they are also detectable in many schizophrenics' asymptomatic family members. However, smooth pursuit abnormalities are also present, although less frequently, in individuals with depression, borderline personality disorders, and other psychiatric disturbances. For example, in depression, they improve with successful treatment.

DIPLOPIA

Diplopia ("double vision") perceived when looking with one eye (monocular diplopia) is usually the result of either ocular abnormalities, such as a dislocated lens, or psychogenic factors. Individuals with monocular diplopia, whatever the cause, lose their diplopia when their affected eye is covered, but

TABLE 12-3 ■ **Common Causes of Smooth Pursuit Abnormalities**

Medications
    Antiepileptic drugs
    Barbiturates and benzodiazepines
    Neuroleptics
Neurodegenerative illnesses
    Alzheimer's
    Huntington's
    Parkinson's
Psychiatric illnesses
    Affective disorders
    Attention deficit hyperactivity disorder
    Borderline personality disorder
    Obsessive-compulsive disorder
    Schizophrenia
Strokes, multiple

regain it when their unaffected eye is covered. Another characteristic is that their diplopia persists in all directions of gaze.

The form of diplopia most characteristic of a neurologic disorder—binocular diplopia—results from misalignment of the two eyes. It is usually present only in certain directions of gaze and covering either eye will abolish it.

When disorders of the nervous system cause diplopia, lesions in the brainstem or further "down" the neurologic ladder are almost always the cause: INO and other brainstem syndromes; oculomotor, trochlear, or abducens cranial nerve injury; neuromuscular junction disorders; or extraocular muscle paresis. In contrast, lesions above the brainstem, such as cerebral and other supranuclear lesions, characteristically cause conjugate gaze palsies not diplopia.

Oculomotor (third cranial) nerve injury results in diplopia that is greatest when the patient looks laterally. The examination, which separates diplopia on lateral gaze from a third nerve injury from other causes, detects ptosis, lateral deviation of the eye, and, most important, a dilated pupil—all of the affected eye (Fig. 12-14). However, one important exception is that third nerve infarctions from diabetes "spare the pupil," that is, the pupil remains reactive to light and the same size as its counterpart. Diplopia will be most pronounced when the patient attempts to adduct the eye (i.e., bring it medially). For example, a patient with damage to the left oculomotor nerve will have difficulty adducting the left eye, and diplopia will be greatest on looking to the right

Abducens (sixth cranial) nerve injury also causes diplopia on looking laterally. However, in contrast to

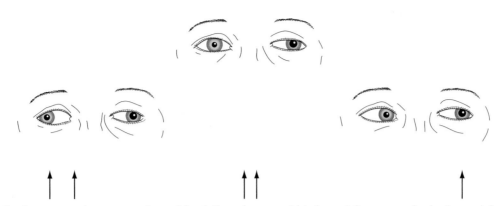

FIGURE 12-14 ■ In the center picture, a patient with a left oculomotor (third cranial) nerve palsy looks straight ahead. The left upper lid is lower, the pupil larger, and the eye deviated slightly laterally. Because the eyes are dysconjugate, the patient sees two arrows (diplopia) when looking ahead. In the picture on the left, the patient looks to the right. Because the paretic left eye fails to cross medially beyond the midline (i.e., it fails to adduct), the eyes are more dysconjugate and there is greater diplopia. In the picture on the right, the patient looks to the left. The eyes are almost conjugate and there is little or no diplopia.

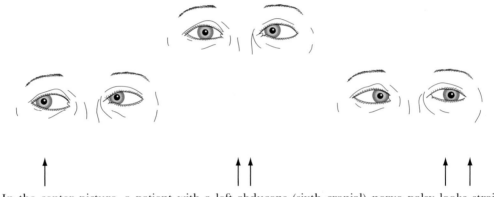

FIGURE 12-15 ■ In the center picture, a patient with a left abducens (sixth cranial) nerve palsy looks straight ahead. The patient's left eye is deviated medially. The eyes are dysconjugate, and the patient sees two arrows when looking ahead. In the picture on the left, the patient looks to the right. The eyes are conjugate, and the patient sees only a single arrow. In the picture on the right, the patient looks to the left. The paretic left eye fails to cross the midline laterally, that is, it fails to abduct. The exaggeration of the dysconjugate gaze increases the diplopia.

a third nerve palsy, the examination finds medial deviation of the affected eye at rest and inability of that eye to abduct. Also in contrast to a third nerve palsy, the examination shows neither ptosis nor pupil dilation (Fig. 12-15).

When myasthenia gravis, the classic neuromuscular junction disorder, causes diplopia, patients have fluctuating symptoms and asymmetric combinations of ptosis and ocular muscle paresis. However, no matter how severe the diplopia and ptosis, patients' pupils are characteristically round, equal, and reactive to light (see Chapter 6).

Although congenital ocular muscle weakness, *strabismus*, causes dysconjugate gaze, children do not have diplopia because the brain suppresses the image from the weaker eye. With continuous suppression of vision

from one eye, that eye will lose vision (i.e., become *amblyopic*). Thus, ophthalmologists patch the "good" eye of babies and children with strabismus for several hours each day. Alternatively, ophthalmologists perform muscle surgery or administer intramuscular botulinum injections to re-establish conjugate gaze to and thereby bring the affected eye into play and stimulate its visual pathways.

Before diagnosing psychogenic diplopia, physicians must not overlook subtle neurologic conditions, especially myasthenia gravis and the MLF syndrome. Psychogenic diplopia is usually intermittent, inconsistent, and present in all directions of gaze. Sometimes the diplopia is monocular. Patients with psychogenic diplopia, of course, have no observable abnormality. A common set of tests consists of the patient reading colored or polarized charts using colored or polarized lenses. In another psychogenic disturbance, *convergence spasm*, children or young adults, as if looking at the tip of their nose, fix their eyes in a downward and inward position, which superficially resembles bilateral sixth nerve palsies. This position is a burlesque that can be overcome by inducing optokinetic nystagmus.

HORNER'S SYNDROME AND ARGYLL-ROBERTSON PUPILS

Contrary to a reasonable expectation that the brain innervates eye muscles through short and direct pathways, the sympathetic tract follows a remarkably long and circuitous route (Fig. 12-16A). Injury to the sympathetic tract leads to *Horner's syndrome*: ptosis, miosis (a small pupil), and anhidrosis (lack of sweating) (see Fig. 12-16B). Given the route of the sympathetic tract, Horner's syndrome can be found in several widely separate injuries, including lateral medullary infarction (see Wallenberg's syndrome; see Fig. 2-10); cervical spinal cord injury; apical lung (Pancoast) tumor; and, because of a carotid artery dysfunction, cluster headache (see Fig. 9-4).

Physicians might confuse Horner's syndrome with a third nerve injury because ptosis is a common manifestation. However, Horner's syndrome's small pupil readily separates it from a third nerve injury, which causes a dilated, unreactive pupil. Anhidrosis of Horner's syndrome, although another clue, is less constant and more difficult to detect.

In a different situation, the astute physician confronting a small pupil must also bear in mind that the real problem may be that the contralateral one is abnormally large. Causes of a dilated pupil include, in addition to an oculomotor nerve injury, other lesions that damage the parasympathetic supply of the pupil sphincter muscles. Lack of parasympathetic innervation leaves the sympathetic innervation unopposed, resulting in a dilated pupil. An acquired benign variation, *Adie's pupil*, exemplifies the pupil-dilating effect of depriving a pupil of its normal parasympathetic innervation (Fig. 12-17). In another example, accidentally rubbing atropine-like substances into the effected eye can cause a dilated pupil. In a notorious variant, which is a manifestation of Factitious Disorder, people—often medical personnel—surreptitiously instill eyedrops containing pupil-dilating substances. The unilateral dilated pupil often triggers hospitalization and a series of investigations.

Argyll-Robertson pupils, which differ in subtle ways from those with other injuries, are irregular, asymmetric, and small (1 to 2 mm). They characteristically

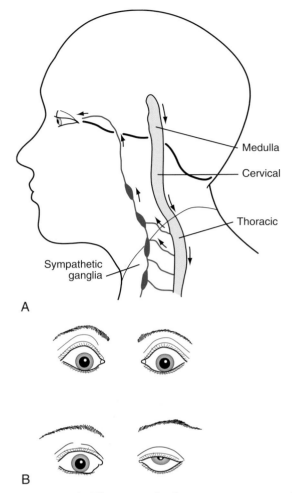

FIGURE 12-16 ■ *A,* The sympathetic nervous system originates in the hypothalamus, passes through the brainstem, and descends into the cervical and then the thoracic spinal cord. Some sympathetic system neurons leave the thoracic spinal cord and, after making a hairpin turn, ascend to form ganglia adjacent to the cervical vertebrae. Postsynaptic neurons ascend further. They wrap successively around the common carotid, and internal carotid. They enter the orbit with the ophthalmic division of the trigeminal nerve (V_1). These neurons innervate the pupil dilator muscles, upper eyelid muscles, and facial sweat glands. *B, Top,* Stimulation of the sympathetic nervous system retracts the eyelid, dilates the pupil, and causes sweating. These cardinal signs of the flight or fright response may also be induced by states of excitement, including amphetamine use. *Bottom,* Sympathetic tract injury causes Horner's syndrome—ptosis, miosis, and anhidrosis—on this patient's left side. A subtle clue to Horner's syndrome is the eyebrow elevation, which is an unconscious maneuver to uncover the pupil.

constrict normally when patients look at closely held objects (i.e., during accommodation) but fail to react to light. The intact accommodation, but impaired light reflex, especially with the historic association with

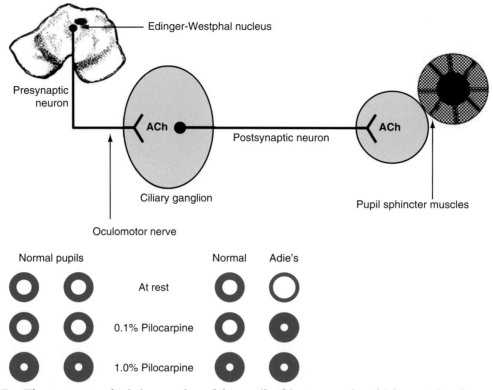

FIGURE 12-17 ■ *Top,* The parasympathetic innervation of the pupil sphincter muscle, which constricts the pupil, originates in the Edinger-Westphal nucleus (also see Fig. 4-2). That nucleus, adjacent to the third cranial (oculomotor) nerve nucleus, sends its parasympathetic fibers along with the oculomotor nerve. These fibers then separate and synapse in the parasympathetic ciliary ganglion. From there, postsynaptic fibers form a neuromuscular junction with the sphincter muscles. Acetylcholine (ACh) is the neurotransmitter in both synapses. Through this pathway, light and various other stimuli cause pupil constriction. *Bottom,* In Adie's pupil, which is typically a unilateral condition, the ciliary ganglion degenerates and the pupil, deprived of parasympathetic innervation, dilates. The loss of the ciliary ganglia subjects the pupil to denervation hypersensitivity. In this case, the left (Adie's) pupil suffers from a congenital impairment of the ciliary ganglion. Without the parasympathetic innervation, the left pupil dilates at rest in room light. In response to bright light, it would constrict only weakly, incompletely, and slowly. A diluted cholinergic eyedrop (0.1% pilocarpine), which has no effect on normal pupils including this patient's unaffected right eye, produces a brisk and long-lasting constriction of the Adie's pupil. The reaction is exaggerated in the Adie's pupil because its denervated postsynaptic neurons are overly sensitive, that is, have denervation hypersensitivity. To a more concentrated solution of pilocarpine (1%), normal pupils as well as the Adie's pupil will constrict. As a seemingly related aspect of this condition, Adie's pupil patients often have lost their quadriceps deep tendon reflexes.

syphilis, has given rise to the saying, "Argyll-Robertson pupils are like prostitutes. They accommodate but do not react." Today's statistics belie that mnemonic: Diabetic autonomic neuropathy and cataract surgery currently cause almost all cases of Argyll-Robertson pupils.

REFERENCES

1. Aldrich MS, Alessi AG, Beck RW, et al: Cortical blindness: Etiology, diagnosis, and prognosis. Ann Neurol 21:149–158, 1987.
2. Craig JE, Ong TJ, Louis DL, et al: Mechanisms of topiramate-induced acute-onset myopia and angle closure glaucoma. Am J Ophthalmol 137:193–195, 2004.
3. Cummings JL, Miller BL: Visual hallucinations: Clinical occurrence and use in differential diagnosis. West J Med 146:46–51, 1987.
4. Damasio AR, Damasio H, Hoesen GWV: Prosopagnosia: Anatomic basis and behavioral mechanisms. Neurology 32:331–341, 1982.
5. Friedman L, Abel LA, Jesberger JA, et al: Saccadic intrusions into smooth pursuit in patients with schizophrenia or affective disorder and normal controls. Biol Psychiatry 31:1110–1118, 1992.
6. Gittinger JW: Functional hemianopsia: A historical perspective. Surv Ophthalmol 32:427–432, 1988.
7. Holbrook JT, Jabs DA, Weinberg DV, et al: Visual loss in patients with cytomegalovirus retinitis and acquired immunodeficiency syndrome before widespread availability of highly active antiretroviral therapy. Arch Ophthalmol 121:99–107, 2003.

8. Keane JR: Neuro-ophthalmologic signs of AIDS. Neurology 41:841–845, 1991.

9. Lieberman E, Stoudemire A: Use of tricyclic antidepressants in patients with glaucoma. Psychosomatics 28:145–148, 1987.

10. Menon GL, Rahman I, Menon SJ, et al: Complex visual hallucinations in the visually impaired. Surv Ophthalmol 48:58–72, 2003.

11. Pomeranz HD, Lessell S: Palinopsia and polyopia in the absence of drugs or cerebral disease. Neurology 54:855–859, 2000.

12. Rovner BW: The Charles Bonnet syndrome. Geriatrics 57:45–46, 2002.

1. Which three findings characterize Argyll-Robertson pupils?
   a. Miosis
   b. Ptosis
   c. Irregular shape
   d. Unresponsiveness to light
   e. Unresponsiveness to accommodation
   f. Failure to dilate with atropine drops

   Answers: a, c, d.

2. Which two medications often produce transient visual impairment because of accommodation paresis?
   a. Butyrophenones
   b. Amitriptyline
   c. Imipramine
   d. Phenobarbital
   e. Phenytoin

   Answers: b, c. Tricyclic antidepressants' anticholinergic side effects lead to visual impairment.

3. Which one of the following does not cause cataracts that impair vision?
   a. Myotonic dystrophy
   b. Diabetes mellitus
   c. Ocular trauma
   d. Chlorpromazine

   Answer: d. Myotonic dystrophy, diabetes, and ocular trauma cause cataracts dense enough to impair vision. Phenothiazines, some atypical neuroleptics, and amiodarone cause lens opacities that do not reach the density of cataracts.

4. A 20-year-old soldier develops loss of vision in the right eye accompanied by retro-orbital pain, especially when looking from side to side. An ophthalmologist finds no ocular or neurologic abnormalities except for a decreased direct light reaction in the right pupil. The right pupil, however, constricts to light shone in the left eye. After 1 week, vision returns, except for a small central scotoma. Which is the most likely diagnosis?
   a. Psychogenic disturbance
   b. Optic neuritis
   c. Left cerebral infarction
   d. Pituitary adenoma
   e. Glaucoma

   Answer: b. The loss of vision, accompanied by an impaired direct light reflex but preserved consensual response, indicates that the origin is in the optic nerve, which is the afferent limb of the light reflex. The pain, which is exacerbated by ocular movement, indicates an inflammatory disturbance. In optic neuritis, the "patient sees nothing, and the ophthalmologist sees nothing" when inspecting the eye. Also, optic neuritis is a relatively common condition among young adults.

5. Which cells produce the covering of optic nerve?
   a. Schwann
   b. Oligodendroglia
   c. Neuron
   d. Microglia

   Answer: b. Oligodendroglia cells produce the myelin that covers the white matter of the CNS, including the optic nerve and a small proximal portion of the acoustic nerve. The optic nerve is actually an extension of the CNS. In contrast, Schwann cells produce the myelin that covers the peripheral nerves and the other cranial nerves. Microglia are supporting cells of the CNS.

6. As individuals age beyond 50 years they typically require reading glasses to discern closely held objects, such as newspapers and sewing. Without their glasses, they must hold such objects at arms length. What accounts for this visual problem?
   a. Cataract formation impairs accommodation.
   b. Retinal degeneration prevents accommodation.
   c. Their lenses lose elasticity and dehydrate.
   d. These visual difficulties are a perceptual problem.

   Answer: c. As people age, their lenses lose elasticity and fluid content. Those lenses are unable to thicken rapidly or fully and thus cannot accommodate to look at closely held objects.

7. A 79-year-old woman who has been blind since cataract surgery 5 years ago discloses that she has been having visual hallucinations. The hallucinations last several minutes to an hour and occur at any time of the day. During them, the patient "sees" her children as babies, her parents, and various real or imagined scenes. She appreciates that the visions are hallucinations. She is not frightened or inclined to act on them. She has no cognitive impairment or

lateralized neurologic signs. What should be the next step?

a. Perform an EEG
b. Obtain an ophthalmology consultation
c. Administer an antipsychotic
d. Administer an antidepressant
e. Obtain an MRI
f. None of the above

Answer: f. She probably has the *Charles Bonnet syndrome,* which is sometimes called "release visual hallucinations," in which elderly, blind individuals, who are not demented or psychologically disturbed, have frequent benign visual hallucinations. The condition probably results from blindness, that is, sensory deprivation. It follows macular degeneration, diabetic retinopathy, bilateral optic nerve lesions, and cortical blindness. Physicians might monitor patients' cognitive status and hearing. The family should provide auditory and tactile sensory clues. If simple measures suppress the hallucinations, physicians do not have to proceed with diagnostic testing and administering medicines. Although reports describe the beneficial effects of antiepileptic drugs and other medicines, atypical antipsychotics, on either an "as-needed" or nightly basis, are the best treatment.

8. Which electroencephalogram (EEG) change characterizes blindness?

a. EEG 8–12 Hz rhythms located over the occipital lobes when the patient rests that persist when the eyes open
b. Absence of these rhythms at rest and when the eyes are open
c. Presence of these rhythms when the eyes are open but not at rest
d. None of the above

Answer: a. These rhythms are normal alpha activity. Individuals at rest with their eyes closed have alpha activity, but when they open their eyes, alpha activity disappears as visual information is transmitted to the occipital lobe. In blind individuals, the alpha activity persists because no visual information is transmitted to the occipital lobe. In contrast, if someone has psychogenic blindness, opening the eyes will abolish alpha activity.

9. Which one of the following statements is false regarding glaucoma?

a. Serotonin reuptake inhibitors are less likely than tricyclic antidepressants to precipitate glaucoma.
b. Marijuana is more effective and carries fewer potential side effects than glaucoma medicines.
c. Beta-blocker topical medications (eyedrops) are often absorbed into the systemic circulation in

concentrations great enough to cause episodic mental changes.
d. Patients being treated for glaucoma may reasonably safely be given tricyclic antidepressants.

Answer: b. Glaucoma medicines are effective and usually produce no side effects. Cogent reasons may be offered for legalizing marijuana, but its use as a glaucoma medicine cannot be one of them.

10–15. Match the usual field loss (10–15) with the underlying illness (a–f). Answers may be used more than once. These drawings follow the common practice of showing visual fields from the patient's perspective.

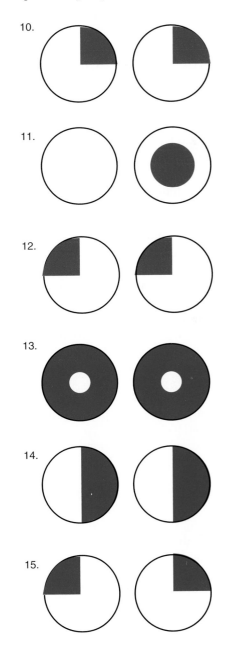

a. A 25-year-old woman has paraparesis and ataxia.

b. A 35-year-old woman has insidious onset of loss of peripheral daytime vision and all night-time vision. Her mother has a similar illness.

c. A 30-year-old man has episodes of seeing the American flag and hearing the first five bars of "America the Beautiful."

d. A 21-year-old man has loss of bodily hair, gynecomastia, and diabetes insipidus.

e. A 70-year-old man has global aphasia, right hemiplegia, and right hemisensory loss.

f. A 75-year-old man has fluent aphasia.

Answers

10-c. The patient may have partial complex (e.g., psychomotor) seizures and a right superior quadrantanopia as the result of a left temporal lobe lesion. *Or* f. Alternatively, the patient may have a left temporal lobe lesion giving him aphasia and a contralateral superior quadrantanopia.

11-a. The patient has spinal cord, cerebellar, and right optic nerve injury, probably as the result of multiple sclerosis (MS).

12-c. The patient may have partial complex seizures and a left superior quadrantanopia as the result of a right temporal lobe lesion.

13-b. The patient and her mother have preservation only of the central vision during daytime. If examination of her fundi showed clumping of retinal pigment, the diagnosis of retinitis pigmentosa would be certain. These visual fields might also be obtained from someone having tunnel vision.

14-e. The patient probably has a dominant hemisphere lesion, such as a cerebrovascular accident or tumor, giving a right homonymous hemianopsia.

15-d. The patient has a large pituitary tumor causing panhypopituitarism and bitemporal hemianopsia.

16–26. Match the characteristics of the visual hallucination or other symptom with its most likely source (a–c).

16. Associated musical hallucinations

17. Flashes of bright lights in the contralateral visual field

18. Associated olfactory hallucinations

19. Rotating blotches of color

20. Formed hallucinations with impaired consciousness

21. Postictal aphasia

22. Throbbing unilateral headache

23. Nausea and vomiting

24. Simple blocks and stars of color

25. Twisting, complicated multicolored lights

26. Faces with distorted features or coloring

a. Seizures that originate in the occipital lobe

b. Seizures that originate in the temporal lobe

c. Migraine with aura (classical migraine)

Answers: 16-b; 17-a, c; 18-b, rarely c; 19-a; 20-b; 21-b, rarely c; 22-c; 23-c; 24-a, c; 25-b, c; 26-b, c.

27–28. Match the symptom (27–28) with the possible origins (a–d).

27. Diplopia when looking to the right

28. Diplopia when looking to the left

a. Left third nerve palsy

b. Left sixth nerve palsy

c. Right third nerve palsy

d. Right sixth nerve palsy

Answers: 27-a, d; 28-b, c.

29–30. Match the actions that cause blindness with the outcome.

29. Staring directly into the sun

30. Drinking adulterated alcohols

a. Methanol-induced optic nerve injury

b. Pigmentary retinal degeneration

c. Retinal burns

Answers: 29-c; 30-a.

31. What four conditions are common causes of ptosis?

a. Third nerve palsy

b. Sixth nerve palsy

c. Pancoast tumor

d. MS

e. Myasthenia gravis

f. Psychogenic disturbances

g. Botulinum treatment of blepharospasm

Answers: a, c, e, g. MS can produce ptosis if a plaque develops in the midbrain, where it would damage the third cranial nerve; however, lesions rarely develop in that location. When injecting botulinum toxin into the orbicularis oculi to treat blepharospasm, physicians avoid the middle of the upper eyelid, which overlies the levator palpebrae. If botulinum toxin enters that muscle, the eyelid weakens.

32. Which two illnesses can cause internuclear ophthalmoplegia?

a. MS

b. Poliomyelitis

c. Muscular dystrophy

d. Psychogenic disturbances

e. Heroin overdose

f. Brainstem strokes

Answers: a, f.

33. Which ocular motility abnormality is associated with schizophrenia?
a. Internuclear ophthalmoplegia
b. Nystagmus
c. Convergence spasm
d. Conjugate gaze paresis
e. Pursuit abnormalities

Answer: e. Schizophrenic patients often have slow, irregular pursuit movements and saccade abnormalities. However, those ocular motility abnormalities are not peculiar to schizophrenia.

34. A 70-year-old man awakens with a right hemiparesis, vertigo, and his eyes deviated to the right. Which condition will also be found?
a. Aphasia
b. Right homonymous hemianopsia
c. Dementia
d. Nystagmus

Answer: d. This patient has an infarction in the left pons. He would have nystagmus because of injury of the vestibular nucleus, which is in the pons. In addition, he might have injury to the left facial and abducens nerve nuclei, which are also in the pons, that would cause left upper and lower facial paresis and medial deviation of the left eye. He would not have signs of cerebral injury, such as aphasia, hemianopsia, or cognitive impairment.

35. Which condition indicates that the dopamine system is involved in conjugate eye movement?
a. Internuclear ophthalmoplegia
b. Nystagmus
c. Pontine gaze center movement
d. Oculogyric crisis

Answer: d. Phenothiazines, including those used for nonpsychotic conditions, such as nausea and vomiting, precipitate oculogyric crises.

36. Which conditions have a predilection for people older than 65 years?
a. Myopia
b. Presbyopia
c. Macular degeneration
d. Classic migraines
e. Temporal or giant cell arteritis
f. Glaucoma
g. Cataracts
h. Optic neuritis

Answers: b, c, e, f, g. Moreover, combinations of these conditions may occur together in the same older patient. Whatever the cause of a visual impairment, it is a major threat to the well-being of patients, especially those with cognitive impairment or loss of other special senses.

37. A 70-year-old man sustained a cerebral infarction. He has a right homonymous hemianopsia, right hemisensory loss, and a mild right hemiparesis. Although he can both say and write the names of objects that he feels, he is unable to name objects that he only sees, even when they are presented to his left visual field. What is the name of this condition?
a. Aphasia
b. Hemi-inattention
c. Visual agnosia
d. Gerstmann's syndrome
e. Balint's syndrome
f. Dementia
g. Alexia

Answer: c. The patient has visual agnosia, a condition in which patients cannot process visually acquired information. Additional testing might reveal Gerstmann's syndrome or alexia without agraphia (see Chapter 8)—conditions also resulting from posterior dominant hemisphere lesions. His problem is not aphasia: Once the examiner circumvents vision, by testing the patient's writing and speaking, language function is revealed to be normal. The lesion causing the visual agnosia is in the left parietal and occipital region.

38. Match the visual disturbance (1–4) with the etiology (a–e).
1. Psychic blindness
2. Night blindness
3. Cortical blindness
4. Transient monocular blindness
   a. Carotid stenosis
   b. Occipital infarction (bilateral)
   c. Conversion reaction
   d. Bilateral temporal lobe injury
   e. Vitamin A deficiency

Answers: 1-d (Klüver-Bucy syndrome), 2-e, 3-b, 4-a (amaurosis fugax). (Night blindness is also a symptom of retinitis pigmentosa.)

39–46. Match the patient's condition (39–46) with the neuropsychologic disorder (a–j).
39. Cannot recognize familiar faces
40. Despite visual loss, willfully but erroneously describes hospital room and physician
41. After cardiac arrest, blindness with intact pupil light reflex
42. Cannot identify a red card, although able to match it to another red card and read a red-colored number on the Ishihara plates

43. Despite only a right homonymous hemianopsia, inability to read; writing ability intact
44. Congenital inability to read Ishihara plates
45. Inability to name common objects under any circumstances
46. Cannot name objects when seen, but can name them when described or grasped
    a. Cortical blindness
    b. Visual agnosia
    c. Color agnosia
    d. Color blindness
    e. Prosopagnosia
    f. Anton's syndrome
    g. Wernicke-Korsakoff syndrome
    h. Alexia without agraphia
    i. Congenital cerebral injury
    j. Anomia

Answers: 39-e, 40-f, 41-a, 42-c, 43-h, 44-d, 45-j, 46-b.

47. Which three conditions cause stereotyped visual hallucinations?
    a. Partial complex seizures
    b. Tonic clonic seizures
    c. LSD ingestions
    d. Occipital lobe seizures
    e. Migraine with aura
    f. Migraine without aura
    g. Hypnagogic hallucinations
    h. Alcohol withdrawal

Answers: a, d, e. Patients with primary generalized—absences (petit mal) and tonic-clonic—seizures have no aura or visual symptoms. Intoxications and withdrawal cause varied symptoms in the context of delirium. Hypnagogic and hypnopompic hallucinations are dreams, which are typically highly variable. When migraine includes an aura, it is stereotyped.

48. Which two varieties of hallucinations appear predominantly or exclusively in hemianopic areas?
    a. Palinopsia
    b. Partial seizures
    c. Migraines
    d. REM-associated dreams
    e. LSD intoxication

Answers: a, b. In palinopsia and partial (elementary and complex) seizures, visual hallucinations often appear exclusively within a hemianopic region. Occipital or temporal lobe lesions often cause such hallucinations. Hallucinations related to migraines, dreams, and intoxications occur randomly and do not respect visual fields.

49. Which of the following is true of slowed smooth pursuit ocular movement?

    a. Abnormal saccades are more indicative of schizophrenia.
    b. Slowed smooth pursuit is sensitive for schizophrenia but not specific.
    c. Slowed smooth pursuit is specific for schizophrenia but not sensitive.
    d. When due to neurologic illness, slowed smooth pursuit is highly indicative of basal ganglia disease.

Answer: b. Slow smooth pursuit ocular movements can result from a wide variety of neurologic diseases, medications, and psychiatric illnesses. This abnormality is a neurophysiologic marker of schizophrenia, but it is not specific (see Table 12-3).

50. Which two of the following statements are true regarding saccades?
    a. Saccades are the smooth, steady tracking movements used to follow moving objects.
    b. They are the quick, conjugate movements that bring images from the periphery to the center of vision.
    c. They are governed by supranuclear centers.
    d. Unlike pursuit movements, they are resistant to structural lesions and degenerative illnesses.

Answers: b, c. Cerebral conjugate gaze centers generate saccades, which are high velocity conjugate gaze movements. Saccades are susceptible to cerebrovascular accidents and other cerebral lesions. Abnormal saccades are a hallmark and an early sign of Huntington's disease.

51. Which two of the following statements are true regarding pursuits?
    a. They are the smooth, steady tracking movements used to follow moving objects.
    b. They are the quick, conjugate movements that bring objects from the periphery to the center of vision.
    c. They are governed by supranuclear centers.
    d. Unlike saccades, they are resistant to structural lesions and degenerative illnesses.

Answers: a, c. Pursuits are relatively slow, smooth conjugate gaze movements. They are susceptible to various illnesses and, along with saccades, are abnormal in schizophrenia and, to a lesser extent, affective disorders.

52. Which two signs are the constituents of Horner's syndrome?
    a. Mitosis
    b. Miosis
    c. Anhidrosis
    d. Tearing
    e. Third cranial nerve palsy

Answers: b, c. In addition to miosis (small pupil) and anhidrosis (lack of sweating), Horner's syndrome includes ptosis. It results from injury to the sympathetic supply of the face and eye.

53. In which four conditions are Horner's syndrome commonly found?
    a. Migraine without aura
    b. Migraine with aura
    c. Cluster headache
    d. Trigeminal neuralgia
    e. Cervical spinal cord injury
    f. Apical lung tumor
    g. Lateral medullary CVAs

    Answers: c, e, f, g. Horner's syndrome may result from lesions in the medulla, upper portion of the spinal cord (the cervical spinal cord), or autonomic nervous system in the chest—anywhere along the circuitous route of the sympathetic innervation of the pupil (see Fig. 12-16).

54. Which cerebral artery supplies the occipital lobes?
    a. Anterior cerebral
    b. Middle cerebral
    c. Posterior cerebral
    d. None of the above

    Answer: c. The posterior cerebral arteries, which are the terminal branches of the basilar artery, perfuse the occipital lobes. Because the occipital lobes contain the visual cortex, occlusion of both posterior cerebral arteries causes cortical blindness.

55. A 33-year-old man claims to have double vision in his right eye after a motor vehicle accident (MVA). When he covers the right eye, the diplopia disappears, but when he covers the left eye, he has persistent diplopia. The visual acuity in the left eye is 20/20 and in the right eye 20/400. Visual fields are normal in the left eye but cannot be determined in the right eye because of the diplopia. Which three statements regarding his situation are true?
    a. His symptom is monocular diplopia.
    b. With the available information, conclusions cannot be drawn concerning the presence of central nervous system (CNS) injury causing the diplopia.
    c. Monocular diplopia is virtually always the result of an ocular injury, such as a dislocated lens or retinal disruption, or psychogenic factors.
    d. The first step in determining the cause of diplopia is to establish whether it arises from a single eye. In other words, determine if covering one eye abolishes the diplopia.

Answers: a, c, d. When the brainstem or cranial nerves III, IV, or VI are injured, patients have diplopia only if both eyes are open. As a general rule, cerebral lesions do not cause diplopia. When diplopia originates from one eye, the patient is said to have monocular diplopia.

56. In which structure is the third cranial nerve nucleus located?
    a. Midbrain
    b. Pons
    c. Medulla
    d. Cerebrum

    Answer: a.

57. In which structure is the fourth cranial nerve nucleus located?
    a. Midbrain
    b. Pons
    c. Medulla
    d. Cerebrum

    Answer: a.

58. In which structure is the sixth cranial nerve nucleus located?
    a. Midbrain
    b. Pons
    c. Medulla
    d. Cerebrum

    Answer: b.

59. A 75-year-old man was shown a picture of his anniversary party that had been held when he was 50 years old. He recognized most friends and family members but could not identify the relationships among them. He could not recall the reason for the party despite a "Happy 25th Anniversary" banner in the background. He looked from one person to another, but he failed to survey the scene and was unable to direct his gaze. He was oriented and had good memory and judgment. His visual acuity and visual fields were within normal limits. Which disorder is impairing his ability to comprehend the picture?
    a. Dementia
    b. Cortical blindness
    c. Bilateral hemi-inattention
    d. Gerstmann's syndrome
    e. Balint's syndrome
    f. Depression

    Answer: e. Balint's syndrome is a neuropsychologic syndrome that consists of psychic paralysis of fixation, optic ataxia, and simultanagnosia. The simultanagnosia prevents him from perceiving objects in the periphery, as well as in the center, of his visual fields. The psychic paralysis refers to someone's inability to shift one's gaze from one object to another, as though the first object was overwhelmingly captivating. The simultanagnosia and psychic paralysis inhibit patients from exploring space. Optic ataxia refers to the inability to look directly from one object to another.

60. If a physician suspects that a patient has psychogenic blindness, which of the following EEG findings will support that diagnosis?
  a. Alpha activity at rest with eyes closed, but loss of alpha activity with the eyes open
  b. Alpha activity at rest with eyes closed and with eyes open
  c. Beta activity with eyes closed, but loss of alpha activity with the eyes open
  d. Beta activity at rest with eyes closed and with eyes open

Answer: a. Alpha activity develops in the occipital region when individuals are at rest with closed eyes. However, if people concentrate, perform simple calculations, preoccupy themselves, or experience anxiety, they will suppress alpha activity. Thus, alpha activity is a popular marker for an anxiety-free state. Unless people are blind, opening their eyes abolishes alpha activity. Thus, individuals with psychogenic blindness will lose their alpha activity when they open their eyes. Beta activity, which is usually present over the frontal regions, suggests that the individual is alert, concentrating, anxious, or under the influence of sedatives and other medications.

61. During her recovery from a lumbar laminectomy, a 35-year-old nurse complains of the sudden onset of poor vision in her right eye. That eye's pupil is dilated. The intraocular pressure is normal. Pilocarpine eyedrops (1%) fail to constrict the pupil. Her extraocular movements are full and the funduscopic examination reveals no abnormalities. The remainder of the neurologic examination is normal. A CT, MRI, and LP all produce normal results. A similar problem had occurred after her hysterectomy the previous year. What is the most likely cause of her visual impairment?
  a. Myasthenia gravis
  b. A left-sided Horner's syndrome
  c. Spinal cord injury from the laminectomy
  d. Adie's pupil
  e. None of the above

Answer: e. The failure of pilocarpine, a strong miotic agent, to constrict the pupil indicates that she or someone else is instilling substances into her eye. Ophthalmologic preparations of cocaine, atropine,

hydroxyamphetamine eyedrops, and several readily available chemicals dilate a normal pupil. Myasthenia gravis does not affect the pupils. A lumbar laminectomy is performed nowhere near the spinal cord. An Adie's pupil, unlike a normal pupil, constricts to a dilute (0.1%) pilocarpine solution.

62. A 27-year-old woman has suddenly lost vision in her left eye. The pupils in room light are equal in size. When a light is shone into the left eye, neither pupil constricts; however, when light is shone into the right eye, both pupils constrict. Which portion of the light reflex is impaired?
  a. Left afferent
  b. Right afferent
  c. Left efferent
  d. Right efferent

Answer: a. Her left optic nerve has been injured.

63. In evaluating another patient with an impaired light reflex, the physician finds that when a light is shone into the left eye, only the right pupil constricts. When light is shone into the right eye, only the right pupil constricts. Which portion of the light reflex is impaired?
  a. Left afferent
  b. Right afferent
  c. Left efferent
  d. Right efferent

Answer: c. Her left oculomotor nerve has been injured. Alternatives include ocular trauma and instillation of eye drops.

64. After open-heart surgery complicated by multiple cerebral emboli, a patient seems unable to watch television news because he cannot follow the video pictures. He can comprehend the audio content. He also has difficulty describing pictures. Although he can name the contents of his room, he is unable to name pictures of a kitchen, bedroom, or backyard. His visual acuity with a hand-held card is approximately 20/30 in both eyes and his visual fields are full. Language, memory, and general cognitive function, although not perfect, are all adequate for these tasks. Which would be the best term for his inability to watch television news?
  a. Simultanagnosia
  b. Cortical blindness
  c. Psychogenic blindness
  d. Glaucoma

Answer: a. Simultanagnosia is perceptual disturbance consisting of inability to integrate and weigh the importance of the various elements of a scene. It prevents the patient from identifying complex scenes and familiar faces (prosopagnosia).

65. A 68-year-old man, a well-respected successful lawyer, remains personable, humorous, and a good ballroom dancer. Years ago he began to forget the names of acquaintances and some colleagues. He consults an ophthalmologist because he has begun to fail to recognize the faces of friends, acquaintances, and historic figures, such as George Washington. However, his visual acuity is 20/20 with glasses. Which is the most likely condition?

a. Mild cognitive impairment

b. Dementia, probably from Alzheimer's disease

c. Visual acuity impairment

d. Prosopagnosia superimposed on mild cognitive impairment

e. Normal age-related cognitive changes

Answer: d. He has developed prosopagnosia, which is a visual perceptual problem consisting of inability to recognize faces, superimposed on mild cognitive impairment. Prosopagnosia is usually attributable to a neurodegenerative illness, such as frontotemporal dementia and Alzheimer's disease, or a lesion of the right temporal lobe. Although the patient may have mild cognitive impairment, he does not have dementia because he still functions.

66. Which of the following is not a normal age-related change?

a. Impaired smooth pursuit eye movements

b. Small pupils

c. Presbyopia

d. Internuclear ophthalmoplegia

Answer: d.

67. A young woman, who was previously entirely healthy, develops optic neuritis without other neurologic or ophthalmologic findings. Her MRI shows several areas of high signal intensity and her cerebrospinal fluid (CSF) contains oligoclonal bands. What is the likelihood of her developing MS?

a. 25% or less

b. 25% to 50%

c. 50% to 75%

d. 90% or greater

Answer: c. The majority of optic neuritis patients with MRI lesions and CSF oligoclonal bands will develop MS.

68. If the patient in the preceding question had a normal MRI and no CSF oligoclonal bands, what would be the likelihood of her developing MS?

a. 25% or less

b. 25% to 50%

c. 50% to 75%

d. 90% or greater

Answer: a. Various viral illnesses, sarcoidosis, vasculitis, and numerous conditions other than MS may cause optic neuritis.

69. With the onset of her menopause, a 59-year-old woman begins to suffer from an increase the frequency of her migraines from once a month to twice weekly. Her neurologist initiates preventative treatment with topiramate. Several weeks later, the woman reports bilateral visual impairment and eye pain. A consulting ophthalmologist finds that she has redness of the eyes, large pupils, and shallow anterior chambers. Which of the following conditions has most likely developed?

a. Open-angle glaucoma

b. Angle-closure glaucoma

c. Optic neuritis

d. Self-inflicted eye injury

Answer: b. She has most likely developed angle-closure glaucoma with abnormally elevated intraocular pressure. Although the glaucoma may have developed spontaneously, the topiramate treatment probably caused it. Giant cell arteritis (temporal arteritis) is unlikely because she is younger than 65 years and, unlike the findings in giant cell arteritis, her eyes are red, and her anterior chambers shallow.

70. Which illness is in the same family as Leber's hereditary optic atrophy (neuropathy)?

a. MELAS

b. MS

c. Huntington's disease

d. Schizophrenia

e. Red-green color blindness

Answer: a. Leber's hereditary optic atrophy (neuropathy), which usually affects young men, causes suddenly occurring severe visual loss in one eye and then the other. This illness and MELAS both belong to the family of mitochondrial disorders. MS belongs to the family of autoimmune inflammatory disorders; Huntington's to the trinucleotide repeat family; and color blindness to the sex-linked genetic family.

71. Which of the following is not a characteristic of an Adie's pupil?

a. Loss of parasympathetic innervation

b. Denervation hypersensitivity to noradrenergic stimulation

c. Denervation hypersensitivity to cholinergic stimulation

d. Constriction to 0.1% pilocarpine

Answer: b. The ciliary ganglion supplies parasympathetic innervation to the pupillary constrictor muscles. If it is damaged, as in the Adie's pupil, unopposed sympathetic innervation dilates the pupil. The unaffected pupil remains normal in size and reactivity. Room light is insufficient to constrict the Adie's pupil. Although bright light constricts it, the movement is slow and incomplete. The distinguishing feature of the Adie's pupil is that, because of parasympathetic denervation, the pupillary constrictor muscles have denervation hypersensitivity to cholinergic stimulation. Thus, a dilute pilocarpine solution (0.1%) constricts an Adie's pupil but not its unaffected counterpart. A more concentrated pilocarpine solution (1%), which is normally used to treat glaucoma, will constrict normal as well as denervated pupils.

72. In a stuporous 1-year-old infant, what further testing does the presence of retinal hemorrhages immediately suggest?
    a. Blood glucose for diabetes mellitus
    b. HIV testing for AIDS-related retinal disease
    c. X-rays of the long bones
    d. Sickle cell determination

Answer: c. Retinal hemorrhages suggest the "shaken baby" syndrome. Physicians should seek other signs of abuse, such as spiral fractures of the long bones. Of course, the physicians should also order a head CT in a stuporous infant with signs of trauma.

Congenital Cerebral Impairments

Many perinatal injuries and genetic abnormalities, which cause cerebral impairments, leave distinct, permanent physical and neuropsychologic deficits. Although usually evident in infancy, these cerebral impairments sometimes produce recognizable deficits only beginning in childhood or adolescence.

CEREBRAL PALSY

Cerebral palsy (CP)—a nonscientific, but generally accepted term—describes the permanent, nonprogressive neurologic *motor system* impairments that result from central nervous system (CNS) injuries of the immature brain. The injuries may occur during fetal development, in *utero*, in the course of delivery (perinatally), during infancy, or in early childhood.

In cases in which physicians can establish the cause, they usually attribute CP to prematurity and low birth weight, particularly weights less than 1.5 kg. Those factors are also associated with vision and hearing disorders, intelligence quotient (IQ) scores less than 85, poor school performance, and impaired social skills.

Other causes of CP include hypoxia before or during labor, prolonged bradycardia, 10- or 15-minute Apgar score of less than 4, and postpartum multisystem organ failure. Over the last 30 years, improved prenatal, obstetric, and postpartum care have reduced the incidence of CP to about 2% of births. However, it has resisted further reductions despite a variety of technical innovations and public health measures.

Although preventable obstetric injuries, such as anoxia, account for less than 10% of cases, unalterable antepartum factors account for more than 70%. For example, CP is often a manifestation of inexplicable congenital malformations, such as microgyria (small cerebral gyri), pachygyria (thickened gyri), hydrocephalus, and porencephaly (see Fig. 20-4). Also, because 5% of CP children have a first-degree relative with a similar condition, as yet undetermined genetic factors undoubtedly contribute to many cases.

The clinical features of CP are usually so apparent to neurologists that they can diagnose most cases "by inspection." Nevertheless, several conditions mimic CP closely enough to represent diagnostic pitfalls.

For example, insidiously advancing leukoencephalopathies (see Chapter 15) may produce spastic paresis indistinguishable from CP. Similarly, dopa-responsive dystonia gives rise to a disorder similar to choreoathetotic CP (see later and Chapter 18). Finally, deafness, which may occur alone or accompanied by other neurologic disabilities, may mimic CP or mental retardation.

Neurologists often divide CP into four varieties. Each one has a characteristic motor impairment, such as *spastic paresis* or *choreoathetosis* (Fig. 13-1), and a correlation with epilepsy and mental retardation. In individual cases, other neurologic problems—hyperactivity and learning disabilities; visual and hearing impairment; and feeding difficulties, dysarthria, and other signs of pseudobulbar palsy—complicate the basic picture.

Neurologists diagnose CP in children who have a nonprogressive or "static" motor impairment following a perinatal cerebral injury (Table 13-1). Their particular impairment must change little or not at all as the affected child grows. In fact, impairments may actually seem to recede as children learn compensatory strategies and benefit from physical therapy. Conversely, progression of symptoms—such as a spreading from paraparesis to quadriparesis—generally precludes a diagnosis of CP.

Although the clinical evaluation emphasizing history and development remains the basis of diagnosis and prognosis, neurologists usually supplement their clinical impression with computed tomography (CT) or

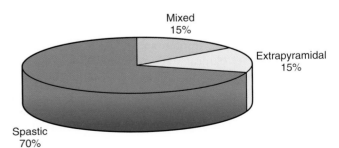

FIGURE 13-1 ■ Most cases of cerebral palsy (CP) are varieties of spastic CP: hemiplegic, diplegic, and quadriplegic. Because studies vary, the percentages are approximations.

TABLE 13-1 ■ Historical Features of Cerebral Palsy
Description of deficit
Motor impairment
Paresis: extent, degree
Movement disorder: nature, age of onset
Delayed acquisition of motor skills
Associated conditions
Mental retardation
Epilepsy
Search for cause
Maternal health
Personal or familial neurologic illness
Prenatal illness or abnormalities
Drug use
Amniocentesis
Delivery
Prematurity
Low weight for date
Prolonged labor, fetal distress
Obstetric complications
Neonatal period
Low Apgar score
Cyanosis, unresponsiveness
Sepsis
Seizures
Jaundice

TABLE 13-2 ■ Physical Findings of Cerebral Palsy (CP)
Motor Deficits
Signs of spastic CP
Gross impairment: paresis/spasticity, growth arrest, pseudobulbar palsy
Subtle impairment: unequal size of hands or feet, toe walking (from shortened heel cords), premature hand preference (e.g., right-handedness) before the age of 18 months
Signs of extrapyramidal CP
Choreoathetosis
Ataxia
Associated conditions
Mental retardation
Epilepsy
Pseudobulbar palsy
Impairment of special senses
Visual: strabismus, myopia, blindness (cortical or ocular)
Auditory: deafness
Vocal: dysarthria

preferably magnetic resonance imaging (MRI). Those studies may identify the etiology and estimate the extent of cerebral damage. In addition, if the history suggests seizures, neurologists also order electroencephalography (EEG). However, they do not routinely order genetic testing or metabolic screening in cases of CP.

Once assured that a child has a stable neurologic deficit rather than a progressive illness, physicians should concentrate on the problem at hand by evaluating the child's potential disabilities—as well as abilities—in intelligence, learning, speech, and hearing as well as motor function (Table 13-2). Because approximately 50% of children with CP have normal intelligence despite major motor deficits, physicians should not label a child as mentally retarded without an individualized evaluation.

In contrast to CP-induced motor impairments and mental retardation remaining stable, epilepsy may complicate the clinical picture. Although epilepsy may not appear during infancy, it usually develops before age 5 years. The incidence of epilepsy in both spastic and extrapyramidal CP corresponds to the severity of physical impairments and mental retardation (Fig. 13-2).

Although mental retardation is prevalent, it does not explain all of their deficiencies. Alternatively,

some CP and epileptic children, with or without mental retardation, are uneducated because they have been unable to attend school. Of children with mental retardation or CP, 10% to 30% have epilepsy. Of mentally retarded children in institutions, 50% have epilepsy. Many CP children have additional impediments, such as learning disabilities, hyperactivity, or hearing problems, that interfere with education.

Spastic CP

In spastic CP, spasticity impairs mobility more than paresis. It causes slow, clumsy, and stiff movements that, most conspicuously, force affected children to walk with extended, unbending legs. The spasticity also precludes them from making normal isolated movements, such as tapping one foot while keeping the other foot immobile. Neurologic examination of children with spastic CP show that the usual signs of upper motor neuron injury—hyperactive deep tendon reflexes (DTRs), clonus, and Babinski signs—accompany the spasticity.

In a signature sign of spastic CP, which results from the cerebral injury occurring prior to childhood and adolescent physical development, affected limbs experience *growth arrest*. Arms or legs, already weak and stiff, fail to develop their proper length and muscle structure. Also, their thumb and great-toe nail beds are smaller on the paretic side, and a short Achilles tendon forces them to walk on the toes of an affected foot.

The most common cause of spastic CP is necrotic areas in the white matter around the ventricles,

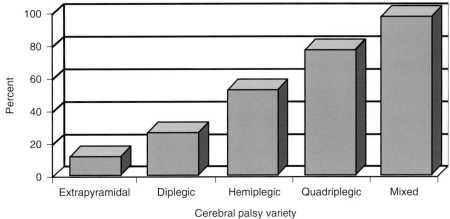

FIGURE 13-2 ■ The proportion of cerebral palsy (CP) patients with mental retardation and epilepsy increases with more extensive cerebral disease. Their incidence of those complications in choreoathetosis or extrapyramidal CP is only approximately 10%; however, the incidence in diplegic CP is 25%; hemiplegic CP 50%; quadriplegic CP 75%; and mixed CP 95%.

periventricular leukomalacia. Ultrasound examinations and MRIs can readily detect it, even in neonates.

Diplegic CP (spastic diplegia) consists of bilateral symmetric paresis characteristically involving the legs more than the arms (Fig. 13-3). This CP variety usually forces children to hold their legs straight, drawn together (adducted), and crossed over each other ("scissored"). It also makes them keep their feet and toes pointed downward (extended). When children begin to walk, this posture obligates them to stand on their toes with their legs brought closely together.

Compared to other varieties of CP, diplegic CP correlates most closely with prematurity and necrotic areas in the white matter around the ventricles, *periventricular leukomalacia.* Ultrasound examinations and MRIs can readily detect periventricular leukomalacia, even in neonates.

Because cerebral damage primarily or exclusively affects the periventricular region, but has relatively little effect on the cerebral cortex, both epilepsy and mental retardation occur in only about 25% of individuals. Although this incidence is substantial, it is less frequent than in other forms of spastic CP. Moreover, many individuals with spastic diplegia have no cognitive impairment. Thus, diplegic CP qualifies, along with amyotrophic lateral sclerosis (ALS) and several other neurologic disorders (see Chapter 18), as a physically devastating condition that may surprisingly allow normal cognition.

Hemiplegic CP consists of spastic hemiparesis that typically affects the face and arm more than the leg (Fig. 13-4). Individuals with hemiplegic CP resemble adults with strokes from middle cerebral artery occlusions, but they have growth arrest of the affected limbs. Another distinguishing feature is premature hand preference (e.g., right-handedness in infancy). In other words, because handedness normally appears only after an age of 2 years, a child's exclusively using one hand suggests plegia of the other.

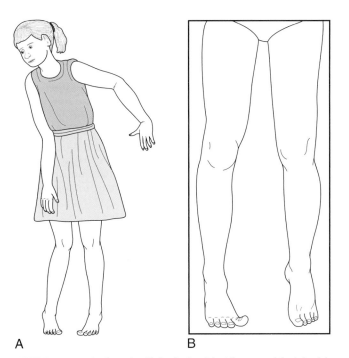

FIGURE 13-3 ■ *A,* Spastic diplegia in this 10-year-old girl with low-normal intelligence causes straightening, inturning, and adduction of her legs; a tiptoe stance; and scissor-like gait. Her uncoordinated, awkward arm movements (posturings) also reflect her cerebral palsy (CP). *B,* Another patient with spastic diplegia, an 18-year-old college engineering student, has typical increased muscle tone, adduction of his legs, and "toe-walking." He also has a subtle, sustained right-sided Babinski sign.

More important, because the right hemisphere can assume dominance in the event of left hemisphere injury during infancy, children with congenital left hemisphere damage tend to develop right hemisphere dominance (see Chapter 8). Those that can manage the change become left-handed and develop normal language function; however, they grow up with right

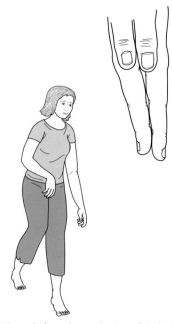

FIGURE 13-4 ■ Spastic hemiparesis since birth, in this 28-year-old woman with normal intelligence, causes weakness of her right arm and leg. She holds the arm, wrist, and fingers in a flexed posture. Growth arrest of her right hand has led to shortened fingers and a less broad thumb nail bed. Similarly, the right leg, especially the heel (Achilles) tendon, is short. The growth arrest causes her to walk on her right toes and circumduct that leg. Her posture and gait are similar to that of adults after a left middle cerebral artery infarction (see Figs. 2-3 to 2-5).

hemiparesis. In contrast, adults who sustain left cerebral hemisphere injuries typically have residual aphasia as well as right hemiparesis.

The underlying cerebral damage in spastic hemiparesis generally surpasses that in spastic cerebral diplegia. Thus, epilepsy is more frequently comorbid with hemiplegic (30%) than diplegic CP (20%). In addition, the severity of the physical disability and presence of epilepsy correlate with other complications, particularly mental retardation.

Quadriplegic CP is paresis of all four limbs usually accompanied by pseudobulbar palsy. Because extensive cerebral damage, often from anoxia during delivery, usually underlies this CP variety, a large proportion—75%—of affected children also suffer from epilepsy and mental retardation. (In contrast, cervical spinal cord birth injury causes quadriplegia without cerebral damage.)

Physical and occupational therapy, bracing, and orthotics can help these children ambulate and effectively usefully use their arms and hands. Surgery that transposes or lengthens tendons; oral medications, such as baclofen and tizanidine; and intramuscular injections of botulinum toxin (see Chapter 18) reduce spasticity and increase patients' mobility.

In these children, epilepsy resists treatment. Seizure control often requires two or more antiepileptic drugs (AEDs), which in turn may produce undesirable side effects, particularly sedation, cognitive impairments, paradoxical hyperactivity, and other behavioral disturbances.

Extrapyramidal CP

Involuntary writhing movements (athetosis) of the face, tongue, hands, and feet punctuated by jerking movements (chorea) of the trunk, arms, and legs—embraced by the term *choreoathetosis*—characterize this variety of CP (Fig. 13-5). Although choreoathetosis may remain subtle throughout patients' lifetime, it often interferes with fine hand movements, walking, and even sitting still. Involuntary larynx, pharynx, and diaphragm movements may lead to incomprehensible dysarthria.

Physicians should distinguish choreoathetotic CP from *dopamine-responsive dystonia*, which produces similar involuntary movements in young children (see Chapter 18). In short, unlike CP, dopamine-responsive dystonia is progressive (albeit slowly), fluctuating in a characteristic diurnal pattern at its onset, and, most important, responsive to small doses of levodopa (L-dopa). Despite the differences, the clinical similarity can be so great that many neurologists routinely suggest a therapeutic trial of L-dopa before accepting a diagnosis of choreoathetotic CP.

Neurologists usually attribute choreoathetotic CP to combinations of low birth weight, anoxia, and neonatal hyperbilirubinemia (*kernicterus*) damage of the basal ganglia. In addition, because these insults also damage the auditory pathways, hearing impairment frequently complicates the clinical picture.

Although the basal ganglia damage occurs during the neonatal period, choreoathetosis might not appear until children are 2 years old. By that time, the children should have developed steady walking and fine motor movements, but the involuntary movements may impair or prevent the normal ones. Similarly, hearing impairment may remain undetected until 1 year of age, when speaking should commence.

On the other hand, probably because kernicterus tends to spare the cerebral cortex, choreoathetotic CP is associated with a low incidence of epilepsy and mental retardation (10%). Despite pronounced physical impediments, many of these CP patients have been able to complete college. Nevertheless, most are liable to be underrated by a superficial academic or medical evaluation. (Physicians should also include

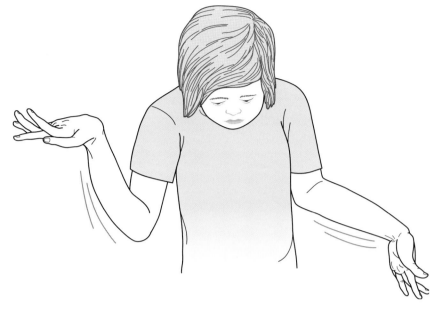

FIGURE 13-5 ■ In a 13-year-old girl, slow sinuous movements (athetosis) of the wrists, hands, and fingers, which have been obvious since age 3 years, signify that she has congenital cerebral palsy (CP)-induced choreoathetosis. Her involuntary movements force her hands into flexion at the wrist and her fingers into extension with overlapping positions.

choreoathetotic CP among devastating neurologic illness that may not affect cognition.)

Most systemic medications provide little relief from the choreoathetosis. Although neurosurgical ablation of deep cerebral structures reduces athetosis, the procedures are risky and not as yet perfected. Experiments involving deep brain stimulation, a less invasive technique, have produced initial success.

Finally, *mixed forms* of CP—combinations of spastic paraparesis and choreoathetosis—account for about 15% of cases. They reflect the most extensive CNS injury, which is naturally associated with the highest incidence of epilepsy and mental retardation (95%).

NEURAL TUBE CLOSURE DEFECTS

During the third and fourth weeks of gestation, dorsal ectoderm normally invaginates to form a closed *neural tube*, situated in the midline, that eventually forms the brain and spinal cord (Fig. 13-6, top). Ectoderm thus gives rise to the CNS as well as the skin, and mesoderm forms the coverings of the CNS—the meninges, vertebrae, and skull.

However, the neural tube sometimes fails to fuse at one or both of its ends. In other words, the neural tube does not close at either the prospective site of the brain or lower end of the spinal cord. Then, because the embryo cannot repair neural tube closure defects, the defects expand during further embryonic development and create malformations of the brain and lower spinal cord. In addition, neural tube closure defects produce abnormalities in the overlying meninges and either vertebrae or skull.

Beyond the neurologic issues, neural tube defects create some of the most public, yet privately heart-wrenching, controversies in medicine, such as harvesting organs in cases in which the brain has failed to develop (see later, anencephaly); parents refusing to allow treatment of severely malformed infants; and the burden of health care costs for infants with a dismal prognosis.

Upper Neural Tube Closure Defects

In an extreme example of a neural tube defect, the entire upper end of the neural tube does not form and the fetus fails to develop a brain. This rare but well-publicized condition, *anencephaly,* is invariably fatal within days of birth. Until then, the organs are ideal for transplantation.

In an *encephalocele,* a skin-covered malformed brain, covered by its meninges and cerebrospinal fluid (CSF), protrudes through an occipital skull defect. In a similar malformation, the *Dandy-Walker syndrome,* the posterior portion of the upper neural tube fails to mature. Posterior brain structures, particularly the cerebellar vermis, remain at an early embryonic stage. Expanding into the empty space, the fourth ventricle grows to resemble a large cyst.

A group of malformations, collectively termed the *Arnold-Chiari malformation,* constitute a variety of upper neural tube closure defects. Usually not obvious by external appearances, the Arnold-Chiari malformation involves downward displacement of the lower portion of the medulla and cerebellum through the foramen magnum (see Figs. 13-6 and 20-22). In older children and adults who may previously have escaped

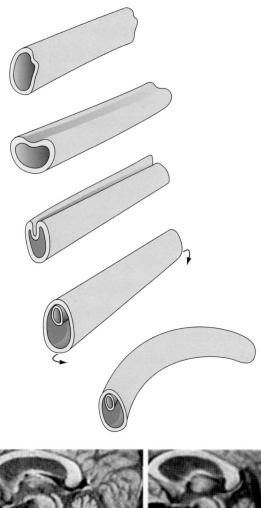

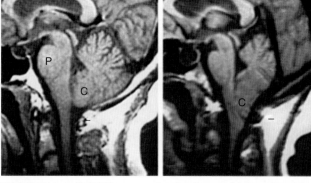

FIGURE 13-6 ■ *Top,* The neural tube forms during the third and fourth weeks of gestation. It begins when the embryo's external layer, the ectoderm, invaginates to form a distinct, midline neural tube that eventually closes at both ends. Once closed, the embryo begins to bend into a curved, fetal shape with the tube on the convex surface. Failure to complete this process results in defects most commonly at the upper and lower ends of the spinal cord. *Bottom left,* The MRI shows the normal relationship of several of the structures contained in the posterior fossa: the pons (P), medulla (unmarked), cerebellum (C), and the fourth ventricle (the black, cerebrospinal fluid [CSF]-filled, triangular area between the pons and middle of the cerebellum). Note that the lower portion of the cerebellum remains above the foramen magnum (indicated by a short horizontal line). *Bottom right,* This MRI shows an Arnold Chiari abnormality. The lower portion of the cerebellum, which includes the tonsils, and the medulla protrudes below the foramen magnum. In addition, in severe cases, aqueductal stenosis causes hydrocephalus.

detection, these malformations produce headaches (especially when bending), bulbar palsy, and neck pain. Patients with compression of the medulla or cerebellum require "unroofing" of the upper cervical spine and occipital portion of the skull.

In many patients, these congenital abnormalities lead to mental retardation and, because of aqueductal stenosis, obstructive hydrocephalus. Those who develop hydrocephalus typically require neurosurgical insertion of a ventriculoperitoneal shunt. In addition, these upper neural tube defects are associated with comparable lower neural tube defects, such as *meningomyelocele* (see later).

Lower Neural Tube Closure Defects

In the most benign case, *spina bifida occulta,* the spine of the lumbar vertebrae simply fails to fuse. With both the underlying spinal cord and cauda equina remaining intact, this disorder usually remains asymptomatic.

In a more serious problem, *meningocele,* the meninges and skin protrude through a lumbosacral spine defect to form a large, CSF-filled bulge. Although this condition may remain asymptomatic, it frequently causes symptoms originating in dysfunction of the lumbar and sacral nerves, such as leg weakness, gait impairment, bladder emptying problems, and thus progressive hydronephrosis. It also deprives the lower CNS of the multiple tissue barriers—intact skin, vertebrae, and meninges—that normally shield it from the environment. To prevent bacteria from entering the CSF through this defect and causing meningitis, infants with meningoceles must undergo neurosurgery for repair.

Meningomyelocele or *myelomeningocele,* the worst case, occurs far more frequently than meningocele. This malformation consists of a tangle of a rudimentary lower spinal cord, lumbar and sacral nerve roots, and meninges protruding into a sac-like structure overlying the lumbosacral spine (Fig. 13-7). The disrupted nerve tissue causes paraparesis, areflexia, and incontinence. In addition, defective meninges place neonates at immediate risk of meningitis. Although hydrocephalus is present in only about 25% of infants with meningomyeloceles, it develops in almost all who survive.

Neurosurgeons usually repair meningomyeloceles during the child's first week. Nevertheless, clinical deficits usually worsen in childhood and particularly during adolescent growth spurts. Although neurosurgery may protect infants from meningitis and reduce the impact of hydrocephalus, most survivors remain mentally retarded and paraplegic. In addition, as affected children physically mature, they often require urinary- and fecal-diversion procedures, revisions of shunts for hydrocephalus, and further surgery on the spine.

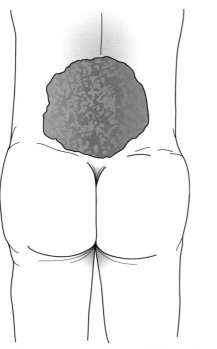

FIGURE 13-7 ■ The meningomyelocele of this newborn infant has a typical broad-based, loose, translucent sac of thin, friable skin arising from the lumbar area. It contains rudiments of a spinal cord and lumbosacral nerves. It weeps a mixture of serum and cerebrospinal fluid (CSF). The infant's legs, lacking innervation, are weak, flaccid, and areflexic. Similarly, the bladder, also lacking innervation, is distended.

Causes

Some studies have implicated genetic factors as a cause of neural tube defects. For example, the risk of a neural tube defect occurring in a sibling of an affected child is 5%, and with two affected children, the risk for a third increases to 10%. Similarly, a frequent occurrence in trisomy 13 and trisomy 18 suggests a genetic basis.

Other studies, which suggest environmental factors, have attributed neural tube defects to carbamazepine and valproate, folic acid deficiency, autoantibodies to folate receptors, radiation, and various toxins, including potato blight. The mechanism by which AEDs cause neural tube defects remains unclear; however, their tendency to reduce serum folate level and thus raise homocysteine levels may be the explanation.

Prenatal testing may provide early warning of a meningomyelocele or other neural tube defect in a fetus. For example, excessive concentrations of α-fetoprotein in amniotic fluid and maternal serum indicate a neural tube defect. Fetal ultrasound examination, a complementary test, may show neural tube defects as well as other congenital malformations.

Women who eat adequate amounts of fruits and vegetables, which contain folic acids and other nutrients, reduce the risk of neural tube defects by 70%. Moreover, studies have found that a folic acid intake of 5 mg daily before conception and during the first month of pregnancy may reduce the incidence of neural tube defects by 85%. Based on this evidence, the U.S. Food and Drug Administration has ordered manufacturers to add folic acid to certain foods, including pasta, breakfast cereals, and cornmeal. In addition, neurologists avoid prescribing carbamazepine or valproate to women who are pregnant or planning to conceive.

NEUROCUTANEOUS DISORDERS

Embryologic defects in the ectoderm also give rise to neurocutaneous disorders that consist of paired abnormalities of the brain and skin. These disorders, in addition, often include abnormalities of other ectoderm and nonectoderm organs. Neurologists often deduce a CNS lesion simply by inspection of a patient's skin.

The neurocutaneous disorders are inherited—with at least one exception—in an autosomal dominant pattern. Although their manifestations usually remain stable through adult life, sometimes the cerebral lesions undergo malignant transformation.

Tuberous Sclerosis

Tuberous sclerosis usually causes conspicuous smooth and firm nodules, *adenoma sebaceum* or *facial angiofibromas*, on the malar surface of the face (Fig. 13-8), but this illness-defining skin lesion usually fails to appear until adolescence. However, during infancy and childhood, the skin shows several other characteristics: subtle hypopigmented splotches, which in about 20% of cases have a feather-like ash leaf shaped configuration; leathery, scaly areas on the trunk (shagreen patches); and periungual fibromas of the fingers.

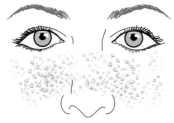

FIGURE 13-8 ■ Adenoma sebaceum (or facial angiofibromas), the cutaneous component of tuberous sclerosis, consist of nodules several millimeters in diameter, firm, and uniformly pale. They spread over the malar surface of the face. Although adenoma sebaceum may resemble acne, acne pimples have a liquid (pus) center surrounded by inflammation. Also acne pimples accumulate on the trunk as well as the face.

TABLE 13-3 ■ Neurologic Syndromes That Include Autism-Like Symptoms
Angelman
Fragile X
Klinefelter's
Rett
Tuberous sclerosis

In addition to the adenoma sebaceum, a classic triad of tuberous sclerosis manifestations, which actually occurs in the minority of affected children, also consists of epilepsy and mental retardation. In some children with tuberous sclerosis, the epilepsy is intractable and the retardation worsens and eventually reaches the severity of dementia. Although mental retardation and epilepsy force many children into institutions, some have a benign form that causes only minimal cognitive impairment and readily controlled epilepsy.

In another important aspect of the illness, some tuberous sclerosis children display autistic behavior. Thus, neurologists consider tuberous sclerosis as one of several neurologic causes of autism-like symptoms (Table 13-3).

The CNS correlate of the skin lesions consists of cerebral *tubers*, which are potato-like brain nodules, 1 to 3 cm in diameter. The tubers frequently grow to compress and irritate the surrounding cerebral cortex and thus cause the epilepsy and, when present, progressive cognitive impairment. Although usually benign, the tubers sometimes undergo malignant transformation. In addition, retinal, renal, and cardiac tumors develop. Especially because cerebral tubers tend to calcify, CT and even plain skull x-rays readily identify them. However, because calcifications, devoid of water, do not emit a signal, MRI often fails to detect them. Neurosurgeons cannot easily remove tubers because they are too numerous and deeply situated.

Although tuberous sclerosis most often occurs spontaneously, many cases are attributable to mutations in either of two tumor suppressor genes: TSC1 (tuberous sclerosis complex 1) on chromosome 9 and TSC 2 on chromosome 16.

Neurofibromatosis

Commonly occurring neurofibromatosis, *neurofibromatosis type 1 (NF1)*—previously called von Recklinghausen's disease or "peripheral type" neurofibromatosis—also causes a triad of readily identifiable manifestations: (1) multiple *café au lait spots*, (2) *neurofibromas*, and (3) *Lisch nodules*. Café au lait spots, the signature of neurofibromatosis, are areas of uniformly light brown, oval, and flat skin (Fig. 13-9). Although

individual café au lait spots are found in at least 10% of normal individuals, the presence of more than six spots, each larger than 1.5 cm, ensures a diagnosis of neurofibromatosis.

Neurofibromas consist of soft, palpable, subcutaneous growths, each a few millimeters to several centimeters in size, that emerge along peripheral nerves (Figs. 13-10 and 13-11). They can also grow from nerve roots within the spinal canal and compress the spinal cord or cauda equina. They occasionally reach grotesque proportions or induce extraordinary growth of an affected limb. However, the famous 19th century "Elephant Man," Joseph Merrick, commonly believed to be an example of neurofibromatosis, actually suffered from a related condition, Proteus syndrome.

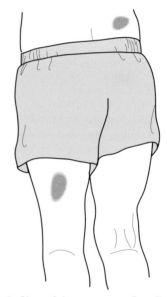

FIGURE 13-9 ■ Café au lait spots are flat, light brown skin lesions. Six or more, each measuring at least 1.5 cm, indicate neurofibromatosis.

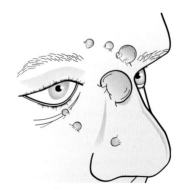

FIGURE 13-10 ■ Neurofibromas often grow to several centimeters of disfiguring protuberances on the face.

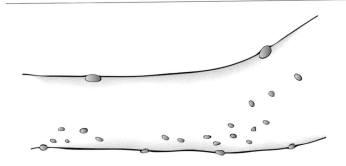

FIGURE 13-11 ■ Neurofibromas are often subtle, multiple, subcutaneous, soft, and typically less than 0.5 cm in size.

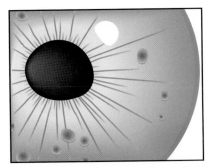

FIGURE 13-12 ■ Lisch nodules, virtually pathognomonic of NF1, are pigmented aggregations on the iris that are often visible with the unaided eye.

Lisch nodules, the least obvious but most common manifestation, are multiple, asymptomatic, macroscopic, yellow to brown nodules (melanocytic hamartomas) situated on the iris (Fig. 13-12). Although a slit-lamp examination may be required to detect Lisch nodules and then differentiate them from inconsequential pigment collections, they are pathognomonic of the disorder.

Excision of neurofibromas, except for those compressing the spinal cord or other vital structures, is impractical because NF1 involves innumerable peripheral nerves. However, laser therapy can blanch café au lait spots.

Although its cutaneous manifestations probably represent the most conspicuous sign of any neurologic disease, NF1 is not entirely peripheral. As with other neurocutaneous disorders, NF1 induces intracerebral tumors. In this case, it induces astrocytomas and optic nerve gliomas.

Moreover, NF1 has a high association with attention deficit hyperactivity disorder (ADHD) and learning disabilities. Some tests detect sustained attention difficulties and learning disabilities in the majority of NF1 children. The IQ of NF1 children is about 5 to 10 points lower than average. Moreover, 5% to 8% of

them may be considered mentally retarded, which is slightly greater than the incidence in the general population (3%). However, psychosis occurs in NF1 patients with the same frequency as in the general population. Moreover, unlike the increased prevalence of autistic behavior in tuberous sclerosis, such behavior is not associated with either variety of NF.

Approximately 50% of patients inherit NF1 in an autosomal dominant pattern, usually because of a gene situated on chromosome 17. In the remainder of patients, NF1 arises sporadically.

Neurofibromatosis type 2 (NF2), which occurs only 10% as frequently as NF1, is an almost completely different disorder. NF2, also called familial acoustic neuroma or "central type" neurofibromatosis, is characterized by bilateral acoustic neuromas (vestibular schwannomas) that steadily impair hearing until deafness ensues. It may induce a few neurofibromas and large, pale café au lait spots, but its hallmark remains the acoustic neuromas (see Fig. 20-27). In fact, NF2 is usually unrecognized until acoustic neuromas are discovered.

This neurocutaneous disorder is associated with the development of meningiomas. Gadolinium-enhanced MRIs can readily detect its two neoplastic complications, acoustic neuroma and meningiomas. Although neurosurgeons can remove those tumors, sometimes they must sacrifice the acoustic nerve or the adjacent cranial nerve. Alternatively, pinpoint radiation or laser treatment may be able to burn away the tumor while sparing the nerve.

Unlike NF1, NF2 does not cause behavioral, learning, or cognitive impairments. Also, NF2 is inherited on chromosome 22 and, in the vast majority of cases, in an autosomal dominant pattern.

Sturge-Weber Syndrome

Sturge-Weber syndrome, also called *encephalo-trigeminal angiomatosis,* consists simply of a vascular malformation of the face (*nevus flammeus*) and underlying cerebral hemisphere. Unlike other the other neurocutaneous disorders, it has no known genetic basis and does not strike multiple family members.

The vascular malformation of the face consists of a deep red discoloration ("port-wine stain") that follows the distribution of one or more divisions of the trigeminal nerve (Fig. 13-13). Clinicians must distinguish that malformation from much more common skin abnormalities, such as small, patchy port-wine stains and small forehead angiomas ("strawberry nevi") in infants, that do not indicate Sturge-Weber syndrome. Whether or not a facial vascular malformation is a manifestation of Sturge Weber syndrome, laser therapy can bleach it.

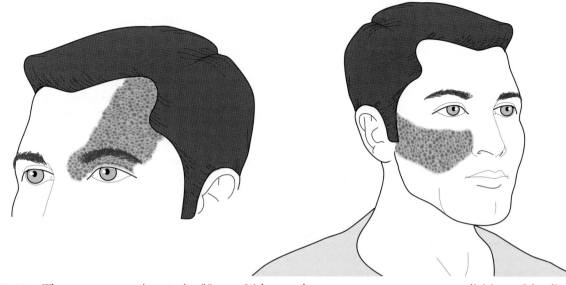

FIGURE 13-13 ■ The cutaneous angiomatosis of Sturge-Weber syndrome encompass one or more divisions of the distribution of the trigeminal nerve (see Fig. 4-12). Because the first division is affected most often, the most common sites of angiomatosis are the anterior scalp, forehead, and upper eyelid. One third of patients have bilateral involvement.

The cerebral component of Sturge-Weber syndrome consists of calcified layers of cortex, accompanied by atrophy, in the hemisphere underlying the facial vascular malformation. As with tubers, CT and plain skull x-rays, but not MRI, readily reveal the calcification.

Sturge-Weber patients tend to have mental retardation, learning disabilities, behavioral disturbances, and refractory epilepsy. Those with seizures have an especially high incidence of developmental delay, cognitive impairment, physical deficits, and unemployability. Depending on the lesion site, patients also have focal neurologic deficits, such as homonymous hemianopsia and spastic hemiparesis. With recurrent epilepsy and the development of sclerosis surrounding the cerebral lesion, physical as well as the cognitive deficits worsen.

Ataxia-Telangiectasia

The cutaneous component of ataxia-telangiectasia consists of aggregations of small, dilated vessels (telangiectasia) on the conjunctiva, bridge of the nose, and cheeks. Neurologic manifestations become evident in children aged 3 to 5 years when degeneration of the cerebellar vermis causes a steadily progressive gait ataxia. Subsequently, they develop cognitive impairment.

Unlike most other neurocutaneous disorders, ataxia-telangiectasia is inherited in a recessive pattern. It is attributable to a genetic abnormality on chromosome 11 that interferes with DNA repair.

Another, almost unique feature of ataxia-telangiectasia is its consistent association with immunodeficiency. Children with ataxia-telangiectasia have both cellular immunity impairment and complete or nearly complete deficiency of immunoglobulin IgA or IgE. Their immunodeficiency leads to severe sinus and respiratory tract infections, which may represent their first symptoms. It also often leads to the development of lymphomas and other neoplasms. (The same association of immunodeficiency with lymphoma also occurs in acquired immunodeficiency syndrome [AIDS] and immunosuppression for organ transplantation.)

OTHER GENETIC NEUROLOGIC DISORDERS

Neurologists group several genetic disorders, each characterized by cognitive impairment and distinctive body habitus. Aside from changes brought on by puberty, their manifestations remain stable throughout life.

Chromosomal Disorders (Autosomal)

Phenylketonuria (PKU) (Chromosome 12)

An autosomal recessive inherited deficiency in *hepatic* phenylalanine hydroxylase produces PKU. In a triumph of medicine, near universal testing and implementation of effective, simple treatment have either almost eliminated PKU or, if it occurs, markedly reduced its consequences.

A deficiency of phenylalanine hydroxylase, which normally converts phenylalanine to tyrosine, would ordinarily lead to a triad of major biochemical ramifications:

1. The deficiency would prevent the normal metabolism of phenylalanine to tyrosine. Thus, affected untreated individuals have elevated plasma concentrations of phenylalanine and little or no tyrosine.
2. The deficiency would also prevent the normal synthesis of "downstream" products, including dopamine, norepinephrine, and melanin (see Chapter 21).

Phenylalanine $\xrightarrow{\text{phenylalanine hydroxylase}}$
Tyrosine $\xrightarrow{\text{tyrosine hydroxylase}}$ DOPA $\xrightarrow{\text{DOPA decarboxylase}}$
Dopamine $\xrightarrow{\text{dopamine }\beta\text{-hydroxylase}}$
Norepinephrine $\xrightarrow{\text{phenylethanolamine N-methyl-transferase}}$
Epinephrine

3. A deficiency of phenylalanine hydroxylase would divert phenylalanine metabolism to secondary metabolic pathways. Those pathways yield phenylpyruvic acid and eventually phenylketones, which would be excreted in the urine. Untreated affected individuals thus have phenylketonuria.

Before the introduction of effective treatment, affected infants, after appearing normal from birth through the next several months, fell behind in all areas of development. In addition, because of reduced melanin, most infants had blond hair, blue eyes, fair complexion, and eczema. Phenylketones turned their urine malodorous.

In untreated children, cognitive delays appeared as early as 8 months of age, and language development lagged. Almost all of them were mentally retarded, and two thirds of them were profoundly retarded. Although occasional children and adults with PKU had little or no mental retardation, evaluations found that many of them had nonspecific, poorly defined "psychiatric illness."

A mutation on chromosome 12 transmits PKU in a classic autosomal recessive pattern. Its incidence varies widely between countries. It is highest in Turkey and lowest in Japan. In the United States, hospitals routinely test all newborns for PKU with screening procedures, such as the Guthrie test, that detect elevated concentrations of plasma phenylalanine. However, these tests may be invalid immediately after birth, when residual maternal enzyme might have metabolized an elevated fetal phenylalanine concentration.

A phenylalanine-free diet usually ameliorates the enzyme deficiency and prevents mental retardation. Noncompliance with the diet, as particularly occurs with adolescents, produces neuropsychologic aberrations. If pregnant women do not strictly adhere to the diet, they accumulate toxic levels of phenylalanine and its metabolic products that easily pass through the placenta. In this case, the fetus, even though heterozygote for the PKU gene, is vulnerable to the toxins and liable to develop mental retardation.

Physicians should be aware that subsisting exclusively on phenylalanine-free foods is difficult and expensive. The diet, which is devoid of artifical sweeteners, leads to short stature, anemia, and hypoglycemia. Experimental therapies attempt to replace the deficient enzyme or provide a substitute gene.

Homocystinuria (Chromosome 21)

Cystathionine beta-synthase, along with vitamin B_6, converts homocysteine to cystathionine (see Fig. 5-8). A deficiency of this enzyme leads to accumulation not only of homocysteine but also its precursor, methionine. The genetic disorder, homocystinuria, is attributable to an abnormality on a gene on chromosome 21. Other conditions that lead to accumulation of homocysteine and possibly some of the same clinical manifestations include vitamin B_{12} deficiency, exposure to nitrous oxide, and use of certain AEDs (such as carbamazepine and phenytoin).

Homocystinuria leads primarily to vascular thrombotic events, particularly strokes in young and middle-aged adults, and mental retardation. The relationship between homocystinuria and strokes is so close that an elevated serum homocysteine level is a risk factor for stroke (see Chapter 11). The other features of homocystinuria, which reflect malformation of multiple organs, include dislocation of the ocular lens, pectus excavatum or carinatum, and a tall, Marfan-like stature. In addition to mental retardation, which is almost universal, homocystinuria patients often have behavior disturbances, obsessive-compulsive symptoms, and personality disorders.

Treatment in the presymptomatic stage reduces the likelihood of patients' developing the illness' major complications, including mental retardation. Administering vitamin B_6, the most common strategy, facilitates the metabolism of homocysteine and reduces levels of methionine and homocysteine in approximately 50% of patients. Although administering vitamin B_6 greatly reduces the risk of stroke in individuals with homocystinuria, administering folate and B_6 have not as yet proven to reduce the stroke risk despite reducing homocysteine levels in adults with idiopathic elevated levels of homocysteine.

Prader-Willi and Angelman Syndromes (Chromosome 15)

In an example in neurology of *genetic imprinting*, the same autosomal dominant abnormality in chromosome 15 produces a pair of different syndromes in affected children.* The abnormality—a deletion of a segment of chromosome 15—produces Prader-Willi syndrome if the father passes it, but Angelman syndrome if the mother passes it. "Prader-Willi is passed in a paternal pattern" serves as the common mnemonic device. Because the gender of the offspring does not affect the phenotype, boys and girls can develop either syndrome.

Most cases of Prader-Willi syndrome are paternally inherited, but some are sporadic. Affected boys and girls have mental retardation and behavior problems, but their characteristic symptoms consist of unapologetic hyperphagia and resultant obesity (Fig. 13-14). Children with Prader-Willi syndrome have more than a voracious appetite. They compulsively and obsessively eat, frequently grabbing food from family members' plates and rummaging through garbage cans.

Children who inherited the same chromosome abnormality from their mother have a very different phenotype—Angelman syndrome, which consists of severe mental retardation and microcephaly, repetitive and purposeless (stereotyped) involuntary movements, jerky-ataxic voluntary movements, a smiling face, and paroxysms of unprovoked laughter. The jerky movements and superficially happy appearance have given rise to the term "happy puppet syndrome." Affected adults require assistance with their daily activities and most of them have epilepsy.

Physicians may initially misdiagnose girls with Angelman syndrome as having Rett syndrome because of those illness' common features, including mental retardation, microcephaly, and involuntary movements (see later). Physicians may also misdiagnose girls with Angelman syndrome as having autism because of their inappropriate behavior and stereotyped movements.

Down Syndrome (Trisomy 21)

The most widely known disorder in this group, Down syndrome, is also, at 1 in 600 births, the most frequently occurring. Affected children have distinctive features (Fig. 13-15). In addition, Down syndrome usually causes mild to moderate degrees of mental retardation, with a median IQ of 40 to 50. An unfortunate but extraordinarily important complication of Down syndrome is that, by the fourth or fifth decade, it uniformly leads to an Alzheimer-like dementia (see Chapter 7). In fact, one theory holds that both Down syndrome and Alzheimer's disease result from a common genetic abnormality on chromosome 21.

Their social skills remain intact and are often an asset that helps to compensate for mild mental retardation.

*Geneticists have borrowed the term "imprinting" from Konrad Lorenz's better-known application in psychology, where it signifies social animals' learning behavior patterns through association with their parents or a substitute.

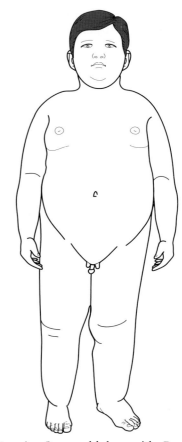

FIGURE 13-14 ■ An 8-year-old boy with Prader-Willi syndrome shows the characteristic obesity, which can reach grotesque proportions, small penis and testicles, short stature, small hands, and short feet. Girls with the syndrome, who also have hypogonadism, usually have small labia majora and no labia minora.

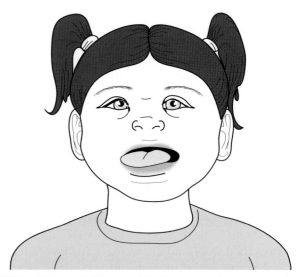

FIGURE 13-15 ■ Children with Down syndrome are short. Their ears are low-set and have small lobes. Their eyes' epicanthal folds are wide and their lids appear to slant upward—thus the outdated term "Mongolism." The bridge of the nose is depressed. The tongue, characteristically large, tends to protrude over a slack jaw. Children's palms are broad with a single midline crease, and their fingers are short and stubby.

Although they do not have psychotic or autistic behavior, Down syndrome children occasionally have behavior that fulfills criteria for ADHD. Curiously, severely affected children may have orofacial dyskinesias unrelated to neuroleptic exposure.

Although the cause in most children is chromosome 21 trisomy, a translocation of that chromosome causes some cases. Nevertheless, because all these patients have the same phenotype, clinicians still call the translocation variety "trisomy 21."

The incidence of Down syndrome correlates with increasing maternal age (especially after 40 years). Because a chromosome analysis of amniotic fluid cells can identify a fetus with Down syndrome, obstetricians urge women older than 40 years to undergo amniocentesis. Even though Down syndrome is genetic, it is not classified as an *inherited* disorder of mental retardation because it is not transmitted from generation to generation. (This distinction allows fragile X syndrome [see later] to be considered the most common form of inherited mental retardation.)

Williams Syndrome (Chromosome 7)

Life-long neuropsychologic impairments and a distinctive facial appearance also characterize Williams syndrome. Children with this disorder have mild to moderate mental retardation and delayed acquisition of motor milestones. In addition, they characteristically have an inordinately poor sense of visual-spatial relationships. However, they do not have gross neurologic abnormalities, such as microcephaly, seizures, or stereotyped movements.

Most striking, the disorder seems paradoxically to enhance other neuropsychologic functions. For example, remarkably and so far inexplicably, affected individuals frequently possess extraordinary talents in music and verbal fluency. Their conversations, although lacking substance, are loquacious, bubbly, and articulate.

Although some Williams syndrome cases have followed an autosomal dominant inheritance pattern, spontaneous mutations have led to most cases. The genetic abnormality, which consists of a minute deletion on chromosome 7, disrupts the elastic properties of the arteries, root of the aorta (causing supravalvular aortic stenosis), and skin. It also explains the children's readily identifiable "elfin" facial appearance (Fig. 13-16).

Chromosomal Disorders (Sex-Linked)

Fragile X Syndrome

The *fragile X syndrome,* like many other genetically determined disorders, consists of mental retardation combined with distinctive non-neurologic physical

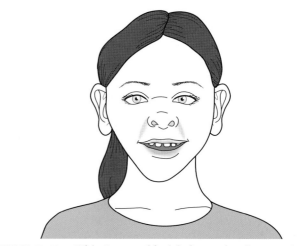

FIGURE 13-16 ■ This 9-year-old girl shows the characteristic elfin (elf-like) appearance of Williams syndrome. She is short. Her forehead is broad and her cheeks are prominent. Her nose has a flat bridge, and its nostrils are full and turned slightly upward. Her teeth are hypoplastic and widely spaced.

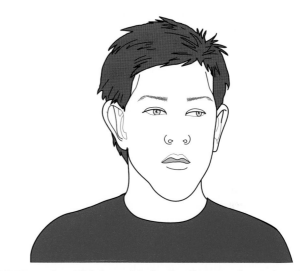

FIGURE 13-17 ■ This boy with the fragile X syndrome has the typical prominent forehead and jaw set against his long, thin face. Another hallmark are his large, everted, low-set, "seashell-shaped" ears. After puberty, his testicles will grow to a disproportionately larger size (*macro-orchidism*) than his penis. Many fragile X syndrome children display autistic behavior, including hand flapping and other stereotypies in addition to mental retardation.

abnormalities (Fig. 13-17). About 70% of boys who inherit the gene have moderate to severe mental retardation. Many of the remainder has only mild retardation, learning disabilities, or language impairment, and approximately 20% seem normal.

Most females carrying a single fragile X gene—including mothers and sisters of affected boys—remain asymptomatic, as if they were carrying other sex-linked abnormal genes, such those for hemophilia, color blindness, and Duchenne's muscular dystrophy (see Chapter 6). However, about one third of females who inherit a fragile X gene express some cognitive impairment. Affected girls often have IQs below 85.

Boys and, to a lesser extent, girls with fragile X syndrome also display behavioral symptoms, including ADHD. These children typically have excessive rates of learning disability, mood disorder, and repetitive, purposeless, involuntary movements (*stereotypies*), such as hand flapping or wringing. About 15% of them have been classified as autistic and meet the criteria for pervasive developmental disorder (PDD).

The defective gene consists of excessive repetitions of the CGG trinucleotide in the X chromosome. Testing can easily detect the DNA abnormality in the blood of affected individuals and, during prenatal screening, in amniotic fluid cells. The normal gene contains 5 to 54 CGG trinucleotide repeats, but the defective gene contains more than 60 repeats. Although individuals with 60 to 200 repeats may have few if any manifestations, those with more than 200 repeats invariably show signs of the disorder. As with other excessive trinucleotide repeat disorders, in successive generations the size of the genetic abnormality increases and symptoms both emerge at an earlier age (anticipation) and are more pronounced.*

Unlike in Down syndrome inheritance, parents regularly and predictably transmit fragile X syndrome to one or more of their children. Occurring in about 1 in 4000 males and half as frequently in females and responsible for as many as 10% of all cases of mental retardation, physicians consider it the most common cause of inherited mental retardation.

Rett Syndrome

Restricted to girls, *Rett syndrome* symptoms start to appear 6 to 18 months after a normal birth and development. Affected girls then begin to regress in virtually all phases of psychomotor development. Over the next several years, they lose language skills, ability to walk, other learned motor activities, and cognitive capacity. In addition, their cognitive skills decline in a pattern similar to the onset of dementia. Whether the underlying problem is a congenital injury or a progressive deterioration, affected children often are left in a state of profound mental retardation. Many victims survive, but their deficits persist throughout life.

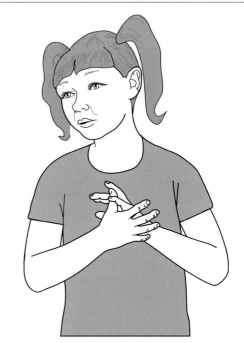

FIGURE 13-18 ■ A 6-year-old girl with Rett syndrome has developed repetitive hand washing and clapping movements and acquired microcephaly. Her head circumference is only 48 cm, which would be normal for a 3-year-old girl, but 2 standard deviations below the mean for her age (51 cm). She has progressively lost her language ability and now cannot speak in a meaningful manner.

Affected girls display two striking neurologic abnormalities: stereotypies and acquired microcephaly (Fig. 13-18). The stereotypies consist typically of incessant hand clapping, flapping, or wringing. The microcephaly is not present at birth, but follows normal head growth from birth to about 6 months. Then, head growth deceleration begins while relatively normal body growth continues. (This pattern of "acquired microcephaly" contrasts with common cases of congenital microcephaly, as occurs with congenital rubella infections, in which the head is small at birth.) In addition, more than 50% of Rett children have seizures.

Rett syndrome is attributable to a faulty gene on the X chromosome. Presumably, the same abnormality is lethal to a male fetus, except for several males who inherit a genetic anomaly, such as a variant of the mutation.

Loss of language, high incidence of epilepsy, and abnormal behavior in Rett syndrome mimic autism and Angelman syndrome. In contrast to autistic children, Rett syndrome children have acquired microcephaly and a progressive loss of motor ability.

Turner's Syndrome (X0)

Individuals with Turner's syndrome, who are phenotypically female, have an abnormality or absence of one of their sex chromosomes. Having only 45 full

*Excessive trinucleotide DNA repeats produce Friedreich's ataxia and other spinocerebellar degenerations, myotonic dystrophy, and Huntington's disease (see Chapters 2, 6, and 18, respectively), as well as fragile X syndrome (Appendix 3D).

chromosomes, Turner's syndrome individuals are usually described as having an "XO" chromosome compliment. From their infancy, when they have congenital edema, Turner's syndrome girls show readily identifiable dysmorphic features (Fig. 13-19).

A minority (10% to 20%) of Turner's syndrome girls has mild to moderate mental retardation and up to 70% have learning difficulties. In general, they have learning disabilities, attention deficit, and greater impairment on performance than verbal IQ testing. Turner's syndrome may be another example—along with Alzheimer's disease and Williams syndrome—of preserved verbal ability despite cognitive impairment.

Klinefelter's Syndrome (XXY)

With an additional X chromosome, Klinefelter's syndrome boys develop a tall stature, but, failing to

mature sexually, they appear eunuchoid after puberty (Fig. 13-20). As young men, their unusual height and lack of secondary sexual characteristics may draw medical attention. In fact, physicians most often diagnose Klinefelter's syndrome only after puberty. Physicians sometimes first diagnose the disorder when an infertility evaluation shows that the man has testicular dysgenesis and lacks sperm.

Klinefelter's syndrome individuals have a below average IQ, typically between 80 and 90. However, only about 25% have any degree of mental retardation, and

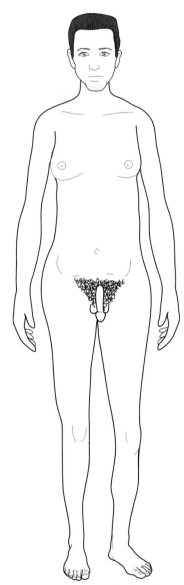

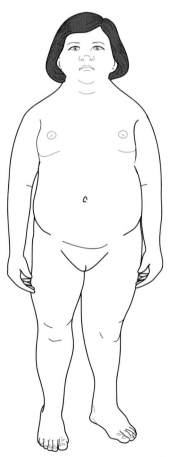

FIGURE 13-19 ■ This 16-year-old girl with Turner's syndrome (XO), with typical mental retardation, has the distinctive short stature, webbed neck, and lack of secondary sexual characteristics. As with other genetic disorders, her ears are low-set but hidden by a low hairline. Her nose is flat and its bridge spreads into broad epicanthal folds. Having failed to undergo normal changes of puberty, she typically lacks breast development and other secondary sexual characteristics. Her elbows' carrying angles are relatively straight, which is the male pattern.

FIGURE 13-20 ■ After a delayed and then incomplete puberty, this 30-year-old man with Klinefelter's syndrome (XXY) has typically grown taller than 6.5 feet, owing in large part to his disproportionately long legs. His body has assumed a eunuchoid shape with gynecomastia, sparse beard, female pattern of pubic hair, and small testicles. Other conditions characterized by excessive height include the XYY and Marfan's syndromes.

it is usually mild. Klinefelter's syndrome boys tend to have dyslexia and other learning disabilities. According to some reports, they have a passive personality and decreased libido.

XYY Syndrome

Individuals who carry an additional Y chromosome are tall—some extremely so—men. Also, they tend to develop severe acne that persists beyond adolescence.

The original studies of this syndrome, which were performed in prisons, suggested that the disorder expressed itself as deviant, violent, and otherwise aggressive behavior. Affected individuals were said to have the "super-male syndrome." In retrospect, the population base for those studies tainted the results.

Modern studies have rejected a causal relationship between a XYY karyotype and violent criminal behavior. However, they found that XYY men had delays in speech acquisition and other neurodevelopmental milestones, characterologic problems, psychiatric difficulties, and average to below normal intelligence.

Heavy Metal Exposure

Lead intoxication, depending on its intensity, causes mental retardation, learning disabilities, and other signs of cerebral impairment in infants and children. The exposure originates in lead-based paint chips, which infants and children ingest, and environmental pollution. Although acute intoxication or heavy exposure causes seizures as well as mental retardation and seizures, the more common low-level exposure leads to subtle intellectual impairment. Chelation therapy may not reverse cognitive impairment in children with mild to moderate lead-induced deficits.

Researchers have only recently recognized mercury toxicity in neonates and infants. Most human mercury intoxication stems from ingestion of methylmercury (CH_3Hg^+). The gastrointestinal tract absorbs almost all ingested methylmercury, which readily crosses the placenta and tends to accumulate in fetal brain tissue. Over time, organic mercury decomposes to inorganic mercury, which causes generalized fetal cerebral damage. Infants exposed to mercury have variable degrees of cognitive impairments.

Aside from mass poisonings from industrial accidents, such as occurred in Japan's Minamata Bay, environmental gases and eating certain fish cause most exposure. Large sea fish, such as swordfish, shark, king mackerel, and tuna, and certain fresh-water fish, such as pike and bass, have relatively high concentrations of methylmercury. Pregnant women should limit their intake of these fish.

On the other hand, the mercury in old-style dental fillings dissolves at such a slow rate that it carries virtually no risk. Even dentists who prepared the fillings on a daily basis had no significant increase in illnesses attributable to mercury. Removing mercury-containing dental fillings offers no benefits to the patient.

Several researchers and many parents proposed an ominous association between the development of autism and the measles, mumps, and rubella (MMR) vaccination. The standard MMR vaccine preparation had contained a preservative, thimerosal, which was composed of ethyl mercury. Because the vaccination may have caused brief but significant mercury exposure in infants, several studies suggested that it subsequently lead to autism and other disorders. Although vaccine manufacturers stopped adding mercury preservatives during the 1990s, the incidence of autism continued to climb. That epidemiologic data and other studies have exonerated both the current and older MMR vaccinations.

REFERENCES

1. Asano E, Chugani DC, Muzik O, et al: Autism in tuberous sclerosis complex is related to both cortical and subcortical dysfunction. Neurology 57:1269–1277, 2001.
2. Ashwal S, Russman BS, Blaso PA, et al: Practice Parameter: Diagnostic assessment of the child with cerebral palsy. Report of the Quality Standards Subcommittee of the American Academy of Neurology and the Practice Committee of the Child Neurology Society. Neurology 62:851–863, 2004.
3. Botto LD, Moore CA, Khoury MJ, et al: Neural-tube defects. N Engl J Med 341:1509–1519, 1999.
4. Canfield RL, Henderson CR, Cory-Slechta DA, et al: Intellectual impairment in children with blood lead concentrations below 10 ug per deciliter. N Engl J Med 348:1517–1526, 2003.
5. Creange A, Zeller J, Rostaing-Rigattieri S, et al: Neurological complications of neurofibromatosis type 1 in adulthood. Brain 122:473–481, 1999.
6. Detrait ER, George TM, Etchevers HC, et al: Human neural tube defects: Developmental biology, epidemiology, and genetics. Neurotoxicol Teratol 27:515–524, 2005.
7. Frank Y (ed): *Pediatric Behavioral Neurology.* New York, CRC Press, 1996.
8. Freund LS, Reiss AL, Abrams MT: Psychiatric disorders associated with fragile X in the young female. Pediatrics 91:321–329, 1993.
9. Fryns JP, Kleczkowska A, Kubien E, et al: XYY syndrome and other Y chromosome polysomies. Mental status and psychosocial functioning. Genet Couns 6:197–206, 1995.
10. Hack M, Taylor G, Drotar D, et al: Chronic conditions, functional limitations, and special health care needs of school-aged children born with extremely low-birth-weight in the 1990s. JAMA 294:318–325, 2005.

11. Hagberg B: Clinical manifestations and stages of Rett syndrome. Ment Retard Dev Disabil Res Rev 8:61–65, 2002.

12. Hankins GD, Speer M: Defining the pathogenesis and pathophysiology of neonatal encephalopathy and cerebral palsy. Obstet Gynecol 102:628–636, 2003.

13. Hyman MH, Whittemore VH: National Institutes of Health Consensus Conference: Tuberous sclerosis complex. Arch Neurol 57:662–665, 2000.

14. Hyman SL, Shores A, North KN: The nature and frequency of cognitive deficits in children with neurofibromatosis type 1. Neurology 65:1037–1044, 2005.

15. Kelly K, Stephen LJ, Brodie MJ: Pharmacological outcomes in people with mental retardation and epilepsy. Epilepsy Behav 5:67–71, 2004.

16. Kerr AM, Belichenko P, Woodcock T, et al: Mind and brain in Rett disorder. Brain Dev 23(Suppl 1):S44–49, 2001.

17. Lann LA, den Boer AT, Hennekam RC, et al: Angelman syndrome in adulthood. Am J Med Genet 66:356–360, 1996.

18. Lenhoff HM, Wang PP, Greenberg F, et al: Williams syndrome and the brain. Sci Am December 68–73, 1997.

19. Leonard H, Silberstein J, Falk R, et al: Occurrence of Rett syndrome in boys. J Child Neurol 16:333–338, 2001.

20. Madsen KM, Hviid A, Vestergaard M, et al: A population-based study of measles, mumps, and rubella vaccinations and autism. N Engl J Med 347:1477–1483, 2002.

21. Matsuishi T, Yamashita Y, Kusage A: Neurobiology and neurochemistry of Rett syndrome. Brain Dev 23(Suppl 1):S58–61, 2001.

22. Mount RH, Hastings RP, Reilly S: Behavioral and emotional features in Rett syndrome. Disabil Rehabil 23:129–138, 2001.

23. North KN, Riccardi V, Samango-Sprouse C, et al: Cognitive function and academic performance in neurofibromatosis 1: Consensus statement from the NF1 Cognitive Disorders Task Force. Neurology 48:1121–1127, 1997.

24. Rossen ML, Sarnat HB: Why should neurologists be interested in Williams syndrome? Neurology 51:8–9, 1998.

25. Sujansky E, Conradi S: Outcome of Sturge-Weber syndrome in 52 adults. Am J Med Genet 57:35–45, 1995.

26. Sybert VP, McCauley E: Turner's syndrome. N Engl J Med 351:1227–1238, 2004.

27. Waisbren SE, Hanley W, Levy HL, et al: Outcome at age 4 years in offspring of women with maternal phenylketonuria: The Maternal PKU Collaborative Study. JAMA 283:756–762, 2000.

28. Wiedemann HR, Kunze J: *Clinical Syndromes,* 3rd ed. London, Times Mirror International Publishers, 1997.

29. Willimas CA, Lossie A, Driscoll D: Angelman syndrome: Mimicking conditions and phenotypes. Am J Med Genet 101:59–64, 2001.

Questions and Answers

1–11. Match the neurocutaneous disorders (a–d) with their primary manifestation (1–11).
   a. Tuberous sclerosis
   b. Neurofibromatosis type 1 (NF1)
   c. Sturge-Weber syndrome
   d. Neurofibromatosis type 2 (NF2)
1. Acoustic neuroma
2. Facial lesions vaguely resemble rhinophyma
3. Progressive dementia
4. Neurofibromas
5. Adenoma sebaceum (angiofibromas)
6. Ash leaf, hypopigmented areas
7. Intractable epilepsy
8. Café au lait spots
9. Facial angiomatosis
10. Optic glioma
11. Shagreen patches

Answers: 1-d, 2-a, 3-a, 4-b, 5-a, 6-a, 7-a, 8-b, 9-c, 10-b, 11-a.

12–17. Which of the following disorders cause inattention or episodic changes in mood in children? (True/False)
12. Migraine
13. Partial complex seizures
14. Antihistamines
15. Cerebral palsy
16. Sedative medications
17. Absence seizures

Answers: 12-True, 13-True, 14-True, 15-False, 16-True, 17-True.

18. Which condition will the Guthrie test detect?
   a. PKU
   b. Trisomy 21
   c. Fragile X syndrome
   d. Turner's syndrome

Answer: a. The Guthrie test detects elevated levels of plasma phenylalanine, which indicate PKU. Karyotyping will reveal Turner's syndrome and other chromosome disorders. Only DNA analysis detects excessive trinucleotide repeats. Culturing chromosomes in folate-deficient media will stress all chromosomes and "break" the X chromosome in fragile X syndrome.

19. Which is the most precise term for an abnormal gene producing different phenotypes depending on whether the mother or father passed the gene to the offspring?
   a. Genetic imprinting
   b. Anticipation
   c. Imprinting
   d. Mitochondrial inheritance

Answer: a.

20. Children who sustain any brain injury until the age of 5 years are eligible for assistance by most programs that serve CP children. (True/False)

Answer: True.

21. Is the following sentence true or false? Children with mental retardation because of a genetic abnormality are usually indistinguishable from those with mental retardation for other reasons.

Answer: False. They usually have overt physical stigmata, such as low-set ears or abnormal habitus, that are often specific for a particular genetic abnormality.

22. Which of the following characteristics of Rett syndrome children are *not* found in autistic children?
   a. Only girls affected
   b. Stereotyped behavior
   c. Loss of language skills
   d. Seizures
   e. Acquired microcephaly

Answers: a, e.

23. Which syndrome carries the lowest incidence of mental retardation?
   a. Klinefelter's
   b. Trisomy 21
   c. Angelman syndrome
   d. Down syndrome
   e. Fragile X
   f. Prader-Willi

Answer: a. Moderate to severe mental retardation is an integral part of all these conditions except for Klinefelter's syndrome. Only about 30% of Klinefelter's syndrome individuals, who are phenotypically male, have mental retardation. In addition, when they have mental retardation, it is usually mild. Often the disorder remains undetected until they undergo an evaluation for infertility.

24. A 1-year-old boy has a stroke because of sickle-cell disease. It results in mild right hemiparesis. Which three of the following conditions will probably be additional consequences?
    a. Chorea
    b. Aphasia
    c. Seizures
    d. Spastic cerebral palsy
    e. Stunted growth (growth arrest) of right arm

    Answers: c, d, e. He will probably not have aphasia because, after an insult to his left hemisphere, the right will emerge as dominant for language and fine motor function.

25–30. Match the disorder (a–d) with its cause (25–30).
25. Choreoathetosis
26. Spastic quadriplegia
27. Spastic hemiparesis
28. Deafness
29. Seizure disorder
30. Cortical blindness
    a. Cervical cord injury
    b. Kernicterus
    c. Cerebral anoxia
    d. Stroke in utero

    Answers: 25-b, 26-a or c, 27-d, 28-b, 29-c or d, 30-c.

31. Which pair of syndromes represents genetic imprinting?
    a. Fragile X and Turner's
    b. Alzheimer's disease and trisomy 21
    c. Prader-Willi and Angelman
    d. Rett and fragile X

    Answer: c. A deletion in chromosome 15 causes both Prader-Willi and Angelman syndromes. In a prime example of genetic imprinting, the phenotype depends on whether the mother or father passes the abnormal gene to the offspring. When the father passes the gene, the child (boy or girl) develops Prader-Willi syndrome. In contrast, when the mother passes the gene, the child (boy or girl) develops Angelman syndrome.

32. Regarding phenylketonuria (PKU), which one of the following statements is false?

    a. The disease is transmitted in an autosomal recessive pattern.
    b. The blood phenylalanine is high and tyrosine is low in affected individuals.
    c. When PKU women conceive, their fetus would most likely be heterozygote for the PKU gene and would therefore be unaffected by the mother's diet.
    d. Diet sweeteners and many other "foods" contain phenylalanine, which individuals with PKU should avoid.

    Answer: c. Women with PKU, who must be homozygous for the disorder, have children who, with rare exception, are heterozygote. (If the father were heterozygote, which is statistically unlikely, the child is 50% likely to be homozygous. If the father had PKU and therefore homozygote for the disorder, 100% of the offspring would also be homozygous.) Assuming that a pregnant woman, who has PKU, strays from her diet and consumes foods with phenylalanine, such as diet soda, she will accumulate excessive concentrations of phenylalanine. The phenylalanine and metabolic products readily cross the placenta. Even though the fetus is heterozygous (or in rare instances homozygous), those substances overwhelm its immature enzyme system and cause severe brain damage.

33. An 8-year-old girl has had delayed acquisition of developmental milestones. She has mild mental retardation and especially poor arithmetic and visual-spatial skills. Her handwriting is difficult to read, and she has impaired fine motor skills. However, she is talkative and has learned several foreign languages that she speaks with a natural accent. She also plays two musical instruments and learns new pieces "by ear." Her facial appearance is "elf-like." Which is the most likely disorder?
    a. Rett syndrome
    b. Turner's syndrome
    c. PKU
    d. Angelman syndrome
    e. Williams syndrome
    f. Klinefelter's syndrome

    Answer: e. Williams syndrome, identifiable by the distinctive elf-like face, causes mild mental retardation, with especially poor visual-spatial relationships. In contrast to their other neuropsychologic deficits, individuals with Williams syndrome often have an outstanding verbal and musical ability.

34. Which condition is likely to be present in the girl in Question 33?
    a. Supravalvular aortic stenosis

b. Microcephaly
c. Stereotypies
d. Hepatosplenomegaly

Answer: a. Williams syndrome involves impaired formation of tissue elastin. Microcephaly results from several conditions: Rett syndrome, Angelman syndrome, congenital rubella infection, and numerous other disorders. Stereotypies—repetitive, involuntary, meaningless movements, usually of the hands—are characteristic of several neurologic conditions, including Rett, Angelman, and fragile X syndromes.

35. Which one of the following statements concerning individuals with the XYY karyotype is false?
    a. They are phenotypically male and referred to as "supermales."
    b. They are tall, often excessively so, and plagued with severe acne.
    c. They frequently have deviant behavior and often commit crimes.
    d. Their karyotype is a valid defense against criminal prosecution.

Answer: d. These men, who are tall and suffer with acne, often have mild mental retardation and deviant behavior, which may be criminal; however, they are cognizant of their activities and considered culpable if they commit a crime.

36. A 10-year-old boy with mental retardation has a tall stature, dislocated ocular lenses, and pectus carinatum. Which enzyme is probably deficient?
    a. Cystathionine synthetase
    b. Hypoxanthine-guanine transferase (HGPRT)
    c. Phenylalanine hydroxylase
    d. Tyrosine hydroxylase

Answer: a. Because of a deficiency in cystathionine synthetase, he had homocystinuria. That illness, caused by a genetic mutation on chromosome 21, causes mental retardation, dislocated lenses, tall stature, and skeletal abnormalities. HGPRT deficiency causes Lesch-Nyhan syndrome. Phenylalanine hydroxylase deficiency causes PKU. Tyrosine hydroxylase leads to parkinsonism.

37. Meningomyeloceles are not associated with which one of the following conditions?
    a. Spastic paraparesis
    b. Mental retardation
    c. Incontinence
    d. Meningitis
    e. Flaccid quadriparesis

Answer: a. A meningomyelocele is a congenital neural tube closure defect. It causes flaccid, not spastic, paraparesis because of malformation of the junction of the lowest portion of the spinal cord and its emerging nerve roots. In addition, meningomyeloceles are associated with comparable defects in the upper neural tube, which often lead to hydrocephalus.

38. Which neurologic condition is associated with immunodeficiency?
    a. Neurofibromatosis
    b. Meningomyelocele
    c. Sturge-Weber syndrome
    d. Ataxia-telangiectasia

Answer: d. Ataxia-telangiectasia is associated with an IgA and IgE immunoglobulin deficiency as well as cellular immunity impairment. Lymphomas develop in ataxia-telangiectasia patients.

39. Match the condition (a–e) with its clinical feature (1–5).
    a. Adrenoleukodystrophy
    b. Rett syndrome
    c. Fragile X syndrome
    d. Down syndrome
    e. Meningomyelocele
    1. In only girls, autistic behavior, repetitive hand slapping, and acquired microcephaly
    2. In only boys, progressive deterioration of mental and motor abilities
    3. In boys and girls, short stature, prominent epicanthal folds, single crease, low-set ears, and mental retardation
    4. In boys and girls with paraparesis, urinary incontinence, hydrocephalus, and mental retardation
    5. In boys, but less commonly in girls, mental retardation and large ears; in boys, macro-orchidism

Answers: a-2, b-1, c-5, d-3, e-4.

40. Match the structures with their origin in the fetal ectoderm or mesoderm.
    a. Brain
    b. Scalp and face
    c. Dura matter
    d. Neural tube
    e. Vertebrae
    f. Spinal cord
    g. Skull

Answers: Ectoderm: a, b, d, f. CNS fetal ectodermal structures include the neural tube and skin. Mesoderm: c, e, g. CNS-associated mesodermal structural elements include the skull, dura matter, and vertebrae.

41. Which two parts of the neural tube does the Dandy-Walker malformation affect?
    a. The bulb

b. Cerebellum
c. Lower spinal cord
d. The frontal lobes

Answers: a, b. In Dandy-Walker malformation, the medulla and cerebellum fail to develop. The malformation usually causes hydrocephalus, including a massively dilated fourth ventricle.

42. Which of the following strategies reduces the incidence of meningomyelocele?
    a. Giving the mother thiamine before and during the first trimester
    b. Giving the mother vitamin A before and during the first trimester
    c. Giving the mother folic acid before and during the first trimester
    d. Screening for toxins in the environment

Answer: c.

43. Match the genetically based disorder (a–c) with its manifestations (1–11).
    a. Rett syndrome
    b. Fragile X syndrome
    c. Down syndrome
       1. Repetitive hand movements
       2. Acquired microcephaly
       3. Associated with trisomy 21
       4. Mental retardation complicated by Alzheimer's-like dementia
       5. Associated with excessive trinucleotide repeats
       6. A single palm crease
       7. Macro-orchidism
       8. Autistic behavior
       9. Cognitive deterioration beginning in childhood
       10. The full syndrome occurs almost exclusively in girls
       11. The full syndrome occurs almost exclusively in males

Answers: 1-a; 2-a; 3-c; 4-c; 5-b; 6-c; 7-b; 8-a, b; 9-a; 10-a; 11-none. Approximately one third of female carriers of the fragile X chromosome show some symptoms of the disorders. Rarely males with certain genetic anomalies will have some features of Rett syndrome.

44. A 14-year-old girl is short, severely obese, and mildly mentally retarded. Her karyotype shows 23 chromosome pairs, including a normal XX, but 15q has a deletion. Which is the most likely syndrome?
    a. Angelman
    b. Turner's
    c. Fragile X

d. Prader-Willi
e. Down
f. Trisomy 21

Answer: d. All these disorders, including fragile X, can occur in girls and cause mental retardation. Of children with mental retardation, the obesity points immediately to Prader-Willi syndrome, which is confirmed by the deletion in 15q. Angelman syndrome also results from the deletion in 15q, but its manifestations include severe mental retardation and hyperactivity. Turner's syndrome, which only occurs in girls, results from an absent sex chromosome, that is XO, leaving only 22 full (autosomal) chromosome pairs.

45. How does Angelman syndrome differ from Prader-Willi syndrome?
    a. Angelman syndrome is inherited from the father.
    b. Angelman syndrome causes greater mental retardation than Prader Willi syndrome.
    c. Angelman syndrome results from excessive trinucleotide repeats.
    d. Angelman syndrome's genotype is determined by genetic imprinting.

Answer: b. Mental retardation is more pronounced in Angelman than Prader Willi syndrome.

46. Which one of the following statements is true regarding fragile X syndrome?
    a. The condition occurs exclusively in girls.
    b. When the trinucleotide repeats range from 60 to 200, the individual may be asymptomatic. However, his or her offspring is likely to have a much greater number of repeats and flagrant symptoms.
    c. Fragile X syndrome is a rare cause of mental retardation.
    d. When it causes mental retardation, the cognitive impairment is unaccompanied by behavioral changes.
    e. The condition is restricted to boys.

Answer: b. Fragile X syndrome occurs in girls who inherit two abnormal X chromosomes, as well as boys who inherit only one. It is the most common cause of inherited mental retardation. Boys with an intermediate number of trinucleotide repeats (60 to 200) may have few if any symptoms, but the abnormal trinucleotide sequence expands with successive generations and their offspring can be predicted to have unequivocal manifestations. The disorder causes hyperactivity and autistic behavior as well as mental retardation.

47. Which of the following syndromes is least likely to include autism-like symptoms?

a. Fragile X
b. Rett
c. Klinefelter's
d. Angelman
e. Tuberous sclerosis

Answer: c.

48. Which of the following treatments will best reduce elevated serum homocysteine levels?
    a. Administering folic acid and vitamins B_6 and B_{12}
    b. Relying on a methionine-free diet
    c. Supplementing the diet with homocysteine
    d. Relying on a phenylalanine-free diet

Answer: a. Although a methionine-free diet will lower serum homocysteine levels, the best strategy is to administer folic acid and vitamins B_6 and B_{12}.

49. Which of the following might expose a fetus to high levels of mercury?
    a. Maternal dental fillings
    b. The mother eating canned tuna every day
    c. The mother eating fresh salmon every day
    d. The mother eating trout every day

Answer: b. Large, predatory fish, such as shark, tuna, king mackerel, and swordfish, have relatively high concentrations of methylmercury, which readily crosses the placenta. Old style mercury-containing dental amalgams cause negligible mercury exposure.

50. In the mid-1990s vaccine manufacturers stopped using ethyl mercury, thimerosal, as a preservative in measles, mumps, and rubella (MMR) vaccinations. What effect did this change in policy have on the incidence of autism?
    a. The incidence continued to rise with no change in rate.
    b. The incidence continued to rise but at a slower rate.
    c. The incidence began to fall.
    d. The incidence immediately fell to zero.

Answer: a. The change in MMR vaccination formulation made no effect on the steadily increasing rate of autism. The brief although intense exposure to mercury did not seem to have caused autism.

51. Which of the following is not associated with a birth weight of less than 1 kg?
    a. Eczema
    b. IQ scores <85
    c. Poor social performance
    d. Visual impairments
    e. Hearing impairments

Answer: a. Extremely low birth weight (<1 kg) is associated with multiple life-long neurologic impairments and asthma but not skin disease.

CHAPTER

14

Neurologic Aspects of Chronic Pain

After a painful bodily injury, "acute pain" resolves as tissue heals. However, with continuous injury or sometimes a healed injury, "chronic pain" extends well beyond the usual healing period or for longer than 3 to 6 months. More than simply endless acute pain, chronic pain is a chronic illness. It interferes with patients' work, activities of daily living, sleeping, and personal relationships. When chronic pain results from cancer, neurologists categorize it as "malignant" pain, but when the pain results from other conditions, "nonmalignant."

Whereas traditional medical approaches to chronic pain emphasized diagnosis, distinguished between psychologic and psychologic components, and sought its eradication, current multidisciplinary pain teams, which usually include psychiatrists, stress symptomatic management—reducing pain's affective component (suffering) and restoring function. As a member of a team or an individual treating physician, psychiatrists should be aware of common chronic pain syndromes and their underlying neuroanatomy, psychiatric comorbidity, and treatments involving long-term use of opioids (narcotics) and adjuvant (primarily nonanalgesic) medications, including antidepressants and antiepileptics.

PAIN VARIETIES

In *nociceptive* disorders, specific nerve receptors (*nociceptors*) detect ongoing tissue damage usually arising from acute painful conditions, such as a metastasis to bone, disease of the viscera, or dental infection. The peripheral nervous system (PNS) and certain cranial nerves then transmit stimuli to the central nervous system (CNS), producing a characteristically dull aching pain at the site of the tissue damage. Diseased viscera, however, may refer pain to another site, such as when gallbladder stones seem to produce pain in the scapula. Removing diseased tissue and other direct treatments reduce or eliminate the pain. Until the injury responds to treatment or heals, analgesics alleviate the pain.

In *neuropathic* disorders, direct PNS, cranial nerve, or CNS injury leads to chronic pain. Some investigators postulate that over time nerve injury reorganizes

CNS pain perception through *plasticity*, a theoretical capacity of the CNS to reorganize its functions. Although plasticity is usually beneficial, in this case it amplifies, distorts, and perpetuates pain.

Neuropathic pain is a symptom of cranial neuropathies, peripheral polyneuropathies (see Chapter 5), lumbar spine disorders, complex regional pain syndrome, thalamic pain syndrome, and other CNS disorders. It is also a symptom of cancer infiltrating a nerve or plexus. The pain in neuropathic conditions is sharp, lancinating, or burning. It is located throughout the distribution of the injured nerves and well beyond them. Unlike nociceptive pain, neuropathic pain is stimulus-sensitive. Patients with neuropathic pain have both pronounced spontaneously occurring painful paresthesias and intensified, distorted, or prolonged responses to painful or even neutral stimuli—allodynia, hyperalgesia, and hyperpathia (see Chapter 5).

Physicians can rarely treat the neuropathic disorders and they cannot remove or repair the injured nerves. Whatever its source, neuropathic pain is common, disabling, and usually unrelenting. Not only does neuropathic pain resist treatment, it carries great psychiatric comorbidity.

The *Diagnostic and Statistical Manual of Mental Disorders, 4th Edition, Text Revision (DSM-IV-TR)* categorizes pain somewhat differently. Its diagnosis of Pain Disorder requires, in short, that pain represents the major focus of the clinical presentation and that it causes distress or functional impairment. It allows psychologic factors to have an important role in the pain's onset, severity, or maintenance. The diagnosis excludes pain better explained by a mood disorder, anxiety, or psychosis. It considers pain resulting from a neurologic or medical condition, such as headaches, peripheral neuropathy, or low back pain, to be a component of those conditions.

The DSM-IV-TR further recognizes Pain Disorders Associated With Psychological Factors and Pain Disorders Associated With Both Psychological Factors and a General Medical Condition. Also, it divides both into durations of shorter (acute) or longer than 6 months (chronic).

The DSM-IV-TR labels individuals as "malingering" who knowingly falsely claim severe and

317

prolonged pain. In addition to financial expectations, incentives to malinger include freedom from work assignments, attention getting, and retribution. Even though the proportion of malingering individuals may be less than 1% of all pain cases, the number of such individuals is quite large.

Despite the existence of clear diagnostic categories, many cases remain ambiguous. Although virtually all neurologic disorders have a psychiatric component, probably none has a greater psychiatric element than chronic pain. Pain management centers report that as many as 50% of patients with chronic pain have dual diagnoses—particularly depression, but also somatoform and personality disorders, substance abuse, and post-traumatic stress disorders. Moreover, chronic pain is linked to drug and alcohol dependency, dysfunctional family relationships, and exaggeration of physical deficits.

The closest association remains between depression and chronic pain, which is almost invariably neuropathic. When it complicates the disorder, depression lowers the threshold for pain, makes it refractory to treatment, and increases disability. In many patients the causal relationship between pain and depression is unclear. For many individuals, painful injuries lead to depression, but, for others, pre-existing depression leads to chronically painful injuries. With respect to chronic pain, major depression is more closely associated with the *number* of painful sites or painful conditions than the severity or duration of pain.

Psychiatric Consultations

Physicians often refer patients with either malignant or nonmalignant chronic pain for psychiatric consultation. The purpose of the referral includes most often evaluation for depression and anxiety, other psychologic disturbances, drug abuse, or failure to respond to the usual treatments. Alternatively, instead of waiting to be consulted as a last resort, psychiatrists encourage referring physicians to send patients for a consultation as an integral part of the initial evaluation. Whether acting individually or as part of a pain-management team, psychiatrists should evaluate patients (1) who have vegetative symptoms, regardless of the apparent connection to the pain; (2) whose pain or disability is refractory to several courses of medical treatment; (3) for whom excessive medications are required; (4) for psychopharmacology consultation; (5) for whom inpatient treatment or surgical procedures have been unsuccessful; or (6) who may have psychopathology that sabotages their treatment.

When possible, psychiatrists should examine the physical location of a patient's pain. An examination involving physical touch of the painful area, where appropriate, probably has therapeutic benefit, albeit a primitive one. Also, in evaluating pain-related functional disability, psychiatrists should watch the patient sit, walk, and, if possible, use the affected part of the body.

With the possible exception of prescribing inadequate amounts of opioids for pain control, physicians tend to overmedicate patients. Where possible, they should consider supplementing or replacing medicines with nonpharmacologic modalities, such as psychotherapy, cognitive-behavior techniques, and physical therapy.

PAIN PATHWAYS

Ascending pathways rapidly bring information from the periphery to the brain. They identify a pain's nature and location, arouse central mechanisms, and activate the limbic system. Analgesic pathways, originating in the brain and descending in the spinal cord, modulate pain perception. This neuroanatomy for pain and analgesia provides the framework for many treatment strategies.

Peripheral Pathways

Painful conditions, such as contusions and menstrual cramps, liberate inflammatory mediators including prostaglandins, arachidonic acid, and bradykinin that stimulate nociceptors. Thus, medicines, such as aspirin and nonsteroidal anti-inflammatory agents (NSAIDs), that inhibit synthesis of prostaglandins or otherwise reduce tissue inflammation, alleviate pain.

If these medicines fail to interrupt the process, nociceptors transmit pain along two types of small diameter PNS fibers, *A-delta* and *C*. These fibers both slowly conduct impulses and are sensitive to local anesthetics. A distinguishing feature is that A-delta fibers are covered with a thin sheet of myelin, and C fibers are unmyelinated (Table 14-1). More important, as the *gate control theory* explains, stimulation of heavily myelinated, large diameter *A-beta* fibers, which ordinarily carry vibration and position sensation, inhibits transmission by the small diameter A-delta and C fibers.

Central Pathways

The PNS fibers enter the CNS at the spinal cord's dorsal horn and, either immediately or after ascending a few segments, synapse in its *substantia gelatinosa* (Fig. 14-1). At many of these synapses, the fibers release an 11-amino acid polypeptide, *substance P*, which

TABLE 14-1 ■ Sensory Fibers of the Peripheral Nervous System

Fiber Type	Diameter	Insulation	Sensations Conveyed
A-delta	Small	Thinly myelinated	Pain and temperature
A-beta	Large	Heavily myelinated	Vibration and position
C	Small	Unmyelinated	Pain and temperature

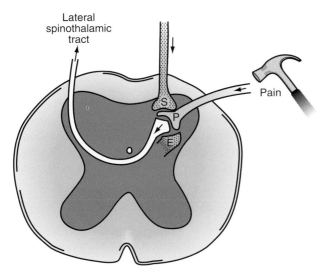

FIGURE 14-1 ■ Painful sensations travel along *A delta* and *C* fibers of the peripheral nerves. These nerves enter the dorsal horn of the spinal cord where, using *substance P* (P), they synapse onto second-order neurons. The second-order neurons cross to the contralateral side of the spinal cord and, comprising the *lateral spinothalamic tract,* ascend to the thalamus. Two powerful pain-dampening or pain-modulating analgesic systems (*stippled*) play on the dorsal horn synapse. One tract descends from the brain and releases *serotonin* (S). The other system is composed of spinal interneurons that release *enkephalins* (E).

constitutes the major neurotransmitter for pain at the spinal cord level.

After the synapse, pain sensation ascends predominantly within the *lateral spinothalamic tract* to the brain (see Figs. 2-6 and 2-15). This crucial tract crosses from the substantia gelatinosa to the spinal cord's other side and ascends, contralateral to the injury, to terminate in specific thalamic segments. Additional synapses then relay the stimuli to the somatosensory cerebral cortex, enabling the individual to locate the pain.

In the *spinohypothalamic tract,* another ascending pain pathway, fibers travel both ipsilateral and contralateral to their origin and terminate directly in the hypothalamus. This pathway may explain pain-induced disturbances in temperature regulation, sleep, and other autonomic functions. The spinal cord also transmits pain in other, less well-defined ipsilateral and contralateral tracts.

In addition to relaying pain to the thalamus and hypothalamus, these tracts convey pain to the limbic system, reticular activating system, and other brainstem regions. This connection partially explains why individuals awaken when given a painful stimulus. It also accounts for chronic pain patients' sleeplessness, loss of appetite, and a tendency to develop anxiety and mood disturbances. On the other hand, loss of this connection explains why patients who are unconscious for any reason cannot feel pain or suffer.

ANALGESIC PATHWAYS

Many analgesic pathways interfere with pain transmission within the brain or spinal cord. Several originate in the frontal lobe and hypothalamus and terminate in the gray matter surrounding the third ventricle and aqueduct of Sylvius (*periaqueductal gray matter*). They contain large amounts of *endogenous opioids,* which are powerful analgesics (Table 14-2). Implanted electrodes that stimulate the periaqueductal gray matter area may provoke the release of endogenous opioids and thereby induce profound analgesia.

Similarly, short neurons located entirely within the spinal cord, *interneurons,* act on incoming PNS fibers. These neurons also release endogenous opioids and other neurotransmitters that reduce pain transmission.

Other analgesic pathways originate in the brainstem and descend in the spinal cord's *dorsolateral funiculus.* These pathways provide "descending analgesia" relief

TABLE 14-2 ■ Glossary

β-endorphin: An endogenous opioid concentrated in the pituitary gland and secreted with adrenocorticotropin (ACTH). It consists of amino acid numbers 61–91 of β-lipotropin and gives rise to the enkephalins (see Fig. 14-2).

β-lipotropin: A 91-amino-acid polypeptide, which may be an ACTH fragment. It gives rise to β-endorphin but has no opioid activity itself (that is, β-lipotropin is not an endogenous opioid).

Dynorphin: An endogenous peptide opioid that binds to kappa opioid receptors.

Endogenous opioids: Polypeptides (amino acid chains) found within the central nervous system (CNS) that create effects similar to those of morphine and other opioids. The effects of both endogenous and exogenous opioids are characteristically reversed by naloxone.

Endorphins: Endogenous morphine-like substances or opioid peptides. This term is virtually synonymous with endogenous opioids.

Enkephalins: Short (5-amino-acid) polypeptide endogenous opioids that include met-enkephalin and leu-enkephalin. They are found primarily in the amygdala, brainstem, and dorsal horn of the spinal cord.

Naloxone (Narcan): A pure opioid antagonist that reverses the effects of endogenous and exogenous opioids.

Substance P: An 11-amino acid polypeptide that is probably the primary pain neurotransmitter at the first synapse of the primary afferent neuron in the spinal cord.

of pain by inhibiting both spinal cord synapses and their ascending pathways. Unlike most other analgesic pathways, they release *serotonin.*

ENDOGENOUS OPIOIDS

Often called *endorphins* (*end*ogenous *morphine*-like substances), endogenous opioids—endorphins, enkephalins, and dynorphins—are powerful analgesic, amino acid chains (polypeptides) synthesized in the CNS (Fig. 14-2). They bind to receptors in the limbic system, periaqueductal gray matter, dorsal horn of the spinal cord, and other CNS sites. Commonly cited examples of endorphins' analgesic effects include the "runner's high" and the initial painlessness described by wounded soldiers.

Synthetic (exogenous) opioids, particularly morphine and other medicines, are virtually identical to endogenous opioids. They bind with the same CNS receptors and produce the same effects—analgesia, mood elevation (euphoria), sedation, and respiratory depression. *Naloxone* (Narcan), an antagonist that competitively binds to the opiate receptor, reverses the effects of endogenous, as well as exogenous, opioids. Indeed, naloxone's opioid antagonist effect is so characteristic that *naloxone-reversibility* serves as a criterion for ascertaining that opioid pathways mediate an analgesic's effect.

TREATMENTS

Physicians prescribe numerous medications and administer them through various routes. Some relieve

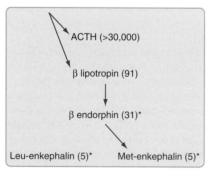

FIGURE 14-2 ■ Endogenous opioids are synthesized and secreted, along with adrenocorticotropin (ACTH), from the pituitary gland in times of stress or acute pain. A large precursor molecule (not pictured) gives rise to ACTH and ß-lipotropin, which are often released together. ß-lipotropin gives rise to ß-endorphin and met-enkephalin, but another precursor gives rise to leu-enkephalin. (The asterisks denote the important endogenous opioids, and the numbers within parentheses are the amino-acid units in the polypeptide chains.)

pain by reducing tissue damage, interrupting pain transmission through peripheral or central pathways, or blunting its impact on cerebral structures. The addition of psychologic treatment and physical therapy may further reduce pain and, as part of a complete care plan, decrease suffering, restore activities of daily living, and return control to patients.

Nonopioid Analgesics

As previously mentioned, aspirin, other salicylates, NSAIDs, steroids, and acetaminophen—nonopioid analgesics—inhibit prostaglandin synthesis at the injury (Table 14-3). Through this mechanism, they relieve acute and chronic pain of mild to moderate severity. In fact, two tablets (650 mg) of aspirin, which remains a standard basis of comparison, produce approximately the same analgesia as two common opioids: 65 mg of propoxyphene (Darvon) or 50 mg of oral meperidine (Demerol).

Nonopioid analgesics generally provide steady analgesia for weeks to months and avoid several potential problems. For example, after completing a course of treatment, patients do not experience withdrawal symptoms. Also, except for high-dose steroids causing psychosis (steroid psychosis, see Chapter 15), these analgesics do not induce mood, cognitive, or thought disorders. (In treatment of acutely herniated lumbar intervertebral disks, injections of steroids and a local anesthetic into the epidural space often provide immediate and long-lasting relief without subjecting the patient to the potential side effects of systemically administered steroids.)

On the other hand, large doses of NSAIDs and aspirin cause gastric irritation or hemorrhage, and prolonged use increases the risk of cardiovascular disease. In addition, nonopioid analgesics provide dose-dependent pain relief, but only up to a point. Once these medicines provide their maximum pain relief, greater doses will not increase the benefit (the "ceiling effect").

TABLE 14-3 ■ **Examples of Nonopioid Analgesics**

Acetaminophen (Tylenol and others)
Aspirin
    Choline magnesium trisalicylate (Trilisate)
    Diflunisal (Dolobid)
Nonsteroidal anti-inflammatory agents
    Ibuprofen (Motrin, Advil)
    Indomethacin (Indocin)
    Ketorolac (Toradol)
    Naproxen (Naprosyn)
Steroids
    Prednisone

Nonopioid analgesics are more effective if patients take them on a prophylactic basis. For example, taking nonopioid analgesics prior to dental procedures or menses will avert much of the pain. They are also more effective if taken in a generous initial, "loading," dose before or after the onset of pain.

Although nonopioid analgesics alone offer little benefit in cases of neuropathic pain, when taken in combination with opioids, they act synergistically. In other words, peripherally acting nonopioid analgesics enhance centrally acting opioid analgesics. For example, even taking two tablets of aspirin increases the pain-relieving effect of methadone in chronic low back pain. Likewise, adding NSAIDs to morphine helps alleviate the pain of metastases to bone. Because nonopioid analgesics allow a smaller dose of opioids to be effective, they are said to have an "opioid-sparing effect."

Opioids

Opioids are unquestionably indicated for moderately to severely painful conditions, such as cancer and acute nonmalignant painful conditions, such as fracture, myocardial infarction, and sickle cell crisis (Table 14-4), which are all typical nociceptive disorders. In addition, an increasing number of studies suggest that opioids are indicated for nonmalignant pain syndromes (see later).

Having no ceiling effect, greater doses or more potent preparations of opioids increase their effect. Their potency can also be enhanced, without increased side effects, by adding NSAIDs or other nonopioid analgesics.

Physicians traditionally prescribed opioids by oral or intramuscular routes. More recently transdermal (skin patches), intranasal (sprays), rectal (suppositories), continuous intravenous, intrathecal (intraspinal injections), and intra-articular (injections) became available. A particularly innovative technique, *patient-controlled analgesia* (PCA), allows patients to regulate continual or intermittent opioid infusions. Through controls in the system, patients regulate the depth of analgesia without causing respiratory depression. Even 6-year-old children can safely and effectively use PCA.

Compared to older analgesics, newer opioids, such as fentanyl (Duragesic), provide more rapid onset of action and greater potency because of their biochemical structures and the new routes of administration. Several opioids are particularly beneficial because of their long duration of action. Parenterally administered opioids maintain analgesia longer than most oral ones because they are spared first pass clearance by hepatic metabolism. Some opioids are long-acting because they are embedded in a matrix, such as a pill or patch, that slowly releases its medication.

Unless opioids are administered continuously by PCA, patches, or long-acting oral preparations, they should be given on a *regular prophylactic* or *time-dependent* basis, such as every 2 to 4 hours, rather than at the onset of pain. Otherwise, the delay makes pain more difficult to alleviate, creates a pattern of undertreatment and overtreatment, and prevents a restful sleep-wake schedule. Moreover, the patient, fearful about pain recurrence, becomes anxious and preoccupied with obtaining drugs. Physicians who prescribe narcotics should select long-acting preparations, such as methadone or transdermal fentanyl (patches), thereby avoiding the pharmacologic "hills and valleys," side effects, and pain recurrence. Also, because various opioids affect different regions of the mu (μ) and related receptors, physicians should vary the opioid for patients with intractable pain.

Physicians should also avoid changing from oral to parenteral form of opioid at a given dose because the substitution will possibly lead to an overdose. If the reverse situation, changing the same dose from an intramuscular or intravenous injection to pills is likely to produce undertreatment, which would cause withdrawal symptoms and recurrence of pain.

"Addiction"

Within weeks of opioid treatment, increasingly greater quantities are required to produce the same level of anesthesia (*tolerance*) as opioids desensitize receptors. Similarly, abruptly stopping opioid treatment produces unpleasant symptoms (*withdrawal*).

Although tolerance and withdrawal characterize physical dependence, physicians in pain management services, as ones in psychiatry, define addiction primarily in behavioral terms, such as potentially harmful drug-seeking activity and overwhelming involvement

---

TABLE 14-4 ■ Examples of Opioid Analgesics

For mild to moderate pain
  Codeine
  Oxycodone (Percocet)
  Propoxyphene (Darvon)
For moderate to severe pain
  Fentanyl (Duragesic)*
  Hydromorphone (Dilaudid)
  Levorphanol (Levo-Dromoran)
  Methadone^
  Morphine+

*Available for transcutaneous (skin patch) and transmucosal (lollipop) administration.
^Long-acting.
+Available in long-acting forms (MS Contin, Oramorph SR).

with use of a drug. They consider tolerance and dependence, which often occur together but can occur independently, as physiologic responses, an expectable aspect of medical treatment, and not peculiar to opioids. They also note that inadequate treatment and development of tolerance drive pain patients to seek larger doses of opioids. Physicians unfamiliar with pain management might misinterpret this behavior as "drug-seeking" and indicative of addiction, but pain management physicians consider it iatrogenic "pseudoaddiction."

In fact, addiction rarely develops in previously opioid-naive individuals who develop an acute painful illness that requires opioids for several weeks. Pain management physicians have been advocating continual opioid treatment of moderate to severe nonmalignant as well as malignant pain.

Other Opioid Side Effects

For the psychiatric consultant, a potential source of confusion is the similarity of opioid-induced mental status changes to those induced by head trauma, metabolic aberrations, and cerebral metastases. Because opioids may cause delirium and depress the level of consciousness, which would obscure the clinical picture, neurologists and neurosurgeons avoid treating head trauma patients with opioids.

Hypoventilation—respiratory depression characterized by slow, shallow, insufficient breathing—is one of the few potentially life-threatening problems associated with opioid use. However, in practical terms, inadvertent combinations of medications and pre-existing pulmonary disease, rather than the opioid overdose, are the usual causes of hypoventilation. Also, patients develop tolerance to hypoventilation and other opioid side effects.

Although depression of sensorium and hypoventilation loom large to physicians as major iatrogenic problems, constipation remains the most troublesome side effect for most patients. It can be managed by a combination of laxatives, such as senna (Senokot), and stool softeners, such as docusate sodium (Colace). Furthermore, to prevent or treat opioid-related nausea, physicians should prescribe antiemetics. However, physicians should cautiously prescribe antiemetics containing phenothiazine or other dopamine-blocking agent because they can cause dystonic reactions or parkinsonism (see Chapter 18). Additionally, synthetic marijuana, dronabinol (Marinol), and related preparations, which have been approved as antiemetics, can cause transient mood and thought disorders.

The use of certain opioids is fraught with difficulties. For example, phenytoin and carbamazepine—whether prescribed for their antiepileptic activity, mood modulation, or pain control—accelerate methadone metabolism. Therefore, giving them to patients on methadone maintenance may precipitate withdrawal symptoms. To avoid that problem, physicians should increase the methadone dose as those medications are added.

Although a frequently prescribed analgesic, meperidine is poorly absorbed when taken orally and changing its route of administration leads to complications. Moreover, when it is given for several days, especially to patients with renal insufficiency, accumulation of its toxic metabolite, normeperidine, often causes dysphoria, cognitive impairment, delirium, tremulousness, myoclonus, and seizures. When taken with monoamine oxidase inhibitors, including deprenyl, meperidine may cause potentially fatal hypertensive encephalopathy. Finally, with chronic use—by pain patients or addicts—meperidine can cause muscle and subcutaneous tissue nodules.

Heroin, another problematic opioid, is no more effective in relieving pain or improving mood than morphine, but its potential for abuse is much greater. Regardless of several medical and nonmedical groups' assertions, heroin has no legitimate use that cannot be better fulfilled by the current array of medicines.

As with other medicines, physicians should discontinue opioids when unnecessary and, in general, taper rather than abruptly stop them. Physicians sometimes replace a short-acting opioid with brief course of methadone to facilitate withdrawal. In the final stages, patients may require a nonopioid analgesic. If withdrawal symptoms develop, benzodiazepines may alleviate some of the physical or mental discomfort, and clonidine (Catapres) may blunt autonomic nervous system hyperactivity (see Chapter 21).

Chronic Opioid Treatment Debate

Physicians routinely prescribe opioids for a preplanned, limited course, such as recovery from surgery, and for indefinite periods and with increasing doses for cancer-related pain. However, long-term opioid treatment of chronic nonmalignant pain remains controversial despite increasing evidence to support its use. Physicians who oppose it foresee several problems related to addiction, side effects, and regulatory issues.

For example, patients may demand opioids for conditions, such as migraine, that usually do not warrant them or when less potent or alternative measures, such as triptans (see Chapter 9), would suffice. Patients may seek opioids for their euphoric effect rather than for pain relief. To obtain opioids patients may falsely report persistent symptoms and thus obscure the course of the underlying illness. Some patients have sold or passed along their medicines. Most important, long-term opioid treatment, especially at high dosage or following a dose increase, may produce sedation, impair cognition, and interfere with psychosocial function. Also, physicians are subject to administrative oversight that may be stringent and punitive.

On the other hand, some physicians have advocated liberally prescribing opioids for pain patients who have otherwise intractable, chronic nonmalignant disorders, and do not display abusive, destructive, drug-seeking behavior. They offer several arguments that are gaining increased acceptance. Opioids are effective, safe, and allow patients to work, use machinery, and drive. They increase functioning, reduce suffering, and help restore sleep. Written, unequivocal, and signed "contracts" greatly reduce, if not eliminate, abuse. Moreover, these physicians claim that, when used to control pain, opioids are not addictive.

Adjuvants

Antidepressants

Adjuvants enhance opioids and nonopioids and modulate the affective component of chronic pain. For example, amitriptyline, nortriptyline, and other tricyclic antidepressants (TCAs) help alleviate neuropathic conditions. In addition, TCAs help restore patients' normal sleep-wake schedule and improve their mood.

TCAs are helpful for chronic pain patients with or without comorbid depression. They are suitable for chronic pain in children. When used to treat pain, TCAs are effective at low doses and have a rapid onset of action. However, even at the low doses, TCAs may cause side effects. Also, unlike with opioid treatment, substituting one TCA for another will probably not improve analgesia.

Selective serotonin reuptake inhibitors (SSRIs), compared to TCAs, have little analgesic effect—surprising given serotonin's crucial analgesic role. However, SSRIs may offer some pain relief in patients with comorbid depression. The mixed reuptake inhibitors, such as duloxetine and venlafaxine, may have greater analgesic potential.

Antiepileptic Drugs

Like antidepressants, antiepileptic drugs (AEDs)—carbamazepine, clonazepam, gabapentin and its congener pregabalin, phenytoin, and valproate—are effective alone or in conjunction with opioids for many neuropathic conditions. For example, carbamazepine and gabapentin relieve trigeminal neuralgia so effectively that a positive response confirms the diagnosis. Not all of their analgesic effects should be attributed to their anticonvulsant properties as many AEDs have a dual action. For example, carbamazepine is structurally similar to TCAs.

Other Adjuvants

Neurologists prescribe other adjuvants to ameliorate comorbid symptoms. If anxiety complicates the picture, benzodiazepines may produce calm, permit sleep, and counteract muscle spasms. By treating those symptoms, they indirectly reduce pain and suffering. On the other hand, benzodiazepines may interact with opioids or other medicines to depress the sensorium or create mental status changes. Similarly, antipsychotic agents alleviate severe anxiety and thus reduce pain and suffering. In addition, those with dopamine-blocking mechanisms also contribute a potentially valuable antiemetic effect.

Finally, many diverse medicines serve as adjuvants. For example, clonidine, an antihypertensive alpha-2 adrenergic agonist, purportedly reduces pain in migraine and various chronic neuropathic conditions. In an apparent paradox, adrenergic alpha-receptor blockers, such as phentolamine, that do not cross the blood–brain barrier have been beneficial for some patients. Even cardiac antiarrhythmics, such as mexiletine, have reduced pain for many patients.

Other Treatments Directed at the Peripheral or Central Pathways

When the skin is affected by postherpetic neuralgia (see later) or other painful condition, applying patches of a long-acting anesthetic agent, such as lidocaine gel (Lidoderm), directly over the lesion interrupts the transmission of pain stimuli. Alternatively, for a region of chronic chest or abdominal pain, physicians may perform a *nerve block* by injecting anesthetic agents into one of the thoracic and lumbar nerve roots, which are readily accessible as they emerge from the spine. Long-acting local preparations provide pain relief for days or, with an alcohol, many months. However, nerve blocks are impractical for chronically painful limbs because they may causes paresis, as well as analgesia. Nor are they useful for facial pain within the first division of the trigeminal nerve (V_1) because analgesia involving the eye leads to corneal ulceration.

Sometimes a sympathetic plexus or ganglion block reduces pain. For example, for patients with pancreatic carcinoma, physicians can deaden the celiac plexus with alcohol injections. Similarly, for patients with the shoulder-hand syndrome, physicians can inactivate the stellate ganglion (the sympathetic ganglion adjacent to the upper cervical vertebrae) with alcohol injections. Nevertheless, their benefit in complex regional pain syndrome remains controversial.

To interrupt pain transmission in the spinal cord, physicians have introduced several different treatments. Capsaicin cream, applied to a painful area, is absorbed though the skin and drawn up along sensory nerves. When it reaches the spinal cord synapse, capsaicin depletes substance P, the crucial neurotransmitter, and thereby impairs pain transmission (Fig. 14-1). This treatment, which complements systemic medicines, helps alleviate pain from arthritis, diabetic neuropathy, and postherpetic neuralgia.

Anesthetics administered intrathecally, the basis of spinal anesthesia, completely block transmission of all sensory and motor nerve impulses. Although suitable for surgical procedures, spinal anesthesia is not selective enough for treatment of chronic pain. However, preliminary studies suggest that certain calcium channel blockers administered intrathecally create anesthesia without producing paresis or incontinence. Another approach to interrupting spinal cord pain transmission, dorsal column stimulation, applies a low intensity current to the spinal cord (see later).

Stimulation-Induced Analgesia

The idea that stimulation of a neurologic pathway inhibits a complimentary one has given rise to attempts at stimulation-induced analgesia. The gate control theory, which embodies this idea, has found practical application in *transcutaneous electrical nerve stimulation* (*TENS*). TENS devices, which stimulate the skin proximal to the painful area, generate low-intensity impulses that stimulate large fibers, which then dampen small pain-transmitting ones (see Table 14-1). Although widely practiced and based on a credible theory, several studies have questioned the effectiveness of TENS. Indeed, in most cases, TENS provides only a small degree of analgesia for several weeks.

A similar but invasive technique, *spinal (dorsal column) cord stimulation*, involves neurosurgeons inserting electrodes into the epidural space overlying the spinal cord. The stimulator, which the patient controls, generates an electric current that presumably interferes with nerve transmission. According to preliminary reports, the device alleviates pain and improves the quality of life in complex regional pain syndrome and chronic low back pain patients.

Along the same line, some studies found that acupuncture provides analgesia in people with mild to moderate pain. Placing the needles in dermatomes (see Fig. 16-2) creates more analgesia than placing them in the traditional regions (meridians). When acupuncture includes electrostimulation, the procedure

TABLE 14-5 ■ Analgesics Mediated by the Endogenous Opioid System*
Acupuncture
Opioids
Placebo
Stimulation^
TENS (transcutaneous electrical nerve stimulation)
Dorsal column stimulation
Periaqueductal gray matter stimulation+

*Because naloxone partially or entirely reverses these analgesics, the endogenous opioid system presumably mediates their actions. In contrast, naloxone does not reverse analgesia induced by tricyclic antidepressants and hypnosis.
^See text regarding efficacy.
+Investigational.

doubles its effectiveness. Because traditional acupuncture induces a rise in cerebrospinal fluid (CSF) endorphins and its benefit is naloxone-reversible, acupuncture presumably works at least in part through the endogenous opioid system (Table 14-5).

In another CNS stimulation technique, neurosurgeons implant electrodes into the periventricular and periaqueductal gray matter and adjacent brainstem regions. As noted earlier, stimulation of these sites, which releases stored endogenous opioids, may induce profound analgesia. Despite the strong rationale, the procedure remains investigational.

For patients with intractable pain confined to a single limb, neurosurgeons have experimented with severing the lateral spinothalamic tract in the spinal cord contralateral to the pain. This procedure, a *cordotomy*, based on the neuroanatomy of the spinothalamic tract, provided profound and almost immediate analgesia. However, because the improvement lasted for only a few months, physicians abandoned the procedure. Neurologists attributed the brevity of its effect to plasticity of central pain pathways. Bilateral cordotomies for extensive pain were also unacceptable because they were complicated by respiratory drive impairment (Ondine's curse) and urinary incontinence.

Placebos, Hypnosis, and Behavioral Therapies

Placebos produce a brief period of analgesia in at least 30% of patients. They suppress severe acute pain, especially with comorbid anxiety, but have little effect on mild continual pain. Contrary to popular belief, a positive response to placebo does not mean that pain is psychogenic. Because the analgesic effect of placebos is partially naloxone-reversible, placebos probably stimulate the endogenous opioid system.

Hypnosis is useful for a limited period in a wide variety of chronic pain conditions, including cancer.

Because patients' susceptibility to hypnosis does not correlate with their response to placebos, neurologists do not equate hypnosis with treatment by placebo. In addition, naloxone does not reverse hypnosis-induced analgesia.

When the usual treatments provide insufficient relief or the pain exceeds the severity or chronicity warranted by the bodily injury, patients may respond to cognitive therapy, behavior modification, operant conditioning, biofeedback, and other psychotherapies. These techniques are also useful in cases of abnormal behavior, opioid abuse, or when family members reinforce maladaptive activities. Pain management services often include psychologic interventions as part of routine care for chronic pain patients.

MALIGNANT PAIN

Cancer can cause unrelenting excruciating neuropathic and nociceptive pain that resists conventional treatment. Such pain may arise from a variety of sources, particularly from metastases in bones, which are richly innervated, and nerves. It can also arise from medical and surgical treatments. Moreover, the combination of pain and underlying illness engenders depression and other psychiatric comorbidity.

Physicians should generally accept patients' accounts of their pain without reservation and monitor pain as regularly as they check the temperature and pulse (Fig. 14-3). In fact, pain has come to be regarded as the "fifth vital sign." Patients should have access to non-pharmacologic treatments, including relaxation techniques, hypnosis, and psychotherapy, as well as the full arsenal of medicines. Physicians should prescribe medicines from the three categories—nonopioid, opioid, and adjuvant—early or preemptively, frequently, and generously. As opioid tolerance develops, physicians should readily increase the doses of opioids.

A three-step treatment plan based on the World Health Organization Guidelines provides relief to as many as 90% of patients:

- Treat with a nonopioid analgesic with or without adjuvants until the ceiling is reached.
- Add a long-acting oral opioid analgesic with or without adjuvants.
- Combine opioids and nonopioids with adjuvants.

NONMALIGNANT PAIN SYNDROMES

Although agonizing pain is generally associated with malignancies, several nonmalignant conditions cause comparable pain, suffering, and disability. In addition, insomnia, drug-seeking behavior, depression, and other psychiatric disturbances are all comorbid with these conditions.

In general, neurologists often successfully apply guidelines for management of cancer-related pain to nonmalignant pain syndromes. Nevertheless, some differences exist. Patients and physicians should acknowledge that although most of these conditions are chronic and incurable, they are not fatal. The goals in these conditions—different from the single-minded one of complete pain relief—should be to reduce suffering, restore ability to work, and allow a return to social roles. They should be clear, acceptable to the patient and caregivers, and attainable within several months.

This chapter continues by discussing six common nonmalignant pain syndromes. The book has already reviewed several other conditions, including painful diabetic neuropathy (see Chapter 5) and trigeminal neuralgia (see Chapter 9). Pharmacologic management of all these conditions usually begins with analgesics, which often includes chronic opioid treatment. Unlike nociceptive pain treatment, TCAs, AEDs, and other adjuvants must supplement neuropathic pain treatment. Supplemental physical and occupational therapy, psychotherapy, hypnosis, and behavioral therapies may further reduce suffering, improve mobility, and increase function.

Physicians should not only strive to alleviate pain. The treatment plan, which usually requires patient cooperation, should aim to minimize suffering, medication side effects, and preoccupation with pain and obtaining medications. Treatment should also restore or maintain mental clarity, function, mobility, sleep, and restfulness.

Postmastectomy Axillary Pain

During a mastectomy, as surgeons explore the axilla and remove lymph nodes, they occasionally damage or sever the cutaneous branch of the first thoracic nerve root, the *intercostobrachial nerve*. Several weeks after the surgery, some women develop searing axillary pain that extends to the inner aspect of the upper arm, well beyond the incision. (In contrast, common incision pain is only mildly to moderately intense, has an itching quality, and is confined to the scar.) Postmastectomy pain, like many painful conditions, worsens at night. Because shoulder movement provokes post-mastectomy pain, it may lead to a "frozen shoulder." Other sources of postmastectomy pain are chemotherapy, radiotherapy, and a variation of phantom limb pain (see later).

Opioid or nonopioid analgesics and adjuvants usually help women with postmastectomy pain. Local treatments, such as lidocaine gel or nerve blocks, provide topical anesthesia complementary to systemic

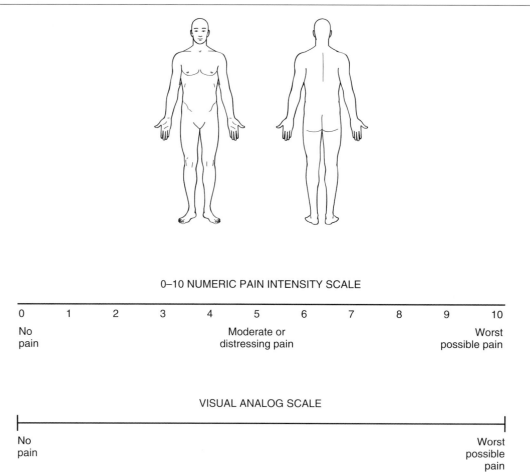

0–10 NUMERIC PAIN INTENSITY SCALE

| 0 | 1 | 2 | 3 | 4 | 5 | 6 | 7 | 8 | 9 | 10 |

No
pain

Moderate or
distressing pain

Worst
possible pain

VISUAL ANALOG SCALE

No
pain

Worst
possible
pain

FIGURE 14-3 ■ Graphics are replacing verbal reports of the site and severity of pain. Patients describe their pain by circling the most painful area on the sketch. Then they circle the single number on the Numeric Pain Scale or mark the Visual Analog Scale at the point that describes the intensity of their pain. Although most children 8 years or older can use the analog scale, physicians for younger children substitute the Wong-Baker smiling-crying faces icons. Although useful for assessing acute pain intensity, these scales are literally one-dimensional and fail to capture suffering, functional impairment, insomnia, or changes in mood. Moreover, these scales do not allow the patient to describe symptoms of neuropathic pain, such as allodynia.(Adapted from Jacox A, Carr DB, Payne R, et al: Management of Cancer Pain: Adults Quick Reference Guide. No 9. AHCPR Publication No. 94–0593. Rockville, MD, Agency for Health Care Policy and Research, U.S. Department of Health and Human Services, Public Health Service, 1994.)

treatment. In addition, physical measures, such as massaging painful skin with a damp cloth after applying a vapor-coolant, for example, ethyl chloride spray, may reduce the pain. Also, patients should increase shoulder mobility and strength through exercise. If conservative measures are ineffective, nerve blocks of the sympathetic ganglion sometimes help.

Even though postmastectomy pain carries little prognostic significance, it intensifies the surgery's psychologic impact. Moreover, it tempts psychologically oriented physicians and nonphysicians to suggest that postmastectomy pain stems from emotional factors.

Postherpetic Neuralgia

Acute *herpes zoster* infection causes a vesicular skin eruption, *shingles,* usually in the distribution of one or two nerve dermatomes. Although any dermatome may be affected, the thoracic dermatomes and then the first branch of the trigeminal nerve, which includes the cornea, are most commonly involved. Reactivated varicella virus that has lain dormant in dorsal (sensory) nerve root ganglia causes the infection. *Herpes zoster* is common in individuals older than 65 years, even those in good health, and especially in patients with immunosuppressive illnesses, such as lymphoproliferative disorders and acquired immunodeficiency syndrome (AIDS). A newly introduced vaccine against this virus may prevent or reduce the severity of this infection and all of its painful sequelae.

The acute infection causes unrelenting moderately severe burning sensations that may precede eruption of the vesicles by several days. In most cases, the pain and skin lesions last for several weeks. During this period, the severe pain justifies the use of opioids.

Antiviral agents, such as acyclovir (Zovirax) and famciclovir (Famvir), may speed healing of vesicles, shorten duration of the pain, and prevent spread of infection to the eye.

Herpes zoster patients are also at risk for developing an even more painful secondary phase, *postherpetic neuralgia,* typically 3 to 6 months after the initial infection has resolved. In an age-related risk pattern, postherpetic neuralgia develops in few individuals younger than 50 years, but in 50% of those older than 60 years and in 75% of those older than 70 years.

Patients with postherpetic neuralgia usually develop a band of numb scarred skin and, if a major motor nerve were involved, muscle weakness and atrophy. The pain has a continual dull quality of excruciating severity with superimposed lancinating paresthesias. It expands to cause anorexia, insomnia, and mood changes. Although it eventually resolves spontaneously, postherpetic neuralgia may torture patients for several years.

Physicians should prescribe generous doses of long-acting opioids, as well as AEDs, particularly gabapentin. If the affected area does not include the eye, they might also prescribe long-acting topical anesthetics, such as the lidocaine gel.

Complex Regional Pain Syndrome

Reflex sympathetic dystrophy (*RSD*), *causalgia,* and *sympathetically maintained pain* (*SMP*) fall under the rubric of complex regional pain syndrome. Type 1 complex regional pain syndrome seems to stem from no definable nerve injury, but type 2 has an underlying definable nerve injury. However, terms suggesting that the sympathetic nervous system is at fault are misleading because studies have demonstrated no consistent abnormalities in it.

Whatever the pathophysiology, patients report pain disproportionately greater than expected from the injury. Often the pain extends far beyond the injury to include the entire limb, but predominantly in its distal portions, and then into adjacent limbs. For example, after several months of left arm pain, a patient may describe similar symptoms in the left leg and then in the right leg. Patients typically describe the pain as relentless burning or lancinating sensations superimposed on irritating numbness. Sometimes their descriptions of the pain seem extravagant. Physicians sometimes diagnose those with lawsuits as having "litigation neurosis."

Neurologists find allodynia, hyperalgesia, and hyperpathia in complex regional pain syndrome patients more often than in any of the other nonmalignant pain syndromes described in this chapter. Because even touching or moving an affected limb increases the pain, patients tend to be preoccupied with the affected limb and protect it with extravagant methods. For example, they assiduously shield an afflicted hand by wearing a sling and glove or protect a foot from weight-bearing by using crutches. The combination of the injury, sensitivity, and protective maneuvers often incapacitate the affected limb.

Fingernails remain uncut and grow thick, long, and brittle. Although the skin may sweat excessively (*hyperhidrosis*), it is usually smooth, shiny, scaly, and dry. Similarly, although the skin of affected regions usually turns pale, it sometimes changes to a dusky color and has a superimposed livedo reticularis. Severe cases can include peripheral edema, muscle wasting (dystrophy), which gave rise to the term RSD, and bone reabsorption. Rare cases involve tremors, dystonia, and other involuntary movement disorders.

Complex regional pain syndrome typically follows major or seemingly minor injuries to a limb. The injuries do not necessarily involve overt nerve damage, but compressive, traction, or penetrating nerve injury may have occurred. Common causes are gunshot wounds, fractures, myocardial infarctions, and peripheral vascular disease.

In addition to the standard treatments for neuropathic pain, physicians prescribe intensive physical therapy to mobilize the affected limb. They also prescribe blockade of regional sympathetic ganglia in carefully selected cases. For example, patients with causalgia of the hand may benefit from blocking the stellate ganglion with an anesthetic agent. Intravenous infusions of bretylium or guanethidine, which block the region's α- and β-adrenergic sympathetic ganglion receptors, occasionally produce dramatic pain relief. Response to such blocks, even though brief, has diagnostic as well as therapeutic value.

Physicians also attempt to block the pain pathways in the spinal cord, but the methods are invasive, dangerous, and remain experimental. Surgically implanted spinal stimulators may suppress the pain. Intrathecal opioids or ziconotide, a new nonopioid voltage gated calcium channel blocker, interrupt the pathways.

Phantom Limb Pain

Phantom limb pain occurs at the site of an amputated limb. For example, a man may have had his leg severed at the thigh in an automobile accident and weeks later may still feel pain as though it were centered in his ankle. The pain is often accompanied by nonpainful sensations. For example, a patient with an amputation will often feel that the limb remains an integral part of the body and sense purposeful movements in an absent hand, finger, or toe. The phenomena of phantom pain are not restricted to limb injuries but may also follow amputation of a breast, ear, or other body part.

Neurologists often classify the pain from phantom limb, as from brachial plexus avulsion and thalamic infarction (see later)—given the sensory deprivation in all of these conditions—as *deafferentation pain*. Whatever their precise origin, abnormal sensations or misperceptions can develop and reach the level of somatic hallucinations. They may resemble the visual hallucinations that stem from visual sensory deprivation, that is, blindness (see Anton's syndrome, Chapter 12).

Pain at the site of a surgical incision, *stump pain*, differs from phantom limb pain because it is confined to the injury and attributable to nerve scars (neuromas). Nevertheless, phantom and stump pain may occur together.

Even in its most typical settings, phantom limb pain varies in quality, severity, and accompanying psychologic symptoms. It usually begins soon after a traumatic amputation and has a self-limited duration of several weeks. However, the pain is even more likely to develop and persist if the affected body part were chronically painful before the amputation (as with osteomyelitis). Because most cases result from war wounds, victims are usually young or middle-aged veterans. In addition to suffering chronic pain, many of them have sustained extensive injuries, including facial disfigurement, loss of several limbs, and castration.

In addition to prescribing usual treatments for nonmalignant pain syndromes, some physicians have claimed benefit from hypnosis that attempts to induce the sensation that the phantom limb is shrinking to the point of disappearing.

Thalamic Pain

Thalamic infarctions initially cause contralateral hemianesthesia but no pain. Depending on which nearby structures are damaged, the hemianesthesia may be accompanied by hemiparesis, hemiataxia, or a homonymous hemianopsia.

Subsequently, many patients develop spontaneous painful sensations on the hemianesthetic side of the body (*Déjérine-Roussy syndrome*). This condition usually involves face and hand pain. As with complex regional pain syndrome, patients are beset with allodynia and hyperpathia and try to ward off pain by wearing hats, long sleeves, and gloves. Fortunately, this pain usually subsides after 6 to 12 months.

Following other CNS injuries, such as spinal cord gunshot wounds, multiple sclerosis, and tabes dorsalis, patients often suffer a similar, although permanent, disturbance, *central pain*. These injuries typically cause lancinating pains, allodynia, and hyperpathia superimposed on paraparesis. Their common underlying pathology is interruption of the spinothalamic tract and possibly other sensory systems.

Low Back Pain

As opposed to acute low back pain from a herniated intervertebral disk (see Chapter 5), chronic low back pain seems to stem from ill-defined injury of the lumbar spine vertebrae, intervertebral disks, or the supporting ligaments. Affecting more than 2 million individuals, it is one of the most prevalent disabling conditions in the United States.

As much as in any neurologic condition, nonmedical factors contribute to persistent pain and prolonged disability. In fact, disability bears little relationship to structural abnormalities visible on magnetic resonance imaging (MRI). Work-related injuries, job dissatisfaction, psychologic distress, outstanding litigation, and other painful conditions portend a poor prognosis. Although depression, distress, somatization, and substance abuse also play a major role, their effects are often hidden. Psychologic screening tests, including the Minnesota Multiphasic Personality Inventory-2 (MMPI-2), cannot reliably predict which chronic low back pain patients will have a satisfactory surgical outcome.

Most patients with chronic low back pain should be advised to accept it as a chronic condition that medical care might ameliorate but not cure. Physicians might shift the goal of treatment to improving function rather than abolishing pain. For example, goals, which should be kept modest, could include completing a 6-hour workday or walking 1 mile.

Although the usual treatments for nonmalignant pain help, severe cases defy treatment. For example, despite obvious MRI abnormalities, surgery on herniated disks, spinal stenosis, and other orthopedic conditions fails in the majority of cases to permanently eliminate pain or enable patients to work. In fact, surgery may even worsen the pain and disability. Also, many popular techniques—acupuncture, back strengthening exercises, massage, spinal manipulation, and sleeping on a firm mattress—produce mild, short-lived, or no improvement. As with complex regional pain syndrome, interrupting pain pathways in the spinal cord may be helpful.

Finally, both physicians and patients should acknowledge, when relevant, that litigation often promises large amounts of money for *permanent* pain, suffering, and disability. This incentive discourages accurate reporting, effective treatment, and a return to work. Many neurologists suggest concluding litigation before expecting successful treatment.

REFERENCES

1. Backonja MM, Krause SJ: Neuropathic pain questionnaire-short form. Clin J Pain 19:315–316, 2003.

2. Ballantyne JC, Mao J: Opioid therapy for chronic pain. N Engl J Med 349:1943–1953, 2003.

3. Bartleson JD: Evidence for and against the use of opioid analgesics for chronic nonmalignant low back pain: A review. Pain Med 3:260–271, 2002.

4. Berde CB, Sethna NF: Analgesics for the treatment of pain in children. N Engl J Med 347:1094–1103, 2002.

5. Carragee EJ: Persistent low back pain. N Engl J Med 352:1891–1898, 2005.

6. Carragee EJ, Alamin TF, Miller JL, et al: Discographic, MRI, and psychosocial determinants of low back pain disability and remission: A prospective study in subjects with benign persistent back pain. Spine J 5:24–35, 2005.

7. Carroll LJ, Cassidy JD, Cote P: Depression as a risk factor for onset of an episode of troublesome neck and low back pain. Pain 107:134–139, 2004.

8. Cherkin DC, Sherman KJ, Deyo R, et al: A review of the evidence for the effectiveness, safety and cost of acupuncture, massage therapy, and spinal manipulation for low back pain. Ann Intern Med 138:898–906, 2003.

9. Dubinsky RM, Kabbani H, El-Chami Z, et al: Practice parameter: Treatment of postherpetic neuralgia. Neurology 63:959–965, 2004.

10. Dworkin RH, Backonja M, Rowbotham MC, et al: Advances in neuropathic pain: Diagnosis, mechanisms, and treatment recommendations. Arch Neurol 60:1524–1534, 2003.

11. Foley KM: Opioids and chronic neuropathic pain. N Engl J Med 348:1279–1281, 2003.

12. Hayden JA, van Tulder MW, Malmivaara AV, et al: Meta-analysis: Exercise therapy for nonspecific low back pain. Ann Intern Med 142:765–775, 2005.

13. Jacox A, Carr DB, Payne R, et al: Management of Cancer Pain: Adults Quick Reference Guide. No 9. AHCPR Publication No. 94-0593. Rockville, MD, Agency for Health Care Policy and Research, U.S. Department of Health and Human Services, Public Health Service, 1994.

14. Jovey RD, Ennis J, Gardner-Nix J, Goldman B, et al: Use of opioid analgesics for the treatment of chronic non-cancer pain—a consensus statement and guidelines from the Canadian Pain Society, 2002. Pain Res Manag 8(Suppl A):3A–28A, 2003.

15. Jung BF, Ahrendt GM, Oaklander AL, et al: Neuropathic pain following breast cancer surgery. Pain 104:1–13, 2003.

16. Kemler MA, Barendse AM, van Kleef M, et al: Spinal cord stimulation in patients with chronic reflex sympathetic dystrophy. N Engl J Med 343:618–624, 2000.

17. Melzack R: Phantom limbs. Sci Am 266:120–126, 1992.

18. Nasreddine ZS, Saver JL: Pain after thalamic stroke: Right diencephalic predominance and clinical features in 180 patients. Neurology 48:1196–1199, 1997.

19. Pappagallo M: Newer antiepileptic drugs: Possible uses in the treatment of neuropathic pain and migraine. Clin Ther 25:2506–2538, 2003.

20. Pincus T, Burton AK, Vogel S, et al: A systemic review of psychological factors as predictors of chronicity/disability in prospective cohorts of low back pain. Spine 27:109–120, 2002.

21. Rowbotham MC, Twilling L, Davies PS, et al: Oral opioid therapy for chronic peripheral and central neuropathic pain. N Engl J Med 348:1223–1232, 2003.

22. Staats PS, Yearwood T, Charapata SG, et al: Intrathecal ziconotide in the treatment of refractory pain in patients with cancer or AIDS. JAMA 291:63–70, 2004.

23. Tubach F, Beaute J, Leclerc A: Natural history and prognostic indicators of sciatica. J Clin Epidemiol 57:174–179, 2004.

24. Williams LS, Jones WJ, Shen J, et al: Outcomes of newly referred neurology outpatients with depression and pain. Neurology 63:674–677, 2004.

25. Woolf CJ, Mannion RJ: Neuropathic pain: Aetiology, symptoms, mechanisms, and management. Lancet 353:1959–1964, 1999.

Questions and Answers

1–7. Match the substance (1–7) with its effect on the pain pathways (a–e). More than one answer may be correct.
1. Morphine
2. Endogenous opioids
3. Serotonin
4. Substance P
5. Enkephalin
6. β-endorphin
7. Nonsteroidal anti-inflammatory drugs (NSAIDs)
   a. Reduces tissue inflammation
   b. Interferes with prostaglandin synthesis
   c. Provides analgesia by acting within the CNS
   d. Acts as a neurotransmitter of pain in the spinal cord
   e. Is liberated in a spinal cord descending analgesic tract

Answers: 1-c, 2-c, 3-c and e, 4-d, 5-c, 6-c, 7-a and b.

8. Which property of morphine is *not* shared with endogenous opioids?
   a. Tendency to cause tolerance
   b. Effectiveness in deep brainstem structures and spinal cord
   c. Ability to cause mood changes, as well as analgesia
   d. Reversibility with naloxone
   e. Commercial availability
   f. Causes respiratory depression

Answer: e. Morphine completely mimics the endogenous opioids.

9–17. Match the substance (9–17) with its composition (a–h).
 9. Leu-enkephalin
10. ACTH
11. Morphine
12. β-endorphin
13. Heroin
14. β-lipotropin
15. Met-enkephalin
16. Serotonin
17. Substance P
   a. 11-amino-acid polypeptide
   b. 5-amino-acid polypeptide
   c. Diacetyl morphine
   d. Greater than 30,000-amino-acid polypeptide
   e. Indole
   f. Alkaloid of opium

g. 91-amino-acid polypeptide
h. 31-amino-acid polypeptide

Answers: 9-b, 10-d, 11-f, 12-h, 13-c and f, 14-g, 15-b, 16-e, 17-a.

18. Which two of these fibers carry pain sensation?
   a. A-delta
   b. C
   c. A-beta
   d. B-delta

Answers: a, b. Of all peripheral nervous system fibers, pain perception is transmitted by certain small diameter nerve fibers (*A-delta* and *C fibers*). Thus, many patients have pain without disruption of other sensory modalities.

19. In which spinal cord tract does most pain sensation ascend?
   a. Fasciculus gracilis
   b. Fasciculus cuneatus
   c. Lateral corticospinal tract
   d. Lateral spinothalamic tract

Answer: d.

20. In which tract do serotonin-based analgesic fibers descend within the spinal cord?
   a. Lateral spinothalamic tract
   b. Dorsolateral funiculus
   c. Fasciculus gracilis
   d. Dentatorubral tract

Answer: b.

21. Which two forms of analgesia are not naloxone-reversible?
   a. Acupuncture
   b. Opioid
   c. Transcutaneous electrical stimulation (TENS)
   d. Aspirin
   e. Hypnosis
   f. Placebo
   g. Stimulation of periventricular gray matter
   h. Intrathecal morphine injections

Answers: d and e.

22. Why would the addition of aspirin or a NSAID increase the effectiveness of opioids?
   a. They are also opioids.

b. They actually do not increase analgesia.

c. They stimulate endogenous opioid release.

d. They interfere with prostaglandin synthesis.

e. They inhibit serotonin reuptake.

Answer: d.

23. Which of the following statements regarding tricyclic antidepressants (TCAs) is incorrect?

    a. TCAs treat depression, which is often comorbid with chronic pain.

    b. TCAs help restore restful sleep patterns.

    c. TCAs increase serotonin levels.

    d. TCAs are less effective than serotonin reuptake inhibitors (SSRIs).

    e. TCAs block reuptake of norepinephrine.

Answer: d. Blocking reuptake of norepinephrine and increasing serotonin levels are both analgesic, but in many conditions, such as diabetic neuropathy, enhancing norepinephrine activity is more effective. However, TCAs' effects on the autonomic nervous system limit their usefulness. Although conventional SSRIs have been disappointing, mixed norepinephrine and serotonin reuptake inhibitors show promise.

24. Which of the following is not a complication of mixed agonist-antagonist opioids, such as pentazocine (Talwin)?

    a. Normeperidine accumulation

    b. Addiction

    c. Delirium

    d. Respiratory depression

    e. Precipitating withdrawal symptoms in patients using meperidine (Demerol)

    f. Skin and subcutaneous scarring (sclerosis)

    g. All of the above

Answer: a.

25. Which of the following is a potential complication of meperidine?

    a. Marked undertreatment when a dose is switched from intramuscular to oral routes

    b. Normeperidine toxicity

    c. Overdose when a dose is switched from intramuscular to oral routes

    d. Stupor

    e. Seizures

    f. Tremulousness

    g. All of the above

Answer: g.

26. Which of the following is *not* characteristic of complex regional pain syndrome?

    a. The sympathetic nervous system is involved.

b. The skin often takes on a shiny and scaly appearance.

c. The pain is usually relieved with blockade of the sympathetic ganglia.

d. The trunk and abdomen are typically involved.

e. The pain spreads beyond the injured nerve.

Answer: d.

27. A 39-year-old headache patient, who has had migraine since childhood, has been taking an aspirin-butalbital-caffeine compound daily for at least 10 years. When the patient attempts to stop the medication, unbearable generalized dull headaches develop. What is the best descriptive term for this phenomenon?

    a. Chronic migraine headache

    b. Rebound headache

    c. Status migrainosus

    d. Addiction

Answer: b. Headaches following withdrawal of analgesics, especially if they are combined with vasoconstrictive medications, represent a major problem in headache management. "Rebound headache" is a form of withdrawal (see Chapter 9).

28. Which of the following is *not* a complication of infarction of the thalamus and its surrounding structures?

    a. Hemianesthesia

    b. Allodynia

    c. Hyperpathia

    d. Abnormal sweating

Answer: d.

29. Which of the following statements regarding the periaqueductal gray matter is incorrect?

    a. Stimulation of the periaqueductal gray matter produces analgesia.

    b. Thiamine deprivation causes hemorrhage into the periaqueductal gray matter.

    c. The periaqueductal gray matter surrounds the aqueduct of Sylvius.

    d. The aqueduct of Sylvius is the conduit for cerebrospinal fluid (CSF) between the lateral and third ventricles.

    e. The aqueduct of Sylvius is the conduit for CSF between the third and fourth ventricles.

Answer: d.

30. Which of the following statements regarding enkephalins is true?

    a. They are tricyclic.

b. They are secondary messengers.
c. Naloxone inhibits them.
d. They are part of the serotonin system.

Answer: c. The enkephalins are peptide neurotransmitters that have a powerful inhibitory effect on spinal cord interneurons. Their effects mimic those of morphine because they are part of the endogenous opioid system.

31. Which of the following statements regarding serotonin's role in pain and analgesia is false?
    a. Serotonin often reduces pain before affecting mood.
    b. Descending serotonin-based spinal cord tracts induce analgesia.
    c. In its analgesic role, serotonin is an inhibitory neurotransmitter.
    d. Serotonin is an endogenous opioid.

Answer: d.

32. Which statement most closely describes the gate control theory?
    a. Descending corticospinal tract pathways inhibit pain.
    b. The periaqueductal gray matter blocks pain transmission to the frontal lobes and limbic system.
    c. Behavioral modification reduces pain-induced suffering.
    d. Stimulation of large-diameter, heavily A-beta myelinated fibers inhibits pain transmission by small unmyelinated and sparsely myelinated A-delta and C fibers.

Answer: d.

33. Which four statements describe NSAIDs?
    a. They often cause gastrointestinal bleeding.
    b. Additional medication produces greater analgesia, that is, they have no "ceiling."
    c. Patients develop a tolerance to the analgesia.
    d. They are as effective as some opioids.
    e. They can be combined with opioids to produce additional analgesia.
    f. Some have been associated with cardiovascular complications.

Answers: a, d, e, f.

34. For a given dose, which route of administration of an opioid provides the lowest blood concentrations?
    a. Intramuscular
    b. Oral release
    c. Intravenous

Answer: b. About 50% of an orally administered opioid is metabolized on its first pass through the liver. Parenteral and transcutaneous administration are generally more effective than oral administration.

35. Which of the following is not an advantage of patient-controlled analgesia (PCA) over analgesia administered on a "by the clock" or an "as needed" basis?
    a. Lower cost
    b. Steadier levels of analgesia that avoid under- and overtreatment
    c. More regular sleep schedules
    d. Earlier hospital discharge

Answer: a. Despite the expense of training, close monitoring, and equipment, PCA is a widely accepted and successful innovation in the management of postoperative and chronic malignant pain. It empowers patients and reduces potential friction between patients, families, physicians, and nurses. However, unless patients have the dexterity and cognitive capacity to adjust the system, PCA may be ineffective or dangerous. As with conventional administration, respiratory depression may complicate PCA administration of opioids in patients with pulmonary disease.

36. Where do pain-carrying peripheral nerves synapse with the lateral spinothalamic tract?
    a. Dorsal columns
    b. Substantia gelatinosa
    c. Limbic system
    d. Thalamus

Answer: b. These peripheral nerves synapse in the spinal cord's substantia gelatinosa with the lateral spinothalamic tract, which ascends a short distance, crosses, and ascends contralateral to the painful site to synapse in the thalamus.

37. Which two of the following painful conditions are considered examples of *deafferentation* pain?
    a. Brachial plexus avulsion
    b. Insect stings
    c. Trigeminal neuralgia
    d. Carcinoma metastatic to bones
    e. Thalamic infarction
    f. Migraine
    g. Postherpetic neuralgia

Answers: a and e. When an injury deprives the brain of normal continual sensory input, the deafferentation produces a variety of neuropathic pain, called deafferentation pain. When conditions, such as in trigeminal neuralgia or postherpetic neuralgia, injure nerves, patients may develop other varieties of neuropathic pain.

38. A passing automobile catches the shirtsleeve of a 40-year-old man and drags him by the arm, dislocating his shoulder. Even after the shoulder has apparently healed, the entire arm develops an intense burning sensation that increases on movement or touching. The patient avoids using the arm and often wears a glove. The skin of the hand becomes smooth, dry, and edematous. He cannot cut his fingernails because the pain is too intense. Which three of the following statements are true concerning this condition?
a. Studies of the hand would likely show bone reabsorption.
b. The skin changes are an integral part of the condition.
c. TENS is usually effective in such cases.
d. Sympathetic blockage usually provides partial, temporary relief in such cases.
e. Shoulder dislocations are painful injuries, but they do not cause nerve damage.

Answers: a, b, d. He has developed complex regional pain syndrome from a traction injury of the brachial plexus. It has caused changes of the skin, nails, and soft tissue and provoked protective maneuvers. Nuclear bone scans and even routine x-rays will probably reveal bone reabsorption.

39. An 80-year-old man sustains a cerebral infarction that initially causes loss of almost all sensation on the left face, trunk, and limbs. Several weeks later, the sensory loss recedes but is replaced by continual burning pain in the left face and arm. Also, the slightest stimulation, including people brushing against his hand or physicians examining it, causes intolerable pain. He carefully shields the hand and arm under a glove and covers his arm with a blanket. What is the name of this condition?
a. Trigeminal neuralgia
b. Thalamic pain
c. Temporal arteritis
d. Postinfarction neoplasm
e. Psychogenic pain

Answer: b. The initial sensory loss indicates that the underlying lesion was a thalamic infarction. The subsequent condition, the thalamic pain syndrome, is a frequently occurring complication. The extraordinary sensitivity, allodynia, gives the aura of a psychogenic disturbance; however, this symptom is a feature of neuropathic pain.

40. Which of the following descriptions of withdrawal is incorrect?
a. Withdrawal symptoms suggest dependence.
b. Abruptly discontinuing regular use of caffeine, tobacco, or alcohol causes withdrawal symptoms.
c. Requiring additional doses of a substance to avoid symptoms is termed withdrawal.
d. Abruptly discontinuing many medications causes withdrawal symptoms.
e. The most common symptom of discontinuing opioids is a flu-like syndrome and anxiety.

Answer: c. Requiring additional doses of a substance is termed tolerance.

41. Match the term with the closest description. More than one answer may be appropriate.
a. Allodynia
b. Deafferentation pain
c. Physical dependence
d. Hyperalgesia
e. Hyperpathia
1. Testing for pain perception with a safety-pin provokes severe pain with crying
2. Spontaneous pain apparently originating from denervated areas, as would follow a brachial plexus avulsion
3. Increasing opioid requirement with disease progression
4. Flu-like symptoms that follow discontinuing opioids
5. Nonpainful stimuli, such as touch with a feather, provokes pain
6. A delayed but exaggerated and prolonged pain in response to safety-pin testing

Answers: a-5, b-2, c-4, d-1, e-6.

42. Which of the following is least likely to occur in patients prescribed opioids for nonmalignant pain?
a. Potentially harmful drug-seeking behavior
b. Need for increasing doses of the narcotic
c. Physical dependence
d. Tolerance

Answer: a. Patients prescribed opioids for nonmalignant pain rarely engage in criminal or other activities potentially harmful to themselves or others. Although they typically develop tolerance and experience symptoms if the opioid were withdrawn, they rarely meet criteria for addiction.

43. Which of the following is an example of nociceptive pain?
a. Postherpetic neuralgia
b. Diabetic neuropathy
c. Painful HIV-associated neuropathy
d. Complex regional pain syndrome
e. Fractured tooth pain

Answer: e. Although quite painful, a fractured tooth causes pain that will subside after it is repaired.

Until then, NSAIDs, opioids, and other analgesics will suppress the pain. The other conditions are examples of neuropathic pain that typically persists despite apparent healing of nerve injury. For them, although analgesics, including opioids, and local treatments will help, antiepileptics and antidepressants—adjuvants—are usually necessary.

44. Which of the following is known as the "fifth vital sign"?
a. Pulse
b. Blood pressure
c. Respiration
d. Temperature
e. Pain

Answer: e.

45. When under treatment with opioids, to which effect is a patient unlikely to develop tolerance?

a. Respiratory depression
b. CNS depression
c. Analgesia
d. None of the above

Answer: d. Opioid treatment leads to tolerance of the side effects as rapidly as the analgesic effects.

46. Which receptor subtype mediates the analgesic effect of opioids?
a. α
b. β
c. κ
d. μ

Answer: d. Opioids characteristically bind to the μ (mu) receptor and sometimes also to related receptors, such as the κ.

Multiple Sclerosis Episodes

Multiple sclerosis (MS) is the most common disabling neurologic illness of North American and European young and middle-aged adults. It is also the primary example of a central nervous system (CNS) autoimmune illness.

The diagnosis of MS traditionally rested on clinical grounds—episodes of neurologic disabilities ("lesions") disseminated in both time and space. Diagnostic criteria, named for the senior member of a 2001 international panel, Dr. W. Ian McDonald, and subsequently revised, now permit certain magnetic resonance imaging (MRI) abnormalities, instead of only the clinical examination, to demonstrate that lesions are disseminated in space. The revised McDonald criteria also allow MRI studies that indicate whether lesions are acute or chronic to establish that episodes are disseminated in time.

Still maintaining a high sensitivity and specificity, neurologists now diagnosis MS during its first episode. They can institute therapy and blunt, if not halt, an abnormal immune process early in its course. The current criteria also allow neurologists to follow patients' subclinical as well as clinical progression and monitor their response to treatment.

ETIOLOGY

MS—usually a chronic recurring illness—typically begins with 1 mm to 3 cm patches of inflammation developing in the oligodendrocyte-generated myelin sheaths of CNS axons. The inflammation strips myelin from (demyelinates) axons and eventually leaves sclerotic (Greek, *sklerosis*, hard) *plaques* scattered throughout the CNS. Plaques disseminated throughout the "white matter" of the cerebrum, cerebellum, spinal cord, ocular motility system, and optic nerves constitute the signature of MS.

When deprived of their myelin insulation, axons transmit nerve impulses slowly or not at all. Some deficits resolve as myelin inflammation spontaneously subsides or anti-inflammatory medications, such as steroids, suppress it. However, with relapses, plaques recur, multiply, and cause permanent neurologic deficits. Over time, the disease usually evolves

from an acute inflammatory to a chronic degenerative condition.

Although MS acts primarily as a CNS demyelinating disorder, its pathology includes prominent axon degeneration. Moreover, axon degeneration, rather than demyelination, produces the permanent mental and physical disabilities.

The illness' mean age of onset is 33 years, with 70% of cases developing between 21 and 40 years. Some patients suffer their first or a subsequent MS attack after a medical insult, such as infection, childbirth, head or spine trauma, intervertebral disk surgery, electrical injury, or psychologic stress. However, most studies have shown that such insults neither cause MS nor precipitate its exacerbations.

The specific cause of MS remains unknown, but some studies suggest that a complex interaction between genetic susceptibility and environmental factors triggers the illness. MS occurs twice as frequently in women than in men, and 20 to 40 times more frequently in first-degree relatives of MS patients than in the general population. Although genetic factors confer susceptibility, they do not constitute the entire explanation. For example, although 25% of monozygotic twins and 5% of dizygotic twins are concordant for MS, those concordance rates, although striking, are far smaller than if the illness resulted from conventional genetic inheritance. Moreover, in affected twins, each tends to display different symptoms and signs. Research has implicated several different chromosomes in causing MS, but none is necessary or sufficient.

Although the apolipoprotein E (Apo-E) gene with the E4 allele (see Chapter 7) does not confer a susceptibility to developing MS, MS patients with the allele suffer a more rapid progression of their illness than MS patients with no E4 alleles.

Epidemiologic studies have found environmental effects. One of the most statistically powerful is the relatively high incidence of MS among people born and raised in cool climates. For example, the incidence of MS is higher in residents of Boston than New Orleans, states north of the 37th parallel in the United States, and Scandinavian countries compared to Italy and Spain. Similarly, the incidence is relatively high in

Australia's cool, southern regions. In Asia, Latin America, and sub-Saharan Africa, the incidence is low. Data complementary to this geographic information indicate that the lack of sun exposure in late childhood represents the risk factor for developing MS.

Related epidemiologic findings suggest that MS patients contract their illness before 15 years of age. Studies in Israel found a higher incidence of MS in patients who emigrated from Northern Europe as adults than as children. In other words, individuals who left Europe during childhood, before they were exposed to an environmental factor, possibly an infectious agent, were unlikely to contract MS. Because spouses are not particularly vulnerable, environmental factors that adults encounter are probably not the cause.

CLINICAL MANIFESTATIONS

Course

The initial episode of MS may range from a single trivial impairment lasting several days to a group of debilitating deficits that remain for several weeks and do not fully recede. Subsequent episodes vary considerably in their manifestations, severity, and permanence. For most MS patients, 2 to 3 years pass before a relapse occurs. During exacerbations, the initial symptoms, accompanied by additional ones, generally reappear.

Almost all MS patients follow one of four reasonably distinct courses, *disease categories,* that consist of multiple attacks, steady deterioration, or several attacks followed by steady deterioration (Fig. 15-1, top). The categories reflect the clinical status as it relates to time. They do not take into account the severity or results of MRIs.

Relapsing-remitting MS, a category that initially includes about 80% of cases, is characterized by discrete attacks followed by partial or complete recovery. Although deficits may accumulate following each attack, patients remain stable between them. Unfortunately, most patients in the relapsing-remitting category eventually change to *secondary progressive* MS, which consists of further, steady deterioration.

Primary progressive MS, characterized by unremitting, steady deterioration from the illness' onset, accounts for only about 20% of cases. Unlike the other disease categories, primary progressive MS first develops in individuals who are in their fifth or sixth decade, rather than their third or fourth decade, and predominantly or exclusively affects the spinal cord. *Progressive-relapsing* MS, the least common category, consists of a steady deterioration with superimposed acute attacks.

In addition to being descriptive, MS categories indicate a patient's prognosis and probable response to immunomodulating treatments. Of the various categories, relapsing-remitting MS is the most amenable to treatment; progressive MS, the least (see later).

Frequent Symptoms

Although numerous symptoms may occur during the illness, the most frequent ones result from the lesions in the white matter tracts of the cerebrum, cerebellum, spinal cord, ocular motility system, and optic nerves (see Fig. 15-1, bottom). Symptoms often arise in combination when they stem from involvement of a critical area of the CNS. For example, during a relapse, an MS patient may have ocular motility impairment and intention tremor from a brainstem lesion's striking the connection between the third and sixth cranial nerves (see later) and cerebellar outflow tracts.

Simultaneous involvement of two separate sites, which produces disparate symptoms, frequently occurs. For example, plaques develop, at the same time, in the cerebellum and thoracic spinal cord, which would cause ataxia and paraparesis. Sometimes plaques simultaneously arise in one optic nerve and the thoracic spinal cord, which would cause monocular blindness and paraparesis, a variant of MS known to neurologists as Devic's disease or neuromyelitis optica.

Cerebellar Signs

As some of their earliest manifestations, MS patients often develop ataxia, intention tremor, and other signs of cerebellar and cerebellar outflow tract injury. When the cerebellum is involved, patients typically develop an ataxic gait (see Fig. 2-13); however, with minimal involvement, patients' gait impairment may consist only of difficulty walking heel-to-toe (*tandem gait*). Cerebellar involvement also typically causes *scanning speech,* a variety of dysarthria analogous to a "speech ataxia," characterized by irregular cadence and uneven emphasis on words. For example, when asked to repeat a pair of short syllables, such as "ba...ga...ba...ga...," the patient might place unequal stress on different syllables, blur them together, or pause excessively. Other manifestations of MS cerebellar involvement include intention tremor (see Fig. 2-11); dysdiadochokinesia; and an irregular, conspicuous, head tremor (*titubation*).

Sensory Disturbances

Both lack of sensation and abnormal sensations occur frequently and prominently. Patients often describe hypalgesia, paresthesias, or dysesthesias in their

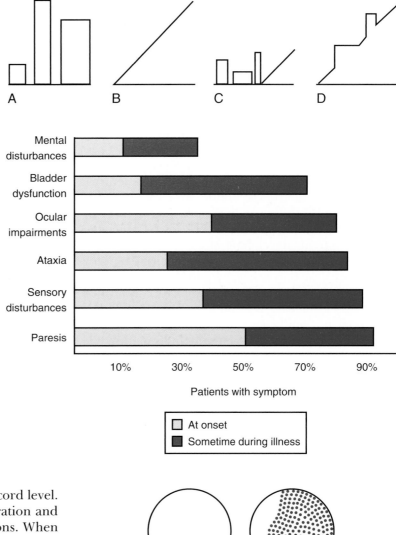

FIGURE 15-1 ■ *Top,* Graphs of different clinical courses—with severity of multiple sclerosis (MS) attacks (vertical axis) plotted against time (horizontal axis)—reveal four patterns or disease categories: *A,* Relapsing-remitting. *B,* Primary progressive. *C,* Secondary progressive. *D,* Progressive-relapsing. *Bottom,* This chart of initial and cumulative manifestations of MS indicates that cognitive impairment develops infrequently at the onset and ultimately less often than physical impairments.

limbs or trunk, or below a particular spinal cord level. They typically lose ability to appreciate vibration and position sensations more than other sensations. When patients without an established diagnosis of MS present with sensory symptoms that are unaccompanied by objective findings and do not conform to commonplace neurologic patterns, physicians may misdiagnose their condition as a psychogenic disturbance.

Ocular Impairments

Impaired visual acuity and disordered ocular motility—which neurologists often call "eye signs"—occur frequently not only at the onset of the illness but also throughout its course. In fact, the absence of such signs in patients believed to have MS prompts neurologists to reconsider the diagnosis (see later).

Visual acuity impairment is usually attributable to inflammation in the retrobulbar portion of the optic nerve, *retrobulbar neuritis* or *optic neuritis* (see Fig. 12-6). It characteristically causes an irregular area of visual loss in one eye, a *scotoma,* that often includes the center of vision (Fig. 15-2). It also leads to *color desaturation,* in which colors, especially red, lose their intensity.

FIGURE 15-2 ■ Optic or retrobulbar neuritis impairs vision in a large, irregular area (*scotoma*) of the affected eye. It also characteristically causes pain, especially when the eye moves. The optic nerve is susceptible to multiple sclerosis (MS) because, unlike almost all other cranial nerves, its covering consists entirely of central nervous system (CNS) myelin. The only other exception consists of the acoustic nerve (cranial nerve 8), and it is the only one partially covered by CNS myelin.

In addition to reducing vision, optic neuritis causes pain in the affected eye. Probably because ocular movement puts traction on an inflamed optic nerve, eye pain increases when patients look from side to side.

Unless the optic disk is swollen, which is difficult to detect, ophthalmoscopic examination usually reveals no abnormality. This discrepancy between visual loss and the normal appearance of the disk has given rise to the saying "The patient sees nothing and the physician sees nothing." As an optic neuritis attack subsides, most vision returns and pain subsides. However, with repeated attacks, progressive visual loss ensues and the disk becomes atrophic.

Statistics vary on the relationship of optic neuritis to MS. Approximately 25% of MS patients have overt optic neuritis as their initial symptom and 80% have it at some time during their illness. On the other hand, only about 30% of young adults who develop optic neuritis as an isolated condition will develop MS during the next 5 years. A single attack of optic neuritis, devoid of other neurologic symptoms, is therefore not diagnostic of MS; however, in the presence of three or more MRI lesions, optic neuritis is closely associated with subsequently developing MS.

Multiple sclerosis also causes ocular motility disturbances, such as *nystagmus* and the characteristic *internuclear ophthalmoplegia (INO)*, which is also called the *medial longitudinal fasciculus (MLF) syndrome*. Either brainstem or cerebellar involvement can lead to nystagmus. Although it is clinically indistinguishable from nystagmus induced by other conditions (see Chapter 12), MS-induced nystagmus typically occurs in combination with dysarthria and tremor (Charcot's triad).

In INO, demyelination or other MLF damage interrupts nerve impulse transmission from the pontine conjugate gaze centers to the oculomotor nuclei (Figs. 15-3 and 15-4). Its primary symptom is diplopia on lateral gaze because of paresis of the adducting eye. In conjunction with other signs of CNS injury, INO is strong evidence of MS; however, systemic lupus erythematosus (SLE or lupus [see later]) and small basilar artery strokes may also cause it. In addition, Wernicke-Korsakoff syndrome, myasthenia gravis, and botulism can produce ocular muscle weakness that mimics INO. From a physiologic viewpoint, INO is analogous to a disconnection syndrome, such as conduction aphasia, in which communicating links are severed but each neurologic center remains intact (see Chapter 8).

Spinal Cord Symptoms and Signs

Patients with spinal cord involvement, which may be the illness' only site in primary progressive MS, have paraparesis with hyperactive DTRs and Babinski signs. They usually have three troublesome, common symptoms (the 3 *Is*)—incontinence, impotence, and impairment of gait. Another troublesome, often incapacitating feature of spinal cord involvement consists of spasticity of the legs. Even in the absence of paraparesis, spasticity impairs patients' gait and causes painful leg spasms. Patients with cervical spinal cord involvement often describe electrical sensations, elicited by neck flexion, that extend from the neck down the spine (*Lhermitte's sign*).

Spinal cord involvement also typically leads to *urinary incontinence* from a combination of spasticity, paresis, and incoordination (*dyssynergia*) of the bladder sphincter muscles (Fig. 15-5). MS patients initially often have incontinence during sleep and sexual intercourse. As the disease progresses, patients develop intermittent urinary retention and then complete loss of control. Many patients must undergo intermittent or continuous catheterization.

Erectile dysfunction, decreased desire, and other forms of sexual impairment plague the majority of MS patients (see Chapter 16). About 40% of women

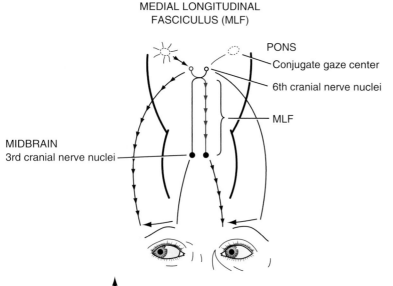

MEDIAL LONGITUDINAL
FASCICULUS (MLF)

PONS
Conjugate gaze center
6th cranial nerve nuclei
MLF

MIDBRAIN
3rd cranial nerve nuclei

FIGURE 15-3 ■ When looking laterally, the pontine conjugate gaze center stimulates the adjacent abducens (sixth) nerve nucleus and, through the *medial longitudinal fasciculus (MLF)*, the contralateral oculomotor (third) nerve nucleus. Thus, when looking to the right, as in this illustration, the right pontine gaze center stimulates the right abducens and the left oculomotor nuclei (also see Fig. 12-12).

INTERNUCLEAR
OPHTHALMOPLEGIA

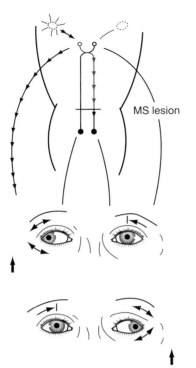

FIGURE 15-4 ■ In *internuclear ophthalmoplegia (INO)*, also called the *MLF syndrome,* an interruption of the MLF prevents impulses from reaching the oculomotor (third) nuclei. Because those nuclei themselves remain intact, the pupils and eyelids are normal in both eyes. However, when looking to the right, because the left oculomotor nucleus is not stimulated, the left eye fails to adduct. The right eye abducts, but nystagmus develops. With bilateral INO, which is characteristic of multiple sclerosis (MS), neither eye adducts and abducting eyes have nystagmus.

with MS do not engage in sexual intercourse. Even before developing erectile dysfunction, men often experience premature or retrograde ejaculation. Sexual dysfunction, with or without urinary incontinence, is attributable to MS involving the spinal cord. With spinal cord damage severe enough to cause paraplegia, men have lowered and abnormal sperm production, but women can conceive and bear children.

Fatigue and Other Important Symptoms

An inexplicable generalized, daily sense of fatigue—sometimes referred to as "lassitude" (weariness of body or mind)—affects about 50% to 80% of MS patients. This symptom, which is entirely subjective, does not correlate with patients' age or whether or not they have paresis. Fatigue, which is aggravated by heat and humidity, reduces work ability, compliance with medical regimens, and quality of life. In addition, it exacerbates other MS manifestations.

BLADDER

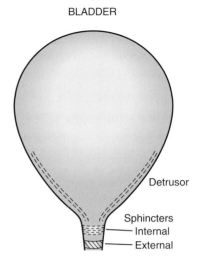

FIGURE 15-5 ■ The urinary outflow of the bladder has two sphincters: an internal sphincter controlled by the autonomic nervous system (ANS), and an external one under voluntary control. Normal urinary bladder emptying (urination) occurs when the detrusor (wall) muscle contracts and *both* sphincter muscles relax. Purposefully urinating requires voluntary action (to relax the external sphincter) and reflex parasympathetic (ANS) activity (to contract the detrusor and relax the internal sphincter). Urinary retention occurs with either anticholinergic medication or excessive sympathetic activity because both inhibit detrusor contraction and internal sphincter muscle relaxation. Urinary retention also occurs with spinal cord injury because the external sphincter is unable to relax because it is spastic and paretic (dyssynergic).

Fatigue may be comorbid with depression and, like depression in MS, interfere with patients' participating in their work and medical regimens; however, fatigue rarely serves as a manifestation of depression. When MS-induced fatigue reaches a state of exhaustion, it represents a physiologic cause of the chronic fatigue syndrome (see Chapter 6). Amantadine may reduce MS-induced fatigue, but, despite expectations generated by initial reports, modafinil does not help.

Common MS symptoms also include various pain syndromes. For example, approximately 2% of MS patients suffer from trigeminal neuralgia (see Chapter 9) and 10% Lhermitte's sign. These pains probably arise from MS plaques irritating CNS pain-transmitting fibers in, respectively, the brainstem and cervical spinal cord. As with other forms of neuropathic pain (see Chapter 14), antiepileptic drugs, such as gabapentin and carbamazepine, are most effective.

Some symptoms occur rarely. Because the cerebral cortical "gray matter," which has little myelin, is relatively spared, MS patients only infrequently develop signs of cerebral cortical dysfunction, such as seizures or aphasia. Similarly, because the basal ganglia are also devoid of myelin, involuntary movement disorders (see Chapter 18) rarely complicate MS.

Pregnancy

Women with MS remain fertile. Oral contraceptives do not affect MS. If women conceive, they do not have an increased rate of miscarriages, obstetric complications, or fetal malformations. Throughout pregnancy, the rates of both first MS attacks and, in established cases, exacerbations significantly fall. In fact, during the third trimester, the exacerbation rate falls to 70% of its baseline. If MS exacerbations occur, they do not affect the pregnancy.

At delivery, MS patients require cesarean sections for only the usual indications. Epidural anesthesia has no affect on the course of MS. Women who are pregnant and those are who breast-feeding infants cannot take interferons and other medications that suppress MS (see later).

Although the pregnancy and delivery pose little or no threat, during the first three postpartum months, mothers with MS have a 20% to 30% incidence of exacerbation. Moreover, those exacerbations are more incapacitating than ones that struck before conception. The rate of exacerbations subsequently returns to its baseline. In the long run, pregnancies do not worsen the course of MS.

PSYCHIATRIC COMORBIDITY IN MS

Depression

Depressive symptoms, often attributable to a nonspecific psychologic response to a chronic, serious illness, occur frequently in MS patients. They correlate with MS-induced physical impairments, loss of bodily function, inability to work, and lack of social support. Although they do not reach the severity or duration of major depression, they tend to interfere with MS patients' following their arduous regimen of self-injecting medicines that have unpleasant side effects, self-catheterization, and participating in rigorous physical therapy programs.

Major depressive illness occurs in 25% to 50% of MS patients during their lifetime. It develops more frequently in patients with MS than in patients with other chronic illnesses (who have a 13% incidence), even if those illnesses produce comparable physical impairments.

Depression tends to complicate MS, from a neurologic viewpoint, mostly in proportion to the severity of the disability. It occurs more when MS involves the cerebrum rather than only the spinal cord. Also, depressive symptoms develop twice as frequently in patients following a relapsing-remitting than a primary progressive course. In general, symptoms arise most frequently at the onset of the illness, during exacerbations, late in the course of the illness, and in conjunction with cognitive impairment. Depression is also associated with cerebral atrophy and the total MS lesion area or volume (*lesion load* or *burden*).

From more of a demographic viewpoint, the risk of developing comorbid depression is greatest for MS patients who were young at the onset of their illness, have recently learned of their diagnosis, have had less education, lack family and social support, and have a history of depression.

Unlike depressive illness that occurs in families without MS, genetic influence in MS-induced depression is negligible. For example, the rate of depression in first-degree relatives of depressed MS patients is considerably lower than the rate of depression in first-degree relatives of depressed individuals who do not have MS.

Largely reflecting the high incidence of depression, the suicide rate of patients in MS clinics is as high as seven times greater than that of comparably aged individuals. Compared to all MS patients, those who have attempted or completed suicide have been younger than 30 years and symptomatic for less than 1 year. In addition, their history includes depression in themselves or their family, alcohol abuse, and limited psychosocial support. However, MS-induced cognitive impairment is not a risk factor for suicide.

Psychopharmacology can improve MS patients' mood, reduce their discomfort associated with immobility, and help restore restful sleep. Depressed patients generally respond to both tricyclics and selective serotonin reuptake inhibitors (SSRIs); however, antidepressants with anticholinergic side effects should be used cautiously because they are liable to cause urinary retention. In addition, SSRIs may increase spasticity.

Antidepressants' effective doses in depression associated with MS are generally lower than in depression not associated with neurologic disease. Electroconvulsive therapy (ECT) is also usually effective, and it can be administered with only the usual precautions, (i.e., MS cerebral lesions are not a counterindication to ECT). Whichever treatment physicians choose, adding psychotherapy, social services, occupational counseling, or physical therapy might be helpful.

In the debate about assisted suicide, MS will undoubtedly become a battleground. Many MS patients will probably seek assisted suicide that will be resisted with more than the usual arguments. Unlike amyotrophic lateral sclerosis (ALS) or terminal cancer patients, for whom the concept is most understandable, MS patients are generally young, have a life expectancy of many years, and rarely have physical pain. Moreover, impairments in their cognitive capacity and depressed mood may arguably cloud their judgment.

Although bipolar affective disorder occurs at twice the rate in MS patients than in the general population, mania rarely develops in MS patients. If it occurs, consultants must watch for steroid treatment of MS causing behavior and thinking that mimic mania (see later).

Consultants should also consider "MS-induced euphoria"—an elevation of mood inappropriate to the illness. Some euphoric patients are masking depression or protecting themselves with denial. Others simply feel relieved as an MS attack subsides. On the other hand, extensive cerebral involvement can cause inappropriate mood or behavior. For example, in as many as 10% of MS patients, pseudobulbar palsy provokes pathologic laughing or crying (see Chapter 4). Such symptoms are associated with physical deterioration, chronicity of the illness, and subtle, if not overt, intellectual impairment.

Psychosis

Unlike depression, psychosis is not significantly more common in MS patients than unaffected individuals. Except for cases described in scattered reports, MS almost never presents with depression or psychosis. Notably, the incidence of psychosis in MS is less than in most other neurologic illnesses, including Alzheimer's disease, head trauma, and epilepsy.

However, MS patients may experience disordered thinking from several sources. If dementia has developed, minor psychologic or physiologic disturbances may trigger an uninhibited, irrational response. MS patients are vulnerable to delirium from infectious illnesses, particularly urinary tract infections, and side effects from steroids and other medications.

On a practical level, psychiatrists should initially assume that in MS patients, psychosis is a manifestation of cerebral demyelination, medications, or concomitant physical illness. Because treatment guidelines for psychosis comorbid with MS have not been established, physicians should treat the psychosis in MS as they would treat it in other neurologic conditions.

Cognitive Impairment

Almost all MS patients—in the initial phase of their illness—have normal cognitive function based on their satisfactorily completing their day-to-day functions, routine mental status examination, and Mini-Mental State Examination (MMSE) (see Fig. 7-1). Nevertheless, neuropsychologic tests, such as the Wechsler Adult Intelligence Scale (WAIS), Selective Reminding Test, and Halstead Category Test, may reveal at least clinically silent deficits in 45% to 65% of MS patients.

Once the illness is established, patients' slow and inarticulate speech, fatigue, and visual impairments impair the testing. When cognitive function declines, memory deterioration occurs first and, throughout the course, most prominently. Language function, in contrast, is comparatively spared. Late in the course of the illness, all cognitive domains deteriorate to the level of dementia.

MS-induced cognitive impairment can hamper activities of daily living, prevent full compliance with medical regimens, and strain interpersonal relationships. Moreover, it can precipitate thought and mood disorders.

In general, MS-induced cognitive impairment correlates with duration of the illness and, to a lesser extent, physical disability. It also correlates with certain MRI abnormalities, particularly enlarged cerebral ventricles, corpus callosum atrophy, periventricular white matter demyelination, and overall lesion load. Of all of them, cognitive impairment correlates most closely with the periventricular region lesion load.

Cognitive impairment in MS differs from that in Alzheimer's disease in several respects. For example, MS produces a subcortical dementia, but Alzheimer's produces a cortical dementia (see Chapter 7). Also, cognitive impairment typically appears late in MS and long after physical disability has developed, but in Alzheimer's disease, intellectual impairment occurs first and becomes profound long before the onset of physical disability. By way of contrast, in vascular dementia, intellectual and physical deficits develop and worsen together.

Physicians attempting to reduce cognitive deficits in MS might institute enhanced structure and strict organization, cognitive rehabilitation, occupational therapy, and psychotherapy. Immunomodulators may prevent or delay the onset of cognitive disabilities (see later). In small studies, the cholinesterase-inhibitor donepezil, often used in Alzheimer's disease treatment, reversed some attention and memory deficits.

LABORATORY TESTS

When patients' symptoms are vague, the neurologic examination shows few objective signs, only a single episode has occurred, or, on MRI, only a single CNS area shows demyelination, several tests are required to diagnose MS and exclude other illnesses. However, no particular test is diagnostic of MS. Moreover, all currently available tests occasionally yield false-negative and false-positive results.

Imaging Studies

Computed tomography (CT) can show atrophy, reveal large areas of demyelination, and exclude large mass lesions that can masquerade as MS. However, it is too insensitive to be useful in diagnosing MS.

MRI—unequivocally the most valuable test—can readily reveal demyelinated areas indicative of MS plaques. The revised McDonald criteria call for combinations of one gadolinium-enhanced lesion or nine T2-weighted hyperintense MRI lesions located in various regions of the brain, particularly in the periventricular area (Figs. 15-6 and 20-25), or spinal cord (Fig. 15-7). Although not pathognomonic, these hyperintensities are detectable in more than 95% of MS patients.

MRI readily detects lesions in large, heavily myelinated tracts of the CNS, such as the corpus callosum, periventricular area, MLF and other brainstem tracts, cerebellum, optic nerves, and spinal cord. It can show asymptomatic as well as symptomatic lesions.

Because gadolinium enhances MS lesions for about 1 month after they develop, gadolinium-enhanced MRI can distinguish between new and old lesions. Neurologists accept the appearance of new MRI lesions, even in the absence of acute symptoms, as a marker of active disease.

In addition to showing lesions, the MRI may reveal atrophy of the corpus callosum and cerebrum. Communicating hydrocephalus or hydrocephalus *ex vacuo*, which occurs commonly, reflects cerebral atrophy and compensatory enlarged ventricles. The cerebral and corpus callosum atrophy correlates with chronicity and cognitive impairment; however, as previously noted, overall lesion load and, more so, periventricular white matter demyelination correlate more closely with cognitive impairment

Despite its reliability, MRI may be misleading. Small T2-weighted hyperintensities, "unidentified bright objects" (UBOs), appear in numerous conditions besides MS, including migraine, hypertensive cerebrovascular disease, and normal age-related changes. When accompanied by neurologic symptoms, MRI UBOs may lead to a misdiagnosis. As another pitfall, the MRI reveals demyelination in neurologic diseases other than MS, such as the leukodystrophies (see later). However, these other diseases usually do not cause the multiple, large, periventricular plaques that characterize MS.

Cerebrospinal Fluid

Routine cerebrospinal fluid (CSF) analysis during an MS attack will usually contain protein concentrations that are either normal (40 mg/100 mL) or only slightly elevated, and a mild, nonspecific gamma globulin elevation (9% or greater). The CSF of 90% of MS patients contains CSF *oligoclonal bands,* which constitute a discrete IgG antibody (Fig. 15-8). Although the association of CSF oligoclonal bands and MS is so close that their presence suggests the illness, they are also detectable in other inflammatory diseases of the CSF, such as lupus and sarcoidosis.

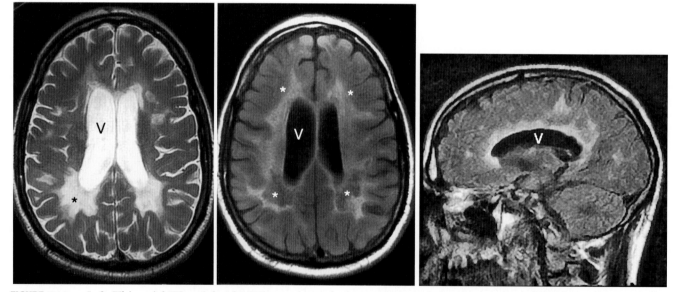

FIGURE 15-6 ■ *Left,* This axial T2-weighted MRI cuts through the cerebrum of a multiple sclerosis (MS) patient and shows multiple plaques (*) concentrated around the ventricles (V), particularly in the posterior regions. The MS plaques are characteristically white (hyperintense), sharply demarcated, and located in the periventricular region. *Center,* This axial T2-weighted, fluid-attenuated inversion recovery (FLAIR) image of the same study also shows hyperintense lesions (*) surrounding the ventricles (V). FLAIR images, in which CSF remains black, allow the demyelinated areas to stand out. *Right,* The sagittal T2 FLAIR image of the same study shows the lateral view of the periventricular hyperintensities surrounding the lateral ventricle (V).

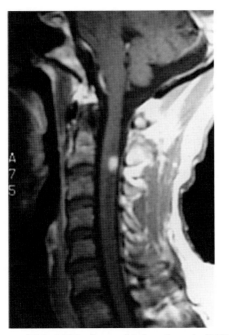

FIGURE 15-7 ■ This MRI of a multiple sclerosis (MS) patient reveals a plaque—the hyperintense lesion—in the high cervical spinal cord.

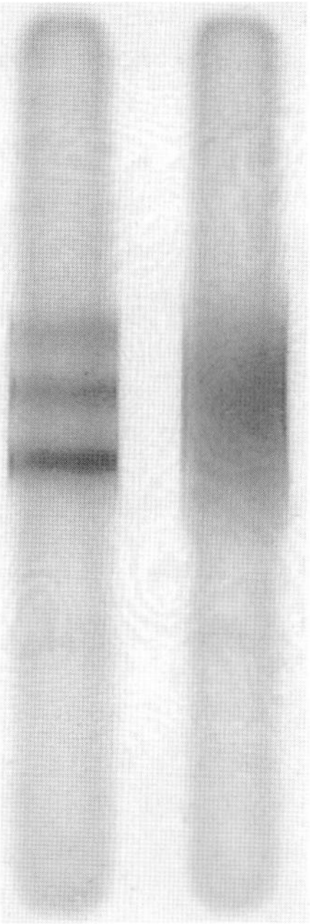

FIGURE 15-8 ■ Electrophoresis of cerebrospinal fluid (CSF) of a patient with multiple sclerosis (MS) (*left*), compared to the CSF of one with no CNS inflammatory disease (*right*), shows three distinct, horizontal oligoclonal bands.

CSF *myelin basic protein*, another protein not present in the CSF of normal individuals, represents a myelin breakdown product. Although CSF of MS patients often contains myelin basic protein, CSF of patients with other chronic inflammatory CNS illnesses—chronic meningitis, sarcoidosis, neurosyphilis, Lyme disease, and acquired immunodeficiency syndrome (AIDS)—also often contain it. Thus, in diagnosing MS, CSF myelin basic protein carries less weight than CSF oligoclonal bands.

Evoked Responses

Although routine electroencephalograms (EEGs) do not help in the diagnosis, related electrophysiologic testing, *evoked response* or *evoked potential tests*, can reveal characteristic interruptions in the visual, auditory, or sensory pathways. Evoked potential testing is based on repetitive stimulation of these pathways, which are heavily myelinated, and then detecting the responses with scalp electrodes similar to those used for EEGs. Normal responses are so small that they are lost in normal cerebral electrical activity and background noise. In evoked testing, hundreds of responses are computer-averaged. After canceling out normal electrical activities, computer averaging displays an otherwise undetectable composite wave pattern. MS injury slows and distorts electrophysiologic conduction. The slowing lengthens the interval between the stimulus and composite response, which is reflected in an abnormally increased *latency*. The injuries also distort the final composite wave pattern.

Evoked response tests are particularly useful in demonstrating lesions that are undetectable on neurologic examination. For example, if a patient has deficits referable only to the spinal cord but evoked response tests reveal a subclinical optic nerve injury, the physician would know that at least two CNS areas were injured and that the illness was disseminated in space.

Visual evoked responses (VERs) reveal visual pathway lesions. The patient stares at a rapidly flashing pattern on a television screen and a computer averages responses detected over the occipital cortex. Optic neuritis increases the latency or distorts the waveform. Because VERs can indicate the site of an interruption in the visual pathway, they are helpful in distinguishing ocular from cortical blindness. When results are entirely normal, VERs help identify psychogenic visual loss (see Chapter 12).

Brainstem auditory evoked responses (BAERs) reveal auditory pathway lesions. By measuring responses to a series of clicks in each ear, BAERs may indicate MS brainstem involvement. They are also useful in a variety of diagnostic tasks related to hearing: characterizing hearing impairments, diagnosing acoustic neuromas, and evaluating hearing in people unable to cooperate, such as infants and those with autism.

Somatosensory evoked responses reveal lesions in the sensory system that extends from the limbs to the cerebral cortex. This test involves stimulating the limbs and detecting the resulting cerebral potentials. In addition to MS lesions, other spinal cord disorders and even nerve injuries in the limbs interfere with neurophysiologic transmission and cause evoked response abnormalities.

THERAPY

For attacks of MS or optic neuritis, with or without other signs of MS, neurologists generally administer high doses of intravenous steroids, such as methyl-prednisolone, that shorten attacks and may reduce residual deficits. Physicians must cautiously administer steroid treatment because it may lead to steroid psychosis (see later) and other potential complications. Fortunately, it almost never produces opportunistic infections, such as tuberculosis or cryptococcal meningitis—as happens with long-term immunosuppression for lupus or renal transplantation rejection.

With the introduction of immunomodulators, neurologists now have the expectation of reducing the frequency, severity, and residue of exacerbations. Immunomodulators also reduce the lesion load and disease activity as determined by the MRI.

Immunomodulator treatment requires that patients inject themselves with recombinant human interferon preparations, such as beta-interferon-1a (Avonex), beta-interferon-1b (Betaseron), beta-interferon-1a (Rebif), or a preparation of four amino acids similar to myelin basic protein (glatiramer acetate [Copaxone]). Depending on the medicine, the regimen requires daily to weekly injections. By interrupting T-cell activity and their migration through the blood–brain barrier, interferons reduce CNS inflammation.

Although helpful, these immunomodulators are not a panacea. They cannot arrest MS, much less cure it. Also, compared to a placebo, they may not even prevent disability at 5 years. After each injection, patients usually experience several hours of fatigue and flu-like symptoms. Immunomodulators are also expensive (see Appendix 2).

Although ultimately unsubstantiated, initial reports indicated that interferons caused or exacerbated pre-existing depression in MS patients. Nevertheless, many neurologists still avoid prescribing interferons to patients with a history of major depression. (*Alpha*-interferon, when used as a treatment for hepatitis, may lead to depression.)

For patients with progressive disease who do not respond to immunomodulators, neurologists administer immunosuppressors that may be cytotoxic or antimitotic, such as azathioprine or mitoxantrone (Novantrone). Although intravenous immunoglobulin suppresses inflammation in several neurologic illnesses, it does not help in MS. Popular "natural treatments," such as snake venom, bee extracts, and vitamins in megadoses, have been ineffective when scientifically tested.

Neurologists treat many individual symptoms. For example, depending on the nature of a patient's bladder dysfunction, either cholinergic medications, such as bethanechol (Urecholine), or anticholinergic ones, such as oxybutynin (Ditropan), might alleviate incontinence; however, patients with advanced disease also often require self-catheterization or sphincter bypass. Although paresis cannot be improved, the accompanying spasticity, which is just as much of an impediment, usually responds to baclofen, diazepam, muscle relaxants, or injections of botulinum toxin (see Chapter 18). Formal exercise programs reduce disability and promote social contacts.

STEROID PSYCHOSIS

Steroid treatment of MS—as with steroid treatment of lupus, organ transplant rejection, and acute asthma—can induce anxiety, euphoria, mania, depressive symptoms, or psychosis. Likewise, Cushing's syndrome and other conditions that generate excessive steroid production can produce similar symptoms. Even athletes who may surreptitiously use steroids for bodybuilding and energy can develop personality and behavioral changes. Even without excessive doses, steroids often produce a ravenous appetite, insomnia, and tremor. The steroid-induced tremor is fine and rapid, which gives it the appearance of anxiety-induced and essential tremors (see Chapter 18).

Glucocorticoid steroids, such as prednisone, are more apt than mineralocorticoid steroids, such as dexamethasone, to induce a steroid psychosis. The incidence of steroid psychosis, which usually begins 1 to 4 days after starting treatment, increases from 4% of patients receiving less than 40 mg of prednisone daily to 20% of patients receiving more than 80 mg daily. When steroid treatment is discontinued, symptoms generally recede. If the euphoria persists and reaches the point of mania, mood-modulating medications, such as valproate, may be required.

Psychosis in a patient with lupus or other systemic inflammatory disease receiving high-dose steroids poses a clinical dilemma. Because these diseases can directly affect the brain, abruptly decreasing the steroids might intensify the illness' cerebral involvement. In addition, at a time when the body is under stress and consequently requires increased dose of steroids, suddenly stopping them may precipitate adrenal insufficiency. As a general rule, in patients with a systemic inflammatory disease, physicians should maintain or increase the steroid dose at least until the evaluation is complete. On the other hand, because steroids are not life-saving in MS, physicians should discontinue them as soon as possible. In the interim, typical or atypical antipsychotic medicines may suppress psychosis. According to a few reports, if the situation requires continued steroid treatment, prophylactic use of lithium may prevent steroid psychosis, but antidepressants may exacerbate it.

CONDITIONS THAT MIMIC MS

Many physically incapacitating neurologic illnesses develop in young people. Several of them can reasonably be confused with MS because of its protean clinical manifestations.

However, physicians much more frequently confuse psychogenic conditions, such as conversion disorder, than these neurologic illnesses with MS. Patients with psychiatric conditions may have clumsiness, sexual impairments, nonspecific sensory loss, fatigue, or even several weeks of paraparesis or blindness. Perhaps some young paraplegic patients described in the original psychoanalytic literature, who improved after a course of psychoanalysis, may actually have had the spontaneous resolution of an MS episode.

Most neurologic disorders that mimic MS today are PNS or CNS demyelinating illnesses. Common symptoms and signs that suggest a disease other than MS ("red flags") include the onset of symptoms before the age of 20 years or after 50 years; multiple family members with the same symptoms; either an explosive or a continually slow course; lack of eye signs; a single manifestation; presence of systemic symptoms; and normal results on MRI, evoked potential, and CSF testing.

Demyelinating Diseases That May Mimic MS

Guillain-Barré Syndrome

Even though it is a demyelinating disease of the peripheral nervous system (PNS) rather than of the CNS, Guillain-Barré syndrome may resemble MS because it generally strikes young and middle-aged adults and causes paraparesis or quadriparesis (see Chapter 5). In contrast to MS, Guillain-Barré syndrome is characterized by a single, monophasic attack, lasting several weeks to months, of symmetric, flaccid, areflexic paresis.

Leukodystrophies

Destruction of CNS myelin, alone or in combination with PNS myelin, is the hallmark of an uncommon group of genetically transmitted illnesses, the *leukodystrophies*. As with MS, the leukodystrophies cause optic nerve, cerebellum, and spinal cord myelin degeneration that leads to progressively severe visual impairment, ataxia, and spastic paraparesis. In contrast to MS, the leukodystrophies are entirely genetically determined and cause unremitting physical and mental deterioration. Their symptoms usually first appear in infants or children but occasionally not until the teen or young adult years. In those older victims, the leukodystrophies may present with behavioral problems, emotional changes, and cognitive impairment. Whether the leukodystrophies appear in infants or young adults, they cause dementia within several years.

Two well-known leukodystrophies are *adrenoleukodystrophy* (*ALD*) and *metachromatic leukodystrophy* (*MLD*; see Chapter 5). ALD, which is transmitted in a sex-linked pattern, typically first produces neurologic symptoms and adrenal insufficiency in boys between 5 and 15 years old. However, sometimes symptoms emerge only when the men carrying the defective gene reach 20 to 30 years. When ALD develops in this older group, CNS demyelination may cause mania, gait impairment, and eventually dementia. In addition to the CNS demyelination, which often has an inflammatory component, MLD causes peripheral neuropathy.

An oxidation enzyme defect in *peroxisomes*, which are intracellular organelles, causes ALD. The defect results in accumulation of saturated unbranched very long chain fatty acids (VLCFAs) in the brain, adrenal glands, other organs, and serum. Lorenzo's oil, a widely publicized therapy developed by two self-trained biochemists whose son inherited the illness, reduces VLCFA concentrations; however, it fails to alter the disease's course. Similarly, treatment by adrenal hormone replacement does not arrest the demyelination. Some research indicates that bone marrow or hematopoietic stem cell transplants, before symptoms develop, may prevent both brain and adrenal damage.

Infections

Several organisms produce demyelination not by an actual infection of the CNS but by provoking an antibody response that invades the CNS and disrupts myelin. For example, *postinfectious* and *postimmunization encephalomyelitis*, which occurs 1 to 4 weeks after an infection or immunization, consists of an extensive and permanent attack on the cerebral and spinal cord myelin. (Postimmunization encephalomyelitis, although rare and unpredictable, imposes a major liability risk on the pharmaceutical industry.)

Progressive multifocal leukoencephalopathy (PML), a true JC virus infection, consists of CNS demyelination. Like MS, PML leads to patchy areas of demyelination throughout the CNS. It is usually a late complication of AIDS and several other illnesses characterized by immunologic impairment. It may also be a complication of medication-induced immunosuppression, such as with organ transplant therapy. In a famous example, a novel immunosuppressant agent for MS that limited the entry of T cells through the blood–brain barrier—natalizumab—when given in combination with an interferon seemed to allow the emergence of PML in several patients.

Several other CNS infections directly or, through antibodies, indirectly attack CNS myelin and mimic MS. In particular, infection with the *human T-lymphotropic virus type 1 (HTLV-1)* causes a demyelinating *myelitis* that particularly affects the corticospinal tracts (see Fig. 2-15). The clinical manifestations of this infection resemble MS when it is restricted to the spinal cord. HTLV-1, a retrovirus related to the *human immunodeficiency virus (HIV)*, is endemic in the Caribbean islands and some areas of Japan. Sexual intercourse, pregnancy, and contaminated blood transmit HTLV-1, just like HIV infections; however, fewer than 5% of individuals infected with HTLV-1 develop symptoms. When it occurs, HTLV-1 myelitis typically produces a slowly evolving, painless, MS-like spastic paraparesis in residents of the Caribbean, where MS is uncommon. HTLV-1 infection rarely causes cognitive impairment or personality change. Antibodies to HTLV-1 are detectable in both CSF, which also has an atypical lymphocytic pleocytosis, and serum of infected individuals.

Toxins

Numerous toxins preferentially attack CNS myelin. For example, *Marchiafava-Bignami syndrome* consists of degeneration of the heavily myelinated corpus callosum. The toxin is probably a contaminant of homemade Italian red wine. Theoretically at least, Marchiafava-Bignami syndrome can damage the corpus callosum severely enough to produce the split brain syndrome (see Chapter 8).

Chronic toluene exposure, whether from inadequate industrial ventilation or recreational volatile substance abuse, damages CNS myelin (see Chapter 5). Although appropriate industrial toluene levels should not produce problems, when individuals regularly inhale high concentrations, they develop cognitive disabilities, personality changes, and MS-like physical findings, such as ataxia, nystagmus, corticospinal tract signs, and even optic nerve impairment. MRI changes from toluene-induced demyelination, which may be more pronounced than ones from MS, correlate with cognitive impairment and physical impairment.

A small group of lawyers and physicians, but not neurologists, have claimed that silicone breast implants cause MS, "multiple sclerosis-like symptoms," chronic fatigue syndrome, cognitive impairment, chronic inflammatory demyelinating polyneuropathy, and other neurologic disorders. However, several major national studies concluded that silicone breast implants do not cause any neurologic disease. Women who reported neurologic disorders after receiving the implants had no consistent pattern of symptoms, virtually no objective signs, and no significant laboratory abnormalities—except in the normal number of women who would be expected to have coincidentally contracted various neurologic illnesses. Also, women with unruptured implants reported the same incidence of postoperative neurologic problems as women with ruptured implants. Women in Sweden and Denmark who had the implants reported essentially the same incidence of neurologic symptoms as those who underwent breast reduction. In other settings, such as its use as cardiac pacemaker coverings, silicone has not been associated with neurologic disease. In individual cases, physicians have established more plausible alternative diagnoses: most often, depression and anxiety, carpal tunnel syndrome, neuropathies, and pre-existing MS.

Lupus Erythematosus

Like MS, vascular inflammatory diseases, such as lupus, may produce sundry neurologic abnormalities that follow a fluctuating course; however, vascular inflammatory diseases more frequently cause mental status abnormalities. At its onset, lupus affects the CNS in only about 5% of cases, but it eventually produces neurologic complications in 25% to 75%—a wide range that reflects different age groups and diagnostic criteria in various studies. Cognitive impairment, thought disturbance, and mood disorder are common and frequently striking manifestations of CNS lupus. These symptoms are often accompanied by physical signs of CNS lupus, such as seizures that are most often tonic-clonic but sometimes partial complex; strokes from cerebral hemorrhage or infarction; chorea; and INO.

Lupus affects the CNS in up to 85% of children hospitalized with the illness. Of children with CNS lupus, approximately 50% develop mental status changes that typically include depression, inattention, memory impairment, or psychosis. They are also frequently beset by headache and delirium. Their physical manifestations are similar to those of adults with CNS lupus.

In individuals with lupus who are older than 50 years, by contrast, less than 20% have CNS involvement. Moreover, their manifestations are relatively mild and responsive to treatment.

In adults, when lupus-induced psychiatric complications occur, they are associated with elevated levels of anticardiolipin antibodies and low serum albumin. MRIs may reveal cerebral infarctions but only in late stages of the illness.

Manifestations of lupus-induced PNS involvement, which occur alone or in conjunction with CNS involvement, include neuropathy and mononeuritis multiplex (see Chapter 5). Both the CNS and PNS neurologic complications have been attributed to immune complexes producing an arteritis, but many complications are clearly manifestations of cardiac valvular disease, a tendency to develop thromboses, opportunistic infections, hypertension, renal failure, or possibly the elaboration of false neurotransmitters.

Other inflammatory illnesses, such as Sjögren's syndrome and sarcoidosis, may damage multiple organs. These illnesses may cause delirium, permanent cognitive impairment, facial nerve injury, and neuropathy. As with lupus, these illnesses' systemic symptoms usually point to the diagnosis; however, in individual cases, these illnesses may involve only the CNS.

Smallpox Vaccinations

A serious inflammatory demyelinating reaction, *postvaccinal encephalomyelitis* (*PVEM*), has consistently complicated smallpox vaccination in a small proportion of individuals. Those affected with PVEM develop paraparesis and other MS-like symptoms 1 to 2 weeks after receiving their primary vaccination; however, sometimes PVEM only complicates revaccination. Compared to the demyelination in MS, the demyelination in PVEM is more extensive, the course more fulminant, and the mortality rate (10%) much greater.

This adverse reaction and the almost complete worldwide eradication of smallpox have halted routine vaccinations. Nevertheless, physicians still vaccinate individuals at risk of smallpox exposure, such as soldiers. Although no reliable data exist, they hesitate to vaccinate MS patients against smallpox.

On the other hand, studies support routinely vaccinating MS patients against influenza, hepatitis B, varicella, and tetanus. On balance, although carrying little risk, these vaccinations protect MS patients against infectious illnesses that might seriously debilitate them.

Spinal Cord Disorders

Insidiously developing, painless paraparesis is a relatively common, important clinical problem.

Numerous diseases in addition to MS that affect the spinal cord can be responsible: combined system disease (B_{12} deficiency), cervical spine degeneration, ALS, HTLV-1 infection, and spinal meningiomas. To diagnose these disorders, neurologists often require an MRI of the spinal cord, serum B_{12} level determinations, electromyographic studies, and various blood and CSF tests.

REFERENCES
Multiple Sclerosis

1. Amato M: Cognitive dysfunction in early-onset multiple sclerosis. Arch Neurol 58:1602–1606, 2001.
2. Amodio P, De Toni EN, Cavalletto L, et al: Mood, cognition and EEG changes during interferon alpha (alpha-IFN) treatment for chronic hepatitis C. J Affect Disord 84:93–98, 2005.
3. Asghar A: Pure neuropsychiatric presentation of multiple sclerosis. Am J Psychiatry 161:226–231, 2004.
4. Bakshi R, Hutton GJ, Miller JR, et al: The use of magnetic resonance imaging in the diagnosis and long-term management of multiple sclerosis. Neurology 63(Suppl 5):S3–S11, 2004.
5. Benedict R: Prediction of neuropsychological impairment in multiple sclerosis. Arch Neurol 61:226–229, 2004.
6. Caine E, Schwid S: Multiple sclerosis, depression and the risk of suicide. Neurology 59:662–663, 2002.
7. Chwastiak L: Depressive symptoms and severity of illness in multiple sclerosis: Epidemiologic study of a large community sample. Am J Psychiatry 159:1862–1868, 2002.
8. Compston A, Coles A: Multiple sclerosis. Lancet 359:1221–1231, 2002.
9. Confavreux C, Hutchinson M, Hours MM, et al: Rate of pregnancy-related relapse in multiple sclerosis. N Engl J Med 339:285–291, 1998.
10. Feinstein A: The neuropsychiatry of multiple sclerosis. Can J Psychiatry 49:157–163, 2004.
11. Fredrickson S, Cheng Q, Jiang GX, et al: Elevated suicide risk among patients with multiple sclerosis in Sweden. Neuroepidemiology 22:146–152, 2003.
12. Goodin DS, Frohman EM, Garmany GP, et al: Disease modifying therapies in multiple sclerosis: Report of the Therapeutics and Technology Assessment Subcommittee of the American Academy of Neurology and the MS Council for Clinical Practice Guidelines. Neurology 58:169–178, 2002.
13. Krupp LB: *Fatigue in Multiple Sclerosis: A Guide to Diagnosis and Management.* New York, Demos, 2004.
14. Kurtzke JF, Page WF: Epidemiology of multiple sclerosis in US veterans. Neurology 48:204–213, 1997.
15. Li J, Johansen C, Bronnum-Hansen H, et al: The risk of multiple sclerosis in bereaved parents: A nationwide cohort study in Denmark. Neurology 62:726–729, 2004.
16. MacAllister WS, Belman AL, Milazzo M, et al: Cognitive functioning in children and adolescents with multiple sclerosis. Neurology 64:1422–1425, 2005.

17. McDonald WI, Compston A, Edan G, et al: Recommended diagnostic criteria for multiple sclerosis: Guidelines from the International Panel on the Diagnosis of Multiple Sclerosis. Ann Neurol 50:121–127, 2001.

18. Mohr DC, Hart SL, Laura J, et al: Association between stressful life events and exacerbation in multiple sclerosis: A meta-analysis. BMJ 328:731, 2004.

19. Noseworthy JH, Lucchinetti C, Rodriguez M, et al: Multiple sclerosis. N Engl J Med 343:938–952, 2000.

20. Patten SB, Francis G, Metz LM, et al: The relationship between depression and interferon beta-1a therapy in patients with multiple sclerosis. Mult Scler 11:175–181, 2005.

21. Polman CH, Reingold SC, Edan G, et al: Diagnostic criteria for multiple sclerosis: 2005 revisions to the "McDonald Criteria." Ann Neurol 58:840–846, 2005.

22. Romberg A, Virtanen A, Ruutianinen J, et al: Effects of a 6-month exercise program on patients with multiple sclerosis. Neurology 63:2034–2038, 2004.

23. Rutschmann OT, McCrory DC, Matchar DB, et al: Immunization and MS: A summary of published evidence and recommendations. Neurology 59:1837–1843, 2002.

24. Solaro C, Brichetto G, Amato MP, et al: The prevalence of pain in multiple sclerosis: A multicenter cross-sectional study. Neurology 63:919–921, 2004.

25. Sirois F: Steroid psychosis: A review. Gen Hosp Psychiatry 25:27–33, 2003.

26. Sperling R: Regional magnet resonance imaging lesions burden and cognitive function in multiple sclerosis. Arch Nerurol 58:115–121, 2001.

27. Stankoff B, Waubant E, Confavreux C, et al: Modafinil for fatigue in MS: A randomized placebo-controlled double-blind study. Neurology 64:1139–1143, 2005.

28. Stenager EN, Stenager E: Suicide and patients with neurologic diseases. Arch Neurol 49:1296–1303, 1992.

29. Swirsky-Sacchetti T, Mitchell DR, Seward J, et al: Neuropsychological and structural brain lesions in multiple sclerosis. Neurology 42:1291–1295, 1992.

30. Therapeutics and Technology Assessment Subcommittee of the American Academy of Neurology: The relationship of MS to physical trauma and psychologic stress. Neurology 52:1737–1745, 1999.

31. Zabad RK, Patten SB, Metz LM: The association of depression with disease course in multiple sclerosis. Neurology 64:359–360, 2005.

32. Zorzon M, de Masi R, Nasuelli D, et al: Depression and anxiety in multiple sclerosis. A clinical and MRI study in 95 subjects. J Neurol 248:416–421, 2001.

Other Illnesses

33. Abrahams BC, Kaufman DM: Anticipating smallpox and monkeypox outbreaks: Complications of the smallpox vaccine. Neurologist 10:265–274, 2004.

34. Angell M: Shattuck Lecture—Evaluating the health risks of breast implants: The interplay of medical science, the law, and public opinion. N Engl J Med 334:1513–1518, 1996.

35. Brey RL, Holliday SL, Saklad AR, et al: Neuropsychiatric syndromes in lupus. Neurology 58:1214–1220, 2002.

36. Burns TM: Neurosarcoidosis. Arch Neurol 60:1166–1168, 2003.

37. Ferguson JH: Silicone breast implants and neurologic disorders: Report of the Practice Committee of the American Academy of Neurology. Neurology 48:1504–1507, 1997.

38. Ferriby D, de Seze J, Stojkovic T, et al: Long-term follow-up of neurosarcoidosis. Neurology 57:927–929, 2001.

39. Monastero R, Bettini P, Del Zotto E, et al: Prevalence and pattern of cognitive impairment in systemic lupus erythematosus patients with and without overt neuropsychiatric manifestations. J Neurol Sci 184:33–39, 2001.

40. Noseworthy JH, Lucchinetti C, Rodriguez M, et al: Multiple sclerosis. N Engl J Med 343:938–952, 2000.

41. Rosebush PI, Garside S, Levinson AJ, et al: The neuropsychiatry of adult-onset adrenoleukodystrophy. J Neuropsychiatry Clin Neurosci 11:315–327, 1999.

42. Sibbitt WL, Brandt JR, Johnson CR, et al: The incidence and prevalence of neuropsychiatric syndromes in pediatric onset systemic lupus erythematosus. J Rheumatol 29:1536–1542, 2002.

43. Steinlin MI, Blaser SI, Gilday DL, et al: Neurologic manifestations of pediatric systemic lupus erythematosus. Pediatr Neurol 13:191–197, 1995.

44. Wolkowitz OM, Reus VI, Canick J, et al: Glucocorticoid medication, memory and steroid psychosis in medical illness. Ann NY Acad Sci 823:81–96, 1997.

Questions and Answers

1–4. Over 4 days, a 25-year-old salesman developed paraparesis. Then his left eye became painful and blind. On examination, his left pupil reacts slowly to light. His legs have hyperactive deep tendon reflexes (DTRs) and bilateral Babinski signs. However, his arms have normal strength, reflexes, and coordination, and he does not have Lhermitte's sign (pain that radiates from the neck down the spine produced by neck flexion.)

1. Which of the following disorders is the most likely cause of his neurologic deficits?
   a. Spinal cord tumor
   b. Psychogenic disturbances
   c. Multiple sclerosis (MS)
   d. Postvaccinal or postinfectious encephalomyelitis
   e. HTLV-1 myelitis

Answer: c. The salesman may have developed MS affecting the optic nerve and spinal cord, which is a common pattern of MS. MRIs will probably reveal lesions in those areas and the CSF will probably show oligoclonal bands. Rare alternative explanations include other demyelinating inflammatory diseases, vasculitis, a toxin, an infection, or reaction to a smallpox vaccination. Spinal cord tumors would create spastic paraparesis but, of course, not visual impairment. Psychogenic disturbances might lead to visual and motor symptoms and possibly feigned Babinski signs; however, people cannot mimic abnormal pupil reactions. HTLV-1 myelitis typically causes spastic paraparesis but does not affect vision or pupil reactions.

2. In regard to the patient, which regions of the CNS are most likely to be affected?
   a. Right occipital lobe and thoracic spinal cord
   b. Thoracic spinal cord and left optic nerve's retrobulbar portion
   c. Sacral spinal cord and left optic nerve's bulbar portion
   d. Left optic nerve's retrobulbar portion and cervical spinal cord

Answer: b. He has retrobulbar neuritis and thoracic myelitis. Unlike the other cranial nerves, the optic nerve (cranial nerve 2) is an outgrowth of the CNS. CNS myelin covers only the optic nerve and a small portion of the acoustic nerve (cranial nerve 8). PNS-type myelin covers the others.

3. After 3 weeks, the patient became ambulatory and had recovered his vision. However, 1 year later, he returned with new symptoms: dysarthria, ataxia, nystagmus, and tremor of the arms. In which two CNS regions are the new lesions probably located?
   a. Cerebrum
   b. Cerebellum
   c. Brainstem
   d. Spinal cord

Answers: b, c. Dysarthria, ataxia, nystagmus, and limb tremor are referable to lesions in the brainstem, cerebellum, or cerebellar outflow tracts.

4. At this visit, what will the head MRI show?
   a. Multiple ring-enhancing lesions
   b. Periventricular demyelination and plaques in the cerebellum and brainstem
   c. Demyelination in the cerebellum and brainstem
   d. None of the above

Answer: b. MS almost always affects the periventricular white matter. MRIs will show demyelination there as well as in clinically affected areas.

5. Of the various MRI abnormalities in MS, which one correlates most closely with cognitive impairment?
   a. Enlarged cerebral ventricles
   b. Corpus callosum atrophy
   c. Lesions seen with gadolinium enhancement
   d. Total lesion area or volume

Answer: d. MS-associated cognitive impairment is most closely associated with total MRI lesion area or volume ("the lesion load"), particularly in the periventricular region.

6. Which three of the following substances produces optic neuritis?
   a. Tobacco
   b. Oral contraceptives
   c. Ethyl alcohol
   d. Methyl alcohol
   e. Penicillin
   f. Heroin

Answers: a, c, d.

7. Which four of these illnesses are associated with optic neuritis?
   a. Rubella

b. Gonorrhea
c. MS
d. AIDS
e. Sarcoidosis
f. Vasculitis
g. Syphilis
h. Lyme disease

Answers: c, e, f, g. Although MS is not the only cause of optic neuritis, it has the closest association. Although the overall risk of subsequently developing MS after an episode of isolated optic neuritis is only about 30%, if the MRI shows three or more cerebral lesions, MS is more than 50% likely to develop during the next five years. In general and particularly in optic neuritis, the diagnosis of MS often hinges on the appearance of the MRI.

8. Which three of the following conditions may lead to internuclear ophthalmoplegia (INO)?
   a. MS
   b. Subdural hematoma
   c. Conversion reaction
   d. Lupus
   e. Brainstem infarctions

Answers: a, d, e. INO, like optic neuritis, is highly suggestive but not pathognomonic of MS.

9–11. A 60-year-old man has gait impairment. He walks with a broad-based gait and excessively lifts his knees. Although his strength in his legs is normal, his DTRs are absent. He has lost position sense (but not pain or touch sense) in the feet. He has small pupils that are unreactive to light.

9. Which one of the following is the most likely cause of his gait disturbance?
   a. Cerebellar damage
   b. Spinal cord compression
   c. MS
   d. Posterior column dysfunction

Answer: d. The gait disturbance is entirely explainable by the loss of proprioception in his legs causing him to have ataxia and a "steppage gait." Neurologists might say that he has "sensory ataxia."

10. Although his pupils are small and unreactive to light, they constrict when he looked at a closely held (regarded) object. What is the pupillary disturbance called?
    a. Argyll-Robertson pupils
    b. Optic neuritis
    c. INO
    d. Miosis

Answer: a. He has small pupils with lack of light reaction but preserved accommodation. This pattern is called "Argyll-Robertson pupils." His neurologic signs indicate tabes dorsalis.

11. What laboratory finding would be most reliable in confirming a diagnosis of CNS syphilis?
    a. A positive CSF MHA
    b. Periventricular white matter changes on an MRI
    c. A positive CSF VDRL
    d. Detecting oligoclonal bands in the CSF

Answer: c. Because many serum and CSF test results are false-negative, the most reliable test for confirming CNS syphilis is a positive CSF VDRL. The CSF MHA is unreliable. Periventricular white matter changes on the MRI indicate MS. CSF oligoclonal bands are found in a variety of CNS infectious or inflammatory illnesses, including MS.

12. Many features of internuclear ophthalmoplegia (INO) are shared by paresis of the oculomotor cranial nerve (CN III). Which of the following distinguishes INO from CN III palsy?
    a. In INO, there is no ptosis or dilation of the pupil.
    b. In INO, the affected eye fails to adduct.
    c. In INO, the adducting eye has nystagmus.
    d. CN III palsy is characterized by ptosis, miosis, and anhidrosis.

Answer: a. Ptosis and dilation of the pupil characterize CN III palsy. In both INO and CN III palsy, the affected eye cannot adduct. In INO, the abducting eye has nystagmus. Horner's syndrome consists of ptosis, miosis, and anhidrosis.

13. During which obstetric period is MS most likely to become exacerbated?
    a. First trimester
    b. Second trimester
    c. Third trimester
    d. First three postpartum months

Answer: d. The first three postpartum months are associated with MS exacerbations. All of pregnancy, especially its third trimester, brings a relief from attacks.

14. What is the effect of one or more pregnancies on the course of a woman's MS?
    a. Her functional status deteriorates with each succeeding pregnancy.
    b. Her functional status is better with each succeeding pregnancy.
    c. Pregnancy has little or no effect.

Answer: c. Contrary to previous thinking, pregnancy and delivery have little or no effect on the mother's MS.

15. Which other statement regarding pregnancy and MS is true?
a. MS causes a high rate of spontaneous abortions.
b. MS frequently causes complications.
c. Fetal malformations in MS patients are common.
d. Cesarean sections are frequently indicated when MS women deliver.
e. Offspring have a greater risk than the general population of developing MS.

Answer: e. Children of MS patients have an increased incidence of the illness. MS does not cause abortions, obstetric complications, fetal malformations, or problems that require cesarean sections.

16. Which MS features are associated with cognitive impairment?
a. Physical impairments
b. Duration of the illness
c. Enlarged cerebral ventricles
d. Corpus callosum atrophy
e. Periventricular demyelination
f. Total lesion area
g. Cerebral hypometabolism
h. All of the above

Answers: h. All of these MS features are associated with cognitive impairment, but total lesion area is the most statistically powerful risk factor.

17. What is the approximate concordance rate of MS among monozygotic twins?
a. 25%
b. 50%
c. 75%
d. 100%
e. 200%

Answer: a. Most studies describe an MS concordance rate for monozygotic twins of only 25% to 30% and for dizygotic twins of only 5%. Moreover, the phenotypes (symptoms) of twins differ when both are affected. These data diminish the importance of genetic factors in MS.

18–24. Match the ocular motility disorder (18–24) with its most likely cause (a–g).
a. Wernicke's encephalopathy
b. Labyrinthitis
c. Psychogenic disorders
d. Myasthenia gravis
e. MS
f. Midbrain infarction
g. None of the above

18. Pupillary dilation, ptosis, and paresis of adduction

Answer: f (oculomotor nerve palsy).

19. Bilateral ptosis

Answer: d (myasthenia gravis).

20. Bilateral horizontal nystagmus

Answers: a, b, e (Wernicke's encephalopathy, labyrinthitis, MS).

21. Bilateral horizontal nystagmus, unilateral paresis of abduction, and areflexic DTRs

Answer: a (Wernicke's encephalopathy).

22. Nystagmus in abducting eye and incomplete adduction of the other eye when looking horizontally

Answer: e (INO or the MLF syndrome from MS).

23. Ptosis bilaterally, paresis of adduction of one eye, and normal pupils

Answer: d (myasthenia gravis).

24. Nystagmus in adducting eye and paresis of abduction of the other eye

Answer: g (none of the above).

25. A 58-year-old man with MS is brought to the emergency room for urinary incontinence. He has a distended bladder, paraparesis, and sensory impairment in his lower trunk and legs. Although fully alert, he is very uncomfortable. Which should be the first step in alleviating his distress?
a. Administer cholinergic medications
b. Do an MRI of the spinal cord
c. Stop any anticholinergic medications
d. Administer analgesics that have no anticholinergic side effects
e. None of the above

Answer: e. He has overflow incontinence and needs to have a catheter inserted into his bladder to drain the urine. However, the drainage should be interrupted after removing each liter to avoid precipitating a hypotensive episode. Not all cases of bladder distention and overflow incontinence in MS are due to the illness. Instead, the cause may be prostatic hypertrophy, other obstructions, anticholinergic medications, or detrusor muscle weakness.

26. A 9-year-old boy has developed social difficulties and then academic difficulties. He has hyperactive DTRs, clumsiness, and an awkward gait. His older brother had similar symptoms and then died of adrenal failure before the correct diagnosis was made. The patient's MRI of the brain shows extensive demyelination. Which of the following statements is correct?

a. Lorenzo's oil will arrest the disease.
b. The illness is transmitted in an autosomal recessive pattern.
c. The illness results from defective mitochondria.
d. The disease is characterized by the accumulation of unbranched saturated very long chain fatty acids (VLCFAs).

Answer: d. The patient, like his brother, has adrenoleukodystrophy (ALD), which is a relatively common leukoencephalopathy. ALD is characterized by accumulation of VLCFAs as the result of defective peroxisomes. The illness is an X-linked disorder that usually presents in boys and runs a fulminant course over 5 years. Neither Lorenzo's oil nor adrenal replacement therapy will arrest the disease.

27. Which one of the following descriptions best characterizes MS-induced MRI changes?
    a. Multiple, white areas scattered in the cerebrum
    b. Conversion of the cerebral hemisphere white matter to gray
    c. Loss of the myelin signal throughout the corpus callosum
    d. Periventricular, high-intensity abnormalities
    e. Periventricular, high-density abnormalities

Answer: d. MS is characterized by multiple, relatively large patches (plaques) in the cerebral periventricular white matter. Plaques are also often routinely detected in other areas of the cerebrum, especially the corpus callosum, and the cerebellum. With high resolution MRI, plaques can even be visualized in the optic nerves and spinal cord. Plaques appear as high-intensity MRI abnormalities. However, scattered, small white matter hyperintense lesions—unidentified bright objects (UBOs)—are a nonspecific finding often confused with MS plaques. MS plaques on MRIs show high intensity on T2 images and low intensity on T1 images.

28. Natives of which of the following cities have the highest MS incidence?
    a. New Orleans
    b. Boston
    c. Philadelphia
    d. Seattle

Answer: b. Boston. Higher latitudes are usually associated with a greater incidence of MS. Cities in Colorado, an exception in terms of latitude but not climate, have a higher incidence than most of the West Coast states.

29. Which of the following regions has the lowest MS incidence?
    a. New England

b. Colorado
c. Scotland
d. Caribbean islands

Answer: d. Caribbean residents have a very low incidence of MS, but they are subject to HTLV1 infection that mimics spinal cord MS.

30. Of the following Israeli groups, which would have the highest incidence of MS?
    a. Native Israelis (Sabras)
    b. Adult European immigrants to Israel
    c. Israeli immigrants raised to age 18 years in Sub-Saharan Africa

Answer: b. Adult European immigrants, like other individuals raised in cool climates, have a relatively high risk of developing MS. The period of vulnerability includes the years from birth to about 16 years. In other words, adults emigrating from one region to another carry the incidence of their homeland. Sabras and sub-Saharan Africans have a low incidence no matter where they emigrate.

31. In which conditions do visual evoked responses (VERs) typically show prolonged latencies or other abnormal pattern?
    a. Asymptomatic optic neuritis
    b. Retrobulbar neuritis
    c. Most patients with long standing MS
    d. Patients with "blindness" from a conversion reaction
    e. Optic nerve gliomas
    f. Deafness

Answers: a, b, c, e. Almost any lesion in the visual pathway slows the nerve action potential, which prolongs the latency, and distorts the waveform.

32. In MS patients, which three findings are most often associated with urinary incontinence?
    a. Leg spasticity
    b. Ataxia
    c. Spasticity of the external sphincter of the bladder
    d. Sexual impairment
    e. MLF syndrome

Answers: a, c, d. Urinary incontinence, sexual impairment, and spastic paraparesis all result from spinal cord involvement. In MS, the spinal cord is often the sole or primary site of involvement. Its pathways are exquisitely sensitive.

33. Which three symptoms typically develop only late or not at all in the course of MS?
    a. Pseudobulbar palsy
    b. INO

c. Optic neuritis

d. Bladder dysfunction

e. Psychosis

f. Depression

g. Sexual dysfunction

h. Dementia

Answers: a, e, h.

34. Which of the following statements is false concerning relapsing-remitting MS?

a. Of the major MS disease categories, relapsing-remitting is the most amenable to immunologic modulation.

b. As with other categories, the clinical course defines the disease category.

c. Relapsing-remitting disease usually evolves into secondary progressive disease.

d. The presence of additional MRI abnormalities in relapsing-remitting disease changes its designation to secondary progressive disease.

e. Immunologic modulation has less effect on progressive than relapsing-remitting disease.

Answer: d. MRI results are not considered in determining the disease category.

35. Which of the following is not an element of the revised McDonald criteria for MS?

a. Certain MRI lesions can substitute for clinical events for lesions being disseminated in space.

b. Certain MRI lesions can substitute for clinical events for lesions being disseminated in time.

c. For diagnostic purposes, depression can serve as an episode of MS.

d. Oligoclonal bands, but not myelin basic protein, in the CSF have reliable diagnostic significance.

Answer. c. The revised McDonald criteria for MS allow substitution of MRI findings to establish that a CNS illness is disseminated in time and space. CSF myelin basic protein is too nonspecific a response to CNS inflammation to carry diagnostic significance; however, CSF oligoclonal bands are closely associated with MS and their presence can support a diagnosis.

36. In the diagnosis of MS, what do the following features share? Onset of symptoms before the age of 20 years or after 50 years, multiple family members with the same illness, either an explosive or a continually slow course, lack of eye signs, a single manifestation, systemic symptoms, and normal results on MRI.

a. They are all consistent with a diagnosis of MS.

b. Although unusual, any three are permissible when making a diagnosis of MS.

c. The presence of any one of them warns against a diagnosis of MS.

d. They all indicate a leukodystrophy.

Answer: c. These findings, "red flags," are each unusual in MS.

37. Which of the following cells produces CNS myelin?

a. Glia cells

b. Neurons

c. Schwann cells

d. Oligodendroglia

e. Lymphocytes

Answer: d. Oligodendroglia produce CNS myelin. Schwann cells produce peripheral nervous system myelin.

38. In regard to the allegation that silicone breast implants cause MS, which of the following statements is true?

a. The incidence of symptoms is greater in women with ruptured than unruptured implants.

b. The incidence of symptoms is greater in women who have had breast implants than in women who have undergone breast reduction surgery.

c. Silicone-covered pacemakers produce similar neurologic problems.

d. Neurologic symptoms associated with silicone breast implants are consistent from patient to patient.

e. None of the above.

Answer: e. There is no credible evidence that silicone breast implants cause neurologic disease.

39. A 22-year-old woman is admitted to a hospital because she has nystagmus, scanning speech, hyperactive DTRs in all limbs, Babinski signs, and a spastic-ataxic gait. She has inappropriate euphoria, impaired recent and remote memory, and impaired judgment. The MRI of her brain shows diffuse loss of myelin in her entire brain and spinal cord. Her HIV test was negative. She smokes 2 packs of cigarettes each day and admits to "huffing" (deliberately inhaling volatile substances for their euphoric effect). Which is the most likely diagnosis?

a. HTLV-1 infection

b. MS

c. Chronic toluene abuse

d. PML

Answer: c. She probably has been inhaling toluene, which is a frequent volatile drug of abuse. Toluene, a hydrocarbon solvent in furniture and shoe manufacturing, acts as a CNS demyelinating agent. When used for recreation, it produces euphoria that has been likened to one produced by Valium. HTLV-1 affects the spinal cord primarily or exclusively and it usually does not produce cognitive changes. PML would have been possible if she had AIDS or other immunodeficiency condition.

40. In MS patients, which is the least likely disturbance?
   a. Psychosis
   b. Inattention and decreased memory
   c. Anxiety
   d. Fatigue
   e. Depression

   Answer: a.

41. Following exposure to a prairie dog infected with monkeypox, public health officials administered smallpox vaccinations to a 19-year-old waitress and a dozen other young adults. Several days later she developed a high fever, stupor, INO, and spastic paraparesis. From which condition does she probably suffer?
   a. Monkeypox
   b. Smallpox
   c. Multiple sclerosis
   d. Postvaccinial encephalomyelitis

   Answer: d. She most likely developed an adverse reaction, postvaccinial encephalomyelitis (PVEM), to the smallpox vaccination. PVEM causes acute MS-like demyelination throughout the CNS. The reaction is explosive, severe, extensive, and associated with a 10% mortality, but it is a monophasic condition. This complication was one of the main reasons that public health officials halted routine smallpox vaccinations. However, smallpox vaccinations are still administered to individuals exposed to cowpox and monkeypox as well as smallpox, which are caused by species of the genus *Orthopoxvirus*, a DNA virus.

42. Why do evoked responses show an increased latency if a MS plaque has damaged the pathway?
   a. The plaque reduces the amplitude.
   b. Demyelinated pathways, deprived of their insulation, conduct impulses more slowly.
   c. Axon damage speeds nerve conduction.
   d. None of the above.

   Answer: b. In MS, slowed or altered conduction by axons that have lost their myelin or have been directly injured causes increased latency and waveform distortion.

43. Which of the following is not a routine pathologic finding in MS?
   a. Demyelination of the periventricular regions of the brain
   b. Loss of axons
   c. Loss of myelin in the optic tracts
   d. Atrophy of the corpus callosum
   e. None of the above

   Answer: e. Although the classic literature has portrayed MS as the quintessential CNS demyelinating disease, recent studies have emphasized the importance of axon damage. With longstanding MS, the major CNS tracts lose their myelin and axons and undergo atrophy.

CHAPTER 16

Neurologic Aspects of Sexual Function

Whatever its underlying psychology, sexual function depends on two complex and delicate neurologic pathways: (1) a connection between the brain and the genitals and (2) a short reflex loop between the genitals and spinal cord. Both involve the central nervous system (CNS), peripheral nervous system (PNS), and autonomic nervous system (ANS).

In the first pathway, the brain converts various stimuli, including sleep-related events, into neurologic impulses that are usually positively, but sometimes negatively, charged. These impulses travel down the spinal cord. Some impulses descend all the way down to its sacral region where they exit to travel through the *pudendal nerve*. In other words, at this juncture, they leave the CNS to join the PNS (Fig. 16-1). Meanwhile, as if diverted to a parallel route, other impulses leave the spinal cord at its low thoracic and upper lumbar regions (T11-L2) to travel through the *sympathetic* division of the ANS. Still others leave the spinal cord's lower sacral segments (S2-S4) to travel through the *parasympathetic* division of the ANS.

Excitatory descending stimuli increase parasympathetic ANS activity, which reduces tone in (relaxes) the wall muscles of genital arteries. As the relaxed arteries dilate, they allow increased blood flow. In men, increased blood flow inflates the penis and produces an erection. In women, it produces clitoral engorgement.

With continued stimulation, a complex series of predominantly sympathetic ANS-mediated events produce an orgasm. Afterward, a return to normal, relatively constricted arterial wall muscle tone reduces blood flow. The resultant reduced vascular engorgement leads to detumescence.

Although the sympathetic and parasympathetic components of the ANS are complementary in sexual function, they depend on different neurotransmitters—acetylcholine in the parasympathetic and monoamines in the sympathetic. Moreover, they have different roles. An admittedly crude mnemonic describes the *para*sympathetic and *s*ympathetic ANS roles in sexual response: "*p*oint and *s*hoot."

In the second pathway, which is shorter and simpler, erotic impulses from genital stimulation pass through the pudendal nerve to the spinal cord. Some impulses, in a *genital-spinal cord reflex*, synapse in the sacral region of the spinal cord and return, via the ANS, to the genitals. Other impulses ascend through the spinal cord to join other cerebral stimuli.

That mnemonic also reflects another point. Current knowledge of sexual function rests primarily on male physiology, evaluation, and treatment. This chapter's predominant references to male function reflect the fact that neurologic aspects of female sexual activity have received much less attention.

NEUROLOGIC IMPAIRMENT

Without accepting a complete distinction between neurologic and psychogenic sexual impairment, certain elements of the patient's history (Table 16-1) and neurologic examination (Table 16-2) reliably indicate a neurologic origin. For example, either spinal cord or peripheral nerve injury might lead to a pattern of weakness and sensory loss below the waist or around the genitals, anus, and buttocks—the "saddle area" (Fig. 16-2). Plantar and deep tendon reflex (DTR) testing will indicate which system is responsible: spinal cord injury causes hyperactive DTRs and Babinski signs, whereas peripheral nerve injury causes hypoactive DTRs and no Babinski signs. Both CNS and PNS impairment lead to loss of the relevant "superficial reflexes": scrotal, cremasteric, and anal (Fig. 16-3).

Signs of ANS impairment, although often subtle, also carry great weight. For example, *orthostatic hypotension*, usually defined as a fall of 10 mmHg in blood pressure on standing, reliably indicates ANS impairment, as might result from diabetes, medications, or idiopathic systemic conditions. Similarly, *anhidrosis*, lack of sweating, indicates ANS impairment. In this condition, *urinary incontinence* and hairless and sallow skin usually accompany dry axillae, groins, and legs. Finally, if microscopic examination of urine obtained after orgasm reveals sperm, the man probably has *retrograde ejaculation*, which usually reflects a disorder of the finely tuned, ANS-based mechanism.

In many conditions, such as spinal cord injury or severe ANS damage, urinary and fecal incontinence accompany neurologic-induced sexual impairment

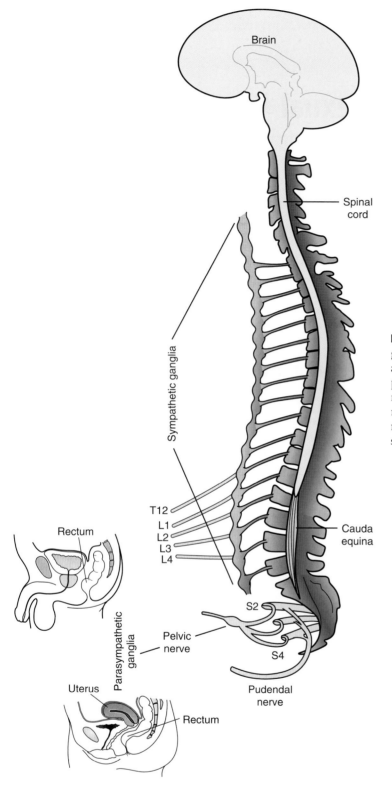

FIGURE 16-1 ■ The sacral (S2-S4) spinal cord segments give rise to the nerves that innervate the genitals. In addition, the sympathetic and parasympathetic components of the autonomic nervous system (ANS) innervate the genitals. The ANS innervates the genitals, reproductive organs, bladder, sweat glands, and arterial wall muscles. Branches of the pudendal nerve supply the genital muscles and skin.

because the bladder, bowel, and genitals share many elements of innervation. The anus, like the bladder, has two sphincters (see Fig. 15-5). Its internal sphincter, more powerful than the external one, constricts in response to increased sympathetic activity and relaxes to parasympathetic activity. The anus' external sphincter is under voluntary control through the pudendal nerves and other branches of the S3 and S4 peripheral nerve roots. Thus, to produce a bowel movement, individuals must deliberately relax their external

TABLE 16-1 ■ Symptoms Suggesting Neurologic Sexual Impairment

Continual erectile dysfunction
  Absence of morning erections
  No erection or orgasm during masturbation or sex with different partners
Related somatic complaints
Sensory loss in genitals, pelvis, or legs
Urinary incontinence
Certain neurologic conditions
  Spinal cord injury
  Diabetic neuropathy
  Multiple sclerosis
  Herniated intervertebral disk
Use of medications

TABLE 16-2 ■ Signs of Neurologic Sexual Impairment

Signs of spinal cord injury
  Paraparesis or quadriparesis
  Leg spasticity
  Urinary incontinence
Signs of autonomic nervous system injury
  Orthostatic hypotension or lightheadedness
  Anhidrosis in groin and legs
  Urinary incontinence
  Retrograde ejaculation
Signs of peripheral nervous system injury
  Loss of sensation in the genitals, "saddle area," and legs
  Paresis and areflexia in legs
  Scrotal, cremasteric, and anal reflex loss

sphincter while the internal sphincter, under involuntary parasympathetic control, simultaneously relaxes.

As could be anticipated, excess sympathetic ANS activity, as in the "fight and flight" response, inhibits both urinating and defecating by constricting the sphincters. Moreover, excess ANS activity, typically caused by anxiety, often impairs sexual arousal, inhibits an erection, and precipitates premature ejaculation.

Laboratory Tests

Sleep-Related Studies

From infancy to old age, normal men have erections and other signs of ANS activity during their rapid eye movement (REM) periods of sleep. The erections develop during dreams, regardless of their overt content. Thus, normal men have three to five erections per night, each lasting about 20 minutes. In a standard test, the *nocturnal penile tumescence (NPT)* study, devices monitor a man's erections and correlate them with REM periods over one to three nights.

Because NPT studies take place in a secluded setting, the testing frees men with erectile dysfunction

from most social and psychologic influences. During NPT studies, some men considered incapable actually develop erections. Those who develop no erections usually have a physiologic disturbance; however, some of them suffer from profound depression, a sleep disorder, or a test-induced artifact.

Other Tests

Physicians may assess men with peripheral vascular disease, atherosclerosis, diabetes, or pelvic injuries by measuring blood pressure and blood flow in the dorsal artery of the penis using a small blood pressure cuff, Doppler ultrasound apparatus, or other devices. Barring vascular disease, an injection of a vasodilator into the penis (i.e., an intracorporal vasodilator injection) produces an erection. In fact, such injections provide a treatment option.

For women as well as men, electrophysiologic studies, such as peripheral nerve conduction velocity, penile nerve conduction velocity, and somatosensory evoked potentials, can disclose underlying polyneuropathy, pudendal nerve damage, or spinal cord injury. These tests help in the diagnosis of patients with diabetes, prostate cancer, pelvic or spine trauma, or multiple sclerosis (MS) (see later).

Individuals with an endocrinologic basis of their sexual dysfunction usually have other signs of hormone imbalance. Relevant screening tests usually measure blood glucose, prolactin, testosterone, estrogen, and gonadotropic hormone concentrations. Many antipsychotic medicines elevate the serum prolactin concentration, although an elevated concentration often otherwise indicates a pituitary adenoma or tumor. Other tests may reveal hypogonadism, hypothyroidism, diabetes, or a disruption of the hypothalamic-pituitary-gonadal axis.

Medical Treatment of Erectile Dysfunction

Several medications can produce erections adequate for sexual intercourse despite neurologic injury or vascular insufficiency. They can also restore erections in men experiencing psychogenic erectile dysfunction and in those taking psychotropic medications.

Many physicians prescribe yohimbine, a centrally acting α-2 adrenergic antagonist (see Chapter 21). It may slightly increase sympathetic vasomotor activity, provide mild psychologic stimulation, and create an aphrodisiac sensation. Although yohimbine may alleviate psychogenic erectile dysfunction, it does not help in cases of sexual function due to medical or neurologic illness. Moreover, it often causes anxiety.

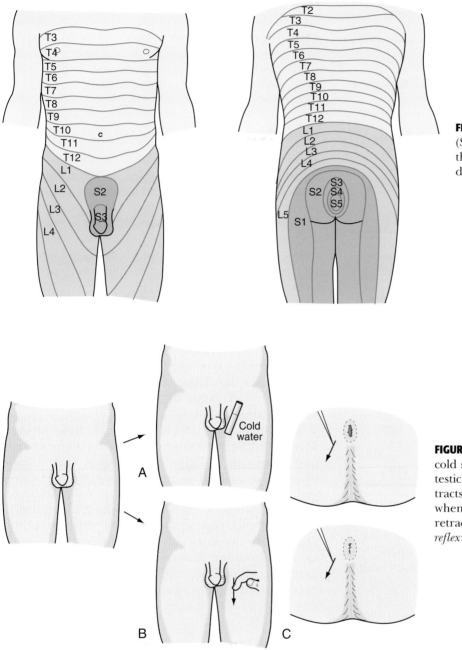

FIGURE 16-2 ■ The sacral dermatomes (S2-S5) innervate the skin overlying the genitals and anus, but the lumbar dermatomes innervate the legs.

FIGURE 16-3 ■ *A,* The *scrotal reflex*: When a cold surface is applied to the scrotum, the testicle normally retracts and the skin contracts. *B,* The *cremasteric reflex*: Likewise, when the inner thigh is stroked, the testicle retracts and the skin contracts. *C,* The *anal reflex*: When scratched, the anus tightens.

Testosterone injections are also popular mostly because they may increase muscle mass, especially in body builders, and provide psychologic stimulation. However, except on cases of hypogonadism, testosterone injections have no effect on sexual function and, in high doses for long periods, they may induce prostate cancer.

In contrast, intracorporeal injections of vasoactive medicines—although briefly painful—are effective. They induce erections in men with spinal cord damage, peripheral neuropathy, or vascular disease. The most effective medicines are papaverine, a nonspecific smooth muscle relaxant; phentolamine, an α-adrenergic antagonist; and alprostadil, a synthetic prostaglandin E1. A man with erectile dysfunction can inject these medicines—individually or as a mixture—into the base of his corpus cavernosum (the vascular erectile tissue of the penis).

Phentolamine-induced erections illustrate an important physiologic distinction. Although α-adrenergic *antagonists,* such as phentolamine, cause erections, α-adrenergic *antagonists,* such as epinephrine (see later), soften erections—by respectively increasing or reducing blood flow into the penis.

Using an alternative treatment, a man inserts a short, thin alprostadil suppository into his urethra. Although initially uncomfortable, it greatly promotes blood flow into the penis, leading to an erection. This method, unlike with sildenafil (Viagra) treatment, does not require stimulation. After an orgasm, the erection usually subsides during the following 1 to 3 hours.

Sildenafil and related medicines—tadalafil (Cialis) and vardenafil (Levitra)—have simplified the treatment of erectile dysfunction. To a greater or lesser degree they assist men with erectile dysfunction from age-related changes, diabetes, MS, spinal cord injury, and nerve damage from prostate surgery. Furthermore, they often correct erectile dysfunction associated with decreased libido, depression, or other psychiatric disturbances. They also partially or completely reverse sexual dysfunction caused by selective serotonin reuptake inhibitors (SSRIs) in both sexes.

These medicines have a well-established, rational mechanism of action. Under normal circumstances, psychologic or tactile sexual stimulation provokes parasympathetic neurons to produce and release the neurotransmitter nitric oxide (NO) within the penis. NO, in turn, promotes the production of cyclic guanylate cyclase monophosphate (cGMP). In turn, cGMP dilates the arteries that promotes blood flow and creates an erection. After an enzyme, cGMP-phosphodiesterase, metabolizes cGMP, the erection subsides.

As their primary mechanism of action, these medicines—"phosphodiesterase inhibitors"—inhibit cGMP-phosphodiesterase. The resulting increased cGMP concentration promotes blood flow in the penis.

Hardly a panacea, phosphodiesterase inhibitors help only about 60% of men with erectile dysfunction. In particular, they are often ineffective in men older than 70 years, with diabetes (especially when it is uncontrolled), undergoing cancer chemotherapy, or who smoke. In addition, they carry some risk. In addition, men taking nitroglycerin, other nitrates, doxazosin, or most other α_1-adrenergic antagonists should not also take phosphodiesterase inhibitors because excess vasodilation may lead to orthostatic hypotension.

Invasive treatments are rarely satisfactory. Delicate and tedious arterial reconstructive procedures are usually disappointing except in men with localized vascular injuries. Surgically implanted devices, such as rigid or semirigid silicone rods or a balloon-like apparatus, can mimic an erection. Unfortunately, implants are costly, unesthetic, and prone to infections and mechanical failures. In contrast, silicone penile implants have never been accused, like silicone breast implants, of causing rheumatologic or MS-like symptoms (see Chapter 15).

UNDERLYING CONDITIONS

Age-Related Changes

In men aged 50 years and older, although their libido generally remains intact, erections decrease in rigidity and duration. Their penis begins to lose sensitivity to touch and vibration, as do other bodily areas in older individuals. Also, older men's refractory period between orgasms, which was 20 minutes when they were in their sexual prime, at age 18 years, lengthens to days to weeks. Their serum testosterone concentration decreases, but changes correlate poorly with erectile function. For example, although restoring testosterone concentrations reverses a diminished libido, it does not improve erectile dysfunction.

One credible explanation for age-related erectile dysfunction implicates increased smooth muscle tone throughout the body. Not only does increased arterial wall smooth muscle tone cause or contribute to essential hypertension but it also leads to reduced blood flow into the penis.

Other factors common among middle-aged and older men that may cause or at least predispose them to erectile dysfunction include hypertension, atherosclerotic disease, smoking, alcohol abuse, and television viewing time. Whether in isolation or as a group, these factors also blunt the response to phosphodiesterase inhibitors.

Spinal Cord Injury

Every year hundreds of teenagers and young adults sustain spinal cord injuries from motorcycle, automobile, diving, horseback riding, and trampoline accidents; knife or bullet wounds; and MS. Some congenital malformations, such as myelomeningocele (see Chapter 13), also damage the spinal cord. Spinal cord injury produces a triad of symptoms that varies according to the injury's level and whether it partially or completely transects the cord:

- Paraparesis or quadriparesis with spasticity, hyperactive reflexes, and Babinski signs
- Sensory loss up to a certain spinal level (see Fig. 16-2)
- Bladder, bowel, and sexual difficulties

In addition, upper cervical cord injuries compromise the respiratory center. They also release the sympathetic nervous system from CNS control.

Cervical and Thoracic Spinal Cord Injury

When injuries sever the cervical spinal cord, patients develop quadriparesis. When injuries sever the thoracic portion, they develop paraparesis. In both of these situations, the injury interrupts ascending sensory impulses, and patients cannot sense genital stimulation. Nevertheless, because the genital-spinal cord loop remains intact, patients retain the capacity for reflex genital arousal. They can achieve an orgasm even though they are unable to perceive it.

In these cases, erections are usually too weak for intercourse. If orgasms occur, they may produce an excessive, almost violent ANS response, called *autonomic hyperreflexia*. This response often causes hypertension, bradycardia, nausea, and lightheadedness. Occasionally the hypertension leads to an intracerebral hemorrhage.

Most spinal cord injury patients develop urinary incontinence and constipation, requiring catheters and enemas. Infections of the urinary tract and decubitus ulcers constantly threaten them. Furthermore, men lose fertility because of inadequate and abnormal sperm production. However, women continue to ovulate and menstruate. They retain their capacity to conceive and bear children.

Incomplete spinal cord damage, as typically occurs in MS and nonpenetrating trauma, causes less pronounced neurologic deficits. Still, because of the delicate nature of the sexual neurologic pathways, even incomplete injuries impair genital arousal and inhibit orgasm.

Lumbosacral Spinal Cord Injury

As with patients who sustain thoracic spinal cord transection, those with lumbosacral spinal cord transection also have paraparesis and incontinence. In addition, because this lower lesion interrupts both the genital-spinal cord reflex and ascending and descending spinal cord tracts, neither genital nor cerebral stimulation produces arousal or orgasm.

Nevertheless, the ANS, which travels in a parallel pathway, may remain undamaged and able to innervate the genitals. This innervation preserves fertility in men and women. Also in contrast to higher spinal cord injuries, sensation of the breasts and their erotic capacity is preserved—and relatively enhanced—because upper chest sensation remains unaffected.

Poliomyelitis and Other Exceptions

Several neurologic illnesses can be so devastating that the untrained physician might assume that their victims have no sexual capacity. However, evaluations may reveal that many patients with these illnesses have retained sexual desire and function.

For example, two relatively common motor neuron diseases, poliomyelitis (polio) and amyotrophic lateral sclerosis (ALS), devastate the voluntary motor system. Polio often left survivors confined to wheelchairs and braces but with stable deficits. ALS, in contrast, causes progressively greater disability that usually results in death after several years (see Chapter 5). Nevertheless, both these illnesses spare victims' intellect, sensation, involuntary muscle strength, and ANS. Thus, they allow patients normal sexual desire and function, genital sensation, bladder and bowel control, and fertility.

Similarly, most extrapyramidal illnesses (see Chapter 18), despite causing difficulties with mobility, do not impair sexual desire, sexual function, or fertility. For example, adolescents with athetotic cerebral palsy and other varieties of congenital birth injury— even those with marked physical impairments—often have intact libido and sexual function. In addition, Parkinson's disease patients have a preserved sexual drive; however, it may remain dormant until dopa-repleting medications allow it to re-emerge. Moreover, illness-induced loss of inhibition, as in frontal lobe trauma and Alzheimer's disease, may lead to sexual aggressiveness.

Diabetes Mellitus

Retrograde ejaculation and erectile dysfunction eventually affect almost 50% of diabetic men. Their sexual impairment results not only from ANS and PNS injury but also from atherosclerosis of the genital arteries (see later). Their erectile dysfunction is associated with age greater than 65 years; duration of diabetes longer than 10 years; obesity; and the common complications of diabetes, such as retinopathy, neuropathy, and arteriopathy. Although sildenafil and related medicines alleviate erectile dysfunction in many men with various illnesses or conditions, they provide uncertain benefits to diabetic men (see later).

The data conflict regarding sexual impairment in diabetic women. Some investigators found that 35% of diabetic women were anorgasmic and that sexual impairment was related to neuropathy; however, others found that diabetic women were not especially prone to sexual impairment and that even those with profound neuropathy experienced full sexual function. All agree, though, that diabetic women are prone to develop vaginal infections. In addition, although diabetic women remain fertile, their pregnancies are often complicated by miscarriages and fetal malformations.

Urinary incontinence often accompanies sexual dysfunction in both men and women because the bladder and genitals share a common ANS innervation. Lack of innervation allows the bladder to dilate excessively and lose its tone (Fig. 16-4). In addition, patients with diabetes-induced sexual dysfunction typically experience other complications of ANS impairment,

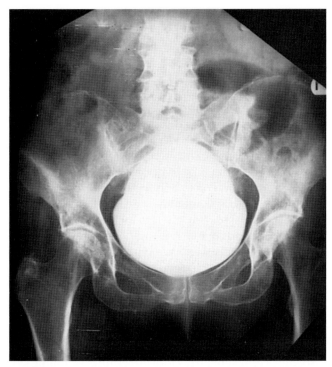

FIGURE 16-4 ■ The patient has diabetes mellitus complicated by urinary incontinence, typically associated with a large, flaccid bladder. An intravenous pyelogram (IVP), a dated but illustrative method, shows his distended bladder (the large white area). In many conditions, including diabetes and multiple sclerosis, urinary incontinence and sexual dysfunction are comorbid. Current studies, such as sonography and computed tomography (CT), provide the same information and do not necessarily subject patients to infusions of a contrast solution.

such as anhidrosis and orthostatic hypotension. However, they do not necessarily have other complications of diabetes, such as retinopathy, nephropathy, or peripheral vascular disease. Although many diabetic men with erectile dysfunction have low testosterone concentrations, testosterone therapy generally provides only a placebo effect.

Multiple Sclerosis

Sexual impairment can be the most bothersome symptom, and it is sometimes even the sole symptom, of MS (see Chapter 15). Patients in an early stage of the disease may have few persistent neurologic deficits, but when attacks develop repeatedly, the incidence of sexual impairment sharply rises. In 90% of cases, sexual impairment is accompanied by urinary bladder dysfunction. It is also often associated with other neurologic impairments, including spasticity, paraparesis, and genital sensory loss. Although MS spinal cord involvement probably underlies most cases, medical and psychiatric factors—anxiety,

depression, and side effects of antidepressants and other medicines—contribute. Whatever the precise mechanism, sexual dysfunction reduces quality of life in MS patients.

Between 70% and 90% of male MS patients experience sexual impairment, particularly erectile dysfunction. Less frequently the illness also causes premature ejaculation, retrograde ejaculation, and anorgasmia. Decreased sperm production, another complication, impairs fertility. Phosphodiesterase inhibitors correct erectile dysfunction and improve quality of life in the majority of affected men.

Among female MS patients, a somewhat smaller proportion (between 50% and 75%) have sexual dysfunction. In these women, MS causes decreased sexual desire, inadequate vaginal lubrication, and anorgasmia. However, they remain fertile.

Medication-Induced Impairment

Reports indicate that more than 100 medications impair sexual function, but only a few categories are consistently responsible. Antidepressant and antipsychotic medications constitute a major category. Another one is standard antihypertensive medicines, such as clonidine, thiazide diuretics, and β-blockers. However, the newer antihypertensive agents, including angiotensin-converting enzyme (ACE) inhibitors and the calcium-channel blockers, cause little or no sexual impairment.

Although many psychiatric patients are prone to sexual dysfunction on account of their disorder, psychotropic medications precipitate or exacerbate sexual dysfunction. In both men and women, such medication-induced sexual dysfunction is primarily dose-related, but it is also closely related to elevated serum prolactin concentrations. Medication-induced sexual dysfunction also correlates with medications' suppression of dopamine activity, increase in serotonin activity, and inhibition of NO synthetase.

In general, antipsychotic medications' sexual side effects are consistent with the hypothesis that decreased dopamine activity, usually accompanied by increased prolactin concentration, leads to sexual dysfunction. Typical antipsychotics, which increase prolactin concentrations, routinely decrease libido, impair erectile function, and cause other sexual problems in both men and women. In contrast, clozapine, olanzapine, quetiapine, and several other atypical antipsychotics, which cause little or no increase in prolactin concentrations, carry a relatively low risk of sexual side effects. Interestingly, almost all typical and atypical antipsychotic agents on rare occasion cause priapism (see later).

Antidepressants—tricyclics, heterocyclics, monoamine oxidase inhibitors, and SSRIs—also lead to sexual dysfunction. This side effect often so troubles patients that they fail to comply with their medication regimen.

SSRIs more so than tricyclic antidepressants delay or prevent orgasm. Furthermore, approximately one third of men taking SSRIs experience erectile dysfunction. These medicines also interfere with vaginal lubrication. For any particular SSRI, the rate of adverse sexual side effects greatly varies among different studies. When an SSRI causes sexual side effects, physicians may prescribe a phosphodiesterase inhibitor, such as sildenafil, which frequently overcomes the problem.

Anticholinergic medications, which psychiatrists often prescribe to counteract antipsychotic medication-induced parkinsonism, also cause sexual impairment. In addition, these medicines cause other bothersome symptoms that reflect ANS dysfunction: dry mouth, orthostatic hypotension, urinary hesitancy, and accommodation paresis (see Chapter 12).

On the other hand, physicians treating men with premature ejaculation may capitalize on certain psychotropic medications' delaying orgasm. For example, clomipramine (Anafranil), sertraline (Zoloft), and trazodone may prolong arousal and delay orgasm in men.

Priapism

In patients who have an unexpected sensitivity, take too large a dose, or have an underlying structural abnormality, phosphodiesterase inhibitor treatments may inadvertently produce an uncomfortable and embarrassing persistent erection (priapism). Prolonged erections may also develop in spinal cord injury patients with denervation hypersensitivity.

Other conditions that lead to priapism include sickle cell crises, leukemia, vascular abnormalities, and venous thrombosis from self-injection of narcotics, blocking the penis' venous drainage and thereby engorge it with blood. In addition, although typical and atypical antipsychotic medications usually dampen sexual function, they occasional produce priapism because they are α-adrenergic antagonists.

In addition to inducing pain, priapism can cause ischemia or, in severe cases, necrosis. Furthermore, repeated bouts lead to fibrosis. Urologists consider priapism an emergency. To stop blood flow into the penis, urologists inject epinephrine, an α-adrenergic agonist, because it acts as an arterial vasoconstrictor (see Chapter 21). Cases that do not respond to epinephrine may require surgical drainage.

THE LIMBIC SYSTEM AND THE LIBIDO

From a neurologic viewpoint, the *limbic system* provides libido. This system consists of a large horseshoe-shaped reverberating subcortical circuit connecting the hippocampal formation and the adjacent amygdala in the temporal lobe, thalamic and hypothalamic structures including the mamillary bodies, midbrain nuclei, and frontal lobe (Fig. 16-5). Among its many functions, the limbic system generates, conveys, or stores memory, emotion, programs for "flight or fight," eating and drinking behavior, and sexual and reproductive urges.

Structural lesions and neurodegenerative illnesses that strike the frontal or temporal lobes often damage the limbic system. For example, head trauma, strokes, or frontotemporal dementia (see Chapter 7) regularly reduce patients' psychic energy, including their sexual appetite. Although most frontal lobe injuries cause apathy and hyposexuality, occasionally they lead to aggressive, sexually charged behavior.

The Klüver-Bucy Syndrome

The *Klüver-Bucy syndrome*, a famous and quite dramatic disorder, represents the closest example of limbic system injury that may occur in humans. In the laboratory experiment that first produced it, neurosurgeons performed bilateral anterior temporal lobectomies, removing both amygdalae (Greek, almond [the shape of the amygdalae]), on rhesus monkeys. Postoperatively, the monkeys displayed aggression and rampant, indiscriminate heterosexual and homosexual activity. In addition, as if they had lost their vision, the monkeys continually grasped objects and placed inedible as well as edible ones in their mouth: Investigators labeled this behavior *psychic blindness* or *oral exploration* (terms related to *visual agnosia*, see Chapter 12).

A human version of the Klüver-Bucy syndrome occasionally develops in both children and adults. The syndrome in them also results from bilateral temporal lobe lesions, but the usual causes consist of *herpes simplex* encephalitis, frontotemporal dementia including Pick's disease, bilateral posterior cerebral artery infarctions, and paraneoplastic limbic encephalitis—conditions that have a predilection for striking the temporal lobes. Additionally, conditions that affect the brain diffusely or nonspecifically, such as anoxia, trauma, and Alzheimer's disease, sometimes predominantly injure the temporal lobes and cause this syndrome.

The manifestations of the human version differ considerably from those that occur in the monkeys. Only about one half of humans show any increase in heterosexual activity or masturbation. Most only speak or gesture in an aggressive or sexually suggestive manner. Showing a version of oral exploration, humans with the Klüver-Bucy syndrome tend to eat excessively and smoke or drink compulsively; however, they

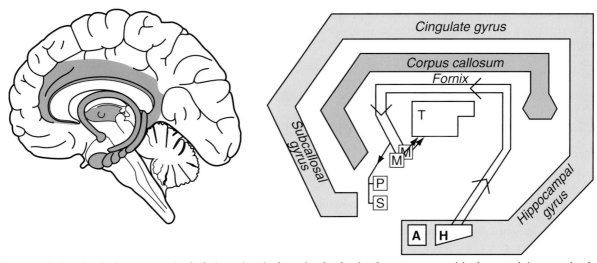

FIGURE 16-5 ■ *Left,* The *limbic system* (shaded) is a circuit deep in the brain that connects with the overlying cerebral cortex. *Right,* This schematic portrayal of the *limbic system* shows its main features:

Hippocampus (H) with the adjacent amygdala (A)

↓

Fornix (*fornix,* Latin arch)

↓

Mamillary bodies (M) that send off a mamillothalamic tract

↓

Anterior nucleus of the thalamus (T)

↓

Cingulate gyrus that connects to the overlying cerebral cortex and back to the hippocampus

↑

rarely become obese. Whatever their behavior, other manifestations of temporal lobe injury, such as amnesia, aphasia, and dementia, place more of a handicap. In particular, children with the Klüver-Bucy syndrome, which usually results from hypoxic cerebral damage, are most impaired by the amnesia.

Other Conditions

Certain medications and drugs of abuse, including hallucinogens, amyl nitrate, "ecstasy," and L-dopa preparations, may increase sexual interest and activity. Although numerous other substances are purported to have aphrodisiac qualities, their effect is minimal or nil, and many may be dangerous. (Sildenafil, despite its ability to enhance sexuality, is not an aphrodisiac because it requires stimulation to be effective and does not affect the libido.)

Similarly, damage to the inhibitory centers of the frontal lobes may unleash suppressed sexual interest and allow some sexual activity. For example, patients with Alzheimer's disease, frontotemporal dementia, or vascular dementia who have lost cerebral inhibition as part of their illness, occasionally increase their sexual activity. Nevertheless, other manifestations of these illnesses—impaired cognitive function, reduced executive ability, and apraxia—often leave their actions rudimentary or clumsy.

On the other hand, most neurologic illnesses decrease libido. Strokes with or without comorbid depression usually limit sexual interest and physical ability. Also, lesions of the pituitary, hypothalamus, and diencephalon of various etiologies usually cause hyposexuality. For example, in Sheehan's syndrome (see Chapter 19), women experience weight loss, amenorrhea, and other manifestations of hypothalamic-pituitary insufficiency, including prominent lack of sexual interest. On the other hand, hypothalamic tumors induce a ravenous appetite without accompanying sexual activity.

Although partial complex epilepsy is usually associated with hyposexuality (see Chapter 10), its seizures sometimes induce activity with sexual overtones. For example, during a complex seizure, patients may engage in rudimentary masturbation or even partially undress; however, the seizures do not cause frank, interactive sexual activity.

Although the libido resists mild fatigue, hunger, and fear, pain almost always dampens it. Patients with chronic pain not only often have comorbid depression but they also take potent analgesics, such as opioids, that reduce sexual interest or function.

REFERENCES

1. Bacon CG, Mittleman MA, Kawachi I, et al: Sexual function in men older than 50 years of age: Results from the health professionals follow-up study. Ann Intern Med 139:161–168, 2003.
2. Basu A, Ryder RE: New treatment options for erectile dysfunction in patients with diabetes mellitus. Drugs 64:2667–2688, 2004.
3. Berman JR, Berman L, Goldstein I: Female sexual dysfunction: Incidence, pathophysiology, evaluation, and treatment options. Urology 54:385–391, 1999.
4. Compton MT, Miller AH: Priapism associated with conventional and atypical antipsychotic medications: A review. J Clin Psychiatry 62:362–366, 2001.
5. Compton MT, Miller AH: Antipsychotic-induced hyperprolactinemia and sexual function. Psychopharmacol Bull 36:143–164, 2002.
6. Fowler CJ, Miller JR, Sarief MK, et al: A double blind, randomized study of sildenafil citrate for erectile dysfunction in men with multiple sclerosis. J Neurol Neurosurg Psychiatry 76:700–705, 2005.
7. Frohman EM: Sexual dysfunction in neurologic disease. Clin Neuropharmacol 25:126–132, 2002.
8. Harrison J, Glass CA, Owens RG et al: Factors associated with sexual functioning in women following spinal cord injury. Paraplegia 33:687–692, 1995.
9. Hulter BM, Lundberg PO: Sexual function in women with advanced multiple sclerosis. J Neurol Neurosurg Psychiatry 59:83–86, 1995.
10. Lilly R, Cummings JL, Benson DF, et al: The human, Klüver-Bucy syndrome. Neurology 33:1141–1145, 1983.
11. Lue TF: Erectile dysfunction. N Engl J Med 342:1802–1813, 2000.
12. Montgomery SA, Baldwin DS, Riley A: Antidepressant medications: A review of the evidence for drug-induced sexual dysfunction. J Affective Disord 69:119–140, 2002.
13. Mota M, Lichiardopol C, Mota E, et al: Erectile dysfunction in diabetes mellitus. Rom J Intern Med 41:163–177, 2003.
14. Nosek MA, Rintala DH, Young ME et al: Sexual functioning among women with physical disabilities. Arch Phys Med Rehabil 77:107–115, 1996.
15. Rudkin L, Taylor MJ, Hawton K: Strategies for managing sexual dysfunction induced by antidepressant medication. Cochrane Database Syst Rev 4: CD003382, 2004.
16. Smith SM, O'Keane V, Murray R: Sexual dysfunction in patients taking conventional antipsychotic medication. Br J Psychiatry 181:49–55, 2002.
17. Tonsgard JH, Harwicke N, Levine SC: Klüver-Bucy syndrome in children. Pediatr Neurol 3:162–165, 1987.
18. Webber R: Erectile dysfunction. Clin Evid 11:1148–1157, 2004.

Questions and Answers

1. A 40-year-old man complains of longstanding erectile dysfunction. He has severe low back pain, mild hypertension, and borderline diabetes. Which of the following is the most likely cause of his sexual dysfunction?
   a. Herniated lumbar intervertebral disk
   b. Antihypertensive medications
   c. Diabetic neuropathy
   d. Mood disorder
   e. Narcotic analgesics
   f. All of the above

Answer: f. Factors a–e may cause erectile dysfunction. Sexual function requires a complex, delicate system that is vulnerable at any of its components: the central nervous system (CNS), peripheral nervous system (PNS), and autonomic nervous system (ANS).

2. A 24-year-old man who complains of premature ejaculation also has episodes of unsteady gait, diplopia, and paraparesis. Which of the following might a neurologic examination reveal?
   a. Internuclear ophthalmoplegia
   b. Absent abdominal reflexes
   c. Ataxia of gait
   d. Babinski signs
   e. Hyperactive deep tendon reflexes (DTRs)
   f. All of the above

Answer: f. The patient probably has multiple sclerosis (MS) with cerebellar, brainstem, and spinal cord involvement. Between episodes, he is likely to retain neurologic impairments (a–e), including sexual dysfunction. Premature ejaculation and erectile dysfunction are frequent symptoms—and possibly the only ones—of quiescent MS involving the spinal cord.

3. Which of the following conditions often causes retrograde ejaculation?
   a. Depression
   b. Diabetic autonomic neuropathy
   c. Psychogenic influence
   d. Yohimbine
   e. Sexual inexperience
   f. All of the above

Answer: b. In retrograde ejaculation, semen is propelled by involuntary mechanisms into the bladder instead of the urethra. It is always the result of neurologic, muscular, or other organic impairment—particularly of the ANS—that diverts the flow of semen.

4. In which illnesses should a physician assume that sexual dysfunction has a neurologic basis?
   a. XYY syndrome
   b. Mild mental retardation
   c. Parkinson's disease
   d. Poliomyelitis
   e. Amyotrophic lateral sclerosis
   f. None of the above

Answer: f. Although each of these illnesses may cause weakness, the patient's sexual drive, genital sensation, and orgasmic reactions are preserved. Physicians should not assume that a patient's physical immobility impairs libido.

5. In which four illnesses is medication-induced sexual dysfunction likely encountered?
   a. Psychosis
   b. Migraine headache
   c. Hypertension
   d. Low back pain
   e. Duodenal ulcer
   f. Glaucoma
   g. Depression
   h. Epilepsy

Answers: a, c, e, g. Medicines prescribed for hypertension, psychosis, and depression—as well as the illnesses themselves—often cause sexual impairments. Also, medicines with systemic anticholinergic properties, particularly ulcer medications and antipsychotics, impair sexual function. Epilepsy is associated with hyposexuality, but it is not iatrogenic.

6. During sleep, when do erections and seminal emissions occur?
   a. NREM stages 1 and 2
   b. NREM stages 3 and 4
   c. REM
   d. All of the above

Answer: c. Erections and emissions occur during REM sleep. As such, erections characteristically remain present on awakening, when the final REM period is waning.

7. In which situation is fertility lost?
   a. Women with cervical spinal cord transection
   b. Men with cervical spinal cord transection
   c. Men with diabetes mellitus and neuropathy
   d. Women with diabetes mellitus and neuropathy

Answer: b. Men with upper spinal cord injury have reduced sperm concentration and abnormalities in their remaining sperm. Women are able to conceive and bear children despite spinal cord injury. Both men and women with diabetes remain fertile.

8. A 43-year-old man describes 2 days of erectile dysfunction each time he completes a several hour bicycle ride. He has no diabetes and takes no medications. Which is the most likely cause of his sexual difficulty?
   a. Compression of the pudendal nerve
   b. Excessive sympathetic autonomic nervous system activity
   c. A muscle disorder
   d. Excessive parasympathetic autonomic nervous system activity
   e. Psychologic factors

Answer: a. When he rides his bicycle, pressure between the seat and his symphysis pubis compresses his pudendal nerve. Additionally, bicycle riders sometimes compress the adjacent blood vessels, which can also cause erectile dysfunction.

9. In which two conditions would cremasteric reflexes be lost?
   a. Diabetic autonomic neuropathy
   b. Anxiety
   c. Sacral spinal cord injury
   d. Frontal meningioma

Answers: a, c. Cremasteric reflexes, which are superficial reflexes rather than DTRs, require that the pudendal nerves, autonomic nervous system, and spinal cord be intact.

10. One month after falling down a flight of stairs, a 35-year-old man complains of low back pain and erectile dysfunction. Examination reveals loss of pinprick sensation below the waist, but intact position, vibratory, and warm-cold sensation. Deep tendon and cremasteric reflexes are intact, and plantar reflexes are flexion. Which is the most likely cause of the erectile dysfunction?
   a. Spinal cord injury
   b. Autonomic nervous system dysfunction
   c. Peripheral neuropathy
   d. Multiple sclerosis
   e. Alcoholism
   f. None of the above

Answer: f. The lack of objective neurologic deficit indicates that no neurologic injury has occurred. In fact, a structural lesion cannot cause the dissociation of pinprick and warm-cold sensation, because both sensations travel in the same nerve pathways. Alcoholism may blunt the libido and cause a neuropathy. In alcoholic peripheral neuropathy, DTRs and sensation are lost.

11. Which is not an aspect of the Klüver-Bucy syndrome in monkeys?
   a. Psychic blindness
   b. Apathy
   c. Frontal lobectomy
   d. Loss of amygdalae
   e. Increased homosexual, heterosexual, and autosexual activity

Answer: c. After temporal lobectomy including removal of the amygdalae, monkeys demonstrate oral exploratory behavior. They are said to have visual agnosia because they do not identify objects by their appearance even though their vision is intact. Moreover, the monkeys characteristically lose extreme emotion. For example, while they may appear fearless, they are actually apathetic. Most striking, they display intermittent aggressive behavior and increased and indiscriminate sexual activity.

12. Which two of the following are almost always found in humans who have sustained bilateral temporal lobe damage?
   a. Memory impairment
   b. Placing food and inedible objects in their mouths
   c. Hypersexuality
   d. Rage attacks
   e. Obesity

Answers: a, b. The human variety of the Klüver-Bucy syndrome is characterized by impaired memory, a tendency to eat excessively, and, as in monkeys, an inclination to place inedible objects in the mouth. Contrary to expectations, affected individuals have little sexual appetite and no violent outbursts.

13. In humans, which one of these conditions does not usually preferentially damage the limbic system?
   a. Herpes simplex
   b. Alcoholism
   c. TIAs of the posterior cerebral arteries
   d. Herpes zoster
   e. Frontotemporal dementia
   f. Paraneoplastic encephalitis

Answer: d. Because the amygdala and hippocampus are situated in the temporal lobes, these limbic system structures are vulnerable to conditions that damage the temporal lobes. *Herpes simplex* virus, which has a predilection for the frontal and temporal lobes, is a frequent cause of encephalitis characterized by memory impairment and partial complex seizures. Although *Herpes zoster* often causes painful neuralgia in the trigeminal nerve distribution, it rarely infects the CNS. Posterior cerebral TIAs cause ischemia of the temporal lobes. These TIAs induce episodes of confusion and memory impairment called "transient global amnesia." Chronic alcohol abuse can cause the Wernicke-Korsakoff syndrome, which is associated with hemorrhage into the mamillary bodies and other parts of the limbic system. Frontotemporal dementia, including Pick's disease, causes early and severe atrophy of the frontal and temporal lobes. An inflammatory remote effect of carcinoma, paraneoplastic limbic encephalitis, typically affects the hippocampus and causes memory impairment, partial complex seizures, and behavioral disturbances that reflect temporal lobe damage.

14. Which two of the following are not consequences of a pituitary microadenoma?
    a. Headaches
    b. Hyperprolactinemia
    c. Optic atrophy
    d. Homonymous superior quadrantanopia
    e. Infertility
    f. Irregular menses

Answers: c, d. Optic atrophy and homonymous superior quadrantanopia are manifestations of large (macroscopic) pituitary adenomas. Microadenomas can cause headaches, hyperprolactinemia, and infertility. Hyperprolactinemia, whether caused by medications or adenomas, causes sexual impairment.

15. In normal males, which of the following is not associated with REM-induced erections?
    a. Dreams with or without overt sexual content
    b. Most dreams, even with frightful or anxiety-producing content
    c. Increased pulse and blood pressure
    d. Increased testosterone level
    e. An EEG that appears, aside from eye movement artifact, as though the patient were awake

Answer: d. During REM sleep, individuals have increased ANS activity and an EEG that has ocular movement artifact superimposed on an "awake" background pattern.

16. Which substance will abort medication-induced erection priapism?
    a. Epinephrine
    b. Phentolamine

c. Papaverine
d. Prostaglandins

Answer: a. In men who have erectile dysfunction because of multiple sclerosis, diabetes, spinal cord injury, or many other illnesses, injections into the dorsum of the penis (intracorporeal injections) of phentolamine, papaverine, or prostaglandins, which are vasodilators, will produce an erection. The injections are so effective that they may be appropriate in some men with psychogenic erectile dysfunction. However, they must be used with caution in men with vascular disease or spinal cord injury. Should priapism occur, an injection of epinephrine, a vasoconstrictor, can terminate it.

17. What is the origin of the sexual organs' sympathetic ANS innervation?
    a. Lower cranial nerves
    b. Cervical and upper thoracic spinal cord
    c. Lower thoracic and upper lumbar spinal cord
    d. Sacral spinal cord

Answer: c.

18. What is the origin of the sexual organs' parasympathetic ANS innervation?
    a. Lower cranial nerves
    b. Cervical and upper thoracic spinal cord
    c. Lower thoracic and upper lumbar spinal cord
    d. Sacral spinal cord

Answer: d.

19. What proportion of men with erectile dysfunction are helped by phosphodiesterase inhibitors, such as sildenafil?
    a. 100%
    b. 75%
    c. 50%
    d. 25%

Answer: c. At most, phosphodiesterase inhibitors help only about 60% of men with erectile dysfunction. They are least effective in men older than 70 years, with uncontrolled diabetes, or who smoke. However, they are helpful in men with erectile dysfunction from minor age-related changes, decreased libido, depression, and SSRIs.

20. What is the mechanism of action of phosphodiesterase inhibitors, such as sildenafil?
    a. They provoke the release of nitric oxide (NO).
    b. They promote the production of cyclic guanylate cyclase monophosphate (cGMP).
    c. They enhance cGMP-phosphodiesterase, which metabolizes cGMP.
    d. By inhibiting cGMP-phosphodiesterase, they increase or prolong cGMP activity.

Answer: d. These medicines inhibit the enzyme cGMP-phosphodiesterase. Increased or prolonged cGMP activity promotes genital blood flow.

21. Which president had survived poliomyelitis (polio)?
    a. J. Carter
    b. T. Roosevelt
    c. F. D. Roosevelt
    d. J. F. Kennedy

Answer: c. As a young man, President Roosevelt contracted polio. He eventually required heavy braces for his legs and eventually was confined to a wheelchair. As in his case, polio caused marked physical disability but spared his intellectual and sexual abilities.

22. Which of the following sequences describes the path of the limbic system?
    a. Fornix, mamillothalamic tract, amygdala, anterior nucleus of the thalamus, cingulate gyrus
    b. Cingulate gyrus, mamillary bodies, mamillothalamic tract, anterior nucleus of the thalamus, hippocampus and adjacent amygdala
    c. Hippocampus and adjacent amygdala, fornix mamillary bodies, mamillothalamic tract, anterior nucleus of the thalamus, cingulate gyrus
    d. Hippocampus and adjacent amygdala, mamillothalamic tract, fornix, hippocampus and adjacent amygdala, mamillary bodies, anterior nucleus of the thalamus, cingulate gyrus

Answer: c.

23. Which of the following acts as the neurotransmitter for *sympathetic* nervous system activity during sexual function?
    a. Acetylcholine
    b. Monoamines
    c. Serotonin
    d. Nitric oxide

Answer: b. Monoamines, such as norepinephrine, are the neurotransmitters in the sympathetic nervous system.

24. Which of the following act as the neurotransmitter for *parasympathetic* nervous system activity during sexual function?
    a. Acetylcholine
    b. Monoamines
    c. Serotonin
    d. Dopamine

Answer: a. Acetylcholine is the neurotransmitter in the parasympathetic nervous system. The actual genital engorgement is mediated by nitric oxide (NO).

24. A 45-year-old diabetic man under evaluation for erectile dysfunction fails to have erections during NPT studies. Which of the following is the least likely explanation?
    a. Profound depression
    b. A sleep disorder
    c. Use of medications or alcohol
    d. Anxiety

Answer: d. Men with anxiety-induced or other psychologic erectile dysfunction, as well as normal men, typically develop erections during REM sleep. Absence of erections on NPT studies, however, does not necessarily indicate a serious neurologic or vascular disease. Depression, a sleep disorder (especially ones that abolish REM sleep), and long-term use of certain medicines or alcohol may also inhibit erections during the test.

25. Which autonomic nervous system effect produces an erection?
    a. Increase in parasympathetic tone
    b. Decrease in parasympathetic tone
    c. Increase in sympathetic tone
    d. Decrease in sympathetic tone

Answer: a.

26. Which autonomic nervous system activity produces ejaculation?
    a. Increased parasympathetic tone
    b. Decreased parasympathetic tone
    c. Increased sympathetic tone
    d. Decreased sympathetic tone

Answer: c. Under normal circumstances, a switch from predominately parasympathetic to sympathetic tone advances the sexual response from arousal to orgasm. In highly anxious individuals, excessive sympathetic activity may suppress an erection or, if one occurs, precipitate a premature ejaculation.

27. At which age do men have the shortest orgasm latency?
    a. 8 years
    b. 18 years
    c. 28 years
    d. 58 years

Answer: b. Men at age 18 are in their sexual prime. Their latency (interval between orgasms) may be as short as 20 minutes. As men age, their latency increases to days to weeks.

28. Which of the following is not a normal age-related sexual change in men older than 50 years?
    a. Erections decrease in rigidity.
    b. The penis loses its sensitivity to touch and vibration.

c. Because of end organ damage, serum testosterone concentrations rise.

d. Erections decrease in duration.

Answer: c. Although their serum testosterone concentrations are frequently low, the decrease correlates poorly with erectile dysfunction. Although testosterone injections will not restore erectile function, they may restore a diminished libido. Erections decrease in rigidity and duration in men older than 50 years. Also, nerves in the penis, like other peripheral nerves, lose sensitivity to touch and vibration, as men age.

29. Which of the following statements concerning α-adrenergic agonists and antagonists is false?

a. α-adrenergic antagonists, such as phentolamine, induce erections.

b. Typical and atypical antipsychotic medications, which have α-adrenergic antagonist properties, occasionally produce priapism.

c. Because epinephrine, an α-adrenergic agonist, reduces blood flow into the penis, it can abort priapism.

d. Men taking phosphodiesterase inhibitors should not simultaneously take α_1-adrenergic antagonists because the combination may lead to generalized vasodilation and profound orthostatic hypotension.

e. All of the above are true.

Answer: e. The general rule is that α-adrenergic agonist activity leads to smooth muscle constriction of the arteries in the systemic circulation and the penis. Epinephrine is a classic α-adrenergic agonist. When urologists inject epinephrine into the penis for treatment of priapism, it constricts the arteries, reduces blood flow into the penis, and allows blood to drain out through the veins. In the opposite situation, α-adrenergic antagonists relax smooth muscle, allowing greater blood flow into the penis. Phosphodiesterase inhibitors, such as sildenafil, promote the accumulation of potentially dangerous concentrations of vasodilators, such as nitroglycerin.

30. A 48-year-old man, under treatment with an SSRI for depression, relates that he has developed erectile dysfunction. On the other hand, the medicine has greatly improved his mood and energy level, and he has returned to work and resumed a social life. What would be the best treatment for the erectile dysfunction?

a. Stop the SSRI.

b. Reduce the dose of the SSRI.

c. Switch to a different class of antidepressant.

d. Add a phosphodiesterase inhibitor.

Answer: d. Although each of the options might be reasonable, the best would be to add a phosphodiesterase inhibitor, such as sildenafil.

31. Which of the following medicines inhibits erections?

a. α-adrenergic antagonists, such as phentolamine

b. α-adrenergic agonists, such as epinephrine

c. Phosphodiesterase inhibitors

d. Synthetic prostaglandin

e. Papaverine

Answer: b. α-adrenergic agonists constrict arteries and restrict blood flow into the penis. In contrast, α-adrenergic antagonists, phosphodiesterase inhibitors (such as sildenafil), and synthetic prostaglandin E1 (such as alprostadil) promote blood flow and induce erections. Papaverine is a nonspecific smooth muscle relaxant, but it may have some phosphodiesterase inhibitory activity.

32. A 34-year-old woman experiences throbbing hemicranial or generalized headaches at the moment of orgasm. Her neurologic examination is normal. Which is the most likely explanation?

a. She has psychogenic headaches.

b. The partner's sildenafil seeps into her circulation.

c. She has repeated subarachnoid hemorrhages.

d. She has a variety of migraine.

Answer: d. She is experiencing orgasmic cephalgia, which is a variety of migraine. Sildenafil may cause mild bilateral headaches, but only in individuals who take it. Subarachnoid hemorrhage is usually a cataclysmic event and victims have nuchal rigidity, photophobia, and prostration. Moreover, it is not an event that repeats.

33. What is the role of nitric oxide (NO) in production of erections?

a. NO acts as a neurotransmitter that promotes the production of cyclic guanylate cyclase monophosphate (cGMP).

b. NO reduces cGMP production.

c. NO promotes the production of cGMP-phosphodiesterase.

d. NO reduces the production of cGMP-phosphodiesterase.

Answer: a. NO acts as a neurotransmitter that promotes the production of cGMP. An enzyme, cGMP-phosphodiesterase, metabolizes cGMP.

34. A 49-year-old man, with diabetes, hypertension, and coronary artery disease, had described having erectile dysfunction. His primary care physician

had prescribed sildenafil. Although the medicine produced satisfactory erections, he developed postcoital severe throbbing headaches and on several occasions postcoital fainting. Very discouraged, he returned. Which of the following medicines would be the best next step?

a. A triptan for medication-induced migraine
b. Tadalafil
c. Vardenafil
d. None of the above

Answer: d. The patient is probably taking an antihypertensive medicine or coronary vasodilator containing a nitrate in addition to the phosphodiesterase inhibitor. The vasodilatory effect of all these medicines causes migraine-like headaches and orthostatic hypotension. To correct this adverse interaction, the physician should change the antihypertensive or coronary vasodilator medicine.

Sleep Disorders

Physiologic information, derived almost entirely from a monitoring system, the *polysomnogram* (*PSG*), defines sleep and its stages. In sleeping individuals, the PSG simultaneously records:

- Cerebral activity through several electroencephalogram (EEG) channels
- Ocular movements through an electro-oculogram (EOG)
- Chin, limb, or other muscle movement and tone through an electromyogram (EMG)
- Oxygen saturation and other vital signs

PSG studies readily distinguish two phases of sleep. In *rapid eye movement* (*REM*) *sleep,* dreaming and flaccid limb paralysis accompany brisk, conjugate, and predominantly horizontal eye movements. *Nonrapid eye movement* (*NREM*) *sleep* consists of relatively long stretches of essentially dreamless sleep accompanied, approximately every 15 minutes, by repositioning movements of the body (Table 17-1).

NORMAL SLEEP

REM Sleep

Because most people awakened during a REM period report that they were having a dream, physicians have come to equate REM sleep with dream-filled sleep. Dreams that occur during REM sleep have an intellectually complexity, at least on a superficial level, and rich visual imagery.

Except for the eye movements and normal breathing, people in REM sleep remain immobile with paretic, areflexic, and flaccid muscles. EMGs recorded from chin and limb muscles, which are a standard placement, show no electric activity (Fig. 17-1). This paralysis is fortuitous because it prevents people from acting on their dreams.

In marked contrast to the muscle paralysis during REM sleep, autonomic nervous system (ANS) activity increases and produces increased pulse, elevated blood pressure, raised intracranial pressure, increased cerebral blood flow, greater muscle metabolism, and, in men, erections. As though defying psychoanalytic interpretation, erections develop regardless of the content of boys' and men's dreams. The discrepancy between intense ANS activity and the immobile body led early researchers to describe REM sleep as "activated" or "paradoxical" sleep. In fact, REM-induced ANS activity has been implicated in the increased incidence of myocardial infarctions and ischemic strokes that strike between 6:00 AM and 11:00 AM.

The EEG also shows surprising activity during REM sleep. Aside from eye-movement artifact, the REM-induced EEG appears similar to the EEG in wakefulness. Overall, REM sleep with its ANS activity and EEG patterns, except for the almost complete absence of EMG activity, resembles wakefulness far more than NREM sleep.

When activated, nuclei in the pons generate the basic physical elements of REM sleep, and the *perilocus ceruleus,* immediately adjacent to locus ceruleus, abolishes muscle tone (see Chapters 18 and 21). In other words, an active process, rather than simply relaxation, produces REM sleep's characteristic atonic paresis.

On a biochemical level, increased acetylcholine (cholinergic) activity seems to promote REM sleep. Cholinergic agonists, such as arecoline, physostigmine, and nicotine, induce or enhance REM activity. Conversely, anticholinergic medications, including antidepressants with anticholinergic activity, suppress it. In addition, REM sleep is associated with decreased activity of monoamine, mostly adrenergic, neurotransmitters: dopamine, norepinephrine, epinephrine, and serotonin.

NREM Sleep

NREM sleep, in contrast to REM sleep, has four stages distinguished primarily by progressively greater depths of unconsciousness and slower, higher-voltage EEG patterns. In addition, during early NREM sleep, eyes roll slowly and cognitive activity consists only of brief, rudimentary, and readily forgotten thoughts or notions. Unlike individuals' ability to recall dreams that occurred during their REM sleep, they can recall little, if anything, of the thought content that developed during their NREM sleep.

TABLE 17-1 ■ Normal Sleep

	Stage	Bodily Movements	Ocular Movements	EMG	EEG
NREM					
1	Light	Persistent face and limb tone with repositioning every 15–20 minutes	Slow, rolling	Continual activity	Loss of alpha (8–12 Hz) activity
2	Intermediate	Same	Slow, rolling	Further reduction	Sleep spindles and K complexes
3	Slow-wave, deep, delta	Same	Slow, rolling	Further reduction	Increased proportion of slow-wave (1–3 Hz) activity
4	Slow-wave, deep, delta	Same	Slow, rolling	Further reduction	Greatest proportion of slow-wave activity
REM	Activated, paradoxical	Flaccid, areflexic paresis, except for brief face and limb movements	Rapid, conjugate	Silent	Low voltage fast with ocular movement artifacts

EMG, electromyogram; EEG, electroencephalogram; NREM, nonrapid eye movement; REM, rapid eye movement.

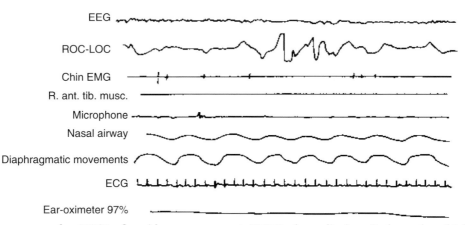

FIGURE 17-1 ■ Polysomnography (PSG) of rapid eye movement (REM) sleep displays 9 channels, which each monitor a physiologic function. Depending on the clinical problem, additional channels may be added. The electroencephalogram (EEG) has low-voltage, fast activity similar to the EEG activity of awake individuals. The electro-oculogram (EOG) channel—ROC-LOC—reflects several REMs by large-scale, quick fluctuations. Electromyograms (EMGs) of the chin and right anterior tibialis muscles show virtually no activity, which indicates an absence of muscle movement and tone (flaccid paresis). The microphone detects a snore. The regular, undulating airway and diaphragm recordings indicate normal breathing and air movement.

Other distinguishing features of NREM sleep relate to the motor system. During NREM sleep, individuals have conspicuous repositioning movements of the body, relatively normal muscle tone, and preserved deep tendon reflexes (DTRs). Their chin and limb muscles display easily detectable EMG activity (Fig. 17-2).

In addition, individuals in NREM sleep, unlike those in REM sleep, have a generalized decrease in ANS activity. The decrease typically leads to hypotension and bradycardia. Similarly, cerebral blood flow and oxygen metabolism fall to about 75% of the awake state, which reaches the level produced by light anesthesia. These physiologic alterations may explain the increased incidence of stroke in the early morning hours.

Nevertheless, important hypothalamic-pituitary (neuroendocrine) activity accompanies NREM sleep. The daily secretion of growth hormone occurs almost entirely during NREM sleep, about 30 to 60 minutes after sleep begins. Likewise, serum prolactin concentration rises to its highest level soon after sleep begins. Also, cortisol secretion occurs in 5 to 7 discrete late night-time episodes, which accumulate to yield the day's highest cortisol concentration at about 8:00 AM.

Overall, the third and fourth stages of NREM sleep, usually called *slow-wave, delta,* or *deep NREM*

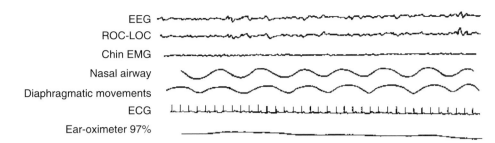

FIGURE 17-2 ■ Polysomnogram (PSG) of stage 1 nonrapid eye movement (NREM) sleep reveals slow electroencephalogram (EEG) activity. Stages 3 and 4 NREM sleep (slow-wave sleep) would show higher-voltage, slower EEG activity. The ROC-LOC channel shows virtually no ocular movement (i.e., no REM activity). Continual, low-voltage EMG activity in the chin muscles reflects persistent muscle tone.

sleep, provide most of the physical recuperation derived from a night's sleep. As if the immediate role of sleep were to revitalize the body, slow-wave sleep occurs predominantly in the early night. After "squeezing in" slow-wave sleep at the beginning of the night, remaining sleep lightens and allows more dreams, that is, naturally shifts to stages 1 and 2 of NREM and REM sleep.

On a biochemical level, whereas REM sleep is associated with increased cholinergic activity, NREM sleep is associated with decreased adrenergic and cholinergic activity. However, wakefulness is associated with increased adrenergic and cholinergic activity.

In summary:

	Cholinergic Activity	**Adrenergic* Activity**
Wakefulness	Increased	Increased
NREM sleep	Decreased	Decreased
REM sleep	Increased	Decreased

*Catecholaminergic and serotoninergic systems.

Patterns

After going to bed, people usually fall asleep within 10 to 20 minutes. That interval, *sleep latency,* is inversely related to sleepiness: The greater the sleepiness, the quicker people fall asleep and the shorter the interval. During daytime, sleep latency reaches its shortest duration during the afternoon, at approximately 4:00 PM, but numerous psychologic and physical factors may alter it. For example, adolescents, who resist sleep, have the longest sleep latency, but elderly people, college students, and individuals with specific sleep disorders have relatively short sleep latencies (Table 17-2).

Once asleep, normal individuals enter NREM sleep and pass in succession through its four stages. After 90 to 120 minutes of NREM sleep, they enter the initial

TABLE 17-2 ■ Sleep Latency* Changes
Shortened sleep latency
Alcohol- and drug-induced sleep
Narcolepsy
Sleep apnea
Sleep deprivation
Prolonged sleep latency
Delayed sleep phase syndrome
Poor sleep hygiene
Psychiatric disorders
Acute schizophrenia
Anxiety
Major depression
Mania
Restless legs syndrome

*Normal sleep latency is approximately 10 to 20 minutes.

TABLE 17-3 ■ Shortened or Sleep-Onset REM Latency*
Depression
Narcolepsy
Sleep apnea
Sleep deprivation^
Withdrawal from alcohol, hypnotics, and TCAs

REM, rapid eye movement; TCAs, tricyclic antidepressants.
*Normal REM latency is approximately 90 to 120 minutes.
^As part of REM rebound.

REM period. Abnormalities in the interval between falling asleep to the first REM period, the *REM latency,* characterize several sleep disorders, particularly narcolepsy (Table 17-3).

The NREM-REM cycle repeats itself throughout the night with a periodicity of approximately 90 minutes. REM periods develop four or five times in total, but in the latter half of the night, they lengthen and occur more frequently (Fig. 17-3). Also, in the latter half, when the tendency toward REM sleep peaks,

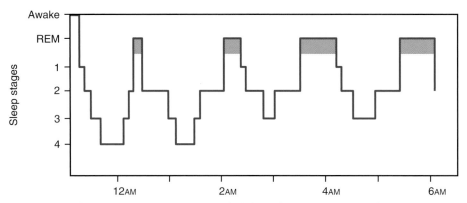

FIGURE 17-3 ■ In the conventional representation of a normal night's sleep pattern—its sleep *architecture*—the first rapid eye movement (REM) period starts about 90 minutes after sleep begins and has a duration of approximately 10 minutes. Later in the night, REM periods recur more frequently and have longer duration. Nonrapid eye movement (REM) sleep progresses through regular, progressively lighter stages.

body temperature falls to its lowest point (the nadir). The final REM period typically merges with awakening. Consequently, surrounding morning household activities may influence a person's final dream, which people can recall. In addition, on awakening, men often have erections.

Without external clues, an "internal biologic clock," centered in the *suprachiasmatic nucleus* of the hypothalamus, would set the daily (*circadian*) sleep-wake cycle at 24.5 to 25 hours (Fig. 17-4). When individuals are forced to rely exclusively on their internal biologic clock, as when they volunteer for experiments that isolate them from their environment and its clues, such as living in caves for months, they gradually lengthen their cycle to almost 25 hours and fall asleep later each day.

Adults average 7.5 to 8 hours of total sleep time, but with a broad range from 4 to 10 hours. Genetic and personal factors probably determine each individual's total sleep requirement; however, environmental light-dark cycles, work schedules, and social plans override it.

Melatonin

Light-dark cycles regulate the sleep-wake cycle in large part through their effect on the pineal gland's synthesis and release of melatonin (*N*-acetyl-5-methoxytryptamine). In turn, melatonin regulates the suprachiasmatic nucleus, which has melatonin receptors on its surface.

The pineal gland synthesizes melatonin, which is an indolamine, through the following pathway:

$$\text{Tryptophan} \rightarrow \text{Serotonin} \rightarrow N\text{-acetyl-} \atop \text{serotonin} \rightarrow \text{Melatonin}$$

Darkness promotes melatonin synthesis and its release into the plasma. Thus, melatonin concentrations rise during night. Similarly, because both natural and artificial light suppress melatonin synthesis and release, its concentration falls during daylight hours. Given its relationship to light, altered melatonin concentrations may play a role in seasonal affective disorder.

Certain medications may change melatonin concentrations. For example, noradrenergic and selective serotonin reuptake inhibitors (SSRIs) and antipsychotics increase melatonin concentration. In contrast, benzodiazepines, monoamine depleting medications, and tryptophan deficiency decrease melatonin concentration.

Melatonin, as a medication, increases sleepiness and REM sleep. It aids in the treatment of insomnia, jet lag, and possibly the delayed sleep phase syndrome (see later). In addition, it may be useful for blind individuals who would benefit from medications that mimic alterations ordinarily induced by light and dark cycles.

Using another strategy to combat insomnia, ramelteon (Rozerem) attempts to promote sleep by binding to melatonin receptors. Stimulation of melatonin receptors inhibits adenyl cyclase activity and thus decreases cyclic AMP. Because fluvoxamine inhibits CYP1A2, concurrent administration of ramelteon and fluvoxamine may lead to increases in ramelteon concentrations that may reach toxic levels.

Sleep Deprivation

When it interrupts a conventional schedule, sleep deprivation causes predictable sleep pattern alterations. Adults who have worked all night and children who skip a customary afternoon nap, for example, have a short sleep latency, increased sleep time, and additional slow-wave sleep. Simply put, after missing sleep, people are tired, fall asleep early, sleep longer, and catch-up on their NREM sleep.

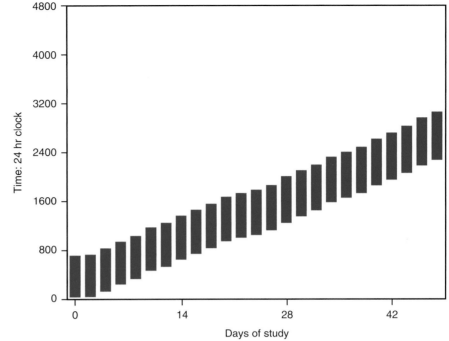

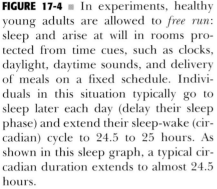

FIGURE 17-4 ■ In experiments, healthy young adults are allowed to *free run*: sleep and arise at will in rooms protected from time cues, such as clocks, daylight, daytime sounds, and delivery of meals on a fixed schedule. Individuals in this situation typically go to sleep later each day (delay their sleep phase) and extend their sleep-wake (circadian) cycle to 24.5 to 25 hours. As shown in this sleep graph, a typical circadian duration extends to almost 24.5 hours.

In another characteristic change, they also have *REM rebound*. This manifestation of sleep deprivation has several major components: The first REM period occurs soon or immediately after falling asleep (*sleep onset REM*), subsequent REM periods are longer than normal, and REM sleep occupies a greater proportion of sleep time. REM rebound translates into sleep-deprived people tending to dream almost as soon as they fall asleep and then plentifully throughout the night.

On some occasions, REM is so abundant and forceful that its final period briefly spills into wakefulness. In those cases, REM-induced paralysis leaves people momentarily unable to move. The same phenomenon occurs in narcolepsy (see later).

REM rebound occurs not only after naturally occurring sleep deprivation, but also following *withdrawal* from REM-suppressing substances, such as alcohol, hypnotics, cocaine and amphetamine, and tricyclic antidepressants (TCAs) (see Table 17-3). People who suddenly stop steady use of these substances often undergo a period of frequent, vivid dreams that can reach the severity of nightmares.

Effects of Age

Sophisticated testing can detect REM-NREM cycles in a 20-week fetus. Neonates sleep 16 to 20 hours a day, with about 50% of that time spent in REM sleep. As individuals mature, they spend less total time sleeping and proportionally less of that time dreaming.

Young children spend 10 to 12 hours sleeping during the night and in afternoon naps, with about 30% in REM sleep. By age 6 years, however, they give up their afternoon nap to consolidate their sleep into the night.

Adolescents and teenagers allow themselves too little time for sleep, despite their great need for it. In addition, social behaviors lead to erratic patterns.

Adults average 6 to 8 hours of total sleep time with a decreased proportion—20% to 30%—in REM sleep. Those adults who are accustomed to relatively little sleep have an increased proportion of slow-wave NREM sleep. In other words, adults preserve slow-wave NREM sleep at the expense of their REM and lighter stages of NREM sleep.

The elderly sleep somewhat less than young and middle-aged adults. Their night-time sleep is relatively short and fragmented by multiple brief awakenings, especially in the early morning. The elderly recoup their sleep during daytime naps after meals, in the late afternoon, and other times of normal sleepiness. In addition, in what is termed *phase-advance*, the elderly, compared to young adults, go to sleep in the earlier evening and awaken earlier in the early morning. Thus, early morning awakening in the elderly does not necessarily constitute a sign of depression.

Decreased total REM time also characterizes sleep in the elderly. Moreover, during REM sleep, often because of their use of hypnotics and certain medications, such as L-dopa, the elderly experience relatively frequent nightmares.

Also, NREM sleep, especially its slow-wave phase, shrinks in the elderly. In fact, slow-wave sleep, as a percent of total sleep time, shows the greatest loss. Slow-wave sleep almost entirely disappears in people older than 75 years. Whereas, in response to reduced total sleep, young adults tend to preserve slow-wave sleep, elderly individuals sacrifice it.

In addition to these normal variations, certain sleep disorders plague the elderly: restless legs syndrome, REM behavior disorder, and sleep apnea syndrome (see later). Also, cardiovascular disturbances and other medical disorders, medication side effects, pain, depression, dementia, and other neurologic illnesses disrupt their sleep.

SLEEP DISORDERS

Neurologists follow the *International Classification of Sleep Disorders* manual, which is, for the most part, consistent with the *Diagnostic and Statistical Manual of Mental Disorders, 4th Edition, Text Revision* (*DSM-IV-TR*). Both are based on the three major categories of sleep disorders (Table 17-4):

- Dyssomnias
- Parasomnias
- Medical/psychiatric disorders

DYSSOMNIAS

The dyssomnias either impair initiating or maintaining sleep (falling asleep or staying asleep) or cause *excessive daytime sleepiness* (*EDS*). This category considers dyssomnias as *Intrinsic, Extrinsic,* and *Circadian Disorders*. Although dyssomnias and other sleep disorders often cause EDS, by far the most common causes of EDS are social and vocation pressures. Other causes, which are also external and non-neurologic, include medicine, illicit drug, and alcohol use; shift-work sleep disorder; and medical illnesses. In quantifying a patient's symptom of sleepiness, physicians often utilize the Epworth Sleepiness Scale (Table 17-5). Nevertheless, by whatever measure, if patients have EDS from sleep apnea, narcolepsy, work-shift sleep disorder, or another condition, it is dangerous. They make mistakes at work, develop mood disorders, and have a markedly increased rate of traffic accidents.

Intrinsic Sleep Disorders

The Intrinsic Sleep Disorders classification includes important, discrete, and well-established neurophysiologic disturbances. Patients typically come to medical attention because of EDS.

TABLE 17-4 ■ Classifications of Sleep Disorders*

American Sleep Disorders Association	DSM-IV-TR
1. Dyssomnias	1. Primary Sleep Disorders
A. Intrinsic	A. Dyssomnias
Insomnia	Primary Insomnia
Psychophysiological	
Idiopathic	
Narcolepsy	Narcolepsy
Sleep Apnea Syndrome	Breathing-Related Sleep Disorder
Periodic Limb Movements	
Restless Legs Syndrome	
Hypersomnias	Primary Hypersomnia
B. Extrinsic	
Inadequate Sleep Hygiene	
Environmental Sleep Disorder	
Hypnotic, Stimulant, Alcohol, and Toxin Dependency	
C. Circadian	Circadian Rhythm Sleep Disorder
Time Zone Change (Jet Lag)	
Shift-work	
Delayed Sleep Phase	
2. Parasomnias	B. Parasomnias
A. Arousal Disorders	
Confusional Arousals	
Sleep Terrors	Sleep Terror Disorder
Sleepwalking	Sleepwalking Disorder
B. Sleep-Wake Transition Disorders	
Rhythmic Movement Disorder	
Sleep Talking	
C. Parasomnias Usually Associated with REM Sleep	
Nightmares	Nightmare Disorder
REM Sleep Behavior Disorder	
D. Other Parasomnias	
Bruxism	
Enuresis	
3. Medical/Psychiatric Disorders	2. Sleep Disorders Related to Another Mental Disorder
A. Psychiatric	
Psychoses	A. Insomnia
Depression	B. Hypersomnia
Alcoholism	
B. Neurologic	3. Sleep Disorder Related to a General Medical Condition ^
Dementia	
Parkinson's disease	
Fatal Familial Insomnia	4. Substance-Induced Sleep Disorder+
Epilepsy	
Headaches	
C. Other	

*Major categories and examples in the classification by the American Sleep Disorders Association, 1991, with their counterparts in the DSM-IV-TR.

^ Including neurologic conditions.

+ Including medication-induced disorders.

TABLE 17-5 ■ The Epworth Sleepiness Scale

How likely are you to doze off or fall asleep in the following situations, in contrast to just feeling tired? This refers to your usual way of life in recent times. Even if you have not done some of these things recently, try to work our how often they would have affected you. Use the following scale to choose the most appropriate number for each situation.

0 = would never doze
1 = slight chance of dozing
2 = moderate chance of dozing
3 = high chance of dozing

Situation	Chance of Dozing
Sitting and reading	
Watching TV	
Sitting, inactive in a public place, e.g., a theater or a meeting	_____
As a passenger in a car for 1 hour without a break	_____
Lying down to rest in the afternoon when circumstances permit	_____
Sitting and talking to someone	_____
Sitting quietly after a lunch without alcohol	_____
In a car, while stopped for a few minutes in traffic	_____
Total Score	_____

This widely used scale allows for a quantitative assessment of sleepiness and determination that an individual has excessive daytime sleepiness. A total score of ≤8 is normal; a total score of 9–12 indicates that the patient is possibly sleepy; a total score of ≥13 indicates that the patient is abnormally sleepy. (From Johns MW: A new method for measuring daytime sleepiness: The Epworth Scale. Sleep 14:540–545, 1991.)

Narcolepsy

Narcolepsy, the most dramatic of the Intrinsic Disorders, affects men and women equally and starts in 90% of patients between their adolescence and 30th year. Its onset, in such young people, often remains undetected or misinterpreted as a neurotic disorder or depression. The most salient feature of narcolepsy, EDS, takes the form of brief, irresistible sleep episodes (attacks). The attacks initially mimic normal daytime naps because they typically occur when patients are bored, comfortable, and engaged in monotonous activities. Each attack usually lasts less than 15 minutes and can be easily interrupted by noise or movement.

As narcolepsy progresses, the attacks evolve into episodes that clearly differ from normal naps but still resemble ones brought on by severe sleep deprivation. Narcolepsy sleep attacks have a relatively abrupt onset and take place when patients are standing, during a lively interchange, or in the middle of activities that require constant attention, including driving. Multiple attacks occur daily. Moreover, they cause momentary amnesia, confusion, and autonomic changes.

The other cardinal symptoms of narcolepsy, *cataplexy, sleep paralysis,* and *sleep hallucinations,* usually develop after the sleep attacks and also reflect disordered REM sleep. Combined with sleep attacks, these symptoms form the *narcoleptic tetrad:*

- Narcolepsy (sleep attacks)
- Cataplexy
- Sleep paralysis
- Sleep hallucinations

Whereas irresistible sleep occurs in several conditions and disables the patient more than any other symptom, cataplexy stands as the unique, almost pathognomonic feature of the syndrome. It begins about 4 years after the onset of narcolepsy and consists of episodes, typically lasting 30 seconds or less, of sudden weakness precipitated by emotional situations. Unless patients have a simultaneous sleep attack, they remain alert during an attack of cataplexy. The three most common situations that lead to an attack are hearing or telling a joke, laughing, or feeling anger. Other situations that provoke cataplexy include being surprised, being frightened, or having sex.

Cataplexy episodes typically occur one to four times daily. The weakness that they cause tends to be symmetric and proximal. For example, the neck, trunk, hips, knees, or shoulders may suddenly lose their strength. Sometimes the eyelids, jaw, or face weaken alone or in combination with the trunk and limbs. In manifestations that physicians could easily dismiss, cataplexy may induce only a brief period of a jaw dropping open or head nodding forward. In only its most sensational but rare form, patients' entire body musculature becomes limp and they collapse to the floor. Whether a group of muscles or the entire musculature weakens, affected muscles become flaccid and areflexic as in REM sleep. Nevertheless, as also in REM sleep, patients breathe normally and retain complete ocular movement.

Sleep paralysis and sleep hallucinations—other components of the tetrad—affect only about 15% of patients. They develop several years after the onset of narcolepsy. In other words, only 10% of narcolepsy patients display the full narcoleptic tetrad. Sleep paralysis and sleep hallucinations may be present on awakening (hypnopompic) or while falling asleep (hypnagogic). In sleep paralysis, patients are unable to move for several seconds on awakening or when falling asleep, but they can breathe and move their eyes. Although sleep paralysis is a characteristic feature of narcolepsy, it is not diagnostic because it routinely occurs in sleep deprived individuals and others with sleep onset REM.

While having hypnopompic or hypnagogic hallucinations, patients essentially experience vivid twilight dreams that qualify as an organic cause of visual hallucinations (see Chapters 9 and 12). As with the other features of narcolepsy, hypnopompic or hypnagogic hallucinations represent REM sleep intruding into people's wakefulness (Fig. 17-5).

In addition to the narcolepsy tetrad, multiple, brief, spontaneous awakenings interrupt night-time sleep. These interruptions cause inadequate night-time sleep that exacerbates the EDS.

Among children, EDS, whether from narcolepsy, sleep apnea, or other disorders, leads to somewhat different symptoms than in adults with the same disorders. Instead of being merely sleepy, children typically develop inattention and often "paradoxical hyperactivity" (increased, usually purposeless, activity). Children with narcolepsy also have behavioral, cognitive, and scholastic disabilities that resemble symptoms of learning disabilities or attention deficit hyperactivity disorder. When combined with cataplexy (see later), these children may appear to have a behavioral disorder.

The *multiple sleep latency test (MSLT)* can confirm a clinical diagnosis of narcolepsy. Using PSG recording techniques, the MSLT determines both sleep latency and REM latency during four or five "nap opportunities" presented at 2-hour intervals during daytime. Compared to the normal adult sleep latency of 10 to 20 minutes, narcoleptic sleep latency usually lasts 5 minutes or less. Also in narcolepsy, the first REM period begins immediately or within 10 minutes of falling asleep rather than following the normal,

preliminary 90 minutes of NREM stages. These short or nonexistent REM latencies fall into the category of *sleep onset REM periods (SOREMPs)*. The majority of narcoleptic patients have two or more SOREMPs during their MSLT.

Although sensitive for the diagnosis of narcolepsy, the MSLT also shows shortened sleep latency and SOREMPs in other conditions characterized by EDS, such as sleep apnea, sleep deprivation, and periodic limb movement disorder. To reduce false-positive results on the MSLT from these conditions, patients suspected of having narcolepsy should first undergo a PSG.

A complementary test measures daytime sleepiness by assessing an individual's ability to remain awake. The *Repeated Test of Sustained Wakefulness (RTSW)* assesses an individual's ability to remain awake in a quiet, dark room throughout the daytime. Those who tend to fall asleep have EDS; however, such a determination does not constitute a diagnosis.

Narcolepsy results, in part, from a genetic predisposition. First-degree relatives have a 20- to 40-fold increased risk of developing the illness. Almost 90% of patients with cataplexy as well as narcolepsy carry a certain major histocompatibility complex, designated human leukocyte antigen (HLA) DQB1, on chromosome 6. However, mostly because approximately 25% of the general population with no symptoms also carries the antigen, it is neither sufficient nor necessary to diagnose narcolepsy-cataplexy.

In a major medical advance that has located its physiologic basis, studies have shown close association between narcolepsy and a deficiency in a pair of polypeptide excitatory neurotransmitters, *hypocretin* 1 and 2, also known as *orexin* A and B. These peptides normally produce wakefulness and activity and stimulate the appetite. Increased concentrations are associated with wakefulness and REM sleep and decreased levels with NREM sleep.

Cells in the hypothalamus normally synthesize hypocretin, which enters tracts to the cerebral cortex and brainstem structures involved with sleep, particularly the locus ceruleus, dorsal raphe nuclei, and substantia nigra. Some hypocretin enters the

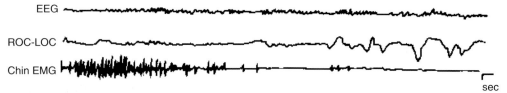

FIGURE 17-5 ■ A narcoleptic attack begins when the electroencephalogram (EEG) channel shows low-voltage fast activity characteristic of rapid eye movement (REM) sleep. The loss of chin electromyogram (EMG) activity indicates that muscles are flaccid. After several seconds, rapid ocular movements begin. The multiple sleep latency test (MSLT) would show similar, characteristic sleep onset REM periods (SOREMPs). However, one SOREMP does not constitute a diagnosis of narcolepsy.

cerebrospinal fluid (CSF). (Different research groups named *hypo*cretin for its location in the *hypo*thalamus, and orexin for *orexis* [Greek, appetite].)

Distinctive findings in narcolepsy-cataplexy consist of absence of hypocretin in the CSF and near or total degeneration of hypocretin-synthesizing cells in the hypothalamus. The absence of CSF hypocretin correlates much more closely with narcolepsy with cataplexy than narcolepsy without cataplexy. Curiously, serum hypocretin concentrations remain normal, which suggests that cells outside the brain also synthesize the polypeptide.

Although a deficiency in hypocretin, perhaps as the result of autoimmune attack on the hypothalamus, seems to underlie most cases of narcolepsy-cataplexy, some have followed head trauma, multiple sclerosis, or tumors. As might be expected, some patients with these conditions have reduced CSF hypocretin concentrations. Narcolepsy with the characteristic hypocretin deficiency also occurs in an autosomal recessive inheritance pattern in certain families of ponies and dogs. Some of them serve as laboratory models of the disorder.

The primary goal in treatment of narcolepsy is for the patient to remain awake at critical times, particularly when driving, attending school, and working. In one approach, methylphenidate (Ritalin) and amphetamines, which enhance adrenergic and dopaminergic activity, reduce EDS and the naps. In a complementary strategy, TCAs and SSRIs, which suppress REM sleep, reduce narcolepsy; however, their benefit is modest, short-lived, and, if abruptly stopped, complicated by rebound cataplexy.

In a newer, superior approach, the nonamphetamine medication, modafinil (Provigil) promotes wakefulness without causing excitation or night-time insomnia. Moreover, unlike stopping amphetamines and other stimulants, stopping modafinil does not lead to a rebound in NREM sleep. In other words, modafinil does not merely keep people awake by postponing sleep. Although modafinil has no discernible effect on melatonin, dopamine, serotonin, or gamma-aminobutyric acid (GABA), it probably activates hypocretin-synthesizing cells and has an α–1 adrenergic agonist (stimulant) effect.

Despite their help in countering narcolepsy and keeping patients awake, these medicines have little effect on cataplexy. Instead, a rapid-acting hypnotic, oxybate (Xyrem), also known as gamma-hydroxybutyrate (GHB) or the "date-rape drug," reduces cataplexy. In addition, it also increases slow-wave sleep but does not affect REM sleep. Illicitly prepared oxybate has caused many complications, including profound amnesia, coma, seizures, and, with continued use, addiction (see Chapter 21). Even pharmaceutical preparations in narcolepsy-cataplexy patients may lead to sleepwalking, enuresis, confusion, and sleepiness but not to addiction or, on stopping it, rebound insomnia.

Whether or not patients use these medicines, they should arrange for regular, strategically placed daytime naps ("nap therapy") after meals and during the late afternoon. The naps should be brief because short naps provide as must rest and recuperation as long ones. Patients should also maintain regular night-time sleep schedules.

Sleep Apnea

Multiple, 10-second to 2-minute interruptions in breathing (apnea) during sleep characterize sleep apnea, one of the most common causes of EDS. Each hour, five or more episodes of apnea produce partial awakenings ("microarousals"), as though the brain interrupts sleep to breathe. Patients remain unaware of the awakenings because they are so brief and incomplete. Nevertheless, the awakenings lead to restless sleep and subsequent EDS.

As breathing resumes at the end of an apneic episode, patients briefly snore loudly and irregularly. That snoring, an audible characteristic of the disorder, represents a resuscitative mechanism. In practice, loud night-time snoring in individuals with irresistible daytime napping and EDS constitutes a diagnosis of sleep apnea.

During the day, because of their EDS, sleep apnea patients succumb to relatively long but unrefreshing naps. Between attacks, patients are often physically fatigued as well as lethargic.

Sleep apnea includes an *obstructive* and *central* variety. Mechanical airway obstructions, such as thickened soft tissues of the pharynx, congenital cranial deformities, hypertrophied tonsils or adenoids, trauma, and other pharyngeal abnormalities, may cause obstructive sleep apnea. In addition, neuromuscular disorders, such as bulbar poliomyelitis, can also produce weakness of the pharynx that may be severe enough to cause it.

The central variety, which is rare, results from reduced or inconsistent central nervous system (CNS) ventilatory effort. Patients who have survived lateral medullary infarctions (see Chapter 2), bulbar poliomyelitis, and other injuries to the medulla, which houses the respiratory drive center, are susceptible to central sleep apnea.

Both varieties can produce arterial blood oxygen desaturation (hypoxia) with oxygen saturation as low as 40%, cardiac arrhythmias, and pulmonary and systemic hypertension. Thus, sleep apnea constitutes a risk factor for stroke. Directly or indirectly, sleep apnea causes morning headache and confusion. It also may cause persistent intellectual impairment and depression.

Sleep apnea develops predominantly but not exclusively in middle-aged men with hypertension and obesity. However, about 30% of patients are not obese. In addition, sleep apnea may develop in older children, adolescents, and young adults. Even young children, who have enlarged tonsils and adenoids, may develop it. However, unlike adults with sleep apnea, children with the disorder usually maintain a normal weight.

A PSG that shows periods of apnea, arousals, and hypoxia confirms a diagnosis of sleep apnea. In the obstructive variety, the PSG detects intermittently loss of airflow despite chest and diaphragm respiratory movements and episodic loud snoring (Fig. 17-6). Because of sleep deprivation, sleep latency and REM latency both shorten and SOREMPs appear. During night-time sleep, apnea episodes occur in either phase but more frequently during REM sleep.

The management of sleep apnea, in most cases, attempts to have patients lose weight, give up smoking, and stop using hypnotics and alcohol. Modafinil (see later) reduces daytime sleepiness. If those strategies do not alleviate the problem, physicians prescribe ventilation by nasal continuous positive airway pressure (CPAP). Although the device is cumbersome, CPAP remains the best specific treatment. Alternative devices that might secure a patent airway include a tongue-retainer, mandibular advancement prosthesis, or a

small nasopharyngeal tube. In the past, tracheostomies were performed to bypass the pharynx, but now surgeons perform other procedures, such as jaw reconstruction or, in children, tonsillectomy. Once popular, uvulopalatopharyngoplasty (UPPP)—a laser-assisted plastic procedure—yielded disappointing results including undesired voice changes. Fluoxetine, protriptyline, or medroxyprogesterone may improve central sleep apnea.

Periodic Limb Movement Disorder

Periodic limb movement disorder, also called *periodic leg movements* when confined to the legs, consists of regular (periodic), episodic movements of the legs or, less often, arms during sleep. Most often individuals move their feet upward in brief (0.5 to 5.0 second) repetitive, stereotyped jerks. In more extensive variations, the entire legs or the arms as well as the legs move. Whatever the pattern, the feet always move. Movements take place at 20- to 40-second intervals, for periods of 10 minutes to several hours primarily during stages 1 and 2 of NREM sleep (Fig. 17-7). Periodic limb movements, like apneas, tend to arouse patients, but this disorder rarely leads to EDS. However, the movements often disrupt the sleep of a bed-partner, who may develop EDS.

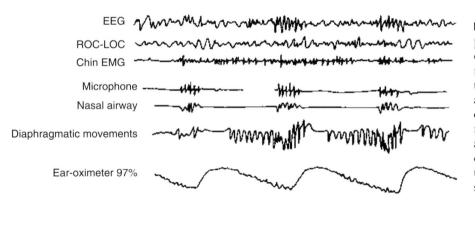

FIGURE 17-6 ■ In sleep apnea, the polysomnogram (PSG) shows that, during a period of nonrapid eye movement (NREM) sleep, oxygen saturation falls. Hypoxia triggers a partial arousal, indicated by faster electroencephalogram (EEG) activity. Diaphragmatic movements reach a crescendo and loud snoring begins. After strenuous diaphragm movements, air moves through the nasal airway and oxygen saturation improves.

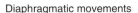

FIGURE 17-7 ■ In periodic limb movements, approximately 30-second intervals of synchronous anterior tibialis contractions cause the patient's ankles to dorsiflex and the electromyogram (EMG) activity.

During periodic limb movements, EMG leads show regular muscle contractions followed by arousals. The disorder usually develops in individuals older than 55 years. It occurs primarily in association with restless legs syndrome but also with sleep apnea and other sleep disorders; use of antidepressants; withdrawal from various medications; and medical illnesses, such as uremia. Benzodiazepines and, as with restless leg syndrome, dopaminergic medications may suppress the movements and restore sleep (see later).

Restless Legs Syndrome

Restless legs syndrome (RLS) consists of involuntary movement of the feet and legs largely in response to an irresistible urge to move or unpleasant sensations. These movements occur predominantly during the early portion of night-time sleep or at other times when patients attempt to rest. To a lesser extent, they also occur during daytime wakefulness.

Characteristically beset by a psychic urge or uncomfortable sensation, RLS patients typically try to obtain relief by walking incessantly or stepping from one foot to the other, moving their feet back and forth while sitting in a chair, or stretching or performing bicycle movements with their legs while lying in bed. Like patients with tics, those with RLS have psychologic discomfort if they fail to respond, but a sense of relief if they do.

Unpleasant sensations (dysesthesias or painful paresthesias), such as burning and aching, deep in patients' feet and legs, almost invariably seem to motivate the movements. In an attempt to reduce these sensations, patients rub, scratch, hit, or stretch their legs. They often attempt to relieve the sensations by walking around the bedroom. Although the family and physicians may see involuntary movements as the problem, patients typically feel that the abnormal sensations and irrepressible urge to move constitute the problem.

Whatever the sequence, the combination of the movements, unpleasant sensations, and attempts to relieve the symptoms cause several problems. The symptoms delay the onset of sleep (prolong sleep latency), later interrupt it, and lead to EDS for both the patient and bed-partner. Moreover, in about 80% of cases, nocturnal periodic leg movements accompany RLS. Despite the frequent comorbidity of RLS and periodic movements, they differ in many respects: Periodic limb movements occur at regular intervals, appear only during sleep, and do not create either an urge to move or sensory symptoms.

Although RLS may develop in young pregnant women and other young adults, it usually first appears in individuals older than 45 years. Several conditions associated with RLS, such as ischemic, diabetic, and uremic polyneuropathies, do not necessarily cause it.

Some patients have iron deficiency anemia characterized by low concentrations of serum ferritin (an iron protein complex). Also, when pregnant women develop RLS, they are usually in their third trimester. During that time, their folate concentrations may be low and their expanded uterus may irritate the adjacent lumbosacral nerves.

An observation that many otherwise healthy individuals with RLS have close relatives with the same problem indicates that RLS has a genetic cause or susceptibility. Decreased D2 receptor binding in the striatum (see Chapter 18) may be responsible for the movements. It also suggests a therapeutic strategy (see later).

Another condition characterized by involuntary nocturnal leg movements, but lacking a sensory component, are the familiar, benign leg thrusts that would appear to protect people when they "fall" asleep. These movements, *sleep starts* or *hypnic* or *hypnagogic jerks*, occur in the twilight of sleep. In view of their time of onset, the classifications consider them a sleep-wake transition disorder parasomnia.

Particularly for psychiatrists, a particularly intriguing aspect of RLS consists of its similarity to *akathisia* (see Chapter 18). The conditions share features—incessant leg movement in response to an urge and common treatments (see later). On the other hand, important differences exist. In akathisia, restlessness but not discomfort occurs throughout the day and subsides when the patient returns to bed in the evening, sensory disturbances do not spur the movements, and periodic limb movements do not routinely complicate the picture. Psychiatrists may also have to consider that both RLS and akathisia may, on at least first glance, mimic agitated depression.

In addition, RLS resembles other involuntary movement disorders (Chapter 18). For example, the illegal substance crack-cocaine sometimes causes *crack dancing*, which consists of incessant and irregular leg and trunk movements accompanied by or in response to psychic agitation. Similarly, chorea, particularly as a component in *Huntington's disease*, leads to incessant involuntary limb movements that interrupt walking, standing, and attempting to lie still in bed.

Finally, RLS is reportedly comorbid with anxiety, depression, and attention deficit/hyperactivity. However, excessive leg movements may be merely a symptom of those disorders rather than a separate condition.

For treatment of idiopathic RLS, dopaminergic medications suppress the movements, reduce the urge to move, and promote restful sleep. In particular, probably because of the decreased D2 receptor binding, dopamine precursors (e.g., L-dopa) and dopamine agonists (e.g., ropinirole) offer the greatest efficacy with the least risk in RLS treatment. With doses as low as 10% of Parkinson's disease treatment, these dopaminergic medicines suppress RLS. For patients with polyneuropathy-induced RLS, medicines that reduce the paresthesias, such as gabapentin and TCAs, help restore sleep. Correcting an iron deficiency anemia frequently reduces the discomfort and movements.

Hypersomnias

The rare Kleine-Levin syndrome, *periodic hypersomnia,* which affects predominantly adolescents, males much more frequently than females, consists of recurrent, 1- to 2-week episodes of sleep (hypersomnia). Patients typically have six episodes, during which they intermittently awaken to eat great quantities of food and display hypersexuality, irritability, and other atypical behavior. When awake, they are confused, withdrawn, and apathetic. However, between episodes, patients have no overt neurologic or psychiatric disorder.

PSGs show only nonspecific frequent awakenings from light, NREM sleep during hypersomnia episodes and none between them. No endocrinologic or other physiologic study shows a consistent, significant abnormality.

In other words, no physical finding, PSG data, or laboratory result can confirm a clinical impression of Kleine-Levin syndrome. Thus, when consulting in cases of suspected Kleine-Levin syndrome, physicians might consider alternatives: depression, drug abuse, focal complex seizures, encephalitis, hypothalamic injuries, and traumatic brain injury (Chapter 22).

Extrinsic Sleep Disorders

Personal, social, or drug- and alcohol-related factors imposed on a normal brain cause *extrinsic sleep disorders.* Circumstances completely outside of the individual, such as a noisy neighborhood, cause *environmental sleep disorder. Inadequate or poor sleep hygiene* includes mostly engaging in activities counterproductive to sleep, such as use of caffeine, alcohol, and certain medications at night or performing exercise, mentally challenging, or anxiety-provoking activities before bed. In most of these conditions, the PSG shows prolonged sleep latency, the physiologic counterpart of "tossing-and-turning" in bed, frequent arousals, and advanced (early morning) awakening. Removing these extrinsic factors from an affected individual's life should restore a normal sleep-wake schedule.

Hypnotic, stimulant, alcohol, or other toxin dependency causes insomnia as well as EDS. The use of these substances for their hypnotic effect defines the condition,

but, cutting a fine line, frank addiction, such as alcoholism, excludes the definition. In the disorder, PSG generally shows short sleep latency, disrupted sleep, and fragmented or suppressed REM phases. Briefly put, people who take bedtime drinks ("nightcaps") rapidly reach deep sleep, but then dependency soon disrupts sleep and subsequently reduces or fragments dreaming.

Just like medicines with hypnotic effects, those with stimulant effects, which are often unappreciated, such as steroids, aminophylline, or pseudoephedrine (Actifed), disrupt sleep. Caffeine, in various preparations, remains the most common and widely known stimulant (Table 17-6). Many Americans easily and often inadvertently ingest so much caffeine (250 to 500 mg per day) that they develop *caffeinism*: insomnia, agitation, tremulousness, palpitations, gastric distress, and diuresis.

When people stop taking medicines or other substances that suppress sleep, they usually fail to sleep properly. During this period of withdrawal, affected individuals not only have insomnia, they have EDS and psychologic agitation. Also, when finally able to fall asleep, they characteristically have REM rebound as though their body recoups lost dream time. With abrupt withdrawal from alcohol or barbiturates, especially short-acting ones, people may develop generalized, tonic-clonic seizures or delirium tremens (DTs).

Circadian Rhythm Disorders

Both neurophysiologic and external factors can alter the sleep-wake schedule to produce *circadian rhythm disorders.* In the best-known example, *time zone change syndrome (jet lag),* people who rapidly traverse at least two time zones develop insomnia and EDS accompanied by changes in digestion and other autonomic behavior. Many travelers feel as though their mind and body have remained on the schedule of their city of origin.

Going east-to-west creates fewer problems than west-to-east because travelers can more easily postpone (delay) their night's sleep than fall asleep earlier (advance it). When going in either direction, travelers can facilitate the transition by shifting their sleep-wake schedule to their destination city's day-night schedule by initiating it *before* the trip or assuming it immediately on arrival. Travelers also can further facilitate the adjustment by exposing themselves to daylight once they have reached their destination. (Light is more powerful than noise in entraining people to a new sleep-wake schedule.) In addition, on long west-to-east flights, the most taxing, travelers can take melatonin or other hypnotic to advance their sleep schedule so that it will conform to the new time zone.

TABLE 17-6 ■ Caffeine Content of Popular Beverages, Medicines, and Foods (in mg)	
Coffees*	
Brewed	
Generic	80–175
Decaf	4
Dunkin' Donuts	143
Expresso^	100
General Foods	
Café Vienna	90
Swiss Mocha	55
Instant, generic	60
Starbucks	200
Teas	
Lipton	
Brewed	40
Peppermint	0
Celestial Seasonings	
Ginseng	50
Herbal	0
Generic	
Black	45
Green	20
White	15
Green tea	30
Snapple	
Black	14
Lemon, Peach	21
Sweet	8
Mistic Lemon	12
Nesta Lemon Sweet	11
Soft Drinks	
7-UP	
Regular	0
Diet	0
AMP Energy Drink	71
Cocoa	2–20
Coca-Cola	
C2	23
Classic	23
Diet	31
Dr. Pepper	28
Jolt	72
Mountain Dew	35
Pepsi-Cola	25
Sprite	
Regular	0
Diet	0
Medicines	
Anacin (2 tablets)	64
Coryban-D Cold	30
Excedrin (2 tablets)	130
NoDoz (1 tablet max.)	200
Vivarin (1 tablet)	200
Miscellaneous	
Ben & Jerry's Coffee	
Frozen Yogurt	85
Chocolate+	
Dark	20

TABLE 17-6 ■ Continued	
Milk	6
Chocolate cake	20–30
Starbucks Coffee	
Ice Cream	40–60

*Although consumers often drink the 12 oz. or larger size of many beverages, this table lists the caffeine content of 8 oz. except for expresso and miscellaneous items. For coffees, caffeine varies by the type of bean, preparation, and fineness of the grind. For teas and coffees, the duration of brewing also determines the caffeine content.
^1.5–2 oz.
+One bar, approximately 1.5 oz.

A related cause of insomnia and EDS caused entirely by external factors is the *shift-work sleep disorder.* This disorder plagues medical house-staff, police officers, factory workers, and other individuals who must work daytime shifts and then rotate to work during evening or night-time shifts. Almost 20% of American workers have schedules that change on a weekly, monthly, or seasonal basis.

Workers starting a new shift typically suffer fatigue and then an inability to fall asleep. They may have a different timing of "daytime sleepiness." Although most workers can make the transition after several days, some may be unsuccessful because their internal schedule is too ingrained or, during weekends or holidays, they continue to follow their old schedule. To supplement conventional strategies, such as drinking coffee and exposure to sunlight, during the transition days when starting a new shift, affected individuals may benefit from taking modafinil. Although imperfect, it reduces extreme sleepiness and improves performance

Whereas factors outside the individual—extrinsic factors—cause the previous disorders, an intrinsic, neurophysiologic delay in falling asleep (prolonged sleep latency) causes the *delayed sleep phase syndrome.* In this disorder, sleep has a delayed start but thereafter a normal quality and duration. The entire sleep cycle, otherwise quite ordinary, merely seems to take place later than customarily in the circadian schedule.

The delayed sleep phase syndrome most commonly first develops in adolescents during a long vacation when they remain active until the early morning. Their late bedtime postpones the time that they awaken. Although the delay may seem benign during a vacation, affected individuals continue to adhere to their new schedule. With their unconventional sleep-wake timing, they cannot attend either school or work without being tardy. When forced to awake "on time," they remain sleep-deprived and perpetually tired. Their delayed sleep-wake schedule, which gives rise to truancy and EDS, resists the usual sleep-altering interventions, such as hypnotics and going to bed earlier.

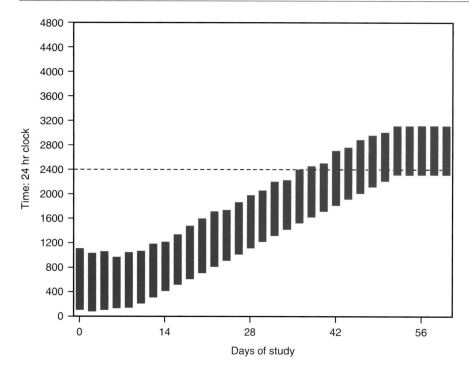

FIGURE 17-8 ▪ A 17-year-old high-school student, with the delayed sleep phase syndrome, has been unable to fall asleep before 1:00 AM or to arise before 9:00 AM. He has been unable to attend school on a regular basis and has gathered friends who have no curfews. Brought into a sleep laboratory, his sleep graph demonstrates a delayed sleep phase during the first week of study. Then each succeeding night, the staff encourages him to remain awake for an additional 30 minutes. By the end of 6 weeks, they have postponed (delayed) his sleep time to 2300 hours (11:00 PM) and then they awaken him at 8:00 AM. For the next week, the 11:00 PM to 8:00 AM is reinforced. The young man stays on this schedule for many months. This strategy, chronotherapy, does not require hypnotics, stimulants, or other medication; a sleep laboratory; or trained personnel.

In a physiologic, nonpharmacologic, and usually successful treatment of the delayed sleep phase syndrome, *chronotherapy*, therapists force affected individuals to delay their sleeptime by 30 minutes to 3 hours successively each night. Using activities, coffee and other stimulants, sunlight, or strong artificial light, this strategy eventually postpones (delays) the sleep onset time by *almost* 24 hours. Patients eventually fall asleep at a conventional time, such as 11:00 PM, and, with effort, maintain that schedule (Fig. 17-8).

PARASOMNIAS

Behavioral or physiologic aberrations, *parasomnias*, intrude into otherwise normal deep, slow-wave NREM sleep. Susceptible individuals usually develop parasomnias during the first 2 hours of sleep if an outside event or internal disorder fully or partially arouses them. Stress and sleep deprivation seem to precipitate most episodes. Immature physiologic mechanisms presumably prevent an orderly transition from deep sleep toward wakefulness.

Aside from parasomnias interrupting their sleep, susceptible individuals usually enjoy normal, restful sleep. In particular, their REM latency maintains normal length (see Tables 17-2 and 17-3), and their days remain free of excessive sleepiness. Parasomnias have no relationship to dreams or REM sleep disturbances.

Arousal Disorders

Confusional Arousals

Confusional arousals consist of disorientation and amnesia when something partly or fully awakens an individual from slow-wave sleep. For example, if a telephone call stirs individuals from deep sleep, they may remain confused during at least the beginning of the conversation. In addition, they will be unable to recall some portions or all of it in the morning.

Sleepwalking

Sleepwalking (somnambulism) usually consists just of sitting or standing but occasionally more complex activities during sleep. In a typical episode, children walk slowly, with their eyes open, along familiar pathways. Although sleepwalking children appear partially awake, their parents cannot completely capture their attention. When questioned, children cannot recall their whereabouts, remember recent events, or converse sensibly.

Sleepwalking and sleep terrors (see later) usually develop in early childhood, affect boys more often than girls, and come to an end before puberty. However, in some individuals episodes of these parasomnias recur through their adult years. Treatment of an episode is neither necessary nor, in view of its brevity, practical; however, episodes occurring several times a week may justify a trial of prophylactic benzodiazepine or imipramine. Until sleepwalking episodes cease, parents should ensure the child's safety by installing night-lights, blocking windows and staircases, and placing alarms in strategic locations.

Children may have more than one variety of parasomnia and display complex behavior during each of them. On the basis of only the parents' description of an episode, physicians might misdiagnose parasomnias as partial complex seizures (see Chapter 10), but these seizures tend to be stereotyped, undergo secondary generalization, and be followed by (postictal) confusion. In children, psychiatric disturbances are not comorbid with parasomnias. However, in adults, various psychiatric disturbances, violence, and CNS pathology are comorbid with parasomnias. PSG, perhaps supplemented by closed circuit EEG monitoring, can distinguish a parasomnia from seizures and abnormal behavior.

Sleep Terrors

Completely different from nightmares (see later), sleep terrors in children consist of episodes in which they suddenly, after a partial awakening from slow-wave sleep, behave as though they were threatened by great danger (Table 17-7). The children stare, moan, and sometimes scream with their eyes fully open and their pupils dilated. They characteristically sweat, hyperventilate, and have tachycardia. They resist their parents' attempts to wake them up, put them back to bed, or comfort them. They often leave their parents' arms to walk aimlessly. The episode lasts for several minutes and ends abruptly with a return to deep sleep. Despite the episode's vivid and awesome features, children do not recall it in the morning.

Sleep terrors usually develop several hours after bedtime and particularly after sleep deprivation. PSG studies show that they arise in slow-wave rather than REM sleep. Noises or other disruptions during slow-wave sleep arouse children and precipitate the episodes. Although frightening events of the day cause nightmares, such events bear no relationship to sleep terrors. Also, although nightmares, like other dreams, occur during REM sleep, night terrors occur during slow-wave NREM sleep. In addition, nightmares occur as often as several times a week, but sleep terrors usually take place only a few times a month.

Night terrors and other parasomnias frequently develop or increase in frequency when children give up their afternoon nap. As they reach this milestone, children are vulnerable because they are "overtired" when they fall asleep and quickly lapse into slow-wave sleep, from which most parasomnias originate.

Parents' enforcing an afternoon nap and avoiding sleep disruptions, such as loud noises, may prevent sleep terrors in some children. Similarly, predisposed children limit themselves to only a few sips of water at bedtime to avoid awakening to urinate. As a last resort, imipramine, benzodiazepines, or paroxetine may help; however, studies have been unable to specify the duration of treatment, likelihood of tolerance developing, or length of post-treatment effectiveness.

Sleep-Wake Transition Disorders

Certain parasomnias have a predilection for appearing during transitions between sleep and wakefulness. In one condition, *rhythmic movement disorder*, infants, children, and occasionally adults have rhythmic, repetitive, stereotyped movements of their head, trunk, or entire body while lying in bed during the initial stages of falling asleep at night or during daytime naps. The condition usually begins in infancy and disappears by age 5 years. The movements usually consist merely of infants slowly rocking their head on the pillow; however, they can increase in forcefulness until they reach the point of *head-banging*. Rhythmic movement disorder can persist into the teenage years and evolve into relatively violent side-to-side rocking of the entire body.

Sleep talking, a common sleep-wake transition disorder, consists of people speaking in their sleep. The term, "talking," however, overstates their verbal

	Sleep Terrors*	Nightmares
Trigger	Partial awakening from deep sleep	Anxiety, fear
Onset	Early in night	Anytime during night
Sleep stage	Stage 3 or 4 NREM (slow-wave sleep)	REM
Verbalization	Crying, screaming	Speaking words, conversing
Autonomic discharge	Marked	Little or none
Behavior after episode	Returns to deep sleep without recall	Awakens, recalls dream content, fearfulness

TABLE 17-7 ■ Sleep Terrors Compared to Nightmares

NREM, nonrapid eye movement; REM, rapid eye movement.
*Other parasomnias frequently accompany terrors.

expression because usually they merely utter a few words. This parasomnia affects both adults and children and takes place in all sleep stages. Sleep talking occurs with no relationship to dreams but sometimes along with sleepwalking and REM sleep behavior (see later).

Parasomnias with REM Sleep

Nightmares

In contrast to sleep terrors, *nightmares* are essentially dreams with frightening content and complex imagery (i.e., "bad dreams"). Children and adults who experience nightmares typically recall them when awake. No bodily movements, except for crying, or autonomic response, other than mild tachycardia, accompany nightmares. Typically, a nightmare ends by itself, but awakening the dreamer can abort it. After becoming fully awake, the dreamer has a slow, difficult return to sleep.

In adults, as in children, nightmares occur during REM periods. Adults tend to have frequent nightmares as a manifestation of REM rebound. Therefore, an evaluation of nightmares in adults should explore not only the circumstances and content of the dreams but also the patient's use of medications, alcohol, and drugs.

REM Sleep Behavior Disorder

During normal REM sleep, even during nightmares, the peri-locus ceruleus nucleus induces motionlessness, flaccidity, and areflexia in limb and trunk muscles. This normal immobility, among other purposes, protects people from participating in their dreams.

In comparison, the *REM sleep behavior disorder* preserves individuals' ability to move and their normal muscle tone during REM sleep. Affected individuals thrash, hit, or make running movements during their REM sleep as though they were participating in their dreams. When awakened from an episode of movement, which can be violent, they typically either recall a dream involving activity or explain that they were only defending themselves against an attack. They deny deliberately aggressive behavior. Individuals with REM sleep behavior disorder, who are usually men older than 65 years, may injure themselves and their bed-partner.

The development of REM sleep behavior disorder often precedes the onset of Parkinson's disease or dementia with Lewy bodies. An accumulation of α-synuclein, as well as Lewy bodies, characterizes these illnesses (see Chapters 7 and 18).

Increased REM activity, especially the REM rebound that follows medication withdrawal, may precipitate attacks. Clonazepam taken at night reduces or eliminates REM sleep behavior disorder. In fact, clonazepam

suppresses it so consistently that a positive response strongly supports the diagnosis. Although SSRIs, TCAs, and, in patients with Parkinson's disease, mirtazapine, suppress REM sleep, they may induce REM sleep behavior disorder. Moreover, these antidepressants allow persistent muscle activity during REM sleep.

Other Parasomnias

Bruxism

Sleep-related, stereotyped, forceful teeth grinding or clenching, *bruxism*, falls into the category of parasomnias. Bruxism makes a loud, disconcerting sound and leads to wearing away of teeth, headaches, and temporomandibular joint dysfunction. Although bruxism occurs in all sleep stages, it develops mainly in the transition from wakefulness to sleep and during light sleep. Individuals with dementia, mental retardation, and Parkinson's disease often have bruxism while awake, as well as when asleep. Night-time dental devices help by cushioning the teeth.

Enuresis

Recurrent involuntary bed-wetting (enuresis), although normal in infants, is considered a parasomnia in girls older than 5 years, boys older than 6 years, and all adults. Enuresis affects boys more than girls, children whose parents had the disorder, and 1% of adults older than 65 years. Like bruxism, enuresis is not restricted to a particular sleep stage or transition; however, it occurs mostly in slow-wave sleep during the first third of the night.

Rather than continuous night-time medications, such as imipramine, behavior modification therapy can best restore night-time bladder control. Evening water restriction, urinary retention control exercises, and "bell and pad" wetness alarm devices alone or in combination suppress enuresis in about 75% of cases. For refractory cases or to avoid potentially embarrassing situations, such having enuresis during a "sleep-over," single injections or nasal sprays of desmopressin (DDAVP), a synthetic form of the antidiuretic hormone (ADH) vasopressin, promotes enough water retention to stop enuresis for one night. However, excessive DDAVP may lead to water retention, even to the point of water intoxication.

PSYCHIATRIC DISORDERS

Mood Disorders

PSG changes in *major depression* are more consistent than in any other psychiatric illness. In *major depression*

PSG studies often show a characteristic triad of abnormalities:

- Short REM latency
- Increased REM density
- Decreased efficiency

However, only a small majority of the patients show the entire triad, no one of the abnormalities is diagnostic, and false-positive findings are common. Thus, although PSGs correlate with major depression, they hold little diagnostic weight.

Specifically, PSGs show REM latency considerably less than 60 minutes or SOREM. REM periods, initially long, occur in quick succession. The large number of REMs per minute (increased REM density) during the early night-time leaves the latter portion of the night almost devoid of REM. The other typical abnormality consists of reduced, fragmented, inefficient slow-wave sleep. That inefficiency accounts not only for reduced total sleep time but also for sleep's failure to restore depressed patients and their EDS.

In addition, depressed individuals have neuroendocrine abnormalities related to their sleep alterations. Their body temperature nadir occurs several hours earlier than normal. Likewise, they have an earlier excretion of cortisol and the norepinephrine metabolite MHPG. Overall, the earlier onset of so many features of sleep—the first REM period, the bulk of REM sleep, the temperature nadir, and nocturnal hormone excretion—results from a forward shift of the normal circadian rhythm (a phase advance). When depressed people fall asleep, they seem to skip into the middle of the normal sleep and neuroendocrine cycle. Sleep disturbances are such an integral part of depression that when it recedes spontaneously or responds to medication, sleep disturbances are one of the last symptoms to improve.

Both TCAs and SSRIs have a hypnotic effect. More important, TCAs postpone the onset of REM (increase REM latency) and reduce REM sleep but increase NREM sleep. Those effects largely reverse those induced by depression. With several exceptions, SSRIs also postpone and reduce REM sleep. Curiously, fluoxetine causes extensive, prominent ocular movements during NREM sleep that mimic REM-induced ocular movements. In another curious aspect, the ocular movements may persist after the fluoxetine has been discontinued. SSRIs may cause myoclonus that has a nocturnal prominence. Also, as previously mentioned, SSRIs and TCAs may exacerbate REM sleep behavior disorder.

In contrast to the effects of depression on sleep latency, *mania* extends sleep latency, sometimes to the point of seeming infinite. Mania can abolish REM sleep and markedly reduce total sleep time.

Psychoses

The data in acute schizophrenia can only provide generalizations. The PSG may show a variety of disturbances including decreased total sleep time, increased sleep latency, and frequent, long awakenings that reflect restlessness ("decreased sleep efficiency"); however, the most consistent finding consists of reduced slow-wave sleep. With chronic schizophrenia, in contrast, PSGs tend to show essentially normal sleep patterns. Interestingly, patients remain able to distinguish their dreams from hallucinations.

Other Psychiatric Disorders

Anxiety disorders also induce a variety of sleep abnormalities. In short, most individuals with anxiety disorder have trouble falling asleep and then staying asleep. The PSG translates those difficulties into prolonged sleep latency and sleep fragmentation. However, their REM latency usually remains normal.

Post-traumatic stress disorder (PTSD) may cause mania-like hypervigilance and insomnia. Although recurrence of the same nightmare and insomnia characterize PTSD, the disorder does not cause frequent, severe, or distinctive sleep alterations on PSG recordings. In other words, psychologic symptoms dwarf physiologic changes.

Alcoholism, also associated with insomnia and EDS, leads, in the first half of the night, to shortened sleep latency, less REM sleep, and increased slow-wave sleep. This pattern mimics alcoholics collapsing into stupor. In the second half of sleep, alcoholics have increased REM and periods of wakefulness, as though they emerged into delirium. The net effect consists of decreased total sleep time and decreased slow-wave sleep. Alcohol withdrawal, which parallels withdrawal from other hypnotic substances, produces insomnia and REM rebound.

Neurologic Disorders

Dementia

Dementia from Alzheimer's disease and related disorders (see Chapter 7), at least in their moderate stages, disrupts patient's sleep-wake cycle and produces night-time thought and behavioral disturbances. During the night, patients tend toward confusion, agitation, and disorientation, especially when brought to new surroundings. For example, Alzheimer's disease patients characteristically wander at night through their house and may actually leave it.

PSGs show increased stage 1 NREM sleep, fragmentations, and decreased efficiency. Patients with dementia typically take many naps of variable length during the day, leading to a "polyphasic sleep" pattern.

Despite an expectation that decreased cholinergic activity in Alzheimer's disease would lead to decreased and delayed REM activity, PSGs do not substantiate such a pattern. Moreover, PSGs do not correlate with any particular etiology of dementia.

Providing daytime exercise, exposure to sunlight, and restricting naps may reduce night-time sleep disturbances in Alzheimer's disease. Nevertheless, early evening administration of tranquilizers, hypnotics, or other medications may help patients and their caregivers have an uninterrupted, restful night of sleep.

Parkinson's Disease

During sleep, *Parkinson's disease* tremor (see Chapter 18) characteristically disappears; however, sleep-related mental disturbances, particularly thought disorders and hallucinations, emerge. Various sleep disorders form an integral part of Parkinson's disease possibly because the disease depigments the locus ceruleus, as well as the substantia nigra. They affect most patients with moderately advanced Parkinson's disease who usually also have comorbid dementia. Of the various symptoms of the illness, caregivers cite sleep-related mental disturbances as the most disruptive one to the family and often the primary reason that they place patients in a nursing home.

In addition to causing sleep-related mental disturbances, Parkinson's disease induces REM sleep behavior disorder (see previous discussion), "sleep reversal" (sleeping during the day and being awake at night), fragmented sleep, and insomnia or hypersomnia. These sleep disorders usually develop in conjunction with Parkinson's disease-induced dementia. In addition, when depression complicates Parkinson's disease, it adds to the sleep disturbances.

Not only does the Parkinson's disease bring about thought disorders, but its medications—both dopamine agonists and L-dopa—often produce vivid dreams that evolve into visual hallucinations. They also lead to EDS, which occurs in men more so than in women and in proportion to the duration and severity of the Parkinson's disease. When patients have severe EDS or ignore premonitory symptoms, the sleepiness can cause "sleep attacks"—episodes of irresistible sleep. Attacks can impair the patient's quality of life and be dangerous, particularly if they occur while patients are driving.

For most patients, reducing the number and dosage of dopaminergic medications and administering them earlier in the evening reduce the sleep-related mental disturbances; however, that strategy may worsen the physical problems in the morning and possibly for the entire day. If tolerated, TCAs may help the patient sleep through the night. Typical antipsychotic agents may reduce night-time hallucinations and agitation, but they also worsen parkinsonism because they block D2 receptors. Clozapine and quetiapine, which produce little or no parkinsonism, suppress serious nocturnal thought and behavioral disturbances.

Other Movement Disorders

As with Parkinson's disease tremor, other basal ganglia-related involuntary movements, such as athetosis and chorea, typically disappear during sleep. In contrast, several involuntary movements occur primarily or exclusively during sleep, such as periodic limb movements, RLS, and hypnic jerks (see previous discussion).

In one special group, disorders commonly evident during the day continue in sleep. This group includes generalized dystonia, tics, blepharospasm, and hemifacial spasm (see Chapter 18). Although partial arousals may precipitate movements, most of them are not confined to a particular sleep stage.

Fatal Familial Insomnia

A recently described illness, *fatal familial insomnia (FFI)*, consists of a progressively severe insomnia, refractory to medicine, that appears on the average at 50 years of age. Neuropsychologic impairments, including inattentiveness, amnesia, sequencing problems, and confusion develop and progress along with the insomnia. Later in their course, patients also suffer hyperactive ANS activity (e.g., tachycardia, hyperhidrosis), endocrine abnormalities (elevated catecholamine and other hormone levels), and motor abnormalities (myoclonus, ataxia). FFI follows a relentless fatal 6- to 36-month course.

FFI, like Creutzfeldt-Jakob disease (see Chapter 7), is a hereditary prion disease caused by a mutation of the prion-protein gene (PRNP) that results in accumulation of abnormal prion protein (PrP^{Sc}). Individuals who are homozygous for the FFI mutation, compared to those who are heterozygous, tend to run a fulminant course characterized by severe sleep disturbances and profound ANS abnormalities. Heterozygous individuals, in contrast, run a longer course with predominantly motor deficits.

Both FFI and Creutzfeldt-Jakob disease present with mental status changes in individuals 50 years old, which is younger than the onset of Alzheimer's disease. In contrast to the pathology of Creutzfeldt-Jakob disease, the thalamus in FFI patients undergoes atrophy. Another difference is that the genetic abnormality entirely determines FFI rather than, as in the case of Creutzfeldt-Jakob disease, merely making individuals susceptible.

Epilepsy

In primary generalized epilepsy compared to focal epilepsy (see Chapter 10), sleep and its NREM stages have a greater role in provoking seizures. About 45% of patients with primary generalized epilepsy have seizures predominantly during sleep. Primary generalized seizures typically develop within stages 1 and 2 of NREM sleep during the first 2 hours of sleep. They also tend to occur at the other end of the sleep cycle—on awakening. REM sleep, in contrast, remains relatively seizure-free.

Focal seizures, compared to primary generalized seizures, occur less frequently during sleep. In addition, when focal seizures occur during sleep, they are less restricted to NREM sleep. When a focal seizure, especially a frontal lobe seizure, develops during sleep, it may resemble a sleep-related disorder, such as a parasomnia, REM sleep behavioral disorder episode, or a nocturnal panic attack. Physicians may require extra EEG electrodes during PSG to distinguish between sleep disturbances and seizures.

Sleep deprivation routinely precipitates seizures in individuals with and sometimes without a history of epilepsy. For example, individuals who have worked all night remain susceptible to tonic-clonic seizures throughout the next day. In more than one third of epileptic patients who have no EEG abnormalities on routine, daytime studies, an EEG obtained during sleep deprivation typically shows sharp waves and a variety of spike-and-sharp wave activity.

Another aspect of epilepsy's interaction with sleep involves its antiepileptic drug (AED) treatment. Even at therapeutic blood concentrations, AEDs may lead to EDS and mood changes. In children and some adults, AEDs may lead instead to hyperactivity. On the other hand, among their many actions, AEDs usually promote normal sleep. In particular, they raise the efficiency of sleep by reducing arousals and increasing slow-wave sleep.

Headaches

REM sleep seems to give rise to migraine and, even more so, cluster headache (see Chapter 9). In some patients, these headache varieties develop only at night during REM periods (nocturnal migraines). For most patients, migraines begin during early morning REM sleep as well as during the day. Thus, excessive sleep or other conditions that increase REM sleep exacerbates them. As would be predicted, medications that suppress REM sleep reduce headaches. Paradoxically, naturally occurring or medication-induced sleep may abort them.

Other Disorders

Sleep may also trigger life-threatening cardiovascular disorders. Angina pectoris and myocardial infarctions take place much more often during REM sleep, when pulse and blood pressure often fluctuate, than during NREM sleep. Thrombotic strokes occur more frequently during NREM sleep, when pulse and blood pressure fall. Family members often discover a stroke only when the individual awakes.

Attacks of asthma, exacerbation of chronic obstructive lung disease, gastroesophageal reflux, and peptic ulcer disease tend to develop during sleep; however, attacks occur with equal frequency in both sleep phases and may be determined by the patient's sleeping position. Whatever their cause, these night-time disturbances interrupt sleep and lead to EDS. In cases of "nocturnal asthma," physicians must not overlook the alternative diagnosis of nocturnal panic attacks.

Violence, in the broadest sense, occurs as an aspect of several conditions: REM sleep behavior disorder, nocturnal focal seizures, head-banging, sleepwalking and other parasomnias, or dementia-induced wandering. In these cases, the physical activity ordinarily consists of poorly directed or self-inflicted flailing or banging but almost never purposeful violence directed at another individual (i.e., aggression) (see Chapter 10). For physicians to accept violence as a manifestation of a sleep disorder, it should have occurred in an individual who has an established history of a sleep disorder. Also, the violence should begin abruptly without provocation, last several minutes or less, and leave little or no residual memory.

Alternatively, several psychiatric disorders, such as dissociative disorders, may express themselves as violence during periods of wakefulness that interrupt sleep. Any episodes of violence that these disorders induce do not constitute sleep-induced violence.

INSOMNIA

Insomnia, a widespread and almost always nonspecific symptom, may be a manifestation of a sleep disorder, a medical illness, substance abuse, other psychiatric disorder, or, in individuals older than 65 years, a normal variant. This book appends a brief discussion of its neurologic aspects.

Treatment of Insomnia

Nonpharmacologic treatments, certainly as part of the initial plan, may alone be sufficient. Individuals should practice good sleep hygiene. They should adhere to a regular sleep schedule even on weekends; exercise on a regular basis, but only during the day; stay away from alcohol, large meals, and stimulants, particularly caffeine and bright light, in the evening; allow themselves, at most, a brief (< 20 minute) early afternoon nap; and use the bed exclusively for sleeping. In addition, individuals with insomnia might try behavior therapies, including relaxation techniques, sleep restriction, and stimulus reduction.

If possible, patients should discontinue insomnia-causing medicines (see previous discussion). Those that neurologists are apt to prescribe include β-blockers, caffeine-containing migraine medications, dopamine precursors and agonists for Parkinson's disease, AEDs, and steroids.

Nonprescription hypnotics commonly can cause sleepiness and confusion the following day. Moreover, they carry several potential worrisome side effects. For example, antihistamines—especially in children—can lead to delirium, confusion, nightmares, and dystonic reactions. Alcohol, when used as a hypnotic, may cause a stuporous sleep that is followed by REM rebound and early morning awakening.

Tryptophan had enjoyed popularity because it is the "active ingredient" in warm milk and a precursor of melatonin. However, as a hypnotic, tryptophan produces little effect. Moreover, one batch of contaminated tryptophan pills caused the eosinophilia-myalgia syndrome (see Chapter 6).

On the other hand, melatonin promotes sleepiness. It decreases sleep latency and increases total sleep time and duration of REM sleep. Moreover, it seems to improve the restfulness of sleep. Unlike other hypnotics, melatonin does not lead to daytime sleepiness or confusion. Melatonin might help in the delayed sleep phase syndrome, jet lag, and age-related insomnia.

Despite their general acceptance, benzodiazepines increase total sleep time only about 10% and decrease valuable slow-wave NREM sleep; however, they reduce sleep fragmentation. Nevertheless, benzodiazepines' potential complications are daunting. Depending on their duration of action and if the patient is elderly, benzodiazepines may cause anterograde amnesia, confusion, insomnia, and EDS. In some cases, they cause patients to fall and sustain a hip fracture. If patients abruptly stop benzodiazepines, they may experience rebound insomnia and, in the extreme, withdrawal seizures.

A group of newer hypnotics, which includes eszopiclone (Lunesta), zaleplon (Sonata), and zolpidem (Ambien), may replace benzodiazepines for treatment of insomnia. Although structurally different from each other and from benzodiazepine, these hypnotics all interact with facets of the benzodiazepine receptor (see Chapter 21). Because they have a short half-life, they do not cause grogginess in the morning. In addition, they have minimal effects on sleep architecture and do not suppress REM sleep. Therefore, when patients stop taking these nonbenzodiazepine hypnotics, REM does not rebound.

INDICATIONS FOR A POLYSOMNOGRAM

Although a thorough medical-psychiatric evaluation will suffice for most patients, the identification of many sleep disorders hinges on the results of a PSG. For example, the clinical diagnosis generally requires PSG confirmation in sleep apnea, abnormal behavior during sleep, REM behavior disorder, periodic limb movements, and potentially injurious parasomnias. In addition, PSG can aid in the diagnosis of seizures that develop exclusively during sleep.

Nonetheless, the study is expensive and applicable in the diagnosis of only certain sleep disorders. For example, the benefit of PSG in evaluating the large number of people with insomnia does not justify the cost. However, PSG may have a role if a patient's insomnia has resisted treatment, induced mental aberrations, or endangered the patient's health.

A MSLT can confirm a clinical diagnosis of narcolepsy provided that a PSG has excluded sleep apnea, sleep deprivation, and periodic limb movement. The implications of the diagnosis of narcolepsy and the expense and side effects of its treatment—amphetamines and other powerful medications—justify the testing. In the future, determination of the CSF hypocretin level will likely supplant both the PSG and MSLT.

REFERENCES

1. Abramowicz M (ed): Gamma hydroxybutyrate (Xyrem) for narcolepsy. Med Lett 44:103–105, 2002.
2. Adler CH, Thorpy MJ: Sleep issues in Parkinson's disease. Neurology 64(Suppl 3):S12–S20, 2005.
3. Allen R, Becker PM, Bogan R, et al: Ropinirole decreases periodic leg movements and improves sleep parameters in patients with restless legs syndrome. Sleep 27:907–914, 2004.
4. American Sleep Disorders Association: *The International Classification of Sleep Disorders Diagnostic and Coding Manual.* Rochester, MN, American Sleep Disorders Association, 1990.
5. Barger LK, Cade BE, Ayas NT, et al: Extended work shifts and the risk of motor vehicle crashes among interns. N Engl J Med 352:125–134, 2005.
6. Boeve BF, Silber MH, Ferman TJ, et al: Association of REM sleep behavior disorder and neurodegenerative disease may reflect an underlying synucleinopathy. Mov Dis 16:622–630, 2001.
7. Brodsky MA, Godbold J, Roth T, et al: Sleepiness in Parkinson's disease: a controlled study. Mov Dis 18:668–672, 2003.

8. Cartwright R: Sleepwalking violence: A sleep disorder, legal dilemma, and a psychological challenge. Am J Psychiatry 161:1149–1158, 2004.

9. Czeisler CA, Walsh JK, Roth T, et al: Modafinil for excessive sleepiness associated with shift-work disorder. N Engl J Med 353:476–486, 2005.

10. Fantini ML, Ferini-Strambi L, Montplaisir J: Idiopathic REM sleep behavior disorder. Neurology 64:780–786, 2005.

11. Gadoth N, Kesler A, Vainstein G, et al: Clinical and polysomnographic characteristics of 34 patients with Kleine-Levin syndrome. J Sleep Res 10:337–341, 2001.

12. Guilleminault C, Kirisoglu C, Bao G, et al: Adult chronic sleepwalking and its treatment based on polysomnography. Brain 128:1062–1069, 2005.

13. Guilleminault C, Palombini L, Pelayo R, et al: Sleepwalking and sleep terrors in prepubertal children: What triggers them? Pediatrics 111:e17–e25, 2003.

14. Herman ST, Walczak TS, Bazil CW: Distribution of partial seizures during the sleep-wake cycle. Differences by seizure onset site. Neurology 56:1453–1459, 2001.

15. Kavey NB, Whyte J, Resor SR, et al: Somnambulism in adults. Neurology 40:749–752, 1990.

16. Kryger MH, Walid R, Manfreda J: Diagnoses received by narcolepsy patients in the year prior to diagnosis by a sleep specialist. Sleep 25:36–41, 2002.

17. Lavie P: Sleep disturbances in the wake of traumatic events. N Engl J Med 345:1825–1832, 2001.

18. Mahowald MW, Schenck CH, Cramer-Bornemann MA: Sleep-related violence. Curr Neurol Neurosci Rep 5:153–158, 2005.

19. Manconi M, Govoni V, De Vito A, et al: Restless legs syndrome and pregnancy. Neurology 63:1065–1069, 2004.

20. Mignot E: Genetic and familial aspects of narcolepsy. Neurology 50(Suppl 1):S16–S22, 1998.

21. Olson EJ, Boeve BF, Silber MH: Rapid eye movement sleep behavior disorder: Demographic, clinical and laboratory findings in 93 cases. Brain 123(Pt 2):331–339, 2000.

22. Scammell TE: The neurobiology, diagnosis, and treatment of narcolepsy. Ann Neurol 53:154–166, 2003.

23. Sevim S, Dogo O, Kaleagasi H, et al: Correlation of anxiety and depression symptoms in patients with restless legs syndrome. J Neurol Neurosurg Psychiatry 75:226–230, 2004.

24. Siegel JM: Hypocretin (orexin): Role in normal behavior and neuropathology. Ann Rev Psychol 55:125–148, 2004.

25. Silber MH: Chronic insomnia. N Engl J Med 353:803–810, 2005.

26. Strollo PJ, Rogers RM: Obstructive sleep apnea. N Engl J Med 334:99–104, 1996.

27. Tandberg E, Larsen JP, Karlsen K: A community-based study of sleep disorders in patients with Parkinson's disease. Move Dis 13:895–899, 1998.

28. Thorpy MJ: New paradigms in the treatment of restless legs syndrome. Neurology 64(Suppl 3):S28–S33, 2005.

29. US Modafinil in Narcolepsy Multicenter Study Group: Randomized trial of modafinil for the treatment of pathological somnolence in narcolepsy. Ann Neurol 43:88–97, 1998.

30. Wagner ML, Walters AS, Fisher BC: Symptoms of attention-deficit/hyperactivity disorder in adults with restless legs syndrome. Sleep 27:1499–1504, 2004.

31. Winkelman JW, James L: Serotonergic antidepressants are associated with REM sleep without atonia. Sleep 27:317–321, 2004.

32. Wise MS: Childhood narcolepsy. Neurology 50(Suppl1):S37–S42, 1998.

33. Wyatt JK: Delayed sleep phase syndrome: Pathophysiology and treatment options. Sleep 27:1195–1203, 2004.

Also, see National Center on Sleep Disorders Web site (http://search.info.nih.gov).

1–15. Is the statement true or false?

1. Normal sleep progresses through the four NREM stages before the first REM sleep period begins.
2. Because REM sleep usually begins about 90 to 120 minutes after the onset of sleep, normal REM latency is 90 to 120 minutes.
3. The bulk of REM sleep occurs in the early night, whereas the bulk of NREM sleep occurs in the early morning.
4. The normal sequence of NREM-REM sleep recurs with a periodicity of about 90 minutes.
5. REM sleep is almost entirely devoid of physical and mental activity.
6. Stages 3 and 4 of NREM sleep provide great physical restfulness.
7. Sleep always begins with stage 1 of NREM sleep.
8. Aside from eye movement artifact, REM sleep EEGs resemble ones during wakefulness.
9. The EEG during NREM sleep is characterized by slow activity.
10. The proportion of REM sleep remains constant from birth to old age.
11. Social and occupational factors, rather than internal, physiologic mechanisms, determine most individuals sleep-wake schedule.
12. The proportion of time spent in slow-wave sleep increases in the elderly.
13. Some productive, vigorous, and well-rested people sleep as little as 5 hours nightly.
14. When an activity, such as falling asleep, shifts to earlier in the daily cycle, the change qualifies as a *phase advance.*
15. Infant boys have penile erections during REM sleep.

Answers: 1-True, 2-True, 3-False, 4-True, 5-False, 6-True, 7-False, 8-True, 9-True, 10-False, 11-True, 12-False, 13-True, 14-True, 15-True.

16. In the night following sleep deprivation, which of the following will probably not occur?
    a. Sleep may begin with a period of REM activity (sleep onset REM, SOREM).
    b. Epileptiform discharges may emanate from the temporal lobe of a patient with partial complex seizures.
    c. Total sleep time will lengthen.
    d. REM sleep time will rebound.

e. Stages 1 and 2 will rebound more than stages 3 and 4 of NREM sleep.

Answer: e. Once allowed to sleep, sleep-deprived individuals will first recoup REM and slow-wave (stages 3 and 4 of NREM) sleep.

17–24. Which of the following characteristics are associated with (a) sleep terrors, (b) nightmares, (c) both, or (d) neither?
17. Onset during stages 1 and 2 of NREM sleep
18. Onset during slow-wave sleep
19. Onset during REM sleep
20. A disturbing variety of common dreams
21. Amnesia for any content
22. Partial arousals during first NREM period often precipitate them
23. Parents cannot interrupt them
24. Are associated with somnambulism

Answers: 17-d, 18-a, 19-b, 20-b, 21-a, 22-a, 23-a, 24-a.

25–37. Which of the following phenomena typically occur during (a) REM sleep, (b) NREM sleep, (c) either phase, or (d) neither phase?
25. Sleepwalking (somnambulism)
26. Areflexic DTRs
27. EEG delta waves
28. Bed-wetting (enuresis)
29. Vulnerability to primary generalized seizures
30. Cluster headache
31. REM sleep behavior disorder
32. Sleep spindles on PSG
33. Body repositioning
34. Low-voltage, fast EEG activity on PSG
35. K complexes
36. Parkinson tremor
37. Hemiballismus

Answers: 25-b, 26-a, 27-b, 28-b, 29-b, 30-a, 31-a, 32-b, 33-b, 34-a, 35-b, 36-d, 37-d.

38. Where are the principle nuclei that generate the rapid eye movements that accompany dreams?
    a. Diencephalon
    b. Midbrain
    c. Pons
    d. Medulla

Answer: c. The pons contains conjugate gaze centers that, when stimulated, produce rapid ipsilateral conjugate ocular movements.

39. Where are the principle nuclei that produce the areflexic quadriparesis that accompanies dreams?
    a. Diencephalon
    b. Midbrain
    c. Pons
    d. Medulla

Answer: c. The pons contains the peri-locus ceruleus. When stimulated, it induces flaccid, areflexic quadriparesis, which is sometimes called "REM atonia."

40. Which of the following statements concerning sleep disturbances following the Oklahoma City bombing and previous, similar events is untrue?
    a. Survivors of the Oklahoma City bombing reported that after 6 months, 70% had insomnia and more than 50% had nightmares.
    b. Trauma-related anxiety dreams are the most consistent symptom of PTSD.
    c. Studies often show a discrepancy between the patients' reports of insomnia and dreaming and the sleep-laboratory data.
    d. Post-traumatic insomnia usually requires medical or psychiatric treatment to prevent development of chronic insomnia.

Answer: d. Most survivors' insomnia resolves without treatment, but a minority of them requires a several-week course of a benzodiazepine or hypnotic. In contrast to widespread symptoms of sleep disturbances, PSG data fail to show frequent or marked sleep disturbances.

41. A 70-year-old man, over 1 year, develops burning in his feet that is so severe at night that it forces him to rub them incessantly. Then he still has to pace about for 1–2 hours. He has no ongoing medical illnesses and takes no medications. Aside from absent ankle reflexes, his neurologic examination is normal. Even given the numerous causes of his illness, which of the following laboratory tests is inappropriate?
    a. Serum ferritin
    b. Blood glucose
    c. BUN or creatinine
    d. Serum β-HCG

Answer: d. He has the RLS, which may be associated with iron deficiency anemia and a low serum ferritin concentration, diabetes, and uremia. RLS also occurs in young women, but usually only in the third trimester of pregnancy. Although many patients have no underlying illness, some of them have a strong family history of RLS.

42. For the patient in the previous question, which of the following is first-line treatment?
    a. Atypical neuroleptics
    b. Dopamine blocking (typical) neuroleptics
    c. Dopamine agonists
    d. Sedatives

Answer: c. Increasing dopamine activity by giving L-dopa or dopamine agonists will reduce both movements and restore a good portion of sleep. Presumably, RLS results from decreased D2 receptor binding in striatum. In the presence of iron deficiency, iron supplements will help. Large doses of sedatives will only force patients to sleep. Although RLS mimics akathisia, neither typical nor atypical neuroleptics will reduce the dysesthesias or their associated movements.

43–47. Is each statement true or false?

43. Narcolepsy typically begins in middle age when normal afternoon fatigue becomes prominent.
44. Sleep apnea is a disorder only of adults.
45. Sleep apnea is associated with morning headaches and cardiovascular disorders.
46. Sleep apnea may lead to cognitive impairments and poor school performance.
47. Hypnopompic refers to phenomena that occur on awakening, and hypnagogic refers to phenomena that occur on falling asleep.

Answers

43-False. About 90% of cases develop between adolescence and age 25 years.
44-False. Children and teenagers, especially ones with nasopharyngeal abnormalities, have the disorder.
45-True. It is also associated with obesity, but the relationship is not invariable. About 30% of patients are not obese.
46-True.
47-True.

48. Which of the following statements concerning melatonin is false?
    a. It is synthesized in the pineal gland.
    b. Serotonin is a precursor in its synthesis.
    c. Its maximum secretion coincides with the brightest time of the day.
    d. Selective serotonin reuptake inhibitors increase melatonin plasma concentration.

Answer: c. Daylight suppresses melatonin synthesis and secretion. Darkness creates the opposite effects.

49. In the synthesis of melatonin, what is the meaning of X tryptophan→X→N-acetyl-X→melation?
    a. Catecholamine
    b. An indolamine

c. An amino acid

d. A steroid

Answer: b. X is serotonin, which is an indolamine. Melatonin is synthesized in the pineal gland through the following pathway: tryptophan → serotonin → N-acetyl-serotonin → melatonin.

50. A 58-year-old man has irregular movements of his legs during the night that prevent him from sleeping and cause excessive daytime sleepiness (EDS). He explains that his legs move because they burn. If he arises from bed and walks 10 times around the room, he can return and go to sleep. However, even when he falls asleep, his wife reports that for the following hour his legs jerk in flurries at approximately 30-second intervals. Both the husband and wife have daytime sleepiness. He takes no medication. He has no underlying medical illnesses. Of the following, which category is the drug of choice?

a. Anticholinergic

b. Opioid

c. Typical neuroleptic

d. Benzodiazepine

e. Dopamine agonist

f. Hypnotic

Answer: e. He has restless legs syndrome (RLS) with superimposed periodic limb movements, which complicate about 80% of RLS cases. Many times, RLS is a manifestation of peripheral neuropathy or iron deficiency. In women, it may complicate the third trimester of pregnancy. Dopamine precursors, such as L-dopa, and dopamine agonists suppress the movements and the underlying dysesthesias. This patient does not have akathisia because the movements occur predominantly when he is in bed and seem to result from dysesthesias rather than a psychogenic urge to move. In addition, he has had no exposure to dopamine-blocking neuroleptics.

51. Which characteristic is common to the sleep patterns of both depression and sleep following sleep deprivation?

a. Increased sleep latency

b. Shortened REM latency

c. Sleep terrors

d. Interruptions in sleep

Answer: b.

52. Which four conditions are characterized by short sleep latency?

a. Alcohol- and drug-induced sleep

b. Narcolepsy

c. Sleep apnea

d. Sleep deprivation

e. Depression

f. Delayed sleep phase syndrome

g. Anxiety

h. Parkinson's disease

Answers: a, b, c, d. As could be anticipated, disorders associated with EDS are generally associated with short sleep latency.

53. Which condition is not associated with sleep onset REM periods (SOREMPs)?

a. RLS

b. Alcohol and hypnotic withdrawal

c. Depression

d. Narcolepsy

e. Sleep apnea

f. Sleep deprivation

Answer: a.

54. Which three physiologic changes are associated with REM sleep?

a. Absent respirations

b. Lower pulse and blood pressure

c. Increased intracranial pressure

d. High-voltage, slow EEG activity

e. Absent limb and chin EMG activity

f. Erections

Answers: c, e, f.

55. In depressed patients, which two of the following are the most typical sleep-related changes?

a. Delay in the night-time body temperature nadir

b. Advance of REM activity

c. Advance of cortisol secretion

d. Delay in MHPG secretion

Answers: b, c.

56. Which one of the following is unusual during alcohol withdrawal?

a. Hallucinations

b. Excessive dreaming

c. Increased REM sleep

d. Tendency to have seizures

e. Insomnia

f. Sleep terrors

Answer: f.

57. Which one of the following conditions usually does not begin before the age 25 years?

a. Delayed sleep phase syndrome

b. Kleine-Levin syndrome

c. Sleep apnea syndrome

d. Narcolepsy

e. REM behavior disorder

Answer: e. REM behavior disorder occurs most commonly in men older than 65 years and almost never in middle-aged and younger adults. More important, the other conditions commonly first appear in teenagers and young adults.

58. Which two of the following are the most effective treatments for the delayed sleep phase syndrome?

a. Continually advancing the bedtime

b. Continually delaying the bedtime

c. Light therapy (phototherapy)

d. Stimulants

Answers: b, c. The object of the treatment is sleep phase delay. Although stimulants, such as amphetamines, are not indicated, innocuous stimulation, such as entertainment and physical activity, will also help in shifting sleep time.

59. Which three conditions will induce SOREMPs during the Multiple Sleep Latency Test (MSLT)?

a. Nightmares

b. Sleep terrors

c. Narcolepsy

d. Sleep apnea

e. REM sleep disorder

f. Sleep deprivation

Answers: c, d, f. In general, conditions that cause EDS lead to short or absent REM latency.

60. Which is the most important factor in determining most individual's sleep schedule?

a. Early learning

b. Social and occupational demands

c. Cerebral cortical "time clocks"

d. Melatonin secretion

e. Suprachiasmatic nucleus of the hypothalamus

Answer: b. The suprachiasmatic nucleus, located in the hypothalamus, serves as the biologic clock. However, social and occupational demands and exposure to light in the environment override the biologic clock. For example, the schedule of people who work at night and sleep during the day determines their behavior.

61. Which is the least likely consequence of hypnotic medication withdrawal?

a. Insomnia

b. EDS

c. REM suppression

d. Heightened awareness

e. Vivid dreams

f. Seizures

Answer: c. REM rebound (excessive REM) is one of the most common and troublesome effects of hypnotic withdrawal.

62. Almost all narcolepsy patients have a major histocompatibility complex antigen in the HLA group. Which one of the following statements regarding this antigen is *false*?

a. It indicates that narcolepsy arises from a genetic predisposition.

b. It is located on the short arm of the chromosome 6.

c. Almost all people with this antigen have narcolepsy.

d. Almost 90% of patients with narcolepsy exhibiting cataplexy carry this HLA antigen.

e. Most monozygotic twins are discordant for narcolepsy.

Answer: c. In the general population, about 25% of people has the antigen, but less than 1% of them has narcolepsy. Of those with narcolepsy, almost all have the antigen. Among monozygotic twins with narcolepsy, the concordance rate is only about 25%. Therefore, although the antigen may be a prerequisite for developing narcolepsy-cataplexy, it does not cause the illness.

63. A 50-year-old man with EDS, restless night-time sleep, and loud snoring undergoes polysomnography (PSG). The PSG shows falls in the blood oxygen concentration that trigger microarousals. What is the best treatment for the daytime sleepiness?

a. Continuous positive airway pressure (CPAP)

b. Tracheostomy

c. Uvula surgery

d. Stimulants

Answer: a. The patient has sleep apnea. CPAP is probably the most effective and least invasive treatment. If possible, he should lose weight. In addition, modafinil will help promote daytime wakefulness.

64. Which feature distinguishes the daytime sleepiness of sleep deprivation from narcolepsy?

a. Falling asleep when sitting and bored

b. Daytime naps are refreshing

c. REM at onset of sleep

d. Falling asleep during the day can occur in potentially dangerous situations

e. Sleep paralysis on awakening from daytime sleep

Answer: b. Although both conditions share all of these features, the most significant difference is that daytime naps are refreshing for sleep deprived individuals but not for those with narcolepsy.

65. Which two sleep changes represent beneficial effects of benzodiazepines?
   a. Increase in total sleep time of 10%
   b. Increase in total sleep time of 30%
   c. Increase in total sleep time of 50% or more
   d. Reduced fragmentation
   e. Increase in slow-wave NREM sleep

Answers: a, d.

66. Which one of the following is not a benzodiazepine side effect?
   a. Hip fractures from an increased tendency to fall
   b. Anterograde amnesia
   c. With long-acting preparations, daytime sleepiness
   d. With short-acting preparations, insomnia in the early morning hours and daytime anxiety
   e. Lowered seizure threshold
   f. Exacerbation of sleep apnea syndrome and chronic obstructive lung disease

Answer: e. Benzodiazepines have a mild to moderate anticonvulsant effect.

67. During the mid-semester break from his freshman year in college, the patient's parents reported that he slept incessantly for six days. He would only awaken to use the toilet and eat large amounts of food—"like a hibernating bear," his mother said. His father observed that the patient masturbated many times. When, asked about his atypical behavior, their normally polite, respectful, studious son was surly and irritable. Also, he seemed to be unable to recall recent events. The previous year, he had experienced a similar event, but it lasted only three days. Neurologic and medical examinations, routine blood tests, MRI, lumbar puncture, EEG, and toxicology studies all showed no significant abnormalities. Which disorder most likely affected their child?
   a. Periodic hypersomnia
   b. A hypothalamic tumor
   c. Encephalitis
   d. Focal complex seizures
   e. Drug abuse

Answer: a. In view of the description of the event, history, and all the negative laboratory tests, he probably has the Kleine-Levin syndrome (periodic hypersomnia). This idiopathic condition affects predominantly adolescent males and consists primarily of periods of hypersomnia that are interrupted by hyperphagia and hypersexuality. When not asleep, they are confused, withdrawn, and apathetic.

68. In which direction is travel most likely to produce jet lag?
   a. East to west
   b. West to east
   c. North to south
   d. South to north
   e. None of the above

Answer: b. Jet lag, time zone change sleep disorder, is greater following eastward travel because individuals cannot as easily advance as delay their sleep schedule. In other words, when going from Los Angeles to New York, most people cannot easily go to sleep 3 hours earlier; however, when returning, most people can easily delay going to sleep by the 3 hours. Travelers who suffer from jet lag should prepare for their trip by changing their own sleep-wake schedule to conform to their destination's schedule several days before the trip. After arriving, they should immediately follow the local time schedule and expose themselves to sunlight in the morning. Eastward travelers can take melatonin or a hypnotic to facilitate their falling asleep earlier than normal.

69. Which statement concerning sleep apnea in children is incorrect?
   a. Affected children have a normal weight.
   b. The most common cause is enlarged tonsils and adenoids.
   c. The disorder can cause paradoxical hyperactivity.
   d. It often causes inattention and academic difficulties.
   e. The diagnosis requires children to have EDS.

Answer: e. Sleep deprivation in children has different manifestations than it has in adults. In children, sleep deprivation often causes inattention, paradoxical hyperactivity, school difficulties, and behavioral disturbances rather than merely EDS. Unlike affected adults, children with sleep apnea usually have enlarged tonsils and adenoids, which cause the problem, and normal weight.

70. By what age do children usually control their bladder during the night?
   a. 3 years
   b. 5 years
   c. 7 years
   d. 9 years

Answer: b. Children usually stop wetting their bed between ages 2 and 4 years. When girls older than 5 years and boys older than 6 years have involuntary bed-wetting, they are considered to have enuresis.

71. Many high functioning, productive individuals exist on relatively little sleep. In general, how do they adjust to 5 to 6 hours of sleep each night?
   a. They increase the proportion of their REM sleep.
   b. They increase the proportion of their stage 1 and 2 NREM sleep.
   c. They increase the proportion of their stage 3 and 4 NREM sleep.
   d. They virtually eliminate REM sleep.

Answer: c. Adults who accustom themselves to relatively little sleep have an increased proportion of deep, slow-wave NREM sleep. In other words, they conserve slow-wave NREM sleep at the expense of REM and light stages of NREM sleep.

72. In which condition are PSG studies most likely to show consistent abnormalities?
   a. Anxiety
   b. Mania
   c. Major depression
   d. Schizophrenia

Answer: c.

73. Which of the following results is least likely to be present in PSG studies in major depression?
   a. Sleep onset or short REM latency
   b. Increased REM density
   c. Decreased efficiency
   d. Greatly increased REM latency

Answer: d. PSG studies in major depression show a characteristic triad of abnormalities—sleep onset or short REM latency, increased REM density, and decreased efficiency. None alone is definitive, but alterations in REM latency and its other characteristics most closely correlate with depression and its treatment.

74. Which component of the narcolepsy-cataplexy tetrad most closely correlates with diminished or absent CSF concentrations of hypocretin?
   a. Narcolepsy
   b. Cataplexy
   c. Sleep hallucinations
   d. Sleep paralysis
   e. None of the above

Answer: b. Cataplexy most closes correlates with diminished or absent CSF concentrations of hypocretin.

75. As individuals age, which of the following changes is most apt to occur?
   a. Increase in REM, slow-wave, and total sleep time

   b. Although a decrease in total sleep time, an increase in REM and slow-wave sleep
   c. Decrease in REM sleep, slow-wave sleep, and total sleep time
   d. None of the above

Answer: c. As individuals age, they have decreased REM, slow-wave, and total sleep time. Moreover, their sleep is phase-advanced and interrupted by frequent awakenings. The early morning awakenings of older people are a manifestation of the normal phase advance. Therefore, early morning awakenings, by themselves, are not an indication of depression.

76. By what age do children consolidate their sleep into night-time and give up their afternoon nap?
   a. 2 years
   b. 4 years
   c. 6 years
   d. 8 years

Answer: c. Children usually give up their afternoon nap by 5 to 6 years old. If loss of their afternoon naps leaves them sleep-deprived, young children may be irritable or hyperactive rather than sleepy.

77. An 18-year-old college freshman, who works part time as a waitress, describes having EDS. On careful questioning, she reveals that she has irresistible urges to sleep about twice daily, a tendency to become weak when laughing, and describes occasional total paralysis when attempting to wake for morning classes. The MSLT recorded 2 naps with sleep latencies of less than 3 minutes. One of them had a REM period after a 2-minute latency. Which one of the following is the least advisable next step for her physicians?
   a. A therapeutic trial of methylphenidate
   b. Repeating the MSLT after she has 3 full nights of sleep
   c. Checking her urine or blood signs of alcohol and drug use
   d. HLA typing
   e. PSG

Answer: a. Her history suggests several symptoms of narcolepsy: EDS, cataplexy, and sleep paralysis. However, she does not nap at inopportune times and her MSLT results were equivocal. Although narcolepsy begins in teenagers and young adults, the entire tetrad rarely develops in such young individuals. She is more likely to have sleep onset REM periods from the most common cause among young adults—sleep deprivation. In addition, she might have one of several other common problems in her age group, including abuse of alcohol, recreational drug use, or depression.

She should have a PSG and repeat MSLT after 3 full nights of sleep.

78. Which of the following is the best treatment for an elderly man who, during REM sleep, flails his arms and frequently strikes his wife. Sometimes, during these episodes, he kicks her. His violence is restricted to REM sleep. He has minimal cognitive impairment but no thought disorder. Which is the best treatment?
    a. Clonazepam
    b. Phenytoin
    c. Carbamazepine
    d. Tricyclic antidepressants

Answer: a. Several disorders can interrupt sleep and cause violent behavior: REM sleep behavior disorder, focal seizures, head banging, sleep walking, other parasomnias, and dementia-induced wandering. Psychotic disturbances, other psychiatric disorders, and purposeful violence can also occur at night. This patient has REM sleep behavior disorder. Clonazepam is the best treatment. In contrast, tricyclic antidepressants, SSRIs, and monoamine oxidase inhibitors are ineffective. Moreover, even though these medicines might suppress REM sleep, they may precipitate the disorder during any remaining REM sleep.

79. Which symptom least justifies requesting a PSG?
    a. EDS
    b. Exclusively nocturnal behavior disturbances
    c. Insomnia
    d. Exclusively nocturnal movement disorders

Answer: c. Of the choices, insomnia is least likely to be a manifestation of a physiologic disorder. Instead, some individuals, who are said to have pseudoinsomnia, report having little or no sleep but, when monitored, have hours and hours of sleep. Also, rare individuals have fatal familial insomnia.

80. A 50-year-old man is brought for psychiatric consultation by his wife because he has become "distant, inattentive, and confused" during the previous several months. He began to develop severe insomnia 4 months before the consultation. A variety of hypnotics, antidepressants, and other psychotropic medicines did not alleviate the insomnia. The patient's older sister died after an 18-month course of a similar illness. The psychiatrist found that the patient had personality changes, cognitive deficits, and subtle myoclonus. An internist found that he had tachycardia and labile hypertension. Of the following, which is the most likely illness?
    a. Creutzfeldt-Jakob disease
    b. Fatal familial insomnia

    c. Iatrogenic sleep disorder
    d. Lewy body disease
    e. Drug or alcohol abuse

Answer: b. He has fatal familial insomnia because he and his sister have had refractory insomnia, dementia, myoclonus, and autonomic nervous system (ANS) dysfunction. This illness, like Creutzfeldt-Jakob disease, is a prion disease characterized by accumulation of PrP^{Sc}.

81. The patient in the preceding question undergoes further evaluation. Which of the following features is unlikely to be found?
    a. Lewy bodies in the cerebral cortex and the basal ganglia
    b. Hyperhidrosis
    c. Atrophy of the thalamus
    d. Spongiform cerebral cortical changes
    e. Elevated catecholamines and other endocrine abnormalities

Answer: a. This patient has fatal familial insomnia, which causes ANS and endocrine system hyperactivity, myoclonus, and other motor abnormalities. The brain would characteristically show atrophy of the thalamus and spongiform appearance of the cerebral cortex. In contrast, widely distributed Lewy bodies indicate dementia with Lewy bodies.

82. When used to treat cataplexy, which is the mechanism of action of chlorimipramine, imipramine, and protriptyline?
    a. They enhance dopamine activity.
    b. They act as alpha-1 adrenergic agonists.
    c. They inhibit adrenergic reuptake.
    d. None of the above.

Answer: c. Tricyclics are helpful in cataplexy because they increase adrenergic activity by inhibiting its reuptake.

83. When used to treat narcolepsy, which is the mechanism of action of methylphenidate and amphetamine?
    a. They enhance dopamine activity.
    b. They act as α-1 adrenergic agonists.
    c. They inhibit adrenergic reuptake.
    d. None of the above.

Answer: a.

84. Which of the following statements concerning using modafinil (Provigil) is false?
    a. It is a nonamphetamine medication with no discernible action on dopamine, serotonin, or GABA systems.
    b. It stimulates hypocretin cells.

c. It promotes wakefulness.

d. As with stopping amphetamines and other stimulants, stopping modafinil leads to a rebound in NREM sleep.

Answer: d. When they are stopped, amphetamines cause a rebound in sleep, but modafinil does not lead to a rebound in total sleep or REM sleep. Probably by stimulating hypocretin-synthesizing cells, modafinil does not keep people awake merely by postponing sleep. It promotes wakefulness in sleep apnea, shift work sleep disorder, and narcolepsy.

85. A 17-year-old student has spent the summer in a band. He went to sleep every night at 4:00 AM. Anticipating the start of school on September 1, he requests an "upper" to help him remain awake during the transition. What would be the best method to change to a sleep schedule of 11:00 PM to 6:30 AM?

a. Use an amphetamine during the transition.

b. Suddenly switch to a new schedule, much like overcoming the change to a new time zone when traveling.

c. Go to bed earlier each night beginning August 16.

d. Delay sleep by one hour beginning August 11.

Answer: d. He has delayed sleep phase syndrome. The best way to reach a conventional schedule would be to delay sleep by 1 hour each night until sleep onset reaches the desired schedule. Going to bed early usually only increases sleep latency, but delaying sleep decreases the latency.

86. Of the following, which is the most effective treatment of cataplexy?

a. Modafinil

b. Oxybate

c. Nortriptyline

d. Amphetamine

Answer: b. Oxybate (Xyrem), the same substance as gamma-hydroxybutyrate (GHB), the "date-rape drug," markedly reduces cataplexy. Oxybate is a rapid acting hypnotic that increases slow-wave sleep but does not affect REM sleep.

87. Which of the following statements concerning normal hypocretin physiology is false?

a. Hypocretin is virtually synonymous with orexin.

b. Hypocretin consists of at least two excitatory polypeptide neurotransmitters, hypocretin 1 and 2.

c. Hypocretin normally produces wakefulness, inhibits REM sleep, and stimulates appetite.

d. Cells in the hypothalamus normally synthesize hypocretin—hence the common prefix.

e. Hypocretin-containing tracts innervate the locus ceruleus and other brainstem tracts involved with sleep and wakefulness, but no hypocretin enters the cerebrospinal fluid (CSF).

Answer: e. Hypocretin-containing tracts innervate the locus ceruleus and other brainstem tracts involved with sleep and wakefulness. Although hypocretin enters the CSF in measurable levels in normal individuals, CSF hypocretin is completely or nearly completely undetectable in narcolepsy patients.

88. What is the relationship between hypocretin and narcolepsy?

a. Almost 100% of narcolepsy patients have complete absence of CSF hypocretin.

b. Patients with narcolepsy have no detectable concentrations of hypocretin in either the serum or CSF.

c. Deficiency of CSF hypocretin is more closely associated with cataplexy than any other element of the narcolepsy-cataplexy tetrad.

d. Deficiency of CSF hypocretin is more closely associated with hallucinations and sleep paralysis than any other elements of the narcolepsy-cataplexy tetrad.

Answer: c. Narcolepsy-cataplexy patients have total or near total loss of CSF hypocretin. The deficiency is less consistent in patients who have only narcolepsy. Examination of the brain of narcolepsy-cataplexy shows degeneration of hypocretin-synthesizing cells in the hypothalamus. Curiously, those patients' hypocretin serum concentrations remain normal, which suggests that cells outside the brain synthesize the polypeptide.

Involuntary Movement Disorders

Involuntary movement disorders occur frequently, provide instructive clinical-anatomic correlations, and cause serious mental and physical disability. In some of them, dementia and depression precede or overshadow the movements, but in others, despite profound physical disability, little or no dementia or depression occurs.

Abnormalities of the basal ganglia underlie the classic movement disorders: Parkinson's disease, athetosis, chorea, hemiballismus, Wilson's disease, and generalized dystonia. In contrast, no known basal ganglia abnormality underlies many other movement disorders, including focal dystonias, essential tremor, tics and Tourette's disorder, and myoclonus. In addition, from time to time movements, particularly ones that mimic tremor or dystonia, stem from psychopathology.

Although laboratory tests can provide a confirmation for many movement disorders, the initial diagnosis and appreciation of their comorbidities rest on clinical grounds. As they do with neurocutaneous disorders, neurologists generally first propose a "diagnosis by inspection."

THE BASAL GANGLIA

Five subcortical, gray matter, macroscopic nuclei (Figs. 18-1 and 18-2) constitute the basal ganglia:

- The *caudate nucleus* and *putamen*, which together form the *striatum*
- The *globus pallidus*
- The *subthalamic nucleus* (*corpus Luysii*)
- The *substantia nigra*

Intricate tracts link the basal ganglia to each other and to the thalamus, conjugate oculomotor circuits, and the frontal lobe. Projections from the basal ganglia constitute the *extrapyramidal* tract, which parallels the *pyramidal* (corticospinal) tract. The extrapyramidal tract modulates the corticospinal tract and promotes, inhibits, and sequences movement. In addition, it maintains appropriate muscle tone and adjusts posture.

Although the extrapyramidal tract seems to play merely a supportive role—indirectly influencing the corticospinal tract by acting on thalamocortical

connections and projecting only within the brain—it has several clinically important divisions. The most important one, from a clinical viewpoint, is its *nigrostriatal tract,* which, as its name suggests, extends from the substantia nigra to the striatum (Fig. 18-3). This division provides dopamine innervation largely through direct and indirect pathways to the globus pallidus internal segment (GPi) of the striatum (see Fig. 21-4). A subdivision travels indirectly, via the subthalamic nucleus, to the GPi.

One of the main differences between dopamine receptors is that, in the striatum, dopamine binding to dopamine 1 (D_1) receptors stimulates adenyl cyclase activity, but dopamine binding to dopamine 2 (D_2) receptors inhibits adenyl cyclase activity (see Table 21-1). A profound dopamine deficiency and concomitant increased inhibition of thalamocortical projections ultimately create the major clinical manifestations of Parkinson's disease.

As with other focal injuries of the brain—except for those in the cerebellum—unilateral injuries of the basal ganglia induce clinical abnormalities in the contralateral limbs. Basal ganglia injuries generally produce combinations of *hypokinesia* (too little movement) and *hyperkinesia* (too much movement). Symptoms of hypokinesia include rigidity, impaired postural reflexes, and *bradykinesia* (slow movement) or *akinesia* (absent movement). Symptoms of hyperkinesia include involuntary movements, such as tremor, hemiballismus, and dystonia.

GENERAL CONSIDERATIONS

The involuntary movement disorders share several clinical features. Anxiety, exertion, fatigue, and stimulants (including caffeine) increase the movements, but willful concentration suppresses them. Relaxation and, in some cases, biofeedback may also suppress them. They disappear during sleep with a few exceptions: hemifacial spasm, myoclonus, palatal tremor, tics, and specific sleep-related disorders, such as restless legs syndrome (RLS) and periodic movements (see Chapter 17).

When illnesses affect only the extrapyramidal tracts, patients have neither signs of pyramidal

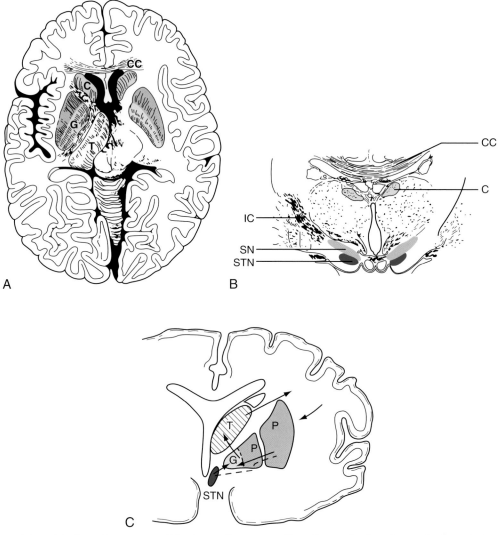

FIGURE 18-1 ■ *A,* This axial view, the one used in CT and MRI studies, shows the basal ganglia in relation to other brain structures. The heads of the caudate nuclei (C) indent the anterior horns of the lateral ventricles. The caudate and putamen (P) constitute the *striatum.* The globus pallidus (G), which has internal and external segments, and the putamen form the *lenticular nucleus,* named for its resemblance to an old-fashioned lens. The posterior limb of the internal capsule (IC) separates the lenticular nucleus from the thalamus (T), which is not a member of the basal ganglia family. *B,* In this coronal view of the diencephalon, the substantia nigra (SN), as well as the subthalamic nuclei (STN), sits below the thalamus. The substantia nigra, because of its black pigment and characteristic shape, serves as a landmark. The lateral ventricles are bounded laterally by the heads of the caudate nuclei (C) and above by the corpus callosum (CC). *C,* This coronal view shows extrapyramidal circuits. The putamen sends a direct and an indirect dopamine tract to the internal segment of the globus pallidus (GP). Dopaminergic neurons in the substantia nigra project to the putamen, where neurons expressing D_1 receptors project directly to the GPi. Putaminal neurons with D_2 receptors project through the globus pallidus external segment (GPe) and subthalamic nucleus and thence to GPi. The GPi innervates the ventrolateral nucleus of the thalamus, which projects to the motor cortex. The cortex, completing a circuit, innervates the putamen.

(corticospinal) tract damage, such as paresis, spasticity, hyperactive reflexes, and Babinski signs, nor signs of cerebral cortex damage (such as dementia and seizures). Although possibly debilitated by uncontrollable movements and inarticulate speech, patients may remain fully alert, intelligent, and, possibly by using unconventional techniques, able to communicate.

Unless physicians are astute, they may misdiagnose these individuals as having mental retardation or dementia.

Another potential error may occur when patients, at first glance, appear to have a psychogenic movement disorder (see later and Chapter 3). In many situations, the lack of a definitive confirmatory

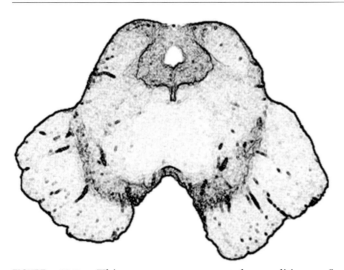

FIGURE 18-2 ▪ This computer-generated rendition of the midbrain should be compared to a photograph (see Fig. 2-9), functional drawings (see Fig. 4-5), and an idealized sketch (see Fig. 21-1). The midbrain, which lies just caudal to the diencephalon, contains in its lower third the pair of horizontal, elongated, stippled pigmented nuclei—the substantia nigra. Parkinson's disease blanches the substantia nigra and other pigmented nuclei. The midbrain also contains the prominent aqueduct of Sylvius, which is the dorsal structure surrounded by the periaqueductal gray matter. Cerebrospinal fluid (CSF) passes from the third ventricle, through the aqueduct, and then to the fourth ventricle. The periaqueductal gray matter develops microscopic hemorrhages in the Wernicke-Korsakoff syndrome.

laboratory test forces neurologists to rely exclusively on their clinical judgment.

PARKINSON'S DISEASE

Although Parkinson's disease ranks as only the second most common of the numerous involuntary movement disorders,* it serves as the prototypical illness. Studies of Parkinson's disease have revealed the underlying neurophysiology of the basal ganglia. Moreover, they have opened the door to understanding many other movement disorders and establishing rational treatments.

Parkinson's disease has three "cardinal features":

- Tremor
- Rigidity
- Bradykinesia

The initial and ultimately most disabling physical feature of Parkinson's disease is bradykinesia or, in the extreme, akinesia. The slow or absent movement produces the classic *masked face* (Fig. 18-4), paucity of

---

*The most common involuntary movement is essential tremor.

trunk and limb movement (Figs. 18-5 and 18-6), and impairment of activities of daily living.

Rigidity typically accompanies bradykinesia (Fig. 18-7). Although one of the cardinal features of Parkinson's disease, rigidity often appears as a manifestation of other extrapyramidal disorders. No matter the context, physicians should not confuse rigidity with spasticity, which signals corticospinal tract disease (see Chapter 2).

Tremor is usually the most conspicuous feature of Parkinson's disease; however, it is the least specific sign, least debilitating symptom, and least associated with dementia and depression. When a manifestation of Parkinson's disease, the tremor usually oscillates in a single plane with a regular rate, although variable amplitude, and primarily involves the hands. Even more characteristically, the affected body part appears predominantly when patients rest quietly with their arms supported. That feature, which gives Parkinson's disease tremor the virtual synonym, *resting tremor* (Fig. 18-8), distinguishes it from cerebellar and essential tremors (see later).

These cardinal features, in contrast to signs of most other movement disorders, typically first develop in an asymmetric or unilateral pattern, termed *hemiparkinsonism*. Even as Parkinson's disease progresses to involve both sides of the body, its manifestations continue to predominate on the side initially involved.

Additional symptoms and signs emerge as Parkinson's disease advances. Patients lose their *postural reflexes*, which are neurologic compensatory mechanisms that adjust muscle tone in response to change in position. Loss of these reflexes, in combination with akinesia and rigidity, results in a certain gait impairment, called *marche à petit pas* or *festinating gait*, characterized by a tendency to lean forward and accelerate the pace (Fig. 18-9A). In a test of postural reflexes, the *pull test*, the examiner pulls the patient from the shoulders (Fig. 18-9B). Normal individuals merely sway. Patients who have mild impairment of their postural reflexes take a few steps (i.e., have *retropulsion*). More severely affected ones rock stiffly backward without flexion or other compensatory movement and topple, *en bloc*, into the examiner's arms.

Parkinson's disease patients' gait abnormality and impaired postural reflexes prevent them from walking safely. Many fall and fracture a hip. These disabilities eventually confine them to bed.

Even at the onset of the illness, patients' handwriting deteriorates to a small and tremulous script, *micrographia* (Fig. 18-10). In a parallel fashion, their voice loses both volume and normal fluctuations in pitch and cadence, that is, their speech becomes *hypophonic* and *monotonous*. Also, because of their illness or the medications used to treat it, Parkinson's disease

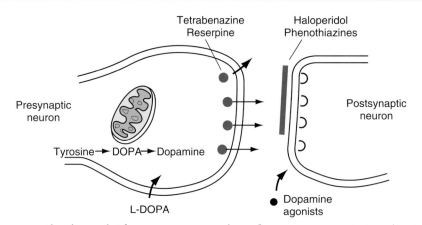

FIGURE 18-3 ▪ In the presynaptic nigrostriatal neuron, a succession of enzymes converts tyrosine to the neurotransmitter dopamine. In Parkinson's disease, the nigrostriatal tract degenerates, but the postsynaptic dopamine receptors remain intact. As a result of the degeneration, an absence of tyrosine hydroxylase leads to insufficient dopa and then markedly reduced synthesis of dopamine. L-dopa, which is given as an oral medication, penetrates the blood–brain barrier and substitutes for the deficient endogenous dopa in dopamine synthesis. (D-dopa is useless as a medication because it does not cross the blood–brain barrier.) Dopamine agonists, such as bromocriptine, pergolide, pramipexole, and ropinirole, act directly on the D_2 receptor and, to a lesser extent, other postsynaptic dopamine receptors. Although dopamine agonists help, especially after the nigrostriatal neurons can no longer synthesize or store dopamine, they produce a less potent effect than L-dopa. Because reserpine or tetrabenazine depletes dopamine from its presynaptic sites, they may reduce hyperkinesia in chorea, tardive dyskinesia, and Tourette's disorder. However, presumably because these dopamine-depleting drugs drain a vital neurotransmitter, they often produce drowsiness and parkinsonism.

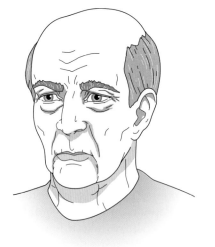

FIGURE 18-4 ▪ Compared to normal individuals of the same age, Parkinson's disease patients blink less frequently, make fewer facial expressions, and less often move their head. Their facial appearance has been called a "stare" or "masked facies" (Latin, face or countenance), but *masked face* has supplanted those terms.

patients characteristically develop several sleep disturbances (see Chapter 17).

Another early but crucial feature of Parkinson's disease consists of treatment with levodopa (L-dopa) reversing the symptoms and signs for several years. In practice, with the absence of a definitive laboratory test,

a positive response to L-dopa serves as a diagnostic criterion. Similarly, a failure to respond should prompt the clinician to reconsider the diagnosis.

With established disease and steady use of the medicines for several years, symptoms intermittently and unpredictable reappear. Inadequate buffering, storage, release, and reuptake of dopamine probably cause fluctuating patterns, termed "on-off," of patients' symptoms. During "on periods," patients remain well-treated and asymptomatic, but during "off periods," which last 30 minutes to 2 hours, rigidity and akinesia incapacitate them. Although patients are almost catatonic in off-periods, they have no change in their consciousness or abnormalities in their electroencephalogram.

Psychiatric Conditions Comorbid with Parkinson's Disease

Depression

For the first several years of Parkinson's disease, before incapacity develops, patients' mood may reflect their failing health, isolation from coworkers and friends, reduced income, and loss of independence. A second, more clear-cut phase of depression emerges as the disease begins to incapacitate them. Depending on the criteria, approximately 30% of all Parkinson's disease patients manifest comorbid depression.

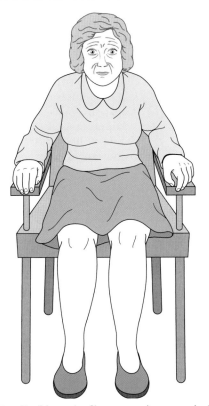

FIGURE 18-5 ■ Parkinson's disease patients typically sit motionless with their legs uncrossed and their feet flat. Their arms remain on the chair or in their lap and rarely participate in normal gestures or repositioning movements. In contrast to normal individuals and especially those with chorea, Parkinson's disease patients do not shift their weight from one hip to another or make any unnecessary movements.

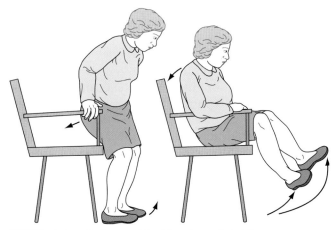

FIGURE 18-6 ■ Patients with akinesia and rigidity cannot rapidly flex their spine, hips, or knees. When sitting, they tend to rock slowly and solidly backward into a chair. Unable to bend rapidly, their feet rise several inches off the floor. Sitting *en bloc* is an early manifestation of parkinsonism. Patients have even a greater difficulty standing without assistance. They may liken their difficulty in moving to slogging through hip-deep mud, wearing lead clothing, or driving a car with its emergency brake engaged.

Despite the frequency of comorbid depression, diagnosing it sometimes requires considerable acumen. For instance, Parkinson's disease patients' obvious physical or cognitive impairments may completely overshadow signs of depression. Even without depression, Parkinson's disease produces hypophonic voice, sleep disturbances, and lack of independence. Physicians may confuse bradykinesia and masked face with psychomotor retardation and apathy. Similarly they may attribute vegetative symptoms, in the absence of overt mood changes, directly to the illness. Also, many manifestations of Parkinson's disease may invalidate certain items on the Beck Depression Inventory and the Hamilton Rating Scales.

Risk factors for comorbid depression include cognitive impairment, akinesia but not tremor, and a history of depression. Onset of the illness at a young age and its having a longer duration constitute additional risk factors.

Comorbid depression worsens cognitive impairment, interferes with sleep, and accentuates physical disabilities, as well as creating its own suffering. Nevertheless, Parkinson's disease with or without comorbid depression generally does not increase the suicide rate. However, an exception occurred in patients who underwent deep brain stimulation (see later) and had a history of depression or prior procedures. Thus, depression currently precludes Parkinson's patients from undergoing the procedure.

Physicians might also keep in mind that patients' caregivers may succumb to depression. If the patient is depressed or has had a lengthy illness, the caregiver is more susceptible to depression.

TREATMENT OF COMORBID DEPRESSION

Psychologic support, social services, and rehabilitation often help, but optimal treatment almost always requires antidepressants. However, before prescribing antidepressants, neurologists should optimize the antiparkinson medication regimen. Insufficient dosages leave the patient incapacitated and discouraged. Excessive dosage or poorly timed administration leads to agitation, sleep disturbances, and hallucinations.

Because administration of antiparkinson medication before bedtime tends to cause nightmares and hallucinations, neurologists prescribe minimal nighttime doses or shift the timing to the early evening. Hypnotics or antipsychotic agents may be necessary to ensure restful sleep for both patient and caregiver.

Although their effect is nonspecific, tricyclic antidepressants (TCAs) and trazodone improve patients' mood and restore restful sleep. However, their anticholinergic side effects may cause or exacerbate problems common in elderly individuals, especially those with Parkinson's disease, such as memory impairments,

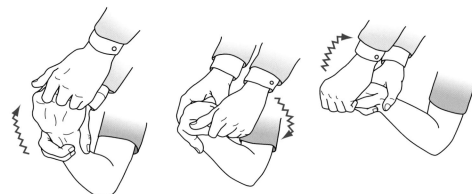

FIGURE 18-7 ■ Physicians typically elicit rigidity by rotating the patient's wrist. When present, rigidity causes an increased tone in all directions of movement. A superimposed tremor adds a ratchet-like resistance to the movement, called *cogwheel rigidity.*

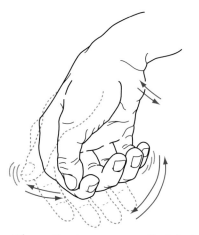

FIGURE 18-8 ■ The *resting tremor*—a cardinal feature of Parkinson's disease—consists of a relatively slow (4 to 6 Hz) to-and-fro flexion movement of the wrist, hand, thumb, and fingers that is most apparent when patients sit comfortably. The cupped hand's appearance of shaking pills gave rise to the name "pill-rolling" tremor. The tremor is exaggerated or sometimes apparent only when patients are anxious. However, it may be momentarily reduced during voluntary movement or by intense concentration. It is absent during sleep. Rigidity and akinesia almost always accompany the resting tremor of Parkinson's disease.

delirium, and physical side effects, such as ocular accommodation impairment, angle-closure glaucoma, and urinary hesitancy or retention.

Selective serotonin reuptake inhibitors (SSRIs), compared to the TCAs, have equal or greater effectiveness and fewer side effects. However, SSRIs and, to a lesser extent, TCAs are less effective in treating depression comorbid with Parkinson's disease than depression without comorbid Parkinson's disease. Moreover, administration of SSRIs in conjunction with selegiline (*deprenyl* [Eldepryl]) can theoretically cause the serotonin syndrome because SSRIs prevent

serotonin reuptake, whereas the monoamine oxidase (MAO) inhibitor selegiline prevents its breakdown (see Chapter 6). Although possible, the actual incidence of serotonin syndrome is very low because selegiline, in the doses used for Parkinson's disease treatment, selectively inhibits MAO-B, which metabolizes dopamine, whereas the serotonin syndrome is mostly a complication of inhibition of MAO-A, which metabolizes serotonin.

Electroconvulsive therapy (ECT) is effective and safe for depression in Parkinson's disease. In addition, it improves the physical impairments for several weeks.

Notably, although L-dopa and other dopaminergic medications readily treat most of the illness' physical features, they do not reverse depression. In other words, although a dopamine deficiency lies at the heart of Parkinson's disease, it probably does not explain one of its main manifestations.

Dementia

Parkinson's disease should not present with dementia. In fact, throughout the first 5 years of the illness, patients typically continue to work (even as physicians), manage a household, and participate in leisure activities. Even when physically incapacitated, some patients retain sufficient cognitive capacity for routine activities.

As Parkinson's disease progresses and patients age, however, dementia increasingly often complicates the illness. Dementia affects about 20% of all Parkinson's disease patients, and 40% of those older than 70 years. Its prevalence increases in proportion to physical impairments, especially bradykinesia, duration of the illness, and the patient's age. Affected patients lose 2.3 points annually on the Mini-Mental State Examination. The cumulative prevalence of dementia in Parkinson's disease eventually reaches 80%. Compared to aged-matched controls, Parkinson's disease patients

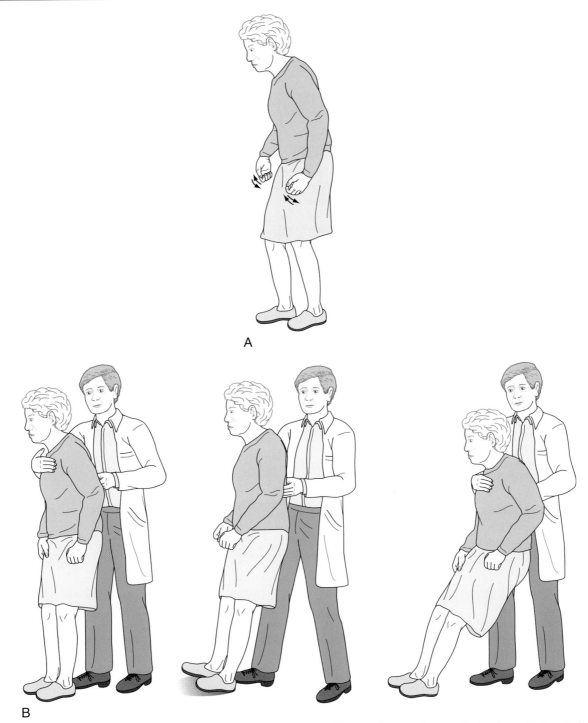

A

B

FIGURE 18-9 ■ *A,* Beyond the initial stages of the illness, Parkinson's disease often produces a *festinating gait,* in which patients take short, shuffling steps and accelerate their pace. When walking, they do not swing their arms, look about, or have other normal accessory movements. Likewise, turning *en bloc,* they simultaneously move their head, trunk, and legs. *B,* The *pull test* consists of the physician's gently but rapidly pulling the patient's shoulders. Unaffected individuals will compensate by taking one or two steps backward. Parkinson's disease patients with impaired postural reflexes will take many steps backward (i.e., have *retropulsion),* because they are unable to stop by righting themselves. In pronounced cases, as the one pictured here, patients unable to alter their posture will tilt backward en bloc and fall into the physician's arms.

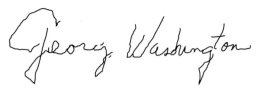

FIGURE 18-10 ■ The handwriting of a Parkinson's disease patient shows a progressive decrease in height, constrained movements in the spiral, and a superimposed tremulousness. This script, micrographia, is a reliable sign of Parkinson's disease. Changes in signatures, such as those on checks, can often date the onset of the illness.

have an approximately five-fold increased incidence of dementia.

Parkinson's disease dementia, which differs clinically from that of Alzheimer's disease dementia, is distinguished by inattention, poor motivation, difficulty shifting mental sets, and *bradyphrenia* (slowed thinking, the cognitive counterpart of bradykinesia). With gait impairment accompanying those deficits, Parkinson's disease dementia serves as a prime example of "subcortical dementia" (see Chapter 7). Dementia in Parkinson's disease often fluctuates throughout the day, probably largely because medications lead to intermittent confusion.

Not only can dementia be the sole psychiatric complication of Parkinson's disease but also it can be comorbid with depression. When both complicate Parkinson's disease, dementia is usually more pronounced, but not qualitatively different, than when it occurs without depression. Moreover, psychosis as an additional comorbid condition frequently complicates the picture (see later).

Although Parkinson's disease medications alleviate the motor disturbances, they do not improve cognitive impairment. Moreover, in advanced cases, they frequently cause confusion, exacerbate dementia, and precipitate a toxic-metabolic encephalopathy or delirium that can resemble psychosis (see later).

The cause of dementia remains unknown. Unlike the motor disabilities, dopamine deficiency is not the cause. However, it shares some pathologic features with Alzheimer's disease. For example, the majority of Parkinson's disease patients with dementia have cerebral cortex histologic changes similar to those of Alzheimer's disease. Also, a cerebral cortex cholinergic deficit in Parkinson's disease patients with dementia is similar but more pronounced than in Alzheimer's disease. Finally, rivastigmine, a cholinesterase inhibitor helpful in Alzheimer's disease, has shown some promise in Parkinson's disease dementia.

A diagnostic hazard consists of overlooking *dementia with Lewy bodies*. In this illness, dementia accompanied by signs of Parkinson's disease constitutes an initial, not a late developing, manifestation (see Chapter 7).

TREATMENT OF COMORBID DEMENTIA

As in the treatment of comorbid depression, strategies that lessen Parkinson's disease motor symptoms do not correct comorbid dementia. For example, L-dopa and dopamine agonists, which are termed *dopaminergic* because they enhance dopamine activity (see later), alleviate tremor and rigidity but fail to improve cognitive function. Moreover, they tend to precipitate hallucinations and psychotic thoughts.

On the other hand, cholinesterase inhibitors may improve cognitive impairment. However, they frequently cause gastrointestinal side effects, particularly, nausea, vomiting, and excessive salivation.

Surgical interventions for Parkinson's disease (see later), which may be otherwise successful, likewise do not reverse dementia. On the other hand, these procedures often allow for reduction in dopaminergic medications and thereby diminish hallucinations and psychotic thoughts. Because these procedures do not improve dementia, criteria for surgical candidates generally exclude Parkinson's patients with dementia.

Psychosis

At least 20%, and perhaps as many as 40%, of Parkinson's disease patients exhibit psychosis. In them, psychosis correlates most closely with dementia, but also with older age, long-standing illness, physical disability, and higher levels of antiparkinson medications. Visual hallucinations represent its most common, consistent manifestation. They typically include complex visions, such as ones of people and animals. Auditory hallucinations rarely occur. The development of visual hallucinations, like psychosis in general, varies directly with the number and strength of dopaminergic medications; physical signs of excessive medication, such as dyskinesias; dementia; sleep disturbances; and visual impairment.

Other characteristics of psychosis in Parkinson's disease include delusions, disordered thinking, chronic confusion, abusive behavior, and a tendency toward paranoid ideation that may involve the treating physicians. The thought disturbances closely resemble those in delirium. For most affected patients, psychosis fluctuates throughout daytime and worsens at night.

Intercurrent illnesses, such as pneumonia, sepsis, and electrolyte imbalance, which commonly complicate Parkinson's disease, precipitate or exacerbate psychotic symptoms. Even more so, medications contribute to or cause this problem. Although medications cause neither the comorbid depression nor dementia, they often cause the psychosis. As a commonly occurring example of iatrogenic symptoms, visual hallucinations closely follow medication administration and often resolve when physicians reduce the dose or number of medications.

As with dementia, psychosis is not a presenting feature but a late-developing comorbidity of Parkinson's disease. Once it develops, psychosis predisposes patients to dementia (which may have already developed), nursing home placement, and death within 2 years. Compared to the physical and cognitive disabilities, psychosis imposes the greatest stress on caregivers.

TREATMENT OF COMORBID PSYCHOSIS

Because of antiparkinson medications' role in causing or exacerbating psychosis, physicians usually first taper or discontinue them. Physicians generally reduce, in order, anticholinergic medications, amantadine, selegiline, dopamine agonists, and lastly L-dopa. Of course, patients can only tolerate elimination of the medicines up to a point, after which motor impairments return; however, patients generally prefer mild rigidity to psychosis.

Caregivers should avoid administering the medications in the late evening or night. Also, they should avoid abruptly stopping dopaminergic medicines, which might lead to irreversible motor deterioration, complications of immobility, or even the neuroleptic-malignant syndrome.

Physicians should prescribe atypical antipsychotic agents rather than typical dopamine-blocking neuroleptics, which are apt to worsen the physical impairments of Parkinson's disease. Despite the slight risk of stroke, several atypical antipsychotic agents greatly help psychosis accompanied or unaccompanied by dementia. Moreover, they alleviate the psychiatric disturbances without exacerbating physical impairments. Quetiapine and clozapine are less likely to exacerbate parkinsonism than are risperidone and olanzapine, probably because they bind less avidly to the D_2 receptor. Although experience is limited, ziprasidone (a relatively weak antagonist at the D_2 receptor) and aripiprazole (a partial D_2 agonist) may also be relatively safer.

After the antipsychotic agents successfully suppress psychotic symptoms, physicians should carefully and tentatively withdraw them. Abruptly stopping the medicines may lead not only to reappearance of symptoms but also, in a rebound, an exacerbation with worsened psychosis.

Other Psychiatric Conditions

In contrast to the frequent occurrence of comorbid depression, manic-depressive illness and schizophrenia rarely complicate Parkinson's disease. Nevertheless, the rare coexistence of schizophrenia and Parkinson's disease contradicts the classic "dopamine hypothesis" of schizophrenia, which predicted that these two conditions, one from decreased dopamine activity and the other from increased dopamine activity, would be mutually exclusive.

Another rare but notable comorbid psychiatric disorder, *dopamine dysregulation syndrome* (*DDS*), may stem from dopaminergic medicines' stimulating desires for pleasure. In the small number of patients with DDS— mostly ones with young-onset Parkinson's disease and premorbid depression—dopamine agonists induce aberrant behavior, such as compulsive gambling, mood swings, and excessive eating, sexual activity, and shopping. Stopping the medicine or treating appropriate patients with deep brain stimulation eliminates much of the problem. Similarly, prescribing Parkinson's disease medications to older individuals debilitated by the illness has unleashed voracious, almost compulsive, inappropriate sexual behavior.

In a related disorder, *hedonistic homeostatic dysregulation*, Parkinson's disease patients not only tend to overmedicate themselves—sometimes enduring toxicity— but they often manifest drug-seeking behavior. Some neurologists find patients' concern for their medication schedule so great that they describe their need as an obsession, addiction, or pseudoaddiction. Whatever its label, this behavior correlates with a history of mood disorder and dopamine agonist treatment.

Pathology of Parkinson's Disease

A well-established synthetic pathway in presynaptic nigrostriatal tract neurons normally converts phenylalanine to dopamine:

$$\text{Phenylalanine} \xrightarrow{\textit{Phenylalanine hydroxylase}}$$
$$\text{Tyrosine} \xrightarrow{\textit{Tyrosine hydroxylase}}$$
$$\text{DOPA} \xrightarrow{\textit{DOPA decarboxylase}} \text{Dopamine}$$

In Parkinson's disease, however, the nigrostriatal neurons slowly degenerate and lose their tyrosine hydroxylase. Degeneration of neurons in Parkinson's disease and other illnesses has given rise to the term "neurodegenerative diseases." Amyotrophic lateral sclerosis (ALS), Alzheimer's disease, Huntington's disease, and several other chronic, progressive illnesses, as well as Parkinson's disease, fall into this category.

The loss of tyrosine hydroxylase represents the critical failure in Parkinson's disease because this enzyme is the rate-limiting enzyme in dopamine synthesis (see

Fig. 18-3). With a deficiency of tyrosine hydroxylase, the ever-shrinking pool of nigrostriatal tract neurons cannot sustain the essential synthetic pathway. Once approximately 80% of these neurons degenerate, the nigrostriatal tract cannot synthesize adequate dopamine and Parkinson's disease symptoms appear.

The illness also impairs synthesis of other neurotransmitters. In particular, it leads to reduced concentrations of serotonin in the brain and cerebrospinal fluid (CSF).

The characteristic neuropathologic finding of Parkinson's disease, which is immediately evident on gross examination of the brain, consists of loss of normal pigment (depigmentation) in certain brainstem nuclei: the substantia nigra (black), locus ceruleus (copper sulfate-like or blue), and vagus (lit. wandering) motor nuclei (black). In addition, neurons in these nuclei accumulate microscopic intracytoplasmic inclusions, *Lewy bodies*, composed of circular, eosinophilic dense cores surrounded by loose fibrils. They contain aggregates of α-*synuclein* and, a less specific substance, *ubiquitin*. (Lewy bodies, which also stain for α-synuclein, located in the cerebral cortex as well as the basal ganglia characterize dementia with Lewy bodies. Thus, both Parkinson's disease and dementia with Lewy bodies fall under the rubric of synucleinopathies [see Chapter 7].)

Positron emission tomography (PET) using fluorodopa shows decreased dopamine activity in the basal ganglia. PET can detect changes in presymptomatic individuals as well as in those with overt Parkinson's disease. Other tests, such as magnetic resonance imaging (MRI), computed tomography (CT), and routine serum and CSF analyses, fail to reveal consistent, readily identifiable abnormalities. The diagnosis therefore remains based on the patient's clinical features and response to treatment.

Possible Causes of Parkinson's Disease

Toxins

The 1917 to 1918 pandemic of influenza, which caused encephalitis as one of its major manifestations, killed tens of millions of people in Europe and North America. Innumerable survivors subsequently developed Parkinson's disease. In fact, until the latter half of the 20th century, the majority of patients with Parkinson's disease had the "postencephalitic" variety.

Current epidemiologic studies have implicated various industrial and environmental toxins rather than infectious agents. For example, studies have found an increased incidence of Parkinson's disease in farmers and other workers with industrial exposure to herbicides and insecticides, but no increase among individuals using these chemicals at home. Studies have also uncovered an increased incidence in miners and welders who probably inhaled manganese. In addition, many case reports describe episodes of cyanide or carbon monoxide intoxication, which destroys the basal ganglia, causing signs of Parkinson's disease.

The most infamous toxin, discovered in a landmark investigation in the 1970s, is *methyl-phenyl-tetrahydropyridine (MPTP)*. This substance, a by-product of the illicit manufacture of meperidine (Demerol) or other narcotics, caused fulminant and often fatal Parkinson's disease in dozens of drug abusers who unknowingly administered it to themselves. Researchers have shown that MPTP selectively poisons nigrostriatal tract neurons and use it to produce the standard laboratory animal model of Parkinson's disease.

In the opposite situation, some otherwise toxic substances fail to produce Parkinson's disease. For example, contrary to initial reports, 3,4-methylenedioxymethamphetamine (*MDMA*), commonly known as *ecstasy*, which depletes serotonin, probably does not cause Parkinson's disease. Although several young adults developed signs of Parkinson's disease after using ecstasy, they may have used other illicit drugs or they may have carried a genetic mutation (see later). Moreover, the small number of cases, compared to the large number of probable ecstasy users, suggests that it is benign in this particular regard. In another curious situation, despite producing various gases, cigarette smoking varies inversely with the incidence of Parkinson's disease, that is, cigarette smoking actually seems to provide a protective effect. Likewise, coffee drinkers also seem to have a lower incidence of Parkinson's disease.

Oxidative Stress

Further research on the neurotoxicity of MPTP led to the *oxidative stress theory*. This theory proposes that defective mitochondria in Parkinson's disease patients cannot detoxify potentially lethal endogenous or environmental oxidants. Endogenous oxidants, by-products of normal metabolism, include hydrogen peroxide and *free radicals*. Free radicals, such as superoxide and nitric oxide, are atoms or molecules that are unstable because they contain a single, unpaired electron. To complete their electron pairs, free radicals snatch away electrons from neighboring atoms or molecules. Loss of electrons oxidizes cells and causes fatally injury.

When naturally occurring MAO acts on MPTP, the oxidized product, methylphenylpyridinium (MPP^+), generates intracellular free radicals that inhibit complex I of the mitochondrial respiratory chain. Pretreatment with MAO inhibitors blocks this reaction and thereby prevents MPP^+ formation and subsequent tissue oxidation. For this reason, pretreatment with MAO inhibitors prevents MPTP-induced Parkinson's disease in laboratory animals.

Similarly, an intravenous infusion of a common insecticide, *rotenone,* which also inhibits complex I of the mitochondrial respiratory chain, causes clinical signs of Parkinson's disease in laboratory animals. In addition, their neurons develop Lewy body-like structures that stain for α-synuclein and ubiquitin.

With a mean age of onset of 60 years, aging—possibly because of its effect on mitochondria—constitutes an unequivocal risk factor for Parkinson's disease. Although children and adolescents rarely develop the illness, pediatric neurologists must first consider several similar and more commonly occurring alternatives before making a diagnosis of childhood Parkinson's disease (see later).

Head Trauma

Unless head trauma is severe enough at least to cause loss of consciousness and post-traumatic amnesia, a single head injury cannot result in Parkinson's disease. Repeated serious head injuries, however, can cause a Parkinson-like syndrome, *dementia pugilistica,* which the public recognizes as the "punch drunk syndrome." Dementia pugilistica consists of insidiously developing intellectual deterioration; dysarthria, stiffness and clumsiness, and spasticity; and striking bradykinesia. It occurs most often in boxers who have been lightweight, alcoholic, or have lost many fights. Their deficits, which often herald the end of the boxer's career, often progress after retirement.

In this disorder, CT and MRI show white matter changes, focal contusions, and cerebral atrophy in proportion to the number of boxing matches. Autopsy studies reveal hydrocephalus and atrophy of the corpus callosum and cerebrum. As in Parkinson's disease, the substantia nigra lose their pigmentation. Histologic examination shows Alzheimer-like neurofibrillary tangles and, with special stains, amyloid plaques. However, despite its similarity to Parkinson's disease, dementia pugilistica does not produce Lewy bodies.

Genetic Factors

Studies have shown only a weak chromosomal link in adults with Parkinson's disease. For example, only 10% and 15% of Parkinson's disease patients have a first-degree relative with the same illness. Even in twins who were older than 50 years at the onset of symptoms, genetic factors played no significant role. However, when the onset of symptoms occurred at a younger age (younger than 50 years), genetic factors played a significant role.

Recent studies have shown that several different mutations, including ones in the *parkin* gene (on chromosome 6) and α-*synuclein* gene (on chromosome 4), caused or allowed Parkinson's disease in some families. These mutations usually lead to early-onset disease in either an autosomal dominant or recessive pattern. Not only does genetically determined Parkinson's disease appear, on the average, as young as 45 years but it may begin in childhood or adolescence. The genetically determined variety also differs because it lacks Lewy bodies. Although the majority of Parkinson's disease patients younger than 20 years harbor a parkin mutation, genetically determined Parkinson's disease cases comprise less than 10% of the total.

Some of the data suggest a variation of the usual pathophysiology. They propose that chromosome mutations produce mitochondrial malfunction that, in turn, produces the disease.

Parkinsonism

The clinical features of Parkinson's disease—in the absence of the illness—constitute the clinical condition *parkinsonism.* For example, when antipsychotic medicines produce tremor, rigidity, and bradykinesia, the patient has parkinsonism not Parkinson's disease. Notably, in several illnesses characterized by parkinsonism—dementia pugilistica, Parkinson-plus diseases, and dementia with Lewy bodies (see later)—dementia may appear as the first or most prominent symptom.

Medication-Induced Parkinsonism

Recent studies have challenged the conventional wisdom that antipsychotic agents, which act primarily on D_2 receptors, constitute the most common cause of parkinsonism. Atypical as well as typical antipsychotic agents cause parkinsonism and other extrapyramidal side effects. As a possible exception, clozapine, which has relatively little affinity for D_2 receptors, rarely if ever produces parkinsonism.

Numerous nonpsychiatric medicines, such as metoclopramide (Reglan), cisapride (Propulsid), trimethobenzamide (Tigan), prochlorperazine (Compazine), and promethazine (Phenergan), which block D_2 receptors, produce parkinsonism. In addition, they can produce other sequelae of dopamine blockade, such as neuroleptic-malignant syndrome, dystonic reactions, oculogyric crisis, and akathisia.

Medication-induced parkinsonism so closely resembles Parkinson's disease that a clinical examination cannot easily distinguish them. However, one feature that separates them is that medication-induced parkinsonism typically causes symmetric, bilateral signs from the onset, whereas Parkinson's disease tends to cause hemiparkinsonism at the onset and to remain asymmetric throughout the course of the illness. Also, antipsychotic medicines often induce akathisia and dyskinesias, as well as parkinsonism.

In general, medication-induced parkinsonism may persist for 3 months to as long as 1 year after patients have stopped taking the medications. Physicians must be careful because at least 10% of patients with persistent symptoms harbor Parkinson's disease. In them, the medicines merely unveil the disorder. Moreover, the group of patients with persistent parkinsonism also probably includes some patients with dementia with Lewy body disease. Their illness not only tends to present with symptoms that require antipsychotic agents but also renders them extremely sensitive to their side effects. Additional potential explanations for persistent parkinsonism following antipsychotic treatment include other conditions that cause parkinsonism in children and young adults (see later).

Reducing or withdrawing the antipsychotic medicine usually reverses parkinsonism. The benefit of using anticholinergics remains controversial because of their immediate side effects, such as memory impairment, and possible role in hastening the development of tardive dyskinesia. If physicians administer anticholinergics, they might try to withdraw them after 3 months to determine if they still seem beneficial. Because antipsychotic agents strongly adhere to dopamine receptors, L-dopa will not reverse the parkinsonism. Worse, it might precipitate a toxic psychosis.

Parkinson-Plus Diseases

A group of related neurodegenerative illnesses—loosely termed *Parkinson-plus diseases*—share many of Parkinson's disease physical signs and its predominantly subcortical dementia. However, other features set them apart them from Parkinson's disease and separate one from another. Compared to Parkinson's disease, Parkinson-plus diseases follow a more rapid course and respond less well to dopaminergic medications.

Limited oculomotor movements and axial rigidity characterize the most commonly occurring Parkinson-plus disease, *progressive supranuclear palsy (PSP)*. *Multisystem atrophy (MSA)*, a family of Parkinson-plus diseases, includes *olivopontocerebellar degeneration*, which is notable for ataxia, and *Shy-Drager syndrome*, notable for pronounced autonomic dysfunction. MSA, like Parkinson's disease, is a synucleinopathy; however, in contrast to Parkinson's disease, MSA causes loss of *postsynaptic* D_2 receptors.

Parkinsonism in Children and Young Adults

Although Parkinson's disease occasionally arises in individuals younger than 21 years, such an early onset is rare and usually the expression of a gene mutation. Among this age group, other conditions more commonly cause parkinsonism. In some of them, dementia, psychosis, depression, a personality disorder, or other psychiatric symptom regularly accompanies the parkinsonism:

- Dopa-responsive dystonia
- Early-onset generalized (DYT1) dystonia
- Juvenile Huntington's disease
- Side effects of medications or illicit drugs
- Wilson's disease

Therapy of Parkinson's Disease

Medications

L-DOPA

The current medical treatment for Parkinson's disease alleviates motor symptoms for many years, but does not reverse neurodegeneration. Medicines maintain normal dopamine activity by enhancing dopamine synthesis, retarding its metabolism, or acting as agonists at the receptors. Enhancing dopamine synthesis, usually the initial treatment, consists of substituting orally administered L-dopa to augment the reduced concentrations of DOPA (see Fig. 18-3).

$$\text{Phenylalanine} \xrightarrow{\textit{Phenylalanine hydroxylase}}$$
$$\text{Tyrosine} \xrightarrow{\textit{Tyrosine hydroxylase}}$$
$$\text{DOPA} \xrightarrow{\textit{DOPA decarboxylase}} \text{Dopamine}$$

To bypass the tyrosine hydroxylase deficiency, L-dopa penetrates the blood–brain barrier and inserts itself into the synthetic chain where it substitutes for DOPA. Like naturally occurring DOPA, L-dopa undergoes decarboxylation to form dopamine:

$$\text{L-dopa} \xrightarrow{\textit{DOPA decarboxylase}} \text{Dopamine}$$

L-dopa remains effective until virtually all the nigrostriatal tract neurons degenerate and the remaining neurons can no longer synthesize sufficient dopamine from it.

In contrast to the degenerating presynaptic neurons, the postsynaptic nigrostriatal neurons, which are coated with the dopamine receptors, remain intact. The receptors respond to naturally synthesized dopamine, dopamine derived from L-dopa, and dopamine agonists.

Prescribing L-dopa, the "precursor replacement" strategy, is highly effective for approximately the first 5 years of the illness. During that time, enough nigrostriatal neurons remain intact to synthesize, store, and release dopamine. This strategy provides the most powerful, easiest to use, and least complicated symptomatic treatment. Neurologists typically prescribe L-dopa as a therapeutic trial and then for routine treatment until deterioration requires supplements.

After 5 years, L-dopa treatment alone is insufficient. Not only does it fail to correct the motor impairments but it begins to cause visual hallucinations, dyskinesias, sleep disturbances, and mental status changes. The dyskinesias consist of buccal-lingual movements, chorea, akathisia, dystonic postures, and rocking. Some of these movements resemble tardive dyskinesia. Despite the problems with dyskinesias, most patients prefer overstimulation, which allows them to walk and move about, to understimulation with its rigidity and immobility.

DOPAMINE-PRESERVING MEDICATIONS

Several medications preserve dopamine by inhibiting enzymes that metabolize it: *dopa decarboxylase* and *catechol-O-methyltransferase (COMT)* (Fig. 18-11). Because they cannot cross the blood–brain barrier in significant concentrations, these enzyme-inhibiting medications do not interfere with the normal nigrostriatal conversion of L-dopa to dopamine. They act in the periphery to prevent conversion of L-dopa to dopamine or other metabolite.

One enzyme-inhibiting medication, *carbidopa,* inactivates dopa decarboxylase. Pharmaceutical firms have marketed fixed combinations of carbidopa and L-dopa as Sinemet. Another enzyme-inhibiting medication, entacapone (Comtan), inhibits COMT. A commercial preparation, Stalevo, combines both enzyme inhibitors—carbidopa and entacapone—with L-dopa.

These dopamine-preserving medications maintain cerebral dopamine concentrations while allowing a reduced L-dopa dosage. Thus, patients avoid systemic side effects, such as nausea, vomiting, cardiac arrhythmias, and hypotension. The most troublesome side effects, nausea and vomiting, resulted from high does of dopamine stimulating the emesis (vomiting) center in the medulla, which is one of the few areas of the brain not protected by the blood–brain barrier. The L-dopa and carbidopa combination Sinemet (Latin, *sine* without, *em* vomiting) almost completely eliminates the nausea and vomiting.

Another strategy consists of blocking the enzymes that metabolize dopamine. For example, selegiline inhibits MAO-B, one of the main enzymes responsible for metabolizing dopamine. Selegiline enhances dopamine activity in Parkinson's disease patients because it reduces the oxidation of both naturally occurring and medically derived dopamine. As an added benefit, it diverts some dopamine metabolism to methamphetamine and then to amphetamine, which provides an antidepressant effect. It may also confer some neuroprotection by reducing free radical formation and providing an antioxidant effect. Although it may not slow the progression of Parkinson's disease, selegiline improves patients' symptoms. Moreover, as previously noted, because it inhibits MAO-B but not MAO-A, selegiline taken in routine (10 mg) doses should not leave patients vulnerable to hypertensive crisis or the serotonin syndrome.

DOPAMINE AGONISTS

Even with L-dopa supplements, dopamine production eventually falls to inadequate levels. As a substitute for dopamine, dopamine agonists—bromocriptine, pergolide, pramipexole, and ropinirole—provide stimulation of postsynaptic dopamine receptors (see Fig. 18-3). They act directly on D_2 receptors and to a lesser extent on other postsynaptic dopamine receptors.

Newly introduced dopamine agonists have particular benefits. Prepared as a self-administered injection to rescue patients from complete, sudden loss of dopamine activity, apomorphine (Apokyn) takes effect within 10 to 20 minutes. Although they relieve immobility, apomorphine injections may cause hypotension, nausea, and vomiting—as might be anticipated from a surge in dopamine activity. If further studies confirm its effect, apomorphine may be enlisted to treat neuroleptic-malignant syndrome (Parkinson-hyperpyrexia).

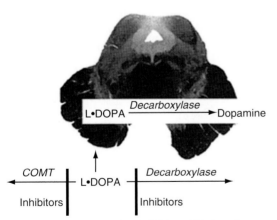

FIGURE 18-11 ■ Medicines that inhibit COMT, such as entacapone, and those that inhibit decarboxylase, such as carbidopa, limit the metabolism of L-dopa. Because the blood–brain barrier prevents these enzyme inhibitors from entering the brain, they do not affect dopamine synthesis in the nigrostriatal tract. Addition of these enzymes to L-dopa permits smaller L-dopa doses, which minimizes systemic side effects.

Another dopamine agonist, rotigotine, comes as a transdermal patch that provides a steady delivery. Because that method greatly reduces fluctuations, it may reduce medication-induced physical and psychiatric complications.

The main advantage of dopamine agonist therapy still lies in its ability to bypass degenerated presynaptic neurons and act directly on the dopamine receptors. Also, compared to L-dopa, agonists may less frequently induce dyskinesias. Some neurologists hoping to reduce young patients' risk of developing dyskinesias after 5 years of treatment prescribe agonists rather than L-dopa from the onset of the illness. However, agonists are less powerful, more expensive, more frequently associated with sleep disorders, and perhaps more closely associated with certain psychiatric disturbances (see previous discussion).

OTHER MEDICATIONS

Coenzyme Q10 plays a vital role in the mitochondrial respiratory chain. Presumably because of its antioxidant effect, pretreatment with coenzyme Q10 greatly reduces the Parkinson-producing potential of MPTP. Preliminary studies suggest that it may slow the progression of Parkinson's disease.

Alpha tocopherol (vitamin E), another antioxidant and free radical scavenger, should protect dopamine from destruction by free radicals and other toxins. Despite the solid rationale, a major study in Parkinson's disease showed that tocopherol, either alone or in combination with selegiline, failed to slow progression of the illness.

Anticholinergics reduce tremor in Parkinson's disease and other forms of parkinsonism. They presumably act by reducing cholinergic activity to maintain the balance with the diminished dopamine activity (Fig. 18-12). On the other hand, they routinely produce anticholinergic side effects—dry mouth, constipation, and urinary retention. More important, anticholinergics can exacerbate cognitive impairments in individuals with mild cognitive impairment (see Chapter 7), Alzheimer's disease, or Parkinson's disease dementia. As previously noted, they may also hasten the development of tardive dyskinesia.

Amantadine enhances dopamine activity by acting on presynaptic neurons to facilitate dopamine release and inhibit its reuptake. In addition, it may antagonize glutamate. Amantadine produces a temporary, modest improvement in rigidity and bradykinesia. It may also ameliorate L-dopa-induced dyskinesias. Unless the patient has underlying dementia, amantadine rarely produces confusion or hallucinations.

Surgery

Several innovative neurosurgical techniques have provided extraordinary therapeutic benefits in Parkinson's disease and revealed aspects of the underlying physiology of the basal ganglia. In addition, similar techniques have been successfully applied in other movement disorders, particularly dystonia and essential tremor.

For Parkinson's disease surgery, the techniques fall into three groups: *ablative procedures, deep brain stimulation (DBS)*, and *transplantation*. The targets consist of two regions: specific thalamic nuclei and the GPi. For hemiparkinsonism, surgeons perform the procedure on the contralateral side of the brain. Bilateral symptoms require bilateral surgery.

In ablative procedures, neurosurgeons place minute lesions in either the thalamus (*thalamotomy*) or GPi (*pallidotomy*) under MRI guidance. Although this procedure has been helpful, it carries risks of serious potential complications, such as cerebral hemorrhage or unintended lesions, particularly ones in adjacent visual tracts. Moreover, bilateral procedures may cause pseudobulbar palsy and cognitive impairment.

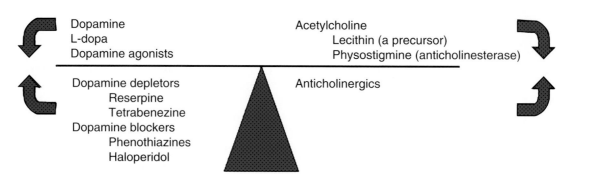

FIGURE 18-12 ■ In a classic but somewhat limited model of a scale, dopamine and acetylcholine activity normally balance each other. When Parkinson's disease reduces dopamine activity, the left side of the scale rises. Dopamine precursors, dopamine agonists, and anticholinergics—Parkinson's disease treatments—restore the balance. Conditions characterized by excessive dopamine activity, such as chorea, push the left side further downward. Substances that either antagonize dopamine or enhance acetylcholine can restore the balance.

In DBS, neurosurgeons insert tiny electrodes in the subthalamic nucleus or GPi. They then connect the electrodes to a pacemaker-like device implanted in the chest. Stimulation probably deactivates neurons by saturating them with high-frequency pulses. DBS has been quite successful in moderate to severe cases. When patients require so much medicine to move that they have dyskinesias, DBS allows them to have greater mobility and greatly reduce or eliminate the dyskinesia-inducing medications dosage. The procedure has several advantages over ablative procedures. Its lesion is smaller, the procedure causes fewer complications, and it does not preclude future treatments, including stem cell transplantation. However, in view of several postoperative suicides, even following successful surgery, and occasional postoperative worsening of cognitive impairments, surgical programs generally exclude patients with either depression or dementia.

In transplantation, neurosurgeons graft dopamine-producing mesencephalic tissue (usually fetal midbrain cells) into the basal ganglia. Transplantation of this tissue has yielded, for the most part, only marginal benefit. In some cases, transplanted cells even grew without restraint and produced greatly excessive dopamine that led to disabling dyskinesias refractory to treatment. Although the blood–brain barrier shields transplanted cells from immunologic rejection by keeping the brain in an "immunologically privileged site," transplanted cells usually survive less than 6 months.

Developing and transplanting stem cells, instead of fetal tissue, particularly to treat Parkinson's disease holds promise, but researchers must overcome many hurdles before realizing this strategy. For example, the cells must survive, grow but only within certain parameters, form synapses, synthesize and appropriately release dopamine, and terminate its action by metabolism and reuptake. Also, the primary cell line or an additional one may have to compensate for deficiencies in other neurotransmitters, such as serotonin.

Supplemental Therapies

Several popular treatments—physical, occupational, speech, and music therapy—would seem benign and beneficial. Individual cases reports, limited studies, and some series have attested to their benefit in Parkinson's disease. However, few studies meeting rigid scientific criteria support their use and their cost-effectiveness remains problematic.

ATHETOSIS

Athetosis consists of involuntary slow, regular, continually changing, twisting movements predominantly affecting the face, neck, and distal limbs (Fig. 18-13).

It sits at one end of a spectrum—athetosis, choreoathetosis, chorea, and hemiballismus—of progressively greater and more irregular movements distinguishable primarily by their clinical features.

In a potentially confusing aspect, additional involuntary movements may coexist with athetosis. For example, chorea may punctuate the slow movements of athetosis and dystonia may override their fluctuations.

Usually a variety of *cerebral palsy* (see Chapter 13), athetosis is often not apparent until early childhood. Most often athetosis results from combinations of perinatal hyperbilirubinemia (kernicterus), hypoxia, and prematurity. Genetic factors are unimportant.

Because athetosis originates in congenital brain injury, seizures and mental retardation frequently accompany the involuntary movements. However, with damage confined to the basal ganglia, some patients have normal intelligence despite disabling movements and garbled speech. These patients represent examples of individuals who retain cognitive capacity despite devastating physical neurologic disabilities.*

Dopamine antagonists may suppress athetosis, but their long-term use may lead to complications. Paradoxically, neurologists often offer an empiric trial of L-dopa to children with athetosis because they may have an element of dystonia or occasionally the underlying problem actually consists of dopa-responsive dystonia (see later) rather than cerebral palsy. According to preliminary reports, neurosurgical procedures akin to those used in Parkinson's disease may also help athetosis. Botulinum toxin injections may temporarily alleviate particularly troublesome involuntary movements in single groups of muscles.

CHOREA

Huntington's Disease

Of the many causes of chorea (Table 18-1), Huntington's disease, previously called "Huntington's chorea," remains the pre-eminent clinical illness. Huntington's disease is a genetic illness with autosomal dominant inheritance characterized by chorea, dementia, and behavioral abnormalities. The mean age when patients' symptoms first become apparent is approximately 37 years. However, approximately 10% of patients develop symptoms in childhood and 25% when they are older than 50 years. Adults with the

---

*Illnesses that produce incapacitating physical disability yet paradoxically allow near normal to even greatly above normal intelligence include ALS, athetotic and spastic diplegia varieties of cerebral palsy, Duchenne's muscular dystrophy, locked-in syndrome, poliomyelitis, and spinal cord transection.

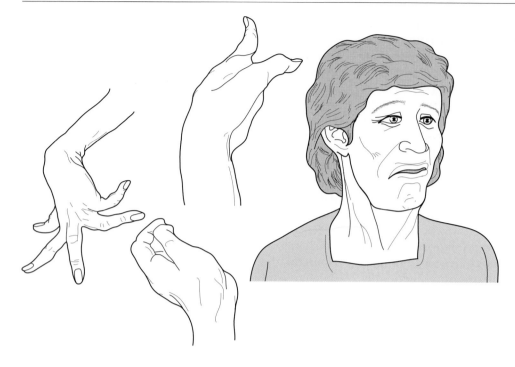

FIGURE 18-13 ■ In athetosis, the face grimaces incessantly. Fragments of smiles alternate with frowns. Pulling of one or the other side distorts the entire appearance. In addition, neck muscles contract and rotate the head. Laryngeal contractions and irregular chest and diaphragm muscle movements cause an irregular cadence, nasal pitch, and dysarthria. Fingers writhe constantly and tend to assume hyperextension postures. At the same time, wrists rotate, flex, and extend. Involuntary limb activity prevents writing, buttoning, and other fine tasks, but it usually allows deliberate, larger scale shoulder, trunk, and hip movement.

TABLE 18-1 ■ Common Causes of Chorea

Basal ganglia lesions
    Perinatal injury (e.g., anoxia, kernicterus)
    Strokes
    Tumors, abscesses, toxoplasmosis*
Genetic disorders
    Huntington's disease
    Wilson's disease
Metabolic derangements
    Hepatic encephalopathy
    Hyperglycemia
    Hyperthyroidism
    Hypocalcemia
Drugs
    Cocaine, amphetamine, methylphenidate
    Dopamine precursors and agonists
    Neuroleptics (tardive and withdrawal-emergent)
    Oral contraceptives^
Inflammatory conditions
    Sydenham's chorea
    Systemic lupus erythematosus (SLE)

---

*Acquired immunodeficiency syndrome (AIDS) causes chorea when toxoplasmosis involves the basal ganglia.
^Estrogens from contraceptives or pregnancy (chorea gravidarum) cause chorea.

illness succumb to aspiration and inanition 1 to 2 decades after the diagnosis.

With 2 and 6 out of 100,000 persons suffering from Huntington's disease, this illness represents a relatively frequent cause of dementia in middle-aged adults. Although it affects individuals from all races and ethnic backgrounds, patients in the United States typically have descended from several 17th-century English immigrants.

The world's largest group of people with Huntington's disease lives in villages near Lake Maracaibo, Venezuela, where more than 100 affected individuals share the same genetic pool, environment, and freedom from exposure to toxins. Extensive studies there have described affected children, heterozygous individuals (carriers) in the presymptomatic state, and patients who are homozygous for the disorder. (Homozygous and heterozygous patients are phenotypically indistinguishable.)

Clinical Features

In contrast to the slow, writhing movements of athetosis, chorea consists of random, discrete, rapid movements that jerk the pelvis, trunk, and limbs (Fig. 18-14). It also includes involuntary face movements that produce brief, meaningless expressions (Fig. 18-15). When individuals with chorea attempt to walk, movements of their trunk and limbs interrupt their cadence and stability (Fig. 18-16).

Movements that comprise chorea, unlike tics, occur with random timing and distribution, do not regularly repeat, and cannot form a pattern. In other words, chorea consists of *nonstereotyped* movements. Also, chorea, as well as other classic movement disorders, comes with no psychic investment in the movements. (In contrast, akathisia, RLS, and tics follow a premonitory urge to move, entail a compulsion to move, and bestow relief if patients move. If patients fail to move, the disorders cause psychologic discomfort [see later].)

In its earliest stage, chorea merely resembles non-specific "fidgety" movements attributable to anxiety, restlessness, discomfort, or clumsiness. It may then consist of only excessive face or hand gestures, weight shifting, leg crossing, or finger twitching (Fig. 18-17). Chorea also impairs the ability to sustain a voluntary muscle contraction, which causes *motor impersistence*. Because of it, patients cannot either sustain a firm

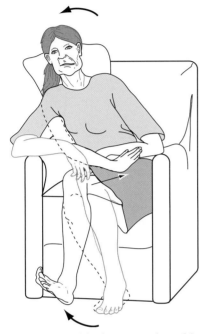

FIGURE 18-14 ■ Patients with chorea, such as this woman who has Huntington's disease, have intermittent and random involuntary movements. Although it usually consists of brisk pelvic, trunk, and limb movements, a mere wrist flick, forward jutting of the leg, or shrugging of the shoulder can constitute the first manifestation of chorea.

grasp or extend their hands or tongue for more than 10 seconds.

Huntington's disease also characteristically interferes with normal eye movements (see Fig. 12-13). In particular, it impairs *saccades,* which are the rapid, almost reflexive, conjugate eye movements that people normally use to glance from one object to another. In Huntington's disease, patients cannot make a rapid, smooth, and accurate shift of their gaze toward an object that suddenly enters their visual field. They routinely first blink or jerk their head to initiate the saccade. Although characteristic, these impaired saccades are not peculiar to Huntington's disease. For example, patients with schizophrenia also have abnormal saccades.

Huntington's disease also interferes with ocular *pursuit movements,* which are the normal, relatively slow conjugate eye movements used in following (tracking) moving objects, such as a baseball thrown into the air or ducks flying across the horizon. Patients typically have irregular, particularly slow, and inaccurate pursuit movements. As with abnormal saccades, abnormal pursuit movements are not peculiar to Huntington's disease.

Dementia typically begins within 1 year of chorea. Even before dementia appears, patients often display inattentiveness, erratic behavior, apathy, personality changes, and impaired judgment. Particularly because of the gait abnormality, neurologists often describe the dementia as subcortical. However, this decision represents another example of the questionable validity of the cortical/subcortical distinction because routine mental status testing, neuropsychologic evaluation, pathologic examination, and other studies reveal cortical as well as subcortical abnormalities.

Almost an integral part of the disease, about 50% of patients have comorbid depressive symptoms,

FIGURE 18-15 ■ Huntington's disease patients characteristically make unexpected, inappropriate, and incomplete facial expressions. Without provocation, they frown, raise eyebrows, and smirk.

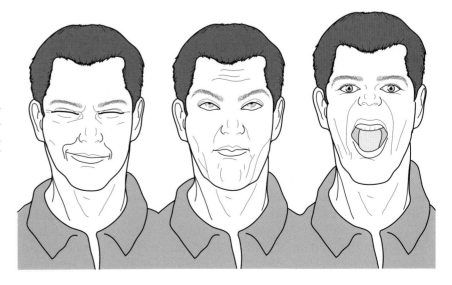

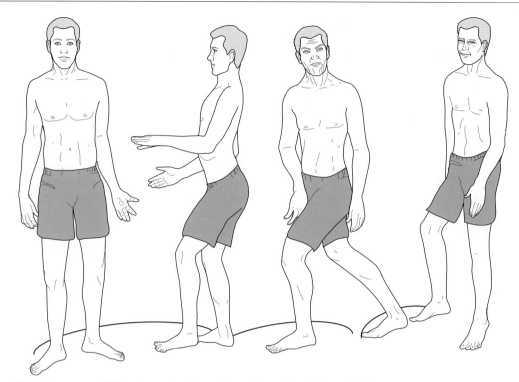

FIGURE 18-16 ■ The signature of Huntington's disease is an irregular, jerky gait that results from intermittent, unexpected trunk and pelvic motions, spontaneous knee flexion, lateral swaying, and a variable cadence. The lack of grace and rhythm belies the origin of *chorea* (Greek, *chorea,* dance).

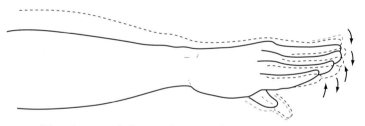

FIGURE 18-17 ■ With their arms and hands extended, Huntington's disease patients fidget with their fingers and wrists, in movements that neurologists describe as "piano playing." When asked by the examiner to squeeze two fingers, patients typically display motor impersistence by exerting inconsistent, variable pressure that they call the "milk maid's sign." Patients also show motor impersistence by intermittently, involuntarily withdrawing the tongue when attempting to protrude it for 30 seconds, "Jack-in-the-box tongue." These classic, graphic terms reflect 200 years of physicians' diagnoses based solely on clinical manifestations.

including either a single episode of major depression or recurrent unipolar depression. Some patients have occasional, transient manic periods. Most have agitation, anxiety, apathy, dysphoria, and irritability. Sometimes these symptoms precede both the dementia and chorea. In addition, about 10% of patients develop psychotic thinking, particularly delusions; however, such aberrations appear only when the other features of the illness have already developed.

Patients tend to commit suicide for several irrational reasons: depression, impaired judgment, and impetuous behavior. They also tend to commit suicide during lucid periods, particularly before learning the results of their genetic testing and when losing their independence. Curiously, the suicide rate immediately before undergoing a diagnostic test exceeds that after receiving a positive result (one that indicates the presence of the disease). Overall, the suicide rate is approximately 10-fold greater than in the general population and higher than in other neurodegenerative illnesses.

Neurologists can base a preliminary diagnosis of Huntington's disease on a patient having chorea, dementia, and a relative with a similar disorder. Readily available DNA testing for patients and potential carriers, including a fetus, can ensure or exclude the diagnosis. However, DNA testing cannot predict the age when symptoms will appear in asymptomatic carriers unless the degree of abnormality is so great that it indicates juvenile Huntington's disease (see later).

Dopamine-blocking neuroleptics or dopamine depletors, such as reserpine, α-methylparatyrosine, and tetrabenazine, may reduce chorea just as they reduce other hyperkinetic movements disorders, such as dystonia and tics. However, they may also cause depression and parkinsonism. If parkinsonism develops, lowering the dose or administering L-dopa may alleviate it.

Typical and atypical antipsychotic agents may control some bizarre thinking and abnormal behavior. Those that block D_2 receptors may, in addition, suppress chorea. In mild cases, benzodiazepines may suffice. Both TCAs and SSRIs may improve mood disturbances, but no treatment reverses the dementia.

Juvenile Huntington's Disease

In 10% of cases, termed the *juvenile variant* of Huntington's disease, symptoms of Huntington's disease appear in individuals younger than 21 years. Their physical signs are different. Unlike adults, who initially show chorea and behavioral abnormalities, children and adolescents first develop rigidity, dystonia, and akinesia (Fig. 18-18). Many of these young Huntington's disease patients resemble children with Parkinson's disease.

In contrast to the adult variety, juvenile Huntington's disease causes seizures and pursues a rapid course. It leads to death twice as rapidly as the adult variety. Also, because the genetic abnormality (excessive trinucleotide repeats [see later]) is more likely to increase if the father rather than mother transmits the gene, the child's father predominantly transmits the juvenile variety. In other words, an affected father is more likely than an affected mother to have a child with juvenile Huntington's disease. The reverse is also true: A child with Huntington's disease is more likely to have a father than mother with Huntington's disease. Nevertheless, despite important clinical differences, the underlying genetic abnormality of the juvenile variety differs quantitatively not qualitatively from the adult variety (see later).

Genetics

The abnormality underlying juvenile and adult varieties of Huntington's disease—as with myotonic dystrophy, fragile X syndrome, and several other genetically transmitted diseases—is a gene containing *excessive trinucleotide repeats* (see Chapter 6 and Appendix 3D). The responsible gene, the *Huntington gene*, located on the short arm of chromosome 4, produces a protein called *huntingtin*. This gene normally consists of 11 to 35 repeats of the trinucleotide base cytosine-adenine-guanine (CAG). Although individuals with between 36 and 39 trinucleotide repeats usually show a *forme fruste* of Huntington's disease, those with 40 or more repeats invariably develop all its manifestations.

In general, the more numerous the trinucleotide repeats, the younger the clinical onset. When the gene contains 60 or more trinucleotide repeats, the juvenile variant develops.

As with other genes containing expanded trinucleotide sequences, the Huntington gene is unstable and tends to increase further in length in successive generations. The progressive expansion of the Huntington gene (*amplification*) explains why carriers of the illness show signs at progressively younger ages in successive generations (*anticipation*). In addition, the gene's trinucleotide sequences enlarge further in sperm than in eggs. Thus, affected fathers are more likely than affected mothers to transmit a Huntington gene amplified enough to cause the juvenile variety.

Pathology

In Huntington's disease, glutamate and other excitatory amino acids excessively stimulate N-methyl-D-aspartate (*NMDA*) receptors. When overstimulated, NMDA receptors become *excitotoxic* (see Chapter 21); they allow calcium to flood neurons, which leads to their death.

The type of cell death that occurs in Huntington's disease, ALS, and several other neurodegenerative illnesses, *apoptosis*, differs from the more common type of cell death, *necrosis*, that occurs in strokes, trauma, and many other brain injuries. Apoptosis, unlike necrosis, is programmed, sequential, and energy requiring. It often occurs as a normal vital process. For example, apoptosis causes closure of the patent ductus arteriosus and involution of the thymus. On a histologic level, unlike necrosis, apoptosis does not provoke inflammation. For example, mononuclear cells do not infiltrate into the area of cells dying of apoptosis.

Pathologists distinguish Huntington's disease by degeneration of the striatal neurons that produce gamma-aminobutyric acid (GABA). In the caudate nuclei portion of the striatum, which shows pronounced atrophy, GABA concentrations fall to less than 50% of normal.

Atrophy of the caudate nuclei, almost a diagnostic macroscopic finding, correlates roughly with the severity of dementia. The atrophy of the caudate

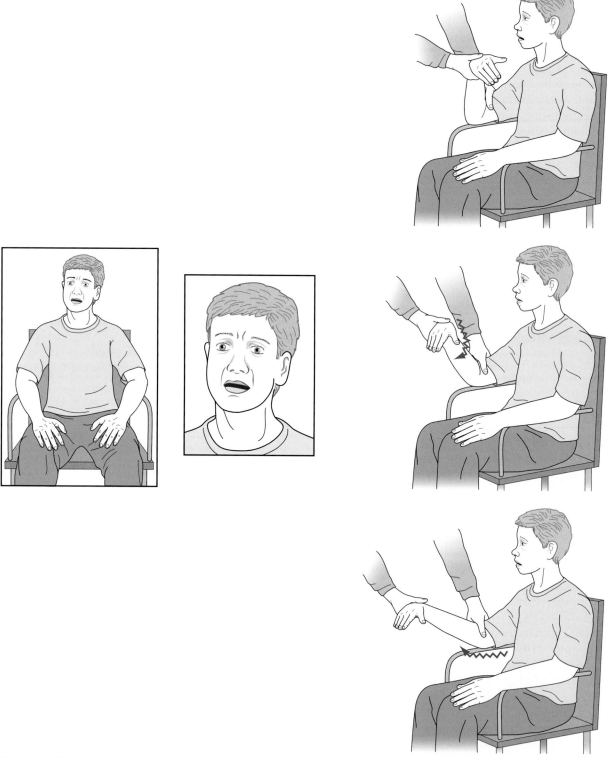

FIGURE 18-18 ■ Having had deteriorating grades and progressively greater isolation from his family and friends, this 18-year-old high-school student came for evaluation. During the interview, he sat motionlessly, had few facial or limb gestures, and moved slowly; however, he had no tremor. He was apathetic and lacked insight. He did not fully cooperate with routine mental status testing, but it seemed to show deficits. When the neurologist flexed and extended his right arm, she detected rigidity. After a routine evaluation, she ordered tests for conditions that cause parkinsonism accompanied by mental deterioration in teenagers—Wilson's disease, drug abuse, and the juvenile variety of Huntington's disease. After she received the report that the genetic testing showed 85 CAG trinucleotide repeats, the neurologist asked to evaluate the father. He displayed subtle but definite chorea and cognitive impairment. His genetic testing also revealed 50 CAG repeats.

nuclei permits the lateral ventricles to balloon outward, that is, develop a convex outline. They expand so much that neurologists call them "bat wing ventricles." CTs and MRIs readily show the caudate atrophy and enlarged, convex ventricles (see Fig. 20-5). As Huntington's disease progresses, the cerebral cortex also undergoes atrophy. PET studies demonstrate caudate hypometabolism early in the illness.

By way of contrast, although normal aging and Alzheimer's disease also cause cerebral atrophy, their atrophy does not preferentially affect the caudate nuclei. In these conditions the caudate nuclei still bulge into the lateral ventricles, which enlarge but maintain a concave outline (see Figs. 20-2, 20-3, and 20-18).

Other Varieties of Chorea

Sydenham's Chorea

Sydenham's chorea, previous known as St. Vitus' dance, is one of the major diagnostic criteria and complications of rheumatic fever with or without carditis. It predominantly affects children between the ages of 5 and 15 years and, of children older than 10 years, girls twice as frequently as boys.

According to the most likely theory of the pathogenesis of Sydenham's chorea, group A β-hemolytic streptococcal infections, which cause rheumatic fever, trigger an autoantibody-mediated inflammatory attack on the basal ganglia.

The chorea usually coincides with rheumatic fever, but it may begin up to 2 to 6 months afterward, when children have recovered their health. It lasts for an average of 2 months, but often complicates recurrences of rheumatic fever. With the decreasing incidence of rheumatic fever and development of various public health measures, Sydenham's chorea and the underlying rheumatic fever seem restricted to small outbreaks occurring mostly in lower socioeconomic neighborhoods.

The chorea begins insidiously with grimaces and limb movements (Fig. 18-19). According to several reports, valproate or carbamazepine suppress it. Sometimes the movements take on a subtle but continual urgency that makes the child seem willfully hyperactive. In that case, neurologists might also consider other causes of hyperactivity in children: attention deficit hyperactivity disorder (ADHD), side effects from medications or illicit drugs, Sydenham's chorea, tics and Tourette's disorders, and withdrawal-emergent syndrome (WES) (see later).

The chorea's significance lies not only in its warning of a life-threatening condition, rheumatic fever, but also because of its comorbid neuropsychiatric symptoms. Obsessive compulsive behavior, obsessive compulsive disorder (OCD), and ADHD occur several-fold

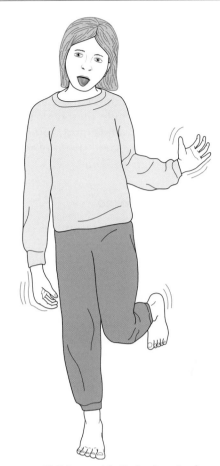

FIGURE 18-19 ■ Children with Sydenham's chorea may appear to have coy smiles and brief grimaces. They seem to walk with a playful sashay. However, the chorea can be made obvious if the children attempt to hold a fixed position, such as standing at attention or standing on the ball of one foot. The chorea lasts for several weeks, but sedating dopamine antagonists can suppress it and allow the child to rest.

more frequently in children with Sydenham's chorea and, to a lesser extent, in children with rheumatic fever without chorea, than in healthy controls (see later). Also, during the 1- to 2-month duration of most cases, OCD parallels the onset and resolution of the chorea. (The opposite may also hold: about one third of children with OCD have *choreiform movements* [mild chorea or movements that mimic chorea].)

Some children reportedly have learning disabilities following Sydenham's chorea; however, in many cases their lower socioeconomic status may have already compromised their premorbid educational status. In any case, despite the serious nature of the illness, Sydenham's chorea does not lead to either frank cognitive impairment or progressive cognitive decline.

Sydenham's chorea's carditis, involuntary movements, and neuropsychiatric symptoms recur under certain circumstances. Most often, repeat streptococcal infections cause recurrent attacks of rheumatic fever, which, in about 20% of cases, give rise to recurrent chorea. Women who contracted rheumatic fever in childhood have a tendency to develop chorea if they start oral contraceptives or conceive (see later). In addition, close relatives and friends of Sydenham's chorea patients frequently develop the illness in "mini-epidemics." Although family members may share a genetic susceptibility, friends and family are also prone to infection by the same strain of streptococcal bacteria because of their proximity.

Estrogen-Related Chorea

Oral estrogen-containing contraceptives on rare occasions produce *oral contraceptive-induced chorea.* This disorder, which is not associated with mental abnormalities other than anxiety, develops in young women several months after starting a contraceptive and resolves after stopping it.

Chorea gravidarum, another rarely occurring disorder, develops almost exclusively in young primigravidas in the first two trimesters of a pregnancy. The disorder often causes motional lability, delirium, and rarely psychotic thinking as well as chorea. When severe, the chorea causes so much exhaustion that a woman often has a spontaneous abortion or must undergo a therapeutic one. Once the pregnancy is terminated, symptoms resolve.

Many women affected by oral contraceptive-induced chorea or chorea gravidarum have had previous episodes of either condition or Sydenham's chorea. Also, their close relatives often have had one of these conditions. However, if chorea develops in a woman who is pregnant or taking oral contraceptives, physicians must still consider conditions other than estrogen-related choreas, such as systemic lupus erythematosus, other rheumatologic disease, hyperthyroidism, or even Huntington's disease.

HEMIBALLISMUS

Hemiballismus consists of intermittent, gross movements of one side of the body. The movements resemble chorea, except that they are more violent, even less predictable, unilateral, and consist of a flinging (ballistic) motion of proximal body parts (Fig. 18-20). On the spectrum of movement disorders, hemiballismus sits, with its greatest amplitude and most intermittent movements, at the opposite end from athetosis with its smallest amplitude and most continuous movements.

Classic papers indelibly associated hemiballismus with lesions in the (contralateral) subthalamic nucleus, but contemporary studies have also attributed hemiballismus to lesions in the caudate nucleus or

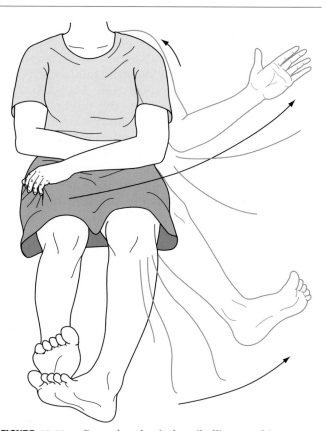

FIGURE 18-20 ■ Beset by classic hemiballismus, this woman has sudden and large-scale movements of the limbs on one side of the body. Even though in most cases, hemiballismus has more modest amplitude, patients use a variety of strategies to suppress it. In this case, the patient uses her left hand to grip her skirt to anchor her moving left arm. Sometimes patients press their body or unaffected limbs against an involuntarily moving limb. They also attempt to camouflage the involuntary movements by converting them into apparently purposeful movements. For example, if her arm were to fly upward, she might incorporate the movement into a gesture, such as waving to someone.

other basal ganglia. In any case, because the responsible lesions are small and situated nowhere near the cerebral cortex, cognitive impairment, paresis, or other corticospinal tract signs do not accompany hemiballismus.

The most common etiology in individuals older than 65 years is an occlusion of a small perforating branch of the basilar artery causing a stroke in the basal ganglia. In individuals infected with human immunodeficiency virus (HIV), toxoplasmosis lesions have a tendency to develop in the basal ganglia and produce hemiballismus (see Fig. 20-11). Similarly, vasculitis can affect the basal ganglia and cause hemiballismus.

Physicians can offer few treatment options. Dopamine-blocking antipsychotic agents can suppress the movements until either a specific medicine takes effect or until the movements spontaneously resolve.

WILSON'S DISEASE

The insidious development of dementia, minor and major psychiatric disturbances, and a variety of involuntary movements, but mostly tremor, in adolescents, teenagers, and young adults characterize Wilson's disease (*hepatolenticular degeneration*). Because early diagnosis and treatment can reverse its symptoms and signs, neurologists often describe Wilson's disease as the quintessential "reversible cause of dementia."

Due to an autosomal recessive mutation of a copper-transporting gene carried on chromosome 13, Wilson's disease leads to insufficient copper excretion that, in turn, allows destructive copper deposits in the brain, liver, cornea, and other organs. As its formal name implies, the illness primarily causes destruction of the liver and the lenticular nuclei of the basal ganglia (see Fig. 18-1A).

Symptoms appear at an average age of 16 years. Unless properly treated, personality changes, conduct disorders, mood disturbances, and thought disorders precede cognitive impairment. The combination of these symptoms, especially when they develop in young individuals, may lead to an erroneous diagnosis of schizophrenia.

The movements consist of rigidity, akinesia, dystonia, or the characteristic *wing-beating tremor* (Fig. 18-21). Other manifestations can be a Parkinson-like tremor and ataxia. The various movements tend to occur in combination and be accompanied by corticospinal or corticobulbar tract signs. With its predominant rigidity and tremor, neurologists often also consider Wilson's disease one of the foremost causes of parkinsonism in children and young adults.

Especially in children, the non-neurologic manifestations of Wilson's disease often overshadow neurologic ones. For example, liver involvement leads to cirrhosis, which is sometimes so severe that it causes hepatic encephalopathy and then liver failure. Copper deposition in the cornea produces a *Kayser-Fleischer ring* (Fig. 18-22).

Physicians consider testing for Wilson's disease, despite its infrequent occurrence (1 per 100,000 persons), in most older children and young adults who develop a wide variety of symptoms, including tremor, parkinsonism, dystonia, atypical psychosis, dementia, and dysarthria, as well as cirrhosis. Because the Kayser-Fleischer ring appears in almost all Wilson's disease patients with neurologic symptoms, individuals with symptoms compatible with the illness should undergo a slit lamp examination. Alternatively, they should also undergo determination of their serum ceruloplasmin (the serum copper-carrying protein) concentration. Even when Wilson's disease does not affect the brain, ceruloplasmin concentrations fall to very low levels. Another test, but a more

cumbersome one, is measurement of the 24-hour urinary copper excretion. In Wilson's disease, the absence of ceruloplasmin greatly increases urinary copper excretion.

Several medications, working through different mechanisms, reduce the body's copper burden. For example, copper-chelating agents, such as penicillamine,

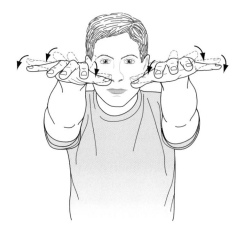

FIGURE 18-21 ■ Although Wilson's disease may induce parkinsonism, dystonia, and dysarthria, it characteristically produces the *wing-beating tremor*. This tremor consists of rhythmic, coarse, up-and-down arm movements centered on the shoulders. Patients with this tremor, as its name implies, flap their arms as though they were attempting to fly.

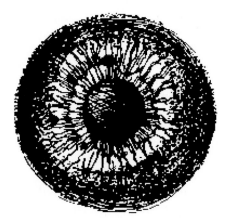

FIGURE 18-22 ■ The Kayser-Fleischer ring, which appears bilaterally, consists primarily of green, brown, or orange copper pigment deposits in the periphery of the cornea. Most obvious at the superior and inferior margins of the cornea, the ring usually obscures the fine structure of the iris. Physicians must use an ophthalmologist's slit lamp to see the Kayser-Fleischer ring in its early stages. Although the ring develops in about 70% of cases when Wilson's disease affects only the liver, it develops in almost all cases that affect the brain. However, because the Kayser-Fleischer ring also develops in primary biliary cirrhosis and several other liver diseases, it is not pathognomic of Wilson's disease. The ring's size and density correlate with the duration of Wilson's disease, and with successful treatment, it resolves.

can reverse some or all of the mental deterioration, movement disorders, and non-neurologic manifestations, including Kayser-Fleisher rings. When cirrhosis refractory to medical treatment threatens permanent brain damage, liver transplantation can rescue the patient.

DYSTONIA

Dystonia consists of involuntary powerful twisting or turning (torsion) movements, sustained at the height of muscle contraction. It can affect one muscle group (*focal dystonia*) or virtually all muscles (*generalized dystonia*). In generalized dystonia, patients' limb (appendicular) muscles and neck, trunk, and pelvis (axial) muscles simultaneously contract and force patients into grotesque dystonic postures. Although focal dystonia usually remains limited to the originally affected region, generalized dystonia progresses over years to involve more and more regions until it encompasses the entire bodily musculature. For the most part, genetic abnormalities play an important role in causing primary and several secondary generalized dystonias (see later) but not focal dystonias.

Compared to other involuntary movements, dystonia usually has several unusual features. It can be suppressed briefly by "tricks," such as skipping, walking backward, dancing (with or without music), or pressing lightly against the affected body part. In addition, dystonia tends to trigger compensatory movements, which sometimes gives patients a bizarre appearance. Probably more frequently than with any other involuntary movement disorder, neurologists misdiagnose dystonia as a psychogenic disturbance because the movements are so unusual and, by using tricks, patients seem to control them. On the other hand, psychogenic movements often mimic dystonia.

In another important clinical feature, primary dystonia (dystonia that is not a symptom of an underlying condition), like several other illnesses previously noted, may cause devastating physical disabilities, but it does not cause dementia. On the other hand, depending on the specific variety of dystonia and degree of disability, depression may be a comorbid condition.

Generalized Dystonias

Early-Onset Primary Dystonia

Early-onset primary dystonia or *idiopathic torsion dystonia,* previously known as dystonia musculorum deformans, develops predominantly among Ashkenazi (Eastern European) Jews. In them, the illness begins typically in 9- to 11-year-old children but almost

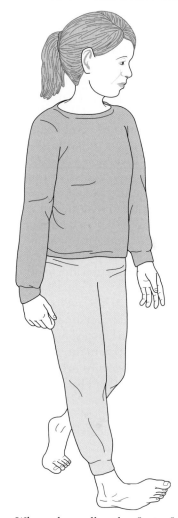

FIGURE 18-23 ■ When she walks, the foot of this girl, with early onset primary dystonia, twists slowly inward and onto its side. Even though incomplete, the twisting causes her to limp. However, using one of her "sensory tricks," she can correct her limp by skipping, dancing, or walking backward.

always by the age of 26 years. The dystonia usually begins with torsion of a hand or foot (Fig. 18-23) and subsequently the other limbs, pelvis (tortipelvis), trunk, and neck (torticollis). It eventually incapacitates its victims (Fig. 18-24). Although early-onset primary dystonia does not impair cognitive function, it is often accompanied by comorbid depression.

An abnormality in the *DYT1* gene, which is located on chromosome 9, carries the illness in an autosomal dominant pattern, but penetrance is only 30% to 40%. In contrast to genes characterized by excessive trinucleotide repeats, this one consists of deletion of the trinucleotide GAG. Several other DYT genes also carry dystonia, but they vary as to whether they express the illness in a dominant or recessive pattern, which ethnic groups carry them, and their physical manifestations.

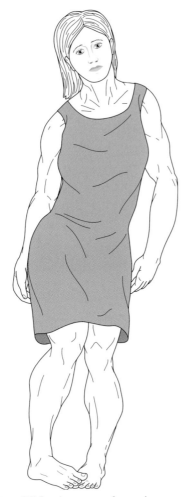

FIGURE 18-24 ■ With time, as dystonia encompasses the remaining limb and axial musculature, patients develop generalized dystonic postures. Because they continually contract, muscles hypertrophy. Patients lose their subcutaneous fat from the incessant exertion. The postures in this condition sometimes resemble those in Wilson's disease and tardive dystonia.

The mechanism by which the DYT genes produce the movements remains unknown. One clue is that, unlike in other movement disorders, studies of CSF and autopsy material found abnormalities in norepinephrine metabolism.

DNA testing for the DYT1 gene can establish the diagnosis. Various tests—blood chemistry, MRI or CT, PET, and brain tissue analysis—reveal no consistent abnormality. Anticholinergics, baclofen, and carbamazepine provide only modest and generally inconsistent benefit. Bilateral thalamotomy, pallidotomy, and, more recently, DBS have greatly relieved the movements in many cases.

Dopa-Responsive Dystonia

In an illness described by Segawa and his Japanese colleagues and often named after them, *dopa-responsive dystonia* (*DRD*) gives rise to dystonia that appears in children and follows a distinctive diurnal pattern. The predominant if not sole symptom, dystonia, becomes evident in children, on the average, when they are 8 years old. Its distinctive pattern consists of diurnal fluctuations. The dystonia is typically absent in the morning but pronounced by the late afternoon and evening (Fig. 18-25). As with early-onset dystonia, DRD first affects children's gait and then progresses to become generalized. In a related feature, DRD sometimes superimposes parkinsonism on the dystonia.

The title, DRD, describes not only the illness' diagnostic test but also its treatment. Small L-dopa doses, typically 10% of those used to treat Parkinson's disease, dramatically ameliorate DRD. Because of the success of L-dopa in DRD, neurologists routinely give it as a therapeutic trial to children who have developed dystonia or almost any movement disorder resembling dystonia. If children improve, genetic testing should confirm the diagnosis of DRD. Unlike treatment of Parkinson's disease, where L-dopa requirements increase, the therapeutic L-dopa dose in DRD remains constant and small throughout life.

In a potential diagnostic pitfall, DRD resembles primary DYT1 dystonia, cerebral palsy, or mental retardation. Even if neurologists believe that one of those conditions, which are essentially untreatable, is most likely, they nevertheless freely administer a therapeutic trial of L-dopa to prevent overlooking the diagnosis of DRD.

DRD exists in all ethnic groups. In affected families, cases usually appear in an autosomal dominant pattern with incomplete penetrance. Several different mutations of a gene, carried on chromosome 14, may impair the synthesis of tetrahydrobiopterin, which is a cofactor for both phenylalanine hydroxylase and tyrosine hydroxylase. The tetrahydrobiopterin deficiency, in turn, eventually leads to serotonin and dopamine deficiencies that are more pronounced after daily activities deplete their stores.

Secondary Generalized Dystonia

Several other neurologic illnesses—Wilson's disease, juvenile Huntington's disease, tardive dyskinesia, and several rare illnesses—can occasionally express themselves as generalized dystonia rather than as their more typical movement. When they produce dystonia, neurologists categorize it as *secondary* or *symptomatic dystonia*.

One of these dystonia-producing illnesses, *Lesch-Nyhan syndrome*, a sex-linked recessive genetic disorder, also serves as prime example of behavioral neurology. In one of neurology's most bizarre symptoms, 2- to 6-year-old children develop ferocious self-mutilation as a manifestation of a biochemical

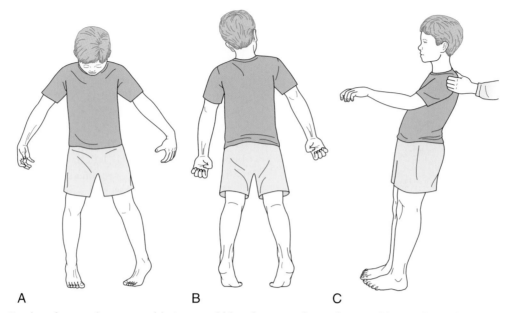

A   B   C

FIGURE 18-25 ■ During the previous year, this 8-year-old boy began to have abnormal leg and trunk movements that forced him to walk on his toes, but only during the afternoon and evening. At those times, his arms and hands showed dystonic posturing and his legs assumed straightened positions, forcing him to walk on his toes. When he awoke in the morning, he walked and ran normally. His parents initially thought that he had developed cerebral palsy (see Fig. 13-3). Pediatric neurologists detected dystonia, more so in his legs than his arms, and found a positive response to the pull test (see Fig. 18-9B). Cognitive testing showed no abnormality. For many reasons, including that cerebral palsy does not develop or become evident after age 5 years, the pediatric neurologists administered a therapeutic trial of a small dose of L-dopa. The boy immediately reverted to normal. Genetic tests later confirmed the diagnosis of dopa-responsive dystonia.

deficit (Fig. 18-26). Children with Lesch-Nyhan syndrome, who are almost all boys, also have mental retardation, corticospinal tract signs, and seizures, as well as dystonia and aberrant behavior.

The basic abnormality in Lesch-Nyhan syndrome consists of a deficiency of a urea metabolism enzyme, hypoxanthine-guanine phosphoribosyl transferase (HGPRT). By late childhood, hyperuricemia, an accumulation of urea in the blood, often leads to renal failure.

Focal Dystonias

In contrast to generalized dystonia, *focal dystonias* typically occur sporadically, develop in middle-aged and older adults, and involve muscles in a single region of the body: the face or head (*cranial dystonia*), neck (*cervical dystonia*), or arm (*limb dystonia*). Because these involuntary movements recur in a particular pattern, neurologists refer to them as stereotyped. A particular action typically causes *task-specific* focal dystonias. For example, such as writing but not drawing or typing, may precipitate writer's cramp. Likewise, job-related motions precipitate *occupational dystonias*. Nevertheless, as with primary generalized dystonia, patients' cognitive capacity remains intact.

Except for one condition, hemifacial spasm, the cause of focal dystonia usually remains unknown. Probably erroneously in almost all cases, neurologists and analysts previously attributed focal dystonias to subconscious conflicts. At one time, they also considered them a form of tardive dyskinesia because they sometimes followed administration of dopamine receptor-blocking medications. However, most patients with focal dystonias have had no exposure to such medications and, aside from disturbances that the movements induce, have normal psychologic backgrounds. In a controversial position, some neurologists attribute cervical and limb dystonia to trauma of the limbs or trunk.

Another feature of focal dystonias is that injections of *botulinum A toxin* (Botox) into affected muscles dramatically reduce the involuntary movements (Fig. 18-27). Botulinum toxin can also treat isolated, overactive, or otherwise troublesome muscle groups in generalized dystonia.

Cranial Dystonias

Blepharospasm, an easily recognizable and frequently occurring focal dystonia, consists of bilateral, simultaneous contractions of the orbicularis oculi (eyelid) and sometimes the frontalis (forehead) muscles

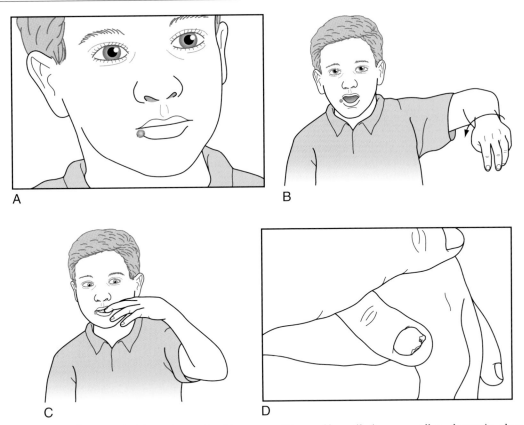

FIGURE 18-26 ■ This mentally retarded boy shows the bizarre, striking self-mutilation, as well as dystonia, that characterizes Lesch-Nyhan syndrome. *A,* His right lower lip has been deeply gnawed even after his front teeth had been removed to stop him from continuously biting his lips. *B,* His limbs writhe and his thumb curls into his palm. *C,* In an apparent compulsion, he uncontrollably chews his fingers and already has amputated the tip of the smallest one. *D,* When the physician pries away his left thumb, deep excoriations are evident.

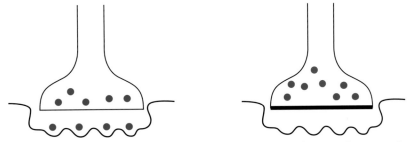

FIGURE 18-27 ■ *Left,* At the normal neuromuscular junction, the presynaptic membrane releases packets of acetylcholine (ACh) (the blue dots) that cross the cleft and bind to postsynaptic membrane receptors, triggering muscle contractions. Focal dystonias are characterized by involuntary segmental muscle contractions. *Right,* Botulinum A toxin, injected directly into affected muscles, binds irreversibly to the presynaptic membrane. It interferes with the release of the ACh packets and thereby weakens the injected muscle. The treatment reduces abnormal contractions for about 3 months. During that period, injected muscles may be weak but they function normally and have little involuntary movement. To maintain the improvement, physicians must repeat the botulinum toxin injections. For cosmetic purposes, physicians sometimes inject small doses of botulinum toxin to relax the facial muscles that cause undesirable furrows and wrinkles of the forehead, eyebrow ("frown lines"), lateral canthus ("crow's feet"), and other areas of the face and neck.

(Fig. 18-28). The muscle spams force the eyelids closed and tend to render patients functionally blind, as well as causing disfiguring facial expressions.

To overcome the involuntary contractions, patients unconsciously learn "sensory tricks" that temporarily suppress the contractions (Fig. 18-29). As with other focal dystonias, botulinum injections reduce or abolish blepharospasm.

Oromandibular dystonia also consists of prominent contractions of the lower facial muscles and jaw

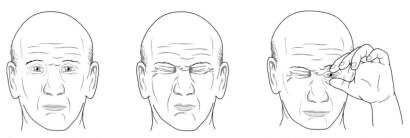

FIGURE 18-28 ■ This elderly man with blepharospasm suffers from unprovoked, bilateral, and prolonged (average duration, 5 seconds) contractions (spasms) of his orbicularis oculi muscles. Because eyelid spasms block his vision, he often resorts to prying them open. (The eyelid contractions in blepharospasm, as opposed to when they occur as a tic, are longer, more forceful, and not provoked by a "need" to close the eyes.)

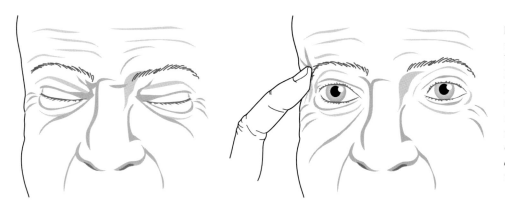

FIGURE 18-29 ■ *Left,* Similarly, this man, during periods of blepharospasm, cannot open his eyelids. He attempts, perhaps unconsciously, to open them by elevating his forehead muscles. *Right,* He has instinctively learned the sensory trick of pressing one eyebrow (a *geste antagoniste*), which suppresses the spasms for several minutes.

muscles. Although oromandibular dystonia, like the oral-buccal-lingual movements of tardive dyskinesia, involves oral-buccal movements, it is distinguishable by the symmetric, predominant upper face involvement, and absence of tongue protrusions. Oromandibular dystonia often accompanies blepharospasm in a condition called *Meige's syndrome* (Fig. 18-30).

Hemifacial spasm, a completely different cranial dystonia, consists of spasms of the muscles on only one side of the face—all those innervated by the ipsilateral facial nerve (the seventh cranial nerve) (Fig. 18-31). In this disorder, spasms occur irregularly, 1 to 10 per minute and disfigure the face. Unlike dystonia and almost all other movement disorders, hemifacial spasm routinely persists into stages 1 and 2 of nonrapid eye movement (NREM) and occasionally into deeper sleep stages.

In addition, unlike other cranial dystonias, hemifacial spam often has an identifiable and correctable cause. In most cases, an aberrant vessel or other structural lesion compresses and presumably irritates the facial nerve at its exit from the pons in the cerebellopontine angle. Sometimes, misdirected regrowth of the facial nerve after an injury, including Bell's palsy, leads to the disorder.

Neurosurgeons can alleviate hemifacial spasm resulting from an aberrant blood vessel by performing a *microvascular decompression.* This procedure consists

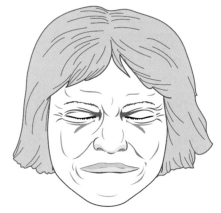

FIGURE 18-30 ■ This patient with Meige's syndrome has contractions of her entire facial musculature, including prominent blepharospasm. In an unconscious sensory trick, patients suppress the movements by talking. Sometimes they talk so much as to appear manic.

of their inserting a cushion between the vessel and the facial nerve, which is a similar to microvascular decompression of the trigeminal nerve (the fifth cranial nerve) for trigeminal neuralgia (see Fig. 9-5). (Generally, trigeminal neuralgia patients suffering from pain will much sooner undergo neurosurgery than hemifacial spasm patients, despite their disfigurement and loss of binocular vision.)

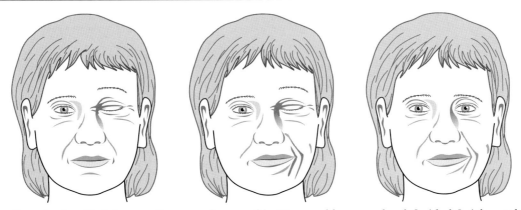

FIGURE 18-31 ■ Beset by hemifacial spasm for several years, this 53-year-old woman has left-sided facial muscle contractions that have a long duration (average duration 7 seconds) and variable forcefulness. The contractions repetitively squeeze shut her left eyelids and pull her mouth to her left side; however, the muscles do not contract synchronously. Muscles sometimes contract only on the side of her mouth or only around her eye. As a compensatory mechanism to uncover her left eye, she often elevates her forehead on that side.

Cervical Dystonias

In *spasmodic torticollis*, the sternocleidomastoid and adjacent neck muscles involuntarily contract to rotate and tilt the head and neck (Figs. 18-32 and 18-33). The contractions initially persist for several seconds to several minutes. As the disease progresses, the abnormal postures becomes continuous and a superimposed tremor may develop. Unlike facial dystonias, spasmodic torticollis is usually painful because of continuous muscle contractions, forceful compression and rotation of vertebra on vertebra, and irritation of the adjacent cervical nerve roots.

Although it usually occurs alone, spasmodic torticollis occasionally serves as a component of primary dystonia. About 10% of cases occur within families. Head and neck injuries, especially "whiplash" from motor vehicle accidents, have allegedly produced isolated cases of spasmodic torticollis and other varieties of focal dystonia. Also, long-term use of dopamine-blocking agents leads to a retrocollis as an aspect of tardive dystonia (see later). Whatever the cause, intramuscular botulinum toxin injections alleviate the movements. Moreover, that treatment also greatly reduces the pain.

Spasmodic dysphonia, previously called "spastic dysphonia," consists of a distinctive speech abnormality caused by a sudden, involuntary contraction of the laryngeal muscles when patients speak. Their voice takes on an intermittently and abruptly strained tone—as if trying to speak while being strangled. Nevertheless, they can shout, sing, and whisper because these varieties of speech bypass the larynx and rely on the lips, mouth, and tongue. Likewise, patients can normally use the appropriate, neighboring muscles to swallow and breathe.

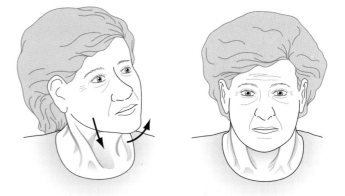

FIGURE 18-32 ■ In spasmodic torticollis, contraction of neck muscles may cause predominant rotation, tilting, and either flexion (*anterocollis*) or extension (*retrocollis*). Shoulder elevation, as though the head and shoulder pull toward each other, accompany the neck movements. Continuous contractions also result in muscle hypertrophy and pain.

Other cranial and cervical dystonias and head tremors often accompany spasmodic dysphonia. Clinical evaluation can distinguish it from related conditions, such as psychogenic voice disorders, vocal cord tumors, and pseudobulbar palsy (see Chapter 4). Electromyography-guided botulinum injections through the anterior of the throat directly into the laryngeal muscles reduce or eliminate their involuntary contractions and restore patients' voice.

Citing several similarities, some investigators have suggested that *stuttering* represents a variety of vocal dystonia. However valid the comparison, treatment with botulinum toxin produces only a hoarse or hypophonic voice without alleviating the stuttering.

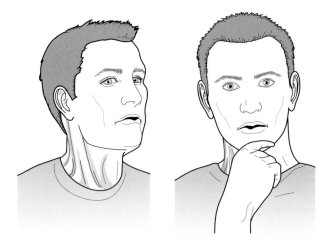

FIGURE 18-33 ■ A concerted effort may temporarily overcome spasmodic torticollis. Alternatively, as with blepharospasm and other focal dystonias, patients instinctively learn sensory tricks, such as applying slight counter-rotational pressure against the chin. These maneuvers not only briefly stop the movement but also camouflage it by striking a studious pose.

Limb Dystonias

Limb dystonias usually affect the hands and arms more than the legs. When hand muscles contract shortly after individuals engage in a repetitive activity that forms the basis of their livelihood, which typically involves manual labor, neurologists term the disorder occupational dystonia, task-specific dystonia, or cramps. The muscle contractions and ensuing pain or discomfort prevent workers from continuing their job. Paradoxically, workers with these disorders can still perform routine functions with their affected hand.

The best example of these disorders is *writer's cramp*. Shortly after a patient begins to write, this disorder provokes spasmodic contraction of finger and hand muscles that distort the hand and prevent individuals from properly grasping a pen or pencil (Fig. 18-34). However, writer's cramp does not prevent eating, buttoning clothing, manipulating small objects, or making other movements that require equal dexterity.

Because affected writers can still dictate or type material that they cannot express by writing, this condition differs fundamentally from the psychologic phenomenon of writer's block. Fatigue-induced cramps also differ from writer's cramp because they occur only after hours of performing the same task and prohibit using the limb or hand for any other purposes.

Comparable occupational dystonias afflict other creative individuals who perform repetitive tasks as part of their work. For example, musicians may develop *pianist's* or *violinist's cramps,* in which repetitive, rapid, and intricate movements of their hands and fingers precipitate performance-interrupting cramps.

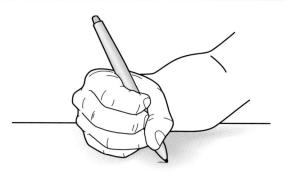

FIGURE 18-34 ■ This author with writer's cramp develops finger and hand muscle spasms several minutes after starting to write. The spasms force her hand into a fist-like position that prevents her from holding a pen. They also cause moderate pain. However, when she uses the same hand to type, eat, or button clothing, she does not develop the cramps.

Similarly, brass and woodwind players are vulnerable to *embouchure dystonia,* in which playing their instrument triggers debilitating lip, jaw, and tongue muscle contractions. Although occupation dystonias that affect creative individuals attract the most attention, they also affect workers in less cerebral occupations, such as bricklaying and sewing.

ESSENTIAL TREMOR

Essential tremor consists of fine oscillations (6 to 9 Hz) of the wrist, hand, or fingers, usually when patients perform particular actions or hold their upper extremities in certain postures (Fig. 18-35). As in other varieties of tremor, the affected region oscillates in one plane. In addition to patients having an essential tremor in their hands, many patients also develop head shaking, usually in a "yes-yes" or "no-no" pattern, and a tremor of their voice.

Essential tremor, the most common involuntary movement disorder, usually develops in young and middle-aged adults. In the majority of cases, it follows a pattern of autosomal dominant inheritance, but with variable penetrance. When the tremor affects multiple family members, neurologists call it *benign familial tremor.* Also, the tremor affects people older than 65 years, but in this case neurologists sometimes label it *senile tremor.* About 50% of affected individuals claim that drinking alcohol-containing beverages suppresses their tremor. In almost all patients with tremor, as with many other neurologic conditions, anxiety precipitates or intensifies the movements. When anxiety affects the tremor, it increases its amplitude but not its frequency.

No completely effective treatment is available. However, β-adrenergic blockers, such as propranolol (Inderal), can suppress most cases of essential tremor

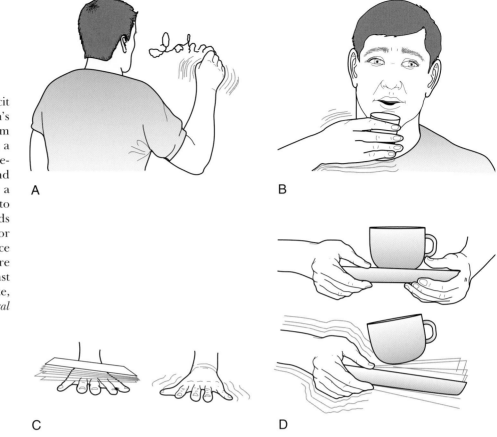

FIGURE 18-35 ■ Physicians elicit this 34-year-old gentleman's essential tremor by having him write his name *(A)*, drink from a filled glass *(B)*, support an envelope on his outstretched and pronated hand *(C)*, or transfer a cup and saucer from one hand to the other *(D)*. When his hands rest in his lap, the tremor completely subsides. Its presence only when hands and arms are held in fixed positions against gravity has led to alternate, descriptive terms, such as *postural* or *positional tremor.*

A

B

C

D

and usually at doses that do not cause depression.* Response to these medicines is consistent with the hypothesis that essential tremor results from excessive β-adrenergic activity. Primidone (Mysoline), an antiepileptic drug, closely related to phenobarbital, alone or in combination with propranolol also often reduces the tremor. Medicines with less efficacy include alprazolam, atenolol, and other β-blockers. In an innovation, DBS directed at the ventral intermediate nucleus of the thalamus, although seemingly highly invasive for a relatively benign condition, dramatically suppresses the tremor.

Other Tremors

Other fine rapid tremors, largely because they also respond to β-blockers, probably originate in excessive adrenergic system activity. These tremors seem to be manifestations of anxiety; stage fright (performance anxiety); hyperthyroidism; excessive caffeine; and many

*Propranolol blocks both β-1 and β-2 adrenergic sympathetic nervous system receptor sites. Metoprolol (Lopressor), which also suppresses the tremor, although less effectively, blocks β-1 adrenergic sites.

medications, including steroids, β-adrenergic stimulating agents, such as isoproterenol and epinephrine, and psychotropics, including amitriptyline, lithium, valproate, and sertraline. In addition, withdrawal from a variety of substances—alcohol, benzodiazepines, or opiates—produces tremor.

By way of contrast, the Parkinson's disease tremor occurs so characteristically at rest that it is the quintessential "resting tremor." It also differs from essential tremor by being "pill rolling," diminished by voluntary movements, and relatively slow (see Fig. 18-8). Cerebellar dysfunction causes a coarse, irregular tremor elicited by movement (see Fig. 2-11). Tremors induced by Wilson's disease remain difficult to categorize, especially because they can appear similar to those of Parkinson's disease, cerebellar disease, or essential tremor. In young adults who develop a tremor, physicians should probably first consider Wilson's disease. The fragile X syndrome includes mental retardation and tremor resembling essential tremor among its manifestations (Chapter 13).

Palatal tremor, which neurologists until recently called *palatal myoclonus,* consists of uninterrupted symmetric, rhythmic contractions of the soft palate. The frequency (120 to 140 times per minute) is consistent from patient to patient. It too persists during sleep or coma. Most cases are caused by small brainstem infarctions that involve the medulla's inferior olivary nucleus or its connections (see Fig. 2-9).

TICS

Tics consist of repetitive, stereotyped, rapid movements that usually involve the face, head, or neck. Neurologists classify tics, depending on their pattern, as *simple* or *complex* and as *motor* or *vocal (phonic)*. *Simple motor tics* include the common head toss, prolonged eye blink, shoulder jerk, and asymmetric smile. *Complex motor tics* consist of actions that utilize several muscle groups, such as touching or hitting oneself, jumping, stomping, or skipping. *Simple vocal tics* are short, inarticulate sounds, such as throat clearing, grunting, and sniffing. *Complex vocal tics* range from words to phrases and include coprolalia (see later). Other varieties of tic can involve the patient's moving in response to an uncomfortable sensation (sensory tics), repeating words (echolalia), or mimicking movements (echopraxia or echokinesis).

Motor tics typically occur with lightning-like rapidity, in succession, and in various combinations. Bursts of tics can persist for several seconds and generate complex movements. Bursts of bursts vary and recur. Within weeks, or months, and years, tic activity develops and subsides.

Tics share many characteristics with other hyperkinetic movement disorders. Excitement, anxiety, fatigue, and use of cocaine and other stimulants increase their frequency and severity, but intense concentration may abolish them for minutes to hours. Also, affected individuals consciously or subconsciously employ various tricks to hide their tics. In fact, affected individuals can suppress tics more than those with any other involuntary movement disorder. However, afterward their tics may rebound in a flurry.

Setting tics apart from most other movement disorders, a nearly universal but hidden urge or premonitory sensation—commonly interpreted as a compulsion—irresistibly provokes the tics. A similar although less intense need occurs with akathisia and RLS. Particularly with tics, patients gain relief if they allow the tic to emerge and suffer anxiety and an unpleasant intensification of the urge if they cannot.

Simple motor tics develop in about 5% to 10% of school-aged children, but, by the end of adolescence, most of them enjoy a spontaneous remission. A disproportionate number of children with tics have a close relative with one or more tics. When their parents or siblings have tics, children are not only more apt to develop tics but also to develop them at a young age.

Tics in Adults

Adults may have motor tics as either a chronic disorder that began in childhood or occasionally as a newly arising condition. Compared to motor tics in children, which usually tend to involve only the head or neck, those in adults often involve the chest, diaphragm, entire trunk, and limb—the more caudal structures.

When tics begin in adults, they are even more of a problem than when they begin in childhood. Those developing in adults tend to have greater forcefulness, duration, frequency, and complexity; occur in combination with other tics; carry psychiatric comorbidity (see later); and impose a great social burden. They are also more resistant to medical therapy. Moreover, they may be a symptom of serious neurologic illnesses, such as encephalitis, Parkinson's disease, tardive dyskinesia (tardive tics), or use of cocaine or other psychoactive substances. Also, dramatic bursts of obscenities that resemble complex vocal tics may stem from either nondominant hemisphere injury or the disordered, frustrated speech of aphasia (see Chapter 8).

Gilles de la Tourette's (Tourette's) Disorder

In general, for a diagnosis of Tourette's disorder, neurologists and psychiatrists require a *combination* of vocal and multiple motor tics that develops in individuals at least younger than 18 years and lasts longer than 1 year (Fig. 18-36). Depending on the specialty, other diagnostic details may differ.

The criteria in the *Diagnostic and Statistical Manual of Mental Disorders, 4th Edition, Text Revision* (*DSM-IV-TR*) for Tourette's disorder require that the patient display both motor and vocal tics but not necessarily concurrently, tics be sudden and rapid, and the disorder develop before age 18 years. In a change from its previous edition, the DSM-IV-TR no longer requires that Tourette's disorder "cause marked distress or significant impairment in social, occupational, or other important areas of functioning."

The DSM-IV-TR also sets criteria for *Chronic Motor or Vocal Tic Disorder*, which allow for single or multiple motor *or* vocal tics, but not both, that begin before age 18 years and have at least a total duration of 1 year. (If both motor and vocal tics are present, the disorder fulfills criteria for Tourette's disorder.) The DSM-IV-TR criteria for *Transient Tic Disorder* are similar, except that the duration is restricted to 1 month to 1 year. As with the DSM-IV-TR criteria for Tourette's disorder, neither of these conditions is required to cause distress or significant functional impairment.

Neurologists, in contrast, generally refer to the condition as Tourette's *syndrome* and have never required

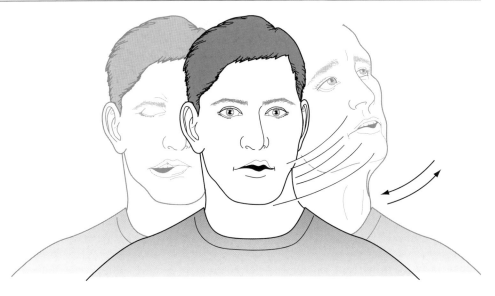

FIGURE 18-36 ■ This young man with Tourette's disorder has multiple motor tics, including head jerking (head toss), grimacing of the right side of his mouth (half-smile), and depression of his forehead (frowning). Vocal tics of throat clearing and a short blowing sound accompany his motor tics. All of his tics continue throughout the day and briefly during sleep. Conversation, eating, and social situations have little influence, but he can suppress them for several minutes by intense concentration.

that it cause distress or social impairment, although it usually does. Moreover, neurologists include cases that have developed in individuals as old as 21 years.

Irrespective of the details of the criteria, Tourette's disorder, as with many neurodevelopmental conditions, such as dyslexia, stuttering, and autism, affects boys multiple times more frequently than girls. Tics appear on average at age 6 to 7 years and in 90% of cases by age 13 years. They generally relapse at the beginning of the school year and remit during the summer months. By their adult years, about 30% of affected children enjoy a complete remission and another 30% a substantial improvement.

At the onset of Tourette's disorder, tics usually involve only the face, eyes, and head, but in succeeding years different tics spread caudally to affect the neck and shoulders, then arms and hands, and finally the trunk and legs. Because each tic may recede or replace another, Tourette's disorder varies in its repertoire, tempo, and intensity from year to year.

Vocal tics, an essential feature of Tourette's disorder, consist of irresistible, repetitive, stereotyped utterances—sounds, words, or, in the extreme, coprolalia (see later). Usually, vocal tics arise several years after the onset of motor tics and remain simple. They typically consist of only inarticulate sounds, such as sniffing, throat clearing, or clicks. However, many vocal tics rise to loud and disconcerting noises, such as grunting, snorting, or honking. Complex vocal tics consist of formed words that can culminate in unprovoked outbursts of obscene words, *coprolalia*. Although most coprolalia consists of only fractions of scatologic words, such as "shi" or "fu," some consist of strings of unequivocal obscenities. Sometimes coprolalia is merely socially reprehensible but occasionally dangerous, such as when a young Chinese girl's vocal tic

belittled Chairman Mao, a Bronx teenager endlessly and uncontrollably repeated the same two words disparaging the New York Yankees, or an otherwise lovely devoutly Catholic adolescent girl incessantly damned her family's priest. Equivalents of coprolalia, such as intrusions of obscene thoughts, *mental coprolalia*, or involuntary obscene movements or gestures, *copropraxia* (Fig. 18-37), may substitute for coprolalia.

Nevertheless, as dramatic and notorious as coprolalia may seem, physicians and the public have overemphasized it ever since the original descriptions of the illness. Coprolalia is not a diagnostic criterion for Tourette's disorder. Less than 10% to 15% of patients exhibit it. Moreover, when it complicates Tourette's disorder, coprolalia does not appear until about 6 years after the onset of motor tics.

Comorbid Psychiatric Conditions

In Tourette's disorder, psychiatric disturbances so frequently complicate the basic clinical picture that tics remain its sole manifestation in less than 20% of patients. These patients, unencumbered by psychiatric comorbidity, enjoy relatively few behavioral disabilities and a better overall outcome. For the majority of patients, however, one or more psychiatric comorbidities often cause marked distress or significant impairment, add a tremendous burden, dominate the clinical picture, and require particular attention.

Nevertheless, physicians exercise caution when diagnosing psychiatric comorbidity. Depending on their perspective, physicians may interpret clinical phenomena as either a psychiatric comorbidity or neurologic morbidity. For example, underlying urges and complex tics lend themselves to labels of either obsessions and compulsions or basic neurologic

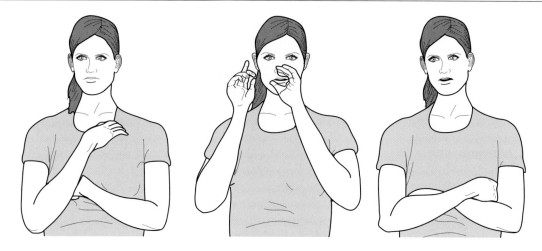

FIGURE 18-37 ■ Furtive and emotionless but compulsive gestures with no sexual or aggressive intention often represent copropraxia.

manifestations. Also, of course, many psychiatric conditions detectable among children with Tourette's disorder occur commonly among their unaffected peers.

The most frequently occurring comorbid psychiatric condition, affecting almost two thirds of boys and one half of girls with Tourette's disorder, is hyperactivity or ADHD. When comorbid with Tourette's disorder, hyperactivity predominantly affects boys and precedes the development of tics by 1 to 2 years.

A concern regarding a hyperactive child with Tourette's disorder had centered on the fear that prescribing stimulants to control hyperactivity would worsen the tics. Neurologists and psychiatrists have found that, although stimulants such as methylphenidate may cause a flare-up in the tics, exacerbations are usually transient and mild. Moreover, their benefits outweigh their risks. Often neurologists prescribe clonidine (Catapres) in conjunction with a stimulant when ADHD is a comorbid condition.

Another psychiatric comorbidity of Tourette's disorder consists of obsessive-compulsive symptoms either alone or as part of OCD. Such symptoms generally occur in about one quarter of both males and females and emerge several years after the onset of tics. Obsessions and compulsions as a manifestation of Tourette's disorder differ somewhat from those that are manifestations of OCD without comorbid Tourette's disorder (pure OCD). For example, obsessions in Tourette's disorder relate to sex, violence, and aggression, but those in pure OCD relate to dirt, germs, and illness. Similarly, compulsions in Tourette's disorders typically consist of checking and ordering, but those of pure OCD consist of more elaborate activities, such as handwashing or housecleaning. Despite these

differences, SSRIs and clomipramine help alleviate these symptoms in both conditions.

Anxieties, phobias, and related disturbances also complicate Tourette's disorder. They affect about 20% of patients of both genders. Their frequency and severity vary directly with the severity of the tics.

Children with Tourette's disorder have normal intelligence and no propensity toward psychosis. Although many of them have learning disabilities, this problem may be an indirect aspect of the disorder. For example, other comorbidities, such as ADHD, or social factors that interfered with children's early education may contribute greatly to learning disabilities. Children with Tourette's disorder also exhibit self-injurious behavior more frequently than unaffected children.

Other Associations

Many patients have soft neurologic signs and minor, nonspecific electroencephalogram (EEG) abnormalities. CT, MRI, and PET do not reveal a consistent, specific abnormality. However, some studies have found increased D_2 receptor activity in the caudate nucleus.

Etiology

Studies have indicated that a single autosomal dominant gene makes children vulnerable to Tourette's disorder. Penetrance is almost complete (100%) in boys but only about 50% to 70% in girls. Because the concordance for Tourette's disorder in monozygotic twins averages only about 85%, nongenetic factors must sometimes override genetic ones.

The theory of *pediatric autoimmune neuropsychiatric disorder associated with streptococcal infections (PANDAS)* proposes, for at least a subpopulation of affected individuals, that *group A β-hemolytic Streptococcus* infections causes or triggers tics, Tourette's disorder, Sydenham's chorea, and other illnesses characterized by hyperkinesias. It also proposes that the infection induces obsessive-compulsive symptoms as well as the movements through "molecular mimicry." In this mechanism, antigens on the streptococcus provoke antibodies directed against the bacteria; however, the antibodies also react with brain tissue possessing similar antigens.

Despite its rationale, studies have seriously challenged the concept of PANDAS. For example, streptococcus antibody titers do not correlate with the symptoms, prophylactic antibiotics do not prevent the development or flare-ups of tics, and the laboratory model is not reproducible. Also, some children initially diagnosed as having developed tics or a flare-up of Tourette's disorder actually had contracted Sydenham's chorea.

Whatever the etiology, several observations indicate that dopamine hypersensitivity leads to the tics. For example, haloperidol suppresses the tics and dopamine-enhancing substances, such as cocaine, exacerbate them. Moreover, as if a feedback loop senses excessive dopamine stimulation, the spinal fluid contains reduced concentrations of the dopamine metabolic product homovanillic acid (HVA).

Treatment

Neurologists often do not prescribe medications for children with a single tic or for adults with either a single tic or multiple motor tics but no accompanying vocal tics. When symptoms require treatment, innumerable approaches, but ones with completely different mechanisms of action, reportedly decrease tics. The most common approach consists of reducing dopaminergic activity. For example, dopamine receptor antagonists, such as haloperidol, fluphenazine, and pimozide, suppress both vocal and most motor tics in about 80% of patients. Likewise, tetrabenazine, which depletes dopamine, greatly lessens tics.

Even antipsychotic agents with relatively little D_2 receptor affinity also suppress tics. Paradoxically, both L-dopa and dopamine agonists, rather than intensifying tics, suppress them at least temporarily.

In an approach not aimed at modifying dopamine activity, physicians sometimes prescribe an α-adrenergic agonist, such as clonidine or guanfacine. Although clonidine may help treat the psychiatric comorbidities, some studies have questioned whether it suppresses tics. Botulinum toxin injections may temporarily eliminate single, particularly bothersome motor tics.

Preliminary work has shown that DBS directed at the thalami suppresses motor and vocal tics as well as numerous other involuntary movement disorders.

Related Conditions

A *stereotypy*, which does not necessarily signify neurologic illness, usually consists of an incessant, repetitive, rhythmic, and complex but relatively slow movement. For example, continual rocking, which may alleviate sensory deprivation in blind or mentally retarded individuals, constitutes a common, benign stereotypy. Some authors include several anxiety-induced activities, such as leg shaking and hair curling. Classic stereotypies subsume the incessant handwashing motions of Rett's syndrome (see Fig. 13-18) and the various movements associated with autism and other pervasive developmental disorders—hand shaking, body rocking, and face slapping. Cocaine use can cause 2 to 6 days of stereotypies ("punding"), tics, chorea, and akathisia-like leg movements ("crack-dancing"). Many of the movements in tardive dyskinesia fall into the rubric of stereotypies (see later). Overall, despite the similar appearance of stereotypies, the underlying neurologic disorders share no other clinical feature or common treatment.

MYOCLONUS

Myoclonus consists of irregular, shock-like, and generalized or focal muscle contractions. It differs from the classic movement disorders in several respects. Myoclonus originates in abnormal discharges from motor neurons in the cerebral cortex, brainstem, or spinal cord rather than the basal ganglia. It may also persist when patients are asleep or comatose. Also, rather than arising spontaneously like chorea or Parkinson's disease, patients' voluntary movements or external stimuli, such as noise, touch, or light, often introduced as part of the neurologic examination, trigger myoclonus (*action* and *stimulus-sensitive myoclonus*).

Not all myoclonus reflects pathology. Benign forms include hiccups, which are merely physiologic shock-like contractions of the diaphragm, and hypnic jerks, which are sudden, generalized muscle contractions that occur at the start of sleep.

On the other hand, a wide variety of disorders, although generally not structural lesions, produce myoclonus. Extensive cerebral cortical damage commonly causes myoclonus. In this case, dementia, delirium, and epilepsy accompany it. For example, myoclonus is one of the most prominent physical manifestations of cerebral anoxia, subacute sclerosing panencephalitis (SSPE), and Creutzfeldt-Jakob disease (see Chapter 7). Also, myoclonic epilepsy or encephalopathy, along with ragged red fibers in muscle, comprises the primary symptoms of the mitochondrial disorder, myoclonic epilepsy with ragged red fibers (MERRF) (see Chapter 6).

Toxic-metabolic aberrations commonly cause delirium accompanied by myoclonus. For example, uremic encephalopathy and toxic levels of medications, including penicillin, meperidine (Demerol), bismuth, lithium, cyclosporin, and SSRIs, all induce myoclonus. In therapeutic as well as toxic levels, lithium, especially when combined with tricyclic antidepressants or clozapine, causes myoclonus, which can be severe and disabling.

In most cases, myoclonus represents a prominent aspect of a serious underlying illness. If physicians can remedy an underlying toxic-metabolic disturbance, the myoclonus will resolve. Treatment with clonazepam or sometimes valproate may suppress myoclonus but, of course, they do not affect the underlying disorder.

MOVEMENT DISORDERS FROM DOPAMINE-BLOCKING MEDICATIONS

As previously discussed, antipsychotic agents and other medicines that block dopamine potentially cause, as extrapyramidal side effects or reactions, parkinsonism and more dramatic involuntary movements. In addition, these medicines may cause the neuroleptic-malignant syndrome (see Chapter 6), lower the seizure threshold, alter the EEG (see Chapter 10), and produce retinal abnormalities (see Chapter 12).

Neurologists divide most of these extrapyramidal side effects into two major groups—*acute* and *tardive dyskinesias* (Table 18-2). In this classification, acute dyskinesias develop within days of either initiating or increasing the dose of the medication, but subside spontaneously or in response to decreasing its dose. Tardive (late) dyskinesias develop at least 3 to 6 months after the onset of treatment. Unlike acute dyskinesias, they rarely subside spontaneously and resist treatment.

Acute Dyskinesias

Parkinsonism and the Parkinson-Hyperpyrexia Syndrome

The most frequently occurring dopamine-blocking, antipsychotic-induced dyskinesia is parkinsonism (see previous discussion). In the extreme, these medications cause the potentially fatal Parkinson-hyperpyrexia syndrome, formerly known as the neuroleptic-malignant syndrome, characterized by extraordinary muscle rigidity, intense fever, and rhabdomyolysis (see Chapter 6).

Acute Dystonias

Acute dystonic reactions consist of the abrupt development of limb or trunk dystonic postures, repetitive jaw and face muscle contractions, tongue protrusion, torticollis, or oculogyric crisis (Fig. 18-38). Each may occur alone or in combination. Compared to middle-aged and older individuals, adolescents and young adults seem more susceptible and more likely to suffer severe reactions. In particular, individuals who have abused cocaine place themselves at a 40-fold increased risk of developing acute dystonic reactions to neuroleptics.

TABLE 18-2 ■ Neuroleptic-Induced Movement Disorders

Acute dyskinesias
  Akathisia
  Oculogyric crisis and other dystonias
Tardive dyskinesias
  Oral-buccal-lingual dyskinesia*
  Dystonia
  Akathisia
  Tics
  Tremor
  Stereotypies
Parkinsonism
Neuroleptic-malignant syndrome
Withdrawal-emergent dyskinesias

*Commonly referred to as tardive dyskinesia.

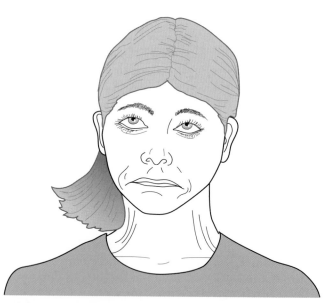

FIGURE 18-38 ■ During an oculogyric crisis, eyes forcefully roll upward but sometimes sideways. Jaw and extensor neck muscle contractions often simultaneously accompany the ocular movements. When dopamine-blocking neuroleptics cause an oculogyric crisis, anticholinergics usually abort it.

Physicians must keep in mind that several serious neurologic disorders—seizures, meningitis, and tetanus—can cause similar postures. Another caveat is that these reactions may complicate treatment of Tourette's disorder or other movement disorder and create a complex clinical picture.

Prophylactic oral anticholinergics may prevent acute dystonic reactions. Once dystonic reactions have begun, intravenous anticholinergic or antihistamine medications can abort them. Common regimens include parenteral diphenhydramine or trihexyphenidyl followed by several days of oral anticholinergics.

The etiology of acute dystonic reactions remains unknown. However, their favorable response to anticholinergics suggests that they result from excessive cholinergic activity. On the other hand, dopamine receptors may cause the problem. For example, brief, excessive dopamine activity when the dopamine blockade initially stimulates dopamine receptors possibly causes the reaction. Alternatively, as the initial dopamine blockade dose falls off, the receptors remain exposed and oversensitive.

Akathisia

Akathisia (Greek, *a* + *kathisis*, without sitting) is continual, almost regular limb and trunk movements that plague patients (Fig. 18-39). Although akathisia can involve the trunk and arms, it predominantly affects the legs. Most important, it forces patients to move about and virtually prohibits them from sitting still or lying quietly in bed. Paradoxically, although akathisia induces excessive leg movement, medication-induced parkinsonism induces arm movement.

As with tics, a psychic urge, in part, drives akathisia. For example, patients with akathisia complain of having restlessness, a need or compulsion to move, or even an intense desire to walk. Because the urge to move can exceed the movements, physicians may reasonably mistake akathisia for anxiety or agitated depression. They may also mistakenly attribute an increase in physical movement to worsening psychosis rather than to akathisia. Thus, psychiatrists must often decide whether to increase or reduce an antipsychotic medicine for a patient with an agitated psychosis. If unable to decide between those options, they might prescribe benzodiazepines as a temporary measure.

In addition to resembling movements induced by agitated depression, akathisia resembles movements induced by fluoxetine, cocaine ("crack dancing"), or excessive L-dopa. Although akathisia also mimics RLS, patients with akathisia experience the urges but not paresthesias that characterize RLS. To emphasize that akathisia, tics, and RLS stem from uncomfortable sensations, one neurologist quipped that patients with most movement disorders are distressed because

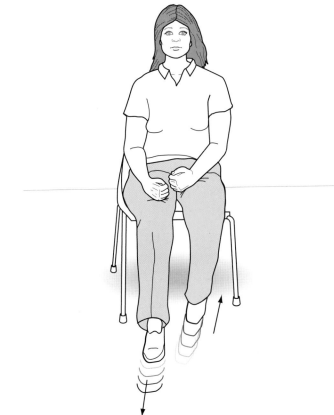

FIGURE 18-39 ■ In a classic example of akathisia, this woman, who just began a regimen of antipsychotic medicines, continually shuffles her legs in regular to-and-fro sliding movements. Although it can lead to repetitive semipurposeful arm movements, such as scratching, hair smoothing, and rubbing, akathisia predominantly affects the legs. In another of characteristic of akathisia, she feels driven to move her legs.

they move, but ones with these disorders move because they are distressed.

As treatment continues or physicians reduce the medication dose or strength, akathisia generally recedes. However, in a small proportion of patients, akathisia persists for more than 6 months or perhaps indefinitely (see later, tardive akathisia). According to some reports, propranolol or benzodiazepines relieve it.

Tardive Dyskinesias

Oral-Buccal-Lingual Variety

Physicians tend to speak of "tardive dyskinesia" when dealing only with its *oral-buccal-lingual*, *choreic*, or *orofacial variety*. However, they should recognize several other varieties of tardive, as well as acute, dyskinesias (see Table 18-2).

Oral-buccal-lingual dyskinesia, the most frequently occurring variety, consists of the well-known tongue,

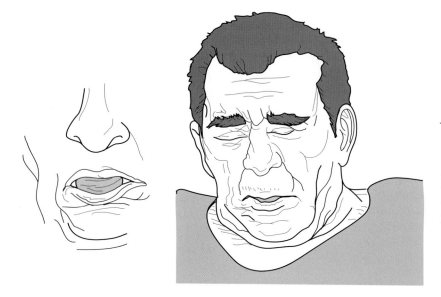

FIGURE 18-40 ■ The oral-buccal-lingual variety of tardive dyskinesia consists of repetitive tongue movements accompanied by continual jaw and facial muscle contractions. These movements typically include tongue darting, lip smacking, kissing, lip puckering, chewing, and sometimes blepharospasm. Unlike the tongue movements in chorea and cranial dystonias, tongue movements in oral-buccal-lingual tardive dyskinesia not only are prominent but lead to tongue enlargement (macroglossia).

jaw, and lower face movements (Fig. 18-40). The movements are painless and not provoked by urges. Physicians often classify these movements and other tardive dyskinesias as stereotypies. However, they must pause before reflexly attributing every case of involuntary facial, tongue, and jaw movement to antipsychotic agents or other variety of medication. For example, neurologists observe similar movements in Huntington's disease, cranial dystonia, tics, jaw tremor, bruxism, spontaneous oral dyskinesia of the elderly, and edentulous orofacial dyskinesia (see later).

Nevertheless, use of dopamine-blocking antipsychotic agents remains the strongest risk factor for developing tardive dyskinesia. Whichever the agent, coadministration of an anticholinergic may increase the likelihood of developing tardive dyskinesia. Pre-existing brain disease also represents a risk factor.

Because the yearly incidence remains constant throughout medication exposure, patients have the same chance of developing this tardive dyskinesia during the first year as during the fifth year of treatment. Prevalence is greater among women than men, especially for individuals older than 65 years and, of course, among individuals with illnesses that have required long-term neuroleptic treatment. Although the dyskinesia persists, even after patients stop medications, it tends to improve over time.

Etiology

Despite its limitations, the *dopamine receptor hypersensitivity theory* remains well-regarded and consistent with several of the condition's major clinical features (Fig. 18-41). For example, tardive dyskinesia begins only after a relatively long time (6 months) from the start of typical dopamine-blocking agents. The dyskinesias resemble, although not perfectly, movements

produced by excessive L-dopa. Maneuvers that expose the postsynaptic neuron to increased dopamine activity—reducing the dosage of the medication, stopping it, or adding L-dopa—worsen the movements. Likewise, increasing the medication dosage, which would reduce dopamine receptor exposure, suppresses them.

An alternative theory attributes the disorder to deficient or abnormal GABA activity in the striatum. Another one posits that the glutamate system triggers excitotoxicity through the NMDA receptors.

Treatment

Physicians should, of course, avoid prescribing or maintain only minimal doses of antipsychotic and other medications associated with tardive dyskinesia. Once they recognize the onset of tardive dyskinesia, physicians should resist a temptation to immediately stop the medicine and should slowly taper it—over weeks or months—because abruptly stopping it may precipitate the WES (see later). Alternatively, switching from a typical to an atypical medication or from one atypical to another sometimes helps. For example, clozapine and quetiapine may suppress tardive dyskinesia and other movement disorders; however, that benefit may take months to materialize.

If the dyskinesia persists, using dopamine-depleting medications to reduce the relatively excessive dopamine activity may reduce the movements. For example, tetrabenazine and reserpine alleviate tardive dyskinesias and other hyperkinetic disorders. However, these medicines frequently cause hypotension, depression, sleep disturbances, or parkinsonism.

Along the same line, but as a last resort, physicians have reinstituted the dopamine receptor blockade by increasing the dosage of a typical dopamine-blocking medication, substituting a more potent one, or

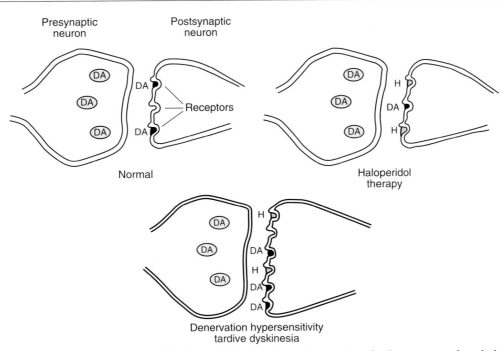

FIGURE 18-41 ■ The denervation hypersensitivity theory proposes that when antipsychotic agents, such as haloperidol, bind to postsynaptic dopamine receptors, the remaining receptors become particularly sensitive and new ones develop. Then, minute quantities of dopamine—either released from the presynaptic neuron or present in the ambient fluid—evade the blockade and trigger these hypersensitive receptors.

restarting it. This strategy obviously may create a vicious cycle in which recurrence of the dyskinesia again requires additional medication.

Using another strategy to reduce dopaminergic activity, branched chain amino acids, possibly by interfering with dopamine synthesis, reportedly alleviate tardive dyskinesia.

A different approach counterbalances enhanced dopamine activity by increasing acetylcholine (ACh) activity. However, except for brief periods, physostigmine, which prolongs ACh activity, and ACh precursors, such as deanol (Deaner), lecithin, or choline, have failed to help. The opposite approach, giving anticholinergics, also does not help and may exacerbate the problem.

Medications that affect other neurotransmitters also fail to help. For example, GABA agonists, such as valproate (Depakote) and baclofen (Lioresal); a calcium channel blocker, diltiazem (Cardizem); lithium; opiates; and clonazepam provide no consistent relief.

Physicians cannot use botulinum toxin injections for dyskinesias that involve the tongue. Injecting its main muscles (genioglossus and geniohyoid) would require a needle to pass through the upper part of the neck, which contains vital delicate structures, and vascular portions of the tongue, which are susceptible to uncontrollable hemorrhage. Moreover, botulinum toxin entails a risk of either tongue or throat muscle weakness, which might occlude the airway.

Tardive Dystonia

Another tardive dyskinesia, *tardive dystonia*, consists of sustained, powerful, and twisting, but predominantly extensor, movements of the neck, trunk, and upper arms (Fig. 18-42). Unlike the rotation and tilting that characterize common, idiopathic spasmodic torticollis, the increased tone of the extensor neck muscles in tardive dystonia produces its characteristic feature, retrocollis. Related movements, including oral-buccal-lingual dyskinesia, blepharospasm, and akathisia, may accompany tardive dystonia. Otherwise, tardive dystonia resembles other secondary dystonias.

A relatively short exposure to dopamine-blocking agents, sometimes as brief as 3 months, can cause tardive dystonia. Thereafter, it complicates exposure at a low but constant yearly rate.

In contrast to the oral-buccal-lingual dyskinesia, tardive dystonia partially responds to anticholinergics and sometimes to dopamine depletors. In addition, botulinum toxin injections may alleviate dystonia in selected, critical muscles groups, such as the neck extensor muscles. In clinically perplexing cases—such as where neck movements may represent spasmodic torticollis, DYT1 dystonia, or tardive dystonia—botulinum toxin injections stop the involuntary muscle contractions whatever the underlying cause. Similarly, preliminary reports indicate that DBS directed at the GPi may ameliorate tardive dystonia as well as DYT1 dystonia.

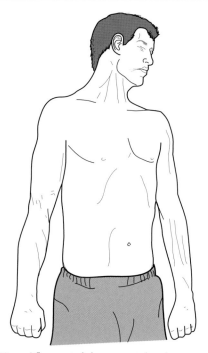

FIGURE 18-42 ■ After receiving neuroleptic treatment for 6 years, this 25-year-old man began to develop prolonged, forceful twisting and extension of his arms, extension of his head and neck (retrocollis), and exaggerated arching of his back. Subsequently, subtle oral-buccal-lingual choreiform movements, blepharospasm, or other varieties of tardive dyskinesia also arose. After excluding Wilson's disease and DYT1 and other varieties of dystonia, his physicians diagnosed his condition as tardive dystonia.

Other Tardive Dyskinesias

Tardive akathisia, which resembles the acutely developing disorder, persists by definition for longer than 6 months. In addition, it may appear only after the patient has stopped the offending medication. Other tardive dyskinesias often accompany tardive akathisia.

Opioids, benzodiazepines, and propranolol can sometimes alleviate tardive akathisia. Reported benefits from reserpine, tetrabenazine, amantadine, anticholinergics, and other medications remain unconfirmed.

As other manifestations of tardive dyskinesia, patients may have *tardive verbal tics,* which involve persistent simple vocalizations, such as grunts, and *respiratory tics,* in which patients make sudden, loud, irregular gasps. They can also have *tardive oculogyric crises, tardive tremors,* and various persistent movements usually associated with acute dyskinesias or other movement disorders. As with tardive dystonia and akathisia, oral movements typically accompany each of these dyskinesias.

Withdrawal-Emergent Syndrome

Involuntary movements sometimes appear for up to 6 weeks after suddenly stopping prolonged treatment with dopamine-blocking agents. These movements, which constitute the WES, usually consist of mild to moderately severe chorea with motor impersistence and restlessness. WES typically affects children and looks like Sydenham's chorea but does not have OCD or ADHD symptoms.

Cases that last longer than 6 months probably represent tardive dyskinesia. For intolerable dyskinesias, physicians might be forced to reinstitute the medication and then slowly withdraw it.

MOVEMENT DISORDERS RELATED TO OTHER PSYCHIATRIC MEDICATIONS

SSRIs

As SSRIs elevate a patient's mood, they may also increase motor activity to abnormal levels, inducing myoclonus, tremor, or akathisia-like leg movements. As discussed previously, SSRIs may cause the serotonin syndrome (see Chapter 6). Despite these caveats, reports of serious adverse reactions to SSRIs refer to a small proportion of patients. Serious reactions usually occur only when SSRIs are administered in extraordinarily high doses or combined with other medications, or patients had a pre-existing neurologic disorder.

Other Medications

About 10% of patients taking TCAs develop a fine tremor that resembles essential tremor and also responds to propranolol. The antidepressant amoxapine, which has dopamine antagonist properties, can induce parkinsonism; however, almost no other antidepressant causes parkinsonism or other sign of extrapyramidal dysfunction.

Lithium, at high therapeutic serum concentrations, can also induce a fine, rapid tremor that resembles essential tremor. At toxic concentrations, it produces a severe, coarse intention tremor often accompanied by ataxia of the trunk—signs of cerebellar dysfunction. Sometimes lithium toxicity causes extrapyramidal signs. Although adding propranolol may suppress a mild tremor, reducing the lithium dose is usually preferable.

Antiepileptic drugs often cause tremors, ataxia, and sometimes asterixis but generally only at serum concentrations greater than necessary for their therapeutic effect. In addition, phenytoin at toxic levels may cause athetosis or chorea. As one exception, valproate may cause a tremor independent of dose.

Noniatrogenic Movements

Abnormal tongue, jaw, and facial movements occur, of course, in conditions other than tardive dyskinesia. In fact, stereotyped movements of the face, mouth, or tongue reportedly appeared in schizophrenic patients before the introduction of neuroleptics. Today, very old individuals, especially those with dementia, sometimes develop *buccolingual dyskinesia of the elderly,* which resembles oral-buccal-lingual dyskinesia. Also, edentulous older individuals may develop a similar disorder, *edentulous orofacial dyskinesia.* In this dyskinesia, the absence of teeth presumably deprives the tongue of its normal proprioceptive feedback. Properly fitting dentures will stop many of these movements.

The *Abnormal Involuntary Movement Scale (AIMS)* allows recording of the presence and severity of abnormal movements (Fig. 18-43). However, this scale has several drawbacks. It attempts to assess dyskinesias that change in intensity during the day; the measurements are gross; it does not recognize akinesia (lack of movement), which carries as much diagnostic weight as hyperkinesia; it does not distinguish between chorea, dystonia, tics, and stereotypies; and it omits tests for akinesia, tremor, and dysarthria.

PSYCHOGENIC MOVEMENTS

Clinical Clues

Many neuroscientists predict that an eventual reunification of neurology and psychiatry will eliminate distinctions between mind and body. Until then, neurologists will probably continue to religiously separate psychogenic from neurologic causes of abnormal movements. They concede, as they do with patients who have psychogenic seizures, that some patients will have psychogenic movements superimposed on involuntary movement disorders. In addition, they will acknowledge that some patients, for a variety of reasons, may exaggerate a genuine movement disorder.

The diagnosis of psychogenic movements rests primarily on neurologists' clinical acumen. They usually cite some of the following factors as indications of a psychogenic movement disorder: (1) the absence of movements when patients believe themselves to be unobserved; (2) relief with nonpharmacologic treatment, such as placebos, physical therapy, and psychotherapy; (3) *incongruency* and *inconsistency* (variability in location, pattern, and intensity of the movements); (4) two or more patterns simultaneously or in succession; (5) disproportionate weakness or sensory loss; and (6) certain characteristics depending on the particular movement (see later).

Common Psychogenic Movements

Neurologists find that psychogenic movements may assume almost any pattern, but they most commonly masquerade as dystonia, tremor, myoclonus, and gait abnormalities. In psychogenic dystonia, the movements appear unique, inconsistent in location, and paroxysmal. Moreover, unlike patients with either focal or generalized dystonia, those with psychogenic dystonia give the impression of having pain, weakness, and sensory loss. Psychogenic tremor characteristically develops abruptly, oscillates in two or more planes, and has a variable frequency. In addition, because of fatigue, it diminishes in amplitude (strength) during long examinations. Despite the movements, the tremor may not interfere with activities requiring the same muscles. Patients with a psychogenic tremor typically display a "selective disability." Their disability often far exceeds the disability of individuals with Parkinson's disease.

Several maneuvers can support a diagnosis of psychogenic tremor. When a psychogenic tremor affects one arm, it often switches sides when the physician restrains that arm. In addition to forcing the tremor to switch sides, the examiner can *entrain* the frequency of a psychogenic tremor using the following maneuver: The examiner asks the patient to shake the affected hand first at a slow speed, then fast speed, and finally back to the slow speed. The examiner often must set an example. The variability in tremor frequency that this maneuver induces reveals its willful origin. Also, placing weights on the wrist of Parkinson's disease patients dampens the amplitude and frequency of their tremor, but weights usually elicit a more forceful psychogenic tremor.

Psychogenic myoclonus imitates shocks that randomly strike different muscle groups. As with true myoclonus, they have variable velocity and intensity of contraction. However, psychogenic myoclonus recedes after a few minutes, presumably as patients tire, but returns after a rest period.

Although they have variable presentations, psychogenic gait impairments all look as if they cause great disability. Overwhelming trembling, dystonia, or myoclonus frequently disrupts the normal walking

EXAMINATION PROCEDURE

Either before or after completing the Examination Procedure observe the patient unobtrusively, at rest (e.g., in waiting room)

The chair to be used in this examination should be a hard, firm one without arms.

1. Ask patient to remove shoes and socks.

2. Ask patient whether there is anything in his/her mouth (i.e., gum, candy, etc.) and if there is, to remove it.

3. Ask patient about the <u>current</u> condition of his/her teeth. Ask patient if he/she wears dentures. Do teeth or dentures bother patient <u>now</u>?

4. Ask patient whether he/she notices any movements in mouth, face, hands, or feet. If yes, ask to describe and to what extent they <u>currently</u> bother patient or interfere with his/her activities.

5. Have patient sit in chair with hands on knees, legs slightly apart, and feet flat on floor. (Look at entire body for movements while in this position.)

6. Ask patient to sit with hands hanging unsupported, if male, between legs, if female and wearing a dress, hanging over knees. (Observe hands and other body areas.)

7. Ask patient to open mouth. (Observe tongue at rest within mouth.) Do this twice.

8. Ask patient to protrude tongue. (Observe abnormalities of tongue movement.) Do this twice.

9. Ask patient to tap thumb, with each finger, as rapidly as possible for 10–15 seconds; separately with right hand, then with left hand. (Observe facial and leg movements.)

10. Flex and extend patient's left and right arms (one at a time). (Note any rigidity.)

11. Ask patient to stand up. (Observe in profile. Observe all body areas again, hips included.)

12. Ask patient to extend both arms outstretched in front with palms down. (Observe trunk, legs, and mouth.)

13. Have patients walk a few paces, turn, and walk back to chair. (Observe hands and gait.) Do this twice.

FIGURE 18-43 ■ Continued

DEPARTMENT OF HEALTH AND HUMAN SERVICES
PUBLIC HEALTH SERVICE
Alcohol, Drug Abuse, and Mental Health Administration
NIMH Treatment Strategies in Schizophrenia Study

**ABNORMAL INVOLUNTARY
MOVEMENT SCALE
(AIMS)**

PATIENT NUMBER	DATA GROUP	EVALUATION DATE
_ _ _ _	aims	_ _ - _ _ - _ _
		M M D D Y Y

PATIENT NAME

RATER NAME

RATER NUMBER

_ _ _

EVALUATION TYPE (Circle)

1 Baseline	4 Start double-blind	7 Start open meds	10 Early termination
2 2-week minor	5 Major evaluation	8 During open meds	11 Study completion
3	6 Other	9 Stop open meds	

INSTRUCTIONS: Complete Examination Procedure (reverse side) before making ratings.
MOVEMENT RATINGS: Rate highest severity observed.

Code: 1 = None
2 = Minimal, may be extreme normal
3 = Mild
4 = Moderate
5 = Severe

			(Circle One)
FACIAL AND ORAL MOVEMENTS:	1. **Muscles of Facial Expression** e.g., movements of forehead, eyebrows, periorbital area, cheeks; include frowning, blinking, smiling, grimacing		1 2 3 4 5
	2. **Lips and Perioral Area** e.g., puckering, pouting, smacking		1 2 3 4 5
	3. **Jaw** e.g., biting, clenching, chewing, mouth opening, lateral movement		1 2 3 4 5
	4. **Tongue** Rate only increase in movement both in and out of mouth. NOT inability to sustain movement		1 2 3 4 5
EXTREMITY MOVEMENTS:	5. **Upper** (arms, wrists, hands, fingers) Include choreic movements, (i.e., rapid, objectively purposeless irregular, spontaneous), athetoid movements (i.e., slow, irregular, complex, serpentine). Do NOT include tremor (i.e., repetitive, regular, rhythmic)		1 2 3 4 5
	6. **Lower** (legs, knees, ankles, toes) e.g., lateral knee movement, foot tapping, heel dropping, foot squirming, inversion and eversion of foot		1 2 3 4 5
TRUNK MOVEMENTS:	7. **Neck, shoulders, hips** e.g., rocking, twisting, squirming, pelvic gyrations		1 2 3 4 5
GLOBAL JUDGMENTS:	8. **Severity of abnormal movements**	None, normal 1 Minimal 2 Mild 3 Moderate 4 Severe 5	
	9. **Incapacitation due to abnormal movements**	None, normal 1 Minimal 2 Mild 3 Moderate 4 Severe 5	
	10. **Patient's awareness of abnormal movements** Rate only patient's report	No awareness 1 Aware, no distress 2 Aware, mild distress 3 Aware, moderate distress 4 Aware, severe distress 5	
DENTAL STATUS:	11. **Current problems with teeth and/or dentures**	No 1 Yes 2	
	12. **Does patient usually wear dentures?**	No 1 Yes 2	

FIGURE 18-43 ■ The *Abnormal Involuntary Movement Scale* (*AIMS*) guides the examiner through inspection for dyskinesias of the face, jaw, tongue, trunk, and limbs. The examiner records observations when the patient is at rest, extending the tongue or limbs, or performing certain activities, such as finger tapping, standing, or walking. In addition, the examiner checks for rigidity. This revision of the original (Guy, 1976) requests that patients remove their shoes and socks, and it does not rate as less severe those movements that are activated by voluntary movements.

pattern in psychogenic gaits. Sometimes the problem rests in psychogenic incoordination that produces apparent unsteadiness or ataxia, in which the patient gives the impression of being on the verge of falling (see astasia-abasia, Fig. 3-4). Sometimes, rather than having abnormal movements, patients with psychogenic gait disturbances display only exaggerated effort or uneconomic postures.

Movements as a Manifestation of Psychiatric Illnesses

Consultation psychiatrists adhering to the DSM-IV-TR often consider psychogenic movements to be similar to psychogenic neurologic deficits (see Chapter 3). Thus, when movements originate in unconscious processes, they are usually classified as manifestations of a *somatoform disorder,* particularly *somatization* or *conversion disorders.* However, in defining somatization disorder, the DSM-IV-TR allows as pseudoneurotic symptoms paralysis, seizures, and impaired coordination or loss of balance, but it does not specifically include psychogenic dystonia, tremors, or other movements. Neurologists typically find underlying comorbid depression in patients with psychogenic movements or deficit. Alternatively, a psychiatric disturbance may consciously but irresistibly drive an individual to imitate a movement or deficit: in both cases the DSM-IV-TR would apply the label of *factitious disorder.* Of course, some individuals feign such disorders in an attempt to reap a benefit, such as entitlements. In this situation, the DSM-IV-TR would apply the label of *malingering.*

Often movement disorders constitute an integral part of certain psychiatric disturbances. For example, autism virtually requires stereotypies, anxiety naturally causes or intensifies a fine tremor, and depression slows most voluntary movement (*psychomotor retardation*). In another example, neurologists diagnose *catatonia* when patients with schizophrenia, major depression, or similar psychiatric disturbance have immobility, mutism, refusal to eat or drink, waxy flexibility, staring, and rigidity. The DSM-IV-TR also allows, as features, "peculiarities of movement," echolalia, and echopraxia. When psychiatric disturbances induce catatonia, an EEG should be normal and a therapeutic trial of a benzodiazepine may interrupt the immobility. On the other hand, a wide variety of neurologic disturbances, such as MPTP- or neuroleptic-induced parkinsonism, off periods in Parkinson's disease, phencyclidine intoxication, and juvenile Huntington's disease, give rise catatonia-like immobility.

Some movements, although also psychogenic in a larger sense of the word, are behavioral, culturally determined, or cultured-bound. Some neurologists call them "folk illnesses." In the best-known example, the *jumping Frenchmen of Maine,* a group of otherwise healthy citizens of French-Canadian descent, respond to unexpected loud noises by leaping upward, screaming, or throwing any object that they might be holding. Similarly, residents of rural Malaysia and Indonesia, *latahs,* sometimes overreact to trivial stimuli by suddenly cursing, laughing convulsively, or moving in exaggerated patterns.

Caveats

On the other hand, making a diagnosis of psychogenic movement disorder carries a risk. As discussed previously (see previous and Chapter 3), neurologists and other physicians may easily misdiagnose movements when they are bizarre or respond to tricks, concentration, anxiety-producing situations, or solitude. In another problem, psychotropic medications may induce unusual yet partly controllable side effects, such as acute dystonic reactions, tardive dystonia, tremors, and akathisia that may appear alone or in combination. In patients with primarily psychiatric symptoms, medication-induced movements may then exacerbate the psychiatric disturbances.

As with the high incidence of psychogenic seizures reported by epilepsy centers (see Chapter 10), the high incidence of psychogenic movement disorders reported by movement disorder centers is partly attributable to their attracting unique cases, having the clinical experience and technology to diagnosis or exclude rare disorders, and willingness to assume the burden of making a probably unwelcome diagnosis. Outside of such centers, the incidence of psychogenic movement disorders is low. In addition, few patients have seen movement disorders that might serve as a model. Even fewer patients have the stamina and determination to sustain a consistent, voluntary movement. (Try it yourself!)

SUMMARY

Physicians may diagnose many involuntary movement disorders exclusively on the basis of their clinical features, family history, patient's age at onset (Table 18-3), presence or absence of dementia (Table 18-4), or exposure to neuroleptics (see Table 18-2). Recent studies have defined their comorbidities. Commercial laboratory or genetic tests are available for Huntington's and Wilson's diseases, SSPE, Lesch-Nyhan syndrome, early onset dystonia, Rett's syndrome, and some familial forms of Parkinson's disease.

TABLE 18-3 ■ Commonly Cited Movement Disorders That May Begin in Childhood or Adolescence

Early childhood
  Athetosis or choreoathetosis
  Lesch-Nyhan syndrome*
Childhood
  Dopa-responsive dystonia*
  Dystonia associated with DYT1 gene*
  Myoclonus from subacute sclerosing panencephalitis (SSPE)
  Parkinson's disease
  Sydenham's chorea
  Tourette's disorder*
  Withdrawal-emergent dyskinesia
Adolescence
  Essential tremor*
  Huntington's disease (juvenile Huntington's disease)*
  Medication- and drug-induced movements
  Tardive dyskinesia
  Wilson's disease*

---

*Genetic transmission.

TABLE 18-4 ■ Movement Disorders Associated with Cognitive Impairment*
Young children
Athetosis or choreoathetosis^
Lesch-Nyhan syndrome
Rett's syndrome
Older children and adolescents
Huntington's disease
Subacute sclerosing panencephalitis
Sydenham's chorea+
Wilson's disease
Adults
Creutzfeldt-Jakob disease#
Huntington's disease
Parkinson's disease

*Dementia, depression, or psychotic behavior.
^Despite incapacitating movement disorders, many choreoathetosis patients have no mental retardation (see Chapter 13).
+Possible learning disabilities.
Myoclonus.

Several recent advances have benefited patients with involuntary movement disorders:

- DBS for Parkinson's disease, dystonia, and probably several other disorders
- Identification of genetic abnormalities in several movements disorders, such as the DNA trinucleotide repeat in Huntington's disease, DYT1 gene in early-onset dystonia, and the parkin gene in Parkinson's disease
- Botulinum toxin treatment for focal dystonias

REFERENCES

Parkinson's Disease and Parkinsonism

1. Aarsland D, Anderson K, Larsen JP, et al: The rate of cognitive decline in Parkinson's disease. Arch Neurol 61:1906–1911, 2004.
2. Bjorklund A: Cell therapy for Parkinson's disease: Problems and prospects. Novartis Found Symp 265:174–186, 2005.
3. Bower JH, Maraganore DM, Peterson BJ, et al: Head trauma preceding PD: A case-control study. Neurology 60:1610–1615, 2003.
4. Burkhard PR, Vingerhoets FJ, Berney A, et al: Suicide after successful deep brain stimulation for movement disorders. Neurology 63:2170–2172, 2004.
5. Castelli L, Perrozo P, Genesia ML, et al: Sexual well being in parkinsonian patients after deep brain stimulation of the subthalamic nucleus. J Neurol Neurosurg Psychiatry 75:1260–1264, 2004.
6. Deane KHO, Ellis-Hill C, Jones D, et al: Systemic review of paramedical therapies for Parkinson's disease. Mov Disord 17:984–991, 2002.
7. Emre M, Aarsland D, Albanese A, et al: Rivastigmine for dementia associated with Parkinson's disease. N Engl J Med 351:2509–2517, 2004.
8. Factor SA, Feustel PJ, Friedman JH, et al: Longitudinal outcome of Parkinson's disease patients with psychosis. Neurology 60:1756–1761, 2003.
9. Fénelon G, Mahieux F, Huon R, et al: Hallucinations in Parkinson's disease: Prevalence, phenomenology and risk factors. Brain 123:733–745, 2000.
10. Fernandez HH, Tabamo REJ, David RR, et al: Predictors of depressive symptoms among spouse caregivers in Parkinson's disease. Mov Disord 16:1123–1125, 2001.
11. Fernandez HH, Trieschmann ME, Burke MA, et al: Long-term outcome of quetiapine use for psychosis among parkinsonian patients. Mov Disord 18:510–514, 2003.
12. Fernandez HH, Trieschmann ME, Okun MS: Rebound psychosis: Effect of discontinuation of antipsychotics in Parkinson's disease. Mov Disord 20:104–115, 2004.
13. Firestone JA, Smith-Weller T, Franklin G, et al: Pesticides and risk of Parkinson's disease. Arch Neurol 62:91–95, 2005.
14. Gage H, Storey L: Rehabilitation for Parkinson's disease: A systemic review of available evidence. Clin Rehabil 18:463–482, 2004.
15. Giovannoni G, O'Sullivan JD, Turner K, et al: Hedonistic homeostatic dysregulation in patients with Parkinson's disease on dopamine replacement therapies. J Neurol Neurosurg Psychiatry 68:423–428, 2000.
16. Goetz CG, Poewe W, Rascol O, et al: Evidenced-based medical review update: Pharmacological and surgical treatments of Parkinson's disease: 2001 to 2004. Mov Disord 20:523–539, 2005.
17. Green J, McDonald WM, Vitek JL, et al: Neuropsychological and psychiatric sequela of pallidotomy for PD. Neurology 58:858–863, 2002.
18. Grosset KA, Reid JL, Grosset DG: Medicine-taking behavior. Neurology 20:1397–1404, 2005.
19. Hughes TA, Ross HF, Musa S, et al: A 10-year study of the incidence of and factors predicting dementia in Parkinson's disease. Neurology 54:1596–1602, 2000.
20. Jankovic J: *Video Atlas of Movement Disorders*. San Diego, Arbor Publishing Co., 1999.
21. Kieburtz K, Kurlan R: Welding and Parkinson's disease: Is there a bond? Neurology 64:2001–2003, 2005.
22. Krack P, Batir A, Blercom NV, et al: Five-year follow-up of bilateral stimulation of the subthalamic nucleus in advanced Parkinson's disease. N Engl J Med 349:1925–1934, 2003.
23. Kish SJ: What is the evidence that ecstasy (MDMA) can cause Parkinson's disease? Move Disord 18:1219–1223, 2003.
24. Marsh L, Williams JR, Rocco M, et al: Psychiatric comorbidities in patients with Parkinson disease and psychosis. Neurology 63:293–300, 2004.
25. Moellentine C, Rumman T, Ahlskog JE, et al: Effectiveness of ECT in patients with parkinsonism. J Neuropsychiatry 10:187–193, 1998.
26. Nutt JG, Wooten GF: Diagnosis and initial management of Parkinson's disease. N Engl J Med 353:1021–1027, 2005.

27. Pate DS, Margolin DI: Cognitive slowing in Parkinson's and Alzheimer's disease patients: Distinguishing brady-phrenia from dementia. Neurology 44:669–674, 1994.

28. Pezella FR, Colosimo C, Vanacore N, et al: Prevalence and clinical features of hedonistic homeostatic dysregula-tion in Parkinson's disease. Mov Disord 20:79–80, 2004.

29. Troster AI, Stalp LD, Paolo AM, et al: Neuropsychologi-cal impairment in Parkinson's disease with and without depression. Arch Neurol 52:1164–1169, 1995.

30. Weintraub D, Morales KH, Moberg PJ, et al: Antidepres-sant studies in Parkinson's disease: A review and meta-analysis. Mov Disord 20:1161–1168, 2005.

31. Witjas T, Baunez C, Henry JM, et al: Addiction in Parkinson's disease: Impact of subthalamic nucleus deep brain stimulation. Mov Disord 20:1052–1054, 2005.

Chorea

32. Friedlander RM: Apoptosis and caspases in neurodegen-erative diseases. N Engl J Med 348:1365–1375, 2003.

33. Maia DP, Teixeria AL, Cunningham MCQ, et al: Obses-sive compulsive behavior, hyperactivity, and attention deficit disorder in Sydenham chorea. Neurology 64:1799–1801, 2005.

34. Martin JB: Molecular basis of the neurodegenerative disorders. N Engl J Med 34:1970–1980, 1999.

35. Meiser B, Dunn S: Psychological impact of genetic test-ing or Huntington's disease: An update of the literature. J Neurol Neurosurg Psychiatry 69:574–578, 2000.

36. Nance MA, Myers RH: Juvenile onset Huntington's dis-ease—Clinical and research perspective. MRDD Res Rev 7:153–157, 2001.

37. Naarding P, Kremer HPH, Zitman FG: Huntington's disease: A review of the literature on prevalence and treatment of neuropsychiatric phenomena. Eur Psychia-try 16:439–445, 2001.

38. Paulsen JS, Hoth KF, Nehl C, et al: Critical periods of suicide risk in Huntington's disease. Am J Psychiatry 162:725–731, 2005.

39. Paulsen JS, Ready RE, Hamilton JM, et al: Neuropsy-chiatric aspects of Huntington's disease. J Neurol Neurosurg Psychiatry 71:310–314, 2001.

40. Penny JB, Young AB, Shoulson I, et al: Huntington's disease in Venezuela: 7 years of follow-up on sympto-matic and asymptomatic individuals. Mov Disord 5:93–99, 1990.

41. Rosenblatt A, Leroi I: Neuropsychiatry of Huntington's disease and other basal ganglia disorders. Psychoso-matics 41:24–30, 2000.

42. Slaughter JR, Slaughter KA, Nichols D, et al: Prevalence, clinical manifestations, etiology, and treatment of depression in Parkinson's disease. J Neuropsychiatry Clin Neurosci 13:187–196, 2001.

Wilson's Disease

43. Akil M, Brewer GJ: Psychiatric and behavioral abnor-malities in Wilson's disease. Adv Neurol 65:1717–1718, 1995.

44. Brewer GJ, Yuzbasiyan-Gurkan V: Wilson disease. Medicine 71:139–164, 1992.

45. Heckmann JG, Lang CJG, Neuduörfer B, et al: Kayser-Fleischer corneal ring. Neurology 55:280, 2000.

46. Portala K, Westermark K, von Knorring L, et al: Psycho-pathology in treated Wilson's disease determined by means of CPRS expert and self-ratings. Acta Psychiatr Scand 101:104–109, 2000.

47. Rathbun JK: Neuropsychological aspects of Wilson's disease. Int J Neurosci 85:221–229, 1996.

Dystonia (Non-Medication Induced)

48. Adler CH, Kumar R: Pharmacological and surgical options for the treatment of cervical dystonia. Neurolo-gy 55(Suppl 5):S9–S14, 2000.

49. Bandmann O, Wood NW: Dopa-responsive dystonia—The story so far. Neuropediatrics 33:1–5, 2002.

50. Frucht SJ, Fahn S, Greene PE, et al: The natural history of embouchure dystonia. Mov Disord 16:899–906, 2001.

51. Heiman GA, Ottman R, Saunders-Pullman RJ, et al: Increased risk for recurrent major depression in DYT1 dystonia mutation carriers. Neurology 63:631–637, 2004.

52. Hallett M: Blepharospam: Recent advances. Neurology 59:1306–1312, 2002.

53. Jankovic J: Can peripheral trauma induce dystonia? Yes! Mov Disord 16:7–12, 2001.

54. Jedynak PC, Tranchant C, de Beyl DZ: Prospective study of writer's cramp. Mov Disord 16:494–499, 2001.

55. Lauterbach EC, Freeman A, Vogel RL: Differential DSM-III psychiatric disorder prevalence in dystonia and Parkinson's disease. J Neuropsychiatry Clin Neu-rosci 16:29–36, 2004.

56. Kaufman DM: Facial dyskinesias. Psychosomatics 30:263–268, 1990.

57. Kiziltan G, Akalin MA: Stuttering may be a type of action dystonia. Mov Disord 11:278–282, 1996.

58. Molho ES, Feustel PJ, Factor SA: Clinical comparison of tardive and idiopathic cervical dystonia. Mov Disord 3:486–489, 1998.

59. Nemeth AH: The genetics of primary dystonia and related disorders. Brain 125:695–721, 2002.

60. Sa DS, Mailis-Gagnon A, Nicholson K, et al: Posttrau-matic painful torticollis. Mov Disord 12:1482–1491, 2003.

61. Schuele S, Lederman RJ: Long-term outcome of focal dystonia in string instrumentalists. Mov Disord 19:43–48, 2003.

62. Vidailhet M, Vercueil L, Houeto JL, et al: Bilateral deep-brain stimulation of the globus pallidus in primary generalized dystonia. N Engl J Med 352:459–467, 2005.

63. Weiner WJ: Can peripheral trauma induce dystonia? No! Mov Disord 16:13–22, 2001.

64. Wenzel T, Schnider P, Griengl H, et al: Psychiatric dis-orders in patients with blepharospasms—A reactive pattern? J Psychosom Res 48:589–591, 2000.

Essential Tremor

65. Deuschl G, Bain P, Brin M, et al: Consensus statement of the Movement Disorder Society on tremor. Mov Disord 13:2–23, 1998.

66. Koller WC, Busenbark K, Miner K, et al: The relationship of essential tremor to other movement disorders: Report on 678 patients. Ann Neurol 35:717–723, 1994.

67. Lou JS, Jankovic J: Essential tremor: Clinical correlates in 350 patients. Neurology 41:234–238, 1991.

68. Rehncrona S, Johnels B, Widner H, et al: Long-term efficacy of thalamic deep brain stimulation for tremor: Double-blind assessments. Mov Disord 18:163–170, 2002.

69. Schuurman PR, Bosch DA, Bossuyt PMM, et al: A comparison of continuous thalamic stimulation and thalamotomy for suppression of severe tremor. N Engl J Med 342:461–468, 2000.

70. Zesiewicz TA, Elble R, Louis ED, et al: Practice parameter: Therapies of essential tremor. Report of the Quality Standards Subcommittee of the American Academy of Neurology. Neurology 64:2008–2020, 2005.

Tics, Tourette's Disorder, and Related Disorders

71. Freeman RD, Fast DK, Burd L, et al: An international perspective on Tourette syndrome: Selected findings from 3500 individuals in 22 countries. Dev Med Child Neurol 42:436–447, 2000.

72. Garvey MA, Giedd J, Swedo SE: PANDAS: The search for environmental triggers of pediatric neuropsychiatric disorders. Lessons from rheumatic fever. J Child Neurol 13:413–423, 1998.

73. Goldenberg JN, Brown SB: Coprolalia in younger patients with Gilles de la Tourette syndrome. Mov Disord 9:622–625, 1994.

74. Jankovic J: Tourette's syndrome. N Engl J Med 345:1184–1192, 2001.

75. Kurlan R: The PANDAS hypothesis: Losing its bite. Mov Disord 19:371–374, 2004.

76. Leckman JF, Cohen DJ: *Tourette's Syndrome—Tics, Obsessions, Compulsions: Developmental Psychopathology and Clinical Care.* New York, John Wiley, 1999.

77. Nass R, Bressman S: Attention deficit hyperactivity disorder and Tourette syndrome: What's the best treatment? Neurology 58:513–514, 2002.

78. Robertson M: Tourette syndrome, associated conditions and the complexities of treatment. Brain 123:425–462, 2000.

79. Singer HS: Current issues in Tourette syndrome. Mov Disord 15:1051–1063, 2000.

80. Swedo SE, Garvey M, Snider L, et al: The PANDAS subgroup: Recognition and treatment. CNS Spectrums 6:419–426, 2001.

81. Tan A, Salgado M, Fahn S: The characterization and outcome of stereotypic movements in nonautistic children. Mov Disord 12:47–52, 1997.

82. Tourette Syndrome Classification Study Group: Definitions and classifications of tic disorders. Arch Neurol 50:1013–1016, 1993.

83. Wojciezek JM, Lang AE: Gestes antagonistes in the suppression of tics. "tricks for tics." Mov Disord 10:226–228, 1995.

Medication-Induced and Related Movement Disorders

84. Blanchet PJ, Abdillahi O, Beauvais C, et al: Prevalence of spontaneous oral dyskinesia in the elderly. Mov Disord 19:892–896, 2004.

85. Burke RE, Fahn S, Jankovic J, et al: Tardive dystonia: Late-onset and persistent dystonia caused by antipsychotic drugs. Neurology 32:1335–1346, 1982.

86. Dolder CR, Jeste DV: Incidence of tardive dyskinesia with typical versus atypical antipsychotics in very high risk patients. Biol Psychiatry 53:1142–1145, 2003.

87. Guy W: Abnormal Involuntary Movement Scale (AIMS). In ECDEU Assessment Manual for Psychopharmacology, U.S. Department of Health, Education, and Welfare, 1976, pp 534–537.

88. Jankovic J, Beach J: Long-term effects of tetrabenazine in hyperkinetic movement disorders. Neurology 48:358–362, 1997.

89. Kaufman DM: Use of botulinum toxin injections for spasmodic torticollis of tardive dyskinesia. J Neuropsychiatry Clin Neurosci 6:50–53, 1994.

90. Lieberman JA, Stroup TS, McEvoy JP, et al: Effectiveness of antipsychotic drugs in patients with chronic schizophrenia. N Engl J Med 353:1209–1223, 2005.

91. Richardson MA, Bevans ML, Read LL, et al: Efficacy of the branched-chain amino acids in the treatment of tardive dyskinesia in men. Am J Psychiatry 160:1117–1124, 2003.

92. Rosebush PI, Mazurek MF: Neurologic side-effects in neuroleptic-naïve patients treated with haloperidol or risperidone. Neurology 52:782–785, 1999.

93. Stacy M, Jankovic J: Tardive tremor. Mov Disord 7:53–57, 1992.

94. Tarsy D, Kaufman D, Sethi KD, et al: An open-label study of botulinum toxin A for treatment of tardive dystonia. Clin Neuropharmacol 20:90–93, 1997.

95. Trottenberg T, Volkmann J, Deuschl G, et al: Treatment of severe tardive dystonia with pallidal deep brain stimulation. Neurology 64:344–346, 2005.

96. Weiner WJ, Rabinstein A, Levin B, et al: Cocaine-induced persistent dyskinesias. Neurology 56:964–965, 2001.

97. Wojcik JD, Falk WE, Fink JS, et al: A review of 32 cases of tardive dystonia. Am J Psychiatry 148:1055–1059, 1991.

Psychogenic Movement Disorders

98. Deuschl G, Koster B, Lucking CH, et al: Diagnosis and pathophysiological aspects of psychogenic tremors. Mov Disorders 13:294–302, 1998.

99. Fahn S, Williams DT: Psychogenic dystonia. Adv Neurol 50:431–455, 1988.

100. Hayes MW, Graham S, Heldorf P, et al: A video review of the diagnosis of psychogenic gait. Mov Disord 14:914–921, 1999.

101. Kirsch DB, Mink JW: Psychogenic movement disorders in children. Pediatr Neurol 30:1–6, 2004.

102. Koller WC, Biary NM: Volitional control of involuntary movements. Mov Disord 4:153–156, 1989.

103. Lang AE: Psychogenic dystonia: A review of 18 cases. Can J Neurol Sci 22:136–143, 1995.

104. Lees A: Jumpers. Mov Disord 16:403–404, 2001.

105. Massey EW: Goosey patients: Relationship to jumping Frenchmen, Myriachit, Latah, and tic convulsif. N C Med J 45:556–558, 1984.

106. Miyasaki J, Sa DS, Galvez-Jimenez N, et al: Psychogenic movement disorders. Can J Neurol Sci 30(Suppl 1): S94–S100, 2003.

107. Owens DG: Dystonia—a potential psychiatric pitfall. Br J Psychiatry 156:620–634, 1990.

108. Rosebush PI, Mazurek MF: Catatonia: Re-awakening to a forgotten disorder. Mov Disord 14:395–397, 1999.

109. Saint-Hilaire MH, Saint-Hilaire JM, Granger L: Jumping Frenchmen of Maine. Neurology 36:1269–1271, 1986.

110. Tanner CM, Chamberland J: Latah in Jakarta, Indonesia. Mov Disord 16:526–529, 2001.

Questions and Answers

1. Which of the following statements concerning obsessive-compulsive symptoms and obsessive-compulsive disorder (OCD) in Tourette's disorder is false?
 a. Symptoms generally occur in about one-quarter of both males and females.
 b. Obsessions and compulsions as a manifestation of Tourette's disorder are indistinguishable from those in pure OCD.
 c. Selective serotonin reuptake inhibitors (SSRIs) and clomipramine help alleviate obsessive-compulsive symptoms and OCD in Tourette's disorder.
 d. Obsessive-compulsive symptoms and OCD emerge several years after the onset of motor tics, generally in late adolescence

Answer: b. Obsessions and compulsions as a manifestation of Tourette's disorder differ somewhat from those that are manifestations of pure OCD. For example, obsessions in Tourette's disorder relate to sex, violence, and aggression, but those in pure OCD relate to dirt, germs, and illness. Similarly, compulsions in Tourette's disorders typically consist of checking and ordering, but those of pure OCD consist of more elaborate activities, such as handwashing or housecleaning.

2. Which of the following statements concerning ADHD in Tourette's disorder is false?
 a. ADHD is the most frequently occurring comorbid psychiatric condition.
 b. It affects boys more frequently than girls.
 c. It develops one to two years before motor tics.
 d. Treating comorbid ADHD with stimulants is contraindicated because they worsen motor and verbal tics.

Answer: d. Neurologists and psychiatrists have found that although stimulants may cause a flare-up in the tics, the exacerbation is usually transient, relatively mild, and worth the risk.

3. Which three descriptions pertain to obscenities in Tourette's disorder?
 a. Vocalizations include only scatologic terms.
 b. Only 15% or less of patients make obscene vocal tics.
 c. Obscene vocal tics usually develop as an initial symptom.
 d. When they occur, obscene vocal tics develop late in the course.

 e. Occasionally patients express obscenities by gestures (copropraxia) rather than speech (coprolalia).

Answers: b, d, e.

4. When Tourette's disorder develops all of its comorbidities, in which sequence does it unfold?
 a. ADHD then motor tics, then vocal tics, then OCD symptoms.
 b. OCD symptoms then motor tics, then vocal tics, then ADHD.
 c. Tics, ADHD, and OCD symptoms occur randomly.
 d. All manifestations arise together.

Answer: a. ADHD is the only psychiatric comorbidity that precedes motor tics. Obsessive-compulsive symptoms and OCD, when they occur, are a late development.

5. Of the following, by which two methods does the nervous system deactivate dopamine?
 a. Decarboxylation
 b. Oxidation
 c. Re-uptake
 d. Hydroxylation
 e. Reduction

Answers: b, c. Most dopamine undergoes re-uptake, but monoamine oxidase (MAO) and catechol-O-methyltransferase metabolize the remainder.

6–9. Match the tremor (6–9) with the examination (a–d) that will elicit it.
6. Essential tremor
7. Cerebellar tremor
8. Parkinson's disease tremor
9. Lithium-induced tremor
 a. Finger-nose test
 b. Psychologic stress
 c. Extending arms and hands
 d. Observing the patient's hands when they are at rest

Answers: 6-c, 7-a, 8-d, 9-c. (Psychologic stress exacerbates most neurologic disorders, including tremors.) The three basic tests to look for tremor are to observe patients resting both arms in their lap; holding their arms and hands extended outward; and moving back and forth between their nose and the examiner's finger. Other tests include handwriting, sipping water, and holding an extended index finger 1 inch from the nose.

10–15. Match the tremor (10–15) with an effective therapy or therapies (a–f). If appropriate, use more than one letter for each number.
10. Essential
11. Cerebellar
12. Parkinson's disease
13. Stage fright
14. Hyperthyroidism
15. Delirium tremens
   a. Levodopa (L-dopa)
   b. Propranolol (Inderal)
   c. Amantadine (Symmetrel)
   d. Trihexyphenidyl (Artane)
   e. Primidone (Mysoline)
   f. None of the above

Answers: 10-b, e; 11-f; 12-a, c, d (L-dopa may be less effective than anticholinergics for Parkinson's tremor); 13-b; 14-b; 15-f.

16. Which three of these statements accurately apply to spasmodic torticollis?
   a. It may consist of retrocollis and anterocollis as well as torticollis.
   b. It develops in childhood.
   c. Surgical sectioning the sternocleidomastoid and adjacent muscles relieves it.
   d. Light pressure to the chin in a counter-rotational direction overcomes it.
   e. Whether a manifestation of tardive dystonia or an idiopathic condition, botulinum toxin injections greatly reduce torticollis.

Answers: a, d, e.

17. A psychiatrist is asked to evaluate an immobile, mute, 21-year-old woman who stares straight ahead and has waxy flexibility. She has an unsubstantiated history of a mood disorder. Which of the following is the least appropriate in the initial management of this patient?
   a. Obtain a blood test for Huntington's disease.
   b. Give a therapeutic trial of a benzodiazepine.
   c. Obtain an EEG to exclude partial complex status epilepticus.
   d. Obtain a blood test and slit-lamp examination to exclude Wilson's disease.
   e. Administer an antipsychotic drug because the patient probably has catatonic schizophrenia.
   f. Screen for illicit drug use.

Answer: e. Catatonia is more likely to be a manifestation of a mood disorder than schizophrenia, but

numerous neurologic conditions can be responsible. The most important neurologic causes of a catatonia-like state include drug abuse, secondary parkinsonism, and focal status epilepticus (psychomotor status epilepticus). Benzodiazepines will briefly reverse psychogenic catatonia.

18. Which statement is false regarding early onset primary dystonia?
   a. The illness usually first affects the lower limb muscles, but patients eventually have involvement of the trunk and neck muscles.
   b. At its onset, the disorder may be confused with Wilson's disease.
   c. Patients may present with tortipelvis.
   d. The inheritance is autosomal dominant with relatively low penetrance.
   e. The disease is most frequent among Eastern European (Ashkenazi) Jews.
   f. Like Huntington's disease, early onset primary dystonia results from excessive trinucleotide repeats.
   g. Affected individuals have no cognitive impairment, despite sometimes devastating physical impairment.

Answer: f. The abnormal gene, DYT1, results from deletion of a trinucleotide.

19. Which feature is least closely associated with the childhood variety of Huntington's disease?
   a. Chorea
   b. Rigidity
   c. More trinucleotide repeats than the adult variety
   d. More rapid demise than the adult variety

Answer: a. The childhood variety of Huntington's disease usually results from an excessively long sequence of trinucleotide repeats, inheritance from the father, more rapid demise, rigidity, and akinesia. The absence of chorea is a hallmark of the juvenile variety of the illness.

20. Chronic dystonia of the head and neck muscles in young adults may result from:
   a. Early onset primary (torsion) dystonia
   b. Wilson's disease
   c. Juvenile Huntington's disease
   d. Antipsychotic medications (i.e., tardive dystonia)
   e. All of the above

Answer: e.

21. For patients with depression comorbid with Parkinson's disease, which treatment will be least effective?

a. SSRIs
b. Tricyclic antidepressants
c. Electroconvulsive therapy (ECT)
d. Add a dopamine agonist to L-dopa

Answer: d. Restoring dopamine to normal concentrations or even providing excessive concentrations does not alleviate depression comorbid with Parkinson's disease.

22. After failing to respond to several antidepressant medications, a patient with advanced Parkinson's disease undergoes ECT. Subsequently, his mood and mobility both improve, but dyskinesias develop. What would be the best treatment to suppress the dyskinesias?
    a. Repeat the ECT
    b. Begin a cholinesterase inhibitor
    c. Reduce dopaminergic medications
    d. Reinstitute a SSRI

Answer: c. He has dopamine-induced dyskinesia because the ECT increases available dopamine. However, excessive L-dopa leads to dyskinesias and may also lead to psychosis. The best treatment would be to reduce dopaminergic medications to reduce their toxicity.

23. Which feature distinguishes dementia as a symptom of Parkinson's disease from dementia as a symptom of diffuse Lewy body disease?
    a. Dementia is one of the first symptoms of Parkinson's disease.
    b. Dementia is one of the first symptoms of diffuse Lewy body disease.
    c. The dementia of Parkinson's disease correlates with the tremor.
    d. The dementia of diffuse Lewy body disease correlates with aggression and loss of inhibition.

Answer: b. Although dementia is characteristically the presenting feature of diffuse Lewy body disease, it usually does not complicate Parkinson's disease until at least 5 years after the disease's onset. When dementia complicates Parkinson's disease, it correlates with rigidity and bradykinesia but not tremor. Aggression and loss of inhibition are associated with frontotemporal dementia.

24. Which one of the following is not a Parkinson-plus syndrome?
    a. Olivopontocerebellar degeneration
    b. Shy-Drager syndrome
    c. Progressive supranuclear palsy
    d. MPTP-induced parkinsonism

Answer: d. A group of several illnesses—loosely termed "Parkinson's plus"—are illnesses that include the cardinal features of Parkinson's disease but are characterized by other disturbances. Olivopontocerebellar degeneration is characterized by ataxia and Shy-Drager syndrome by hypotension and incontinence—illnesses that belong to the category of multisystem atrophies. Progressive supranuclear palsy, a Parkinson's-plus syndrome, is characterized by ocular motility limitations. MPTP-induced parkinsonism, a neurotoxic disorder, significantly affects only the extrapyramidal system.

25. An 8-year-old girl, who had been entirely well, began to develop dystonic movements of her legs that interfered with her athletic activities most afternoons. Then she had gait impairments every evening. She remained undiagnosed for 2 years. By then, she clearly had dystonia that was present almost throughout the day, but it fluctuated in a diurnal pattern. The dystonia worsened in the afternoon, but it was almost absent in the morning. No family member has a similar problem. Of the following, which is the most likely illness that has affected her?
    a. Duchenne's muscular dystrophy
    b. Dopa-responsive dystonia
    c. Cerebral palsy
    d. Early onset primary (torsion) dystonia

Answer: b. Dopa responsive dystonia (DRD) is characterized initially by dystonia that interferes with gait and, unlike primary dystonia, has diurnal fluctuations. Small doses of L-dopa, which serves as a diagnostic trial as well as treatment, correct the gait impairment and involuntary movements. DRD may resemble cerebral palsy (CP), especially the athetotic variety. Duchenne's muscular dystrophy affects only boys and does not cause involuntary movements.

26. What is the biochemical deficiency in dopa-responsive dystonia?
    a. Loss of the cofactor for synthesis of tyrosine hydroxylase
    b. Loss of dopa-decarboxylase
    c. Absence of the substrate phenylalanine
    d. Abnormal DOPA

Answer: a. Dopamine responsive dystonia is due to insufficient synthesis of tetrahydrobiopterin, which is an essential cofactor for phenylalanine and tyrosine hydroxylases.

27. Which statement is correct regarding the development of oral-buccal-lingual dyskinesia from typical dopamine-blocking antipsychotic agents?
    a. The incidence is greater in the first year of use.
    b. The incidence is greater in the fifth year of use.

c. The incidence is equal in the first and fifth years.

Answer: c. The annual rate of the development of this complication for each person at risk (the incidence) is constant. With time, any individual patient is more likely to develop the complication.

28. A psychiatrist is asked to evaluate a 70-year-old retired waiter, who has developed visual hallucinations. An ophthalmologist had found only mild visual impairment. During the past year, the patient had developed cognitive impairments, which seemed to fluctuate from day to day. The patient has mild slowness and generally increased tone. His neurologic examination is otherwise normal. The psychiatrist prescribes small doses of haloperidol. Several days later, the patient becomes rigid, akinetic, and unable to speak or eat. Of the following, which is the most likely underlying pathology?
    a. He has been overmedicated with haloperidol, relative to the requirements of older patients.
    b. He has Parkinson's disease that was made overt by the haloperidol.
    c. He probably has an illness that causes excessive plaques and tangles in the cerebral cortex.
    d. He probably has an illness that causes Lewy bodies in the cerebral cortex.

Answer: d. He probably has dementia with Lewy body disease, which causes fluctuating cognitive impairment early in the illness; visual hallucinations; and mild parkinsonism. Because the illness renders patients unusually sensitive to dopamine-blocking medications, the haloperidol produced severe parkinsonism in him.

29. Which one of the following enzymes increases the concentration of L-dopa?
    a. COMT
    b. MAO
    c. Decarboxylase
    d. Tyrosine hydroxylase

Answer: d. Tyrosine hydroxylase converts tyrosine to L-dopa, but the other enzymes metabolize L-dopa.

30. Which one of the following is characteristic of necrosis but not apoptosis?
    a. Energy-requiring
    b. Programmed
    c. Infiltration of mononuclear cells into the area of cell death
    d. Normal mechanism of development for some organs
    e. Cell death

Answer: c. Both apoptosis and necrosis are forms of cell death. Apoptosis is programmed cell death, which occurs in the normal development of certain organs, such as the thymus gland, as well as in several degenerative illnesses, such as Huntington's disease and ALS. It is sequential and requires energy. Apoptosis, however, does not cause inflammation, which is a characteristic of necrosis.

31. A 70-year-old man is comatose 1 week after sustaining a brainstem infarction. Among other abnormalities, his soft palate contracts regularly and symmetrically at a rate of 120 times per minute. The palate elevates, as though the patient were saying "ah." Which feature is untrue?
    a. As the coma lightens, the movements will persist during sleep as well as wakefulness.
    b. Connections to the inferior olivary nuclei, the paired scalloped-shaped structures in the medulla, have sustained damage.
    c. The regular movements in one plane define the disorder as a tremor.
    d. The disorder is really a variety of myoclonus.

Answer: d. He has palatal tremor, which was reclassified from myoclonus, because it consists of regular, rhythmic movements in a single plane. Palatal tremor results from lesions, usually in the medulla, of pathways that involve the inferior olivary nuclei. Unlike most movement disorders, palatal tremor persists during sleep and coma.

32–35. Match the illness (32–35) with its inheritance pattern (a–d).
32. Huntington's disease
33. Red-green color blindness
34. Wilson's disease
35. DYT1 dystonia
    a. Recessive sex-linked
    b. Autosomal recessive
    c. Autosomal dominant
    d. None of the above

Answers: 32-c, 33-a, 34-b, 35-c, with variable penetrance.

36. One strategy in the treatment of hyperkinetic movement disorders, such as tics, chorea, and the oral-buccolingual variety of tardive dyskinesia, is to deplete dopamine from presynaptic neurons. Which two medications may deplete dopamine and treat such disorders?
    a. Carbidopa
    b. COMT inhibitors
    c. Reserpine
    d. Risperidone
    e. Tetrabenazine

Answers: c, e. Both tetrabenazine and reserpine deplete dopamine from the storage vesicles of the presynaptic neurons and reduce the movements in hyperkinetic disorders. Carbidopa blocks the synthesis of dopamine from DOPA, but because it does not cross the blood–brain barrier, carbidopa would be ineffective in reducing basal ganglia dopamine stores.

37. What is the implication of a patient falling backward during the pull test?
    a. Cerebellar dysfunction
    b. Gait apraxia
    c. Gait ataxia
    d. Impaired postural reflexes

Answer: d. A patient having retropulsion during the test has the same significance as falling. Whichever the underlying illness, impaired postural reflexes indicate basal ganglia disease. The finding is typical in moderately advanced Parkinson's disease.

38. Which of the following statements regarding dementia in Parkinson's disease is false?
    a. In Parkinson's disease, the prevalence of dementia increases in proportion to physical impairments, especially bradykinesia, and its cumulative prevalence eventually reaches 80%.
    b. Affected patients lose 2.3 points annually on the Mini-Mental State Examination.
    c. Bradyphrenia characterizes Parkinson's disease dementia.
    d. Parkinson's disease dementia is an example of cortical dementia.

Answer: d. The gait impairment accompanying Parkinson's disease dementia renders it a prime example of subcortical dementia.

39. A 30-year-old woman, recovering from cocaine addiction, has suddenly developed incessant movements of her feet. She claims that she must walk constantly. When forced to sit, she continually moves her legs together and apart. She is belligerent, but alert and without cognitive impairment. Which of the following is the most likely cause of her movements and walking?
    a. Sydenham's chorea
    b. Obsessive-compulsive disorder
    c. Huntington's chorea
    d. Tourette's disorder
    e. Active cocaine use

Answer: e. She has cocaine-induced "crack dancing," in which an urge to walk compels incessant movements in the feet. Cocaine provokes release of dopamine from presynaptic storage sites and thus increases dopamine activity. Akathisia and the restless leg syndrome similarly cause involuntary movements of the legs and a compulsion to walk. Chorea causes arm and trunk as well as leg movements, but unlike these other conditions, it does not provoke an irresistible urge to move.

40. Which is the rate-limiting step in dopamine synthesis?
   a. Phenylalanine to tyrosine
   b. Tyrosine to DOPA
   c. Tyrosine to dopamine
   d. DOPA to dopamine
   e. Dopamine to norepinephrine
   f. None of the above

Answer: b. The rate-limiting step in dopamine synthesis is dependent on tyrosine hydroxylase, which converts tyrosine to DOPA.

41–49. Match the underlying abnormality (41–49) with the associated condition (a–g).
41. Cerebral cortical anoxia or uremia
42. Toxoplasmosis
43. Perinatal kernicterus
44. Low serum ceruloplasmin
45. Infarction of the subthalamic nucleus
46. Nigrostriatal depigmentation
47. Prion infection
48. Atrophy of the caudate heads
49. Cavitary lesions of the globus pallidus and putamen
   a. Huntington's disease
   b. Wilson's disease
   c. Hemiballismus
   d. Creutzfeldt-Jakob disease
   e. Choreoathetotic cerebral palsy
   f. Parkinson's disease
   g. Myoclonus

Answers: 41-g; 42-c; 43-e; 44-b; 45-c; 46-f; 47-d; 48-a; 49-b.

50. A 70-year-old man, who has moderately severe Parkinson's disease, resides in a nursing home. Its medical director sought a psychiatry consult because the patient stopped attending rehabilitation and occupational therapy. On questioning, the patient was alert but apathetic and states that these programs do not help. Which of the following statements regarding depression is correct?
   a. When it complicates Parkinson's disease, depression worsens cognitive impairment.
   b. Comorbid depression is a potential explanation for a Parkinson's disease patient responding poorly to medical and physical therapy.
   c. Comorbid depression interferes with patients' sleep.
   d. Comorbid depression interferes with patients' ability to adjust to the illness or its demands.
   e. All of the above.

Answer: e. Depression frequently complicates Parkinson's disease and worsens patients' mood, sleep cycle, cognitive capacity, and motor function.

51. Which of the following is not a risk factor for comorbid depression in Parkinson's disease?
   a. Cognitive impairment
   b. Akinesia
   c. Tremor
   d. History of depression
   e. Young age at onset of the illness
   f. Long duration of the illness

Answer: c.

52. Which of the following statements regarding familial Parkinson's disease is false?
   a. The parkin and α-synuclein mutations give rise to familial Parkinson's disease.
   b. Mutations usually lead to early onset Parkinson's disease.
   c. The majority of Parkinson's disease patients younger than 20 years harbor the parkin mutation.
   d. Genetically determined Parkinson's disease cases comprise less than 1% of the total.
   e. Autopsy studies of the genetically determined Parkinson's disease show that the basal ganglia lack Lewy bodies.

Answer: d. Genetically determined Parkinson's disease cases comprise up to 10% of the total cases.

53. A 29-year-old man has been hospitalized on several occasions during the previous 3 years for progressively severe schizophrenia. He was readmitted because of paranoid hallucinations and dopamine-blocking antipsychotic agent treatment was reinstituted. Several weeks later, a visiting physician notices that the patient has intermittent, forceful contractions of all the head and neck muscles that last several seconds. His neck tends to retrovert (extend). Likewise, his limbs involuntarily extend forward. His tongue protrudes intermittently for several seconds. The patient remains alert during these bizarre movements that appear "psychotic" to a neurology consultant. Which condition is the least likely to be the cause of this individual's movement disorder?
   a. Wilson's disease
   b. Tardive dystonia due to chronic neuroleptic use
   c. Huntington's disease
   d. Cerebellar disease, such as multiple sclerosis

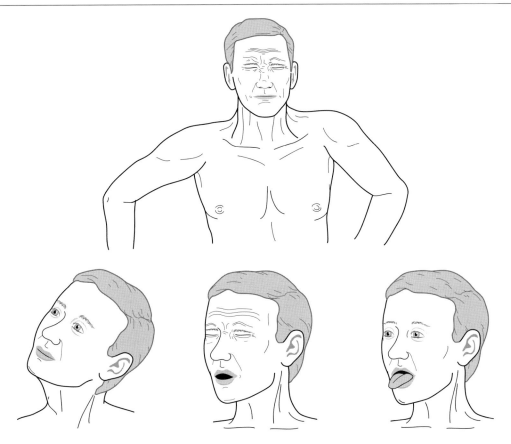

Answer: d. Wilson's and Huntington's diseases both cause thought disorders, which may be misdiagnosed as schizophrenia, and involuntary movement. Tardive dystonia often develops in individuals who already have schizophrenia. Cerebellar disease does not cause either thought disorder or involuntary movements. Except for multiple sclerosis, which almost never produces a movement disorder because it affects white matter, each of the conditions might be responsible.

54. Which three of the following neurodegenerative disorders are labeled "tauopathies" by neurologists?
    a. Alzheimer's disease
    b. Frontotemporal dementia
    c. Progressive supranuclear palsy (PSP)
    d. Dementia with Lewy bodies
    e. Multisystem atrophy (MSA)
    f. Parkinson's disease

    Answers: a, b, c.

55. In the previous question, which three of the disorders are labeled "synucleinopathies" by neurologists?

    Answers: d, e, f. Neurologists label dementia with Lewy bodies, MSA, and Parkinson's disease as synucleinopathies.

56. Which single statement is true regarding the trinucleotide (CAG) repeats in Huntington's disease?
    a. The pathologic sequence is located on chromosome 4.
    b. Normal individuals do not have trinucleotide (CAG) repeats.
    c. The repeats in affected individuals are stable.
    d. An affected mother's gene would be more unstable than an affected father's.

    Answer: a. Normal individuals have about 20 repeats of the CAG trinucleotide. Huntington's disease patients have 37 or more repeats. Because the DNA in the father's sperm is unstable, the father is more apt than the mother to have an offspring with juvenile Huntington's disease.

57. Which three illnesses result from excessive trinucleotide repeats?
    a. Myotonic dystrophy
    b. Depression
    c. Fragile X syndrome
    d. Alzheimer's disease
    e. Huntington's disease
    f. Duchenne's muscular dystrophy

    Answers: a, c, e.

58. What is the term applied when a genetic illness produces symptoms in younger victims in successive generations?
   a. Anticipation
   b. Suppression
   c. Disinhibition
   d. None of the above because it does not happen

Answer: a. *Anticipation* occurs in Huntington's disease, myotonic dystrophy, and several other illnesses. It results from unstable trinucleotide repeats.

59. Which four disorders often develop in adolescence and are associated with dementia?
   a. Creutzfeldt-Jakob disease
   b. Wilson's disease
   c. Choreoathetotic cerebral palsy
   d. Huntington's disease
   e. Subacute sclerosing panencephalitis (SSPE)
   f. Variant Creutzfeldt-Jakob disease
   g. Dopamine-responsive dystonia

Answers: b, d, e, f. These illnesses cause dementia that, in adolescents, might initially appear as personality change.

60. Which patients are most apt to cause depression in their caregivers?
   a. Patients with depression
   b. Patients with acute, devastating illness
   c. Patients with physical impairments
   d. Patients who require complicated medical regimens.

Answer: a. Caregivers are most apt to develop depression when the patient has depression and a chronic illness.

61–65. Match the patients' description (61–65) with the neurologic disturbances (a–h).
61. A 70-year-old man develops a high-pitched, squeaky voice that forces him to speak in a whisper. Nevertheless, he can sing in a normal volume and pitch.
62. An actor begins to have hand tremor while on stage.
63. Continual forced bilateral eyelid closure prevents a 70-year-old man from seeing.
64. A middle-aged woman develops continual face, eyelid, and jaw contractions.
65. An author develops hand cramps when writing with a pen, but he can use a computer keyboard, play tennis, and button his shirts.
   a. Blepharospasm
   b. Writer's cramp
   c. Spasmodic dysphonia
   d. Meige's syndrome

   e. Oromandibular dystonia
   f. Anxiety-induced tremor
   g. Aphasia
   h. Spasmodic torticollis

Answers: 61-c, 62-f, 63-a, 64-d, 65-b. Blepharospasm, Meige's syndrome, oromandibular dystonia, and spasmodic dysphonia are varieties of cranial dystonia. Spasmodic dysphonia and spasmodic torticollis are varieties of cervical dystonia. Neuroleptic exposure often precedes the development of cranial and cervical dystonias; however, many patients have no history of medicine exposure, psychiatric illness, or other indication that their movements are a variety of tardive dyskinesia. Stage fright is an example of anxiety-induced tremor.

66. Which two structures constitute the striatum?
   a. Caudate
   b. Putamen
   c. Globus pallidus
   d. Subthalamic
   e. Substantia nigra

Answers: a, b.

67. Which one of the following characteristics does not apply to the nigrostriatal tract?
   a. It links the substantia nigra to the striatum.
   b. The substantia nigra is normally black, but in Parkinson's disease, it is hypopigmented.
   c. It produces about 80% of the dopamine of the brain.
   d. Tyrosine is converted to DOPA in its presynaptic neurons.
   e. When it undergoes neurodegeneration, the lateral ventricles balloon outward.
   f. Its major metabolic end product is homovanillic acid (HVA).
   g. Degeneration of most of the presynaptic neurons leads to Parkinson's disease.

Answer: e. Atrophy of the head of the caudate nuclei allows the lateral ventricles to balloon outward. They expand in a convex shape, often called "batwing," which is characteristic of Huntington's disease.

68. Sinemet is a combination of L-dopa and which other substance?
   a. Carbidopa
   b. Bromocriptine (Parlodel), a dopamine agonist
   c. Anticholinergics
   d. Selegiline, an MAO-B inhibitor

Answer: a. Carbidopa, a dopa decarboxylase inhibitor, impedes metabolism of L-dopa in the systemic circulation. Because it cannot cross the blood–brain barrier, carbidopa does not interfere with the nigro-striatal tract conversion of L-dopa to dopamine.

69. Since infancy, a 25-year-old man has had involuntary slow, twisting movements of his face, mouth, trunk, and limbs. The neck muscles have hypertrophied. He performs poorly on standard intelligence tests. Which two of the following statements regarding his condition are true?

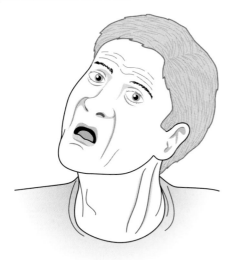

  a. His children might inherit this condition.
  b. He probably performs poorly on standard intelligence tests, in part, because he is dysarthric and unable to use his hands.
  c. He probably has congenital abnormalities in the basal ganglia.
  d. His condition is not associated with cognitive impairments.

Answers: b, c. He probably has congenital athetosis, which is a variety of cerebral palsy (CP) that becomes apparent between infancy and ages 2 and 4 years. It is often, but not necessarily, associated with mental retardation. Superficial clinical examinations and standard intelligence tests tend to underestimate children with cerebral palsy, especially the athetotic and choreoathetotic varieties, because of their motor impairments and dysarthria. Early onset primary dystonia (torsion dystonia or dystonia musculorum deformans), which appears in childhood, is carried on the DYT1 gene and inherited as an autosomal dominant condition. It is not associated with cognitive impairment. Dopa-responsive dystonia, which resembles cerebral palsy, appears during childhood and has a diurnal fluctuation. It, too, is not associated with cognitive impairment.

70. Which of the following statements concerning the Lesch-Nyhan syndrome is false?
  a. Its symptoms include dystonia and other movements in children aged 2 to 6 years.
  b. It is transmitted as an autosomal dominant genetic illness.
  c. Lesch-Nyhan syndrome children have often bitten off parts of their lips and fingertips.
  d. The basic deficit is a deficiency of HGPRT.
  e. The enzyme deficiency often leads to renal failure.

Answer: b. Lesch-Nyhan syndrome, characterized by self-mutilation, is transmitted as a sex-linked recessive illness. Its underlying HGPRT deficiency causes hyperuricemia, which often leads to renal failure.

71. In which conditions is myoclonus found?
  a. Cerebral anoxia
  b. SSPE
  c. Creutzfeldt-Jakob disease
  d. Use of SSRIs
  e. Use of meperidine (Demerol)
  f. Uremia
  g. Use of typical dopamine-blocking antipsychotics
  h. Use of atypical dopamine-blocking antipsychotics

Answers: a, b, c, d (occasionally), e, f.

72. What is the mechanism of action that permits propranolol to suppress essential tremor?
  a. It reduces cardiac output.
  b. It is a mild sedative.
  c. It blocks adrenergic sympathetic nervous system receptor sites.
  d. It suppresses synthesis of norepinephrine.

Answer: c. Propranolol is a relatively nonspecific adrenergic blocker that is useful in suppressing essential tremor and migraines headaches, as well hypertension and angina. However, it may precipitate asthma and congestive heart failure. Some recent data have questioned the tendency of propranolol to cause depression.

73. Which one of the following is *not* a characteristic of MPTP-induced parkinsonism?
  a. MPTP provides a laboratory model of Parkinson's disease.
  b. Pre-treatment with monoamine oxidase inhibitors protects animals.
  c. Patients respond, at least temporarily, to L-dopa replacement.
  d. MPTP is toxic only when oxidized by a monoamine oxidase.

e. MPTP is a by-product of hydrocarbon manufacturing.

Answer: e. Methyl-phenyl-tetrahydro-pyridine (MPTP), a meperidine analogue, is a by-product of illicit narcotic manufacturing. MPTP is actually not the toxin. MAO must first convert it to MPP$^+$. However, MAO inhibitors can prevent the reaction.

74. By which mechanism does botulinum toxin treat blepharospasm, Meige's syndrome, and other focal dystonias?
    a. Botulinum toxin, like tetrabenazine, depletes dopamine.
    b. Botulinum toxin binds to the postsynaptic neuron.
    c. Botulinum toxin prevents release of acetylcholine (ACh) from the presynaptic neuromuscular junction neuron.
    d. Botulinum toxin, like myasthenia gravis antibodies, binds to the postsynaptic ACh receptors.

Answer: c.

75. After developing personality changes and slowed thinking for 1 to 2 years, a 39-year-old man presents for evaluation. He relates that his father died at 60 years of age of Huntington's disease, but his mother is alive and well. A neurologic examination shows subtle chorea, motor impersistence, and jerky saccades. After the neurologist offers a clinical diagnosis of Huntington's disease, the patient agrees to undergo genetic testing. Which of the following patterns of his genes will the test most likely show?
    a. Maternal gene, 20 CAG repeats; paternal gene, 45 repeats
    b. Maternal gene, 30 CAG repeats; paternal gene, 30 repeats
    c. Maternal gene, 45 CAG repeats; paternal gene, 20 repeats
    d. Maternal gene, 20 CAG repeats; paternal gene, 80 repeats
    e. Maternal gene, 80 CAG repeats; paternal gene, 20 repeats

Answer: a. The patient's father, who died relatively late of Huntington's disease, probably had a relatively low elevation of CAG repeats. Because the mother is not affected, her CAG complement level is probably normal. Had the father carried a gene with more than 60 repeats (answer d), he would have developed the illness and died at a young age, probably before fathering any children. If the mother's CAG complement had been elevated (answers c and e), she would have been the affected parent. If both sets of genes show normal CAG repeats (answer b), the neurologist must consider another illness.

76. Which statement about saccades is false?
    a. Saccades are rapid, accurate, conjugate eye movements.
    b. Saccadic eye movement is abnormal in Huntington's disease and schizophrenia.
    c. Abnormal saccades are an early sign of Huntington's disease.
    d. In Huntington's disease, patients may initiate saccades by jerking their head or blinking.
    e. Neurologists consider saccadic eye movement normal if the eyes eventually come to rest on the target, whether or not they initially undershoot or overshoot it.
    f. In Huntington's disease, in addition to patients' initiating ocular movement by head movement or blinking, their saccades are jerky.

Answer: e. Normal saccades shoot directly and accurately from one target to another.

77. Which statement is false regarding the NMDA receptor?
    a. It is a glutamate receptor.
    b. Its inactivity is causally related to Huntington's disease.
    c. It is probably causally related to neurologic damage in epilepsy and stroke.
    d. It is a receptor for excitatory neurotransmitters.

Answer: b. In Huntington's disease, excessive NMDA activity probably leads to excitotoxicity and apoptosis.

78. Several members of a French-Canadian family, currently living in northern Maine, were found to have an unusual response to stimulation. To unexpected noises, they and many of their relatives leap upward, scream, and throw any object in their hands. Which is the most likely explanation for their response?
    a. Culture-bound behavior
    b. Stimulus-sensitive myoclonus
    c. Anxiety
    d. Hyperacusis

Answer: a. They are jumping Frenchmen of Maine who demonstrate culture-bound behavior or folk-illnesses. Similarly, *latahs* of rural Malaysia and Indonesia and myriachit of Siberia tend to overreact to trivial stimuli by suddenly cursing, laughing convulsively, or moving in exaggerated patterns.

79. At the suggestion of the psychiatric consultant, emergency room physicians administered a small

intramuscular dose of haloperidol to an intravenous drug addict with dangerous agitation and psychotic thinking. Shortly thereafter, all the physicians noticed that muscles throughout his entire body were having intermittent but powerful contractions. His temperature was 103°F. The physicians found a deep infection in his left thigh. As the evaluation continued, laryngeal and pharyngeal contractions made his breathing difficult, his face intermittently grimaced, and his jaw pulled clinched. As physicians examined him further, they seemed to trigger violent muscle contractions. The physicians started broad-spectrum antibiotics for the infection, but anticholinergics and antihistamines did not correct the muscle contractions. Which condition best explains the muscle contractions?

a. Acute dystonic reaction to haloperidol
b. Seizures
c. Meige's syndrome
d. The thigh infection

Answer: d. Trismus (lockjaw), prominent involuntary face and jaw muscle contractions, and the examination provoking muscle contractions, in a drug addict, indicate that he has tetanus from the thigh infection. Drug addicts are prone to tetanus because they use contaminated needles. Tetanus immunity lasts for only about 10 years. When it wears off, patients can develop either generalized tetanus or "regional tetanus," in which only the infected limb is affected. The neuroleptic-malignant syndrome is less likely because the emergency room staff administered only a small dose of haloperidol and the rise in temperature was explainable by the abscess.

80. Which of the following medicines elevates the serum prolactin concentration?
    a. Clozapine
    b. Risperidone
    c. Haloperidol
    d. L-dopa

Answer: c. Classic dopamine-blocking antipsychotic agents provoke prolactin release. In addition, primary generalized and some partial complex seizures, and pituitary adenomas also provoke prolactin release. Prolactin is a pituitary hormone but not a neurotransmitter. Its secretion into the systemic circulation is normally inhibited by dopamine. Dopamine agonists and L-dopa, as well as dopamine, inhibit its secretion. In contrast, dopamine blockade, as occurs with many classic antipsychotic agents, enhances prolactin secretion, which produces elevated serum prolactin levels.

81. A 50-year-old woman, who has been taking various SSRIs for 10 years, states that her face has begun to pull to the left. The movements are more intense during anxiety and last for several seconds, but they are not painful. The eyelid closure prevents her from driving her car. Which one of the following conditions is probably causing her movements?

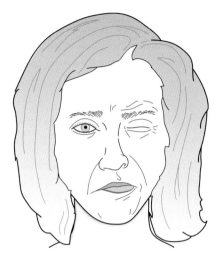

a. An aberrant blood vessel at the cerebellopontine angle
b. Partial complex seizures
c. Dopamine-blocking neuroleptics
d. Anxiety
e. Antidepressants

Answer: a. She has hemifacial spasm. In many cases, an aberrant blood vessel that compresses the facial nerve as it exits from the brainstem causes it.

82. Which two structures constitute the lenticular nuclei?
    a. Caudate
    b. Putamen
    c. Globus pallidus
    d. Subthalamic nucleus
    e. Substantia nigra

Answers: b, c. The putamen and globus pallidus form the lenticular nuclei, which bear the brunt of hepatolenticular degeneration (Wilson's disease).

83. Which one of the following nuclei is not part of the set of the others?
    a. Substantia nigra
    b. Locus ceruleus
    c. Dorsal motor
    d. Anterior thalamic

Answer: d. Thalamic nuclei are not pigmented. Moreover, they are mostly sensory relay nuclei. Substantia nigra, locus ceruleus, and dorsal motor nuclei are normally pigmented but lose their color in Parkinson's disease and are constituents of the motor system.

84. A family brings its 72-year-old patriarch for evaluation of dementia that developed during the previous 4 to 6 months. The neurologic examination reveals mild rigidity and bradykinesia, as well as a nonspecific dementia. Which one of the following statements is best applied to this case?
    a. His substantia nigra probably contains Lewy bodies.
    b. His cerebral cortex, as well as substantia nigra, probably contain Lewy bodies.
    c. He probably has depression.
    d. He probably has Alzheimer's disease.

Answer: b. He probably has dementia with Lewy body disease in view of the extrapyramidal signs (rigidity and bradykinesia). Parkinson's disease, at its onset, generally does not cause depression or dementia. Alzheimer's disease does not present with either pyramidal or extrapyramidal signs.

85. In the treatment of depression in Parkinson's disease patients, which of the following statements are false?
    a. Psychotherapy is not only essential, it is often sufficient.
    b. ECT is contraindicated.
    c. Selegiline has an antidepressant effect.
    d. Tocopherol is often helpful.

Answers: b, d. ECT is often indicated for depression in Parkinson's disease patients, in whom it will temporarily relieve the motor symptoms as well as the depression. Tocopherol (vitamin E) has no benefit on either the mental or physical manifestations of Parkinson's disease. Selegiline is metabolized, in part, to amphetamine. Although physicians should use caution when administering an SSRI together with selegiline, the actual incidence of serotonin syndrome is very low because selegiline at the usual doses selectively inhibits MAO-B, which metabolizes dopamine. In contrast, the serotonin syndrome is mostly a complication of inhibitors of MAO-A, which metabolize serotonin.

86. Which of the following complications is the most common reason why families place Parkinson's disease patients in nursing homes?
    a. Hallucinations and delusions
    b. Depression
    c. Rigidity
    d. Akinesia

Answer: a. Psychosis, not physical incapacity or incontinence, is the most frequent reason that families place Parkinson's disease patients in nursing homes. The family's disturbed sleep, which usually results from patient's behavior, is the particular reason.

87. With which of the following dopamine receptor subtypes do all dopamine agonists effective in the treatment of Parkinson's disease interact?
    a. D_1
    b. D_2
    c. Both
    d. Neither

Answer: b. Effective antiparkinson dopamine agonists stimulate D_2, but they may either stimulate or inhibit D_1.

88. With which cardinal feature of Parkinson's disease is dementia least associated?
    a. Older age
    b. Rapid progression of the illness
    c. Poor response to dopamine medications
    d. Tremor
    e. Akinesia

Answer: d. Dementia is least closely associated with tremor. If dementia occurs at the onset of an illness with parkinsonism disease in individuals older than 50 years, consider dementia with Lewy body. In young adults, consider Wilson's disease, juvenile Huntington's disease, and drug abuse.

89. A 70-year-old man, under treatment for depression for 10 years, has begun to develop intermittent contractions of the orbicularis oculi. His medications included a tricyclic antidepressant (TCA) until 2 years ago when a serotonin reuptake inhibitor was substituted. He had a good response to the change. He has undergone two courses of ECT. The involuntary movements impair his ability to read and intensify the depression. What would be the best treatment?
    a. Return to a TCA.
    b. Prohibit any further ECT.
    c. Reduce the dose of the serotonin re-uptake inhibitors.
    d. Add anticholinergic medications.
    e. None of the above.

Answer: e. The patient has developed blepharospasm, but it is probably not a side effect of either the antidepressants or ECT. Although blepharospasm may follow treatment with dopamine-blocking

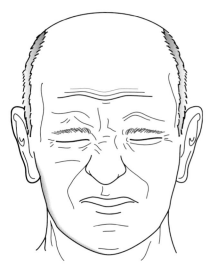

antipsychotic agents, it is almost always an idiopathic condition. Regardless of its origin, botulinum toxin injections into the affected muscles will alleviate the blepharospasm and permit antidepressant treatment to continue.

90–92. Match the neurotransmitter (90–92) with its metabolic product(s) (a–c).
90. Norepinephrine
91. Dopamine
92. Serotonin
  a. HVA
  b. 5-Hydroxyindoleacetic acid (5-HIAA)
  c. Vanillylmandelic acid (VMA)

Answers: 90-c, 91-a, 92-b.

93. Which one of the following movement disorders is not accompanied or preceded by an urge to move?
  a. Tics
  b. Akathisia
  c. Tremor
  d. Restless legs syndrome movements

Answer: c. Such sensations do not precede tremor, athetosis, hemiballismus, dystonia or most other movements. However, tics, akathisia, and restless legs movements seem to stem from irrepressible, sometimes indescribable, sensations, urges, or psychic tension, which are sometimes termed a compulsion. Patients can suppress these movements for several minutes, but when the movements break through, they return in a flurry.

94. Which of the following medicines is not associated with myoclonus?
  a. Lithium at toxic levels
  b. Lithium coadministered with TCAs
  c. Lithium coadministered with clozapine

  d. Dopamine-blocking antipsychotic agents
  e. Bismuth
  f. Meperidine (Demerol)
  g. Cyclosporine
  h. SSRIs

Answer: d. Dopamine-blocking antipsychotic agents cause many problems, which generally involve dopamine transmission in the basal ganglia, but myoclonus, which originates in irritability of motor neurons, is not one of them. Clonazepam or valproate can suppress medication-induced myoclonus.

95. Unlike typical antipsychotic agents, clozapine does not induce parkinsonism. Sparing of which receptor explains this freedom?
  a. D_1 dopamine
  b. D_2 dopamine
  c. D_3 dopamine
  d. NMDA
  e. GABA

Answer: b.

96. Which of the following does not describe free radicals?
  a. They contain single, unpaired electrons.
  b. They are stable.
  c. They snatch away electrons from neighboring atoms or molecules.
  d. Removal of electrons oxidizes atoms or molecules.
  e. Methylphenylpyridinium (MMP^+) is a free radical.

Answer: b. Because they lack an unpaired electron, they capture one as soon as possible, which leads to oxidation.

97. Which three characteristics distinguish visual hallucinations in Parkinson's disease from those in schizophrenia?
  a. In Parkinson's disease, visual hallucinations often arise independent of psychotic thought.
  b. In Parkinson's disease, visual hallucinations are almost never accompanied by auditory hallucinations.
  c. In Parkinson's disease, visual hallucinations are often accompanied by dyskinesias.
  d. In Parkinson's disease, visual hallucinations are a symptom at the onset of the illness.

Answers: a, b, c. Visual symptoms in Parkinson's disease are precipitated or caused by dopaminergic medications, such as L-dopa and dopamine agonists. They typically occur in older patients with long-standing Parkinson's disease, already complicated by dementia. Although visual hallucinations are usually not an early symptom of Parkinson's disease, they are an early symptom of dementia with Lewy body disease.

98. Which two of the following characteristics accurately describe dementia in Parkinson's disease?
    a. It responds to L-dopa.
    b. It responds to dopa agonists.
    c. Thought processes are typically slow.
    d. Patients have difficult shifting mental sets.
    e. Aphasia and apraxia are common manifestations of the dementia.

Answers: c, d. Bradyphrenia and lack of initiative are frequently occurring manifestations of the dementia of Parkinson's disease; however, these cognitive impairments and commonplace, generalized dementia do not respond to dopaminergic medications. (Comorbid depression also does not respond to dopaminergic medications.) The incidence of dementia in Parkinson's disease increases with age. Although the dementia conforms more to a subcortical than cortical pattern, a valid distinction is often impossible because of the frequent coexistence of Alzheimer's and Parkinson's diseases, the possibility that the illness is actually Lewy body disease, and the general unreliability of the dichotomy.

99. Which three of the following Parkinson's disease symptoms do not respond to dopaminergic medications?
    a. Dementia
    b. Tremor
    c. Rigidity
    d. Bradykinesia
    e. Depression
    f. Hallucinations

Answers: a, e, f. Mental aberrations are unaffected by restoring dopamine activity. In fact, excessive dopamine activity precipitates hallucinations, especially in the later states of the illness.

100. A neurologic examination of a 17-year-old boy, who has had declining schoolwork, reveals dysarthria, tremor, and a brown-green ring at the periphery of each cornea. Which of the following laboratory abnormalities is most likely to be found?
    a. Little or no copper-transporting serum protein
    b. Metachromatic granules in the urine
    c. Periodic EEG complexes
    d. MPTP metabolic products in the urine

Answer: a. In view of the history, tremor, and Kayser-Fleisher ring, he probably has Wilson's disease (hepatolenticular degeneration). It is an autosomal recessive disorder associated with a marked reduction in ceruloplasmin, the copper-transporting serum protein, and visible copper deposits in the periphery of the cornea, the Kayser-Fleisher ring.

101. Which is the effect of dopamine stimulating D_1 receptors?
    a. The interaction stimulates adenyl cyclase activity.
    b. The interaction inhibits adenyl cyclase activity.
    c. The interaction has no effect on adenyl cyclase activity.

Answer: a. Dopamine-D_1 receptor interaction stimulates adenyl cyclase activity, but dopamine-D_2 receptor interaction inhibits adenyl cyclase activity.

102. Why do typical dopamine blocking neuroleptics produce parkinsonism?
    a. They block D_1 receptors.
    b. They block D_2 receptors.
    c. They stimulate D_1 receptors.
    d. They stimulate D_2 receptors.

Answer: b. Their tendency to induce parkinsonism results from their affinity for (tendency to block) D_2 dopamine receptors.

103. In Huntington's disease and several other neurologic disorders that result from excessive trinucleotide repeats, the abnormal genetic segment tends to undergo amplification. Which one of the following statements concerning amplification is true?
    a. Amplification of trinucleotide repeats leads to the genetic abnormality appearing in additional chromosomes.
    b. Amplification of trinucleotide repeats is more apt to occur in eggs than sperm.
    c. Amplification leads to anticipation.
    d. Amplification is equivalent to anticipation.

Answer: c. In amplification, the expanded trinucleotide segment expands further in successive generations. Because this defect is more unstable in sperm than eggs, amplification is more likely when the abnormality is transmitted from the father than from the mother. In addition, the greater the amplification, the younger the age of onset of symptoms in offspring who inherit the abnormal chromosome. Anticipation refers to symptoms appearing at a younger age.

104. What is the net effect of reducing dopaminergic input to the striatum?

a. Increased GPi activity
b. Decreased GPi activity
c. Inability to replete the deficiency with medications
d. All of the above

Answer: a. Increased GPi activity leads to increased inhibition of thalamocortical pathways.

105. A 60-year-old man who has had Parkinson's disease for 4 years has begun to develop several minute episodes of kicking and punching during his sleep. The episodes differ from each other and do not include incontinence or tongue biting. The man has no recollection of them in the morning. Which of the following tests would most likely reveal the diagnosis?
a. Electroencephalogram (EEG)
b. Magnetic resonance imaging (MRI)
c. Polysomnogram (PSG)
d. None of the above

Answer: c. A PSG would probably show that he has REM sleep behavior disorder. Parkinson's disease and diffuse Lewy body disease are associated with REM sleep behavior disorder. His episodes are probably not seizures because they vary and the activity is semipurposeful.

106. In the preceding question, which would be the best treatment?
a. Clonazepam
b. Phenytoin
c. Carbamazepine
d. Choral hydrate
e. Clonidine

Answer: a. Clonazepam is highly effective. Given at bedtime, clonazepam suppresses most episodes of REM sleep behavior disorder. Antiepileptic drugs will have little or no benefit.

107. A 70-year-old man has begun to gamble for the first time in his life. Moreover, although he has neither won nor lost much money, he has spent inordinate time in casinos. Although he feels compelled to gamble, he enjoys all of its aspects. He had had depression 10 years ago, but currently has no symptoms of depression. He has had Parkinson's disease for about 5 years. Which is the most likely explanation for his newly developed pastime?
a. Dopamine dysregulation syndrome (DDS)
b. Depression
c. Dementia

d. OCD

Answer: a. His behavior, the dopamine dysregulation syndrome (DDS), probably stems from dopaminergic medicines' stimulating award systems. In this disorder, which is similar to hedonistic dysregulation, dopamine agonists induce aberrant behavior, such as compulsive gambling, and excessive eating, sexual activity, shopping, and mood swings. Simply stopping the medicine eliminates the problem.

108. Which of the following characteristics does not indicate that a tremor has a psychogenic basis?
a. Tremors in both upper extremities oscillate synchronously.
b. Following the example of the examiner, the patient's affected hand oscillates at a slow speed, then fast speed, and then back to the slow speed.
c. When stressed, a tremor increases in amplitude.
d. A physician holding the arm affected by a tremor may see it shift to the other arm.

Answer: c. Stress precipitates many neurologic and medical illnesses, such as asthma, Parkinson's disease tremor, and essential tremor. Psychogenic tremors, when *coherent*, affect both arms with identical movements. The examiner can frequently *entrain* a psychogenic tremor to follow a variable frequency. Also, a psychogenic tremor often switches sides when the physician restrains the affected arm.

109. Which of the following statements concerning dementia in Parkinson's disease is false?
a. It can be the sole comorbid psychiatric condition.
b. It can be comorbid with depression.
c. When comorbid with depression, dementia assumes different features.
d. When comorbid with depression, dementia has more pronounced deficits.

Answer: c. Not only can dementia be the sole psychiatric complication of Parkinson's disease, but also it can be comorbid with depression. In such cases, dementia is more pronounced, although not qualitatively different, than when it occurs without depression.

110. Regarding dementia pugilistica, which one of the following statements is untrue?
a. It mimics Parkinson's disease: tremors, rigidity, and depigmentation of the substantia nigra.
b. Histologic examination shows Alzheimer's-like cerebral plaques and tangles.

c. It occurs most frequently in lightweight boxers and alcoholics.
d. Gross examination shows atrophy of the corpus callosum and the cerebrum.
e. As in Parkinson's disease, histologic examination shows Lewy bodies in the basal ganglia in dementia pugilistica.

f. Paradoxically, dementia is not a component of dementia pugilistica.

Answer: e. Although dementia pugilistica shares many clinical and histologic features with Parkinson's disease, Lewy bodies occur only in Parkinson's disease.

CHAPTER 19

Brain Tumors and Metastatic Cancer

With their unpredictable onset and potentially tragic consequences, brain tumors command unique attention. Moreover, they frequently develop insidiously in young and middle-aged adults in whom they may produce depression, thought disorders, or cognitive impairment accompanied or unaccompanied by physical symptoms. Brain tumors epitomize organic causes of psychiatric disturbances.

VARIETIES

Primary Brain Tumors

Primary brain tumors, which are named after their original cell line, develop within the brain or spinal cord tissue (*parenchyma*) or their coverings (*meninges*) (Table 19-1). The numerous, mostly small, *glial cells*, which normally provide the structural, biochemical, and immunologic support for the central nervous system (CNS), give rise to most parenchymal tumors—*gliomas*. Malignant proliferation of the meningeal cells gives rise to *meningiomas*. However, CNS neurons rarely undergo malignant transformation in adults.

Of the various potential etiologies of primary brain tumors, data have established only that ionizing radiation, certain neurocutaneous disorders (see Chapter 13), and various genetic mutations constitute risk factors for brain tumors. In contrast, data do not support the fear that cellular telephone use constitutes a risk factor.

Gliomas

The group of parenchymal tumors, gliomas, includes *oligodendrogliomas*, *astrocytomas*, and, its most malignant variety, *glioblastoma multiforme*. *Oligodendrocytes*, which normally produce the myelin covering that insulates CNS neurons,* may give rise to *oligodendrogliomas*. These tumors, which occur infrequently and grow slowly, produce similar manifestations as the more commonly occurring astrocytomas (see later).

Astrocytomas, which arise from *astrocytes*, strike children as well as adults, do not invade surrounding

*Schwann cells produce the myelin insulation for the peripheral nervous system (PNS).

tissue when they are low-grade, and develop anywhere in the CNS. In children, astrocytomas tend to develop as cystic, noninvasive tumors in the cerebellum, but infiltrative ones in the brainstem. Because neurosurgeons can readily remove an entire cerebellar astrocytoma, the cure rate reaches almost 90%.

In adults, astrocytomas occur predominantly in the cerebrum, infiltrate extensively, and often degenerate into glioblastomas. Total surgical removal is practical when the surrounding brain can be sacrificed. For low-grade astrocytomas, combined surgery and radiotherapy prolong life for approximately 10 years.

Glioblastomas, highly aggressive and infiltrating tumors, develop predominantly in the cerebrum. They grow rapidly and invade across the corpus callosum (Figs. 19-1A, 20-8, and 20-20). Contrary to many physicians' expectations that brain tumors, like most other cancers, arise in the elderly, the age of patients at the time of a glioblastoma diagnosis averages only 54 years.

Although radiotherapy, steroids, and chemotherapy may reduce glioblastomas and other high-grade astrocytomas' growth rate and provide a brief (6 month to 1 year) physically comfortable period, surgical excision rarely eliminates them. In fact, many patients, especially the elderly and those with pronounced neurologic deficits, gain little or nothing from such treatments. Glioblastoma patients survive, on average, only 1 year. Moreover, persistence of the tumor and side effects of radiotherapy often produce progressive cognitive and emotional deterioration.

TABLE 19-1 ■ Primary Brain Tumors

Gliomas
    Astrocyte tumors
        Astrocytoma
        Glioblastoma
    Oligodendroglioma
Meningioma*
Lymphoma
Medulloblastoma
Pituitary adenoma*
Acoustic neuroma*

*Relatively benign histology.

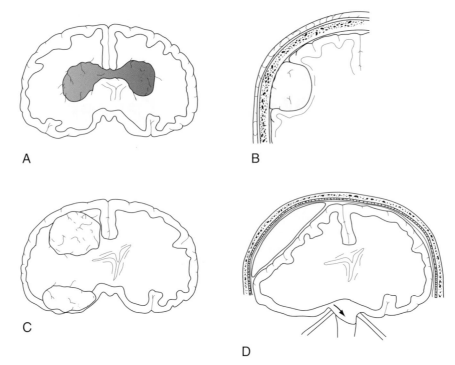

A

B

C

D

FIGURE 19-1 ■ *A, A glioblastoma* is a highly malignant tumor that typically infiltrates along white matter tracts. Sometimes it spreads through the heavily myelinated corpus callosum in a "butterfly" pattern (see Figs. 20-8 and 20-20). *B, Meningiomas* arise from the meninges overlying the brain or spinal cord and grow slowly (see Fig. 20-10). They compress and irritate but do not infiltrate the central nervous system (CNS). *C, Metastatic tumors,* usually multiple and surrounded by edema, destroy large areas of brain and raise intracranial pressure (see Fig. 20-8). *D, A subdural hematoma,* a nonmalignant mass lesion, typically located over one cerebral hemisphere (see Fig. 20-9), compresses the underlying brain. Acute subdural hematomas, which expand rapidly, force the brainstem and ipsilateral oculomotor (third cranial) nerve through the tentorial notch. Such *transtentor-ial herniation,* which also occurs with epidural hematomas (see Chapter 22), constitutes an immediately life-threatening condition. In contrast, small or slowly growing meningiomas and small, chronic subdural hematomas cause relatively few physical symptoms because they are "extra-axial," that is, situated outside of the brain.

Meningiomas

Meningiomas arise from cells of the meninges, which form the coverings of the CNS, rather than from actual brain or spinal cord tissue. Although their etiology is rarely known, meningiomas are an integral part of neurofibromatosis type 1 (see Chapter 13).

Meningiomas usually create symptoms by compressing the underlying brain or spinal cord (see Figs. 19-1B and 20-10). They grow slowly and develop almost exclusively in adults. If their expansion is insidious, they may grow quite large before they produce symptoms.

Neurologists often detect small meningiomas as an incidental finding on imaging studies. These tumors usually remain innocuous and asymptomatic and rarely require surgical removal. Even moderate-sized meningiomas located in certain areas may not produce symptoms. For example, meningiomas over the right frontal lobe can grow to an extraordinary size before they cause

problems. When necessary, surgeons can successfully remove most meningiomas.

Primary Cerebral Lymphoma

In contrast to systemic lymphoma, which commonly spreads to the CNS, *primary cerebral lymphoma* develops exclusively within the brain, where it tends to arise simultaneously in multiple sites. Because lymphomas often result from an impaired immune system, primary cerebral lymphomas typically develop in patients with the acquired immunodeficiency syndrome (AIDS) and those receiving immunosuppressive therapy for renal and cardiac transplants.

On computed tomography (CT), and magnetic resonance imaging (MRI), primary cerebral lymphoma resembles cerebral toxoplasmosis (see Figs. 20-11 and 20-21) and cytomegalic inclusion disease. Indeed, the clinical features of cerebral toxoplasmosis sometimes parallel those of the lymphoma. Although surgery cannot remove lymphomas, steroids often produce dramatic, although temporary, remissions.

Metastatic Tumors

Because the brain does not have a lymphatic system, systemic tumors metastasize to the brain and spinal cord by hematogenous routes. Metastatic tumors tend to be multiple, surrounded by edema, and rapidly growing. Although individual tumors are small, in total, they constitute a burdensome intracerebral mass (see Figs. 19-1C and 20-8).

Cancer of the lung, breast, kidney, and skin (malignant melanomas) most often give rise to cerebral metastases. In contrast, because the portal vein diverts metastases to the liver, gastrointestinal, pelvic, and prostatic cancers spread to the brain rarely or only late in their course.

At this time, approximately 15% of all cancer patients develop symptoms of cerebral metastases, but as treatment forces systemic tumors into long remissions, cerebral metastases, which are usually unaffected, will persist and cause symptoms in a greater proportion of patients. Metastases survive systemic chemotherapy because the blood–brain barrier ironically blocks most medications from attacking them. Moreover, chemotherapy and radiotherapy have relatively little effect against metastatic tumors because, compared to the primary tumor, they are poorly differentiated. On the other hand, the discovery of a metastatic brain tumor is occasionally the first indication that a person has cancer.

Whatever the origin of cerebral metastases, conventional treatments, such as steroids, which dramatically reduce the edema, and radiotherapy, provide only palliative care. In cases involving a single metastasis, surgeons can help the patient, at least temporarily, by removing it.

INITIAL SYMPTOMS

Local Signs

By damaging tissue surrounding the region where they have arisen, brain tumors usually produce lateralized neurologic deficits, often called "local signs," such as hemiparesis, seizures, and dominant or nondominant hemisphere neuropsychologic disorders (see Chapter 8). When just forming, tumors arising in "eloquent" regions—cerebral cortex areas critical to motor or neuropsychologic function, such as Broca's or Wernicke's areas—produce obvious impairments. Tumors that are small, slowly growing, or located in "silent" regions of the brain, such as the right frontal lobe or either of the anterior temporal lobes, notoriously fail to produce symptoms.

In contrast, tumors that arise from cranial nerves, although rare, almost immediately result in readily recognizable deficits. For example, optic nerve gliomas cause visual loss and optic atrophy. Similarly, acoustic neuromas cause unilateral progressive hearing loss and tinnitus (see later).

Seizures in individuals older than 60 years are frequently the presenting feature of cerebral tumors. However, because strokes cause seizures nearly as often as tumors, a 60-year-old individual presenting with the first seizure is approximately equally likely to have sustained a stroke as have developed a brain tumor. When the etiology is either a brain tumor or stroke, seizures typically begin as a partial seizure that undergoes secondary generalization (see Chapter 10).

A brain tumor's tendency to cause seizures also pertains to electroconvulsive therapy (ECT). For example, if a patient harboring a brain tumor were to undergo ECT, the procedure might give rise to multiple, uninterrupted, life-threatening seizures (*status epilepticus*). Large brain tumors constitute another problem regarding ECT. Not only might they explain depressive symptoms but also, in certain circumstances, large brain tumors might precipitate transtentorial herniation (see Fig. 19-1D). Thus, before their patients undergo ECT, neurologists order either an MRI or a CT to exclude tumors and other mass lesions.

Signs of Increased Intracranial Pressure

In addition to damaging brain tissue, tumors raise intracranial pressure when they grow rapidly, reach a large size, accumulate surrounding edema, obstruct the flow of cerebrospinal fluid (CSF) through the ventricles, or impede its reabsorption through the arachnoid villi. Whichever its cause, increased pressure (pressures exceeding 200 mm H_2O) creates symptoms and signs that may add to or supersede local ones.

Headaches, although the most common manifestation of increased intracranial pressure, still occur in only one half of patients. Although brain tumor-induced headaches lack distinctive features, they usually resemble tension-type headaches because they consist of diffuse, dull, relatively mild pain that initially responds to mild analgesics, including aspirin. Sometimes, a predominantly localized or unilateral headache points to a tumor's location and mimics migraine. In any case, as pressure rises, headaches worsen, especially in the early morning hours, and begin to awaken patients from sleep. Increasing intracranial pressure eventually produces nausea and vomiting, as well as further intensifying the headache.

On the other hand, both patients and physicians frequently express great concern that any headache may indicate a brain tumor. Nevertheless, less than 1 out of 1000 people with headache has developed a tumor.

Another manifestation of increased intracranial pressure, *papilledema,* occurs as pressure is transmitted along the optic nerve to the optic disks (Fig. 19-2). Although papilledema has a notorious association with brain tumors, the triad of headache, vomiting, and papilledema occurs late, if at all, in their course. In fact, among young adults, especially overweight females with menstrual irregularity, *idiopathic intracranial hypertension (pseudotumor cerebri)* is much more likely than a brain tumor to explain papilledema (see Chapter 9). Overall, because only a small proportion of brain tumor patients has papilledema during an initial examination, its absence should not be taken as evidence against the presence of a brain tumor.

In considering manifestations of brain tumors, meningiomas constitute a special category. Unlike gliomas, as discussed previously, small meningiomas are common and usually innocuous. Even large, slowly growing ones may remain asymptomatic. Also, they begin and usually remain entirely in extra-axial locations.

Also unlike gliomas, meningiomas have a predilection to develop in certain locations and produce characteristic signs. For example, a meningioma arising from the falx, a *parasagittal meningioma,* can compress the medial motor cortex and cause spastic paresis of one or both legs. A meningioma arising from the sphenoid wing can damage the adjacent temporal lobe and, because of its proximity to the orbit, cause proptosis and paresis of eye movement. Likewise, an *olfactory*

groove meningioma can compress the immediately adjacent olfactory and optic nerves and the overlying frontal lobe (see Foster-Kennedy Syndrome, Chapter 4). This tumor characteristically causes anosmia, unilateral blindness, and, when large, frontal lobe dysfunction (see Chapter 7).

INITIAL MENTAL SYMPTOMS

Direct Effects of Tumors

Depending on numerous factors, tumors may create neuropsychologic syndromes, cognitive impairments, or personality changes. For example, tumors in eloquent areas may cause aphasia or various nondominant hemisphere syndromes (see Chapter 8). Most tumor-related cognitive impairments or personality changes that would bring a patient first to a psychiatrist result from a glioblastoma.

Those in the frontal lobe produce a characteristic picture, often labeled "frontal lobe personality changes," consisting of psychomotor retardation, emotional dulling, loss of initiative, poor insight, and reduced capacity to execute complex mental tasks. This clinical picture naturally resembles frontotemporal dementia (see Chapter 7). In both conditions, disturbances in behavior and affect overshadow cognitive impairments, and those disturbances overshadow local signs.

In a somewhat opposite effect, frontal lobe tumors sometimes impair normal inhibitory systems. Patients with lack of inhibition, or *disinhibition,* may overreact to any irritation, tend to use profanities, cry with little provocation, and jump excitedly from topic to topic. However, parietal or occipital lobe, as well as right-sided anterior frontal tumors, unless they cause increased intracranial pressure, have relatively little effect on mood or cognitive function.

Even without destruction of critical neuropsychologic centers, tumor-induced increased intracranial pressure generally impairs cerebral function, which often leads to mood and cognitive changes. At this point, patients usually also have headache.

Overall, with numerous potential explanations, brain tumor patients develop depression. Depressive symptoms not only arise soon after diagnosis but increase in frequency and strength during the ensuing course of the patient with a brain tumor. Along with physical debility, treatment-induced fatigue, cognitive impairments, and other emotional changes, depression predicts a poor quality of life.

In brain tumor cases, a psychiatrist might attempt to determine the patient's mood, cognitive capacity, neurologic deficits, and iatrogenic factors (Table 19-2). With no standard guidelines for prescribing antidepressants

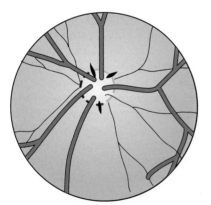

FIGURE 19-2 ■ The main features of papilledema consist of reddening of the optic disk, which loses its distinct margin, and distention of the retinal veins. In addition, the disk is elevated and hemorrhages appear at its edge. (Compare this disk to the normal optic disk in Fig. 4-4.)

CT, computed tomography; MRI, magnetic resonance imaging.
*Cancers that tend to metastasize.

TABLE 19-2 ■ Evaluation of Cancer Patients with Mental Aberrations

What is the primary tumor?
  Lung, breast, kidney, malignant melanoma*
Where are metastases known to be present?
  Brain, liver, lung, spine
Does the patient have symptoms or signs of a cerebral lesion?
  Headache, seizures, hemiparesis, papilledema
What treatments have been given?
  Radiation: total dose
  Chemotherapy: medications and antiemetics
  Analgesics: daily dose, route, indication, recent changes
  Psychotropics: antidepressants, hypnotics, tranquilizers
  Others: steroids, cimetidine
What is the patient's general status?
  Level of awareness
  Mood, cognitive mental status, insight
  Pain control
  Sleep schedule and restfulness
  Nutrition, weight change, and appetite
  Temperature
What are the results of important laboratory tests?
  Complete blood count
  Liver and renal function tests
  Serum calcium concentration
  CT or MRI

In addition to symptoms from cerebral metastases, cancer patients may develop neurologic problems from metastases to the peripheral nervous system (PNS) or non-neurologic organs, remote effects of systemic cancer, or adverse reactions to many treatments.

or other psychotropics for brain tumor patients, psychiatrists must approach each situation entirely on an individual basis. In addition to prescribing psychotropic medications, if the situation warrants them, psychiatrists might provide psychologic support, advise on alterations in mental status, guide pain management, assist in appointing a health care proxy, and help with decisions about end of life care.

Medication and Other Treatment

Medications, notoriously opioids, can cause delirium and other signs of toxic-metabolic encephalopathy. In an extreme example, accumulation of normeperidine, which is the metabolic product of meperidine (Demerol), results in a toxic psychosis and myoclonus. On the other hand, insufficient opioids can lead to relentless suffering, restless sleep, and drug-seeking behavior. Benzodiazepines and hypnotics present a similar quandary. They help control pain, anxiety, and insomnia, but can themselves cause mental dullness, confusion, and disruption of the sleep-wake cycle.

Other medications likely to induce mental status changes in cancer patients are antiepileptic drugs (AEDs), steroids, psychotropics, antiemetics, and antihistamines. Although physicians can usually predict common medications' potential physical side effects, their mental side effects in cancer patients often develop insidiously and unexpectedly. For example, patients might have undiagnosed liver metastases that slow metabolism of medications and allow their unsuspected accumulation. Similarly, because cancer patients often have lost body mass, physicians may prescribe relatively too large doses of their medications. When cancer involves several organs, various specialists may each order different medications that not only cause mental status abnormalities but also interact adversely.

Chemotherapy agents generally do not cause mental status changes because they cannot penetrate the blood–brain barrier. However, when physicians administer methotrexate intrathecally (into the subarachnoid space, usually through a lumbar puncture [LP]), it often causes adverse CNS effects. Although intrathecal methotrexate, which is frequently administered in conjunction with cranial radiotherapy, may protect children from leukemic cells invading the CNS, it often induces short-term confusional states and occasional permanent learning disabilities and other intellectual impairments.

Another debilitating aspect of chemotherapy is its tendency to induce nausea and vomiting (chemotherapy-induced emesis). This problem usually stems from chemotherapy agents triggering the brain's chemoreceptor zone and its adjacent vomiting center. These zones are located in the area postrema of the medulla, which is one of the only regions of the brain unprotected by the blood–brain barrier. The absence of an overlying blood–brain barrier leaves the chemoreceptor zone freely accessible to any blood-borne substance. Thus, if people inadvertently ingest many toxins, such as in poisonous foodstuff, they will vomit. On a medical level, morphine, heroin, and high doses of L-dopa, as well as several chemotherapeutic agents, readily activate the chemoreceptor zone and trigger regurgitation. On the other hand, both dopamine blocking agents and 5-HT$_3$ antagonists prevent chemotherapy-induced nausea and vomiting (see Chapter 21).

In contrast to partial brain fractionated radiotherapy, cranial (whole brain) radiotherapy routinely causes long-term cognitive impairment. MRIs of patients with radiation-induced cognitive impairments typically reveal white matter changes (leukoencephalopathy). Although radiotherapy adds only an additional burden to the cognitive impairments brought on by the tumor and various medications, it often precipitates a flagrant delirium or, in extreme cases, eventually leads to a subcortical dementia (see Chapter 7). Moreover, whole brain radiation administered to children for acute leukemia or brain tumors can result not only in mental retardation or cognitive impairment but also in signs of hypothalamic-pituitary deficiency, particularly growth retardation and failure to develop secondary sexual characteristics. Young children, compared to young and middle-aged adults, are more susceptible to radiation-induced cognitive impairment.

Radiotherapy, when delivered in high doses over a short period of time, causes the leukoencephalopathy by creating necrosis of small cerebral arteries, termed *radiation necrosis* or *radiation arteritis*. Beginning about 6 to 18 months after a course of radiotherapy, affected patients develop a series of small, stroke-like cerebral infarctions. The infarctions lead to a stepwise progression of cognitive impairment, hemiparesis, and dysarthria that resembles vascular dementia.

In an analogous complication, radiotherapy of the spine or mediastinum can cause spinal cord radiation necrosis, *radiation myelitis*. Similarly, radiation of pituitary tumors may lead to necrosis of the remaining pituitary gland, which would cause panhypopituitarism. Scatter of radiation might also cause necrosis of the nearby medial-inferior temporal lobes, which may lead to memory impairment and partial seizures.

Sepsis and Organ Failure

Immunosuppressive agents, radiotherapy, and various open ports, such as intravenous lines and urinary catheters, leave cancer patients susceptible to systemic infection. Bacteria, fungi, and opportunistic organisms frequently invade, proliferate without an immunologic response, and cause sepsis. In addition, systemic cancer and its treatments often cause renal, pulmonary, or hepatic failure.

Alone or together, sepsis and organ failure lead to toxic encephalopathy. Although these insults typically cause delirium with fluctuating sensorium, confusion, and disorientation, in cancer patients they may instead produce a subtle, muted version. Perhaps also owing to a concurrent depression, cancer patients' delirium may consist only of apathy, reticence, and sleep disturbance but little overt cognitive impairment or fluctuations in consciousness.

In addition, toxic encephalopathy may trigger seizures. In that case, neurologists usually add an AED, at least until they exclude a metastatic tumor and restore a normal metabolic state. Unfortunately an AED may, directly or through an interaction with another medicine, alter a patient's mental state.

Paraneoplastic Syndromes

Systemic cancer can provoke antibody-mediated immune disorders of the CNS or PNS, termed *paraneoplastic syndromes* or *remote effects of carcinoma*. In the majority of cases, these disorders, which often disable and sometimes kill the patient, precede the discovery of the cancer by several months.

The most common paraneoplastic syndrome consists of cerebellar degeneration associated with gynecologic cancers, small cell tumors of the lung, or lymphoma. Another relatively common paraneoplastic condition, the Lambert-Eaton syndrome, affects the PNS and resembles myasthenia gravis (see later). Blood tests, in these and most other paraneoplastic syndromes, reveal antibodies directed against the relevant CNS or PNS neurons. When neurologists diagnose one of these syndromes in someone otherwise apparently in good health, they suggest further evaluation, which might eventually include positron emission tomography (PET), for an occult malignancy.

Another paraneoplastic syndrome, *limbic encephalitis*, consists of antibody-mediated limbic system inflammatory degeneration. Although this disorder rarely occurs, it often heralds small cell carcinoma of the lung or testicular cancer. Typically, over several days to several weeks, individuals with this disorder develop pronounced memory impairment combined with a wide variety of psychologic changes, such as depression, personality changes, irritability, and behavioral disturbances. They may also have partial complex seizures. Sometimes the symptoms consist solely of amnesia. (However, because the amnesia develops slowly and usually persists, neurologists do not include it among the causes of "transient amnesia" [see Table 7-1].)

MRIs in cases of limbic encephalopathy commonly show atrophy of the mesial temporal lobes. Similarly, electroencephalograms (EEGs) typically show spikes or slow waves emanating from the temporal lobes. Serum often contains antibodies, of the anti-Hu or anti-Ma2 varieties, that react with limbic system neurons.

When treatment removes or shrinks the underlying tumor, limbic encephalopathy may subside, but it usually persists. Likewise, immunosuppressive treatments, such as steroids, plasmapheresis, or intravenous immunoglobulin, inconsistently relieve the symptoms.

Other paraneoplastic syndromes consist of certain cancers' synthesizing various hormones, "ectopic hormones," that endocrine glands would normally synthesize and excrete in a regulated pattern and quantity. For example, tumors may induce excessive parathyroid hormone production, which causes hypercalcemia, and tumor-induced inappropriate antidiuretic hormone (ADH) secretion causes hyponatremia. Because tumors can produce enough ectopic hormone to cause clinically significant chemical aberrations, neurologists consider them in the differential diagnosis of metabolic encephalopathy.

CNS Infections

In cancer patients, infective agents sometimes invade the CNS but not other organs. When cancer patients cannot respond with fever or leukocytosis to the infection, which is often the case, patients may have inexplicable changes in their mental status. For example, *progressive multifocal leukoencephalopathy* (*PML*), which probably results from a papovavirus infection, attacks CNS myelin (see Chapters 7, 15, and 20). Usually late in the course of an illness, PML causes dementia and variable physical impairments but not delirium. In addition to developing in cancer, it also complicates AIDS and immunosuppression therapy, including one aborted multiple sclerosis treatment (see Chapter 15).

DIAGNOSTIC TESTS FOR BRAIN TUMORS

Physicians should consider brain tumors and related conditions without waiting for a patient to have florid physical or mental deficits. They should not rely exclusively on the mental status examination to distinguish between psychiatric disorders and brain tumors. In addition, commonplace complaints of fatigue, weight loss, menstrual irregularity, or infertility might prompt evaluation for pituitary insufficiency, as well as a general medical evaluation.

Neurologists generally order CT or MRI of the brain, admittedly liberally, for any patients who have intellectual decline; those older than 50 years who develop substantial emotional changes; and most adults with headaches not attributable to migraine, cluster, or giant cell arteritis (see Chapter 9). Neurologists often also suggest CT or MRI for patients who develop any new psychiatric illness severe enough to warrant hospitalization or ECT. Finally, when a patient worries about harboring a brain tumor, a CT or MRI might resolve that concern and permit appropriate therapy to begin.

CT remains a satisfactory screening procedure in many situations (see Chapter 20). It is sensitive to most tumors and other mass lesions, rapidly performed, relatively inexpensive, and permissible for patients with pacemakers. It remains preferable for detecting acute intracranial bleeding, including subarachnoid hemorrhage, subdural hematomas, and intracerebral hemorrhages. CT will also detect fractures and other abnormalities of the skull.

Nevertheless, MRI, especially with gadolinium infusion, remains superior in locating lesions that are small or located in areas encased by bone, such as optic gliomas, acoustic neuromas, pituitary adenomas, and some posterior fossa tumors. It can detect nonmalignant white matter abnormalities, such as PML. If CT suggests a tumor, MRI still remains necessary to determine its exact location, internal structure, and involvement of surrounding brain. PET can help differentiate cerebral radiation necrosis from tumor recurrence.

For detecting tumors or other mass lesions, an EEG, especially in comparison to CT and MRI, is simply inappropriate. Nevertheless, in brain tumor and other cancer patients, it remains a good diagnostic test for delirium, particularly hepatic encephalopathy, as well as seizures.

Neurologists generally do not perform an LP to analyze CSF when they suspect a brain tumor or other intracranial mass lesion because, in such cases, the CSF profile lacks a distinctive profile and rarely reveals malignant cells (see Chapter 20). More important, with large, expanding supratentorial mass lesions, an LP can precipitate transtentorial herniation (Fig. 19-3). However, neurologists perform an LP when patients may have either carcinomatous or chronic infectious meningitis. To diagnose those conditions, physicians must examine large volumes of CSF, which may require a series of LPs, for neoplastic cells, chemistry studies, fungi, and bacterial and fungal antigens.

RELATED CONDITIONS

Pituitary Adenomas

Although clinicians often view pituitary adenomas as brain tumors, their symptoms, histology, and treatment differ considerably from those of glioblastomas, astrocytomas, and meningiomas. In classic studies, the usual manifestations of pituitary adenomas included major mental, physical, and visual abnormalities; however, those symptoms resulted from massive pituitary tumors that produced extraordinary levels of hormones, expanded out of the sella to encroach on the adjacent temporal lobes and optic chiasm, and obstructed the flow of CSF through the third ventricle. Physicians now routinely diagnose pituitary adenomas early in their course, while they remain microscopic in size, by using MRI and blood tests for hormone levels, which represent practical applications of two Nobel Prize-winning concepts.

Most pituitary adenomas are either *prolactinomas*, which secrete prolactin, or *chromophobe adenomas*, which do not. Although prolactinomas usually remain microscopic, chromophobe adenomas typically grow large enough to exert pressure on surrounding structures (Fig. 19-4). Their upward pressure on the diaphragm sellae usually causes bitemporal and generalized headache. Compressing the optic chiasm, which is above the diaphragm, also causes characteristic

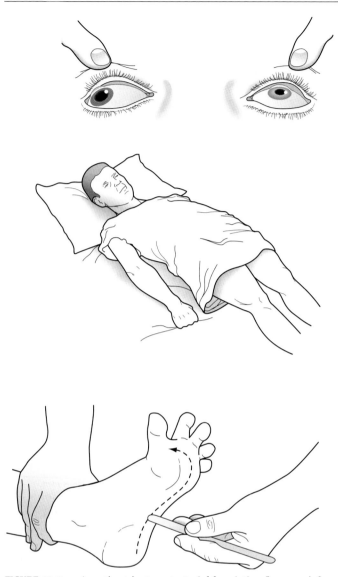

FIGURE 19-3 ■ A patient in *transtentorial herniation* from a right-sided subdural hematoma, as in Fig. 19-1*D*, has coma, decerebrate (extensor) posture, Babinski signs, and a dilated right pupil. The right temporal lobe compressing the right-sided oculomotor nerve and brainstem through the tentorial notch causes this catastrophe.

visual field cuts: bitemporal superior quadrantanopia and, with further enlargement, bitemporal hemianopsia (see Fig. 12-9).

Even before causing visual field defects, however, pituitary adenomas may insidiously lead to pituitary hormone insufficiency. Thus, their early symptoms include infertility, amenorrhea, decreased libido, and galactorrhea. Eventually pituitary hormone failure results in a lack of energy, apathy, and listlessness. Although patients with these symptoms seem depressed, they usually retain their cognitive capacity.

MRI reveals almost all pituitary adenomas. Serum prolactin level determination, another diagnostic test, usually shows elevations with prolactinomas and some chromophobe adenomas. Visual field testing helps detect pituitary adenomas that have expanded out of the sella. Treatment varies with tumor type, symptoms, and institutional expertise, but the usual options include radiation, trans-sphenoidal microsurgery, and, with prolactin-secreting tumors, a dopamine agonist, such as bromocriptine. As in a previous caveat, treating large tumors with radiation or craniotomy risks causing panhypopituitarism and, from temporal lobe damage, memory impairment and seizures.

Less commonly occurring pituitary growths secrete *growth hormone,* which can cause *acromegaly,* or *adrenocorticotropin hormone (ACTH),* which can lead to *Cushing's syndrome.* In addition to disfiguring patients, the endocrine changes produce various psychologic symptoms, including depression and psychosis. However, these growths usually remain as collections of hyperplastic cells, rather than coalesce into adenoma-like masses, and rarely grow large enough to encroach on the optic chiasm or cause severe headache.

In contrast to these relatively benign pituitary lesions, *craniopharyngioma,* a tumor that occurs in children as well as in adults, frequently requires extensive surgery and radiotherapy that still leave patients in a debilitated state. Craniopharyngioma is a calcified, cystic, congenital lesion derived from Rathke's pouch. Unlike pituitary adenomas, craniopharyngiomas grow within the hypothalamus, located above the diaphragm sellae (see Fig. 19-4). Because theses tumors cause endocrine deficiency, affected children have delayed or incomplete physical, sexual, and mental development; adults tend to have impaired libido, amenorrhea, and apathy; and both children and adults develop diabetes insipidus. Large craniopharyngiomas press downward on the optic chiasm. The pressure causes optic atrophy and, like pituitary tumors, bitemporal hemianopsia. If they compress the third ventricle, patients develop obstructive hydrocephalus, which leads to papilledema with headache, nausea, and vomiting—classic signs of increased intracranial pressure.

Postpartum pituitary necrosis, more widely known as *Sheehan's syndrome,* also causes pituitary insufficiency. Although radiotherapy and several other conditions might cause pituitary infarction with necrosis, Sheehan's syndrome typically results from obstetric deliveries complicated by hypotension from massive blood loss. In overt cases, postpartum women fail to lactate, remain hypotensive, lose weight, and undergo regression of secondary sexual characteristics. In subtle cases, several months to several years after delivering,

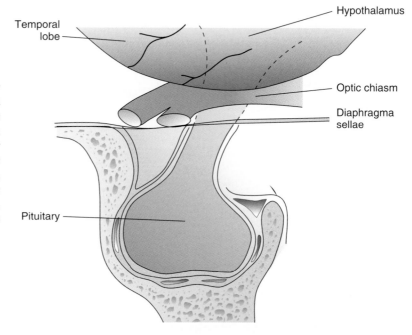

FIGURE 19-4 ■ Pituitary adenomas grow laterally and inferiorly against the walls of the sella turcica and upward against the *diaphragm sellae*. Large adenomas compress the optic chiasm, which causes a distinctive bitemporal hemianopsia or bitemporal superior quadrantanopia (see Fig. 12-9). The suprasellar region of the brain, situated above the diaphragm sellae, contains the hypothalamus. Lesions that destroy this area, such as craniopharyngiomas, also cause diabetes insipidus.

women develop scant menses, diminished libido, and constant weakness. Physicians may misinterpret their symptoms as delayed postpartum depression or chronic fatigue syndrome.

Acoustic Neuromas

If the cells covering the acoustic (eighth cranial) nerve proliferate, they form a distinctive tumor—the *acoustic neuroma* or *schwannoma*. (The term "acoustic neuroma," however, contains an inaccuracy because Schwann cells, not neurons, proliferate.) The tumor develops in the internal auditory canal and cerebellopontine angle where it may compress adjacent structures, particularly the fifth (trigeminal) and seventh (facial) cranial nerves. Although relatively benign, this tumor first causes hearing impairment with predominant loss of speech discrimination, and then tinnitus, imbalance, and vertigo. If the acoustic neuroma grows to compress the fifth cranial nerve, patients experience sensory symptoms in their face, ranging from sensory loss to trigeminal neuralgia-like pain. If the tumor compresses the seventh cranial nerve, patients can lose facial muscle strength.

Most acoustic neuromas develop unilaterally and spontaneously. Bilateral acoustic neuromas, in contrast, characteristically represent neurofibromatosis type 2 (NF2), an autosomal dominant disorder of chromosome 22 (see Chapter 13). Gadolinium-enhanced MRI (see Fig. 20-27), auditory tests, and brainstem auditory evoked responses (see BAERs, Chapter 15) detect acoustic neuromas. Neurosurgeons, performing stereotactic radiosurgery with a gamma knife or linear accelerator, can remove acoustic neuromas while preserving most if not all hearing and facial strength.

Spine Metastases

Lung, breast, and other cancers often metastasize to the vertebrae and then grow into the spinal epidural space (Fig. 19-5). *Epidural metastases* characteristically cause severe pain not only in the affected region (local pain) but also along the path of the affected nerve roots (radicular pain). For example, patients with thoracic spine metastases typically have interscapular spine pain that radiates around the chest in a band-like pattern. Similarly, patients with lumbar spine metastases suffer from lower back pain that, unlike simple musculoskeletal pain, radiates down the legs.

If cervical or thoracic epidural metastases grow large enough, they compress the spinal cord. Metastatic spinal cord compression causes not only local and radicular pain but also quadriplegia or paraplegia, loss of sensation below the site of the lesion, and incontinence of urine and feces (see Chapters 2 and 16). In addition, although patients typically retain their cognitive capacity, their pain, incapacity, and undeniable progression of their illness often lead to depression.

Early diagnosis and treatment may prevent this dreaded complication; however, once paraplegia occurs, patients almost never regain their ability to walk. Neurologists usually rely on an MRI to confirm a clinical impression. Therapy usually consists of steroids, radiation, and, sometimes, decompressive laminectomy.

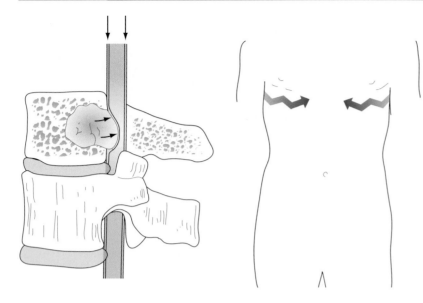

FIGURE 19-5 ■ *Left*, Vertebral metastases typically grow posteriorly to encroach on the spinal *epidural space* (*arrows*), which contains the spinal cord and its nerve roots. These *epidural metastases* cause spinal cord compression, which results in paraplegia or quadriplegia, loss of sensation (hypalgesia) below the level of the lesion, and incontinence of feces and urine. *Right*, Patients have "local pain" from destruction of the vertebrae and band-like "radiating pain," which follows the course of the nerves (*jagged arrows*). The location of the pain and level of the hypalgesia indicate the site of an epidural metastatic tumor (see Fig. 2-15).

Other Causes of Limb Weakness

Certain cancers trigger paraneoplastic inflammatory conditions that affect the PNS as well as the CNS. For example, lung, breast, ovarian, gastric, and other solid tumors provoke *dermatomyositis,* which consists of diffuse, proximal muscle weakness, muscle tenderness, and a heliotrope rash on the face and extensor skin surfaces.

In another PNS paraneoplastic disorder, *Lambert-Eaton syndrome,* small cell lung cancer provokes antibodies directed against the presynaptic side of the neuromuscular junction (see Chapter 6). The antibody-induced neuromuscular junction dysfunction causes weakness, but with different qualities and in a different distribution than myasthenia gravis, the most widely known neuromuscular junction disorder. Patients with the Lambert-Eaton syndrome, in contrast to those with myasthenia gravis, present with proximal limb muscle weakness, which they partly overcome with repetitive actions, and they retain extraocular muscle strength.

The Lambert-Eaton syndrome, like botulism and botulinum toxin, causes the weakness by impairing the release of acetylcholine (ACh) from the *presynaptic* neuromuscular junction neuron. By way of contrast, in myasthenia, abnormally rapid ACh inactivation at the *postsynaptic* site causes weakness. Nevertheless, immunosuppressive treatments may alleviate the symptoms of Lambert-Eaton syndrome as they do with myasthenia gravis.

Cancer-related iatrogenic myopathies and neuropathies commonly cause debilitating weakness. Prolonged use of steroids, whether as a medication or an illicit bodybuilding supplement, may result in *steroid myopathy* or hip or vertebral body collapse.

Similarly, long-term use of diuretics without potassium supplements results in *hypokalemic myopathy.* Various chemotherapy agents, such as vincristine, cause *polyneuropathy.* Not only does chemotherapy-induced polyneuropathy often include a disturbing sensory component (see Chapter 5) but it can arise so suddenly and cause such profound, extensive weakness that it may resemble metastatic spinal cord compression; however, it lacks the spine pain characteristic of metastatic disease. Fortunately, in most cases, the polyneuropathy symptoms subside several months after completion of chemotherapy.

In contrast to the generalized weakness of these polyneuropathies, cancer-induced injuries of individual peripheral nerves, *mononeuropathies,* cause paresis and sensory loss involving the distribution of only a single nerve (see Table 5-1). With cancer-induced loss of muscle bulk and subcutaneous fat, mild to moderate pressure—even as light as the patient's own weight—compresses peripheral nerves deprived of their protective cushion. Compression injuries most often damage the sciatic, peroneal, and radial nerves when bedridden patients are moved onto stretchers or secured in wheel chairs. Sometimes misplaced injections or other accidents injure these nerves.

Direct tumor infiltration of a nerve plexus may produce excruciating pain. For example, when lung and breast cancer invades the brachial plexus or pelvic cancer invades the lumbosacral plexus, patients develop severe, almost intractable pain as well as paresis. Because tumor cells invade the nerves, routine treatments, such as radiotherapy and opioids, provide only limited analgesia. To reduce the pain and alleviate the suffering from this and other cancer-related pains, physicians must enlist powerful pain control measures (see Chapter 14).

DISORDERS THAT RESEMBLE BRAIN TUMORS

Strokes, as well as tumors, occur predominantly in older people and cause physical deficits, seizures, and cognitive impairment. However, the course, many symptoms, and results of imaging studies of strokes and tumors differ so much that, in the final analysis, physicians almost always arrive at the correct diagnosis. Although strokes usually occur acutely or occasionally develop over several days, brain tumors usually evolve over at least several weeks. In addition, even when strokes cause extensive physical and intellectual deficits, patients usually remain alert and free of headaches. For example, a patient with a stroke may remain fully alert despite sustaining aphasia, hemiparesis, homonymous hemianopsia, and hemisensory loss. To produce a comparable extensive deficit, a tumor would have to grow throughout the entire left cerebral hemisphere. It would then increase the intracranial pressure so much that stupor would ensue. Even if the history and examination were equivocal, CT and MRI can almost always differentiate between these conditions.

Subdural hematomas also occur frequently and may mimic brain tumors. Typically, head trauma induces intracranial bleeding in the potential space between the dura (the thick layer of the meninges) and the underlying brain (see Figs. 19-1D and 20-9). Because the bleeding originates from the intracranial venous system, its pressure is low and volume relatively small. Nevertheless, it slowly leads to a hematoma over a period of several weeks. Arising either unilaterally or bilaterally, subdural hematomas accumulate fluid and progressively enlarge. They exert a mass effect that presses broadly against one or both cerebral hemispheres. The pressure produces headaches, confusion, personality change, dementia, and other signs of generalized cerebral dysfunction—much more so than focal signs.

For several reasons, older individuals are especially vulnerable to developing subdural hematomas. They often take aspirin or other medicines that have an anticoagulant effect. In them, trivial head injuries often lead to intracranial bleeding. Once bleeding starts, it continues unchecked because an atrophied brain cannot compress the bleeding vessels. Also, because subdural hematomas typically produce slowly developing nonspecific symptoms and signs, rather than lateralized ones, the patient and family may fail to appreciate the significance of headaches and other changes.

Neurosurgeons may easily evacuate subdural hematomas, but frequently a conservative approach, often using steroids, suffices. Prompt diagnosis and treatment usually restore cerebral function. In other words, subdural hematomas, which frequently occur in the elderly, represent a correctable form of dementia.

Arteriovenous malformations (AVMs) and brain abscesses also resemble brain tumors (see Fig. 20-15). AVMs consist of congenital vascular anomalies of large veins and arteries directly joined without the normal intervening capillary bed. If these vessels rupture, the AVM causes intraparenchymal hemorrhage, lateralized signs, and seizures.

Bacterial abscesses usually result from sepsis originating in intravenous drug abuse, dental procedures, sinusitis, endocarditis, or immunodeficiency. They usually present with signs of a cerebral mass lesion or seizures. Abscesses, in their clinical appearance and imaging studies, resemble brain tumors.

Although bacteria are the infecting organisms in most cases of abscess, *toxoplasmosis* is usually responsible but in AIDS cases. Cerebral toxoplasmosis differs from ordinary bacterial abscesses in that it tends to develop in multiple sites but concentrate in the basal ganglia. Thus, unlike almost all other infectious or malignant mass lesions, toxoplasmosis routinely presents with chorea, hemiballismus, or other involuntary movement disorder.

Patients with *neurocysticercosis,* the neurologic component of *cysticercosis,* usually have developed multiple intracerebral cysts from a primary gastrointestinal infestation by the tapeworm *Taenia solium.* Although each may be small, the numerous cysts, in total, occupy considerable volume. They also tend to block CSF flow, which causes obstructive hydrocephalus. Moreover, as they die, their fluid contents leak and provoke an inflammatory response in the surrounding brain. Thus, patients with neurocysticercosis may present with dementia, symptoms and signs of increased intracranial pressure, or, most often, seizures. Because cysticercosis is endemic in Central and South America, immigrants from these areas often harbor neurocysticercosis. In addition, neurocysticercosis has also increased in frequency among citizens of the Indian subcontinent. CT and MRI readily detect the cysts (see Fig. 20-12). The treatment remains controversial, but neurologists almost always prescribe AEDs.

Tuberculosis causes intracerebral masses, *tuberculomas,* particularly in AIDS patients and citizens of the Indian subcontinent. CT and MRI can also detect these lesions, even when the clinical evaluation does not suggest the diagnosis.

As another alternative to brain tumor, pseudotumor cerebri, which results from excessive fluid accumulation in the brain, produces headache, papilledema, constricted visual fields, and sometimes sixth cranial nerve palsies; however, it does not affect cognitive capacity or produce seizures (see Chapter 9).

REFERENCES

1. Armstrong CL, Hunter JV, Ledakis GE, et al: Late cognitive and radiographic changes related to radiotherapy. Neurology 59:40–48, 2002.
2. Christensen HC, Schuz J, Kosteljanetz M, et al: Cellular telephones and risk for brain tumors: A population-based, incident case-control study. Neurology 64:1189–1195, 2005.
3. Darnell RB, Posner JB: Paraneoplastic syndromes involving the nervous system. N Engl J Med 349:1543–1554, 2003.
4. DeAngelis LM: Brain tumors. N Engl J Med 344:114–122, 2001.
5. Duffner PK: Long-term effects of radiation therapy on cognitive and endocrine function in children with leukemia and brain tumors. Neurology 10:293–310, 2004.
6. Gultekin SH, Rosenfeld MR, Voltz R, et al: Paraneoplastic limbic encephalitis. Brain 123:1481–1494, 2000.
7. Litofsky NS, Farace E, Anderson F, et al: Depression in patients with high-grade glioma: Results of the Glioma Outcomes Project. Neurosurgery 54:358–366, 2004.
8. Pelletier G, Verhoef MJ, Khatri N, et al: Quality of life in brain tumor patients: The relative contributions of depression, fatigue, emotional distress, and existential issues. J Neurooncol 57:41–49, 2002.
9. Peterson K, DeAngelis LM: Weighing the benefits and risks of radiation therapy for low-grade glioma. Neurology 56:1255–1256, 2001.
10. Ross L, Johansen C, Dalton SO, et al: Psychiatric hospitalization among survivors of cancer in childhood or adolescence. N Engl J Med 349:650–657, 2003.
11. Scharf D: Neurocysticercosis: Two hundred thirty-eight cases from a California hospital. Arch Neurol 45:777–780, 1988.
12. Taphoorn MJ, Klein M: Cognitive deficits in adult patients with brain tumors. Lancet Neurol 3:159–168, 2004.
13. Torres IJ, Mundt AJ, Sweeney PJ, et al: A longitudinal neuropsychological study of partial brain radiation in adults with brain tumors. Neurology 60:1113–1118, 2003.
14. Tuma R, DeAngelis LM: Altered mental status in patients with cancer. Arch Neurol 57:1727–1731, 2000.
15. Wallin MT, Kurtzke JF: Neurocysticercosis in the United States: Review of an important emerging infection. Neurology 63:1559–1564, 2004.
16. Zaidat OO, Ruff RL: Treatment of spinal epidural metastasis improves patient survival and functional state. Neurology 58:1360–1366, 2002.

Questions and Answers

1. An 8-year-old boy, with a 6-week history of progressively greater difficulty with athletic activities, develops a severe headache, nausea, and vomiting. His examination shows papilledema and ataxia. Of the following, which is the most likely cause?
   a. Migraine
   b. Pseudotumor cerebri
   c. Glioblastoma
   d. Astrocytoma of the cerebellum

   Answer: d. The combination of headache, nausea, vomiting, and, most significantly, papilledema suggests hydrocephalus. The preceding ataxia, as evidenced by diminished athletic ability, suggests that the problem originated in the cerebellum. Most likely, a cerebellar astrocytoma grew large enough to block CSF flow through the fourth ventricle, causing obstructive hydrocephalus. Among children with brain tumors, cerebellar astrocytomas occur frequently. Although basilar migraine attacks can cause nausea, vomiting, and ataxia, they do not last for 6 weeks or cause papilledema. Pseudotumor cerebri is a condition almost exclusively of young women. Glioblastomas develop almost only in older adults.

2. A 60-year-old man, who has smoked two packs of cigarettes daily since he was 20 years old, develops partial complex seizures. He has headaches, a left superior quadrantanopia, and a mild left hemiparesis. In addition, he has right-sided dysmetria and intention tremor. Of the following conditions, which is the most likely illness?
   a. Subdural hematomas
   b. Metastatic carcinoma in the right temporal lobe and right cerebellar hemisphere
   c. Glioblastoma of the left temporal lobe
   d. Strokes in the right temporal lobe and right cerebellar hemisphere
   e. Multiple sclerosis

   Answer: b. Although neurologists first try to assign all symptoms to a single lesion or illness, this patient's symptoms require separate explanations. His partial complex seizures, visual field loss, and hemiparesis are attributable to lesions in the right frontal and temporal lobes. In addition, he has right-sided coordination impairments attributable to a right cerebellar lesion. These multiple lesions are probably manifestations of metastatic cancer, but alternative explanations include multiple embolic strokes and abscesses. Strokes cause

mild, transient headaches. Subdural hematomas rarely cause seizures or cerebellar dysfunction. In addition, although subdural hematomas often occur over both cerebral hemispheres, they rarely occur in the posterior fossa. He is too old to have developed multiple sclerosis (MS). Moreover, headaches and seizures are not initial symptoms of MS.

3. Which of the following patients is most likely to develop cerebral gliomas?
   a. A 30-year-old woman with multiple *café au lait* spots
   b. A 21-year-old woman with bilateral acoustic neuromas
   c. A 21-year-old man with mental retardation, epilepsy, and adenoma sebaceum
   d. A 30-year-old man with a vascular malformation in the distribution of the trigeminal nerve

   Answer: c. The patient with the mental retardation, epilepsy, and adenoma sebaceum has tuberous sclerosis. The cerebral tubers in this illness often undergo malignant transformation into gliomas. The woman with the *café au lait* spots has neurofibromatosis type 1 (NF1), which is often complicated by meningiomas, as well as neuromas of peripheral nerves. The woman with the acoustic neuromas probably has neurofibromatosis type 2 (NF2). The man with the vascular malformation has Sturge-Weber syndrome, which is not associated with neoplasms.

4. A 50-year-old woman has an impaired ability to hear when she places her telephone receiver against her right ear. She also has right-sided tinnitus and loss of auditory acuity. Her neurologic examination is otherwise normal. Of the following, which one is the most likely illness?
   a. Left temporal lobe meningioma
   b. Psychogenic factors
   c. MS
   d. A cerebellopontine angle tumor

   Answer: d. Acoustic neuroma, the most common cerebellopontine angle tumor, typically causes speech discrimination impairment, tinnitus, and the gradual loss of auditory acuity. Because they develop slowly, acoustic neuromas do not cause vertigo. Lesions of the cerebral hemispheres or the brainstem, such as MS, do not cause auditory disturbances. As noted in the previous case, bilateral acoustic neuromas are a typical manifestation of NF2.

5. During the previous two years, a 55-year-old woman with multiple *café au lait* spots developed slowly increasing severe paresis of the left leg, which had hyperactive DTRs and a Babinski sign. Before undergoing further evaluation, she had a seizure that began with clonic movements of the left foot, then leg, and finally the arm. On examination, she has left hemiparesis, hyperactive DTRs, and a Babinski sign. Of the following, which is the most likely illness?
   a. Right cerebral glioblastoma
   b. Right cerebral meningioma
   c. Left cerebral glioblastoma
   d. Left cerebral meningioma

Answer: b. The evolution of a hemiparesis over a relatively long time, especially when it is accompanied by a partial (motor) seizure, suggests a cerebral tumor. In view of the chronicity of the hemiparesis and her probably having NF1, a meningioma is more likely than a glioblastoma. Moreover, meningiomas are more common in women than men.

6. Which of the following is least likely to cause headaches in the elderly?
   a. Subdural hematomas
   b. Open-angle glaucoma
   c. Brain tumors
   d. Temporal arteritis
   e. Nitroglycerin and other vasodilator medications

Answer: b. Open-angle glaucoma is not associated with headaches. The other conditions often cause headaches in the elderly.

7. Brain tumors often produce headaches that are worse in the early morning, waking patients from sleep. Which four of the following headaches also typically begin in the early morning?
   a. Muscle contraction tension
   b. Pseudotumor cerebri
   c. Migraine
   d. Trigeminal neuralgia
   e. Postconcussive syndrome
   f. Cluster headache
   g. Sleep apnea-induced headache
   h. Caffeine withdrawal

Answers: c, f, g, h. Migraine and cluster headaches characteristically develop during REM sleep, which occurs predominantly in the early morning. Hypoxia and carbon dioxide retention also cause headache.

8. An obese 22-year-old woman has moderately severe, generalized headaches. She has papilledema and paresis of abduction of her right eye but no other neurologic abnormalities. Routine blood and chemistry tests are normal. A CT shows small ventricles but no mass lesion. What would be the most appropriate next step?
   a. MRI
   b. EEG
   c. Lumbar puncture (LP) to measure the pressure and withdraw CSF
   d. None of the above

Answer: c. The patient almost certainly has pseudotumor cerebri. The increased intracranial pressure stretches the sixth nerve and immobilizes the abducens muscle. However, because the sixth nerve injury does not reflect a mass lesion or damage to one side of the nervous system, it is called a "false localizing sign." Given the clinical situation and normal CT, MRI is not indicated. Instead, physicians should perform an LP to diagnosis pseudotumor cerebri and exclude the unlikely possibility of chronic meningitis. In pseudotumor, the CSF pressure is usually above 300 mm H_2O, which is a marked elevation. Prolonged papilledema, for any reason, will lead to optic atrophy and then blindness. Pseudotumor is one of the rare situations in which an LP is performed despite papilledema.

9. A 45-year-old police officer with various emotional difficulties has become obsessed with the thought that he has a brain tumor. Careful medical and neurologic examinations are normal. What would most neurologists do next?
   a. Offer reassurance
   b. Suggest psychotherapy
   c. Give an antidepressant
   d. Treat him for obsession
   e. Order an MRI

Answer: e. Even though brain tumors are uncommon in middle-aged people and almost unheard of in those with a normal neurologic examination, most neurologists would order a MRI or CT for several reasons. At the onset, about 50% of the patients with tumors have no overt physical neurologic deficits. Other structural lesions, such as an AVM or subdural hematoma, could be responsible for the patient's symptoms. Furthermore, with a normal study, a neurologist can give more secure reassurance, feel protected in the event of a medical-legal problem, and refer the patient to a psychiatrist who will probably feel more confident in accepting the patient.

10. A 60-year-old man with lung cancer develops confusion and agitation. He refuses a full neurologic examination, but physicians determine that he has no hemiparesis, papilledema, or nuchal rigidity. A noncontrast head CT is normal. Which one of

the following is the least likely cause of an alteration in the mental status of such a patient?
a. Hyperkalemia
b. Pneumonia
c. Liver metastases with hepatic encephalopathy
d. Increased intracranial pressure
e. Inappropriate ADH secretion
f. Hypercalcemia
g. Liver metastases with slowed metabolism of medications

Answer: a. The normal neurologic examination, although rudimentary, and normal noncontrast head CT indicate that he does not have cerebral metastases. Except for hyperkalemia, all these disorders frequently complicate lung cancer even when it has not spread to the brain. (The superior vena cava syndrome causes increased intracranial pressure.)

11. Two months later, the man in the previous case undergoes a CT that reveals two ring-shaped lesions with surrounding lucency. When he became combative during the evaluation, his primary care physicians solicited a psychiatry consultation. Which two medications should be recommended?
a. A neuroleptic
b. An antidepressant
c. Steroids
d. Hypnotics
e. An anticonvulsant (antiepileptic drug)

Answers: a, c. A neuroleptic will reduce the patient's behavioral disturbances. Because steroids, such as dexamethasone, will reduce the edema and thus the volume of the lesions, they will bring about a rapid and dramatic, although short-lived, improvement. Some neurologists would also prophylactically suggest an antiepileptic drug because cerebral metastases often cause seizures and the neuroleptic might lower the seizure threshold.

12. A 65-year-old woman with the onset of dementia over 9 months has no physical or neurologic abnormalities except for frontal release signs and hyperactive DTRs. A complete laboratory and EEG evaluation reveals no specific abnormality. A CT shows atrophy and a small meningioma in the right parietal convexity. Which would be the most appropriate next step?
a. Have the tumor removed.
b. Tentatively diagnose Alzheimer's disease and repeat the clinical evaluation and CT in 6 to 12 months.
c. Obtain an MRI.

Answer: b. The meningioma is irrelevant to the dementia. These tumors grow so slowly that they can

be followed with periodic scans. They might be removed if they are large enough to compress brain tissue or become symptomatic. Because a meningioma has a paucity of water and a great deal of calcium-containing material, MRIs will be less helpful than CTs in confirming that a lesion is a meningioma and following its course.

13. A 75-year-old man, who has had dementia for 6 years, suddenly develops increased irritability and behavioral disturbances. He has no lateralized signs or indication of increased intracranial pressure. He is treated with a major tranquilizer. One week later, he becomes somnolent and has a seizure. He remains comatose with a left hemiparesis. No abnormalities are found on a general medical examination or routine laboratory tests, but a CT shows an extra-axial lucency containing dense regions and a shift of midline cerebral structures. Before any treatment can be instituted, the patient dies. An autopsy discloses cerebral atrophy and a large chronic subdural hematoma with recent hemorrhage. Which of the following statements concerning subdural hematomas is false?
a. Subdural hematomas are apt to occur in the elderly, especially in those individuals who have a history of dementia and cerebral atrophy.
b. The location of subdural hematomas is outside or overlying the brain (i.e., extra-axial).
c. Unless they are large or rapidly expanding, subdural hematomas may not cause lateralized signs or greatly raise intracranial pressure.
d. In chronic subdurals, CT portrays blood as less radiodense than brain. With superimposed acute bleeding, densities appear within these lucent regions. In other words, chronic hematomas are black (radiolucent), and fresh ones are white (radiodense).
e. The trauma required to cause a subdural hematoma is usually so great that it causes loss of consciousness for 1 hour or longer.

Answer: e. In the elderly, little or no trauma is required. On the other hand, subdural hematomas in the elderly may be a sign of deliberate trauma, as might occur in "elder abuse."

14. Which structure is *not* located in the posterior fossa?
a. Sphenoid wing
b. Chemoreceptors for vomiting
c. Vertebrobasilar artery system
d. Cerebellum
e. Fourth ventricle

Answer: a.

15. Match the brain lesion (1–6) with the group(s) with the greatest risk (a–j).
1. Chronic subdural hematoma
2. Cerebellar astrocytoma
3. Cerebral lymphomas
4. Neurocysticercosis
5. Tuberculomas
6. Acoustic neuromas
   a. Drug addicts
   b. Elderly individuals
   c. Homosexuals
   d. Children
   e. Residents of Central America
   f. Residents of India
   g. Neurofibromatosis type 1
   h. Neurofibromatosis type 2
   i. Trisomy 21
   j. AIDS patients

Answers: 1-b; 2-d; 3-a, c, j; 4-e; 5-f; 6-h.

16. Which one of the following does not usually indicate a pituitary adenoma?
a. Increased serum prolactin level
b. Cognitive impairment
c. Galactorrhea
d. Bitemporal hemianopsia
e. Decreased libido
f. Menstrual irregularity
g. Headaches
h. Bitemporal superior quadrantanopia
i. Infertility

Answer: b. Because pituitary tumors can grow upward to compress the optic chiasm and hypothalamus, they lead to headaches, visual field impairments, and panhypopituitarism. Also, certain pituitary tumors secrete prolactin.

17. Which of the following pituitary conditions is most likely to emerge in a 14-year-old child and delay growth, puberty, and social maturity?
a. Chromophobe adenoma
b. Prolactinoma
c. Cushing's syndrome
d. Craniopharyngioma

Answer: d. Unlike other pituitary region tumors, craniopharyngiomas are congenital lesions that produce symptoms in children and adults. They are typically cystic, located in the hypothalamic region, and contain calcium. They can be visualized on skull x-rays as well as CT, MRI, and histologic studies. In children, craniopharyngiomas cause delayed puberty and poor school performance. When craniopharyngiomas are large, they cause visual impairments characteristic of pituitary tumors (e.g., bitemporal hemianopsia or superior quadrantanopia and optic atrophy). They also cause diabetes insipidus if they grow into the hypothalamus and obstructive hydrocephalus if they occlude outflow from the third ventricle.

18. Of the following statements regarding paraneoplastic syndromes, which is false?
a. They often appear before the underlying cancer has been detected.
b. They are frequently associated with small cell carcinoma of the lung.
c. Immunosuppression relieves the symptoms.
d. Neurologic paraneoplastic syndromes include Lambert-Eaton syndrome, cerebellar degeneration, and limbic encephalitis.

Answer: c. Paraneoplastic syndromes resist treatment; however, they occasionally remit if the underlying cancer is cured.

19. A 65-year-old man with metastatic prostate carcinoma has been in agony from bone metastases. He is agitated, loud, and threatening in his demands for narcotics. He has become a major management problem, and his family is also becoming disruptive. Tests have shown that the patient has no cerebral metastases, hypercalcemia, or other metabolic aberrations. Which two steps should a psychiatry consultant take as an initial response to this situation?
a. Help the primary physician control the patient's pain with as much narcotic (opioid medication) as he requires. Once the pain is controlled, the situation can be reassessed.
b. Stop all medications because they can be the cause of the behavioral disorder.
c. Immediately administer minor or major tranquilizers.
d. Before treating further, check with an MRI and LP for signs of cerebral metastases or opportunistic infections.

Answer: a and possibly c. Prostatic cancer rarely spreads to the brain, but it commonly spreads to bone where metastases cause agonizing pain. However, hormone manipulation, radiotherapy, and opioids can partly or fully control it. If medicines do not alleviate the pain, drug-seeking behavior ensues. Long-acting opioids, such as methadone, and ones delivered by patch or continuous intravenous infusion are particularly effective. Breakthrough pain may be alleviated by rescue doses of parenteral opioids, such as morphine. Judicious use of antidepressants, antiepileptic drugs, and tranquilizers may provide additional analgesia, mood improvement, and restful sleep.

20. What mechanism has been proposed to explain limbic encephalitis and other paraneoplastic syndromes?
a. Antibody formation
b. Viral infection
c. Endocrine disturbance
d. Toxins secreted by the tumor

Answer: a. The etiology of paraneoplastic cerebellar degeneration, limbic encephalitis, and other paraneoplastic syndromes has been attributed to antibodies that react with neurons.

21. Of the following lesions, which three tend to be located extra-axially?
a. Butterfly gliomas
b. Astrocytomas
c. Meningiomas
d. Epidural hematomas
e. Subdural hematomas
f. Medulloblastomas

Answers: c, d, e.

22. Which two of the following are not functions of glial cells?
a. To provide structure for the spinal cord
b. To provide structure for the brain
c. To clear debris from infections and CVAs
d. To generate a myelin coat for CNS neurons
e. To generate a myelin coat for PNS neurons
f. To generate electrochemical potentials

Answers: e, f. Schwann cells generate the myelin coat for PNS neurons. Neurons generate electrochemical potentials.

23. Which three are actions of oligodendrocytes?
a. Occasionally become oligodendrogliomas
b. Generate myelin for the CNS
c. Generate myelin for the PNS
d. Generate action potentials
e. Act as a glial cell

Answers: a, b, e. Oligodendrocytes are also the target of the demyelinating process in multiple sclerosis.

24. In which three aspects do brain tumors in children differ from those in adults?
a. Childhood tumors usually develop in posterior fossa structures.
b. Childhood astrocytomas are usually resectable.
c. In children, tumors often present with signs of hydrocephalus.
d. Metastatic tumors in children are as common as primary brain tumors.
e. Meningiomas are relatively common in children.

f. Pituitary adenomas are relatively common in children.

Answers: a, b, c.

25. Match the condition that causes weakness (1–5) with the impairment of ACh transmission (a–d).
1. Myasthenia gravis
2. Lambert-Eaton syndrome
3. Botulism
4. Guillain-Barré syndrome
5. Botulinum toxin
   a. Impaired ACh release from the presynaptic surface of the neuromuscular junction
   b. Inactivation at the postsynaptic surface of the neuromuscular junction
   c. Enhanced reuptake
   d. None of the above

Answers: 1-b, 2-a, 3-a, 4-d, 5-a.

26. Which statement is false regarding the chemoreceptor area of the brain?
a. It is located in the superior surface of the medulla.
b. It is located in the area postrema.
c. It is unprotected by the blood–brain barrier.
d. The area is inaccessible to most chemicals.

Answer: d. The chemoreceptor area of the brain, devoid of the blood–brain barrier, is almost completely exposed to blood-borne substances. Morphine, heroin, many chemotherapeutic agents, numerous toxins and, in large doses, L-dopa that circulate in the blood provoke vomiting as soon as they contact the superior surface of the medulla, which houses the chemoreceptor area.

27. Serum prolactin levels that are transiently elevated above the baseline are a useful diagnostic test for seizures. Which five of the following conditions or medicines elevate the baseline serum prolactin level?
a. Chromophobe adenoma
b. Prolactinoma
c. Phenothiazines
d. Butyrophenones
e. Estrogens
f. Bromocriptine
g. Dopamine
h. Quetiapine
i. L-dopa

Answers: a–e. In contrast, bromocriptine, dopamine, and L-dopa reduce prolactin secretion.

28. Which two are complications of performing ECT on a patient with an undetected meningioma?
a. Skin necrosis

b. Status epilepticus
c. Transtentorial herniation
d. Exacerbating Parkinson's disease

Answers: b, c.

29–31. Match the varieties of hemorrhage with the most likely cause.
29. Subarachnoid hemorrhage
30. Subdural hematoma
31. Epidural hematoma
   a. Middle meningeal artery laceration
   b. Rupture of a berry aneurysm
   c. Trauma of bridging meningeal veins

Answers

29-b. Although trauma and mycotic aneurysms may cause a subarachnoid hemorrhage, the most frequent and important cause is rupture of an aneurysm arising from one of the arteries that comprise the circle of Willis.
30-c. Bleeding from small meningeal veins are the usual cause of subdural hematomas.
31-a. Lacerations of the middle meningeal artery, which often result from a fracture of the skull's temporal bone, usually cause epidural hematomas.

32. A 46-year-old woman with metastatic breast cancer develops a disconcerting numbness in the skin over the right lower chin. She has no weakness of face or jaw muscles and the remainder of her neurologic examination is normal. However, x-rays of her jaw reveals a lytic lesion in the right lower mandible. What is the diagnosis?
   a. Mental neuropathy
   b. Mononeuritis multiplex
   c. A remote effect of carcinoma
   d. A facial nerve injury

Answer: a. The mental nerve, a branch of the trigeminal nerve, provides sensation from the skin overlying the chin. Damage to this nerve, "mental neuropathy"—an unfortunate coincidence of words—causes numbness of the skin of one side of the chin, that is, the "numb chin sign." In this case, a metastasis to the jaw at the site where the mental nerve passes through its foramen has caused the mental neuropathy. Trauma to the same region could also produce the same sensory defect.

33. A family brings a 59-year-old man for a consultation because he has become apathetic and markedly forgetful but intermittently and inexplicably irritable. An examination confirms that he has amnesia and personality changes. One month before this consultation, his physicians

diagnosed small cell carcinoma of the lung. An MRI of the head and 3 LPs show no sign of metastases. The results of all his clinical chemistry tests are within normal limits. However, an EEG shows focal slowing and spikes over the temporal lobes. Which is the most likely explanation for his memory deficit and other abnormalities?
   a. A depressive disorder
   b. An inflammatory condition affecting the temporal lobes
   c. Temporal lobe metastases that have remained undetected by the MRI
   d. Partial complex seizures

Answer: b. He has limbic encephalitis, which is a paraneoplastic syndrome associated with small cell carcinoma of the lung and testicular carcinoma. It is characterized primarily by memory impairment and personality changes, but it may also lead to generalized cognitive impairment and seizures.

34. Which of the following organs is most resistant to ionizing radiation?
   a. Bone marrow
   b. Brain
   c. Gastrointestinal tract
   d. Lung

Answer: b. The CNS is relatively resistant to ionizing radiation; however, ionizing radiation, in large or sustained doses, may lead to the development of brain tumors. On the other hand, cell phone and radiofrequency emissions do not lead to brain tumors.

35. A 59-year-old active professor of English presents with a 3-week history of progressively more pronounced dulled affect, sleeplessness, and mild morning headaches. Aspirin relieves the headaches. His past medical history includes an episode of depression. On examination, he scores 28/30 on the MMSE, but he is inattentive and reticent. He has psychomotor impersistence but no lateralized neurologic deficit. An MRI reveals a single large ring-shaped mass lesion in the right frontal lobe that compresses the anterior horn of the lateral ventricle and shifts midline structures to the left. Which is the most likely nature of the lesion?
   a. Glioblastoma multiforme
   b. Meningioma
   c. Bacterial abscess
   d. None of the above

Answer: a. Unfortunately, the most likely etiology of the symptoms, which seem to have appeared rapidly, is a glioblastoma multiforme. Meningiomas grow slowly and arise in the extra-axial compartment. Although the clinical and MRI features are consistent with a bacterial abscess, a single infectious mass lesion would be much less common. However, standard practice would be to request a biopsy. If the tumor, such as this one, were situated in the nondominant frontal lobe, a wide excision would provide the patient with several additional months of life and reduction of headaches.

36. In evaluating patients suspected of harboring a mass lesion, for which condition would a CT provide more useful information than a MRI?
    a. Acoustic neuroma
    b. Pituitary adenoma
    c. Low-grade glioma
    d. Radiation necrosis
    e. Acute subdural hematoma

Answer: e. CTs, which perform imaging studies more rapidly and less expensively than MRIs, also show acute hematomas, subarachnoid hemorrhages, skull fractures, and calcified lesions more reliably than MRIs. However, MRIs better visualize acoustic neuromas, pituitary adenomas, low-grade gliomas, acute strokes, radiation necrosis, and other leukoencephalopathies.

37. Which of the following statements concerning depression comorbid with brain tumors is true?
    a. Depression develops before surgery and subsides after tumor resection.
    b. Depression rarely occurs in brain-tumor patients.
    c. Depression arises immediately after surgery and subsequently increases in severity.
    d. The presence of comorbid depression does not affect the patient's quality of life.

Answer: c. In brain tumor patients, depression not only arises immediately after surgery but increases in severity during the ensuing course. Along with physical debility, treatment-induced fatigue, cognitive impairments, and other emotional changes, depressive symptoms predict a poor quality of life.

38. The surgical service solicits a psychiatric consultation because the patient, a 79-year-old man, suddenly became "depressed." The psychiatrist determines that he had been making an uneventful recovery for the preceding 3 weeks following resection of extensive colon cancer. When the psychiatrist examines the patient, she finds that he is intermittently lethargic and often inattentive. When she captures his attention for further examination, she finds that he is incompletely oriented and has a poor memory. Although his white count is elevated, he has no fever, asterixis,

nuchal rigidity, papilledema, or lateralized neurologic findings. A head CT shows no abnormality. Which is most likely responsible for his change in mental state?
    a. Toxic-metabolic encephalopathy
    b. Paraneoplastic limbic encephalitis
    c. Cerebral metastases
    d. Major depression

Answer: a. The patient probably has delirium from a toxic-metabolic encephalopathy, which has several potential explanations, including sepsis, electrolyte imbalance, and metastases to the liver. Even minimal toxic-metabolic aberrations in elderly patients cause marked changes in their mood and level of consciousness. Another potentially misleading aspect is that overwhelming sepsis sometimes fails to raise the white blood count. After the surgeons correct the encephalopathy and determine the extent of tumor spread, they can reconsult the psychiatrist to evaluate the patient for depression that the medical illnesses may have overwhelmed.

39. A family brings their 74-year-old patriarch to the neurologist because he has been offending guests in his restaurant and forgetting important information about orders. Although he rarely drinks alcohol, he has smoked 2 packs of cigarettes daily since he came to this country as a teenager. He takes no medications. He has lost 20 lb. His neurologic examination shows pronounced memory impairment but no lateralized signs or papilledema. An MRI detected no mass lesions but the medial temporal lobes are smaller than normal. Routine blood tests show only mild anemia. An EEG contains temporal spikes. Which test should the neurologist now order?
    a. CT of the head
    b. CT of the chest
    c. CSF analysis by a spinal tap
    d. Brain biopsy

Answer: b. A man with a more than a 100 pack-year history of smoking cigarettes and an unexplained 20 lb weight loss deserves a CT of the chest for investigation of lung cancer. His amnesia, MRI, and EEG point to temporal lobe damage. Most likely he has developed limbic encephalitis as the presenting feature of a small cell carcinoma of the lung. In addition to ordering the chest CT, his physician should order an anti-Hu serum antibody determination. However, CSF analysis would probably not reveal useful information in this situation, except possibly for suggesting Creutzfeldt-Jakob disease (where it may detect 14-3-3 protein). Creutzfeldt-Jakob disease is a reasonable alternative diagnosis, but he has amnesia, systemic symptoms, and no myoclonus.

40. A 29-year-old intravenous drug addict comes to the emergency room with uncontrollable involuntary, uncoordinated, large-scale jerky movements of his left arm and leg. He remains alert and free of headache. Which of the following is an MRI most likely to show?
   a. A mass lesion tracking across the corpus callosum and infiltrating both frontal lobes
   b. Multiple cerebral cortical cysts
   c. A single, large ring-enhancing cerebral lesion in the right frontal area
   d. Multiple small ring-enhancing lesions predominantly in the basal ganglia

Answer: d. He has toxoplasmosis, which typically develops in the basal ganglia and causes movement disorders, including, as in this case, hemiballismus. A mass lesion tracking across the corpus callosum and infiltrating both frontal lobes, in a "butterfly" pattern, suggests a glioblastoma invading both frontal lobes. Multiple cerebral cortical cysts indicate neurocysticercosis.

41. Neurosurgeons are naturally reluctant to excise "eloquent"—physically or neuropsychologically critical—regions of the brain while resecting a seizure focus or tumor. Which of the following is the most eloquent region of the brain?
   a. The anterior section of the right frontal lobe
   b. The posterior section of the left frontal lobe
   c. The anterior section of the right occipital lobe
   d. The posterior section of the left occipital lobe

Answer: b. Broca's area, one of the most eloquent areas of the brain, is situated in the posterior section of the left frontal lobe. The occipital lobes contain the visual cortex, which is important but not as crucial as the language cortex. Almost the entire right frontal lobe, anterior to the motor strip, and the anterior tips of the temporal lobes are "silent"—devoid of readily recognizable function. Surgeons may remove these areas with little consequence.

42. Which is the most frequently occurring complication of radiation leukoencephalopathy in adults?
   a. Cognitive impairment
   b. Psychosis
   c. Convulsions
   d. None of the above

Answer: a. Sometimes immediately but more frequently after a several-year interval, whole brain radiotherapy causes cognitive impairment because it induces leukoencephalopathy.

43. When administered to children, radiation therapy may prevent the spread of acute leukemia to the CNS or obliterate unresectable tumors. However, the treatment has many potential complications. Which of the following is untrue?
   a. Young children, compared to young and middle-aged adults, are resistant to radiation-induced cognitive impairment.
   b. In young children, radiation therapy may lead to mental retardation.
   c. In children, radiation therapy can lead to panhypopituitarism.
   d. In children, radiation therapy can lead to growth retardation.

Answer: a. Young children are more vulnerable to radiation-induced cognitive impairment.

44. A close friend brings a 68-year-old retired nurse for psychiatric evaluation for depression. They both state that she has lost her liveliness, energy, and interest in other people during the previous 3 to 6 months. However, she denies memory and other cognitive impairments, headaches, and systemic symptoms. On examination, she scores 28 on the MMSE and has no physical neurologic abnormalities, but she has psychomotor retardation, emotional dulling, and reduced capacity to execute complex mental tasks. During the examination and more so afterward, she spoke excessively, loudly, and aggressively. With which two conditions is her clinical presentation most consistent?
   a. Frontal lobe tumor
   b. Alzheimer's disease
   c. Dementia with Lewy body disease
   d. Frontotemporal dementia
   e. Creutzfeldt-Jakob disease
   f. Vascular dementia

Answers: a and d. Her dulling of affect, loss of inhibition, and loquaciousness, with relatively normal memory and cognitive capacity, indicate frontal lobe dysfunction rather than simply dementia. Also, she has no physical abnormalities that would point to Creutzfeldt-Jakob or dementia with Lewy body diseases or vascular dementia. MRI would distinguish a frontal lobe tumor from frontotemporal dementia.

CHAPTER 20

Lumbar Puncture and Imaging Studies

LUMBAR PUNCTURE

Neurologists often obtain cerebrospinal fluid (CSF) by performing a lumbar puncture (LP)—one of the oldest neurologic tests still employed—under a variety of clinical circumstances. When patients have at least two elements of the relatively common triad of headache, fever, and nuchal rigidity, neurologists usually perform an LP to look for meningitis, subarachnoid hemorrhage, or other inflammatory condition affecting the central nervous system (CNS). They also perform an LP in cases of dementia attributable to infectious illnesses. In Creutzfeldt-Jakob disease (CJD), CSF almost always contains 14-3-3 protein; in subacute sclerosing panencephalitis (SSPE), it contains antimeasles antibodies; in acquired immunodeficiency syndrome (AIDS), retrovirus markers; and other infectious illnesses, such as cryptococcal or tuberculous meningitis, *herpes simplex* encephalitis, and neurosyphilis, specific antigens or DNA detectable by polymerase chain reaction (PCR). Neurologists also test the CSF of patients suspected of having multiple sclerosis (MS) for oligoclonal bands and myelin basic protein (see Chapter 15); however, those markers are inconsistent for initial diagnosis and do not correlate with disease progression.

In Alzheimer's disease, the CSF contains increased levels of tau protein but decreased levels of β-amyloid and Aβ42 peptide. Although those findings are interesting, they are too insensitive and nonspecific for diagnostic purposes.

Diagnosing neurologic illnesses sometimes rests on abnormalities of the CSF *profile*, which comprises the CSF color, red and white blood cell count, and concentrations of protein and glucose (Table 20-1). For example, most infectious or inflammatory CNS illnesses cause a CSF *pleocytosis* (increase in the CSF white blood cell count). In these illnesses, a rise in protein concentration parallels CSF pleocytosis, and, in their hallmark, glucose concentration falls to abnormally low levels. Bacterial meningitis accentuates that profile: CSF pleocytosis is markedly elevated, with a predominance of polymorphonuclear instead of lymphocytic cells, and the glucose concentration can fall to undetectable levels. Cultures of virus, fungus, and

Mycobacterium may require 1 to 3 weeks to identify an organism, but sometimes antigen testing can immediately indicate bacterial and nonbacterial organisms. As an exception to the general observation that infectious and inflammatory conditions produce CSF pleocytosis, in Guillain-Barré syndrome, CSF contains a markedly elevated protein concentration but little or no increase in the white cell content (the "albumino-cytologic disassociation," see Chapter 5).

Despite the potential contribution of CSF examination, certain circumstances are a contraindication to performing an LP. For example, neurologists do not perform one when patients have an extensive sacral decubitus ulcer because the LP needle might drive bacteria into the spinal canal and infect the CSF. In addition, neurologists insert the LP needle only below the first lumbar vertebra, which is the lower boundary of the spinal cord, to prevent spinal cord injury.

An intracranial mass lesion is one of the most common contraindications to an LP. This prohibition is based on the fear that an LP could suddenly reduce pressure in the spinal canal, allowing the unopposed force of a cerebral mass to lead to transtentorial herniation (see Fig. 19-3). Moreover, a CSF examination would not help in diagnosing most mass lesions, such as brain tumors, strokes, subdural hematomas, and toxoplasmosis abscesses, because their CSF profiles are not distinctive. Although increased intracranial pressure without an associated mass lesion defines pseudotumor cerebri (idiopathic increased intracranial hypertension, see Chapter 9), in this setting neurologists perform LPs with impunity for diagnosis and occasionally for treatment. Overall, unless neurologists suspect acute bacterial meningitis or subarachnoid hemorrhage, in which case rapid diagnosis is crucial, they usually do not perform an LP or they postpone it until after imaging studies have excluded an intracranial lesion.

Another potential problem with an LP occurs when trauma during the procedure allows blood to mix with the CSF, which may falsely indicate a subarachnoid hemorrhage or other intracranial source. To distinguish blood induced by the procedure, laboratories centrifuge bloody CSF. A xanthochromic supernatant means that intracranial bleeding took place several

TABLE 20-1 ■ Cerebrospinal Fluid (CSF) Profiles*

	Color	WBC/mL	Protein (mg/dL)	Glucose (mg/dL)	Miscellaneous
Normal	Clear	0–4[+]	30–45	60–100	
Bacterial meningitis	*Turbid*	100–500[°]	75–200	*0–40*	Gram-stain may reveal organisms
Viral meningitis	*Turbid*	*50–100[+]* [&]	50–100	0–60	
TB and fungal meningitis^	*Turbid*	*100–500[+]*	100–500	40–60	Cryptococcus antigen should be ordered
Neurosyphilis	Clear	5–200[+]	45–100	40–80	VDRL positive[$]
Guillain-Barré syndrome	Clear	*5–20[+]*	*80–200*	60–100	
Subarachnoid hemorrhage	*Bloody[#]*	45–80	60–100		Supernatant usually xanthochromic

WBC, white blood cell; TB, tuberculosis; VDRL, Venereal Disease Research Laboratory.

*Characteristic abnormalities in italics.

[+] Mostly lymphocytes.

[&] In encephalitis from *herpes simplex virus*, the CSF also contains red blood cells.

[°] Mostly polymorphonuclear cells.

^ In carcinomatous meningitis, the CSF profile is similar to fungal meningitis but malignant cells may be detected on cytologic examination.

[$] About 40% of neurosyphilis cases have a false-negative VDRL CSF test (see Chapter 7).

[#] White and red cells are in same proportion as in blood (1:1000).

hours before the LP and that the red blood cells gave rise to the yellow pigment. In contrast, a clear supernatant means that the LP gave rise to the blood in the CSF.

IMAGING STUDIES

Although imaging studies—computed tomography (CT) or magnetic resonance imaging (MRI)—should not enslave physicians, they undeniably provide extraordinarily accurate diagnoses. Each technique has given clinical neurology a quantum leap forward. In fact, Drs. Allan M. Cormack and Godfrey N. Hounsfield garnered Nobel prizes in 1979 for the development of CT, and Dr. Paul C. Lauterbur and Sir Peter Mansfield garnered Nobel prizes in 2003 for their discoveries concerning MRI.

Neurologists, readily conceding that in many situations these imaging studies surpass the reliability of their neurologic examination, routinely order them to evaluate patients with common neurologic conditions, including dementia, delirium, aphasia, other neuropsychologic deficits, headaches in elderly individuals, seizures, and postconcussion syndrome. They also use imaging studies to follow the course of certain illnesses, such as brain tumors and multiple sclerosis, because their clinical manifestations often fail to reflect disease progression as accurately as imaging studies. On the other hand, neurologists do not routinely order imaging studies in evaluating patients with sleep disturbances, absence seizures, cluster and migraine headaches, Parkinson's disease, tics, or essential tremor.

When neurologists consult on psychiatric patients, they often recommend imaging studies, among other tests, for patients who have a first episode of psychosis, atypical psychosis, major depression after age 50 years, episodic behavioral disturbances, and, in some cases, anorexia. They also suggest imaging studies for patients prior to electroconvulsive treatment (ECT) to detect lesions that either could explain the psychiatric symptoms or cause ECT-induced complications, such as status epilepticus or cerebral herniation. Although helpful in many circumstances, imaging studies fail to clarify the relationships between psychiatric symptoms and many common abnormalities that the studies uncover, including cerebral atrophy, mild communicating hydrocephalus, small cerebral lesions, subcortical hyperintensities, and congenital abnormalities.

COMPUTED TOMOGRAPHY

Using beams of ionizing radiation, which are essentially x-rays, CT generates images of the brain, other soft tissues, and skull. CT displays structures increasingly *more* radiodense than brain, such as tumors, blood, bone, calcifications, and surgical devices, in gradations increasingly closer to white than black. Similarly, it shows structures increasingly *less* radiodense than the brain, particularly the CSF-filled ventricles, in gradations increasingly closer to black. Thus, it shows in dark to black gradations several common lesions characterized by the absence of blood, such as cerebral infarctions, chronic subdural hematomas, edema surrounding tumors, and the center of cystic lesions.

Likewise, it shows in light to white gradations several common lesions characterized by calcium or excessive blood, such as calcifications in the choroid plexus or meningiomas; acute subarachnoid, subdural, or intracerebral hemorrhages; and intraventricular shunts. By manipulating the software, CT and MRI can display the brain from three major perspectives: transaxial (axial, the conventional top-down view), coronal (front-to-back view), and sagittal (side view).

Although lacking fine detail, CT can clearly reveal changes in major structures (Fig. 20-1). It shows generalized cerebral atrophy, such as occurs in advanced age or Alzheimer's disease (Figs. 20-2 and 20-3), and atrophy of a particular region, such as with porencephaly (Fig. 20-4), Huntington's disease (Fig. 20-5), and frontotemporal dementia (Fig. 20-6). Similarly, it shows expansion of the ventricles—hydrocephalus—not only as a consequence of generalized atrophy (hydrocephalus ex vacuo) (see Fig. 20-3), but also from normal pressure hydrocephalus (Fig. 20-7) and CSF obstructions (obstructive hydrocephalus) (see later). Although MRI better detects and characterizes most mass lesions, CT readily detects large lesions, such as primary and metastatic tumors (Fig. 20-8) and, except perhaps for isodense ones, subdural hematomas (Fig. 20-9). CT is even superior at finding dense, calcium laden meningiomas (Fig. 20-10). It can show numerous small lesions, such as in toxoplasmosis (Fig. 20-11) and cysticercosis (Fig. 20-12), with the detail necessary for a

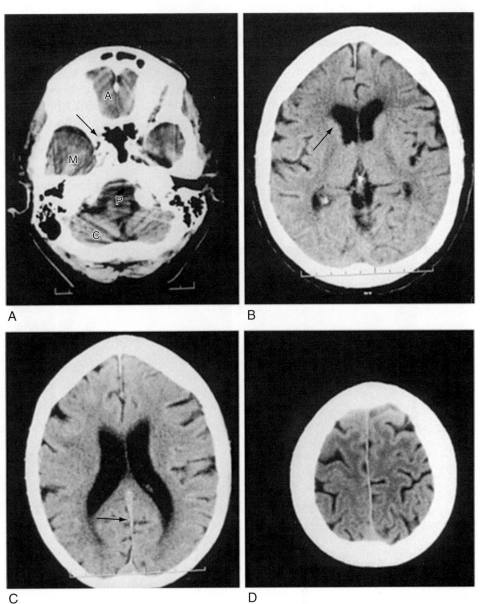

FIGURE 20-1 ■ These CTs show progressively higher axial images of a normal brain. *A,* The anterior cranial fossae (*A*) contain the anterior frontal lobes and the olfactory nerves. The middle fossae (*M*) contain the anterior temporal lobes, which are situated behind the sphenoid wing (*arrow*). The posterior fossa contains the cerebellum (*C*) and the medulla and pons (*P*)—main components of the bulb. The linear black streaks that cut across the posterior fossa are artifacts from the skull. *B,* The head of the caudate nucleus (*arrow*) indents the anterior horn of the lateral ventricle. *C,* The lateral ventricles, spread lengthwise in the hemispheres, are separated by the white, straight sagittal sinus (*arrow*). *D,* The cerebral cortex rests against the inner table of the skull. Thin sulci separate the gyri.

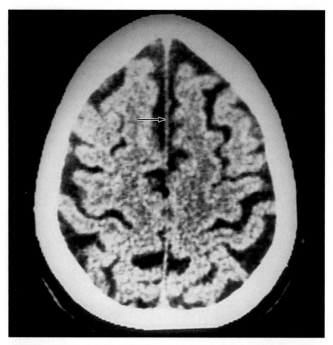

FIGURE 20-2 ■ This CT illustrates cerebral atrophy. (See Fig. 20-18 for MRI appearance of cerebral atrophy). Because of atrophy, the gyri shrink, sulci expand, the cerebral cortex retracts from the inner table of the skull and from the sagittal sinus (*open arrowhead*), and ventricles expand (see later). Cerebral atrophy, as pictured in this case, is a normal concomitant of old age. Although cerebral atrophy is associated with Alzheimer's disease, trisomy 21, alcoholism, neurodegenerative illnesses, and treatment-resistant schizophrenia, it is not invariably associated with dementia.

firm diagnosis. (Cysticercosis, which is caused by the parasite *Taenia solium,* is the most common cerebral mass lesion in South and Central America. CT suffices for a clinical diagnosis.)

CT can also show strokes that are large established infarctions and those that are hemorrhagic (Fig. 20-13); however, MRI can better locate ones that are small or acute. CT is invaluable in the special situation of cerebellar hemorrhage, where rapid diagnosis is essential to prevent brainstem compression and obstructive hydrocephalus (Fig. 20-14).

The administration of an intravenous contrast solution during CT increases the density of blood-filled structures and whitens their image. This technique, *contrast enhancement,* highlights vascular structures, such as arteriovenous malformations (AVMs), glioblastomas, and membranes surrounding chronic subdural hematomas and cystic lesions (Fig. 20-15).

Although MRI holds many advantages, CT remains clinically indispensable, less expensive than MRI, and highly reliable. It is particularly valuable during emergencies, when speed is critical and gross anatomic pictures suffice. For example, the procedure, which may take as little as 10 minutes, satisfactorily reveals lesions that require immediate attention, such as epidural and acute subdural hematomas, large cerebellar hemorrhages, obstructive hydrocephalus, and subarachnoid hemorrhage. Also, patients with pacemakers, defibrillators, and other indwelling metallic devices, and those with claustrophobia can undergo CT but not MRI.

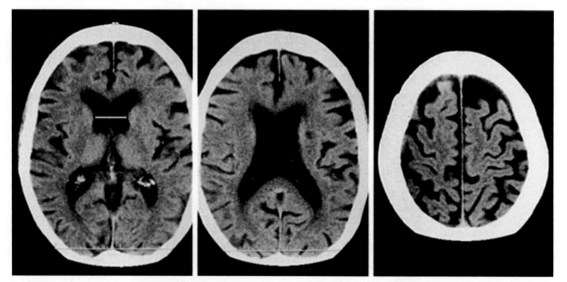

FIGURE 20-3 ■ These three progressively higher CT images (left to right) show that cerebral atrophy leads to expansion of the lateral ventricles and widening of the third ventricle (*line* in the left-most image)—*hydrocephalus ex vacuo*—as well as thinning of cerebral gyri and widening of sulci (right-most image). Nevertheless, as the left-most image shows, the head of the caudate nucleus maintains its normal volume and continues to indent the lateral border of the lateral ventricle. In Huntington's disease, by way of contrast, the characteristic atrophy of the head of the caudate nuclei allows the ventricles to bow outward (see Fig. 20-5).

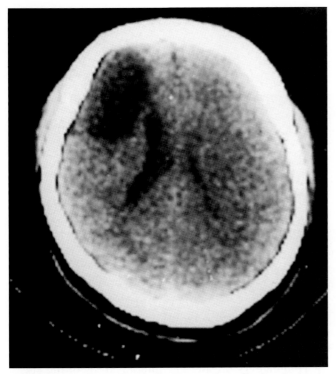

FIGURE 20-4 ■ CT and MRI, by convention, display the brain with its lateral, but not vertical, sides reversed. For example, the left cerebral hemisphere appears on the right side of the CT image while the frontal lobes still appear on the top on the image. In this CT, the oval region filled with cerebrospinal fluid (CSF) in the frontal lobe represents a congenital absence of brain tissue, called a *porencephaly*, in the patients' right frontal lobe. The porencephaly displays the opposite effect of a mass lesion. In particular, the absence of mass effect draws the adjacent lateral ventricle and midline structures shift toward it.

MAGNETIC RESONANCE IMAGING

In MRI, a powerful magnet forces protons to spin with their axes parallel to the magnetic field. Then radio-frequency (RF) pulses align the axes. After each RF pulse, the protons resume their original alignment ("relax") within the magnetic field and thereby emit energy. Different tissues emit characteristic, identifiable energy signals.

In the brain, hydrogen nuclei (protons) in water-containing tissues emit most of the signal. The differences in water content of tissues in various areas of the brain result in signals of different intensity. Sophisticated software converts them into images (the scans).

MRI offers several advantages over CT (Table 20-2). Because the resolution of MRI surpasses that of CT, its images provide finer detail (Fig. 20-16), more vivid

displays of neuroanatomy (Fig. 20-17), and better illustrations of large common structural changes, such as atrophy (Fig. 20-18) and hydrocephalus (Figs. 20-5, 20-7, and 20-19). It also shows fine detail of mass lesions, such as glioblastomas (Figs. 20-20, 20-21, 20-22, and 20-23). With certain sequences, MRI can show cerebral infarctions not only with fine detail, but, unlike CT, also almost immediately after their onset (Fig. 20-24). MRI, but not CT, can support the diagnosis of illnesses that alter cerebral or spinal cord white matter, that is, leukoencephalopathies, such as many congenital storage disease, MS (Fig. 20-25), progressive multifocal leukoencephalopathy (PML), and hydrocarbon solvent abuse. In MS, neurologists rely on MRI to confirm the diagnosis, establish the extent, and subsequently detect subclinical as well as clinical progression. It also shows characteristic changes, although not diagnostic ones, in prion illnesses, such as CJD and fatal familial insomnia (see Chapter 17).

MRI holds another advantage because most of the skull is composed of cortical bone, which contains no water: the skull does not produce linear streak artifacts that obscure images—a common problem in CT. The lack of artifact allows MRI to generate detailed images of structures in bony casings, such as the acoustic nerves, cerebellum, and other posterior fossa contents; the pituitary gland; and the spinal cord. Neurologists require MRI in diagnosing medial temporal sclerosis (Fig. 20-26) and planning epilepsy surgery. It is also indispensable in identifying acoustic neuromas (Fig. 20-27). However, because it does not detect lesions with little or no water content, MRI may fail to display meningiomas and skull fractures.

Administration of "paramagnetic" contrast solutions, such as gadopentetate (gadolinium), can enhance intracranial abnormalities. Although they do not cross the intact blood–brain barrier, contrast solutions highlight lesions that disrupt the barrier, such as neoplasms, abscesses, active MS plaques, and acute infarctions.

Despite its greater resolution, MRI is no more effective than CT in diagnosing several important illnesses, including Alzheimer's disease. Moreover, it has some disadvantages (Table 20-3). One problem is that for 30 to 40 minutes, patients remain entirely within the bore of the MRI magnet—an intimidating long, narrow tunnel, with a diameter only slightly wider than their body. Even excluding patients with known claustrophobia, at least 10% of the remainder, sometimes in utter panic, abort the procedure. Taking a benzodiazepine and wearing a sleep mask alleviates enough anxiety to allow many mildly claustrophobic patients to remain in the machine.

A potentially life-threatening problem with MRI is that the magnet forcefully attracts ferrous metals.

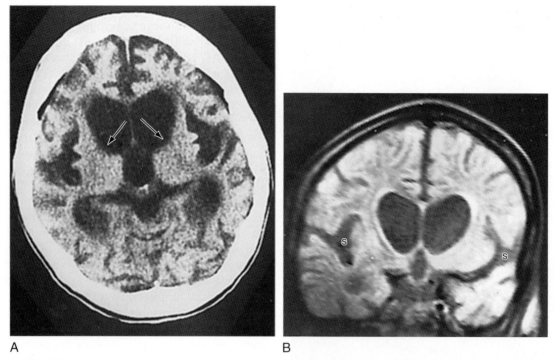

A   B

FIGURE 20-5 ■ *A,* This CT shows the characteristic abnormality of Huntington's disease: the anterior horns of the lateral ventricles are convex (bowed outward) because of atrophy of the caudate nuclei (*arrows*). Contrast that convex shape of the ventricles in Huntington's disease to the concave shape seen in normal individuals (Figs. 20-1B and 20-17) and in those with cerebral atrophy and hydrocephalus ex vacuo (Figs. 20-2, 20-3, and 20-18). In addition to the caudate atrophy, Huntington's disease, like many other neurodegenerative illnesses, causes cortical atrophy with widened sulci and enlarged ventricles. *B,* This *coronal* view of the MRI of the same patient also shows the convex expansion of the lateral ventricles, large sulci, and widened sylvian fissures (*S*).

Metallic objects inadvertently brought into the room have formed deadly missiles. Pacemakers, implanted hearing devices, intracranial aneurysm clips manufactured before 1993, and other medical devices might be dislodged or destroyed if the patient were exposed to the intense magnetic field.

Other Applications of Magnetic Resonance

With the appropriate software, magnetic resonance can generate images of intracranial and extracranial cerebral vessels. This technique, magnetic resonance angiography (MRA), can display highly accurate images of the carotid and vertebral arteries (see Figs. 11-2 and 20-28). It can detect aneurysms, AVMs, and other vascular malformations. Because it can outline internal carotid artery stenosis, plaques, and dissections, MRA eliminates the need for conventional carotid angiography, which can be hazardous and painful, in most cases.

The remarkable sensitivity of MRI has led to *functional MRI (fMRI),* a technique that displays gross metabolic activity. fMRI exploits small increases in blood flow and oxygenation during cerebral activity. It can highlight areas of the brain receiving sensory stimuli, initiating physical activity, imagining sensory or physical experiences, and performing cognitive processes. For example, it can detect the location of the language circuits in patients who are epilepsy surgery candidates. It may eventually replace the Wada test, which is invasive (see Chapter 8).

Magnetic resonance spectroscopy (MRS) detects the chemical composition of cerebral tissues and lesions. The technique's software suppresses water-generated signals and then analyzes the remaining signals to determine the presence and concentration of choline, creatine, N-acetylaspartate, lactic acid, lipids, and other chemicals. Preliminary work has shown that MRS can characterize tumors, abscesses, other lesions, mitochondrial encephalopathies, and degenerative diseases by the presence and relative concentrations of these substrates.

POSITRON EMISSION TOMOGRAPHY

In contrast to CT and MRI, which can provide exquisitely detailed images of CNS anatomy, *positron*

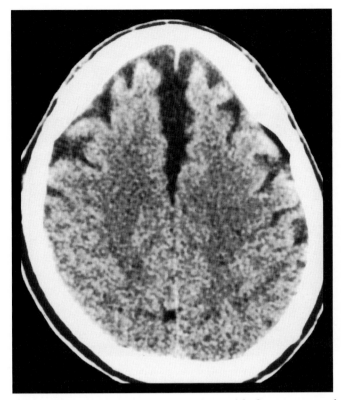

FIGURE 20-6 ■ This CT from a patient with frontotemporal dementia shows that the frontal lobes have undergone atrophy and retracted both from each other and from the inner table of the skull. Other views, which are not shown, reveal comparable changes in the temporal lobes; however, characteristically, the parietal and occipital lobes remain unchanged.

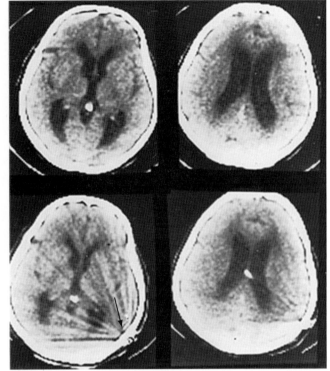

FIGURE 20-7 ■ *Top two scans,* CT, from a patient with normal pressure hydrocephalus (NPH), shows widening of the third and lateral ventricles with little or no cerebral atrophy. (See Fig. 20-19 for MRI of NPH.) *Bottom two scans,* Insertion of a shunt (*open arrow*) into the lateral ventricles has decreased their size. Linear artifacts spread from the shunt and obscure some of the anatomy.

emission tomography (*PET*) provides a rough picture of metabolic activity, chemistry, and physiology of the brain. PET relies on positron-emitting, biologically active radioisotopes (*radioligands*) produced in cyclotrons and incorporated into organic molecules. The radioligands, which are inhaled or injected intravenously, undergo metabolism in the brain and emit positrons. The reaction between positrons and electrons produces photons, which PET detects and transforms into images.

Most PET studies measure the metabolism of a substitute for glucose, fluorine-18 labeled fluorodeoxyglucose (FDG). Like glucose, FDG is absorbed into the brain and metabolized. The metabolism of FDG emits positrons at a rate that parallels cerebral glucose metabolism. Similarly, metabolism of oxygen-15 labeled water reflects cerebral blood flow and metabolism of fluorine-18 labeled fluorodopa reflects dopamine metabolism.

PET using radioligands for serotonin, gamma-aminobutyric acid (GABA), and acetylcholine (ACh) permits visualization of the distribution and activity of their receptors. All these radioligands have a brief half-life. For example, oxygen-15 has a half-life of 2 minutes and fluorine-18 less than 2 hours.

Neuroscientists use PET to analyze cerebral metabolism during normal activities, administration of medications, and several illnesses. PET images have shown that, in partial complex epilepsy, the affected temporal lobe is generally hypoactive in the interictal period but hyperactive during seizures. Determining whether the temporal lobe is epileptogenic by this method, which is complementary to electroencephalography, helps decide if a temporal lobectomy would benefit a patient with intractable epilepsy (see Chapter 10).

PET is also helpful in studying Parkinson's and Huntington's diseases. In these illnesses, abnormalities may appear before either clinical signs or MRI abnormalities have appeared. PET studies have also tracked basal ganglia changes in individuals exposed to methyl-phenyl-tetrahydro-pyridine (MPTP) before and after they developed in parkinsonism.

In Alzheimer's disease, PET shows decreased cerebral metabolism, especially in the parietal and frontal lobes' association areas. In vascular dementia, in contrast, PET studies show multiple, random areas of decreased metabolism. PET can also distinguish between recurrent brain tumors and radiation necrosis.

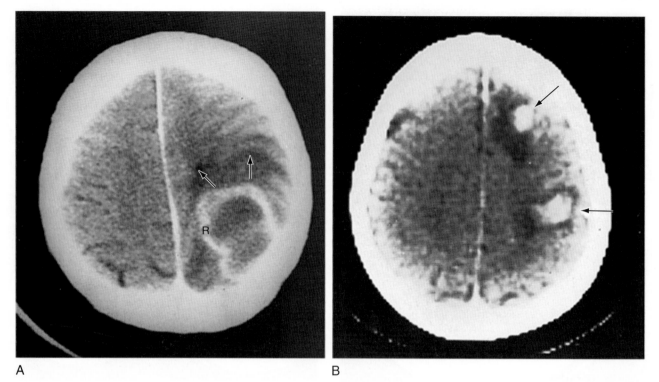

FIGURE 20-8 ■ *A,* CT shows a glioblastoma with its characteristic white, contrast-enhanced ring (*R*) and black border of edema (*open arrows*). (See Fig. 20-20 for MRI showing a glioblastoma.) *B,* With contrast-enhancement, CT shows two metastatic cerebral tumors (*arrows*). It is their being radiodense, relatively solid, and surrounded by edema, as well as their multiplicity, that identifies them as metastases. However, distinguishing between a glioblastoma and a single metastatic lesion is often difficult.

PET has come to play a crucial role in investigations of epilepsy, neurodegenerative diseases, and cerebral ischemia. However, it remains prohibitively expensive and impractical for routine clinical neurologic diagnosis.

SINGLE PHOTON EMISSION COMPUTED TOMOGRAPHY

Compared to PET, *single photon emission computed tomography (SPECT)*, although similar, lacks precision and fine spatial resolution. On the other hand, it is simpler to operate, less expensive, and suitable for many clinical studies.

SPECT uses readily available, stable radioligands, such as radioactive xenon, that do not require a cyclotron for preparation. The radioligands emit only a single easily detectable photon.

SPECT, like PET, portrays changes in cerebral function. It can map cerebral blood flow and, to a certain extent, neurotransmitter receptor activity. It can show major changes in cerebral blood flow, which reflects metabolic activity, in strokes, seizures, migraine, recurrent brain tumors, and neurodegenerative diseases. It demonstrates somewhat different patterns in dementia from Alzheimer's disease, vascular disease, or head injury. However, neurologists do not consider SPECT a part of the routine evaluation of patients with dementia.

INTERVENTIONAL RADIOLOGY

In the past decade, neuroradiologists have introduced dramatic therapies for several neurologic diseases. They offer MRI-guided needle biopsies of cerebral and spinal lesions, which are often deep-seated or otherwise unapproachable, that spare patients invasive and painful surgery. Neuroradiologists have been able to dilate stenoses of external carotid arteries and insert stents to maintain their patency (see Chapter 11). They also have been able to treat abnormalities in small intracerebral vessels. They can float epoxy resins or particles into inoperable AVMs or aneurysms and can correct stenoses of intracranial arteries. Similarly, they can direct catheters to deliver chemotherapy to brain tumors.

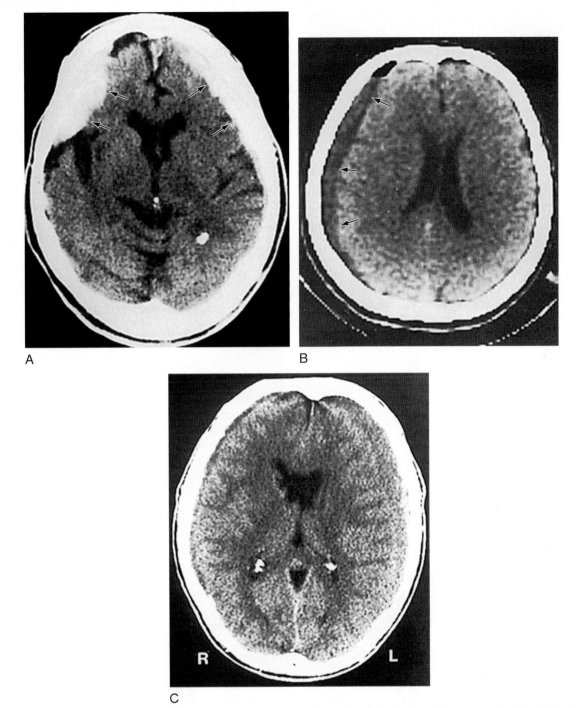

FIGURE 20-9 ■ *A,* The *acute* subdural hematoma (*arrows*) overlying the patient's right frontal lobe, contains fresh blood, which is radiodense compared to normal brain tissue. *B,* The *chronic* subdural hematoma (*arrows*), overlying this patient's right cerebral hemisphere, contains aged, liquefied blood that is less radiodense than brain. Chronic subdural hematomas are typically black on a CT and bordered by a radiodense, contrast-enhancing membrane. *C,* As acute subdural hematomas evolve into chronic ones, their density decreases to that of the underlying brain's density. When they become isodense, subdurals are indistinguishable. This CT shows a barely visible isodense subdural overlying this patient's left cerebral hemisphere. However, the membrane, compression of the gyri-sulci pattern, and shift of midline structures reveal its presence.

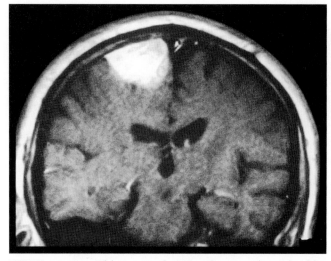

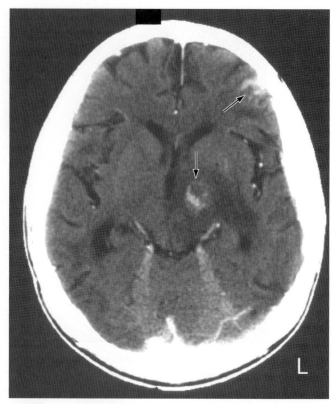

FIGURE 20-10 ■ This coronal CT, of a previous healthy 59-year-old man shows a large, rounded radiodense right frontal lesion, with a dural margin, that compresses the adjacent anterior horn of the lateral ventricle. The lesion is a typical, chronic, and slowly growing meningioma. As this CT exemplifies, frontal meningiomas often reach a large size before producing seizures, neuropsychologic changes, such as apathy or disinhibition, or other symptoms.

FIGURE 20-11 ■ A CT shows two toxoplasmosis lesions (arrowheads), enhanced by contrast infusion, in the left cerebrum in a patient with AIDS. As in this study, toxoplasmosis has a predilection for developing in the basal ganglia in AIDS patients with CD_4 counts less than 200 cells/mm^3. The infection's propensity to develop in the basal ganglia explains why AIDS patients who develop involuntary movement disorders, such as hemiballismus or chorea, are likely to be harboring toxoplasmosis.

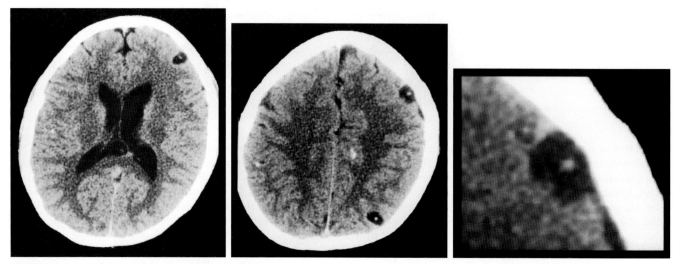

FIGURE 20-12 ■ This CT shows multiple cerebral cysticercosis lesions in views through the cerebrum (*left*) and cerebral cortex (*middle*) and an enlargement of the frontal cortex lesion (*right*). These lesions, in contrast to toxoplasmosis (Fig. 20-11), are usually situated in the cerebral cortex, contain calcification, and lack surrounding edema. Even though each cyst is small, together they exert a substantial cumulative mass effect and irritate the surrounding cerebral cortex. Their tendency to irritate the cerebral cortex explains why patients with cysticercosis often first come to medical attention because of seizures.

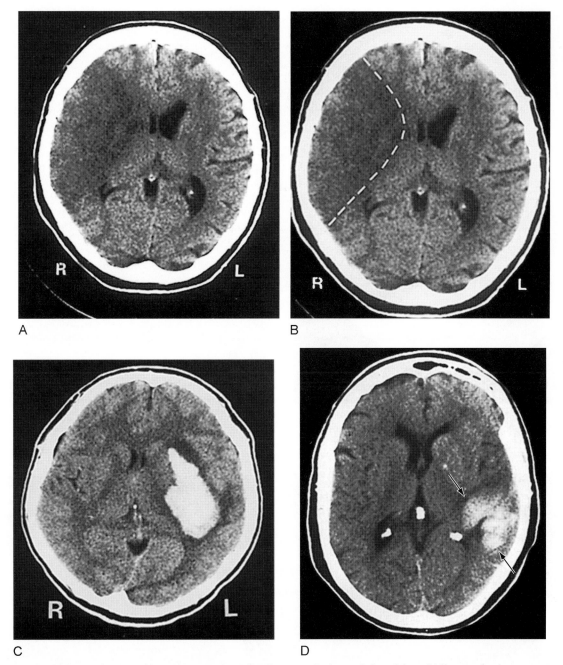

FIGURE 20-13 ■ *A,* This CT image shows an acute stroke from occlusion of the *right* middle cerebral artery. Because the infarcted area of the brain is deprived of blood, which is normally radiodense, it is darker (more hypodense) than the adjacent normal brain. In addition, its mass effect compresses the adjacent lateral ventricle and shifts midline structures. *B,* An outline of the stroke on the same image shows its pie-shaped area in the lateral portion of the right cerebral hemisphere, containing the origin of the corticospinal tract for the left face and arm. *C,* This image shows a cerebral hemorrhage that originated in the left thalamus and extended into the lateral ventricle. The blood, denser than the brain, forms the white plume. *D,* In this image, a hemorrhage (*arrows*) involves the left parietal lobe and compresses the occipital horn of the left lateral ventricle. The three small white objects are, laterally, the normally calcified choroid plexus of the lateral ventricles and, medially, the pineal gland.

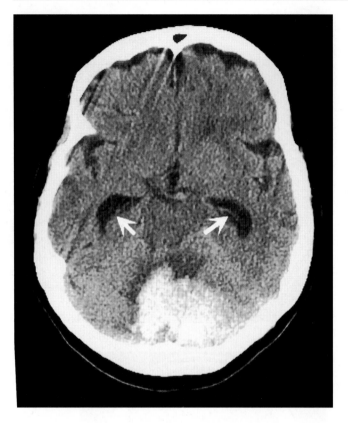

FIGURE 20-14 ■ This CT shows a large white mass lesion in the posterior fossa. The lesion is a cerebellar hemorrhage that has completely compressed the fourth ventricle and blocked cerebrospinal fluid (CSF) passage. The resulting obstructive hydrocephalus has caused dilation of the temporal horns of the lateral ventricles (*arrows*).

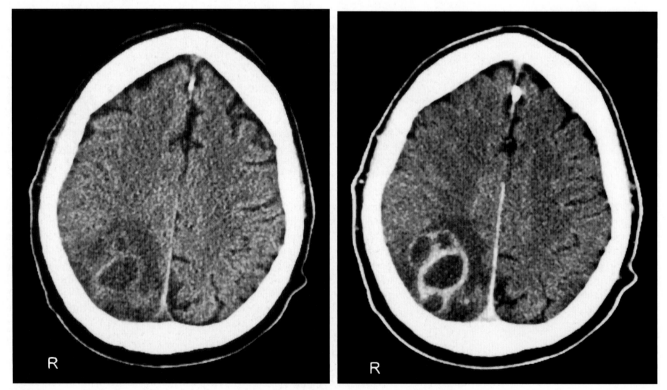

FIGURE 20-15 ■ CT before (*left*) and during (*right*) infusion of contrast material highlights a lobulated abscess in a patient's right parietal-occipital region. Disruption of the blood–brain barrier allows the contrast material to concentrate in the lesion's membranes.

TABLE 20-2 ■ Advantages of MRI Over CT

Greater imaging ability
  MRI has greater resolution enabling it to capture smaller objects
  Distinguishes white from gray matter
  Routinely displays images in three planes: coronal, axial, and sagittal
  Contrast medium is water-based not iodine-based
No distortion from bone
  Can display posterior fossa structures, pituitary gland, and optic nerves
  Can image the spinal cord
Does not utilize ionizing radiation
Can visualize intracranial and extracranial arteries and their abnormalities
Can indicate certain conditions
  White matter plaques of MS and PML
  Mesial temporal sclerosis, AVMs, and small gliomas

MS, multiple sclerosis; PML, progressive multifocal leukoencephalopathy; AVMs, arteriovenous malformations.
*Common findings in partial complex seizures.

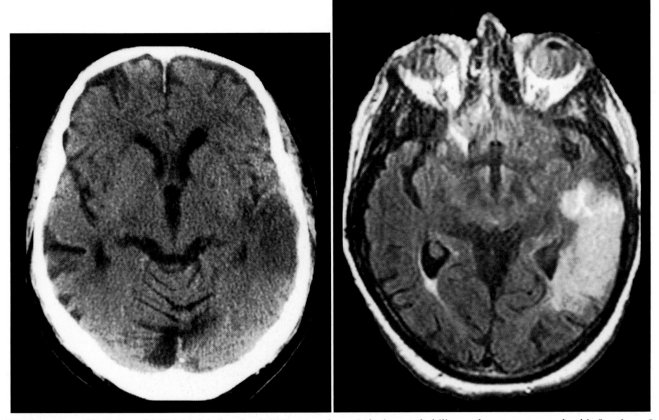

FIGURE 20-16 ■ CT (*left*) and MRI (*right*) showing MRI's superior resolution and ability to detect acute cerebral infarctions. In this case, a left temporal lobe infarction, barely discernible on CT, is obvious on MRI.

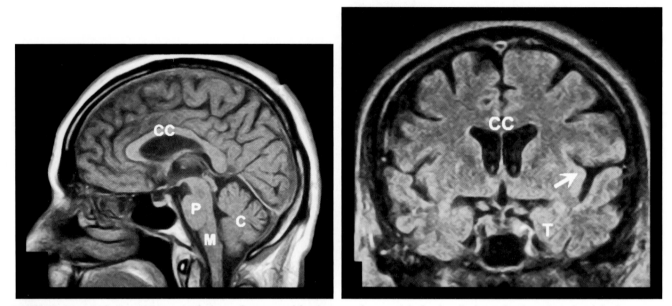

FIGURE 20-17 ■ *Left,* An MRI *sagittal* view of a normal brain reveals exquisitely detailed cerebral gyri and sulci, the corpus callosum (*CC*), and three major structures of the posterior fossa, the pons (*P*), medulla (*M*), and cerebellum (*C*). The anterior portion of the corpus callosum is the genu (*G*), and its posterior portion, the splenium (*S*). In addition, it shows the cervical-medullary junction and various non-neurologic soft tissue structures. Note that the medulla remains above the foramen magnum. *Right,* The *coronal* view reveals the corpus callosum (*CC*), the "great commissure," which spans and interconnects the cerebral hemispheres. The white matter of the corpus callosum and subcortical cerebral hemispheres is distinct from the ribbon of overlying gray matter. The anterior horns of the lateral ventricles, with their concave lateral borders, are beneath the corpus callosum and medial to the caudate nuclei (see Fig. 18-1A). The cerebral cortex around the left (dominant) sylvian fissure (*arrow*), including the planum temporale, is usually more convoluted than that around the right (nondominant). The convolutions confer greater cortical area for language function on the dominant hemisphere. The frontal lobe is above the sylvian fissure, and the temporal lobe is below. The medial-inferior surface of the temporal lobe (*T*), which is the origin of most partial complex seizures, is sequestered by the bulk of the temporal lobe above and the sphenoid wing anteriorly. It is far from the sites of conventional scalp electroencephalogram (EEG) electrodes.

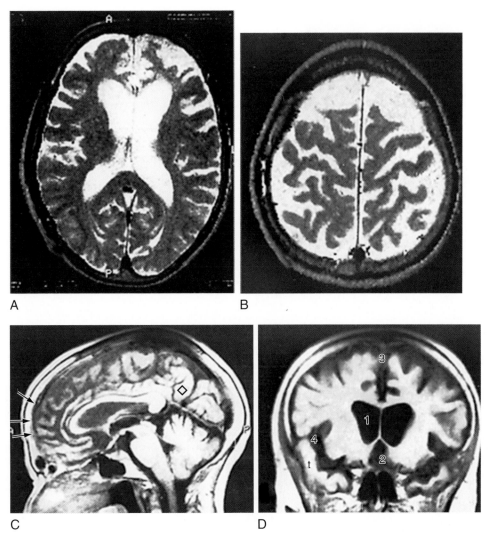

FIGURE 20-18 ■ Four MRI images of cerebral atrophy can be contrasted to the normal brain (see Fig. 20-17). MRI emphasizes cerebral atrophy because it does not detect the cortical bone of the skull, which emits almost no signal because it contains virtually no water. However, the scalp emits a signal because it contains blood, fat, and other water-containing soft tissues. *A,* In this axial view through the cerebral hemispheres, the cerebrospinal fluid (CSF), which is white, fills the dilated lateral ventricles and sulci. *B,* In a view that shows the surface of the brain, CT demonstrates the thin gyri. To fill the void left by the atrophied gyri, copious amounts of CSF fill the sulci and cover the cortex. *C,* In a sagittal view, where the sequence disregards the CSF signal, the MRI shows thin, ribbon-like frontal lobe gyri (*arrowheads*) and the less atrophied parietal lobe gyri (*diamond*). The corpus callosum, pons, and cerebellum stand out. The tentorium, appearing as a straight line, is situated above the cerebellum. *D,* This coronal view through the frontal lobes shows typical manifestations of cerebral atrophy: (1) dilated lateral ventricles, (2) an enlarged third ventricle, (3) enlargement of the anterior interhemispheric fissure because of separation of the medial surfaces of the frontal lobes, and (4) dilated sylvian fissures with the atrophic temporal lobe (*t*) below and the atrophic frontal lobe above.

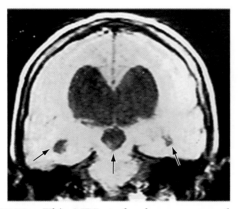

FIGURE 20-19 ■ This MRI study shows a coronal view of the brain of a patient with NPH. (See Fig. 20-7 for a comparable CT.) It demonstrates the classic findings: dilation of the lateral ventricles, their temporal horns (*black arrows*), and the third ventricle (*open arrow*), and absence of cerebral atrophy.

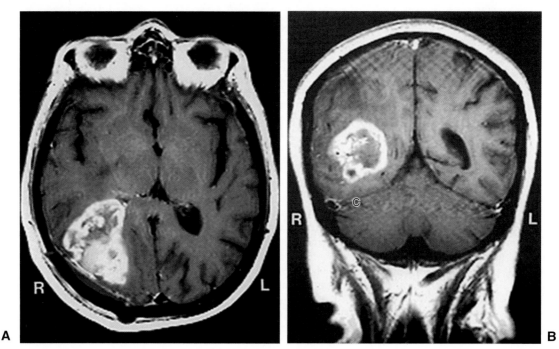

FIGURE 20-20 ■ Transaxial (axial) *(A)* and coronal *(B)* projections of an MRI show a large lobulated hyperintense, right posterior parietal glioblastoma. Its mass effect has obliterated the occipital horn of the lateral ventricle and shifted midline structures to the patient's left side. The coronal view shows the cerebellum (*C*) as well as the posterior cerebrum.

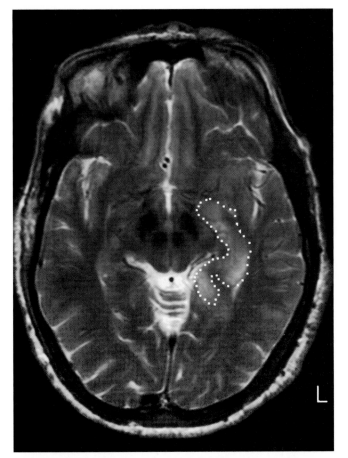

FIGURE. 20-21 ■ An axial projection of an MRI of a young man with acute *herpes simplex* encephalitis shows hyperintensity in inferior gyri of the left temporal lobe (*outlined*). As in this case, *herpes simplex* infection typically causes hemorrhagic inflammation in the inferior surface of the temporal and frontal lobes. Permanent temporal lobe damage, which is often bilateral, subjects survivors to memory impairment (amnesia), partial complex seizures, and the Klüver-Bucy syndrome.

FIGURE 20-22 ■ *Left*, In this sagittal view of the normal neuroanatomy, the cerebellum and medulla sit above the foramen magnum (*arrow*). *Right*, In the Arnold-Chiari malformation, the cerebellar tonsils and the medulla are situated below the foramen magnum (*arrow*), as though they were pulled downward. The malformation has also caused aqueductal stenosis that will lead to hydrocephalus (not seen).

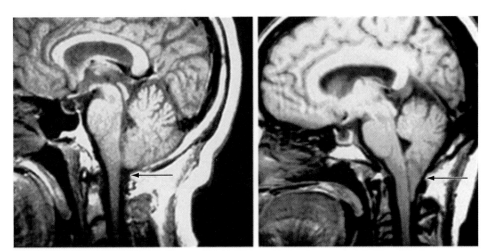

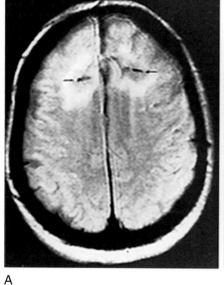
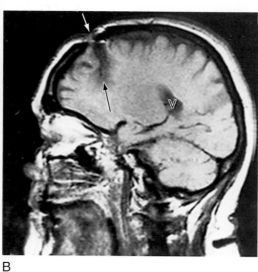

A

B

FIGURE 20-23 ■ This MRI, from a patient who had undergone a frontal lobotomy, shows the results of drilling a hole through the skull above each frontal lobe and severing their white matter tracts. *A*, The axial view shows black horizontal slits, which represent the incisions (*arrows*) and their surrounding scar tissue. *B*, The sagittal view, through the right cerebral hemisphere, shows the skull defect (*white arrow*) and lowermost extent of the incision (*black arrow*). The frontal lobe anterior to the incision has undergone atrophy. The radiolucent area in the posterior cerebrum (*V*) is the right posterior lateral ventricle.

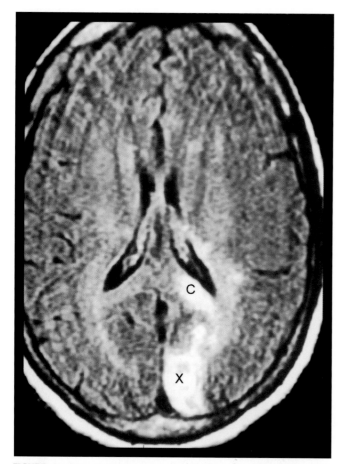

FIGURE 20-24 ■ From a case of with alexia without agraphia (see Fig. 8-4), this MRI shows a stroke (*X*) in the patient's left occipital lobe that extends anteriorly to the splenium (posterior corpus callosum, *C*). As in this case, occlusions of the left posterior cerebral artery most often cause this stroke.

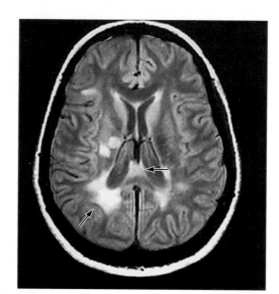

FIGURE 20-25 ■ This MRI, from a patient with multiple sclerosis (MS), shows multiple areas of demyelination. MS lesions, often called plaques, are typically high signal (*white*) and clustered in the white matter deep of the cerebral hemispheres, and tend to spread outward from the ventricles. In this image, a large lesion is situated in the patient's right occipital lobe, posterior to the lateral ventricle (*arrowhead*). Another involves the splenium (*arrow*). Because MS plaques generally first develop in the periventricular white matter and spare the cerebral cortex, cognitive impairments are not an early manifestation of MS.

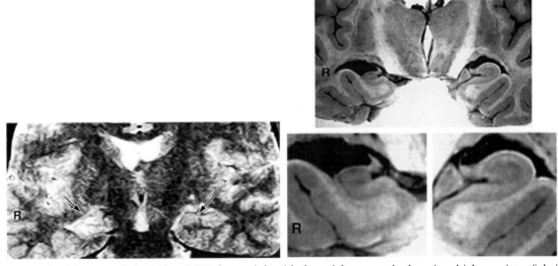

FIGURE 20-26 ■ *Left,* This coronal view of an MRI shows right-sided mesial temporal sclerosis, which consists of shrinkage and scarring of the hippocampus and underlying amygdala. Comparing the medial temporal lobes (*arrows*), the patient's left-sided medial temporal lobe is round and broad, but the right-sided one, beset by sclerosis, is contracted and poorly demarcated. Moreover, because of the sclerosis, it emits a brighter (*white*) signal. *Right,* The brain, at approximately the comparable level as the MRI, shows that the patient's normal, left medial temporal lobe is round and has a well-demarcated cortex. In the enlarged sections (*below*), the patient's left medial temporal lobe appears as a duck's head facing medially. The lateral ventricle's rounded temporal horn overlies the temporal lobe. In contrast, the patient's right medial temporal lobe is shrunken and contracted inferiorly and laterally. The overlying ventricle's temporal horn is much larger than its counterpart because atrophy allowed it to expand.

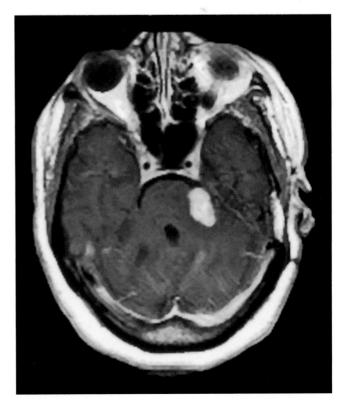

FIGURE 20-27 ■ A large acoustic neuroma, originating from the patient's left cerebellopontine angle, compresses the pons and shifts the fourth ventricle. In contrast to being obvious on this MRI, cerebellopontine angle lesions may escape detection on CT because they are usually small and sequestered in a corner of the skull base where artifacts obscure them. Neurofibromatosis type 2 patients, who tend to develop bilateral acoustic neuromas, routinely undergo MRI with views of the internal auditory canals.

TABLE 20-3 ■ Disadvantages of MRI Over CT
Cost is approximately two to three times greater than CT
Requires at least 30 minutes, more than twice as long as CT
Being in the magnet often precipitates a claustrophobic reaction
Metal devices cannot be placed near the MRI magnet:
Patients cannot have a pacemaker, intracranial aneurysm clips manufactured before 1993, cochlear implants, or many other implanted ferrous metal devices
Respirators and most other life-support machinery, unless specially designed, cannot be near the magnet

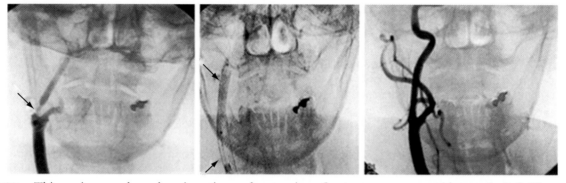

FIGURE 20-28 ■ This angiogram shows how insertion and expansion of a stent corrects carotid stenosis. *Left,* The angiogram demonstrates the right common carotid artery ascending and dividing into the external and internal carotid artery, which has a severe stenosis (*arrow*). *Middle,* The stent (*arrows*) has been inserted and expanded. *Right,* A follow-up angiogram shows a patent and smooth internal carotid artery.

REFERENCES

1. Atlas SW: MRI of the Brain and Spine on CD-ROM. Hagerstown, MD, Lippincott-Raven, 1998.
2. Grossman R, Yousem DM: *Neuroradiology.* 2nd ed. Philadelphia, Mosby, 2004.
3. Osborn AG: *Diagnostic Imaging: Brain.* Philadelphia Saunders, 2004.
4. Beek DVD, Gans JD, Tunkel AR, et al: Community-acquired bacterial meningitis. N Engl J Med 354:44–53, 2006.

Web sites for Neuroimaging

1. American Academy of Neurology: http://www.aan.com
2. Johnson KA, Becker JA: The Whole Brain Atlas: http://www.med.harvard.edu/AANLIB/home.html

Questions and Answers

1. Why do laboratories centrifuge blood-tinged CSF?
   a. Concentrating cells allows for easier counting.
   b. It permits detection of xanthochromia.
   c. It restores the balance between cells and protein.
   d. The proteins separate from the glucose.

   Answer: b. Centrifuging separates the cells from the CSF and thus permits detection of xanthochromia. If present, xanthochromia indicates that bleeding occurred in the CSF more than several hours before a spinal tap. Its origin was likely trauma or a subarachnoid hemorrhage, not merely a traumatic spinal tap.

2–3. During the 12 hours before his family brought him for evaluation, a 50-year-old man developed fever, confusion, headache, and lethargy. His neurologic examination showed memory loss and inattention but no nuchal rigidity or lateralized findings. During his general medical examination, which revealed no abnormalities, he had repetitive lip-smacking movements, shaking movements of his right hand, and then loss of consciousness for 15 minutes. A chest x-ray and head CT showed no abnormalities.

2. Which profile is his CSF apt to show?
   a. WBC 80, 90% lymphocytes; glucose 50 mg/dL; protein 60 mg/dL
   b. WBC 200, 80% polymorphonuclear cells; glucose 15 mg/dL; protein 90 mg/dL
   c. WBC 3; glucose 80 mg/dL; protein 35 mg/dL
   d. WBC 300, 100% lymphocytes; glucose 5 mg/dL; protein 300 mg/dL

   Answer: a. He probably has developed *herpes simplex* encephalitis in view of the amnesia and partial complex seizure, which reflect temporal lobe damage. The lack of nuchal rigidity indicates the absence of meningitis. Profile *b* indicates bacterial meningitis; profile *c* is normal; and profile *d* suggests a chronic nonbacterial process, such as tuberculous meningitis.

3. If further testing confirms the clinical diagnosis of *herpes simplex* encephalitis, which is the most common variety of nonepidemic encephalitis, what is the MRI most likely to show?

   a. No abnormalities
   b. Hemorrhagic regions in one or both temporal lobes
   c. Multiple circular lesions in the cerebral cortex
   d. Multiple circular lesions in the deep cerebrum

   Answer: b. *Herpes zoster* causes hemorrhagic encephalitis that affects the base of the brain, particularly the temporal and base of the frontal lobes.

4–7. Match the disease with the CSF marker.
4. Alzheimer's disease
5. Creutzfeldt-Jakob
6. Multiple sclerosis
7. Subacute sclerosis panencephalitis
   a. 14-3-3 protein
   b. Antimeasles antibodies
   c. Increased levels of tau protein and decreased levels of Aβ42 peptide
   d. Oligoclonal bands

   Answers: 4-c, 5-a, 6-d, 7-b.

8. A 30-year-old woman with a history of depression develops increasingly severe generalized headaches. Neurologic examination shows florid papilledema and bilateral sixth cranial nerve palsies, but she remains fully alert and with no cognitive impairment, paresis, or ataxia. An MRI shows small ventricles and no mass lesions. Which profile is her CSF apt to show?
   a. Pressure 300 mm H_2O; WBC 80, 90% lymphocytes; glucose 50 mg/dL; protein 60 mg/dL
   b. Pressure 200 mm H_2O; WBC 200, 80% polymorphonuclear cells; glucose 15 mg/dL; protein 90 mg/dL
   c. Pressure 550 mm H_2O; WBC 1; glucose 65 mg/dL; protein 20 mg/dL
   d. Pressure 100 mm H_2O; WBC 300, 100% lymphocytes; glucose 5 mg/dL; protein 300 mg/dL

   Answer c. She probably has pseudotumor cerebri with high enough intracranial pressure to stretch the sixth nerves, creating a classic false localizing sign. In this condition, the CSF protein and glucose concentrations are often lower than normal, as if by dilution.

9. Why does contrast infusion during CT highlight brain tumors and abscesses?
   a. Inflammatory cells absorb contrast material.
   b. Osmotic forces pull the material into the lesion.
   c. Breakdown of the blood–brain barrier surrounding the lesion allows contrast material to highlight its periphery.
   d. Neoplastic and infectious cells metabolize contrast material.

Answer: c. These and other lesions disrupt the blood–brain barrier, allowing contrast material to surround them.

10. Which of the following intracranial objects will be readily recognizable on CT but almost invisible on MRI?
   a. Temporal lobe hematoma
   b. Porencephaly
   c. Calcified pineal gland
   d. Toxoplasmosis

Answer: c. Calcified objects that lack water, such as some meningiomas, calcium in a choroid plexus, congenital infections, and a calcified pineal gland, will emit little or no signal on MRI. However, their calcium, which is radiodense, blocks the ionizing radiation of CT and thus allows for their detection.

11–12. A 30-year-old man with progressive cognitive impairment for 3 years and a family history of a similar disorder has this MRI.

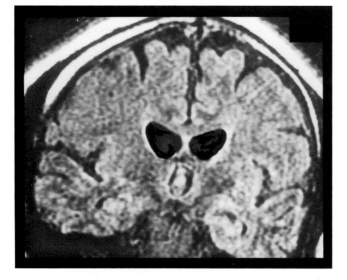

11. Which view of the brain does this scan portray?
   a. Axial
   b. Transaxial

   c. Coronal
   d. Sagittal

Answer: c. This is a *coronal* view, which is readily identifiable by displaying simultaneously the frontal and temporal lobes and the lateral and third ventricles. *Axial* and *transaxial* are equivalent terms.

12. Although the image is not definitive, which cause of dementia does it suggest?
   a. Alzheimer's disease
   b. Frontotemporal dementia
   c. Huntington's disease
   d. Diffuse Lewy body disease
   e. A structural lesion

Answer: c. This image shows diffuse cerebral atrophy, which is nonspecific. More important, it shows convex expansion of the lateral ventricles because of atrophy of the head of the caudate nuclei. That change strongly suggests Huntington's disease.

13–14. A 65-year-old man's wife reports that over 6 months he has lost his liveliness. She states that, "The situation has gone from bad to worse." He sold his business 4 months before the visit because of his disinterest and then financial miscalculations. On examination, he has mild cognitive impairment and apathy but no lateral signs. This is his CT.

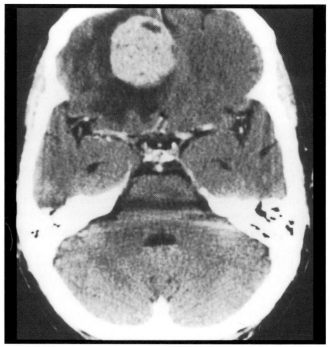

13. Where is the lesion located?
   a. Left frontal
   b. Right frontal
   c. At the junction of the middle and anterior fossae
   d. None of the above

Answer: b. In this CT axial view, as is customary, the left and right sides are reversed. A large radiodense (white) circular lesion sits in the medial portion of the patient's right frontal lobe. Its black border, posterior and lateral to the lesion, indicates edema. Structural lesions of the frontal lobes, especially those that grow slowly on the right side, may reach extraordinary size before they produce symptoms. Frontal lobe lesions frequently dull the patient's personality, drain initiative and creativity, and sometimes reduce inhibitions. Compared to the psychologic changes, frontal lobe lesions may cause little cognitive impairment or physical defects.

14. What is the most likely etiology of the lesion?
   a. Abscess
   b. Glioblastoma
   c. Meningioma
   d. Stroke

Answer: c. The lesion's extra-axial location, circular shape, and relatively uniform, high density indicate that it is a meningioma. Altering the image would probably reveal that it contains calcium, which is a characteristic of meningiomas. The patient's progressive decline also suggests a slowly developing lesion, such as a meningioma, rather than an abscess or glioblastoma. Also, abscesses and glioblastomas usually have hyperintense borders and nonuniform density. Large strokes generally conform to the distribution of a cerebral artery and have a pie-shaped appearance.

15–16. Performed as part of the evaluation of a 30-year-old man who presented after his first seizure, an MRI showed several ring-shaped lesions.

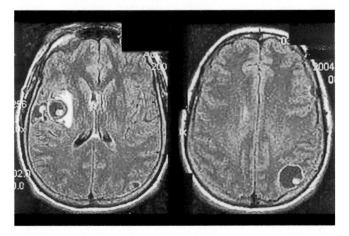

15. Which of the following conditions do not typically cause multiple ring-shaped lesions?
   a. Abscess
   b. Toxoplasmosis
   c. Cysticercosis
   d. Metastases
   e. Primary brain tumors

Answer: e. Primary brain tumors, such as meningiomas, glioblastomas, and astrocytomas, typically cause only single lesions. The other conditions typically cause multiple ring-shaped lesions. The history, non-neurologic findings, or, if necessary, a biopsy will usually allow a diagnosis.

16. In this case, which is the most likely diagnosis?
   a. Abscess
   b. Toxoplasmosis
   c. Cysticercosis
   d. Metastases

Answer: c. The two MRI images show three ring-shaped lesions at the gray-white matter junction. The lesions have rims with a high signal and a small high signal lesion in their periphery. In the left image, the broad white streak medial to the lesion is edema. The appearance of these lesions is characteristic of cysticercosis, which is one of the most common causes of seizures, especially among recent immigrants from South and Central America.

17. A 39-year-old man, who has been under immunosuppressive treatment for 12 years to preserve a renal transplant, has developed cognitive impairment and mild left hemiparesis. Based on the history and MRIs, which of the following is the most likely diagnosis?
   a. Multiple sclerosis (MS)
   b. Progressive multifocal leukoencephalopathy (PML)
   c. Toluene abuse
   d. Metachromatic leukodystrophy (MLD)

Answer: b. The MRI images show multiple regions of high signal intensity in the white matter in both cerebral hemispheres, but in his right more so than his left hemisphere. The lower cut (*Left*) shows an enlarged right lateral ventricle and high signal emanating from the subcortical white matter. The higher cut (*Right*) shows the cerebral cortex with the signal changes in the subcortical white matter of the patient's right hemisphere and anterior and posterior regions of the left hemisphere. The images also show cerebral atrophy, which has led to ventricular enlargement and loss of cerebral volume. Patients with chronic immunosuppression from chemotherapy (for malignancy or

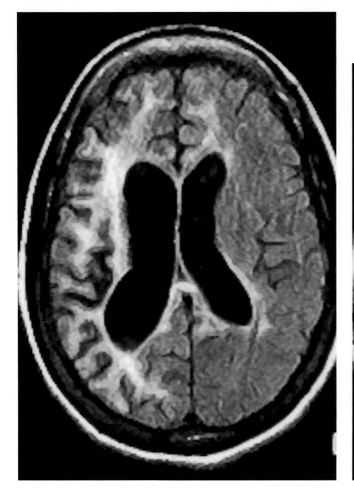

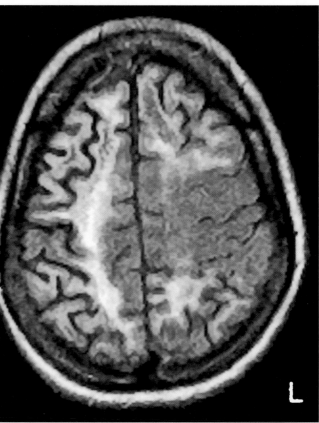

organ transplantation) or acquired immunodeficiency syndrome (AIDS) are prone to develop PML and cerebral atrophy. MS, toluene abuse, and MLD also cause white matter damage, but the history more strongly suggests PML.

18. A 75-year-old man came to his physician because, for 6 weeks, he had had an increasingly severe left-sided headache. A neurologic examination showed inattention, apathy, word-finding difficulties, and a mild right-sided hemiparesis. Before the onset of these symptoms, he had been in good health and a general medical examination disclosed no significant abnormalities. Which condition does the CT indicate?
   a. Glioblastoma
   b. Acute subdural hematoma
   c. Chronic subdural hematoma
   d. Stroke
   e. Porencephaly

   Answer: c. The CT reveals a large, radiolucent mass lesion, with a surrounding radiodense membrane,

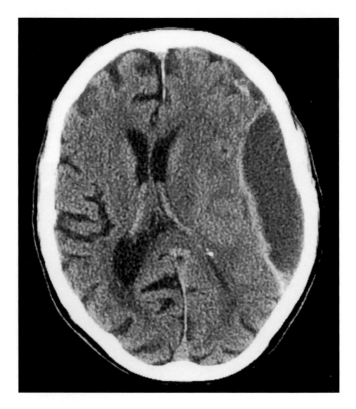

overlying the patient's left cerebral hemisphere. The lesion compresses and shifts structures contralaterally. Because it is extra-axial, the lesion is most likely a subdural hematoma. Also, because the hematoma is radiolucent, it is chronic. Subdural hematomas are relatively common in older individuals because their pre-existing cerebral atrophy does not allow their brain to compress any bleeding that might occur and they often take aspirin or other medicine that inhibits coagulation.

Neurotransmitters and Drug Abuse

This chapter, recapitulating and expanding information that this book introduced in previous chapters, focuses on the major neurotransmitters' synthesis, metabolism, functional anatomic pathways, and the mechanism of action at cellular receptors. In addition, it reviews their altered activity in important neurologic disorders and treatments. With few exceptions, it restricts the discussion of neurotransmitters' role in the central nervous system (CNS) diseases and does not address psychopharmacology. This chapter reviews the following neurotransmitters:

- Monoamines
  - Catecholamines: dopamine, norepinephrine, and epinephrine
  - Indolamines: serotonin
- Acetylcholine
- Neuropeptides
  - Inhibitory amino acids: gamma-aminobutyric acid (GABA)
  - Excitatory amino acids: glutamate
- Nitric oxide

MONOAMINES

Dopamine

Synthesis and Metabolism

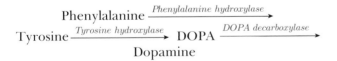

Neurologists hold dopamine synthesis in preeminence, treasuring each substrate, synthetic and metabolic enzyme, and by-product. Each day they capitalize on its synthesis when they treat Parkinson's disease and several other neurologic illnesses.

Dopamine synthesis begins with the amino acid, phenylalanine, and proceeds sequentially through tyrosine, DOPA, and then dopamine. *Tyrosine hydroxylase* is the rate-limiting enzyme in this pathway. Another important enzyme is *DOPA decarboxylase,* which decarboxylates DOPA to form dopamine. That same

enzymatic acts on both naturally occurring DOPA and L-dopa (levodopa), the Parkinson's disease medicine.

Several different processes terminate dopamine activity at the synapse. The primary one consists of dopamine reuptake into the presynaptic neuron. In another termination process, two different enzymes metabolize dopamine. *Catechol-O-methyltransferase* (*COMT*), mostly an extracellular enzyme, and *monoamine oxidase* (*MAO*), mostly an intracellular enzyme, both metabolize dopamine. Some medicines for Parkinson's disease and other conditions defined by dopamine deficiency preserve dopamine by inhibiting these enzymes (see later).

When these enzymes metabolize dopamine, the main product consists of *homovanillic acid* (*HVA*). Some studies indicate that the concentration of this metabolite in the cerebrospinal fluid (CSF) roughly corresponds to dopaminergic activity in the brain.

Anatomy

Three "long dopamine tracts" hold the greatest clinical importance in neurology:

1. The *nigrostriatal tract,* the major component of the extrapyramidal motor system, synthesizes most dopamine in the brain. This tract projects from the substantia nigra, the crescentic pigmented nuclei in the midbrain (Fig. 21-1), to the predominantly D_2 receptors of the striatum (the caudate nucleus and putamen [see Chapter 18]).

2. The *mesolimbic tract* projects from the ventral tegmental area, which is in the inferior medial portion of the midbrain, to the amygdala and other portions of the limbic system. The receptors are predominantly D_4. This tract appears to propagate the positive symptoms of psychosis and antipsychotic agents reduce psychotic symptoms by blocking dopamine transmission in this tract, thereby attenuating dopamine activity in the limbic system.

3. The *mesocortical tract* also projects from the ventral tegmental area, but it terminates primarily in the frontal cortex. In addition, it terminates

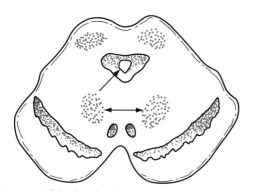

FIGURE 21-1 ■ This sketch shows a coronal view of the midbrain, which gives rise to several dopamine-producing tracts—including the nigrostriatal, mesolimbic, and mesocortical. The nigrostriatal tract begins in the substantia nigra (*SN*), the large curved black structures in the base of the midbrain (also see Fig. 18-2). Above the substantia nigra sit the red nuclei (*RN*), which receive cerebellar outflow tracts. The upper portion of the midbrain, the tectum (Latin, roof; *tego*, to cover), contains the aqueduct of Sylvius (*A*), which is surrounded by the periaqueductal gray matter and the superior colliculi (SC). The oculomotor nuclei (*III*), which give rise to the third cranial nerves, lie midline, just below the aqueduct.

in the cingulate and prefrontal gyrus, creating an overlap with the mesolimbic system. The mesocortical tract likely propagates negative symptoms of psychosis. Also, because illicit drugs affect the mesolimbic and mesocortical tracts, these tracts serve as the neural substrates for drug addiction.

In addition to these long tracts, several "short dopamine tracts" carry some clinical significance. The *tubero-infundibular tract* connects the hypothalamic region with the pituitary gland. Dopamine in this tract suppresses prolactin secretion and thus inhibits galactorrhea. (Its absence promotes galactorrhea.) Another short tract exists within the retina.

Receptors

Although neuroscientists have identified numerous dopamine receptors, the most important groups consist of D_1-like and D_2-like receptors. The D_1-like receptor group includes D_1 and D_5 receptors, and the D_2-like receptor group includes D_2, D_3, and D_5 receptors. These receptors are coupled to guanine nucleotide-binding protein (G-proteins). Because they exert their effects through second messengers, such as cyclic AMP, neuroscientists consider them "slow" neurotransmitters.

The D_1 and D_2 receptors remain the most important in extrapyramidal system disorders (Table 21-1). Both of these are plentiful in the striatum, but D_1 receptors are more abundant and more widely distributed.

When antipsychotics block D_2 receptors, the blockade induces parkinsonism, raises prolactin production, initiates galactorrhea, and may eventually lead to tardive dyskinesia. Some atypical antipsychotic agents, particularly risperidone, raise prolactin concentration more than typical antipsychotic agents. In contrast, clozapine, which has little or no D_2 receptor affinity, does not.

Conditions Due to Reduced Dopamine Activity

PHENYLKETONURIA (PKU)

Deficiencies in dopamine synthesis enzymes underlie several well-known neurologic disorders. A congenital absence of *phenylalanine hydroxylase*, the initial enzyme in the synthetic pathway, leads to *phenylketonuria* (*PKU*). In PKU, an autosomal recessive disorder, a lack of phenylalanine hydroxylase results in the accumulation of phenylalanine. As a result, alternative pathways convert the excess phenylalanine to phenylketones, which are excreted and readily detectable in the urine.

Unless corrected, PKU leads to severe mental retardation and epilepsy. In addition, because the enzyme deficiency prevents synthesis of tyrosine, which is also a melanin precursor, affected children lack color pigment in their hair and irises. The absence of color gives them a fair complexion, blond hair, and blue eyes.

If research in gene replacement therapy succeeds, it will be able to replace phenylalanine hydroxylase. Until then, affected individuals must remain on a phenylalanine-free diet.

DOPAMINE RESPONSIVE DYSTONIA (DRD)

Dopamine responsive dystonia (*DRD*), a multifactorial genetic deficiency of both phenylalanine hydroxylase and tyrosine hydroxylase, leads to a dopamine deficiency in children. Characteristically, in the afternoon, after dopamine stores have been depleted, dystonia and other abnormal involuntary movements, which may mimic cerebral palsy, develop in affected children. In the morning, after the brain has replenished dopamine stores, these children have regained full mobility and show no involuntary movements. Thus, a diurnal fluctuation of an involuntary movement disorder characterizes DRD.

L-dopa, even in small amounts, inserts itself into the synthetic pathway. It bypasses the enzyme deficiencies and allows the nigrostriatal neurons to synthesize enough dopamine to reverse the symptoms (see Chapter 18). Small doses of L-dopa restore normal mobility throughout the entire day. The response to L-dopa is so reliable that it serves as a preliminary diagnostic test for DRD.

TABLE 21-1 ■ Pharmacology of D₁ and D₂ Receptors

	D₁	D₂
Effect of stimulation on cyclic AMP production	Increased	Decreased
Greatest concentrations	Striatum, limbic system, and cerebral cortex	Striatum, substantia nigra
Effect of dopamine	Weak agonist	Strong agonist
Effects of dopamine agonists	Vary with agonist	Strong
Effect of phenothiazines	Strong antagonists	Strong antagonists
Effect of butyrophenones	Weak antagonists	Strong antagonists
Effect of clozapine	Weak antagonist	Weak antagonist

PARKINSON'S DISEASE

In Parkinson's disease, the progressive degeneration of dopaminergic neurons in the substantia nigra leads to an increasingly severe dopamine deficiency. Neurologists attempt to replace dopamine activity by administering exogenous precursors, such as L-dopa; inhibiting the metabolism of naturally occurring and medicine-induced dopamine precursors; and providing receptor agonists.

During the early stages of the disease, administration of the *dopamine precursor* L-dopa corrects the deficiency. At the same time, although it is not as clinically evident, Parkinson's disease patients have a cholinergic deficit (see later). As long as enough nigrostriatal (presynaptic) neurons remain intact, DOPA decarboxylase converts L-dopa to sufficient quantities of dopamine to reverse the symptoms (see Fig. 18-3).

As the disease progresses, the presynaptic neurons degenerate beyond the point at which they can convert dopa to dopamine, store dopamine, or appropriately release it. As a substitute or supplement for L-dopa, *dopamine agonists,* such as pramipexole, ropinirole, and apomorphine, can stimulate dopamine receptors and replicate a dopamine effect to alleviate symptoms.

As long as dopamine synthesis continues, medicines that slow L-dopa metabolism in the periphery allow remaining L-dopa to continue to form dopamine centrally. Working in that way, two Parkinson's disease medications—*carbidopa* and *entacapone*—inactivate enzymes that metabolize L-dopa and thereby enhance dopamine activity (see Fig. 18-11). Carbidopa inactivates DOPA decarboxylase, and entacapone inhibits COMT, which usually would inactivate L-dopa by converting it to 3-O-methyldopa. Both enzyme inhibitors act almost entirely outside the CNS because they have little ability to penetrate the blood–brain barrier. Therefore, they do not interfere with basal ganglia dopamine synthesis. Giving these enzyme-inhibitors along with L-dopa enables small doses of L-dopa to be effective. Moreover, the small doses of dopamine reduce its systemic side effects, such as nausea, vomiting, cardiac arrhythmias, and hypotension.

Commercial preparations combine enzyme inhibitors with L-dopa to prevent its metabolism outside of the brain. For example, Sinemet combines carbidopa with L-dopa and Stalevo adds entacapone to carbidopa and L-dopa. As compared to L-dopa alone, L-dopa-carbidopa combinations, such as Sinemet (Latin, *sine* without, *em* vomiting), almost completely eliminate the side effects of nausea and vomiting.

Another therapeutic option entails protecting dopamine itself from metabolic enzymes, particularly MAO. Selegiline (deprenyl [Eldepryl]) inhibits MAO-B, one of the two major forms of MAO. Selegiline readily penetrates the blood–brain barrier and, by inhibiting MAO-B, preserves both naturally occurring and L-dopa derived dopamine. It also diverts some dopamine metabolism to amphetamine-like byproducts that partially offset Parkinson's disease-related fatigue and depression.

Although antidepressant MAO inhibitors inactivate both MAO-A and MAO-B or only MAO-A, selegiline inhibits only MAO-B. In its usual therapeutic dose (<10 mg) for Parkinson's disease treatment, selegiline preserves dopamine but does not place patients, even if they eat tyramine-containing foods, at risk of a hypertensive crisis. Nevertheless, neurologists cautiously use serotonin-enhancing medicines, such as triptans for headaches and selective serotonin reuptake inhibitors (SSRIs) for Parkinson's disease-induced depression, in patients taking selegiline.

MEDICATION-INDUCED PARKINSONISM

In contrast to Parkinson's disease, in which presynaptic neurons have degenerated, medication-induced parkinsonism results from blockade of basal ganglia D₂ receptors. This distinction holds great clinical importance when a patient, who is under treatment with an antipsychotic agent, develops Parkinson's disease symptoms. Giving L-dopa, when antipsychotic agents block D_2 receptors, may still increase dopamine synthesis, but the dopamine will not affect the receptors or correct the symptoms. More important, excess dopamine will be diverted to stimulate frontal cortex and limbic system dopamine receptors, which may provoke or exacerbate a psychosis. Thus, when a patient who has been treated with an antipsychotic agent—even as recently as 1 month—appears to have developed Parkinson's disease, physicians should generally maintain that the patient has iatrogenic parkinsonism; search for alternative diagnoses that can cause both psychosis and parkinsonism, such as dementia with Lewy bodies or Wilson's disease; and postpone administering medicines that enhance dopamine.

NEUROLEPTIC MALIGNANT SYNDROME

In addition, apomorphine and other dopamine agonists may compensate for the absence of dopamine activity underlying the Parkinson-hyperpyrexia or central dopaminergic syndrome (more commonly known as the neuroleptic malignant syndrome, see Chapter 6). Patients usually require parenteral treatment, such an intramuscular injections of apomorphine, because the severe muscle rigidity prevents their swallowing pills and the urgency of the situation demands treatment with rapid onset of action.

Conditions Due to Excessive Dopamine Activity

Of the several mechanisms that lead to excessive dopamine activity, the most common is the administration of L-dopa. Cocaine and amphetamine also cause excessive dopamine activity because they provoke dopamine release from its presynaptic storage sites and then block its reuptake. Some psychiatric medications, such as bupropion (Wellbutrin), also block dopamine's reuptake. In a different mechanism, which may underlie some cases of tardive dyskinesia, increased sensitivity of the postsynaptic receptors results in excessive dopaminergic activity.

Whatever the cause, excessive dopamine activity produces visual hallucinations and thought disorders that can reach psychotic proportions. For example, patients with Parkinson's disease who take excessive L-dopa commonly experience hallucinations and delusions. Excessive dopamine activity also produces hyperkinetic movement disorders, such as chorea, tremor, tics, dystonia, and the oral-buccal-lingual variety of tardive dyskinesia. For example, individuals who have taken cocaine or Parkinson's disease patients taking too much L-dopa often develop chorea and dyskinesias.

On the other hand, with a small increase in dopamine activity, as occurs with bupropion, individuals enjoy a sense of well-being. With a surge of dopamine activity, as with modest doses of cocaine or amphetamine, individuals feel euphoric.

In addition to their effects on movements, dopamine and its agonists, acting through the tubero-infundibular tract, inhibit prolactin release from the pituitary gland. On the other hand, dopamine receptor blockade of the tubero-infundibular tract by typical neuroleptics and risperidone—but not clozapine or quetiapine—may enhance prolactin release and raise its serum concentration. For example, in cases of pituitary adenomas, which can either secrete prolactin or stimulate other cells to secrete it, the dopamine agonist, bromocriptine, suppresses prolactin production and reduces the size of adenomas.

Norepinephrine and Epinephrine

Synthesis and Metabolism

$$\text{Dopamine} \xrightarrow{\textit{Dopamine } \beta\textit{-hydroxylase}}$$
$$\text{Norepinephrine} \xrightarrow{\textit{Phenylethanolamine N-methyl-transferase}}$$
$$\text{Epinephrine}$$

A continuation of the dopamine pathway synthesizes norepinephrine and then epinephrine. These neurotransmitters, as well as dopamine, are *catecholamines*, a subcategory of the monoamines. As with dopamine synthesis, tyrosine hydroxylase remains the rate-limiting enzyme in their synthesis. Also, as with dopamine activity, reuptake and metabolism by COMT and MAO terminate their actions. However, in contrast to dopamine metabolism, most norepinephrine metabolism takes place outside the CNS. Moreover, its primary metabolic by-product, which is readily detectable in the urine, is *vanillylmandelic acid* (*VMA*).

Anatomy

CNS norepinephrine synthesis takes place primarily in the *locus ceruleus*, which is located in the dorsal portion of the pons (Fig. 21-2). Neurons from the locus ceruleus project to the cerebral cortex, limbic system, and reticular activating system. In addition, whereas dopamine tracts remain confined to the brain, norepinephrine tracts project down into the spinal cord.

Norepinephrine also serves as the neurotransmitter for the sympathetic nervous system's postganglionic neurons. In the adrenal gland, a synthetic pathway converts norepinephrine to epinephrine.

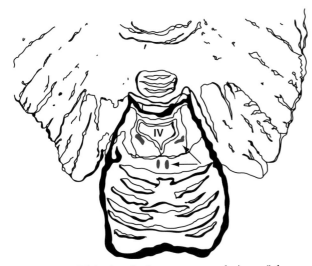

FIGURE 21-2 ■ This sketch shows a coronal view of the pons, fourth ventricle (IV), and cerebellum. This portion of the brainstem contains paired locus ceruleus (*diagonal arrow*) and dorsal raphe nucleus (*horizontal arrow*). Each locus ceruleus, which sits lateral and inferior to the fourth ventricle, gives rise to norepinephrine tracts. Each dorsal raphe nucleus gives rise to serotonin tracts that spread cephalad, to the diencephalon and cerebrum. A caudal raphe nucleus, in the pons and medulla (not pictured), gives rise to serotonin tracts that spread to the spinal cord.

Receptors

Norepinephrine receptors are located in the cerebral cortex, brainstem, and spinal cord. The α_2 and β_2 receptors, termed "autoreceptors," are situated on presynaptic neurons. Through a feedback mechanism, these presynaptic receptors modulate norepinephrine synthesis and release (Fig. 21-3). Postsynaptic receptors are also of two varieties, α_1 and β_1, and produce varied and sometimes almost opposite effects (Table 21-2).

Conditions Due to Changes in Norepinephrine Activity

In Parkinson's disease, the locus ceruleus, in addition to the substantia nigra, degenerates and loses its pigment. Loss of norepinephrine synthesis by the locus ceruleus often leads to orthostatic hypotension, sleep disturbances, and depression.

In the opposite situation, excessive stimulation of β_2 adrenergic sites leads to tremor and bronchodilatation. For example, isoproterenol and epinephrine, particularly when used for asthma, cause tremor as they alleviate bronchospasm. Conversely, β-blockers, which are contraindicated in asthma patients, suppress essential tremor (see Chapter 18).

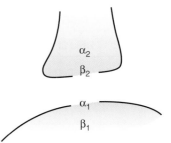

FIGURE 21-3 ■ In norepinephrine and epinephrine synapses, the postsynaptic neuron has α_1 and β_1 receptors, which initiate the sympathetic "flight or fight" response. The presynaptic neuron has α_2 and β_2 autoreceptors that modulate sympathetic responses (see Table 21-2).

Although rare, pheochromocytomas are the best known example of excessive norepinephrine and epinephrine activity. Continually or in erratic bursts, these tumors secrete norepinephrine or epinephrine. Depending on the pattern, patients have hypertension, tachycardia, and, in a small percent of cases, convulsions.

Serotonin

Synthesis and Metabolism

$$\text{Tryptophan} \xrightarrow[\textit{hydroxylase}]{\textit{Tryptophan}}$$
$$\text{5-Hydroxytryptophan} \xrightarrow[\textit{decarboxylase}]{\textit{Amino acid}}$$
$$\text{5-Hydroxytryptamine (5-HT, Serotonin)} \xrightarrow{\textit{MAO}}$$
$$\text{5-Hydroxyindoleacetic acid (5HIAA)}$$

Serotonin (5-hydroxytryptamine, 5-HT) is another monoamine, but an *indolamine* rather than a catecholamine. The synthesis of serotonin parallels the synthesis of dopamine—hydroxylation followed by decarboxylation. Although the rate-limiting enzyme in serotonin synthesis is *tryptophan* hydroxylase rather than tyrosine hydroxylase, hydroxylation remains the rate-limiting step in its synthesis. Also, reuptake and, to a lesser extent, oxidation terminate serotonin activity. One difference is that the availability of the initial substrate, tryptophan, may represent a more significant rate-limiting factor in synthesis than tryptophan hydroxylase.

MAO-A metabolizes serotonin to 5-hydroxyindoleacetic acid (5-HIAA). Although platelets and various non-neurologic cells synthesize more than 98% of the body's *total* serotonin, CSF concentrations of HIAA may reflect CNS serotonin activity. Other enzymes metabolize serotonin to melatonin.

TABLE 21-2 ■ Pharmacology of Epinephrine and Norepinephrine Receptors

Receptor*	Effect of Stimulation	Agonists	Antagonists
Presynaptic			
α_2	Vasodilation, hypotension	Clonidine	Yohimbine
β_2	Bronchodilation	Isoproterenol	Propranolol
Postsynaptic			
α_1	Vasoconstriction	Phenylephrine	Phenoxybenzamine, phentolamine
β_1	Cardiac stimulation	Dobutamine	Metoprolol

*See Fig. 21-3.

Anatomy

Serotonin-producing neurons originate predominantly in the *dorsal raphe nuclei,* which are located in the midline of the dorsal midbrain and pons (see Figs. 21-2 and 18-2). Serotonin tracts project rostrally (upward) to innervate the cortex, limbic system, striatum, and cerebellum. They also innervate intracranial blood vessels, particularly those around the trigeminal nerve.

Other serotonin-producing nuclei, the *caudal raphe nuclei,* are located in the midline of the lower pons and medulla. They project caudally (downward) to the dorsal horn of the spinal cord to provide analgesia (see Chapter 14).

Receptors

Studies have identified numerous CNS serotonin receptors ($5HT_1$-$5HT_7$) and many subtypes. Serotonin receptors differ in their function, response to medications, effect on second-messenger systems, and excitatory or inhibitory capacity. Several, such as $5\text{-}HT_{1D}$, are presynaptic autoreceptors that suppress serotonin synthesis or block its release. Whereas $5HT_1$ promotes production of adenyl cyclase and is inhibitory, $5HT_2$ promotes production of phosphatidyl inositol and is excitatory. Other serotonin receptors are usually G-protein linked and excitatory.

Conditions Due to Changes in Serotonin Activity

Serotonin plays a major role in the daily sleep-wake cycle. The activity of serotonin-producing cells reaches its highest level during arousal, drops to quiescent levels during slow-wave sleep, and disappears during REM sleep (see Chapter 17).

Depression is the disorder most closely associated with low serotonin activity. Cases of suicide by violent means are characterized by low postmortem CSF concentrations of HIAA, the serotonin metabolite. This finding, one of the most consistent in biologic psychiatry, reflects low CNS serotonin activity. Similarly, individuals with poorly controlled violent tendencies, even those

without a history of depression, have low concentrations of CSF HIAA.

Brain serotonin levels are also decreased in individuals with Parkinson's or Alzheimer's disease. Among Parkinson's disease patients, the decrease is more pronounced in those with comorbid depression.

Sumatriptan and other triptans, a mainstay of current migraine therapy, are selective $5\text{-}HT_{1D}$ receptor agonists. Once stimulated, these serotonin receptors inhibit the release of pain-producing vasoactive and inflammatory substances from trigeminal nerve endings.

A series of powerful antiemetics, including dolasetron and ondansetron, are $5HT_3$ antagonists. By affecting the medulla's *area postrema,* one of the few areas of the brain unprotected by the blood–brain barrier, they reduce chemotherapy-induced nausea and vomiting.

Although increased serotonin activity is often therapeutic, excessive activity may be dangerous. For example, combinations of medicines that simultaneously block serotonin reuptake and inhibit its metabolism lead to serotonin accumulation. These combinations may cause toxic levels and the *serotonin syndrome* (see Chapters 6 and 18).

In another dangerous situation characterized by excessive serotonin activity, D-lysergic acid diethylamide (LSD) induces hallucinations by stimulating $5\text{-}HT_2$ receptors. Similarly, although it also enhances dopaminergic activity, the hallucinogen "ecstasy" (methylenedioxymethamphetamine [MDMA]) greatly enhances serotonin activity by creating a presynaptic outpouring.

ACETYLCHOLINE (ACH)

Synthesis and Metabolism

$$\text{Acetyl CoA} + \text{Choline} \xrightarrow{\textit{Choline acetyltransferase}} \text{ACh}$$

The combination of acetyl coenzyme A and choline form acetylcholine (ACh). Although ACh synthesis depends on the enzyme *choline acetyltransferase (ChAT)*, the rate-limiting factor is the substrate, choline.

Unlike monoamines, ACh does not undergo reuptake. Instead, *cholinesterase* terminates its action in the synaptic cleft. This enzyme hydrolyzes ACh back to acetyl coenzyme A and choline.

Anatomy

In the CNS, most ACh tracts originate in the *nucleus basalis of Meynert* (also known as the *substantia innominata*) and adjacent nuclei situated in the *basal forebrain* (a rostral portion of the brainstem) (Fig. 21-4). These nuclei project their cholinergic tracts throughout the cerebral cortex but particularly to the hippocampus, amygdala, and cortical association areas. In addition, ACh serves as the autonomic nervous system and neuromuscular junction neurotransmitter (see Fig. 6-1).

Receptors

ACh receptors fall into two categories, *nicotinic* and *muscarinic*, which predominate in either the cerebral cortex or the neuromuscular junction, produce excitatory or inhibitory actions, and remain vulnerable to different blocking agents (Table 21-3).

Conditions Due to Reduced ACh Activity at the Neuromuscular Junction

In the peripheral nervous system, decreased neuromuscular ACh activity—from either impaired presynaptic ACh release or blockade of postsynaptic ACh

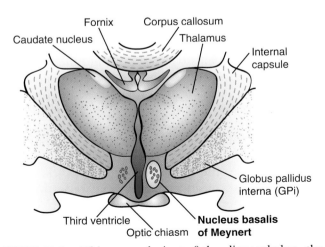

FIGURE 21-4 ■ This coronal view of the diencephalon, the uppermost brainstem region, shows the nucleus basalis of Meynert, which is situated adjacent to the third ventricle and the hypothalamus.

receptors—leads to muscle paralysis. Although some of their features may overlap, conditions that interfere with ACh activity have different etiologies and induce distinctive patterns of weakness. For example, in Lambert-Eaton syndrome, the paraneoplastic disorder, antibodies impair the release of ACh from presynaptic neurons and cause weakness of limbs (see Chapters 6 and 19). Similarly, although botulinum toxin also impairs ACh release from the presynaptic neuron, when ingested as a food poison (botulism), it primarily causes potentially fatal weakness of ocular, facial, limb, and respiratory muscles. When injected into affected muscles for treatment of focal dystonia, medicinal botulinum toxin inhibits forceful muscle contractions because it slows or prevents ACh release from the presynaptic side of the neuromuscular junction (see Chapter 18).

At the postsynaptic side of the neuromuscular junction, curare, other poisons, and antibodies, such as those associated with myasthenia gravis, block ACh receptors. The pattern of weakness in myasthenia gravis is distinctive: Patients have asymmetric paresis of the extraocular and facial muscles but not the pupils. To overcome the ACh receptor blockade in myasthenia gravis, neurologists administer *anticholinesterase* medications, such as edrophonium (Tensilon) and physostigmine, to inhibit cholinesterase and thereby reduce the breakdown of ACh in the synaptic cleft (see Chapter 6 and Fig. 7-6). The reliability of edrophonium in temporarily reversing myasthenia-induced paralysis has led to its great diagnostic value in the "Tensilon test" (see Fig. 6-3).

Conditions Due to Reduced ACh Activity in the CNS

In Alzheimer's disease, the cerebral cortex has markedly reduced cerebral ACh concentrations, ChAT activity, and muscarinic receptors (see Chapter 7). In addition, some nicotinic receptors are depleted.

To counteract the ACh deficiency in Alzheimer's disease, neurologists have attempted several strategies to enhance its synthesis or slow its metabolism. In hopes of driving ACh synthesis, they have administered precursors, such as choline and lecithin (phosphatidylcholine). Although well-conceived—along the line of providing a dopamine precursor (L-dopa) in Parkinson's disease treatment—this plan did not succeed. A complementary strategy has been to slow ACh metabolism by administering long-acting cholinesterase inhibitors that cross the blood–brain barrier. Several such cholinesterase inhibitors, such as donepezil, slow the progression of dementia in Alzheimer's disease and several other illnesses (see Chapter 7).

TABLE 21-3 ■ Cerebral Cortex and Neuromuscular Junction ACh Receptors

	Cerebral Cortex	Neuromuscular Junction
Predominant ACh receptors	Muscarinic	Nicotinic
Main action	Excitatory or inhibitory	Excitatory
Agents that block receptor	Atropine, scopolamine	Curare, α-bungarotoxin

ACh, acetylcholine.

Reduced ACh concentrations also characterize trisomy 21, which shares many clinical and physiologic features of Alzheimer's disease, and Parkinson's disease. In fact, Reduced ACh activity leading to cognitive impairment may occasionally have an iatrogenic basis. For example, scopolamine and other drugs that block muscarinic ACh receptors interfere with memory and learning—even in normal individuals. Similarly, anticholinergic medicines, including some used for movement disorders, can produce cognitive impairment.

Chlorpromazine, other typical antipsychotic agents, and tricyclic antidepressants may block muscarinic ACh receptors and cause physical anticholinergic side effects, such as accommodation paresis (see Chapter 12), drowsiness, dry mouth, urinary hesitancy, and constipation. Anticholinergic activity may rise to dangerous levels in individuals taking substances with strong anticholinergic effects, including medicines, such as atropine, scopolamine, benztropine, or trihexyphenidyl; and plants, such as jimson weed. These individuals may develop a full-scale *anticholinergic syndrome,* which consists of dilated pupils, elevated pulse and blood pressure, dry skin and hyperthermia, and delirium that may progress to coma. Physostigmine, an anticholinesterase that crosses the blood–brain barrier, restores ACh activity and thus can reverse an acute anticholinergic syndrome.

Antipsychotic agents rarely produce life-threatening anticholinergic side effects. Nevertheless, those with the greatest tendency to produce anticholinergic side effects have the least tendency to produce extrapyramidal side effects, such as parkinsonism. Conversely, antipsychotic agents with the least anticholinergic side effects have the greatest extrapyramidal side effects.

NEUROPEPTIDES

GABA—An Inhibitory Amino Acid Neurotransmitter

Synthesis and Metabolism

$$\text{Glutamate} \xrightarrow{\textit{Glutamate decarboxylase} + B_6} \text{GABA}$$

GABA and, to a lesser extent, glycine are the brain's major inhibitory neurotransmitters. Glutamate, decarboxylated by the enzyme *glutamate decarboxylase (GAD),* forms GABA. An important aspect of the synthesis is that GAD requires vitamin B_6 (pyridoxine) as a cofactor. GABA undergoes reuptake or metabolism by several enzymes.

Metabolism of GABA yields, in part, gamma-hydroxybutyrate (GHB) or oxybate. GHB, in turn, activates GABA receptors and modulates other categories of neurotransmitters.

Anatomy

Reflecting its widespread and critical role in inhibition, GABA is distributed throughout the entire CNS. However, it is concentrated in the striatum, hypothalamus, spinal cord, and temporal lobe.

Receptors

The two GABA receptors, $GABA_A$ and $GABA_B$, are complex molecules. $GABA_A$ receptors, which are more numerous and important than $GABA_B$ receptors, are gated to various molecules called *ligands.* The receptors have binding sites for benzodiazepines, barbiturates, alcohol, and some antiepileptic drugs (AEDs).

When activated by these ligands, $GABA_A$ receptor opens chloride channels, which allows negatively charged chloride ions (Cl^-) to flow into the cell. The influx of these negative charged ions into neurons lowers (makes more negative) their resting potential, which is normally -70 mV. GABA-induced lowering of the resting potential, which hyperpolarizes the membrane, has an inhibitory effect on the cell. Because of the rapidity of this hyperpolarization, which is based on changes in the permeability of ion channels, neuroscientists consider GABA and several other neurotransmitters as "fast."

The $GABA_B$ receptor, a G-protein coupled to calcium and potassium channels, is also inhibitory. Baclofen, which inhibits spasticity, binds to this receptor. However, the large numbers of ligands that bind to the $GABA_A$ receptor fail to interact with the $GABA_B$ receptor.

Conditions Due to Changes in GABA Activity

GABA deficiency is characterized by a lack of inhibition leading to excessive activity. For example, Huntington's disease, which leads to chorea, depletes GABA concentrations in the basal ganglia and CSF. The resulting lack of inhibition in the basal ganglia presumably leads to excessive involuntary movement, typically chorea. Tetanus and strychnine poisoning, which impair presynaptic GABA release, provide even more dramatic examples of the effects of increased motor activity attributable to GABA deficiency. In these disorders, spontaneous movement or minimal stimuli, such as sound or light, trigger uninhibited, painful muscle spasms.

In the *stiff-person syndrome*, formerly known as the stiff-man syndrome, antiGAD antibodies reduce GABA synthesis. The reduced GABA activity in this disorder leads to muscle stiffness and gait impairment that physicians might mistake for catatonia; however, the symptoms are not so acute or severe that neurologists might diagnose tetanus or strychnine poisoning. Neurologists typically diagnose the stiff-person syndrome, which is associated with underlying neoplasms, such as breast cancer, and various autoimmune diseases, by finding antiGAD antibodies in the serum and CSF. Immunomodulation and diazepam alleviate the stiffness of the stiff-person syndrome.

Similarly, diets deficient in pyridoxine, the cofactor for GAD, impair GABA synthesis and cause seizures. Likewise, overdose of isoniazid (INH), which interferes with pyridoxine, occasionally leads to seizures. In both cases, the seizures respond to intravenous pyridoxine.

Several AEDs are effective, in part, because they increase GABA activity. For example, valproate (Depakote) increases brain GABA concentration. Tiagabine inhibits GABA reuptake. Topiramate (Topamax) enhances $GABA_A$ receptor activity. Vigabatrin* increases GABA concentrations by reducing GABA-transaminase.

GHB, a metabolite of GABA, which gained notoriety as the "date rape drug," remains an addictive, popular drug of abuse. As an intoxicant, GHB induces an almost immediate—within 15 minutes after ingestion—deep sleep-like state. After about 2 hours, victims rapidly return to full consciousness with little or no recall. Studies of its hypnotic capacity in narcolepsy patients showed that by taking GHB at bedtime, these patients enjoyed sound sleep and, more important, greatly reduced cataplexy (see Chapter 17).

In a different situation, flumazenil, a benzodiazepine antagonist, blocks the actions of GABA at its receptor and reverses benzodiazepine-induced stupor and hepatic encephalopathy. In the case of hepatic encephalopathy, flumazenil presumably displaces false, benzodiazepine-like neurotransmitters from GABA receptors (see Chapter 7).

Glutamate—An Excitatory Amino Acid Neurotransmitter

Synthesis, Metabolism, and Anatomy

$$\text{Glutamine} \xrightarrow{\textit{Glutaminase}} \text{Glutamate}$$

Glutamate, a simple amino acid synthesized from glutamine, is the most important excitatory neurotransmitters. Reuptake into presynaptic neurons and adjacent support cells terminates glutamate activity. To a lesser extent, glutamate undergoes nonspecific metabolism. Its tracts project widely throughout the brain and spinal cord.

Aspartate is another excitatory amino acid. However, compared to glutamate, its anatomy and clinical importance are less well established.

Receptors

Of several glutamate receptors, N-methyl-D-aspartate (*NMDA*) is the most important. It has binding sites for glycine, phencyclidine (PCP), and a PCP congener, ketamine (see later). Through its interactions with NMDA receptors, which regulate calcium channels, glutamate acts as a fast neurotransmitter.

Conditions Due to Changes in NMDA Activity

Excessive NMDA activity floods the neuron with potentially lethal concentrations of calcium and sodium in several disorders. Through this process, termed *excitotoxicity*, glutamate-NMDA interactions lead to neuron death through apoptosis. Excitotoxicity may be intimately involved in the pathophysiology of epilepsy, stroke, neurodegenerative diseases (such as Parkinson's and Huntington's diseases), head trauma, and, conceivably, schizophrenia.

Consequently, one approach to stemming the progression of neurodegenerative diseases has been to use medicines that block glutamate-NMDA interactions. Despite the sound rationale, such medicines provide only a modicum of neuroprotection. For example, riluzole (Rilutek), which decreases glutamate

---

*Vigabatrin, an AED, remains an investigational drug in the United States.

activity, only transiently interrupts the progression of amyotrophic lateral sclerosis (ALS). Similarly, memantine (Namenda), an NMDA receptor antagonist, blocks its deleterious excitatory neurotransmission and slows the progression of Alzheimer's disease by approximately 6 months. Also, the glutamate antagonists, such as gabapentin and lamotrigine, are also clinically useful because they act as AEDs.

Deficient NMDA activity can also be harmful. For example, PCP and ketamine may block the NMDA calcium channel and cause psychosis.

Other Neuropeptides

Endorphins, enkephalins, and substance P, which are situated in the spinal cord and brain, provide endogenous analgesia in response to painful stimuli (see Chapter 14). Substance P and, to a lesser degree, other neuropeptides are depleted in Alzheimer's disease. Other neuropeptides include somatostatin, cholecystokinin, and vasoactive intestinal peptide (VIP).

A pair of neuropeptides, hypocretin-1 and -2, also known as orexin A and B, are excitatory neurotransmitters that play a crucial—but as yet not clearly defined—role in integrating locomotion, metabolism, appetite, and the sleep-wake cycle (see Chapter 17). Synthesized in the hypothalamus, where they are cleaved from a large precursor protein, these neuropeptides increase during wakefulness and rapid eye movement (REM) sleep, and decrease during nonrapid eye movement (NREM) sleep. Unlike normal individuals, narcolepsy patients have little or no hypocretin in their CSF and their hypothalamus is devoid of hypocretin-producing cells.

NITRIC OXIDE

Synthesis and Metabolism

$$\text{Arginine} + \text{Oxygen} \xrightarrow{\textit{Nitric oxide synthase}} \text{Nitric oxide} + \text{Citrulline}$$

Nitric oxide (NO), the product of a complex synthesis, is an important neurotransmitter for endothelial cells and the immunologic system. NO should not be confused with nitrous oxide (N_2O), which is a gaseous anesthetic ("laughing gas"). N_2O, when inhaled daily as a form of drug abuse, leads to vitamin B_{12} deficiency, which results in peripheral neuropathy and spinal cord damage.

Important in many roles, NO inhibits platelet aggregation, dilates blood vessels, and boosts host defenses against infections and tumors. However, from a neurologic viewpoint, its main functions include regulating cerebral blood flow and facilitating penile erections. In the CNS, NO may have a neuroprotective effect.

Receptors

NO diffuses into cells and interacts directly with enzymes and iron-sulfur complexes; however, it has no specific membrane receptors.

Conditions Due to Changes in NO Activity

The best-known role of NO is in generating erections (see Chapter 16). With sexual stimulation of the penis, parasympathetic neurons produce and release NO. NO then promotes the production of cyclic guanylate cyclase monophosphate (cGMP), which dilates the vascular system and creates an erection. Sildenafil slows the metabolism of cGMP and increases blood flow in the penis, which, in turn, produces, strengthens, and prolongs erections.

NEUROLOGIC ASPECTS OF DRUG ABUSE

Cocaine

Pharmacology

Cocaine and amphetamine (see later) act primarily as CNS stimulants through sympathomimetic mechanisms. Cocaine provokes a discharge of dopamine from its presynaptic storage vesicles and then blocks its reuptake. Although resulting more from the blocked reuptake than forced discharge, dopamine synaptic concentration greatly increases and overstimulates its receptors, especially those in the mesolimbic system.

Cocaine similarly blocks the reuptake of serotonin and norepinephrine. The enhanced serotonin activity presumably produces euphoria. The excess norepinephrine activity causes pronounced sympathomimetic effects, such as arrhythmias, hypertension, vasospasm, and pupillary dilation. (Similarly, following instillation of 2% to 10% cocaine eye drops, normal pupils widely dilate because cocaine leads to local α_1 stimulation.)

Cocaine also blocks peripheral nerve impulses. Thus, when cocaine is applied or injected at a specific site, it produces local anesthesia.

Individuals who use cocaine sometimes inject it, but usually they smoke its solid alkaloid form (*crack*). Although cocaine users rarely swallow it, however, couriers ("mules") occasionally have cocaine-filled condoms break open in their intestines, prompting a massive absorption of the drug.

Plasma and liver enzymes rapidly metabolize cocaine, giving it a half-life as brief as 30 to 90 minutes. However, urine toxicology screens may detect cocaine's metabolic products for about 2 days.

Clinical Effects

The immediate effects of cocaine typically consist of a short period of intense euphoria accompanied by a sense of increased sexual, physical, and mental power. Individuals using cocaine remain fully alert—even hypervigilant. Their heightened awareness is a prominent exception to the general rule that patients in delirium or a toxic-metabolic encephalopathy are lethargic or stuporous and have a fluctuating level of consciousness (see Chapter 7). In contrast to the miosis produced by opioids, such as heroin, cocaine users have dilated pupils.

Cocaine, like other stimulants, not only reduces sleep time, it particularly suppresses rapid eye movement (REM) sleep, often to the point of eliminating it. Another characteristic effect follows individuals' discontinuing cocaine: They experience a rebound in REM sleep as if to compensate for the loss of REM during intoxication (see Chapter 17).

Overdose

When taking greater than their usual dose, cocaine users may become agitated, irrational, hallucinatory, and paranoid. Moreover, cocaine's sympathomimetic and dopaminergic effects may produce permanent neurologic damage, such as strokes, myocardial infarctions, and seizures.

Cocaine-induced strokes usually occur within 2 hours of cocaine use. Although some cocaine-induced strokes are nonhemorrhagic ("bland") cerebral infarctions, most are cerebral hemorrhages related to cocaine-induced hypertension or vasculitis.

Cocaine-induced seizures, which also occur within 2 hours of drug use, disproportionately follow first-time exposure. Sometimes they are the presenting sign of a cocaine-induced stroke. In fact, seizures related to those substances constitute a marker of dependency. For practical purposes, the development of a seizure disorder in a young adult should prompt an investigation for drug abuse.

In contrast, even an overdose of barbiturates or benzodiazepines rarely causes strokes or seizures. Withdrawal from either of these substances or alcohol, however, frequently precipitates not only seizures but also status epilepticus (see Chapter 10).

Probably because it suddenly increases dopamine activity, cocaine use also produces involuntary movements, such as tic-like facial muscle contractions,

chorea, tremor, dystonia, and repetitive, purposeless behavior (stereotypies, see Chapter 18). Cocaine also exacerbates tics in individuals with Tourette's or other tic disorder. When cocaine induces chorea, patients' legs and feet move incessantly, and they cannot stand at attention. Neurologists label these movements "crack dancing" and point out that they mimic chorea, restless legs syndrome, akathisia, and undertreated agitation.

In addition, cocaine seems to increase sensitivity to neuroleptic-induced dystonic reactions. For example, hospitalized cocaine users, compared to other inpatients, have a many-fold increase in dystonic reactions to neuroleptics.

Studies have not established the frequency, nature, or severity of cocaine-induced cognitive impairment. However, some studies indicate that individuals repeatedly using cocaine have cognitive defects that consist of impairments in attention, verbal learning, and memory. When these deficits are present, a stroke and other brain damage are probably responsible.

Computed tomography (CT) of habitual cocaine users shows cerebral atrophy. With its superior resolution, magnetic resonance imaging (MRI) also shows demyelination, hyperintensities, vasospasm, and stroke-like defects. Functional imaging, such as single photon emission computed tomography (SPECT), shows multiple patchy areas of hypoperfusion (a "Swiss cheese" pattern).

Treatment of Intoxication and Overdose

Behavioral and cognitive aspects of cocaine overdose generally resolve spontaneously. Rest, seclusion, and, if necessary, benzodiazepines will moderate agitation and related symptoms. Dopamine-blocking antipsychotic agents will reduce or eliminate psychosis and violent behavior; however, because these neuroleptics, as well as cocaine itself, lower the seizure threshold, physicians must administer them judiciously. Potentially life-threatening hypertension may require aggressive treatment with an α-blocker antihypertensive medication, such as phentolamine (see Table 21-2).

Withdrawal

When deprived of cocaine, habitual users often suddenly lose their energy and ability to appreciate their normally pleasurable activities (i.e., they "crash"). While typically craving the stimulation, they languish in a dysphoric mood. Vivid, disturbing dreams, which probably represent REM rebound, disturb their sleep.

Reflecting the lack of dopamine receptor stimulation during withdrawal, dopamine agonists and other dopamine-enhancing medications often alleviate some withdrawal symptoms. Probably by restoring depleted serotonin stores, antidepressants may also help.

Amphetamine

The term "amphetamine" commonly refers to illicit stimulants, particularly methamphetamine (crystal, ice, speed), and stimulant medications, such as dextroamphetamine (Dexedrine) and methylphenidate (Ritalin). Like cocaine, amphetamine provokes a powerful presynaptic dopamine discharge and then blocks its reuptake. To a lesser degree, it also increases norepinephrine activity that produces sympathomimetic effects and complications, including strokes. Because the half-life of amphetamine, in general, is about 8 hours, its effects persist much longer than those of cocaine.

When given to children and adults with attention deficit hyperactivity disorder (ADHD), amphetamine paradoxically suppresses physical and mental hyperactivity. One theory suggests that amphetamine stimulates inhibitory neurons but does not affect the less sensitive excitatory ones.

Amphetamines produce cocaine-like effects, including a hyperalert state, decreased total sleep time, and reduced proportion of REM sleep. However, its effects last longer than cocaine's. For example, methamphetamine, which is lipophilic and therefore readily crosses the blood–brain barrier, has a half-life of 12 hours.

Overdose

As with cocaine, amphetamine often causes bland or hemorrhagic strokes from hypertension or vasculitis. Also like cocaine, amphetamine precipitates dyskinesias and stereotypies. However, an overdose rarely causes seizures.

During an amphetamine overdose, thought disorders, which may be accompanied by hallucinations, can reach psychotic proportions. Similarly, chronic amphetamine use might lead to long-lasting cognitive impairment and psychiatric disturbances.

Because the pharmacology of amphetamine is similar to cocaine's, treatment of amphetamine overdose also relies on dopamine blocking neuroleptics. Likewise, symptoms of withdrawal from these substances and their treatment are similar.

MDMA

MDMA, commonly known as ecstasy, also acts predominantly as a stimulant. MDMA creates its effect by suddenly emptying presynaptic serotonin stores to create a wave of serotonin. The MDMA-induced increase in serotonin activity contrasts to the cocaine and amphetamine-induced increase in dopamine activity. With continued use, MDMA destroys serotoninergic neurons and creates cognitive impairments.

Opioids

Pharmacology

Opioid is a broad term encompassing medicinal narcotics, "street" narcotics, and endogenous opiate-like substances (see endorphins, Chapter 14). Although opioids may inhibit the reuptake of monamines and affect other neurotransmitters, their primary action is directly on a group of specific opioid receptors that are situated in the brain and spinal cord. Of the several opioid receptors, the *mu* receptors mediate opioid-induced euphoria.

Clinical Effects

Medicinal opioids may relieve pain and suffering and reduce anxiety. Higher doses, usually associated with the early stages of abuse, lead to a burst of euphoria, a sense of well-being, and then sleepiness. Sometimes opioids produce paradoxical agitation, psychosis, and mood changes. Intravenously administered opioids routinely lead to nausea and vomiting, which presumably result from opioids directly stimulating the medulla's chemoreceptor trigger zone. Either directly related to intravenous drug abuse or indirectly to their lifestyle, drug abusers suffer brain damage from vasospasm, bacterial endocarditis, acquired immunodeficiency syndrome (AIDS), foreign particle emboli, and head trauma.

Overdose

Opioid overdose causes a characteristic triad of coma, miosis, and respiratory depression. The respiratory depression takes the form of slowed rate rather than shallower depth, and often causes neurogenic pulmonary edema. The coma routinely leads to nerve compression from prolonged, static positioning of the body (see Chapter 5). In contrast to the complications of stimulants, opioid-induced strokes or seizures rarely occur.

If an overdose leads to cerebral hypoxia, which particularly damages the basal ganglia and cerebral cortex, it can result in cognitive impairment. However, formal studies have failed to demonstrate cognitive impairment with chronic, well-controlled opioid use. For example, individuals on methadone maintenance programs, patients treated with opioids for chronic pain, and well-known intellectuals who abused opioids do not show signs of cognitive decline.

Several antagonists, which displace morphine and other medicinal opioids from their receptors, reverse opioid-induced respiratory depression and other life-threatening effects. On the other hand, in the case of patients under treatment with opioids for severe pain, opioid antagonists also reverse the analgesia and allow patients' pain and agony to return. Sometimes administering an opioid antagonist, such as naloxone (Narcan), precipitates narcotic withdrawal. Another antagonist, naltrexone (ReVia), an oral opioid maintenance or detoxification medication, also prevents opioids from reaching their receptors and thus blocks their usual effects.

Withdrawal from Chronic Use

Symptoms of opioid withdrawal typically consist of intense drug- or medication-seeking behavior, dysphoric mood, lacrimation, abdominal cramps, piloerection, and autonomic hyperactivity. Heroin withdrawal symptoms begin within several hours after the last dose and peak at 1 to 3 days. Because of its longer half-life, withdrawal symptoms from methadone begin after 1 to 2 days after the last dose and peak at about 6 days. Clonidine, the α_2 norepinephrine agonist, may alleviate autonomic symptoms of opioid withdrawal.

Other Clinical Aspects

Physicians should be aware of several miscellaneous aspects of opioid use. Medical personnel, including physicians, dentists, nurses, and other health care workers, are particularly at risk for surreptitious opioid abuse. They have been prone to develop illicit dependancy on readily available, highly addictive opioids, particularly meperidine (Demerol) and fentanyl (Sublimaze).

Physicians should avoid prescribing several medicines, for any reason, to patients enrolled in methadone-maintenance programs. For example, phenytoin (Dilantin) and carbamazepine (Tegretol), but not valproate (Depakote), enhance methadone metabolism or interfere with its receptor. When given to individuals taking daily methadone, these medicines will likely precipitate opioid withdrawal symptoms. Increasing the methadone dose when these medicines are added will greatly reduce or even prevent the problem.

Compared to morphine, heroin more easily penetrates the blood–brain barrier. It does not have a specific CNS receptor, but, like morphine and other opioids, attaches to the mu receptor and produces the same effects. Contrary to some popular pronouncements, heroin holds no medically distinguishable advantage as a treatment for cancer patients.

Phencyclidine (PCP)

PCP is simultaneously a central analgesic, depressant, and hallucinogen. Individuals usually either snort, swallow, or smoke it, often with marijuana or tobacco. In its primary mechanism of action, PCP blocks the NMDA receptor and prevents glutamate from interacting with it. The PCP-NMDA receptor interaction thus prevents the normal glutamate-induced influx of calcium.

In small doses, PCP causes symptoms and signs similar to alcohol intoxication, such as euphoria, dysarthria, ataxia, and nystagmus. At higher doses, it causes disorganized and bizarre thinking, negativism, and visual hallucinations.

Moreover, PCP may cause not only delusions, paranoia, and hallucinations (the positive symptoms of schizophrenia) but also psychomotor retardation and emotional withdrawal (the negative symptoms). With its capacity to produce the full range of schizophrenia symptoms, PCP stands apart from LSD and other psychomimetic drugs, which usually produce only the positive symptoms. Because it has this feature, PCP serves as a laboratory model of the illness.

Overdose

PCP overdose causes combinations of muscle rigidity, characteristic bursts of horizontal and vertical nystagmus, stereotypies, and a blank stare. The muscle rigidity may evolve into rhabdomyolysis that mimics the neuroleptic malignant syndrome. Individuals who have taken an overdose have been described as existing in "PCP coma"—with their eyes open, unaware of their surroundings, and oblivious to pain. In addition, PCP overdose often causes seizures that progress to status epilepticus; however, PCP rarely causes strokes. Another important aspect of PCP overdose is that the drug-induced psychosis often leads to violent incidents, such as motor vehicle accidents, confrontations with police, and drowning.

Multiple exposures to PCP, according to individual reports, may produce chronic memory impairment and confusion. In addition, one study found that about one fourth of individuals who experienced a PCP-induced psychosis returned in about 1 year with the diagnosis of schizophrenia.

Treatment

Unlike opioid antagonists, no particular medicine acts as an antagonist for PCP. Treatment usually includes seclusion, sedation with benzodiazepines for mild intoxications, and other symptomatic treatments. Because PCP often causes muscle rigidity, physicians should reserve antipsychotic agents, such as haloperidol, which might further increase muscle rigidity, for extreme situations. If muscle rigidity develops, muscle relaxants, such as dantrolene, may prevent rhabdomyolysis. Benzodiazepines will abort seizures.

Ketamine

Ketamine is a legitimate general veterinarian anesthetic. It has a chemical structure similar to PCP and also blocks NMDA receptors. Although ketamine produces many of the same mood and thought disturbances as PCP, its effects are briefer and less likely to include hallucinations, agitation, and violence.

Marijuana

Marijuana (cannabis) is a cannabinoid that contains several psychoactive ingredients, but the most potent is Δ9-THC. The cerebral cortex, basal ganglia, hippocampus, and cerebellum all contain specific Δ9-THC receptors.

In mild, recreational doses, marijuana produces euphoria, and pleasantly altered perceptions, but it slows thinking and impairs judgment. Its effects usually last 1 to 3 hours, but heavy use can result in symptoms that last from 1 to 2 days. As with other illicit drugs, marijuana reduces REM sleep.

Overdose

Large dose of marijuana can cause severe anxiety or psychosis that includes hallucinations and delusions. If these symptoms do not spontaneously recede, benzodiazepines or, if necessary, antipsychotic agents can control them. Unlike overdoses of other drugs of abuse, marijuana overdoses are not fatal. Moreover, they rarely if ever cause acute neurologic problems, such as seizures or strokes.

Other Considerations

Albeit to a minor degree, marijuana possesses several properties that serve as the springboard in attempts at legalization. For example, in addition to its mood-elevating properties, marijuana purportedly possesses anticonvulsant activity, reduces intraocular pressure, reduces chemotherapy-induced nausea and vomiting, and provides analgesia for multiple sclerosis-induced pain.

On the other hand, advocates overstate its medicinal benefits. Conventional medicines are more effective for all these purposes. D_2 dopamine and $5HT_3$ serotonin antagonists, for example, are much more effective than marijuana as antiemetics. Also, although marijuana lowers intraocular pressure, its effect is too mild and short-lived to constitute a useful, reliable treatment for glaucoma patients.

Moreover, marijuana has some unequivocal deleterious effects. It is associated with an inordinate number of motor vehicle accidents. Also, drug enforcement agencies, attempting to kill marijuana plants, spray them with toxic chemicals (herbicides). Those herbicides remain on the leaves of surviving plants and smokers inhale their residue.

For most marijuana exposures, cognitive impairments, if they occur at all, are mild and transient. However, heavy, long-term use causes dose-related impairments in memory, executive function, and psychomotor speed that last for more than 4 weeks. Long-term marijuana use also probably induces cerebral atrophy. On the other hand, studies have been unable to attribute either dementia or an "amotivational syndrome," consisting of lack of energy and drive to work, to marijuana use.

Nicotine

Nicotine affects mesolimbic nicotinic receptors, which represent a minority of cerebral cortex cholinergic receptors. As with other drugs of abuse, nicotine probably stimulates the release of mesolimbic dopamine to provide pleasure and modulate affect. However, the main impetus for chronic tobacco use lies more in suppressing withdrawal symptoms—anxiety, restlessness, tremulousness, and craving—than providing pleasure.

Virtually all individuals who use nicotine obtain it from cigarettes, which, as the tobacco industry has acknowledged, serve primarily as nicotine delivery devices. Although nicotine in cigarettes has no appreciable cognitive effect, individuals going through withdrawal may have temporary cognitive impairment because of anxiety, poor concentration, and preoccupation with their lack of cigarettes.

During attempts to stop cigarette smoking, other nicotine delivery systems may alleviate withdrawal symptoms. For example nicotine chewing gum, nasal spray, and transdermal patches can provide blood nicotine concentrations equal to or greater than those from cigarettes. Alternatives or supplements to cigarette-derived nicotine, bupropion (Wellbutrin) or sustained-release bupropion (Zyban), may also help in withdrawal because, like nicotine, they increase dopamine concentration in the mesolimbic system.

REFERENCES

Neurotransmitters

1. Ackerman MJ, Clapham DE: Ion channels—Basic science and clinical disease. N Engl J Med 336:1575–1586, 1997.
2. Cooper JR, Bloom FE, Roth RH: *The Biochemical Basis of Neuropharmacology*, 8th ed. New York, Oxford University Press, 2003.

3. Hilker R, Thomas AV, Klein JC, et al: Dementia in Parkinson's disease: Functional imaging of cholinergic and dopaminergic pathways. Neurology 65:1716–1722, 2005.

4. Murinson BB: Stiff-person syndrome. Neurologist 10:131–137, 2004.

5. Stahl SM, Munter N: *Essential Psychopharmacology: Neuroscientific Basis and Practical Applications,* 2nd ed. Cambridge, Cambridge University Press, 2000.

Drug Abuse

6. Abramowicz M (ed): Acute reactions to drugs of abuse. Med Lett 44:21–24, 2002.

7. Bolla KI, Brown K, Eldreth D, et al: Dose-related neurocognitive effects of marijuana use. Neurology 59:1337–1343, 2002.

8. Bolla KI, McCann UD, Ricaurte GA: Memory impairment in abstinent MDMA ("ecstasy") users. Neurology 51:1532–1537, 1998.

9. Burst JCM: *Neurologic Aspects of Substance Abuse*, 2nd ed. Boston, Butterworth-Heinemann, 2004.

10. Cami J, Farré M: Drug addiction. N Engl J Med 349:975–986, 2003.

11. Derlet RW, Rice P, Horowitz BZ, et al: Amphetamine toxicity: Experience with 127 cases. J Emerg Med 7:157–161, 1989.

12. Herning RI, Better W, Tate K, et al: Neuropsychiatric alterations in MDMA users. Ann N Y Acad Sci 1053:20–27, 2005.

13. Iversen L: Cannabis and the brain. Brain 126:1252–1270, 2003.

14. McCarron MM, Schulze BW, Thompson GA, et al: Acute phencyclidine intoxication: Incidence of clinical findings in 1,000 cases. Ann Emerg Med 10:237–242, 1981.

15. Pascual-Leone A, Dhuna A, Anderson DC: Cerebral atrophy in habitual cocaine abusers: A planimetric study. Neurology 41:34–38, 1991.

16. Qureshi AI, Akbar MS, Czander E, et al: Crack cocaine use and stroke in young patients. Neurology 48:431–345, 1997.

17. Snead OC, Gibson KM: γ-hydroxybutyric acid. N Engl J Med 352:2721–2732, 2005.

18. Spivey WH, Euerle B: Neurologic complications of cocaine abuse. Ann Emerg Med 19:1422–1428, 1990.

19. Weiner WJ, Rabinstein A, Levin B, et al: Cocaine-induced persistent dyskinesias. Neurology 56:964–965, 2001.

20. Zakzanis KK, Young DA: Memory impairment in abstinent MDMA ("ecstasy") users: A longitudinal investigation. Neurology 56:966–969, 2001.

1. Which are the effects of opioids?
   a. Block reuptake of dopamine into presynaptic neurons
   b. Routinely cause agitation
   c. Cause hypertension
   d. Slow respiratory rate
   e. Stimulate the area postrema
   f. Cause miosis
   g. Reduce the depth of respiration
   h. Cause vomiting

   Answers: d, e, f, h.

2. Which features frequently complicate opioid overdose?
   a. Cerebral hemorrhage
   b. Respiratory arrest
   c. Seizures
   d. Radial nerve palsy
   e. Tics
   f. Stereotypies
   g. Psychotic thinking
   h. Pulmonary edema

   Answers: b, d, h.

3. Which three causes of seizures are disproportionately more common in 15- to 50-year-old individuals than in older adults?
   a. Marijuana use
   b. Head trauma
   c. Drug abuse
   d. Sleep deprivation
   e. Brain tumors
   f. Strokes

   Answers: b, c, d.

4. Which substance's primary active ingredient is Δ9-THC?
   a. Cocaine
   b. Phencyclidine (PCP)
   c. Amphetamine
   d. Cannabis
   e. Heroin

   Answer: d. Cannabis is marijuana.

5. When the patient develops unilateral miosis, ptosis, and anhidrosis, which neurotransmitter is most likely deficient?

   a. Acetylcholine
   b. Dopamine
   c. Norepinephrine
   d. Serotonin

   Answer: c. The patient has Horner's syndrome, which is a manifestation of sympathetic denervation.

6. A former heroin addict in a methadone maintenance program develops a seizure for which he is hospitalized and treated with phenytoin (Dilantin). A psychiatry consultation is solicited when the patient becomes combative. The psychiatrist finds that he has piloerection, muscle cramps, nausea, and abdominal pain. Clinical chemistry and hematology laboratory results are normal. Which is the best course of action?
   a. Administer a minor tranquilizer.
   b. Administer a major tranquilizer.
   c. Increase the dose of phenytoin.
   d. Increase the dose of methadone.
   e. Demand CT and EEG results before making a diagnosis.
   f. None of the above.

   Answer: d. Opioid addicts often undergo withdrawal when hospitalized and given inadequate methadone. In addition, phenytoin increases the metabolism of methadone.

7. Which is the primary mechanism of action of acute cocaine administration?
   a. It enhances dopamine activity.
   b. It enhances serotonin metabolism.
   c. It reduces serotonin metabolism.
   d. It reduces gamma-aminobutyric acid (GABA) levels.

   Answer: a. Cocaine suddenly increases dopamine activity by triggering its release from presynaptic nerve endings and then blocking its reuptake.

8. Which is not a sign of excessive sympathetic activity?
   a. Tachycardia
   b. Eyelid retraction
   c. Hypertension
   d. Miosis
   e. Anxiety

   Answer: d. With excessive sympathetic activity, pupils dilate.

9. Which one of the following is not a manifestation of amphetamine use?
   a. Weight loss
   b. Insomnia
   c. Psychosis similar to cocaine-induced psychosis
   d. Parkinsonism
   e. Stereotypies

Answer: d. Use of synthetic narcotics, particularly MPTP, but not amphetamines, has been routinely complicated by parkinsonism. MPTP destroys nigrostriatal neurons.

10. The police bring a comatose young man to the emergency room. He has a weak and thready pulse, infrequent and shallow respirations, and miosis. A chest x-ray shows pulmonary edema. After securing an airway, which should be the staff's next treatment?
    a. Naloxone
    b. Thiamine
    c. Haloperidol
    e. Glucose

Answer: a. He probably has a narcotic overdose, which typically causes coma, depressed respirations, and miosis. In severe cases, it also causes pulmonary edema. Naloxone, a narcotic antagonist, is the best treatment. Because its half-life is often shorter than the half-life of narcotics, patients often require repeated naloxone treatments. One caveat is that naloxone may precipitate withdrawal in narcotic addicts.

11. Which statement regarding vomiting is false?
    a. Opioids typically induce vomiting.
    b. Marijuana reduces nausea and vomiting induced by chemotherapy.
    c. The blood–brain barrier protects the brain's vomiting center.
    d. Lesions located in posterior fossa structures are more apt to induce vomiting than those in the other parts of the brain.

Answer: c. Vomiting is induced by stimulation of the chemoreceptor trigger zone (CTZ), which is located in the area postrema of the medulla. Although it generally covers almost the entire brain, the blood–brain barrier does not protect this particular region. D_2 dopamine blockers and $5HT_3$ antagonists have tremendous antiemetic potential. Marijuana has relatively weak antiemetic effects that do not justify its popular support as a chemotherapy adjunct.

12. After physicians revive a 29-year-old man from an opioid overdose, they find that he has paresis of his right wrist extensor muscles and impairment of his ability to make a fist. He is alert and has normal mental and language ability. The strength in his other arm and both legs is normal. Babinski signs are absent. His gait is normal. Where is the most likely location of his injury?
    a. Left cerebral hemisphere
    b. Left internal capsule
    c. Near the right humerus spiral groove
    d. Near the right wrist

Answer: c. He has a "wrist drop" from compression of his right radial nerve as it winds around the spiral groove of the humerus. Because he cannot extend his wrists, he cannot make a fist. Radial nerve and other nerve compressions, known as "pressure palsies," are frequent complications of alcohol and drug overdose. The normal language function indicates that the lesion is not located in the cerebrum.

13. Which metabolic product of dopamine is measurable in the CSF?
    a. Monoamine oxidase (MAO)
    b. Homovanillic acid (HVA)
    c. Catechol-O-methyltransferase (COMT)
    d. Vanillylmandelic acid (VMA)

Answer: b. MAO and COMT are metabolic enzymes of dopamine. VMA is a metabolic product of norepinephrine that is excreted in the urine.

14. Which is the rate-limiting enzyme in the synthesis of dopamine?
    a. DOPA decarboxylase
    b. Tyrosine hydroxylase
    c. MAO
    d. COMT
    e. Dopamine β-hydroxylase

Answer: b.

15. Of the enzymes listed in Question 14, which converts dopamine to norepinephrine?

Answer: e.

16. Of the choices listed in Question 14, which is the rate-limiting enzyme in the synthesis of norepinephrine?

Answer: b.

17. Which two statements about stimulating D_1 and D_2 dopamine receptors are correct?
    a. Stimulation of the D_1 receptor increases cyclic AMP activity.
    b. Stimulation of the D_2 receptor decreases cyclic AMP activity.
    c. Stimulation of the D_1 receptor decreases ATP to cyclic AMP production.

d. Stimulation of the D_2 receptor increases ATP to cyclic AMP production.

Answers: a, b. A characteristic difference between these two receptors is that D_1 receptor activity increases ATP to cyclic AMP production through adenyl cyclase.

18. Which dopamine tract is responsible for the elevated prolactin concentration induced by many antipsychotic agents?
    a. Nigrostriatal
    b. Mesolimbic
    c. Tubero-infundibular
    d. None of the above

Answer: c. The tubero-infundibular tract connects the hypothalamus and the pituitary gland. Dopamine D_2 blockade provokes prolactin release and elevates serum prolactin concentration. However, dopamine blockade of the mesolimbic system accounts for these medicines' antipsychotic effect.

19. Which is the primary site for conversion of norepinephrine to epinephrine?
    a. Locus ceruleus
    b. Striatum
    c. Adrenal medulla
    d. Nigrostriatal tact

Answer: c.

20. Which is the major pathway for serotonin metabolism?
    a. Metabolism by COMT to 5-hydroxyindole-acetic acid (5-HIAA)
    b. Metabolism by MAO to 5-HIAA
    c. Metabolism by decarboxylase to HVA
    d. Metabolism by HVA to 5-HIAA

Answer: b. Although serotonin mostly undergoes reuptake, MAO metabolizes the remainder to 5-HIAA.

21. Where is the main site of serotonin production?
    a. Dorsal raphe nuclei
    b. Regions adjacent to the aqueduct in the midbrain
    c. Striatum
    d. None of the above

Answer: d. Almost all serotonin is produced in platelets and various non-neurologic cells. Within the brain, serotonin-producing neurons are located predominantly in the dorsal raphe nuclei, which are adjacent to the aqueduct in the dorsal midbrain. Although plentiful, these neurons produce only 2% of the body's total serotonin.

22. A 48-year-old man, with a history of major depression, commits suicide by igniting several sticks of dynamite. Which neurotransmitter abnormality would investigators most likely find on postmortem examination?
    a. Low concentrations of CSF HVA
    b. Low concentrations of CSF HIAA
    c. Low GABA concentrations in the basal ganglia
    d. High dopamine concentrations

Answer: b. Low concentration of CSF HIAA, which may reflect decreased CNS serotonin activity, characterizes violent suicides. Low GABA concentrations in the basal ganglia are characteristic of Huntington's disease.

23. Which two statements are false regarding ACh receptors in the cerebral cortex?
    a. They are predominantly muscarinic.
    b. They are predominantly nicotinic.
    c. Atropine blocks muscarinic receptors.
    d. Scopolamine, which antagonizes muscarinic receptors, induces memory impairments that mimic Alzheimer's disease dementia.
    e. Botulinum toxin penetrates the blood–brain barrier to block cholinergic receptors and cause memory impairments.

Answers: b, e. Cerebral cortex ACh receptors are predominantly muscarinic. Blocking CNS muscarinic receptors, with scopolamine for example, causes memory impairments, even in normal individuals. Botulinum toxin, which impairs release of ACh from the presynaptic neuron at the neuromuscular junction, does not penetrate the blood–brain barrier or cause memory impairments.

24. In the reaction, acetyl-CoA + choline to acetylcholine, which is the rate-limiting factor?
    a. Choline acetyltransferase (ChAT)
    b. Acetyl CoA
    c. Choline
    d. None of the above

Answer: c.

25. Which two comparisons of Lambert-Eaton syndrome and myasthenia gravis are true?
    a. Lambert-Eaton syndrome is a paraneoplastic syndrome, whereas myasthenia gravis is an autoimmune disorder.
    b. Lambert-Eaton syndrome is associated with decreased ACh production, whereas myasthenia gravis is associated with excess ACh production.
    c. Lambert-Eaton syndrome is characterized by impaired presynaptic ACh release, whereas

myasthenia gravis is characterized by defective ACh-receptor interaction.

d. Lambert-Eaton syndrome is alleviated by botulism, whereas myasthenia gravis is alleviated by anticholinesterases.

Answers: a, c.

26. When gamma-aminobutyric acid (GABA) interacts with postsynaptic $GABA_A$ receptors, which four events are likely to occur?
    a. Sodium channels are opened.
    b. Chloride channels are opened.
    c. The electrolyte shift depolarizes the neuron.
    d. The electrolyte shift hyperpolarizes the neuron.
    e. Hyperpolarization leads to inhibition.
    f. The electrolyte shift in polarization leads to excitation.
    g. Glutamate provokes a similar response.
    h. Glycine provokes a similar response.

Answers: b, d, e, h. The $GABA_A$ receptor is a ubiquitous, multifaceted complex sensitive to benzodiazepines and barbiturates as well as GABA. When stimulated, the $GABA_A$ receptor permits the influx of chloride. The electrolyte shift hyperpolarizes the neuron's membrane and inhibits depolarization. Glycine, like GABA, is an inhibitory amino acid neurotransmitter.

27. Which is the approximate normal resting potential of neurons?
    a. +100 mV
    b. +70 mV
    c. 0 mV
    d. −70 mV
    e. −100 mV

Answer: d. The normal resting potential is −70 mV. When the resting potential is −100 mV, the neuron is hyperpolarized and thereby inhibited.

28. Which two roles does glycine play?
    a. Glycine is an inhibitory amino acid neurotransmitter.
    b. Glycine modulates the N-methyl-D-aspartate (NMDA) receptor.
    c. Glycine is the rate-limiting substrate in glutamate synthesis.
    d. Glycine raises the resting potential (i.e., makes it less negative).

Answers: a, b. Glycine is an inhibitory amino acid neurotransmitter that modulates the NMDA receptor. Inhibitory neurotransmitters generally make the resting potential more negative.

29. Which two roles do nitric oxide (NO) play?
    a. It leads to cerebral vasodilation and, when the penis is stimulated, generates erections.
    b. Like aspirin (ASA), it promotes platelet aggregation.
    c. Excessive NMDA activity leads to increase in NO activity, which leads to neuron death.
    d. When used excessively, NO causes a peripheral neuropathy.

Answers: a, b. Both NO and ASA inhibit platelet aggregation. Nitrous oxide (N_2O) is a gas anesthetic that, when used daily, causes a peripheral neuropathy.

30. Which neurotransmitter is confined almost entirely to the brain?
    a. Dopamine
    b. ACh
    c. Glycine
    d. Norepinephrine
    e. Serotonin
    f. Glutamate

Answer: a. Dopamine is found in the adrenal medulla, but its primary tracts are confined to the brain. The other neurotransmitters are found in high concentrations in the spinal cord, as well as in the brain.

31. Which are two effects of glutamate-NMDA interaction?
    a. Intracellular neuron calcium concentration increases.
    b. Inhibition occurs through hyperpolarization.
    c. Excitation occurs under normal circumstances.
    d. Excitotoxicity occurs under normal circumstances.
    e. Inhibition occurs under normal circumstances.

Answers: a, c. Glutamate, the principal CNS excitatory neurotransmitter, interacts with the NMDA and other receptors to open calcium channels. With excessive activity, in a process termed "excitotoxicity," the calcium influx raises intracellular concentrations to lethal levels.

32. Of the following, which is the best treatment for atropine poisoning?
    a. Scopolamine
    b. Edrophonium
    c. Neostigmine
    d. Physostigmine

Answer: d. Atropine is an inhibitor of muscarinic cholinergic receptors. Physostigmine crosses the blood–brain barrier and restores acetylcholine concentration.

33. In Alzheimer's disease, which of the following receptors is most severely depleted?
   a. Muscarinic acetylcholine
   b. Nicotinic acetylcholine
   c. Nigrostriatal dopamine
   d. Frontal dopamine

Answer: a. In Alzheimer's disease, muscarinic acetylcholine receptors are depleted, especially in the limbic system and association areas. Although they are also present in the brain, nicotinic acetylcholine receptors are located predominantly in the spinal cord and the neuromuscular junction.

34. Which one of the following inhibits dopamine metabolism and creates some amphetamine-like metabolites?
   a. Haloperidol
   b. Selegiline (deprenyl)
   c. Amitriptyline
   d. Bromocriptine

Answer: b. Although the neuroprotective role of selegiline remains controversial, it provides an antidepressant effect partly through diverting dopamine metabolism to amphetamine.

35. What effect does tetrabenazine have on dopamine transmission?
   a. It stimulates dopamine transmission by acting as a precursor.
   b. It substitutes for dopamine by acting as an agonist.
   c. It interferes with dopamine transmission by blocking D_2 receptors.
   d. It reduces dopamine transmission by depleting dopamine from its presynaptic storage sites.

Answer: d. Tetrabenazine, like reserpine, depletes dopamine from its presynaptic storage sites and reduces involuntary movements. Both tetrabenazine and reserpine are useful, although to a limited extent, in the treatment of hyperkinetic movement disorders, such as chorea, Tourette's syndrome, and oral-buccolingual tardive dyskinesia.

36. A 50-year-old man is hospitalized for alcohol withdrawal. Clonidine and a β-blocker are administered prophylactically. Which of the following complications will be unaffected?
   a. Tachycardia
   b. Tremor
   c. Agitation
   d. Seizures
   e. Hypertension

Answer: d. During alcohol withdrawal, these medicines will reduce cardiovascular and some psychologic manifestations; however, they will not prevent alcohol-withdrawal seizures. The α2 norepinephrine agonist, clonidine, may alleviate autonomic symptoms of opioid withdrawal but offers little benefit in alcohol detoxification.

37. On the third day of withdrawal, the man in Question 36 develops several seizures. Which treatment should be administered while further evaluation and treatment are undertaken?
   a. Lorazepam
   b. Valproate
   c. Carbamazepine
   d. Phenobarbital

Answer: a. Lorazepam is probably the most rapidly acting, effective antiepileptic medicine in this situation. Because valproate and carbamazepine cannot be given as a "load," they require too much time to be effective in acute situations. Physicians often administer phenobarbital, but it sedates patients and has a very long half-life.

38. Which one of the following characterizes fast neurotransmitters?
   a. They work through ion channels.
   b. They work through G-proteins.
   c. They work through second messengers.
   d. They include dopamine and norepinephrine.

Answer: a. Fast neurotransmitters, such as GABA and glutamate, work through ion channels. Slow neurotransmitters, such as the catecholamines, work through G-proteins and second messengers, such as adenyl cyclase.

39. To which process do excessive glutamate-NMDA interactions lead?
   a. Hyperpolarization
   b. Excitotoxicity
   c. Apoptosis
   d. Involution

Answer: b. Excessive NMDA activation—excitotoxicity—leads to flooding of the neurons with lethal concentrations of calcium.

40. Which of the following statements is false regarding serotonin?
   a. Serotonin is a monoamine but not a catecholamine.
   b. Depending on the receptor class, serotonin interactions may lead to increased adenyl cyclase activity.
   c. Serotonin is a slow neurotransmitter that works through G-proteins and second messengers.
   d. Depending on the receptor class, serotonin may result in inhibitory or excitatory actions.

e. The antimigraine medications, "triptans," are 5-HT$_{1D}$ receptors antagonists.

Answer: e. In one of neurology's most effective therapies, sumatriptan and other triptans, which are 5-HT$_{1D}$ receptor agonists, consistently abort migraines. Serotonin is not a catecholamine but a monoamine with either slow inhibitory or excitatory actions. It works through G-proteins and second messengers.

41. Which one of the following statements concerning neurotransmission is false?
    a. Glutamate-NMDA interactions are fast and excitatory.
    b. Glutamate-NMDA interactions affect the calcium channel.
    c. Benzodiazepine-GABA$_A$ receptor interactions are fast and inhibitory.
    d. Benzodiazepine-GABA$_A$ receptor interactions affect the chloride channel.
    e. Benzodiazepine-GABA$_A$ receptor interactions, which promote the influx of chloride, reduce the polarization of the resting potential.

Answer: e. Benzodiazepine-GABA$_A$ receptor interactions promote the influx of chloride, which makes the resting potential more negative. Hyperpolarized neurons are refractory to stimulation (inhibited).

42. Which of the following is a second messenger?
    a. Cyclic AMP
    b. Serotonin
    c. Endorphins
    d. Thyroid hormone
    e. Glutamate

Answer: a. Cyclic AMP, like phosphatidyl inositol, is a common second messenger.

43. Which dopamine tract is most likely responsible for positive symptoms in psychosis?
    a. Nigrostriatal
    b. Mesolimbic
    c. Tubero-infundibular
    d. Mesocortical

Answer: b.

44. Which dopamine tract is most likely responsible for negative symptoms in psychosis?
    a. Nigrostriatal
    b. Mesolimbic
    c. Tubero-infundibular
    d. Mesocortical

Answer: d.

45. Which of the following pairs are inhibitory amino acid neurotransmitters?
    a. GABA and glycine
    b. Glutamate and aspartate
    c. Epinephrine and norepinephrine
    d. L-dopa (levodopa) and carbidopa

Answer: a. GABA and glycine are inhibitory amino acid neurotransmitters. Glutamate and aspartate are excitatory amino acid neurotransmitters.

46–51. Match the medication (46–51) with the enzyme (a–e) that it inhibits.
46. Selegiline
47. Carbidopa
48. Entacapone
49. Edrophonium
50. Tranylcypromine
51. Pyridostigmine
    a. Dopa decarboxylase
    b. COMT
    c. MAO-B
    d. Acetylcholinesterase
    e. MAO-A

Answers: 46-c, 47-a, 48-b, 49-d, 50-e, 51-d.

52–56. Match the illness (52–56) with the deficient enzyme(s) (a–d).
52. Phenylketonuria
53. Parkinson's disease
54. Dopamine responsive dystonia
55. Alzheimer's disease
56. Huntington's disease
    a. Phenylalanine hydroxylase
    b. Tyrosine hydroxylase
    c. Glutamate decarboxylase
    d. Choline acetyltransferase

Answers: 52-a, 53-b, 54-a and b, 55-d, 56-c.

57. Which of the following is not a characteristic of nicotinic ACh receptors?
    a. They are neuromuscular junction receptors.
    b. Curare and α-bungarotoxin block them.
    c. They are inhibitory.
    d. They are one of two main ACh receptors in the nervous system.

Answer: c. Nicotinic ACh receptors are excitatory.

58. Which of the following is not a characteristic of muscarinic ACh receptors?
    a. Cerebral cortex ACh receptors are predominantly muscarinic.
    b. They are entirely inhibitory.

c. Atropine and scopolamine block them.

d. They are depleted in Alzheimer's disease.

Answer: b. Muscarinic ACh receptors can be excitatory as well as inhibitory.

59. Which of the following is not an effect of increased GABA-GABA$_A$ receptor activity?

a. Chloride ions flow into the channel.

b. The resting potential, which is normally −70 mV, is furthered lowered (made more negative).

c. Calcium ions flow into the channel.

d. Lowering their resting potential hyperpolarizes neurons.

e. The speed of the reaction has allowed GABA to be termed a "fast neurotransmitter."

Answer: c. Calcium influx characterizes NMDA activity.

60. Which of the following is false regarding the GABA$_B$ receptor?

a. GABA$_B$ receptors are more numerous and more widely distributed than GABA$_A$ receptors.

b. GABA$_B$ receptors are G-protein linked channel inhibitors.

c. Baclofen binds to GABA$_B$ receptors.

d. Compared to the number and diversity of ligands that bind to GABA$_A$ receptors, relatively few bind to GABA$_B$ receptors.

e. Like GABA$_A$ receptors, GABA$_B$ receptors are complex molecules.

Answer: a.

61. A 40-year-old man has been under treatment for major depression for several years. After he contracted tuberculosis (TB), his physicians prescribed isoniazid (INH). Although the TB began to respond, his depression recurred. In a suicide attempt, he took an overdose of INH and developed status epilepticus. Which would be the most specific, effective treatment?

a. Phenytoin

b. Thiamine

c. Lorazepam

d. Pyridoxine (B$_6$)

e. Topiramate

Answer: d. Pyridoxine-deficient states lead to seizures. For example, infants inadvertently fed pyridoxine-deficient diets developed seizures. In this case, INH interferes with pyridoxine, which is the cofactor for glutamate decarboxylase. Glutamate decarboxylase is a crucial enzyme in GABA synthesis. Thus, large doses of INH deplete GABA, which causes seizures. Intravenous pyridoxine aborts pyridoxine deficiency-induced seizures. Doctors prescribing INH should combine it with pyridoxine. Topiramate enhances GABA$_A$ receptor activity, but it is ineffective without GABA.

62. Which is a false statement regarding the NMDA receptor?

a. The NMDA receptor has binding sites for ketamine as well as phencyclidine.

b. Excessive NMDA receptor activity leads to excitotoxicity, which purportedly causes cell death in Huntington's disease, stroke, and possibly schizophrenia.

c. Lamotrigine and riluzole decrease glutamate activity but not necessarily at the NMDA receptor.

d. Excessive NMDA activity floods the neuron with excessive concentrations of chloride.

e. The NMDA receptor's activity is modulated by glycine, which is an inhibitory neurotransmitter.

Answer: d. Excessive NMDA activity floods the neuron with excessive concentrations of calcium.

63–67. Match the neurotransmitter (63–67) with the region of the nervous system (a–e) where it is synthesized.

63. Dopamine

64. Norepinephrine

65. Epinephrine

66. Serotonin

67. Acetylcholine

a. Locus ceruleus

b. Adrenal medulla

c. Dorsal raphe nuclei

d. Substantia nigra

e. Nucleus basalis of Meynert

Answers: 63-d, 64-a, 65-b, 66-c, 67-e.

68–73. Match the site of neurotransmitter synthesis (68–73) with the region(s) of the nervous system (a–e) where it is located.

68. Locus ceruleus

69. Dorsal raphe nuclei

70. Adrenal medulla

71. Substantia nigra

72. Nucleus basalis of Meynert

73. Caudal raphe nuclei

a. Basal forebrain bundle

b. Midbrain

c. Pons

d. Medulla

e. Adrenal gland

Answers: 68-c, 69-b and c, 70-e, 71-b, 72-a, 73-c and d.

74. A woman, who is 5 months pregnant, asks for methadone maintenance because detectives have interrupted her heroin supply. Which action would best preserve her health and that of the baby?
  a. Do not accept her into a methadone maintenance program until after she delivers.
  b. Have her undergo heroin detoxification to avoid exposing the fetus to methadone.
  c. Enroll her in a methadone maintenance program as soon as possible.
  d. None of the above.

Answer: c. The fetus, as well as the mother, is probably addicted to heroin. Attempting to abruptly stop the mother's opioid use would probably be futile; however, physicians could probably switch her from heroin to methadone. After she delivers, physicians could detoxify both the mother and infant.

75. To which receptors do ketamine and PCP bind?
  a. Dopamine
  b. Norepinephrine
  c. Serotonin
  d. $GABA_A$
  e. NMDA

Answer: e. Ketamine and PCP affect the ion channels of NMDA receptors and interfere with their action.

76. What is the effect of ketamine and PCP binding on the NMDA receptor?
  a. Inhibition of the influx of calcium
  b. Promotion of the influx of calcium
  c. Inhibition of the influx of chloride
  d. Promotion of the influx of chloride
  e. None of the above

Answer: a. Ketamine and PCP inhibit the influx of calcium, which is usually provoked by interactions of glutamate or aspartate with the NMDA receptor.

77. What is the pathophysiology of strychnine and tetanus toxins?
  a. They both inhibit inhibitory neurotransmitters.
  b. They both activate inhibitory neurotransmitters.
  c. They both inhibit excitatory neurotransmitters.
  d. They both activate excitatory neurotransmitters.

Answer: a. Strychnine and tetanus toxin inhibit release of presynaptic GABA and glycine, which are inhibitory neurotransmitters. Their absence allows unbridled motor activity that leads to involuntary motor spasms in response to minimal or no stimulation.

78. Of the following dopamine receptors, which is most stimulated by cocaine?
  a. D_1
  b. D_2 mesocortical
  c. D_2 mesolimbic
  d. D_3

Answer: c. Cocaine mostly affects the D_2 mesolimbic receptors.

79. Which is the best treatment for cocaine-induced psychosis and violent behavior?
  a. Dopamine-blocking neuroleptics
  b. Benzodiazepines
  c. Seclusion and, if necessary, restraints
  d. None of the above

Answer: a. Because the main effect of cocaine is to increase dopamine activity by blocking its reuptake, the best treatment for excessive dopamine activity is dopamine-blocking neuroleptics. However, in this situation, physicians should cautiously use these neuroleptics because most of them lower the seizure threshold.

80. Which are the least common neurologic complications of cocaine use?
  a. Nonhemorrhagic strokes
  b. Hemorrhagic strokes
  c. Seizures during withdrawal
  d. Seizures during overdose
  e. Increased incidence of neuroleptic-induced dystonic reactions

Answer: c. Seizures are apt to complicate withdrawal from alcohol, barbiturates, and benzodiazepines. With cocaine, seizures complicate withdrawal only from chronic, frequent, high-dose use. However, seizures are a common complication of cocaine intoxication and may signify an underlying stroke. Hemorrhagic and, to a lesser extent, nonhemorrhagic strokes complicate cocaine use.

81. Which is the best treatment for cocaine-induced severe hypertension?
  a. Diuretics
  b. Calcium channel blockers
  c. ACE inhibitors
  d. Phentolamine

Answer: d. An α-blocker, such as phentolamine, will be the most rapid and effective antihypertensive therapy. Controlling blood pressure may forestall a cerebral hemorrhage.

82. Which is the effect of amphetamines on sleep?
  a. Decreases proportion of NREM stages 1 and 2
  b. Decreases proportion of NREM stages 3 and 4
  c. Decreases proportion of REM
  d. Displaces REM from night-time to daytime

Answer: c. Not only does cocaine reduce total sleep time but also it almost abolishes REM sleep.

83. What is the effect of opioids on respiration?
  a. They reduce the respiratory rate.
  b. They reduce the depth of respirations.
  c. They increase the rate but reduce the depth.
  d. They reduce the depth but increase the rate.

Answer: a. Opioids reduce the respiratory rate. In severe overdoses, opioids lead to pulmonary edema and respiratory arrest.

84. What is the effect of PCP-NMDA receptor interaction?
  a. A PCP-NMDA receptor interaction stabilizes the ion channel.
  b. It leads to an influx of negatively charged chloride ions, which hyperpolarizes the neuron.
  c. It triggers an influx of calcium, which leads to excitotoxicity.
  d. It prevents the influx of calcium that glutamate would ordinarily trigger.

Answer: d.

85. Which of the following is a common effect of marijuana?
  a. A fatal reaction to overdose
  b. Seizures
  c. Strokes
  d. Reduced REM sleep

Answer: d.

86. Which of the following statements concerning nicotine is false?
  a. It affects CNS cholinergic receptors.
  b. Its receptors are located in the mesolimbic pathway.
  c. Bupropion may help smokers through withdrawal because, like nicotine, it increases dopamine concentrations.
  d. Nicotinic receptors are the predominant CNS receptors.
  e. Nicotinic receptors are the predominant neuromuscular junction receptors.

Answer: d. Although both muscarinic and nicotinic receptors are present in the CNS, muscarinic receptors are predominant. Nicotinic receptors predominate at the neuromuscular junction.

87. Which are four characteristic features of cocaine use?
  a. Blocks reuptake of dopamine into presynaptic neurons
  b. Agitation or delirium
  c. Hypertension
  d. Slowed respiratory rate
  e. Stimulation of the area postrema
  f. Miosis
  g. Chorea in some cases

Answers: a, b, c, g. In contrast, slowed respiratory rate, stimulation of the area postrema, and miosis are characteristic features of heroin or other opioid overdose.

88. Which five are potential complications of cocaine administration?
  a. Cerebral hemorrhage
  b. Cerebral anoxia
  c. Seizures
  d. Radial nerve palsy
  e. Tics
  f. Stereotypies
  g. Psychotic thinking
  h. Pulmonary edema

Answers: a, c, e, f, g. Cerebral anoxia and radial nerve palsy may follow respiratory depression from opioids or other drugs that depress consciousness. The development or exacerbation of tics characteristically follows cocaine use. Pulmonary edema characteristically follows heroin, methadone, or other opioid overdose.

89. In comparing heroin to morphine in terms of their use in cancer-induced pain, which of the following are heroin's advantages?
  a. Like benzodiazepine, heroin has its own receptor.
  b. Because it more rapidly penetrates the blood–brain barrier, it has a more rapid onset of action.
  c. It does not induce vomiting.
  d. It improves affect to a greater degree.

Answer: b. Compared to morphine, heroin penetrates the blood–brain barrier more rapidly. Like other opioids, it attaches to the *mu* receptor. Its effects are virtually indistinguishable from morphine's.

90. When used in the treatment of Parkinson's disease, what is the role of entacapone?
  a. It inhibits DOPA decarboxylase.
  b. It readily penetrates the blood–brain barrier and preserves dopamine.
  c. It inhibits MAO.

d. It acts as a dopamine agonist.
e. It inhibits COMT.

Answer: e. Entacapone penetrates the blood–brain barrier but slowly and in small quantities. In its main action, entacapone inhibits COMT. Usually combined with carbidopa, which inhibits DOPA decarboxylase, entacapone slows COMT metabolism and preserves L-dopa in the systemic circulation.

91. Which of these medicines is not like the others?
    a. Apomorphine
    b. Ropinirole
    c. Pramipexole
    d. L-dopa
    e. Bromocriptine

Answer: d. Although all these medicines alleviate the symptoms of Parkinson's disease, only L-dopa is a dopamine precursor. The others are dopamine agonists.

92. In its fluctuations during the sleep-wake cycle, when is serotonin concentration highest?
    a. Slow-wave sleep
    b. REM sleep
    c. Arousal
    d. None of the above

Answer: c.

93. In its fluctuations during the sleep-wake cycle, when is serotonin concentration lowest?
    a. Slow-wave sleep
    b. REM sleep
    c. Arousal
    d. None of the above

Answer: b. Serotonin concentration falls during slow-wave sleep and almost disappears during REM sleep.

94. Which enzyme is most important in serotonin metabolism?
    a. MOA-A
    b. MAO-B
    c. COMT
    d. DOPA decarboxylase

Answer: a. In general terms, MAO-A metabolizes serotonin and MAO-B metabolizes dopamine. Selegiline, the Parkinson's disease medicine, inhibits MAO-B. In the doses that neurologists prescribe (10 mg/daily), patients do not develop hypertensive crises from tyramine-containing food. Also, because selegiline does not interfere with serotonin metabolism, it should not cause the serotonin syndrome.

95. Which of the following is not a manifestation of anticholinergic medicines?
    a. Miosis
    b. Tachycardia and hypertension
    c. Dry skin and low grade fever
    d. Constipation and urinary retention
    e. Toxic encephalopathy (with high doses)

Answer: a. Because anticholinergic medications reduce parasympathetic activity, thereby allowing sympathetic activity to predominate, they dilate pupils, cause tachycardia and hypertension, and reduce bowel and bladder activity. At high concentrations, they interfere with CNS ACh transmission and cause confusion, hallucinations, and depressed sensorium. Pharmacologic agents that might cause toxic levels of anticholinergic activity include atropine, trihexyphenidyl, tricyclic antidepressants, and dopamine-blocking antipsychotic agents. Physostigmine, an anticholinesterase that crosses the blood–brain barrier, restores ACh activity and thus can reverse excessive anticholinergic activity.

96. Which of the following is not a manifestation of medicines that increase cholinergic activity?
    a. Miosis
    b. Rash
    c. Profuse salivation
    d. Abdominal cramping and diarrhea
    e. Fasciculations
    f. Bradycardia

Answer: b. Because cholinergic medications increase parasympathetic activity, they counteract sympathetic activity. They constrict pupils and slow the heart rate, but increase gastrointestinal activity. At high doses, they interfere with the neuromuscular junction ACh transmission and cause fasciculations. Pharmacologic agents that might cause toxic levels of cholinergic activity include anticholinesterases (cholinesterase inhibitors) used for Alzheimer's disease and those used for myasthenia gravis, organophosphates in insecticides, and nerve gases.

97. Which of the following is not a manifestation of medicines that increase sympathetic activity?
    a. Asthma
    b. Tachycardia and hypertension
    c. Tremor
    d. Large pupils

Answer: a. Sympathomimetic medicines, such as epinephrine, abort asthma attacks. They cause tremor and the "flight or fight" signs, such as tachycardia, hypertension, and large pupils. They also cause tremor. Psychoactive drugs that have sympathomimetic properties include cocaine, amphetamine, and PCP.

98. What is the mechanism of action of MDMA (ecstasy) producing euphoria?
   a. Dopamine release and blocked reuptake
   b. Serotonin surge
   c. Mild glutamate toxicity
   d. Mu receptor stimulation

Answer: b. Cocaine and other stimulants increase dopamine activity. Opioids stimulate mu receptors.

99. Which is the most prevalent excitatory neurotransmitter?
   a. Norepinephrine
   b. ACh
   c. Glutamate
   d. Dopamine
   e. GABA

Answer: c.

100. When used in the treatment of Alzheimer's disease, what is the mechanism of action of memantine?
   a. It interferes with cholinesterase.
   b. It antagonizes NMDA receptors.
   c. It acts as ACh.
   d. It dissolves amyloid.

Answer: b. Unlike standard therapies for Alzheimer's disease, which attempt to restore ACh concentrations by inhibiting cholinesterase, memantine antagonizes NMDA receptors.

101. Which of the following is untrue regarding oxybate (γ-hydroxybutyrate [GHB])?
   a. GHB rapidly induces deep sleep and profound amnesia.
   b. GHB is a product of GABA metabolism.
   c. GHB suppresses cataplexy.
   d. GHB assists night-time sleep in narcolepsy.
   e. GHB reduces dopamine activity.

Answer: e. GHB, a product of GABA metabolism, induces sleep, which is beneficial in narcolepsy, in which night-time sleep is inadequate, but dangerous, as when sexual predators intoxicate potential victims. Used judiciously, it suppresses cataplexy.

102. Through which systems do all illicit drugs act?
   a. Mesolimbic and mesocortical dopamine
   b. Nigrostriatal dopamine
   c. Dorsal raphe serotonin
   d. Locus ceruleus

Answer: a. Although illicit drugs may act on several systems, they all increase dopamine activity in the limbic system and cerebral cortex.

103. A 30-year-old man presented to a neurologist because of increasingly severe and prolonged low and middle back pains. When upright, he had hyperlordosis and limited range of movement about the low back and legs. He had begun to walk like a "tin soldier." Extensive testing revealed antibodies to glutamic acid decarboxylase (GAD) in the serum and spinal fluid. What is the most likely diagnosis?
   a. Parkinson's disease
   b. Tetanus
   c. Stiff-person syndrome
   d. Catatonia

Answer: c. He has stiff-person syndrome, which neurologists previously called "stiff-man" syndrome. This disorder is often a paraneoplastic syndrome or comorbid with various autoimmune diseases. It is associated with anti-GAD antibodies, which impair the synthesis of GABA. Decreased GABA activity and resulting abnormally increased muscular tone is common to tetanus and stiff-person syndrome.

104. Which of the following is untrue regarding hypocretins?
   a. Hypocretin-1 and -2 are equivalent to orexin A and B.
   b. They are inhibitory neuropeptides.
   c. They are increased during wakefulness and REM sleep.
   d. In normal individuals, specific cells in the hypothalamus synthesize hypocretins and secrete them into the CSF.
   e. Narcolepsy patients lose hypocretin-producing hypothalamic cells and have little or no CSF hypocretin.

Answer: b. They are excitatory neuropeptides.

Traumatic Brain Injury

MAJOR HEAD TRAUMA

The nature and severity of head trauma determine the manifestations of *traumatic brain injury* (*TBI*). In a somewhat arbitrary separation, neurologists distinguish major from minor head trauma. They consider that major head trauma results in at least 1 hour of post-traumatic unconsciousness and leaves permanent residual neurologic deficits.

Neurologists further divide major head trauma along etiologic lines into *penetrating* injuries, such as gunshot wounds (GSWs), and *blunt* or *nonpenetrating* injuries, such as falls. However, in many circumstances this division again seems arbitrary. For example, with a depressed skull fracture, blunt head trauma can lead to penetrating injury.

Common causes of major head trauma in civilians include motor vehicle accidents (MVAs), bicycle accidents, work-related accidents, violent assaults, and GSWs. In the elderly, common causes are falls, abuse, and trauma precipitated by use of various medicines. Alcohol plays a major role in TBI because it impairs judgment, coordination, and wakefulness. Overall, individuals most at risk for TBI are 15- to 24-year-old men and those older than 75 years.

How Does Head Trauma Cause Brain Injury?

Direct Force

A blow—by its direct mechanical force (a *coup* injury)—may destroy the underlying delicate brain tissue (the *parenchyma*). As with strokes, trauma causes cell death by necrosis with its accompanying monocular cell infiltration and other inflammatory changes. (In contrast, neurodegenerative diseases, such as Huntington's disease and amyotrophic lateral sclerosis [ALS], cause cell death by apoptosis [see Chapter 18].)

Head trauma, in addition, throws the brain against the opposite inner table of the skull and injures that side of the brain (a *contrecoup* injury). Often the damage from contrecoup injuries surpasses that from the coup injury. In particular, contrecoup injuries damage the temporal lobe and the anterior-inferior surface of

the frontal lobes because they abut sharp edges of the skull's anterior and middle cranial fossae (Fig. 22-1). Depending on its severity, frontal and temporal lobe damage characteristically leads to memory impairment and personality changes.

In one exception to this mechanism, frontal trauma rarely leads to countercoup occipital lobe injuries because the occipital skull is relatively flat and smooth. Thus, TBI rarely causes long-lasting visual impairments.

Diffuse Axonal Shearing

Another mechanism that leads to brain injury consists of *diffuse axonal shearing*. This process consists not only of trauma to long subcortical white matter axons, but also damage to cells' cytoskeletal components and fatal intracellular influx of calcium. Although computed tomography (CT) cannot detect axonal shearing, magnetic resonance imaging (MRI) often suggests it while revealing petechia in the brainstem and cerebral white matter. A definite diagnosis of diffuse axonal shearing requires a postmortem pathologic examination, but neurologists, on the basis of the clinical examination and MRI results, often attribute post-traumatic cognitive dysfunction and personality changes to it.

Intracerebral Bleeding

Blunt trauma causes intraparenchymal hematomas and petechiae, especially in the brainstem. In addition,

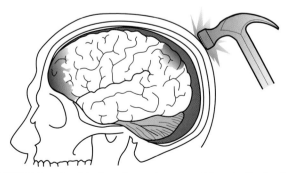

FIGURE 22-1 ■ In this drawing, a hammer blow to the back of the head inflicts a *coup* injury to the occipital region and through the *contrecoup*, a more extensive injury to the tips of the frontal and temporal lobes.

it causes diffuse *cerebral edema,* which increases intracranial pressure. Hematomas within the brain and over its surface exert pressure on the surrounding brain. If they expand beyond a certain size, they force transtentorial herniation (see later).

Bleeding Within the Skull, but Outside the Brain

Head injury, ruptured aneurysms, and other insults often cause bleeding in the spaces between the meninges, which are readily recalled using the mnemonic *PAD—pia, arachnoid,* and *dura mater.*

- Pia mater, the innermost layer, is a thin, almost transparent, vascular membrane adherent to the cerebral gyri. It follows gyri into sulci and thus allows a generous region, the *subarachnoid space,* between it and the immediately overlying layer—the arachnoid mater.

- Arachnoid mater, also thin, represents the middle layer of the meninges. It spans the tops of gyri to cap the sulci. The subarachnoid space, which contains the cerebrospinal fluid (CSF), surrounds the brain and, continuing downward within the spinal canal to the sacrum, the spinal cord and cauda equina. Neurologists performing a spinal tap or lumbar puncture (LP) insert a special needle into the subarachnoid space below the *conus medullaris* (lower end of the spinal cord), which is situated between the T12 and L1 vertebrae, to sample CSF.

- *Dura mater,* the outermost layer of the meninges, is a thick fibrous tissue adherent to the interior surface of the skull. Two of its infoldings, the *falx* and *tentorium,* support the brain and contain most of its venous drainage. Neurologists designate the space between the skull and dura as the *epidural space,* and between the dura and arachnoid as the *subdural space.* Major head trauma may cause hematomas in either or both of these areas.

Epidural hematomas, which typically result from temporal bone fractures with concomitant middle meningeal artery lacerations, are essentially rapidly expanding, high-pressure, fresh blood clots (Fig. 22-2). They compress the underlying brain and force it through the tentorial notch, that is, they produce *transtentorial herniation* (see Fig. 19-3). Unless surgery can immediately arrest the bleeding, epidural hematomas are usually fatal.

In contrast, *subdural hematomas* usually result from slowly bleeding bridging veins, under relatively low pressure, into the subdural space (see Fig. 20-9). Dark, venous blood generally oozes into the extensive subdural space until the expanding hematoma encounters underlying brain. Resisting further expansion, the

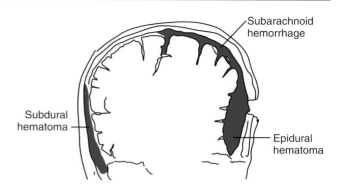

FIGURE 22-2 ■ Meningeal arterial bleeding, which generally results from blows forceful enough to cause skull fractures, causes *epidural hematomas.* In contrast, venous bleeding, usually slower and less forceful, causes *subdural hematomas.* Hematomas in either location may produce potentially fatal mass effects, including compression of the gyri and shift of midline structures. Ruptured aneurysms and head trauma often cause subarachnoid hemorrhage (SAH). In SAH, blood usually spreads through the subarachnoid space at the base of the brain, over the convexities, between the gyri, into the interhemispheric fissure, and down into the spinal canal. A lumbar puncture (LP) usually shows blood-tinged cerebrospinal fluid (CSF) within the first few days and xanthochromia thereafter.

brain dampens bleeding. However, if the hematoma continues to expand, it may lead to transtentorial herniation. Survivors often have permanent brain damage either from the initial trauma or the pressure from the subdural hematoma.

Chronic subdural hematomas, ones that have persisted for weeks, usually have spread extensively in the subdural space. They typically give rise to insidiously developing headaches, changes in personality, cognitive impairment, and dementia but only subtle focal physical deficits (see Chapters 19 and 20). Although the circulation may spontaneously absorb subdural hematomas, neurologists often suggest surgical evacuation. Because successful treatment usually reverses the patient's symptoms and signs, neurologists often designate subdural hematomas as a potentially reversible cause of dementia.

People older than 65 years are especially susceptible to chronic subdural hematomas for several reasons. They have a tendency to fall. They are often taking aspirin, anticoagulants, and other medications that increase their tendency to bleed. Most important, age-related cerebral atrophy enlarges the subdural space: The capacious space allows hematomas to reach considerable size before they encounter the resistance of the underlying brain.

Foreign Bodies

In addition to the disruption of brain tissue and intraparenchymal bleeding, GSWs and other penetrating injuries leave bone, shrapnel, and other foreign bodies in the brain. These foreign bodies may act either as a focus that generates seizures or a nidus for brain abscesses. Although desirable, neurosurgeons cannot remove all foreign bodies because many lodge in inaccessible areas.

Post-Traumatic Coma and Delirium

Following head trauma, as well as at other times, neurologists often classify patients' level of consciousness as *alert, lethargic, stuporous,* or *comatose*. Alternatively, they use the *Glasgow Coma Scale (GCS)*, which measures three readily obvious neurologic functions: eye opening, speaking, and moving (Table 22-1). In major head trauma, the GCS correlates closely with survival and neurologic sequelae; however, in minor head trauma, it correlates poorly. Moreover, physicians cannot appropriately include the GCS as part of a standard mental status examination for patients suspected of having dementia or circumscribed neuropsychologic deficits.

By the first day after TBI, of patients who score 3 on the GCS, which is the lowest possible score, 90% have a fatal outcome and most of the remaining never regain consciousness. Major TBI victims usually remain in coma for less than several days, but some linger in a comatose state for as long as 3 to 4 weeks. When in coma or another condition causing unconsciousness, such as the vegetative state, individuals cannot perceive pain and do not suffer. By 4 weeks, almost all comatose patients either die, partially recover and regain consciousness, or evolve into the vegetative state (Chapter 11).

As patients surviving major TBI emerge from coma, their mental state usually fluctuates and cognitive and personality disturbances emerge. These patients are often confused, disoriented, agitated, and combative. Their mental disturbances may be so disrupted that they warrant treatment with antipsychotic agents.

During this time, physicians must keep in mind the role of drug and alcohol use in trauma and its aftermath. Not only may substance abuse have caused the trauma but also the effects of drugs and alcohol may linger so long that on admission to a hospital and for the next day, patients may show signs of substance-induced delirium as well as TBI. Subsequently, alcohol or drug withdrawal may cause abnormal behavior, seizures, and a markedly lower pain threshold. Throughout their recovery, substance abuse may remain a source of continued disability for TBI victims.

Pre-existing dementia also leaves patients particularly susceptible to post-traumatic altered levels of consciousness, behavioral disturbances, and increased cognitive impairment. In fact, dementia may have led to the trauma, as when a patient with Alzheimer's disease causes a MVA.

Even without major TBI, numerous conditions may produce post-traumatic delirium, such as painful extracranial injuries; adverse reactions to antiepileptic, opioid, and other medications; and complications of bodily trauma, including hypoxia, sepsis, electrolyte disturbances, and fat emboli. These conditions, alone or superimposed on TBI, worsen delirium, further depress the level of consciousness, and leave the patient prone to seizures.

TABLE 22-1 ■ The Glasgow Coma Scale (GCS)		
Category		**Score**
Eyes opening	Never	1
	To pain	2
	To verbal stimuli	3
	Spontaneously	4
Best verbal response	None	1
	Incomprehensible sounds	2
	Inappropriate words	3
	Disoriented and converses	4
	Oriented and converses	5
Best motor response	None	1
	Extension*	2
	Flexion^	3
	Flexion withdrawal	4
	Patient localizes pain	5
	Patient obeys	6
Total		3–15

*Decerebrate rigidity (see Fig. 19-3).

^Decorticate rigidity (see Fig. 11-5).

This standard scale quantitates the level of consciousness, with the lower scores indicating less neurologic function. Neurologists interpret scores of 3–8 as signifying severe traumatic brain injury (TBI) or coma; 9–12, moderate TBI; and 13–15, mild TBI. However, the GCS is not readily applicable to patients who have sustained cerebral hypoxia and, because they cannot make a verbal response, those who are intubated. Adapted, with kind permission, from Teasdale G, Jennett B: Assessment of coma and impaired consciousness: A practical scale. Lancet 2:81–84, 1974.

Physical Sequelae

TBI characteristically causes focal neurologic deficits, such as hemiparesis, spasticity, and ataxia. Some studies, which remain controversial, claim that TBI may also cause involuntary movement disorders, such as Parkinson's disease.

Recovery from physical deficits, to the extent that it occurs, usually reaches a maximum within six months. During that period and afterward, patients can increase their functional abilities with physical and occupational therapy, braces, other mechanical devices, and modifications of their environment. Neurologists

TABLE 22-2 ■ The Glasgow Outcome Scale (GOS)

Good recovery: resumption of normal life despite minor deficits
Moderate disability: disabled but independent
Severe disability: conscious but disabled
Persistent vegetative state: unresponsive and speechless
Death

Adapted, with kind permission, from Jennett B, Bond M: Assessment of outcome after severe brain damage. Lancet 5:480–484, 1975.

and physiatrists often monitor patients' progress using the *Glasgow Outcome Scale (GOS)* (Table 22-2).

Damage to the special sensory organs, such as the eye, ear, or nose and their cranial nerves, although not strictly speaking "brain injury," adds to patients' neurologic disability. It also leads to sensory deprivation, disfigurement, and functional impairment. Frontal head trauma, which is probably the most common injury, often shears the filaments of the olfactory nerves as they pass through the cribriform plate. Thus, patients sustaining frontal head trauma develop combinations of anosmia and personality and cognitive impairments. In addition, major TBI that damages patients' hypothalamus disrupts their sleep-wake cycle, causing insomnia, inattention, and, sometimes, a requirement for additional medicines (see later).

Post-Traumatic Epilepsy

Cerebral scars and residual foreign bodies routinely form epileptic foci. They generate post-traumatic epilepsy, which is one of the most commonly occurring complications of major TBI. As time passes after an injury, the prevalence of post-traumatic epilepsy increases, eventually reaching 50%. The prevalence is greater following penetrating rather than blunt trauma, and among patients who abuse alcohol. In contrast, post-traumatic epilepsy rarely complicates minor TBI.

Post-traumatic epilepsy usually takes the form of partial complex seizures that undergo secondary generalization (see Chapter 10). Not only does post-traumatic epilepsy cause disability and carry the risk of further head injury, side effects of antiepileptic drugs (AEDs) may exacerbate TBI-induced cognitive and personality changes.

Cognitive Impairment

The period of coma due to TBI usually lasts less than 4 weeks. By then, depending on many factors, most patients either succumb to their injuries or recover some or occasionally almost all their cognitive function. However, some TBI patients remain unconscious

and devoid of thought, although with their eyes open; incapable of communication or deliberate, purposeful movement; and unable to perceive pain or suffering. Most patients in this last group exist permanently in the *persistent vegetative state* (see Chapter 11).

Some TBI patients who regain consciousness still face incapacitating cognitive impairments. They remain reticent, responsive to only simple requests, and capable of initiating only rudimentary bodily functions. Moreover, they usually also have comorbid debilitating physical impairments and post-traumatic epilepsy. Even without the physical deficits, the *Diagnostic and Statistical Manual of Mental Disorders, 4th Edition, Text Revision (DSM-IV-TR)* would label their condition Dementia Due to Head Trauma.

More severely injured patients naturally have more pronounced cognitive deficits. To some extent their deficits correlate with their immediate post-traumatic depth of coma, as measured by the GCS. However, their deficits more strongly correlate with the duration of the post-traumatic amnesia, which includes the patient's time in coma. Cognitive deficits include not only memory impairment (see later) but also apraxia, impulsivity, inattention, and slowed information processing. Surprisingly, the lesion's location, with one important exception, correlates relatively poorly with cognitive impairment. Left temporal lobe injuries, the exception, produce vocabulary deficits similar to anomic aphasia (see Chapter 8).

Just as with medications' causing or adding to delirium in the immediate post-traumatic period, numerous AEDs, muscle relaxants, and opioids may further depress cognitive function. They even may alter the patient's personality, mood, and sleep-wake cycle. Similarly, comorbid post-traumatic stress disorder (PTSD) may contribute to cognitive impairments and other post-traumatic mental changes (see later).

Whereas recovery of motor and language skills usually reaches a maximum within 6 months, intellectual recovery may not reach its maximum until 18 months. Older patients generally recover more slowly and less completely than younger ones.

In addition to TBI causing debilitating cognitive impairments, some epidemiologic studies suggest that it also constitutes a risk factor for Alzheimer's disease. Pathologic studies have shown that severe head trauma causes amyloid protein deposition in the brain that might act as a nidus for plaques, one of the hallmarks of Alzheimer's disease. Several, but not all, studies also suggest that moderately severe head trauma in individuals with two Apo-E4 alleles correlates with a several-fold increased risk of developing Alzheimer's disease (see Chapter 7). Finally, following mild head trauma, individuals carrying at least one Apo-E4 allele, but not those carrying only other alleles, showed deterioration on neuropsychologic testing. (A confounding issue for some of these studies is that individuals with Alzheimer's disease are prone to cause an accident in which they sustain TBI.)

Memory impairment or *post-traumatic amnesia,* the most consistent neuropsychologic TBI-induced deficit, includes memory loss for the trauma and immediately preceding events (retrograde amnesia) and, to a less extent, for newly presented information (anterograde amnesia). Most important, the duration of post-traumatic amnesia provides the most accurate prognosis for overall outcome, cognitive impairments, and other neuropsychologic sequelae. It is even more reliable than either the depth or duration of coma.

The *DSM-IV-TR* includes post-traumatic amnesia as an Amnesic Disorder Due to TBI. It calls the disorder "transient" if the duration is shorter than one month and "chronic" if longer.

Treatment Strategies for Post-Traumatic Cognitive Impairment

No psychopharmacologic approach to post-traumatic dementia has restored cognitive function. Neurologists, naturally assuming that loss of brain tissue meant loss of neurotransmitters, administer dopamine agonists, such as bromocriptine, and cholinesterase inhibitors to restore dopamine and acetylcholine activity. They have also prescribed stimulants, such as dextroamphetamine, methylphenidate, and pemoline. Although the stimulants have increased patients' memory, attentiveness, concentration, and daytime wakefulness, their benefit derived mostly from improving patients' mood and energy. Similarly, treatment of comorbid PTSD, if present, may improve cognitive impairments and other post-traumatic mental changes.

Neurologists and physiatrists also refer patients for cognitive, behavioral, physical, and occupational rehabilitation. In most programs, multidisciplinary teams aim to restore patients' intellectual functioning and return them, as much as possible, to their place in the family and work. Classic strategies—physical, occupational, and speech therapy; identification and treatment of depression, anxiety, and insomnia; and social interactions with peers—enhance remaining functions, reduce impediments, and provide compensatory mechanisms for injured ones.

Other Mental Disturbances

Intermittent Explosive Disorder

Many severe TBI patients, particularly those with frontal lobe damage, remain reticent, docile, and dependent. On the other hand, some patients tend toward agitation. When minimal provocation provokes episodes of impulsive violence, it is best termed *Intermittent Explosive Disorder* (previously known as "episodic dyscontrol syndrome"). Because patients with impulsive violence are unusually sensitive to alcohol, TBI patients' consuming a few alcoholic drinks may trigger violent outbursts. AEDs, especially ones with mood-stabilizing effects, such as valproate and carbamazepine, may suppress violent outbursts.

Personality Changes

Personality changes, presumably from frontal and temporal lobe damage, often lead to patients' developing an abrupt, suspicious, or argumentative manner. In some cases, frontal lobe damage impairs inhibitory centers. The lack of inhibition—*disinhibition*—allows unbridled aggressiveness, loquaciousness, impulsivity, and hyperactivity.

In addition to altering patients' personality and possibly cognitive capacity, frontal lobe injury may disable their executive abilities. Just as with patients who sustain anterior cerebral artery infarctions, those who sustain frontal lobe trauma have impaired ability to solve abstract problems, plan sequenced actions, or execute responses. Moreover, patients who develop pseudobulbar palsy, another complication of frontal lobe trauma, may display emotional incontinence with easily precipitated fits of *pathologic laughing* or *crying* and unpredictable immediate switches between them (see Chapter 4).

Depression

Post-traumatic depression, which the *DSM-IV-TR* classifies as a Mood Disorder Due to TBI, consists of an ill-defined combination of depressive symptoms. It develops in about 25% of TBI patients, but sometimes appears decades after the inciting head trauma and has a weak correlation with its severity. Some studies have attributed post-traumatic depression, along with poststroke depression (see Chapter 11), to left anterior cerebral hemisphere injury. Several pre-existing factors—particularly drug and alcohol abuse, previous depression, and poor baseline social functioning—predispose TBI patients to post-traumatic depression. In addition, trauma-induced cognitive impairments, epilepsy, and impaired physical, occupational, and social skills place TBI patients at risk for depression.

If it develops, post-traumatic depression interferes with patients' rehabilitation, compliance, and socialization. It also reduces patients' likelihood of making a complete recovery.

Depressed TBI patients invariably require psychopharmacology. They may benefit from selective serotonin reuptake inhibitors (SSRIs), mood stabilizers, and anxiolytics. They also often need a full array of ancillary services, such as physical and occupational therapy, financial assistance, and psychologic support.

Overall, various combinations of cognitive, personality, and mood impairments—nonphysical sequelae of TBI—cause or greatly contribute to post-traumatic unemployment; social isolation and divorce; medicine, alcohol, and drug abuse; and self-injurious behavior.

Psychosis

Although depression, substance abuse, and personality disorders are considerably more common as sequelae of TBI, post-traumatic psychosis occasionally occurs. Probably best considered by the DSM-IV-TR as Psychotic Disorder Due to TBI, post-traumatic psychosis takes the form primarily of delusions, paranoia, and auditory hallucinations. In addition, impairments in cognition, especially memory, and executive ability typically accompany the psychotic disorder.

Most cases of post-traumatic psychosis develop in male victims, within the first 2 years after the trauma, and usually in the aftermath of moderate to severe brain injury. Risk factors include a family history of psychosis and a long duration of unconsciousness.

Treatment usually entails not only typical or atypical antipsychotics but also sometimes the addition of antidepressants or AEDs. As with depressed TBI patients, those with psychosis require extensive ancillary services.

Trauma in Childhood

Compared to TBI in adults, TBI in children has somewhat different features. For example, children are frequent victims of nonaccidental head injury (see later). Also, children with attention deficit hyperactivity disorder (ADHD), compared to unaffected ones, are more likely to have suffered deliberately inflicted injuries or to have engaged in dangerous activities. The high proportion of childhood trauma survivors who are hyperactive partly reflects their preinjury status, suggesting that ADHD children are more likely than non-ADHD children to suffer abuse.

Similarly, children with learning disabilities, compared to those without such disabilities, are more apt to sustain sports-related TBI. Then, in a reciprocal relationship, TBI is likely to exacerbate learning disabilities (see later).

The prognosis for children with TBI, in general, surpasses that for adults who have survived comparable TBI. The severity and extent of brain damage in children largely determine their prognosis, but the GCS is not a suitable guide. Other prognostic factors include the family's socioeconomic status and psychiatric history.

As with adults, children's memory is particularly vulnerable to TBI and the duration of their post-traumatic amnesia correlates with their ultimate cognitive impairment and behavioral disturbances. In addition, TBI-induced social problems and behavioral disturbances handicap children as well as adults. Sometimes their residual injuries do not appear until they confront the increasing academic and social demands of successive school years. As children "grow into their deficits," TBI may limit their cognitive and psychosocial development.

When TBI occurs before growth spurts, affected limbs may fail to achieve their normal, expected size. This pattern resembles the spastic hemiparesis with foreshortened limbs that characterizes congenital cerebral injuries (see Fig. 13-4). If dominant hemisphere injury were to occur before age 5 years, the opposite hemisphere would usually assume control of language. For example, a left-sided cerebral injury in a 4-year-old child will probably not result in aphasia because the plasticity of the brain allows the right cerebral hemisphere to develop language centers. If TBI affects the dominant hemisphere of someone age 5 years or older, it is likely to cause language impairment, if not severe aphasia.

In another potential consequence, TBI in children may damage hypothalamic-pituitary hormone secretion. These endocrine disturbances may result in obesity, precocious puberty, or delayed puberty.

Nonaccidental Head Injury

Nonaccidental head injury (NAHI), a recently introduced euphemism and more legally palatable term, generally means child abuse. It often takes the form of a closed head injury unaccompanied by outward signs of trauma, such as face or scalp abrasions, spiral fractures of long bones, or damage to internal organs. For example, rages of violent shaking often injure the brain, retinae, and internal organs but do not cause obvious external injuries. Of all the organs, the brain of an infant, compared to that of an adult, is especially vulnerable to trauma because it has a greater water content, much less myelin, and a covering of only the soft, thin skull.

In the *shaken baby syndrome*, violent back-and-forth throws, without any direct impact, injure the brain parenchyma by rotational (angular) deceleration and diffuse axonal shearing. Severe shaking also produces hemorrhages in the brain's delicate parenchyma, subdural space, and retinae.

Although children may accidentally fall backward and injure their occiput, if they fall forward, they reflexively extend their arms to shield their face and eyes. Therefore, facial, ocular, and anterior skull injuries more strongly suggest NAHI than occipital injuries. Limb injuries accompanying head injuries also indicate NAHI. Because abuse tends to recur, physicians may discover injuries in different stages of development and resolution during an evaluation.

MRIs may detect and approximate the chronicity of intracranial bleeding. They can show hemorrhages in the subarachnoid, subdural, and epidural spaces and in the cerebrum and brainstem. They may also indicate diffuse axonal shearing. Nevertheless, as in most acute head trauma, neurologists and neurosurgeons usually first obtain a head CT because hospitals can perform it more rapidly, which is a great advantage for unstable patients.

Physicians must perform a funduscopic examination to find retinal hemorrhages. In the absence of external injuries, this finding may be the sole clinical indication that a child has sustained NAHI. However, retinal hemorrhages are not pathognomonic. For example, bleeding diatheses, spontaneous subarachnoid hemorrhages, arteriovenous malformations, and sepsis, as well as genuine accidental trauma, may also cause retinal hemorrhages.

Children who survive NAHI often have residual cognitive impairment, behavioral difficulties, learning disabilities, developmental delay, and seizures. Sometimes neuropsychologic sequelae may not appear for several years. As discussed previously, many NAHI survivors have either had ADHD before abuse or develop it afterward.

Elder Abuse

Elder abuse, child abuse's geriatric counterpart, usually results from family members or other caregivers violently mistreating older individuals. Chronic neurologic and psychiatric disorders, particularly dementia, are risk factors. Older individuals are prone to falls and, even with minimal trauma, subdural hematomas. TBI from elder abuse easily leads to greater cognitive impairment and reduced life expectancy.

MINOR HEAD TRAUMA

Neurologists usually define minor TBI, including *concussions*, as trauma-induced impairment or loss of consciousness for less than 30 minutes and a GCS no lower than 13. If amnesia also occurs, it must last less than 24 hours. Although MVAs and occupational injuries frequently cause minor TBI, neurologic studies have concentrated on sports-induced TBIs because they are numerous, predictable, and, by studying pre-injury academic records, amenable to thorough analysis.

Head Trauma in Sports

Sports-induced TBIs usually consist of concussions, the most common form of minor head trauma. When assessing injured athletes, neurologists describe the severity of a concussion on a scale ranging from Grade 1 to Grade 3. Grade 1 consists of transient confusion without loss of consciousness, lasting less than 15 minutes; Grade 2, transient confusion without loss of consciousness, lasting longer than 15 minutes; and Grade 3, loss of consciousness lasting seconds to minutes. Even when alert, athletes who have suffered a concussion generally have inattention, slowed responses to inquiries, disorientation, and impaired memory. They frequently report headache and nausea. Examining physicians typically elicit dysarthria, impairment of tandem gait, and loss of dexterity.

Sometimes head trauma damages one or both trochlear (fourth) cranial nerves, which each supply the ipsilateral superior oblique muscle. Affected individuals find that they have diplopia when looking at closely held objects, such as when reading a newspaper, but not when looking into the distance. With unilateral nerve damage, tiling the head away from the injured side reduces the diplopia.

Head trauma may also damage the inner ear's labyrinthine system. This injury causes vertigo, which patients may describe as "dizziness." Patients' rapidly moving their head or changing position induces this symptom. A neurologic examination of vertiginous patients may show nystagmus.

Initial physical deficits usually diminish by 1 week after the injury. Afterward, only subjective problems comprise the postconcussion picture.

At 1 week, athletes with a headache, the most common postconcussion symptom, will also typically show impairments in memory and other neuropsychologic functions. Their other postconcussion symptoms may include irritability, mood changes, and sleep disturbances. Physicians assess injured athletes with various bedside or computerized tests, but the Mini-Mental Status Examination (MMSE) (see Chapter 7) is less valuable than instruments especially designed for this situation.

Most postconcussion symptoms clear within 1 week. However, during the time that they persist, which may extend to several months, neurologists routinely bar athletes from returning to play. Following concussions that involved loss of consciousness, neurologists disallow athletes from playing for the entire season.

Studies justify such a stringent policy. They show that athletes who sustain a concussion are more apt than uninjured ones to have additional concussions. Even allowing for a full recovery from a concussion, subsequent concussions have a cumulative effect. For a variety of reasons, athletes often under-report symptoms. Although perhaps unaware of some deficits, they tend toward stoicism and denial of obvious problems. Most important, athletes having received a concussion are vulnerable to the *second impact syndrome,* in which an additional blow, received within days of the original injury, may lead to destructive and potentially fatal brain swelling.

The intercollegiate sports with the greatest risk of concussion include ice hockey, football, and both men's and women's soccer. High school TBI risks are the greatest for football, but also significant for wrestling, basketball, field hockey, and soccer. The risk in soccer probably relates to players, unlike those in most other contact sports, not wearing helmets despite their routine head-to-head collisions and "heading" the soccer ball.

Professional and amateur soccer players have subtle but undeniable impairments in memory, visual perception, and other cognitive functions. College football players develop neuropsychologic impairments and exacerbation of pre-existing learning disabilities.

Patients, parents, and psychiatrists should weigh the risks of TBI in contact sports against those in other equally vigorous noncontact ones. At the least, parents and psychiatrists should steer children with learning disabilities and other academic impediments away from such danger.

Dementia Pugilistica

Boxers (pugilists) generally receive blows to the head that frequently leave them dazed. Repeated episodes of such TBI lead to cognitive impairment, often reaching the severity of dementia, and Parkinson's disease-like physical deficits (see Dementia Pugilistica, Chapter 18).

Postconcussion Syndrome

The sequelae of minor head trauma often consist of various symptoms that neurologists group into the catch-all condition, *postconcussion syndrome.* Lacking a strict definition in the neurologic literature, a diagnosis of postconcussion syndrome usually rests on several core problems—headache, memory impairment, and insomnia—lasting more than 2 to 3 months. Otherwise, symptoms tend to be nonspecific, variable, and occasionally unending. They usually remain entirely subjective. Moreover, some symptoms, such as "dizziness," are not only trivial but commonplace in the general, healthy population.

The *DSM-IV-TR* lists research criteria for Postcussional Disorder as a diagnosis for further study but not a defined clinical entity. Its diagnosis rests on loss of consciousness and post-traumatic amnesia, but also requires several other symptoms, including insomnia, easy fatigability, headache, and dizziness. The disorder

must begin shortly after the trauma and last for more than 3 months.

Neurologists find that postconcussion syndrome patients have a normal physical neurologic examination, CT, and MRI. Although the electroencephalogram (EEG) often shows minor abnormalities, the changes are generally inconsistent, insignificant, and often attributable to medications and normal variations. Similarly, neuropsychologic tests often reveal minor and uneven abnormalities, but those changes may be attributable to inattention, depression, exaggeration, lack of education, or even malingering.

Proposed etiologies of the postconcussion syndrome include diffuse axonal shearing, excitatory neurotransmitter imbalance, and subtle cerebral contusions. In addition, any coexistent whiplash injury (see later) may cause head and neck pain. No matter which ones predominate, postconcussion symptoms distract patients, interfere with their sleep, and require them to take medicines that may impair their mood and cognition.

Although neurologists routinely diagnose and treat patients with the postconcussion syndrome, individual patients regularly provoke their skepticism. Prolonged symptoms are associated with psychiatric and socioeconomic factors as much as with neurologic injury and do not correlate with either the estimated force of impact or the usual neurologic parameters of TBI—GCS scores and duration of amnesia. Among compensation claimants, effort may have more of an effect than severity of TBI on neuropsychologic test scores. In contrast to assembly line workers dissatisfied with their workplace, children, soldiers, self-employed workers, and professionals rarely report prolonged or incapacitating symptoms. Finally, treatment that is usually effective in most circumstances often fails to alleviate common post-traumatic symptoms, particularly headache and insomnia.

The postconcussion syndrome sometimes persists for extraordinarily long periods, especially in patients with abnormal premorbid intellectual and personality traits. For some patients, symptoms seem inextricably linked to potential monetary rewards and other aspects of unsettled litigation. If minor neurologic sequelae persist, some individuals exaggerate the deficits or allow themselves to be overwhelmed.

On the other hand, some reports indicate that the postconcussion syndrome results predominantly from neurologic injury. Support for this position is that postconcussion symptoms are similar from patient to patient. In addition, the syndrome develops in many self-employed and highly motivated people, including physicians. Also, according to some data, symptoms correlate poorly with outstanding litigation and persist after legal claims are settled.

Many children and some adults may not report postconcussion symptoms because they are unable to describe them, have a stoic disposition, cannot readily admit to pain, or substitute other symptoms for post-concussion disturbances. For example, rather than complaining of post-traumatic headaches, children may have somnolence, inattention, or hyperactivity. Professionals unable to describe their feelings may develop unusual irritability.

Finally, normal neurologic examinations and laboratory test results do not necessarily exclude a neurologic illness. For example, neurologists routinely diagnose many illnesses—migraines, trigeminal neuralgia, chronic pain, and dementia—in the absence of physical and laboratory abnormalities. Postconcussion syndrome may fall into this category.

Headache

The essential feature of postconcussion syndrome is a dull, generalized, continuous headache. Movement, bending, work, and alcohol use exacerbate it. In 50% of patients, postconcussion headache lasts longer than 1 year, and in 25%, longer than 3 years. Surprisingly, postconcussion headache occurs more frequently in mildly injured than in severely injured individuals.

Physicians should not dismiss such headaches. When post-traumatic headaches are hemicranial or throbbing, develop in a context of migraines, or are accompanied by autonomic nervous system dysfunction, they may represent *post-traumatic migraine* (see Chapter 9). However, head trauma does not seem to provoke cluster headache or trigeminal neuralgia. Also, patients might have headaches from a slowly developing subdural hematoma. Another alternative cause, partly iatrogenic, results from daily use of analgesic or vasoactive medications leading to "rebound" or "withdrawal" headaches (see Chapter 9).

Memory Impairment

Patients with postconcussion symptom characteristically have mild or intermittent amnesia accompanied by slowed information processing, inattention, and difficulty completing complex mental tasks. As with other postconcussion symptoms, the amnesia shows little correlation with the severity of trauma.

One potential explanation for amnesia in postconcussion syndrome is frontal and temporal lobe damage from having been thrown against the bony inner surfaces of the anterior and middle cranial fossae. Comorbid PTSD might also explain some of the impaired recollection of events surrounding the trauma.

Insomnia

Postconcussion syndrome patients regularly report inability to fall or remain asleep. They also describe excessive daytime sleepiness (EDS) that causes fatigue and forces them to nap (see Chapter 17); however, neither night-time sleep nor daytime naps restore their full normal wakefulness.

For patients with insomnia, one potential explanation sometimes lies in their tendency to consume excessive caffeine, alcohol, opioids, and other medications. In addition, sometimes anxiety, depression, and PTSD exacerbate if not cause insomnia.

On the other hand, whatever the cause, physicians might consider that a pre-existing sleep disorder actually led to the TBI. For example, patients with sleep apnea, narcolepsy, or sleep deprivation might cause a MVA or be unable to avoid one (see Chapter 17).

Other Symptoms

Postconcussion syndrome patients often report that they have dizziness. In most cases, their symptom is not authentic vertigo but a nonspecific sensation with variable, idiosyncratic meanings that possibly substitutes for lightheadedness, anxiety, unsteadiness, or lassitude. Except for patients who have vertigo because they sustained labyrinth damage, post-traumatic dizziness remains difficult to define and almost impossible to treat.

Patients also commonly have exquisite sensitivity to light (photophobia) and sound (phonophobia). They cannot tolerate even everyday levels of sunlight, street noise, or workplace activity. The hypersensitivity intensifies patients' headaches, distracts them from work-related tasks, and drives them into seclusion.

In addition, patients often describe symptoms of depression, anxiety, irritability, and moodiness, but perhaps not in a few words. They also frequently report that their injuries reduce their desire for sex and other previously enjoyable activities. That post-traumatic anhedonia may also overlap with symptoms of depression.

In contrast, some patients with the postconcussion syndrome may consciously or subconsciously minimize their symptoms. Whether stoic or in denial, they fail to acknowledge memory impairments, other cognitive deficits, personality changes, or physical impediments. Relying on poor judgment, they may attempt to fulfill all their commitments and work at demanding jobs.

Treatment and Recovery

Neurologists attempt to educate the patient and family about the nature, extent, and course of postconcussion syndrome. Many urge patients with minor or vague symptoms to return to work, perhaps with a reduced load, but those with demanding or dangerous jobs to remain on a medical leave. With a patient completely refractory to treatment, neurologists often decide not to challenge the patient's and family's beliefs but agree that symptoms exist without necessarily accepting that they originate in permanent brain injury.

For headaches, neurologists prescribe often mild, nonaddicting analgesics similar to those used for muscle contraction headaches. Sometimes, even when only a minimal migraine component exists, antimigraine medicines help (see Chapter 9). Neurologists also prescribe nonsteroidal anti-inflammatory drugs (NSAIDs) and tricyclic antidepressants. These medications may alleviate insomnia and neck pain as well as headaches.

Psychotherapy and antidepressants often reduce anxiety and improve depression. However, cognitive retraining remains controversial and biofeedback has shown no demonstrable benefit.

Physicians must cautiously treat insomnia. They should avoid prescribing hypnotics because they may easily lead to EDS, mimic symptoms of TBI, or worsen depression and cognitive impairment. In addition, physicians should prohibit alcohol because it may induce disturbances in personality, behavior, sleep, and judgment.

Almost all patients improve to a greater or lesser extent. About 85% fully recover and none deteriorates. Although recovery from postconcussion symptoms often follows a nonlinear and uncertain course, it should take place by 3 months in uncomplicated cases.

However, some patients have symptoms that persist, recur under certain circumstances, or, in a small proportion of cases, incapacitate the patient. Risk factors for incomplete recovery from postconcussion syndrome include the following:

- The patient has a history of attention deficit disorder, learning disability, or neurosis.
- Before the accident, the patient was in a low socioeconomic status, an unskilled or semiskilled worker, dissatisfied with the job, or in danger of being fired.
- A MVA caused the concussion.
- The symptoms are multiple and include bodily pains.

WHIPLASH

Mechanism of Action

In the common rear-end MVA, the sudden impact throws the head and neck of the driver and passengers backward and then forward. The forceful movement causes *flexion-extension* neck injury or *whiplash* because, when the anterior neck muscles cannot resist, the neck extends beyond its normal range (hyperextends), but then, in a rebound, the neck rapidly flexes excessively forward (hyperflexes) (Fig. 22-3). The rapid, uncontrolled hyperextension-hyperflexion wrenches the neck's soft tissues, including ligaments, tendons, and the trapezius, paraspinal, and numerous, small, delicate muscles.

Whiplash not only injures cervical soft tissues, but it may aggravate degenerative spine disease and herniate intervertebral disks (see Chapter 5). A severe rear-end MVA may fracture or dislocate cervical vertebrae, which can even transect the spinal cord.

If MVA victims wear their seatbelt, they should not sustain concomitant direct head trauma. However, because whiplash often jostles the brain within the skull, some MVA patients develop the postconcussion syndrome superimposed on whiplash symptoms.

Symptoms

As in the postconcussion syndrome, the development, severity, and duration of whiplash symptoms do not correlate with the forcefulness of the MVA, as calculated from its speed. The primary symptom is neck pain of variable severity with radiation upward toward the head and downward toward the shoulders, arms, and lower back. With simultaneous head trauma and whiplash, symptoms multiply. Even without head trauma, whiplash patients also often describe cognitive impairments, mood changes, inattention, dizziness, and fatigue. Despite the large number of people involved and regularity of psychiatric

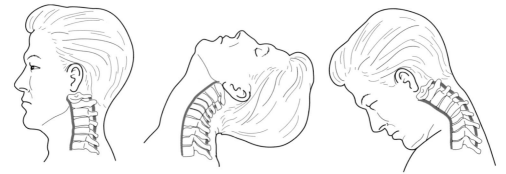

FIGURE 22-3 ■ Cervical flexion-extension injuries, popularly called "whiplash," may tear the anterior and posterior longitudinal ligaments (blue) and other soft tissues, herniate intervertebral disks, and exacerbate cervical spondylosis (see Chapter 5).

sequelae, the *DSM-IV-TR* does not offer a description of this disorder.

When trauma herniates cervical intervertebral disks, patients typically have pain that radiates along the nerve roots (radicular pain), weakness, and loss of deep tendon reflexes in their arms. MRI can detect herniated disks as well as fractures and dislocations. Electromyograms (EMGs) may establish the presence, nature, severity, and extent of a nerve or nerve root injury. However, numerous other techniques, such as thermography, surface EMGs, and ultrasound, which have crept into the field, lack diagnostic reliability.

Approximately 50% of whiplash patients recover by 3 months and 75% by 6 months. Still, 20% have symptoms for 2 years or longer. Risk factors for prolonged disability include middle age, pre-existing degenerative spine disease, persistent headache, and psychiatric comorbidity, such as anxiety, depression, or PTSD. In addition, compensation and other forms of litigation, looking at the population at large, constitute one of the most powerful risk factors. For example, after Saskatchewan, Canada converted its tort-compensation system to a no-fault plan, its citizens enjoyed a markedly reduced incidence of whiplash and, if it developed, a better prognosis.

Treatment

Treatment of whiplash injury remains largely empiric and variable. In fact, patients may improve with little or no treatment. Many respond to reassurance, rest, at-home exercising, or simple physical measures, such as massage and heat. However, patients should avoid vigorous cervical manipulation, as occurs as part of chiropractic treatment, because it may lead to spinal cord injury or vertebral artery dissection. Although protecting the head and neck from further abrupt movement is obviously reasonable, the purported benefits of a restraining soft cervical collar remain controversial. Medications for whiplash pain include muscle relaxants, NSAIDs, nonopioid analgesics, and—for their analgesic and sedative, as well as their mood-altering, effects—antidepressants. Migraine medications, according to some reports, may help.

Good "neck hygiene" would probably help whiplash patients. For example, if they frequently speak on a telephone during multitasking, whiplash patients should wear a headset or separate earpiece. They should also keep the computer monitor at or below eye level so that looking at it does not require neck hyperextension. They should use only one pillow and should curtail tennis, golf, and other activities that cause neck strain.

REFERENCES

1. Arciniegas DB, Harris SN, Brousseau KM, et al: Psychosis following traumatic brain injury. Int Rev Psychiatry 15:328–340, 2003.
2. Barnes BC, Cooper L, Kirkendall DT, et al: Concussion history in elite male and female soccer players. Am J Sports Med 26:433–438, 1998.
3. Cassidy JD, Carroll LJ, Côté P, et al: Effect of eliminating compensation for pain and suffering on the outcome of insurance claims for whiplash injury. N Engl J Med 342:1179–1186, 2000.
4. Diaz-Olavarrieta C, Campbell J, Garcia de la Cadena C, et al: Domestic violence against patients with chronic neurologic disorders. Arch Neurol 56:681–685, 1999.
5. DiScala C, Lescohier I, Barthel M, et al: Injuries to children with attention deficit hyperactivity disorder. Pediatrics 102:1415–1421, 1998.
6. Fleminger S, Oliver DL, Lovestone S, et al: Head injury as a risk factor for Alzheimer's disease: The evidence 10 years on; a partial replication. J Neurol Neurosurg Psychiatry 74:857–862, 2003.
7. Fujii D, Ahmed I: Characteristics of psychotic disorder due to traumatic brain injury. J Neuropsychiatry Clin Neurosci 14:130–140, 2002.
8. Grafman J, Jonas BS, Martin A, et al: Intellectual function following penetrating head injury in Vietnam veterans. Brain 111:169–184, 1988.
9. Green P, Rohling ML, Lees-Haley PR, et al: Effort has a greater effect on test scores than severe brain injury in compensation claimants. Brain Inj 15:1045–1060, 2001.
10. Jennett B, Bond M: Assessment of outcome after severe brain damage. Lancet 5:480–484, 1975.
11. Jennett B, Teasdale G, Braakman R, et al: Prognosis of patients with severe head injury. Neurosurgery 4:283–289, 1979.
12. Koponen S, Taiminen T, Kairisto V, et al: APO-ε4 predicts dementia but not other psychiatric disorders after traumatic brain injury. Neurology 63:749–750, 2004.
13. Kleinschmidt KC: Elder abuse: A review. Ann Emerg Med 30:463–472, 1997.
14. Koponen S, Taiminen T, Portin R, et al: Axis I and II psychiatric disorders after traumatic brain injury: A 30-year follow-up study. Am J Psychiatry 159:1315–1321, 2002.
15. Lovell MR, Collins MW, Iverson GL, et al: Recovery from mild concussion in high school athletes. J Neurosurg 98:296–301, 2003.
16. Max JE, Robertson BAM, Lansing AE: The phenomenology of personality change due to traumatic brain injury in children and adolescents. J Neuropsychiatry Clin Neurosci 13:161–170, 2001.
17. McAllister TW, Ferrell RB: Evaluation and treatment of psychosis after traumatic brain injury. NeuroRehabil 17:357–368, 2002.
18. McCrea M, Guskiewicz KM, Marshall SW, et al: Acute effects and recovery time following concussion in collegiate football players: The NCAA Concussion Study. JAMA 290:2556–2563, 2003.

19. NIH Consensus Development Panel: Rehabilitation of persons with traumatic brain injury. JAMA 282:974–983, 1999.

20. Obelieniene D, Schrader H, Bovim G, et al: Pain after whiplash: A prospective controlled inception cohort study. J Neurol Neurosurg Psychiatry 66:279–283, 1999.

21. Quality Standards Subcommittee, American Academy of Neurology: Practice parameter: The management of concussion in sports. Neurology 48:581–585, 1997.

22. Radanov BP, DiStefano G, Schnidrig A, et al: Cognitive functioning after common whiplash. Arch Neurol 50:87–91, 1993.

23. Radanov BP, Sturzenegger M, DiStefano G, et al: Factors influencing recovery from headache after common whiplash. Br Med J 307:652–655, 1993.

24. Roberts GW, Allsop D, Bruton C: The occult aftermath of boxing. J Neurol Neurosurg Psychiatry 53:373–378, 1990.

25. Rohling ML, Allen LM, Green P: Who is exaggerating cognitive impairment and who is not? CNS Spectrums 7:387–395, 2002.

26. Rosenthal M, Christensen BK, Ross TP: Depression following traumatic brain injury. Arch Phys Med Rehabil 79:90–103, 1998.

27. Saper JR: Posttraumatic headache: A neurobehavioral disorder. Arch Neurol 57:1776–1778, 2000.

28. Satz P, Forney DL, Zaucha K, et al: Depression, cognition, and functional correlates of recovery outcome after traumatic brain injury. Brain Inj 12:537–553, 1998.

29. Schmans B, Lindboom J, Schagen S, et al: Cognitive complaints in patients after whiplash injury: The impact of malingering. J Neurol Neurosurg Psychiatry 64:339–343, 1998.

30. Schwab K, Grafman J, Salazar AM, et al: Residual impairments and work status 15 years after penetrating head injury: Report from the Vietnam Head Injury Study. Neurology 43:95–103, 1993.

31. Sachdev P, Smith JS, Cathcart S: Schizophrenia-like psychosis following traumatic brain injury: A chart-based descriptive and case-control study. Psychol Med 31:231–239, 2001.

32. Siddall OM: Use of methylphenidate in traumatic brain injury. Ann Pharmacother 39:1309–1313, 2005.

33. Silver JM, McAllister TW: Forensic issues in the neuropsychiatric evaluation of the patient with mild traumatic brain injury. J Neuropsychiatry 9:102–113, 1997.

34. Spitzer WO, Skovron ML, Salmi LR, et al: Scientific monograph of the Quebec Task Force on whiplash-associated disorders: Redefining "whiplash" and its management. Spine 20(Suppl 8S):1S–73S, 1995.

35. Sundström A, Marklund P, Nilsson LG, et al: *APOE* influences on neuropsychological function after mild head injury: Within-person comparisons. Neurology 62:1963–1966, 2004.

36. Tateno A, Jorge RE, Robinson RG: Clinical correlates of aggressive behavior after traumatic brain injury. J Neuropsychiatry Clin Neurosci 15:155–160, 2003.

37. Tateno A, Jorge RE, Robinson RG: Pathologic laughing and crying following traumatic brain injury. J Neuropsychiatry Clin Neurosci 16:426–434, 2004.

38. Teasdale G, Jennett B: Assessment of coma and impaired consciousness: A practical scale. Lancet 2:81–84, 1974.

39. Warner JS: Posttraumatic headache—A myth? Arch Neurol 57:1778–1780, 2000.

40. Wenzel HG, Haug TT, Mykletun A, et al: A population study of anxiety and depression among persons who report whiplash traumas. J Psychsom Res 53:831–835, 2002.

Questions and Answers

1. Physicians use the Glasgow Coma Scale (GCS) to assess three parameters of a patient's level of consciousness following head trauma. Which of the following functions is not assessed by the GCS?
   a. Vital signs
   b. Eye opening
   c. Speaking (best verbal response)
   d. Moving (best motor response)

   Answer: a. Vital signs, except for spontaneous respirations, may be normal in deeply comatose patients. Physicians using the GCS rate three functions that reflect responsiveness and score patients on a scale of 3 to 15.

2. At the scene of a high-speed, single-vehicle, motor vehicle accident (MVA), emergency workers found a stuporous 24-year-old man. As they cared for his head and bodily wounds, they gave him a GCS score of 9. During transfer to the hospital, he lapsed into coma while developing decerebrate posture and a left third cranial nerve palsy. On arrival at the emergency room, his GCS had fallen to 3. Skull x-rays showed a fracture through his left temporal bone. Which is the most likely cause of his deterioration?
   a. Subdural hematoma
   b. Alcohol intoxication
   c. Middle meningeal artery laceration
   d. Subarachnoid hemorrhage

   Answer: c. The temporal skull fracture probably lacerated the middle meningeal artery, which led to an epidural hematoma. His GCS score of 3, as well as developing decerebrate posturing, reliably predicted a fatal outcome. In another aspect of this case, a high-speed, single-driver, single-vehicle MVA may represent a suicide.

3. Which statement is untrue regarding chronic subdural hematomas?
   a. On CT, they frequently appear as extra-axial, long, curved, radiolucent (black) lesions.
   b. They are a correctable cause of dementia.
   c. They cause few lateralized deficits, such as hemiparesis, compared to nonspecific generalized symptoms, such as headaches and personality changes.
   d. The elderly are prone to subdural hematomas because they have cerebral atrophy and a tendency to fall.
   e. Many chronic subdural hematomas are reabsorbed without the need for surgery.
   f. On CT, they are typically radiodense.

   Answer: f. *Acute* subdural hematomas, which contain fresh blood, are radiodense (white) lesions. Chronic ones are radiolucent (black). However, between its acute and chronic stages, blood in the subdural hematoma is isodense to the brain. Then, the CT shows the subdural hematoma, as well as the brain, as gray. Although indistinguishable from the brain parenchyma, the isodense subdural still exerts a mass effect. It compresses the adjacent ventricles and shifts midline structures to the opposite side.

4. Which condition is most likely to follow TBI causing a GCS score of 7?
   a. Anterograde amnesia
   b. Postconcussion syndrome
   c. Chronic neck pain
   d. Seizures

   Answer: a. The most common sequela of moderately severe TBI consists of anterograde amnesia. TBI less often and less severely produces retrograde amnesia. Seizures, postconcussion syndrome, and neck pains are also associated but less closely.

5. To which injury does the term *contrecoup* most appropriately apply?
   a. Injury of temporal lobe, especially the temporal tip, after an occipital blow
   b. Blindness after an occipital lobe blow
   c. Diffuse axonal shearing after localized head trauma
   d. Neck pain after head injury

   Answer: a. Head trauma that damages the opposite side of the brain is a *contrecoup* injury. These injuries can be envisioned as resulting from the brain "bouncing against the other side of the skull." They are most apparent in areas where the brain strikes rough or sharpened inner surfaces of the skull, such as in the middle cranial fossa, which cradles the temporal lobes. Temporal lobe injuries characteristically result in post-traumatic amnesia.

6. Neurosurgeons frequently cannot remove all shrapnel and other fragments from penetrating head wounds. Which are two consequences of retained foreign bodies?

a. They may act as a scar focus for post-traumatic epilepsy.
b. They envelop themselves with calcium and remain benign scars.
c. They may act as a nidus for a brain abscess.
d. They can dislodge and enter the general circulation.

Answers: a, c. Foreign bodies may be so numerous or situated in inoperable areas that neurosurgeons cannot remove all of them. Each retained foreign body may act as a nidus for an abscess or a scar focus for post-traumatic epilepsy.

7. Which injury suggests the shaken baby syndrome?
   a. Periventricular intracranial calcifications
   b. Retinal hemorrhages
   c. Tram tract calcifications
   d. Dislocated optic lens

Answer: b. Violent shaking of infants and young children causes nonaccidental head injury (NAHI), a common form of child abuse. Shaken babies often develop raised intracranial pressure and intracranial bleeding; however, the only visible sign on clinical evaluation, which requires funduscopic examination, is retinal hemorrhages. Periventricular intracranial calcifications are a sign of *in utero* infection with cytomegalovirus. Scattered intracranial calcifications are a sign of *in utero* infection with toxoplasmosis. Calcifications in layers of the cerebral cortex, tram tract calcifications, are a manifestation of Sturge-Weber syndrome. Homocystinuria causes dislocated lens.

8. Which cognitive function is most susceptible to head trauma?
   a. Judgment
   b. Language function
   c. Memory
   d. Constructional ability

Answer: c. Head trauma is most apt to cause amnesia for the period immediately before the trauma (retrograde amnesia) as well as amnesia for the trauma.

9. Of the following varieties of seizure, which is the most common sequela of TBI?
   a. Psychogenic
   b. Partial with secondary generalization
   c. Petit mal
   d. Primary generalized

Answer: b. Because of its component of cerebral cortex injury, TBI typically causes partial (focal) seizures, including partial complex seizures, that undergo secondary generalization, that is, post-traumatic epilepsy. TBI does not cause primary generalized seizures—petit mal (absences) or tonic-clonic seizures.

10. After falling forward and striking his head, a 72-year-old gentleman describes being unable to read because he sees double. To alleviate the problem, he covers one eye, avoids looking at closely held objects, or tilts his head to the left. The visual acuity in each eye is normal. Which is the most likely site of injury?
    a. Medial longitudinal fasciculus
    b. Left trochlear nerve
    c. Right trochlear nerve
    d. Left abducens nerve
    e. Right abducens nerve

Answer: c. Head trauma may damage one or both trochlear (fourth) cranial nerves, which supply the ipsilateral superior oblique muscle. Affected individuals cannot intort the eye when it is adducted. Thus, they have diplopia when looking at a closely held object, such as when reading a newspaper. With unilateral nerve damage, tilting the head away from the injured side reduces the diplopia.

11. Of the following, which is the most reliable indicator of TBI sequelae?
    a. GCS score
    b. Duration of retrograde amnesia
    c. Duration of anterograde amnesia
    d. Blood alcohol level
    e. Delta waves on the EEG immediately after the trauma

Answer: b. The duration of retrograde amnesia, which includes the duration of the patient's coma, correlates with the functional outcome and neuropsychologic impairments. It provides a more reliable prognosis than either the GCS or duration of coma.

12. Of the following regions of the brain, which two are most likely to be damaged by a coup-contrecoup blow?
    a. Frontal lobe
    b. Parietal lobe
    c. Occipital lobe
    d. Temporal lobe tips
    e. Cerebellum
    f. Brainstem

Answers: a, d. Coup-contrecoup injuries have their greatest impact on the temporal lobe and frontal lobes' anterior-inferior surfaces because they abut against the sharp, rough surfaces of the anterior and middle cranial fossae.

13. Which three of the following are typically found in the subarachnoid space?
    a. Cerebrospinal fluid (CSF)
    b. Urine

c. Purulent CSF in cases of meningitis

d. Epidural hematomas in cases of major head trauma

e. Blood from ruptured berry aneurysms

f. Aqueous humor

Answers: a, c, e. The subarachnoid space, which is situated between the arachnoid and the pia layers of the meninges, normally contains crystal clear CSF. However, the CSF becomes purulent in bacterial meningitis, bloody with subarachnoid hemorrhage from ruptured berry aneurysms or trauma, and filled with mononuclear cells in viral meningitis. The subarachnoid space surrounds the brain and extends down into the lumbar sac. To sample the CSF, neurologists insert LP needles into the lumbar subarachnoid space.

14. Regarding post-traumatic cognitive impairment, which of these statements is false?

a. Cognitive recovery is slower and less complete in patients older than 65 years compared to younger patients.

b. Recovery of motor and language skills usually reaches a maximum within 6 months after the injury.

c. Cognitive recovery, to the extent that it occurs, takes place sooner than motor recovery.

d. Cognitive impairment correlates with low GCS scores.

Answer: c. Maximum motor recovery usually is completed during the first 6 months after trauma, but cognitive recovery does not reach its maximum until 18 months. In addition, cognitive recovery may be further delayed in individuals older than 65 years and by other factors.

15. Regarding post-traumatic cognitive impairment, which of these statements is false?

a. Cognitive impairment correlates with the lesion's size.

b. Cognitive impairment correlates with the lesion's location.

c. Use of alcohol may add to post-traumatic cognitive impairment.

d. Use of antiepileptic drugs may add to post-traumatic cognitive impairment.

Answer: b. With one exception, the traumatic lesion's location does not correlate with the presence or severity of cognitive impairment. Left temporal lesions, the exception, are associated with aphasia-like difficulties.

16. Of the following statements, which one best describes postconcussive headaches?

a. Their severity is proportional to the duration of unconsciousness.

b. Their severity is proportional to the severity of the head trauma.

c. Of common postconcussive symptoms, headaches are most closely associated with memory and concentration impairment.

d. They are a risk factor for post-traumatic epilepsy.

Answer: c. As with the other postconcussive symptoms, headaches show little correlation with the duration of unconsciousness or severity of trauma. Concussions, in contrast to penetrating TBI, carry a negligible risk for post-traumatic epilepsy.

17. Regarding NAHI, which of the following statements is false?

a. Survivors have an increased incidence of developmental delay and learning disabilities.

b. Survivors have an increased incidence of epilepsy.

c. Neuropsychologic sequelae are always detectable during the period of abuse.

d. Many survivors develop post-traumatic ADHD or have had pre-existing ADHD.

Answer: c. Neuropsychologic sequelae may not appear for several years.

18. Which of the following statements best describes diffuse axonal shearing?

a. Head MRI, but not CT, can readily detect diffuse axonal shearing.

b. It predominantly affects long subcortical white matter axons.

c. It explains post-traumatic headache.

d. The EEG can reliably diagnose diffuse axonal shearing.

e. It predominantly affects long cortical gray matter neurons.

Answer: b. Diffuse axonal shearing, which predominantly affects long subcortical white matter axons, is a pathologic diagnosis that includes much more than shearing of long axons. It includes damage to cytoskeletal structures and affects an intracellular influx of calcium. Although MRI may show petechia, that is not a diagnostic finding. Similarly, EEG, and neuropsychologic testing cannot reliably diagnose it. Only an autopsy can confirm the diagnosis.

19. Which is the order of the layers of the meningeal mater, from innermost to outermost?

a. Arachnoid, pia, dura

b. Dura, pia, arachnoid

c. Pia, arachnoid, dura

d. Pia, dura, arachnoid

Answer: c. The mnemonic is PAD.

20. Of the following statements, which one most accurately describes post-traumatic depression?
    a. It develops in almost all patients who have had a GCS score of 3 to 7.
    b. Pre-existing drug and alcohol abuse, depression, and poor social functioning are risk factors for post-traumatic depression.
    c. It closely correlates with the severity of the head trauma.
    d. Although post-traumatic depression affects mood, it does not impede recovery of function.

Answer: b. Post-traumatic depression develops in about 25% of TBI patients, but correlates weakly with the severity of the head trauma and the GCS score. Not only are drug and alcohol abuse, previous depression, and poor social functioning risk factors for depression but so are trauma-induced cognitive impairments, epilepsy, and impaired physical, occupational, and social skills. When it complicates TBI, depression interferes with patients' rehabilitation, compliance, and socialization and it reduces patients' likelihood of making a complete recovery.

21. Which histologic change characterizes TBI?
    a. Vacuoles in the cerebral cortex
    b. Infiltration of monocular cells and other inflammatory changes
    c. Degenerating neurons without a monocular infiltrate
    d. Loss of myelin in the periventricular region

Answer: b. Inflammatory changes characterize cell necrosis, which is the mechanism of action of cell death from strokes and TBI. Vacuoles characterize spongiform changes, the hallmark of prion infections, such as Creutzfeldt-Jakob disease. Degenerating neurons

without a monocular infiltrate signify apoptosis, a form of cell death that occurs in amyotrophic lateral sclerosis and other neurodegenerative conditions. Demyelination, especially in the periventricular region, characterizes multiple sclerosis.

22. Of the following complications of TBI, which is the most infrequent?
    a. Depression
    b. Substance abuse
    c. Personality disorders
    d. Psychosis

Answer: d. In descending order of their frequency, TBI psychiatric complications include post-traumatic depression, substance abuse, personality disorders, and psychosis.

23. Regarding TBI, what is the second impact syndrome?
    a. Contrecoup injuries causing greater damage than coup injuries
    b. Frontal head injuries causing cervical spine injuries that may sever the spinal cord
    c. A second head injury, occurring several days to several weeks after a concussion, causing catastrophic brain swelling
    d. Head trauma causing intracerebral and subarachnoid hemorrhage

Answer: c. Although all of these combinations occur, the second impact syndrome refers to a second head injury, occurring several days to several weeks after a concussion, causing catastrophic, potentially fatal brain swelling. Even though the second impact syndrome rarely occurs, its effects are so devastating that neurologists and other physicians forbid athletes from returning to play for weeks to months following a concussion.

Patient and Family Support Groups

The following organizations provide patients and their families with educational, legal, medical, and personal assistance. However, because these groups often consist disproportionately of incapacitated patients, a personal visit may be discouraging. Some organizations also provide educational materials for physicians.

GENERAL RESOURCES

Neurology: Official Journal of the American Academy of Neurology
www.neurology.org
National Institutes of Health
www.nih.gov

ACQUIRED IMMUNODEFICIENCY SYNDROME (AIDS)

Gay Men's Health Crisis
www.gmhc.org

ALZHEIMER'S DISEASE

Alzheimer's Association
www.alz.org

AMYOTROPHIC LATERAL SCLEROSIS (ALS)

Amyotrophic Lateral Sclerosis Association
www.alsa.org

APHASIA AND RELATED DISORDERS

American Speech-Language Hearing Association
www.asha.org

AUTISM

Autism Society of America
www.autism-society.org

BLEPHAROSPASM

Benign Essential Blepharospasm Research Foundation
www.blepharospasm.org

BLINDNESS

American Foundation for the Blind
www.afb.org

BRAIN TUMORS

American Brain Tumor Association
www.abta.org
Children's Brain Tumor Foundation
www.cbtf.org
National Brain Tumor Foundation
www.braintumor.org

CEREBRAL PALSY

United Cerebral Palsy Association
www.ucp.org

DYSTONIA

Dystonia Medical Research Foundation
www.dystonia-foundation.org

EPILEPSY

Epilepsy Foundation of America
www.epilepsyfoundation.org

FRAUDULENT THERAPIES

www.quackwatch.org

GUILLAIN-BARRÉ SYNDROME

Guillain-Barré Syndrome Foundation International
www.guillain-barre.com

HEAD INJURY

Brain Injury Association
www.biausa.org

HUNTINGTON'S DISEASE

Huntington's Disease Society of America
www.hdsa.org

MIGRAINE AND HEADACHE

American Council for Headache Education
www.achenet.org
National Headache Foundation
www.headaches.org

MULTIPLE SCLEROSIS

National Multiple Sclerosis Association of America
    (MSAA)
www.msaa.com
National Multiple Sclerosis Society
www.nmss.org

MUSCULAR DYSTROPHY AND RELATED DISORDERS

Muscular Dystrophy Association, Inc.
www.mdausa.org

MYASTHENIA GRAVIS

Myasthenia Gravis Foundation of America
www.myasthenia.org

NEUROFIBROMATOSIS

National Neurofibromatosis Foundation
www.nf.org

PAIN

American Chronic Pain Association
www.theacpa.org
International Association for the Study of Pain
www.iasp-pain.org/defsopen.html
American Pain Foundation
www.painfoundation.org
National Pain Foundation
www.painconnection.org
American Academy of Pain Medicine
www.painmed.org

PARAPLEGIA

See spinal cord injury

PARKINSON'S DISEASE

National Parkinson Foundation
www.parkinson.org
Parkinson's Disease Foundation
www.pdf.org

POSTPOLIO SYNDROME

International Polio Network
www.post-polio.org

RETT SYNDROME

International Rett Syndrome Association
www.rettsyndrome.org

SLEEP DISORDERS

American Academy of Sleep Medicine
www.aasmnet.org

SPASMODIC DYSPHONIA

See dystonia

SPASMODIC TORTICOLLIS

National Spasmodic Torticollis Association
www.torticollis.org

SPINA BIFIDA

Spina Bifida Association of America
www.sbaa.org

SPINAL CORD INJURY

American Paralysis Association
www.apacure.org
National Spinal Cord Injury Association
www.spinalcord.org
Paralyzed Veterans of America
www.pva.org

STROKE

American Heart Association
www.americanheart.org
National Stroke Association
www.stroke.org

TOURETTE SYNDROME

Tourette Syndrome Association
www.tsa-usa.org

TUBEROUS SCLEROSIS

Tuberous Sclerosis Alliance
www.tsalliance.org

TREMOR

International Tremor Foundation
www.essentialtremor.org

WILSON'S DISEASE

Wilson's Disease Association International
www.wilsonsdisease.org

APPENDIX

2

Costs of Various Tests and Treatments*

Tests	Cost
Computed tomography (CT):	
Head	$2250
Spine	2250
Genetic tests:	
APO genotype	450
Duchenne's muscular dystrophy	5000
Dystonia (DYT1)	650
Fragile X DNA test	400
Huntington's disease	500
MERRF mtDNA	1400
Myotonic dystrophy	1200
Electroencephalogram (EEG)	350
EEG video monitoring per day	3700
Electromyography (EMG)	500
Evoked response testing	450

Continued

Tests	Cost
Lumbar puncture (spinal tap)	350
Magnetic resonance imaging (MRI) of head	2200
Nerve conduction velocity (NCV), per nerve	90
Typical cost for a study	1200
Sleep studies	
Multiple sleep latency test (MSLT)	1500
Polysomnography (PSG) for 2 nights	1500
Positron emission tomography (PET)	4200
Syphilis tests	
Fluorescent treponemal antibody absorption (FTA-ABS)	35
Rapid plasma reagin (RPR)	15
Treponema microhemagglutination assay (MHA-TP)	40

Treatments	Cost
Deep brain stimulation for essential or Parkinson's tremor	45,000
Lumbar spine fusion	35,000
Medications' monthly wholesale cost:	

Continued

Test and Treatments	Cost (in $)
Alzheimer's Disease	
Donepezil (Aricept) 10 mg, 30 pills	250
Memantine (Namenda) 10 mg, 60 pills	270
Rivastigmine (Exelon)	250
Epilepsy	
Valproate (Depakote) 500 mg, 90 pills	225
Lamotrigine (Lamictal) 150 mg, 60 pills	260
Levetiracetam (Keppra) 500 mg, 90 pills	300
Phenytoin (Dilantin) 100 mg, 90 pills	25
Topiramate (Topamax) 100 mg, 90 pills	450
Erectile Dysfunction	
Sildenafil (Viagra) 50 mg, 8 pills	85

Continued

Tests and Treatments	Cost (in $)
Migraine	
Sumatriptan (Imitrex) 50 mg, 8 pills	80
Parkinson's Disease	
L-dopa with carbidopa 25/250, 120 pills	45
Ropinirole (Requip) 1 mg, 120 pills	220
Nursing home care, annual	75,000–150,000
Plasmapheresis (for Guillain-Barré syndrome or myasthenia gravis):	
Six-exchange course	12,000
Vagus nerve stimulation	20,000

*Approximate costs of representative tests and treatments in New York City, 2006.

APPENDIX

3

Diseases Transmitted by Chromosomes or Mitochondria Abnormalities*

A. Chromosomes and the Diseases They Transmit

1 Alzheimer's disease, presenilin 2
3 von Hippel-Lindau disease
4 Huntington's disease
  Parkinson's disease parkin gene
5 Infantile and juvenile spinal muscular atrophy
  (Werdnig-Hoffmann and Kugelberg-Welander diseases)
  Tay Sachs
6 Narcolepsy
  Parkinson's disease α-synuclein gene
  Spinocerebellar degeneration (Type 1)
7 Williams syndrome
9 Dystonia (early onset primary dystonia [DYT1])
  Friedreich's ataxia
  Tuberous sclerosis (TSCI)
10 Metachromatic leukodystrophy
11 Acute intermittent porphyria
  Ataxia telangiectasia
12 Phenylketonuria
  Tuberous sclerosis
13 Wilson's disease
14 Alzheimer's disease, presenilin 2
  Dopamine responsive dystonia
  Porphyria variegata
  Presenillin 1 (14)
15 Angelman syndrome
  Dyslexia
  Prader-Willi syndrome

  Tay-Sachs disease, GM2 gangliosidosis
16 Tuberous sclerosis (TSC2)
17 Charcot-Marie-Tooth disease
  Frontotemporal dementia/Tau
  Neurofibromatosis type 1 (NF1), "peripheral," von Recklinghausen
18 Tourette syndrome
19 Alzheimer's disease, familial, late onset
  Apolipoprotein E (Apo-E)*
  Familial hemiplegic migraine
  Malignant hyperthermia (ryanodine receptor)
  Myotonic dystrophy
20 Creutzfeldt-Jakob, familial prion disease
  (Gerstmann-Schenker-Strauss)
21 Alzheimer's disease, early onset familial
  Amyloid precursor protein (APP)
  Amyotrophic lateral sclerosis (ALS), familial
  Homocystinuria due to cystathionine beta-synthase deficiency
  Progressive myoclonic epilepsy
22 Metachromatic leukodystrophy
  Neurofibromatosis type 2 (NF2), familial acoustic neuroma
  X Adrenoleukodystrophy
  Becker's muscular dystrophy
  Duchenne's muscular dystrophy
  Fragile X
  Lesch-Nyhan syndrome
  Mental retardation, nonspecific
  Spastic paraplegia

*Risk factor for Alzheimer's disease.

Continued

B. Diseases Transmitted by Chromosomes (Number or X) or Mitochondria (M)

Acute intermittent porphyria (11)

Adrenoleukodystrophy (X)

Alzheimer's disease, presenilin 1 and 2 (14, 21)

Alzheimer's disease, late onset familial (19)

Amyloid precursor protein (APP) (21)^

Amyotrophic lateral sclerosis (ALS), familial (21)

Angelman syndrome (15)

Apolipoprotein E (Apo-E) (19)

Ataxia telangiectasia (11)

Becker's muscular dystrophy (X)

Charcot-Marie-Tooth (17)

Creutzfeldt-Jakob, familial prion disease (20) (Gerstmann-Schenker-Strauss)

Cytochrome c oxidase deficiency (M)

Dopamine responsive dystonia (14)

Duchenne's muscular dystrophy (X)

Dyslexia (15)

Dystonia, early onset primary dystonia, DYTI (9)

Familial hemiplegic migraine (19)

Fragile X (X)

Friedreich's ataxia (9)

Frontotemporal dementia (17)

Homocystinuria due to cystathionine beta-synthase deficiency (21)

Huntington's disease (4)

Kugelberg-Welander disease (spinal muscular atrophy Type III) (5)

Leigh's syndrome (M)

Lesch-Nyhan syndrome (X)

Malignant hyperthermia (ryanodine receptor) (19)

MELAS (mitochondrial encephalomyopathy, lactic acidosis, stroke) (M)

Mental retardation, nonspecific (X)

MERRF (myoclonic epilepsy, ragged red fibers) (M)

Metachromatic leukodystrophy (10)

Myotonic muscular dystrophy (19)

Narcolepsy (6)

Neurofibromatosis NF1, peripheral, von Recklinghausen disease (17)

Neurofibromatosis NF2, familial acoustic neuroma (22)

Parkinson's disease α-synuclein gene (4), parkin gene (6)

Phenylketonuria (12)

Prader-Willi syndrome (15)

Porphyria variegata (14)

Presenilin 1 (14)

Presenilin 2 (1)

Progressive external ophthalmoplegia (M)

Progressive myoclonic epilepsy (21)

Spastic paraplegia (X)

Spinal muscular atrophy (5)

Spinocerebellar degeneration, Type 1 (6)

Tau (17)

Tay-Sachs disease (5)

Tay-Sachs disease, GM2, gangliosidosis (15)

Tourette's syndrome (18)

Tuberous sclerosis (9, 16)

Von Hippel-Lindau disease (3)

Werdnig-Hoffmann disease (spinal muscular atrophy type I) (5)

Williams syndrome (7)

Wilson's disease (13)

C. Diseases Transmitted by Mitochondria

Cytochrome c oxidase deficiency

Leigh's syndrome

MELAS (mitochondrial encephalomyopathy, lactic acidosis, stroke)

MERRF (myoclonic epilepsy, ragged red fibers)

Progressive external ophthalmoplegia

D. Diseases Transmitted by Excessive Trinucleotide Repeats

Disease	Transmission	Chromosome	Trinucleotide
Fragile X syndrome	Sex linked	X	CGG
Friedreich's ataxia	Autosomal recessive	9	GAA
Huntington's disease	Autosomal dominant	4	CAG
Myotonic dystrophy	Autosomal dominant	19	CTG
Spinocerebellar atrophies (SCAs)			
Type 1	Autosomal dominant	6	CAG
Type 2	Autosomal dominant	12	CAG
Type 3*	Autosomal dominant	14	CAG

*Machado-Joseph disease.

*For additional and continually updated information visit www.genetests.org.

^ Risk factor for Alzheimer's disease.

Chemical and Biologic Neurotoxins

Condition	Mechanism of Action	Effects
Atropine, scopolamine	Blocks cerebral ACh receptors	Delirium, amnesia, systemic autonomic anticholinergic effects
Botulinum toxin poisoning	Impairs release of ACh from *presynaptic* neurons	Paresis, especially of ocular, pharyngeal, and respiratory muscles
Curare, α-bungarotoxin	Blocks neuromuscular ACh receptor	Paralysis of voluntary muscle
Ciguatera fish poisoning	Prolongs opening of voltage-gated Na^+ channels in nerves and muscles	Acute painful neuropathy, loss of sensation in limbs, victims perceive hot objects as cold
Lambert-Eaton syndrome	Impairs release of ACh from *presynaptic* neurons	Weakness of limb muscles
Myasthenia gravis	Impairs function of *postsynaptic* ACh receptors	Weakness of ocular, bulbar, and proximal limb muscles
Organophosphate insecticides/nerve gas exposure	Inhibits cholinesterase, which increases ACh concentration, causing *postsynaptic* dysfunction	Brief stimulation then paresis of all muscles; increased parasympathetic activity; confusion, seizures
Tetanus or strychnine poisoning	Inhibits GABA* and glycine* receptors	Spasmodic, tetanic muscle contractions from uninhibited motor system

ACh, acetylcholine; GABA, gamma-aminobutyric acid.
*Inhibitory neurotransmitters.

Additional Review Questions and Answers

1. Which portion of the brain is shown in this picture?
   a. Diencephalon
   b. Midbrain
   c. Pons
   d. Medulla

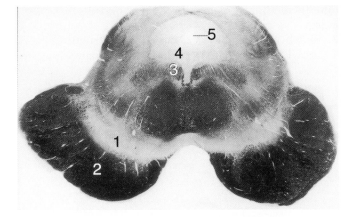

Answer: b. The midbrain, one of the four sections of the brainstem, is situated between the diencephalon and the pons. Neurologists identify the midbrain by its silhouette and sometimes quip that the midbrain, held upside-down, looks like Mickey Mouse. Other features are the curved horizontal stripe in the lower third (1) and the passageway in the topmost section (5).

2. Match the description (a–j) to the area of the midbrain (1–5) pictured in Question 1. If appropriate, use more than one letter for each number.
   a. Origin of the nigrostriatal tract
   b. Passageway for cerebrospinal fluid (CSF)
   c. Periaqueductal gray matter
   d. Sixth cranial nerve nucleus
   e. Third cranial nerve nucleus
   f. Descending corticospinal tract
   g. Ascending corticospinal tract
   h. Site of dopamine synthesis
   i. Aqueduct of Sylvius
   j. Cerebral peduncle

Answers: a, h-1: The curved area, lightly stained in this section, is the substantia nigra, which is the origin of the nigrostriatal tract and synthesizes dopamine. b, i-5: This small, completely unstained area represents the aqueduct of Sylvius, which is the CSF passageway from the third to fourth ventricles. c-4: The gray area surrounding the aqueduct is the periaqueductal gray area. d: The sixth cranial nerve nuclei are located in the pons and are not included in this picture. e-3: The third cranial nerve nuclei, like most other brainstem motor nuclei, are paired and midline. The third and fourth cranial nerve nuclei are situated in the midbrain and the sixth cranial nerve nuclei are situated in the pons. f, j-2: The corticospinal tracts descend in the dark, heavily myelinated cerebral peduncle. In the midbrain they are ipsilateral to their origin, but, in the medulla, they cross in the pyramids. g: No ascending corticospinal tract exists.

3. Which portion of the brain is shown in this picture?
   a. Diencephalon
   b. Midbrain
   c. Pons
   d. Medulla

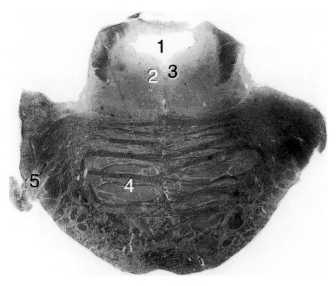

Answer: c. The pons, another of the four sections of the brainstem, is situated between the midbrain and the medulla. The bulbous silhouette, large CSF passageway in its top, and prominent crossing fibers in its lower portion identify it.

4. Match the description (a–h) to the area of the pons (1–5) pictured in Question 3.
   a. Corticobulbar and corticospinal tract fibers
   b. Basis pontis
   c. Seventh cranial nerve exiting the brainstem

d. Upper portion of the fourth ventricle
e. Medial longitudinal fasciculus (MLF)
f. Third cranial nerve nucleus
g. Sixth cranial nerve nucleus
h. Site of norepinephrine synthesis

Answers: a, b-4: The corticobulbar and corticospinal tract fibers, as well as the cerebellar fibers, are the main constituents of the basis pontis, which is the large bulbous lower portion of the pons. c-5: The seventh cranial nerve exits laterally from the pons and joins the fifth and eighth cranial nerves in the cerebellopontine angle. d-1: The fourth ventricle overlies the pons and medulla. e-2: The MLF, upper midline heavily myelinated tracts, extends from the pons to the midbrain and coordinates activity of the third and sixth cranial nerves. f: The third cranial nerve nuclei are located in the midbrain. g-3: As with the third cranial nerve nuclei, the abducens cranial nerve nuclei are paired midline structures, but they are situated in the pons. h: Each locus ceruleus, sites of norepinephrine synthesis, is situated inferiorly and laterally to the fourth ventricle, but they are not identifiable in this picture.

5. Which portion of the brain is shown in this picture?
   a. Diencephalon
   b. Midbrain
   c. Pons
   d. Medulla

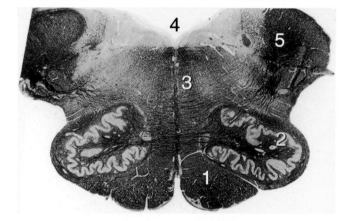

Answer: d. The medulla, the most caudal (lowermost) section of the brainstem, is readily identifiable by its lateral, inferiorly pointing, scalloped structures.

6. Match the description (a–f) to the area of the medulla (1–5) pictured in question 5.
   a. Cerebellar outflow tract
   b. Inferior olivary nuclei
   c. Fourth ventricle
   d. Decussation of the medial lemniscus

e. Corticospinal tracts
f. Pyramids

Answer: a-5: Cerebellar inflow and outflow tracts pass through the medulla. b-2: The inferior olivary nuclei are the scalloped structures. c-4: The fourth ventricle sits above the medulla and below the cerebellum. The hypoglossal motor nuclei (not numbered) sit in the midline of the medulla below the floor of the fourth ventricle. d-3: The posterior columns of the spinal cord, conveying position and vibration sensations, ascend into the medulla, where they cross in the decussation of the medial lemniscus. e, f-1: The corticospinal tracts descend into the medulla and cross in the pyramids.

7. Match the numbers (1–4) with the structures (a–i) shown on this axial MRI (magnetic resonance image).

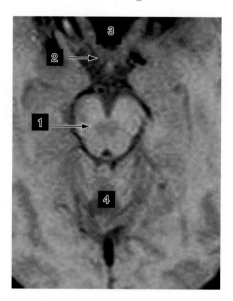

   a. Diencephalon
   b. Midbrain
   c. Pons
   d. Medulla
   e. Optic tract
   f. Optic chiasm
   g. Optic nerves
   h. Cerebrum
   i. Cerebellum

Answers: 1-b: This view of the midbrain shows the Mickey Mouse silhouette and aqueduct of Sylvius. 2-f and 3-g: The optic nerves exit from the eyes and travel posteriorly to merge in the optic chiasm. 4-i: This slice also captures the anterior medial portion of the cerebellum, which contains the vermis.

8. Match the numbers (1–4) with the structures (a–i) shown on this MRI.

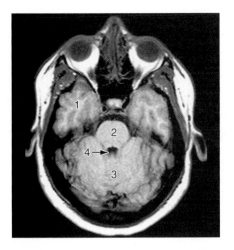

a. Midbrain
b. Pons
c. Medulla
d. Cerebellum
e. Frontal lobe
f. Temporal lobe
g. Occipital lobe
h. Third ventricle
i. Fourth ventricle

Answers: Compared to the previous MRI, this one shows a more caudal (lower) slice of brain. 1-f: The temporal lobe occupies most of the middle fossa. 2-b: The bulbous shape defines the pons. 3-d: The cerebellum, with gyri much thinner than cerebral gyri, is posterior to the pons. 4-h: The fourth ventricle sits between the pons and the cerebellum.

9. Match the numbers (1–5) with the structures (a–r) shown on this MRI.

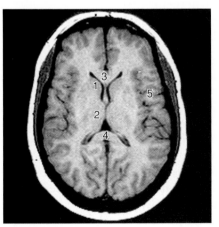

a. Diencephalon
b. Midbrain
c. Pons
d. Medulla
e. Thalamus

f. Globus pallidus
g. Putamen
h. Head of the caudate nucleus
i. Genu of the corpus callosum
j. Splenium of the corpus callosum
k. Planum temporale
l. Prefrontal cortex
m. Parietal lobe
n. Cingulate gyrus
o. Cerebellum
p. Optic nerve
q. Fourth ventricle
r. Occipital lobe

Answers: This MRI shows a more cephalad (higher) axial slice of brain. It cuts through the cerebrum and uppermost brainstem. 1-h: The head of the caudate nucleus indents the lateral ventricle and forms its lateral border. With the putamen (not numbered), it constitutes the corpus striatum. 2-a and e: The thalamus, a large sensory nucleus, forms the lateral border of the third ventricle. It is a major component of the diencephalon, which includes the thalamus, hypothalamus, and subthalamus. 3-i and 4-j: This slice captures the anterior (3) and posterior (4) portions of the corpus callosum, the great commissure. 5-k: The dominant hemisphere planum temporale includes many more infoldings than the nondominant one. The greater cortex area of the dominant hemisphere accommodates the requirements for language. Following convention, the MRI shows the dominant hemisphere (left-sided) planum temporale on the right side.

10. Match the numbers (1–11) with the structures, listed in the previous question, in this MRI.

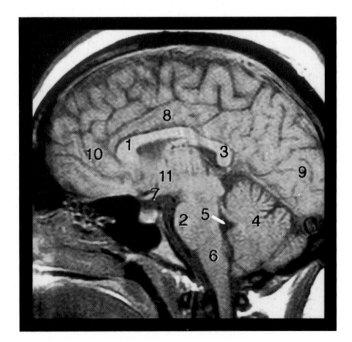

Answers: This is a sagittal view of the brain. 1-i and 3-j: It shows the anterior (genu) and posterior (splenium) corpus callosum. 2-c. 4-o: The cerebellum, occupying most of the posterior fossa, overlies the fourth ventricle and sits above the foramen magnum (not pictured). 5-q. 6-d. 7-p. 8-n: The cingulate gyrus is a component of the limbic system. 9-r. 10-l. 11-a: This portion of the diencephalon includes the hypothalamus and subthalamus, but it is too inferior to include the thalamus.

11. An aunt has taken her 5-month-old nephew, who has recently been brought to the United States from an underdeveloped country, to the emergency room because his right arm and left leg had become weak. In the emergency room, the child is lethargic, in pain, and febrile. His neck is rigid. The entire right arm has flaccid paresis and absent deep tendon reflexes (DTRs). He has no rashes. A lumbar puncture (LP) discloses cerebrospinal fluid (CSF) with 100 lymphocytes/mm^3, glucose of 35 mg/dL, and protein of 80 mg/dL. Which of the following conditions is the most likely diagnosis?
    a. Abuse or other form of trauma
    b. Brachial plexus inflammation ("plexitis") following a vaccination
    c. Werdnig-Hoffman disease
    d. Poliomyelitis

Answer d. Although poliomyelitis has been almost entirely eradicated, small epidemics still occur in the Middle East and Africa. Several patients in the United States have also contracted the illness. As in this case, poliomyelitis causes a viral meningitis picture, characterized by flaccid, areflexic weakness in an asymmetric pattern, fever and nuchal rigidity, and a lymphotic pleocytosis in the CSF. Werdnig-Hoffman disease is an autosomal recessive genetic motor neuron disease that appears insidiously, painlessly, and symmetrically in infants. Physicians should consider trauma in infants and children with limb injuries and x-ray apparently normal limbs as well as the injured ones. Vaccinations occasionally lead to an immunologic cross-reaction with the adjacent brachial or lumbosacral plexus. Postvaccinial inflammation often causes a plexitis with fever, pain, and flaccid limb weakness but not nuchal rigidity or CSF abnormalities.

12. Three years following kidney transplantation, the 44-year-old recipient required constant powerful immunosuppression. When he developed malaise, headache, and confusion, his nephrologist solicited a neurologic consultation. In addition to cognitive impairment, the neurologic examination showed fever, blurred optic disk margins, nuchal rigidity, and bilateral sixth cranial nerve palsies. A CT showed dilation of all the ventricles, but no mass lesions. The CSF, under a pressure of 400 mm H$_2$O, was turbid. It contained 400 WBC/mL (86% lymphocytes), 250 mg/dL protein, and 40 mg/dL glucose. Microscopic inspection revealed encapsulated organisms. Which organism has most likely caused the meningitis?
    a. Cryptococcus
    b. Pneumonia
    c. Herpes simplex
    d. Tuberculosus
    e. None of the above

Answer: a. Immunosuppressed or immunodeficient patients are susceptible to opportunistic infections. Fungal and tuberculous meningitis prevents CSF reabsorption through the arachnoid, which causes communicating hydrocephalus. The resulting increased intracranial pressure stretches the sixth cranial nerves to give a "false localizing sign." The CSF profile suggests a tuberculous or fungal rather than a bacterial or viral infection (see Table 20-1). The finding of encapsulated organisms indicates that the infective agent was cryptococcus. A CSF antigen determination would confirm the diagnosis of cryptococcal meningitis.

13. For decades, inadequate ventilation has probably exposed a worker in an old-fashioned factory to toxic levels of inorganic mercury vapor. Which of the following symptoms cannot be attributed to his work environment?
    a. A dark line along the gums
    b. Constriction of visual fields
    c. Tremors and tremulousness
    d. Polyneuropathy
    e. Personality changes, fatigue, gastrointestinal disturbances

Answer: b. Organic and inorganic forms of mercury have great affinity for the nervous system. In his case, inorganic mercury neurotoxicity caused polyneuropathy, tremors and tremulousness, and changes in mentation. The body also deposits mercury compounds in the gums that form horizontal lines at the base of the upper and lower teeth. In contrast to neurotoxicity from the inorganic form of mercury, neurotoxicity from the organic form, which has usually resulted from industrial contamination of fisheries or seeds, characteristically leads to constriction of visual fields that may culminate in blindness. Organic mercury poisoning may also cause ataxia, tremor, and mental aberrations.

14. A 68-year-old recently retired businessman began to develop erratic behavioral and brief periods of elation and depression several months before his

family brought him for a psychiatric consultation. Aside from intermittently loud and boisterous speech, with sexual innuendoes, his neurologic examination was normal. His Mini Mental Status Examination (MMSE) score was 23. This is his

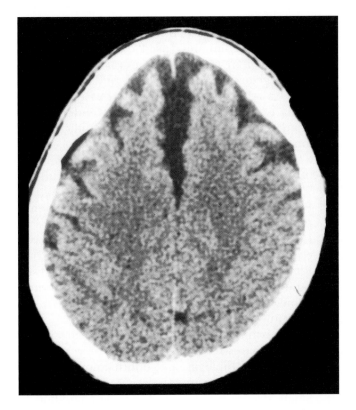

head CT. Which of the following conditions is most likely responsible for his cognitive and behavioral symptoms?

a. Alzheimer's disease
b. Depressive illness
c. Frontotemporal dementia
d. Vascular dementia
e. Subdural hematomas

Answer: c. This patient shows uninhibited behavior and labile affect. His recent retirement and the MMSE score of 23 suggest only a relatively mild cognitive impairment. The symptoms indicate a diagnosis of frontotemporal dementia. The CT showing atrophy of only the frontal lobes, with no sign of infarctions or mass lesions, confirms the diagnosis of frontotemporal dementia.

15. A 70-year-old man reported that he was suddenly unable to see. He was so upset that he refused to let physicians examine him. Nevertheless, he consented to undergo a CT (*left*) then MRI (*right*) of his head. When he allows it, what will a clinical examination most likely reveal?

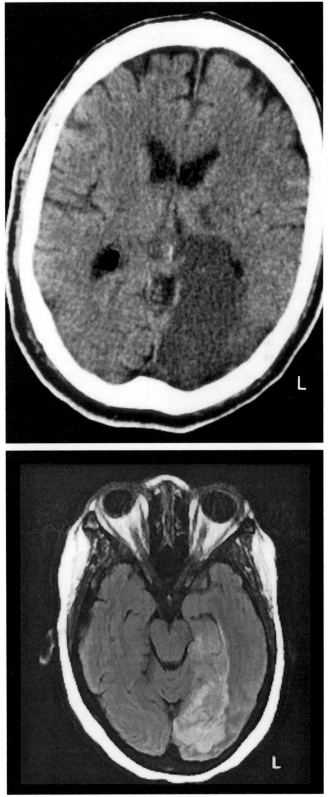

a. Left homonymous hemianopsia
b. Right homonymous hemianopsia
c. Aphasia
d. Dementia

Answer: b. The CT and MRI both show an infarction in the distribution of the left posterior cerebral artery (PCA) that includes the left occipital lobe. In the CT, the infarction is black because the lack of blood and necrotic brain render the tissue radiolucent. In this MRI sequence, increased signal indicates the ischemic region.

The left occipital infarction will cause a right homonymous hemianopsia. In addition, if the infarction includes the posterior corpus callosum (the splenium), it may also cause alexia without agraphia. Note that the MRI, compared to the CT, can detect more extensive involvement. Moreover, it shows that the PCAs supply the medial-inferior surface of the temporal lobes. With ischemia of both PCAs, the portion of the limbic system housed in the temporal lobes cannot function and amnesia results. This mechanism may explain why ischemia of the basilar artery, which gives rise to the PCAs, causes transient global amnesia.

16–20. Match the visual field loss (16–20) most closely associated with each condition (a–k). If appropriate, use more than one letter for each number.
16. Left homonymous hemianopsia with macular sparing
17. Fortification scotoma
18. Central scotoma, lasting for 2 weeks
19. Bitemporal hemianopsia
20. Unilateral superior quadrantanopia
  a. Retinal injury, for example retinal detachment or embolus from carotid artery
  b. Psychogenic disturbance
  c. Migraine with aura
  d. Diabetes insipidus
  e. Loss of libido
  f. Optic atrophy
  g. Amaurosis fugax
  h. Internal capsule infarction
  i. Aphasia
  j. Occipital infarction
  k. Optic or retrobulbar neuritis

Answers: 16-j, 17-c, 18-k, 19-d, e, f (all associated with pituitary tumors), 20-a.

21. An 80-year-old man, who is being treated for depression, has developed right-sided frontal headaches, pain on chewing, diffuse muscle aches, and intermittent, low-grade fevers. Examination shows that the vision in his right eye is 20/200, but in the left eye 20/30. His temporal arteries are prominent but not especially tender. There is no papilledema, hemiparesis, or other neurologic sign. Which condition is most likely?
  a. Open-angle glaucoma
  b. Metastases to the skull

  c. Meningioma
  d. Optic neuritis
  e. Temporal arteritis
  f. Narrow-angle glaucoma

Answer: e. The headache, jaw claudication, and systemic symptoms indicate temporal arteritis. Physicians should diagnose this condition rapidly because, if untreated, it can cause blindness or cerebral infarction. The most commonly used diagnostic tests are the sedimentation rate and temporal artery biopsy. Untreated glaucoma (both narrow- and open-angle) can also rapidly lead to blindness, but open-angle glaucoma is not associated with either tenderness or pain, and neither is associated with jaw claudication or systemic symptoms.

22–30. Match the ocular abnormality (22–30) with the most probable cause (a–k).
22. Right third cranial nerve paresis and left hemiparesis
23. Left sixth cranial nerve paresis and right hemiparesis
24. Right Horner's syndrome, right facial hypalgesia, right limb ataxia, and left limb and trunk hypalgesia
25. Internuclear ophthalmoplegia
26. Right sixth and seventh cranial nerve paresis and left hemiparesis
27. Ptosis, facial diplegia, and ophthalmoplegia with normally reactive pupils
28. Small, irregular pupils that accommodate but do not react
29. Fever, agitated confusion, and dilated pupils
30. Stupor, miosis, and pulmonary edema
  a. Neuromuscular junction impairment
  b. Anticholinergic intoxication
  c. Right pontine lesion
  d. Left pontine lesion
  e. Left midbrain lesion
  f. Right midbrain lesion
  g. Midline, dorsal brainstem lesion
  h. Left lateral medullary lesion
  i. Right lateral medullary lesion
  j. Syphilis
  k. Opioids

Answers: 22-f, 23-d, 24-i, 25-g, 26-c, 27-a (myasthenia gravis), 28-j (Argyll-Robertson pupils), 29-b (scopolamine intoxication), 30-k (heroin or methadone overdose).

31. Which three of the following are found in Alzheimer's disease but not in normal elderly individuals?
  a. Loss of brain weight
  b. Increase in sulci width

c. Expansion of the lateral ventricles

d. Major loss of large cortical neurons

e. Marked reduction of choline acetyltransferase in the hippocampus

f. Cerebral atrophy

g. Multiple neurofibrillary tangles

h. Senile plaques

Answers: d, e, g. Cerebral atrophy (a, b, c), plaques (h), neurofibrillary tangles, and granulovacuolar degeneration are found in normal brains. However, they are present in greater concentrations and different distributions in Alzheimer's disease brains.

32. A 60-year-old man with dementia has a gait abnormality in which he excessively raises his legs. He seems to climb as he walks. His pupils are small (miotic), poorly reactive, and irregular. What is the gait abnormality?

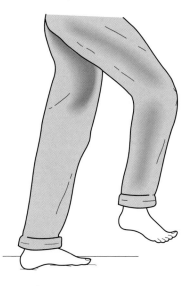

a. Gait apraxia

b. Congenital spastic paraparesis

c. Steppage gait from posterior spinal cord degeneration

d. Astasia abasia

Answer: c. The patient has a steppage gait because he has lost position sense. He must raise his legs to avoid catching the tips of his toes when he walks and especially when he steps onto curbs. He has lost his position sense because he has tabes dorsalis and Argyll-Robertson pupils as a manifestation of tertiary syphilis. Loss of position sense from combined system disease and spinocerebellar ataxia also damage the posterior columns and cause steppage gait. In addition, severe diabetic neuropathy may impair position sense and cause a similar gait abnormality.

33–35. Match the confabulation (33–35) with the lesion (a–c) that might produce it.

33. A blind patient "describes" the examiner's clothing. His pupils are round and reactive to light.

34. A man with recent onset of left hemiparesis claims that he cannot move his left arm and leg because he is too tired.

35. An agitated, diaphoretic middle-aged man describes bizarre occurrences and experiences visual hallucinations. When asked to repeat six digits, he seems to select random numbers.

a. Nondominant parietal lobe infarction

b. Bilateral occipital lobe infarctions

c. Hemorrhage into the limbic system

Answers

33-b. In cortical blindness, some patients implicitly deny their lack of vision by confabulating (Anton's syndrome). Cortical blindness usually results from infarction or trauma of both occipital lobes. The pupils react normally because the optic and oculomotor nerves and the brainstem synapses are unaffected.

34-a. In anosognosia, patients with hemiparesis from a nondominant hemisphere infarct often confabulate, deny, and use other defense mechanisms in not recognizing their hemiparesis. The lesion typically involves the right parietal lobe.

35-c. In alcohol withdrawal, alone or as part of delirium tremens, patients may confabulate. Petechiae in the mamillary bodies, which are a cornerstone of the limbic system, constitute the underlying neuropathology.

36. A lethargic and disoriented young man staggers into the emergency room. The medical staff finds that he has nystagmus, gait ataxia, and finger-to-nose dysmetria. Which is the most likely illness?

a. Subdural hematoma

b. Cerebral infarction

c. Wernicke-Korsakoff syndrome

d. Psychogenic disturbance

Answer: c. The immediate treatment is thiamine 50 mg IV.

37. An 11-year-old boy is admitted because of headache, nausea, and vomiting. He has had clumsiness for the 2 weeks before admission. He has papilledema, ataxia, bilateral hyperactive DTRs, and Babinski signs. Which is the most likely diagnosis?

a. MS

b. Drug abuse

c. Cerebellar tumor

d. Spinocerebellar degeneration

Answer: c. Cerebellar astrocytomas, which are relatively common in children, block the aqueduct of Sylvius, creating obstructive hydrocephalus. The hydrocephalus increases intracranial pressure, which causes headaches, nausea, vomiting, and papilledema.

38. Which four of the following symptoms constitute the narcoleptic tetrad?
a. Inability to move on awakening (sleep paralysis)
b. Hunger or anorexia
c. Vivid dreams when falling asleep (hypnagogic hallucinations)
d. Attacks of daytime sleep (narcolepsy)
e. Night terrors (pavor nocturnus)
f. Episodic loss of muscle tone (cataplexy)
g. Snoring

Answers: a, c, d, f.

39. During the first week of hospitalization for acute psychosis, an adolescent began to drink large quantities of water and other fluids. After 1 week, he developed a seizure. Which two of the following conditions would be most likely to have caused the seizure?
a. Steroid abuse
b. Valproic acid
c. Diabetes mellitus
d. Parkinson's disease
e. Huntington's disease
f. Psychogenic polydipsia

Answers: c, f. Polydipsia, whatever its etiology, frequently leads to hyponatremia that, in turn, causes seizures. Alternatively, diabetes mellitus leads to hyperglycemia, which causes hyponatremia. Carbamazepine and oxcarbazepine lead to hyponatremia, particularly in patients older than 65 years and those taking diuretics. In addition, young adults who take ecstasy and drink water while at all-night dance parties are at risk for developing hyponatremia-induced seizures.

40. Whenever a 40-year-old man heard a good joke or was surprised, his jaw would drop open and often his neck muscles would lose their tone, and his head would fall forward. Although he tolerates those reactions, when frightened or very excited, his entire body also feels weak. On several occasions, he collapsed into a chair. Aside from excessive daytime sleepiness, obesity, and mild hypertension, he is in good health. Which is probably the best medicine for this patient?
a. An anxiolytic
b. Oxybate
c. Modafinil
d. Beta-blocker
e. None of the above

Answer: b. He probably has cataplexy as a component of the narcolepsy-cataplexy tetrad. As in this patient's case, cataplexy sometimes consists only of an inconspicuous loss of tone in a limited muscle group, such as those of the jaw or neck. Also, the cataplexy occasionally creates more of a problem than the sleep attacks (narcolepsy). Oxybate (Xyrem), the same substance as gamma-hydroxybutyrate (GHB), often called the "date-rape drug," will suppress the cataplexy. Modafinil reduces excessive daytime sleepiness. Sometimes antihypertensive agents lead to orthostatic hypotension and then loss of body tone.

41. A 23-year-old woman presents to a hospital with a 6-year history of a progressively severe involuntary movement disorder. She has no history of exposure to neuroleptics or any family member with similar symptoms. Her limbs, trunk, and neck continuously contort into sustained, twisted, and sometimes grotesque postures. Her muscles are hypertrophied. She has lost her body fat. In contrast to her physical disability, her cognitive function remains normal. Of the following, which is the most likely cause of her movement disorder?
a. Huntington's disease
b. Conversion disorder
c. Dystonia, early onset, DYT1
d. Tardive dystonia
e. Factitious illness
f. Cerebral palsy

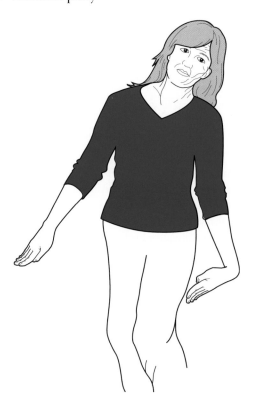

Answer: c. She has dystonia. The muscle hypertrophy and lack of bodily fat indicate its chronicity and "organic" basis. The most common causes of dystonia in young adults are DYT1 early onset primary dystonia (torsion dystonia), tardive dystonia, Wilson's disease, the juvenile form of Huntington's disease, or, in children, dopa-responsive dystonia. Of the choices offered, the most likely is early onset dystonia from DYT1. Her physicians should inquire if her relatives are Ashkenazi Jews, which is the population that most commonly carries the DYT1 gene, and send her blood to the appropriate genetic test. Because of incomplete penetrance, only 30% of DYT1 carriers show symptoms.

42. A 20-year-old sailor, who has a history of "glue sniffing," develops paresthesias and mild weakness in his hands and toes. Of the following, which single portion of the nervous system has been damaged?
    a. Spinal cord
    b. Corpus callosum
    c. Peripheral nerves
    d. Spinal cord
    e. Neuromuscular junction

    Answer: c. Major components of glue, which carries a great potential for abuse, include N-hexane and other volatile hydrocarbon solvents. These constituents, which are lipophilic, permeate and dissolve or otherwise damage the lipid-rich myelin cover of peripheral nerves. Chronic exposure causes peripheral neuropathy.

43. Three weeks after recovering from an apparently successful repair of a ruptured anterior communicating artery aneurysm, a patient remains apathetic and almost mute but not aphasic. When walking, his steps are short and hesitant. He has never regained bladder control. A CT shows lucencies in both frontal lobes but normal size ventricles. Which one of the following is most likely to have complicated the aneurysm or surgery?
    a. After surviving the rupture of an aneurysm and the neurosurgery, he has developed post-traumatic stress disorder.
    b. He has developed depression.
    c. The surgery or subarachnoid hemorrhage-induced vasospasm occluded both anterior cerebral arteries and caused bifrontal infarctions.
    d. The hemorrhage has led to communicating then normal pressure hydrocephalus (NPH).
    e. Brain damage from the aneurysm and the surgery has lead to dementia.

    Answer: c. The anterior communicating arteries supply a large portion of the frontal lobes, including the medial surface of the motor cortex, which controls the voluntary function of the legs and bladder. Infarction of these arteries, from the aneurysm rupture or

surgery, creates personality changes, gait impairment, and urinary incontinence. Communicating hydrocephalus sometimes follows subarachnoid hemorrhage because blood in the subarachnoid space impairs reabsorption of CSF. It often leads to NPH. The CT in this case would show enlarged ventricles.

44. Which three of the following conditions often lead to patients reporting "putrid smells" that the physician cannot detect?
    a. Seizures that originate in the uncus
    b. Sinusitis
    c. Migraines
    d. Seizures that originate in the parietal lobe
    e. Valproic acid
    f. Dental infections

    Answers: a, b, f. Migraines, curiously, often include visual but rarely auditory or olfactory auras. Infections in the sinuses and mouth are the most common causes of putrid smells.

45. For which conditions might an LP be indicated?
    a. Subdural hematoma
    b. Brain abscess
    c. Brain tumor
    d. Unruptured arteriovenous malformation (AVM)
    e. Idiopathic intracranial hypertension (pseudotumor cerebri)
    f. MS
    g. Bacterial meningitis
    h. Subacute sclerosing panencephalitis
    i. Viral encephalitis
    j. Sexual impairment

    Answers: e, f, g, h, i. Intracranial mass lesions usually preclude an LP because CSF analysis will not be helpful and the procedure might precipitate transtentorial herniation.

46. A 68-year-old man with metastatic prostate cancer controls his pain with morphine tablets that he takes exactly at intervals of every 6 hours. When leaving the house for a daytime trip with his family, he counts and recounts the number of pills that he must take. Then during the trip, he recounts the remaining pills. Which term would most accurately describe his behavior?
    a. Obsessive-compulsive ritual
    b. Hoarding
    c. Addiction
    d. None of the above

    Answer: d. Anticipating a recurrence of severe pain from metastatic cancer if he exhausts his supply of opioids, the patient carefully schedules himself. Although his behavior appears to reflect addiction or obsessive-compulsive ritual, it is best termed pseudoaddiction. His behavior also suggests that his medicine dose is too meager and that he has no margin. With his restrictions, he cannot pursue attempts to maintain a normal life. His physicians should prescribe more generous doses and switch him to long-acting oral or transdermal preparations.

47. Many individuals with disabling neurologic illnesses retain normal cognitive capacity. Of the following illnesses, which three may be characterized by a normal cognitive capacity despite quadriparesis and respiratory distress?
   a. Guillain-Barré syndrome
   b. Locked-in syndrome
   c. Persistent vegetative state
   d. Cervical spinal cord gunshot wound

   Answers: a, b, d.

48. The parents of an 11-year-old girl bring her to the pediatrician because she has developed twitchy, restless movements. The parents, as well as the girl, are distraught, and the excitement intensifies each other's anxiety; however, the patient's orientation, judgment, and language functions are normal. When her arms are extended, at the pediatrician's request, the girl's fingers have individual flexion or extension movements. Her face grimaces and smirks. Her walking is irregular and clumsy. She is unable to protrude her tongue for 10 seconds. Which four tests would be most appropriate?
   a. VDRL
   b. Inquiries about oral contraceptives
   c. Antistreptolysin O titer (ALSO)
   d. Pregnancy test
   e. Lupus preparation
   f. LP for CSF oligoclonal bands

   Answers: b, c, d, e. Chorea in adolescents may be a sign of rheumatic fever (Sydenham's chorea), lupus, pregnancy (chorea gravidarum), or a reaction to oral contraceptives. CSF oligoclonal bands might suggest MS or other inflammatory neurologic diseases, but MS rarely develops in such young children and rarely causes movement disorders.

49. Which four procedures would be most helpful in determining the dominant hemisphere?
   a. Positron emission tomography (PET)
   b. Computed tomography (CT)
   c. EEG with sphenoidal electrodes
   d. Functional magnetic resonance imaging (fMRI)
   e. Intracarotid sodium amobarbital injection
   f. Wada test
   g. Visual evoked responses (VER)
   h. Brainstem auditory evoked responses (BAER)

   Answers: a, d, e, f. In the Wada test, intracarotid amobarbital injections perfusing the dominant hemisphere induce aphasia. fMRI, but not standard MRI, can detect the dominant hemisphere.

50. When women take nonsteroidal anti-inflammatory drugs (NSAIDs) for menstrual cramps, which substances do these medicines inhibit?
   a. Enkephalins
   b. Endorphins
   c. Prostaglandins
   d. Serotonin
   e. Dopamine

   Answer: c.

51. Which two statements are true regarding the dorsal raphe nucleus?
   a. It contains high concentrations of endorphins.
   b. Pain is caused by stimulating it.
   c. Analgesia is produced by stimulating it.
   d. Behavioral changes are produced by stimulating it.
   e. Its destruction causes analgesia.
   f. It contains high serotonin concentrations.

   Answers: c, f.

52. Several friends brought a stuporous 14-year-old boy to the emergency room. The physicians find that he is apneic and his pupils are miotic. Which condition is most likely responsible?
   a. Brainstem stroke
   b. Heroin overdose
   c. Hypoglycemia
   d. Postictal stupor
   e. Psychogenic disturbance

   Answer: b. Heroin overdose typically causes stupor, miosis, and apnea. It should be treated with naloxone (Narcan). Brainstem strokes, particularly ones with damage to the pons, may cause this constellation; however, they rarely occur in this age group.

53–55. A 29-year-old woman reports that she has developed a tremor when she writes, drinks coffee, and lights a cigarette.

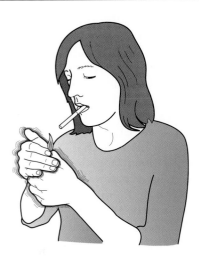

53. Which five of the following conditions can lead to such a tremor?
 a. Essential tremor
 b. Wilson's disease
 c. Anxiety
 d. Huntington's chorea
 e. Athetosis
 f. Benign familial tremor
 g. Dystonia
 h. Rett syndrome
 i. Use of valproate

Answers: a, b, c, f, i. Essential tremor and benign familial tremor are probably varieties of the same condition. Wilson's disease is a rare but important condition that might be considered in young adults who develop a tremor. Anxiety can produce a tremor that is virtually indistinguishable from essential tremor and also responds to β-adrenergic blockers. Numerous medications, including tricyclic antidepressants and valproate, cause or exacerbate tremor.

54. Which two tests should be performed to exclude Wilson's disease when only mild tremors are evident?
 a. MRI
 b. SPECT
 c. PET
 d. Serum ceruloplasmin
 e. Serum copper concentration
 f. Slit lamp examination

Answers: d, f.

55. Of the following medications, which is most effective for essential tremor?
 a. Anticholinergics
 b. Dopamine agonists
 c. Neuroleptics
 d. Propranolol
 e. Antiviral agents
 f. α-adrenergic blockers

Answer: d. In addition to this beta-blocker, primidone (Mysoline), which undergoes metabolism to phenobarbital, may suppress the tremor. For selected cases, benzodiazepines may be appropriate. For severe cases, deep brain stimulation alleviates the tremor.

56. Of the following, which two characteristics distinguish classic neurotransmitters from endocrine hormones, such as thyroxine?
 a. Classic neurotransmitters or their metabolic products circulate in detectable quantities in the blood.
 b. They are produced and stored at a site adjacent to the target organ.
 c. Classic neurotransmitters or their metabolic products are often present in detectable concentrations in the CSF, but not in the blood.
 d. They are steroids.

Answers: b, c.

57. To which feature of neurons does the term "plasticity" refer?
 a. Mechanical properties
 b. Ability to reorganize
 c. Ability to resist change
 d. Chemical constituents

Answer: b. Plasticity, in general, means the capacity to be altered or molded. In neurologic terms, plasticity refers to the ability of the CNS to be reorganized. Ordinarily, the CNS is not plastic and reorganization does not take place. For example, the corticospinal tract always crosses. However, CNS plasticity has been postulated to develop under certain circumstances, such as perpetuation of pain and partial recovery of some function after strokes.

58. After embarking on a stringent program of vigorous exercise, taking large quantities of "megavitamins," and abstaining from red meat and alcohol, a 28-year-old woman notes paresthesias in her feet and unsteadiness while walking. On examination, she has marked sensory loss and absent DTRs in all limbs, but her strength is normal. She cannot walk heel-to-toe. Which one of the following conditions is most likely to be responsible for her symptoms?
 a. Cervical spondylosis
 b. Myopathy
 c. Vitamin toxicity
 d. Iron-deficiency anemia

Answer: c. Pyridoxine (vitamin B_6) in large daily doses—toxic quantities—creates a neuropathy that impairs sensation. After eliminating vitamins, this pyridoxine-induced neuropathy resolves.

59. A 68-year-old house painter has weakness, atrophy, and areflexic DTRs in his arms. The biceps and triceps muscles have fasciculations. He has sensory loss in his right hand, brisk DTRs in his legs, and a right Babinski sign. Which one of the following features suggests that he has cervical spondylosis rather than amyotrophic lateral sclerosis (ALS)?
    a. Hand atrophy
    b. Hyperactive DTRs
    c. Sensory loss
    d. The Babinski sign

Answer: c. House painting requires prolonged neck hyperextension, which may lead to cervical spondylosis. Whatever its cause, cervical spondylosis leads to sensory impairment, fasciculations, lower motor neuron loss in the arms and hands, and upper motor neuron loss in the legs. Cervical spondylosis is a much more frequently occurring condition than ALS. ALS, like other motor neuron diseases, typically does not cause sensory loss.

60. Which cerebral lobes are superior to the Sylvian fissure?
    a. Frontal and parietal
    b. Parietal and occipital
    c. Frontal and temporal
    d. Parietal and temporal

Answer: a.

61. Which cerebral lobe is inferior to the Sylvian fissure?
    a. Frontal
    b. Parietal
    c. Occipital
    d. Temporal
    e. None of the above

Answer: d.

62. As people age, what is the most common EEG change?
    a. Loss of amplitude
    b. Slowing of the background activity
    c. Fragmentation of background
    d. Episodic β activity

Answer: b.

63. At the suggestion of his sister, a 45-year-old man with testicular cancer consults with a neurologist

because, although the tumor is in remission, he has developed a short temper, apathy, and irritability. He takes no medications and does not use alcohol or drugs. His neurologic examination shows no abnormalities except for pronounced memory loss and a flattened affect. An MRI with gadolinium shows atrophy of the mesial temporal lobes and an EEG shows spikes and slow waves emanating from that same region. Routine blood tests, including HIV testing, show no abnormalities. Which of the following tests is most likely to reveal the diagnosis?
    a. Serum anti-Hu antibodies
    b. CSF for 14-3-3 protein
    c. ACh receptor antibodies
    d. CT of the head

Answer: a. Even though the tumor may be in remission, he probably has developed limbic encephalitis. This paraneoplastic syndrome, which consists of limbic system inflammation, often represents the initial symptom or sign of recurrence of small cell carcinoma of the lung or testes. Individuals with this disorder, develop pronounced memory impairment combined with irritability, behavioral disturbances, personality changes, and focal complex seizures over several days to several weeks. Their serum often contains antibodies, of the anti-Hu or anti-Ma2 varieties, that react with limbic system neurons.

64. Which structure contains 80% of the brain's dopamine content?
    a. Third ventricle
    b. Thalamus
    c. Cerebral cortex
    d. Corpus striatum

Answer: d.

65. After a 29-year-old man reported having incapacitating hemicranial headaches five times a month, a neurologist switched his preventative treatment from propranolol to topiramate. The morning after the patient started to take 25 mg twice a day, he awoke with markedly impaired visual acuity. Although he was able to discern closely held objects, such as the newspaper print, his visual acuity on a wall chart was 20/400 OU. His visual fields were full. The eyes were not painful or injected. Pupils were equal and reactive to light. His discs and fundi were normal. The remainder of the neurologic examination revealed no abnormalities. What is the most likely cause of the sudden loss of vision?
    a. Acute angle-closure glaucoma
    b. Acute myopia

c. Pseudotumor cerebri
d. Migraine-induced blindness

Answer: b. Topiramate, which neurologists prescribe for migraine and seizure prevention, can cause acute angle-closure glaucoma and acute myopia. Acute myopia, particularly his preserved ability to see closely held objects, explains this man's visual loss. The absence of ocular pain and injection and the normal pupil reactivity exclude acute angle-closure glaucoma. When migraine induces blindness the visual obscuration is limited to a scotoma and its duration is limited to a maximum of several hours.

66. One week after a right cerebral infarction that caused a mild left hemiparesis, a 60-year-old man describes an intense burning sensation in the left side of his face and arm. He has a marked sensory loss to all modalities in these regions. What is the origin of the patient's symptom?
    a. Parietal lobe injury
    b. Brachial plexus injury
    c. Lateral spinothalamic injury
    d. Thalamic injury

Answer: d. The patient really has thalamic pain, which is a distressing consequence of an infarction in the thalamus. Its characteristic burning sensation results from loss of sensory input to the brain, which is often called *deafferentation*. Amputations (phantom limb) and brachial plexus avulsion also cause similar unpleasant sensations. Thalamic pain frequently responds to AEDs but generally not to analgesics. Deafferentation pain should be distinguished from neuropathic pain, in which pain results directly from nerve injury, such as in postherpetic neuralgia.

67. Which two of the following tests rely on ionizing radiation?
    a. CT
    b. MRI
    c. Isotopic brain scan
    d. EEG
    e. EMG
    f. VER
    g. BAER

    Answers: a, c.

68. In patients with the human variety of the Klüver-Bucy syndrome, which symptom is least common?
    a. Oral exploration
    b. Amnesia
    c. Uncontrollable sexual activity
    d. Placid demeanor
    e. Anger

Answer: c. All these symptoms may occur as features of the Klüver-Bucy syndrome in humans, as well as in monkeys. Although humans may have increased sexual desire, they express only inappropriate verbal outbursts and abide by most social conventions. Their affect is usually bland, as with frontal lobe injury, but bursts of anger may punctuate it. Herpes encephalitis, contusion of the temporal lobes, and multiple strokes are the most common causes of the Klüver-Bucy syndrome in humans.

69. Medical treatments occasionally produce neurologic complications. Which one of the following statements is false?
    a. Creutzfeldt-Jakob disease has complicated human growth hormone injections given to correct short stature in children.
    b. Smallpox vaccinations rarely cause an attack of disseminated MS-like CNS demyelination.
    c. Measles vaccinations occasionally cause subacute sclerosing panencephalitis (SSPE).
    d. Artificial insemination with donor semen has induced acquired immunodeficiency syndrome (AIDS).

Answer: c. Although the CSF of SSPE patients (who are usually children) usually contains elevated measles antibody titers, measles virus has not been proven to be its cause. Measles vaccination programs have been followed by a marked reduction in the incidence of SSPE.

The development of Creutzfeldt-Jakob disease in children given growth hormone extracted from human pituitary glands led to the use of genetically engineered growth. Creutzfeldt-Jakob disease has also been transferred by the use of depth EEG electrodes and corneal transplantation. Smallpox vaccinations occasionally cause postvaccinal demyelination, a condition that resembles MS; however, attacks of postvaccinal demyelination are single events. Postvaccinal demyelination has been one of the major reasons that smallpox vaccinations are given sparingly. AIDS transmission has resulted from artificial semen transfer.

70. REM sleep behavior disorder is often a precursor of which disorders?
    a. Synucleopathies
    b. Tauopathies
    c. Vascular dementia
    d. Prion illnesses

Answer: a. REM sleep behavior disorder often presages Parkinson's disease and dementia with Lewy body disease—synucleopathies. However, it does not presage either Alzheimer's disease or frontotemporal dementia—tauopathies. Also, it bears no relationship to vascular dementia or prion illnesses.

71. In Alzheimer's disease, which region has a pronounced neuron loss associated with an acetylcholine (ACh) deficit?
a. Frontal lobe
b. Frontal and temporal lobe
c. Hippocampus
d. Nucleus basalis Meynert

Answer: d. The brain has a marked loss of neurons in the hippocampus, with the most pronounced neuron loss in the nucleus basalis of Meynert.

72. A 15-year-old waiter has episodes of feeling dizzy and dreamy that last 3 to 5 minutes. During them, he also has paresthesias in his fingertips and around his mouth. Sometimes his wrists bend, his fingers cramp together, and his foot flexes. An EEG during an episode showed slowing of the background activity and bursts of high voltage 3-Hz activity. Of the following conditions, which one is most likely affecting the patient?
a. Partial complex seizures
b. Focal dystonia
c. Petit mal (absence) seizures
d. Occupational cramps
e. None of the above

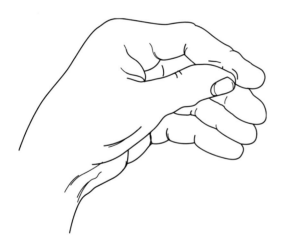

Answer: e. He is probably having episodes of hyperventilation with carpopedal spasm and EEG slowing. A clinical diagnosis of hyperventilation can be confirmed if patients reproduce their symptoms by hyperventilating for 2 to 4 minutes.

73. The patient in the preceding question is asked to hyperventilate. After 90 seconds, he becomes giddy and then irrational. What is the best way to abort the test?
a. Intravenous benzodiazepine
b. Having the patient breathe into a paper bag
c. Offering reassurance
d. Inhaling oxygen

Answer: b. He probably has developed cerebral hypoxia because of a reduction in carbon dioxide tension in the blood, which reduces cerebral blood flow. Physicians should have him breathe into a paper bag to increase his carbon dioxide blood tension, which will increase cerebral blood flow.

74. A 32-year-old woman is referred to a psychiatrist for postpartum depression. For 5 months after the delivery of her fifth child, which was complicated by hemorrhage, she finds herself unable to cope with the family. She describes having insufficient energy to do her share of the housework. She is unable to return to her usual occupation (dentistry). She never resumed her menses or regained her libido. She has anorexia and slight weight loss. She has a mild continual headache but no cognitive loss, visual changes, or other neurologic symptoms. Her obstetrician, internist, and a neurologic consultant find no physical signs of illness. Nevertheless, which condition is most likely responsible?
a. MS
b. Lupus
c. Sheehan's syndrome
d. Pregnancy

Answer: c. Deliveries complicated by hypotension occasionally cause postpartum pituitary necrosis (Sheehan's syndrome). Its symptoms, which may not develop for several months to several years postpartum, include failure of lactation, scanty or no menses, sexual and generalized indifference, and being easily fatigued. Except for a subtle loss of secondary sexual characteristics, patients may have no physical abnormalities.

75. A 27-year-old man with a history of intractable seizures and violent behavior has had numerous EEGs that have shown only equivocal abnormalities. His serum phenytoin concentration has always been below the therapeutic range, despite a 500 mg/day prescription. He is suspected of abusing phenobarbital and other barbiturates, which he obtains on the basis of his diagnosis of epilepsy. After seriously injuring a friend during a fistfight in a bar, his lawyer attributed the violence to the seizure disorder. As part of forensic evaluation, an EEG was performed (see p. 573). During the study, the patient became rigid and then had symmetric motor activity of all his limbs. Afterward, he remained unresponsive for several minutes and then became confused and amnestic. He was found to have had urinary incontinence. Evaluate the case in view of the history and the EEG.

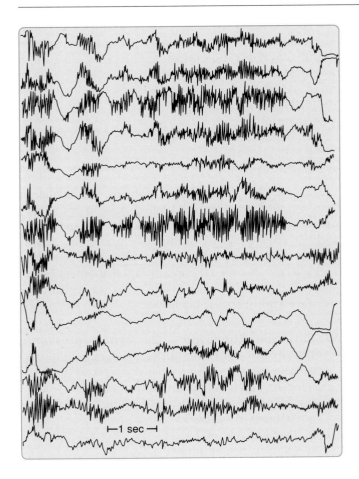

Answer: The most prominent features of this EEG are bursts of high-voltage activity in the first and middle third of the sample. Although impressive, this activity is only muscle artifact, which can be caused by either voluntary or involuntary muscle contraction. The diagnostic feature of this EEG is the α and β activity. This activity, which is normal, occurs during a pause in the muscle artifact that can be seen above and below the 1-second marker. Muscle artifact cannot

distinguish between epileptic and psychogenic seizures; however, normal (α) EEG activity, in the midst of apparent generalized tonic-clonic movements, clearly indicates that the activity is psychogenic.

Individuals can convincingly mimic seizures. Alternatively, a patient with genuine seizures might allow them to become intractable by failing to take AEDs. The most common explanation for low serum concentrations of AEDs is neither impaired absorption nor rapid metabolism but failure to take the prescribed dosage (noncompliance). Aggression that occurs in bars more likely results from alcohol consumption than epilepsy.

76. A 45-year-old woman has developed frequent blinking and involuntarily closure of her left eye (see below). The eyelid closure is forceful, has a duration of 4 to 6 seconds, and is intensified by anxiety. She has no ocular abnormality, change in intellectual capacity, prior neurologic conditions, or medical illnesses. With which area is her problem associated?
    a. Corpus striatum
    b. Lenticular nuclei
    c. Facial nerve at the cerebellopontine angle
    d. Autonomic nervous system
    e. Trigeminal nerve at the cerebellopontine angle
    f. Unknown regions

Answer: c. The patient has hemifacial spasm, not blepharospasm. Note that in addition to the closure of her left upper and lower eyelids, the muscles of the left side of her mouth contract, pulling it laterally and deepening the nasolabial fold. Hemifacial spasm, which develops in middle-aged and older individuals, is associated with an aberrant vessel compressing the facial nerve as it emerges from the brainstem. Hemifacial spasm can be treated with botulinum toxin injections or neurosurgical microvascular decompression

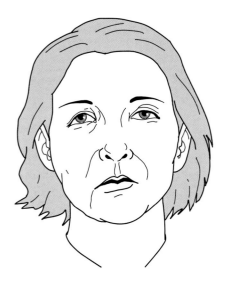

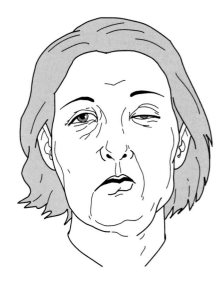

of the facial nerve as it exits from the brainstem at the cerebellopontine angle. Tics may involve one eye, but they are momentary. Tardive dyskinesia may cause facial movements, but it does not cause such unilateral movements.

77–78. A teenage couple attempted suicide by sitting in a car with the engine running in a closed garage. They were discovered in a comatose state.

77. Three months later, the young man was alert, but bedridden, and always remained in a flexed posture, mute, and unresponsive to stimulation. From which condition does he most likely suffer?
   a. Dementia
   b. Global aphasia
   c. Persistent vegetative state
   d. Depression
   e. Isolation aphasia
   f. Conduction aphasia
   g. Multiple strokes
   h. None of the above

Answer: c. Carbon monoxide poisoning probably caused generalized cerebral cortex destruction that resulted in the persistent vegetative state. He has permanent dementia, unconsciousness, unresponsiveness, and lack of voluntary movements.

78. Three months later, the young woman also failed to recover. Although she could sit in a chair with her eyes open, she was unable to follow verbal requests, initiate conversation, or respond purposefully. However, she would repeat incessantly whatever questions or phrases she heard from visitors, television, and nearby casual conversations. Of the choices in Question 77, from which disorder did she most likely suffer?

Answer: e. In her case, incomplete cortex damage resulted in isolation aphasia (also called "mixed transcortical aphasia"). Characteristically, she has lost all her intellectual functions, except for a tendency—sometimes compulsion—to repeat (echolalia). Her isolation aphasia results from hypoxia of the large watershed area of the cerebral cortex with sparing of the perisylvian language arc.

79. While recovering from abdominal surgery for a gunshot wound, a 25-year-old drug addict complains of persistent severe postoperative pain. When moderate doses of various opioids fail to alleviate the pain, his surgeons administer pentazocine. After he becomes agitated, severely anxious, irrational, and diaphoretic, the surgeons request a psychiatric consultation. Which one of the following medicines would reduce the symptoms and allow further investigation?
   a. A major tranquilizer
   b. Methadone
   c. Alcohol
   d. Phenobarbital
   e. Steroids
   f. Benadryl
   g. Pentazocine
   h. Butorphanol

Answer: b. Pentazocine (Talwin), butorphanol (Stadol), and other mixed opioid agonist-antagonist preparations may precipitate withdrawal in opioid addicts. (Being aware of their vulnerability, opioid addicts often claim, with some justification, that they are allergic to mixed opioid agonist-antagonists.) Methadone or other opioids will abort the withdrawal symptoms and provide analgesia.

80. Physicians hospitalize a 22-year-old previously healthy nurse for the sudden onset of generalized muscle weakness. An internist diagnoses hypokalemic myopathy. What are four causes of hypokalemic myopathy that develop in young adults?
   a. Adrenal insufficiency
   b. Pernicious anemia
   c. Diuretic use or abuse
   d. Vomiting
   e. Diarrhea from laxative use or abuse
   f. Steroid use
   g. Excessive vitamin use

Answers: c, d, e, f. Hypokalemic myopathy in previously healthy young adults may be iatrogenic, a sign of underlying illness, or self-induced. Hypokalemia is especially likely to be self-induced by health care workers who surreptitiously take diuretics. Steroids may cause weakness by a direct muscle injury (steroid myopathy) or indirectly by depleting serum potassium (hypokalemic myopathy). Weakness from steroid myopathy is an occasional paradoxical result of bodybuilders' using steroids.

81. Which two of the following statements concerning prions are true?
   a. They contain RNA.
   b. They contain reverse transcriptase.
   c. They are infective agents.
   d. They cause Creutzfeldt-Jakob disease.
   e. Prion-markers are identifiable in cerebral biopsy tissue of Alzheimer's disease patients.

Answers: c, d. Prions are protein-containing infective agents that contain neither DNA nor RNA. They cause Creutzfeldt-Jakob disease and other spongiform encephalopathies. Prion-markers can be identified in cerebral biopsies of patients with Creutzfeldt-Jakob, but not Alzheimer's, disease. The human immunodeficiency virus (HIV) is an RNA virus that contains reverse transcriptase.

82–87. Match the clinical description of patients with mental status changes and the appropriate CT.

82. A 23-year-old woman, who had just delivered a baby boy after an uneventful pregnancy, had the sequential development of personality changes, agitation, garbled speech, seizures, and right hemiparesis. She did not use alcohol, tobacco, or drugs, but her boyfriend is a former drug addict.

83. Following mild head trauma the previous day, an 85-year-old man develops stupor and a mild left hemiparesis.

84. The family of a 65-year-old man has noticed that for several weeks he has had difficulty reading newspapers and books, but he can repeat phrases, comprehend spoken statements, and even transcribe entire sentences. His memory and other aspects of general intellect remain intact.

85. An 80-year-old man has malaise, a frontal headache, and progressively severe cognitive impairment with prominent anomias. Otherwise, he has no abnormalities on neurologic or general medical examination. Routine laboratory tests, including a sedimentation rate, are normal.

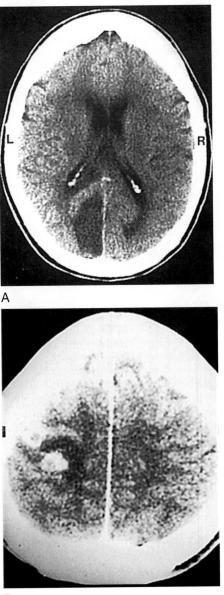

A

B

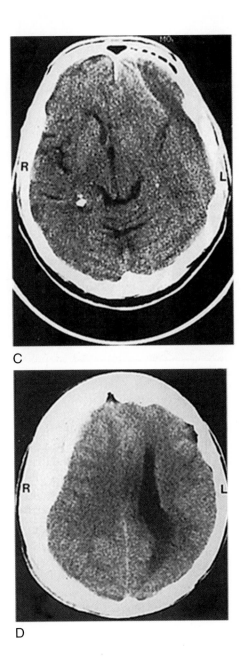

C

D

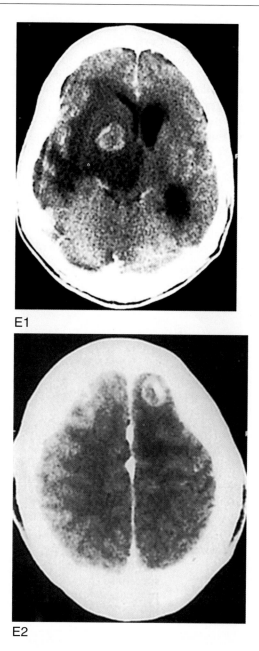

E1

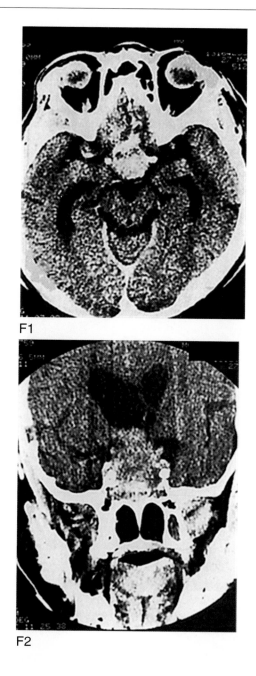

F1

E2

F2

86. A 50-year-old architect is unable to complete his work. On examination, he seems inattentive and cannot make simple drawings, but his cognitive capacity is grossly normal.

87. A 38-year-old woman, who has been infertile, has the onset of headaches and bitemporal hemianopsia.

Answers

82-e. The two CTs show two circular lesions that are each enhanced by contrast infusion. The use of contrast can be surmised by seeing that the falx, a thick, linear vascular structure, is white (more apparent on E2 than E1). A large lesion, surrounded by extensive edema, is situated in the basal ganglia (Scan E1) and another in the contralateral frontal lobe (E2). The basal ganglia lesion compresses the anterior and occipital horns of the lateral ventricle, and shifts midline structures (E1). In the higher cut (E2), the falx, which acts as a rigid barrier, prevents a shift of midline structures. The multiple masses, enhanced by contrast and located in the basal ganglia, are consistent with toxoplasmosis, bacterial abscesses, and metastatic tumors. However, because the patient's sexual partner is a drug addict, the most likely diagnosis is AIDS-related cerebral toxoplasmosis.

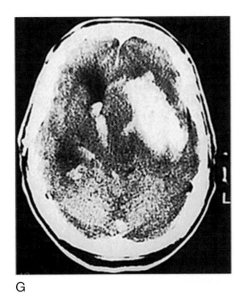

G

83-d. Note that this CT follows the convention: CTs and MRIs generally portray the brain with the left and right sides reversed. This CT shows the lesion, which is a right-sided acute subdural hematoma, as a thick white border overlying the right side of the brain that exerts considerable mass effect. It compresses the right cerebral hemisphere and almost obliterates its lateral ventricle. Fresh blood, as in an intracerebral hemorrhage (G), as well as in this acute subdural hematoma, is more radiodense than brain tissue and therefore white on a CT.

84-a. This CT shows a large, dark, semicircular area adjacent to the posterior falx in the left occipital lobe. Its lucency and pattern indicate that the lesion is an infarction of the left posterior cerebral artery. Because of the infarction, the patient has the interesting and important neuropsychologic condition alexia without agraphia. He probably also has a right homonymous hemianopsia.

85-c. This CT shows an abnormality overlying the left frontal lobe that has a white border in its anterior portion. The mixed black and gray intensities indicate that its density is less than that of the brain. CSF, edema fluid, aged blood, and necrotic brain—all portrayed as black on the CT—are the most common hypodense tissues. The frontal horn of the left lateral ventricle is compressed, and the left frontal lobe is shifted slightly to the right. This CT indicates a chronic subdural hematoma.

86-b. The CT shows a lesion located in the posterior portion of the right cerebral hemisphere that has a white center and fragments of a surrounding white ring. The white falx indicates infusion of contrast material. The lesion is probably a tumor or other mass lesion. Lesions in the nondominant parietal lobe,

whatever their etiology, produce constructional apraxia, hemi-inattention, and anosognosia. This patient's presenting symptom is probably a manifestation of constructional apraxia. Because symptoms of right hemisphere lesions are often accompanied by anosognosia, patients may ignore their difficulties or describe them only in imprecise terms.

87-f. *Left,* This axial view, a contrast-enhanced CT shows a midline circular radiodense lesion, just anterior to the midbrain. *Right,* In this coronal view, the lesion can be seen to be arising from the sella and growing into the hypothalamus. The lateral ventricles are pushed aside and dilated, which suggests that blockage of the third ventricle has caused hydrocephalus. In the axial view, the white, upside-down, wishbone-shaped structure in the posterior portion of the axial CT is the normal venous drainage. In adults, pituitary lesions are usually adenomas that cause endocrine disturbances, including elevated prolactin concentrations, headaches, and, when large, bitemporal hemianopsia.

88–89. A physician is called to see a colleague, known to be hypertensive and seriously depressed, who has developed severe headache, nausea, and vomiting. She finds that he is stuporous and diaphoretic with nuchal rigidity and bilateral Babinski signs. His blood pressure is 210/130 mm Hg. His family reports that they found bottles of chlorpromazine, isocarboxazid, propranolol, meperidine, and hydrochlorothiazide.

88. What are the two most likely diagnoses?
   a. Medication interaction
   b. Meningitis
   c. Intracranial hemorrhage
   d. None of the above

Answers: a, c. The patient has classic signs of an intracranial hemorrhage: headache, stupor, nausea, vomiting, and nuchal rigidity. The illness may be a hypertensive cerebral hemorrhage despite his use of antihypertensive medications. Alternatively, the etiology may have been a drug-induced hemorrhage from the isocarboxazid (Marplan). That medication, like tranylcypromine (Parnate), phenelzine (Nardil), and others, is a monoamine oxidase inhibitor (MAOI). Meperidine (Demerol) and dextromethorphan will cause similar, potentially fatal interactions. MAOIs cause acute, severe hypertension if certain foods, such as aged cheese, are eaten. Sometimes depressed people purposefully take prohibited foods or medicines in suicide attempts.

89. If an MAOI caused a hypertensive reaction, which of the following medications might reduce the blood pressure?

a. Meperidine
b. Chlorpromazine
c. Propranolol
d. Hydrochlorothiazide
e. Phentolamine
f. Dibenzoxazepine

Answer: e. The most specific treatment for a hypertensive reaction to an MAOI is the α-adrenergic blocking agent, phentolamine (Regitine), at a dose of 5 mg slowly given intravenously. Of the medications that are readily available, propranolol or chlorpromazine would be most helpful. Although the headache may be agonizingly severe, meperidine (Demerol) is contraindicated.

90. Which structure connects the hippocampus and the hypothalamus?
    a. Corpus callosum
    b. Cingulate gyrus
    c. Fornix
    d. None of the above

Answer: c. The fornix connects the hippocampus with the mamillary bodies, which are an extension of the hypothalamus. The mamillary bodies communicate through the mamillothalamic tract with the anterior nucleus of the thalamus.

91. After rescue from a high-speed motor vehicle accident (MVA), the driver was stuporous and had facial contusions. After regaining consciousness, emergency room physicians found that he had paresis of his right arm and leg, which also had decreased position sensation. The left arm and leg had decreased sensation to pin prick. He had a right-sided Babinski sign. The paresis persisted even though he fully regained consciousness and had no language, ocular, or visual impairment. Where would the lesion have to be located to explain the paresis?
    a. Frontal lobe
    b. Brainstem
    c. Cervical spinal cord
    d. Lumbar spinal cord

Answer: c. He has hemitransection of the cervical spinal cord. The cervical spinal cord is vulnerable in MVAs because, when the forehead strikes the wheel or dashboard, the head and neck snap backward (hyperextends). Drivers involved in a high-speed MVA, especially if they display behavioral abnormalities, should be evaluated for drug and alcohol use, as well as head trauma.

92. Which statement concerning the cerebellum is false?

a. MS frequently involves the cerebellum.
b. Lesions in the cerebellum may cause scanning speech.
c. In adults, strokes and tumors involve the cerebellum less frequently than the cerebrum.
d. A lesion in a cerebellar hemisphere causes contralateral limb ataxia.

Answer: d. A lesion in a cerebellar hemisphere causes ipsilateral limb ataxia. Possibly because the cerebellum receives about 10% of the brain's blood supply, only about 10% of strokes and tumors involve the cerebellum.

93. Which sign is not found with the others?
    a. Fasciculations
    b. Spasticity
    c. Babinski signs
    d. Clonus

Answer: a. Spasticity, Babinski signs, and clonus are all manifestations of upper motor neuron injury. Fasciculations are a manifestation of lower motor neuron injury.

94. In Parkinson's disease, which tract undergoes degeneration?
    a. Nigrostriatal
    b. Geniculocalcarine
    c. Spinothalamic
    d. Corticospinal

Answer: a. The nigrostriatal tract, which undergoes degeneration in Parkinson's disease, originates in the substantia nigra and terminates in the striatum (caudate and putamen). The geniculocalcarine tract conveys the visual pathways from the lateral geniculate bodies to the calcarine cortex of the occipital lobes. The spinothalamic tract conveys pain pathways from the dorsal horn of the spinal cord to the contralateral thalamus. (Crossing shortly after it originates, the spinothalamic tract ascends in the spinal cord contralateral to the side of its origin.) The corticospinal tract originates in the motor strips of the cerebrum and descends, after crossing in the medulla, in the spinal cord to the contralateral anterior horn cells of the spinal cord. It conveys voluntary motor system signals.

95. Of the following substances, which one is most likely to produce seizures during an acute intoxication?
    a. Cocaine
    b. Phencyclidine (PCP)
    c. D9-TCH
    d. Heroin
    e. Valium
    f. Amphetamine

g. Alcohol

h. Morphine

Answer: a. Cocaine, whether smoked, inhaled, injected, or swallowed, readily causes seizures. Almost one-half of the cases of cocaine-induced seizures occur in first-time users. Phencyclidine (PCP) and amphetamine cause seizures less frequently. Overdose of heroin and other opioids usually does not cause seizures, except if it leads to hypoxia. Benzodiazepines and alcohol rarely cause seizures during intoxication; however, withdrawal from these substances often produces seizures that are sometimes intractable. The active agent in marijuana, D9-TCH, actually has a mild antiepileptic drug (AED) effect.

96. Which two of the substances listed in Question 95 are associated with seizures after several days of abstinence?

Answers: e, g. Although adult opiate addicts do not develop seizures during either withdrawal or detoxification, neonates develop seizures during opiate withdrawal.

97. Which one of the substances listed in Question 95 is most likely to cause a stroke?

Answer: a. Cocaine often causes cerebral hemorrhages and bland infarctions. Moreover, seizures often complicate cocaine-induced strokes. Amphetamine produces similar mental changes, but less often strokes or seizures.

98. Immediately after a 19-year-old college student developed physical and mental agitation, vivid hallucinations, and combative behavior, her roommates bring her to the emergency room. The story eventually emerged that she had smoked marijuana; however, when she previously used it, she never developed such a reaction. She was hypertensive, oblivious to a laceration, and kept her eyes wide open. She made repetitive, purposeless kissing movements. She had three-directional nystagmus. Which of the substances listed in Question 95 is probably responsible?

Answer: b. Pronounced nystagmus is characteristic of PCP intoxication. Somebody probably laced her marijuana with PCP.

99. Which are two effects of the normal gamma-aminobutyric acid (GABA)-induced influx of chloride ions?
   a. Neurons are inhibited.
   b. Neurons are excited.
   c. The resting potential is made more negative.
   d. The resting potential is made more positive.
   e. NMDA receptors are activated.

Answers: a, c. The normal resting potential is $-70\,mV$. An influx of chloride ion (Cl^-), which makes the resting potential more negative, inhibits neuron activity.

100. One dozen unrelated middle-aged individuals have found that, when exposed to various everyday chemicals or merely their odors, they develop asthma-like reactions, skin rashes or pruritus, anxiety, seizures, migraine headaches, paresthesias, and other neurologic problems. They have banded together and formed a community that prohibits the use of all perfumes, carpet and other fabric cleaners, dry cleaning, deodorants, and other synthetic and some naturally occurring volatile chemicals. When encountered individually, each seems thoughtful, reasonable, friendly, cheerful, and well-dressed. Which condition would best describe these individuals' condition?
   a. Mass hysteria
   b. Multiple chemical sensitivity syndrome
   c. Neurotoxic exposure
   d. Asthma

Answer: b. Multiple chemical sensitivity syndrome is a prime example of a psychiatric-based pseudoneurotoxic disease. Studies have shown that when odors are masked or presented unknowingly to "victims," they do not cause a reaction. This condition occurs among individuals who tend to draw together. Sometimes they establish communities free of as many volatile and other potentially harmful chemicals as possible. In matters unrelated to these concerns, they are free of overt psychiatric disorders.

101. Insert the proper enzyme (a–d) into the synthetic steps for epinephrine synthesis.

$$\text{Tyrosine} \xrightarrow{1} \text{DOPA} \xrightarrow{2} \text{Dopamine} \xrightarrow{3}$$
$$\text{Norepinephrine} \xrightarrow{4} \text{Epinephrine}$$

   a. DOPA decarboxylase
   b. Phenylethanolamine N-methyl-transferase
   c. Dopamine β-hydroxylase
   d. Tyrosine hydroxylase

Answers: 1-d, 2-a, 3-c, 4-b.

$$\text{Tyrosine} \xrightarrow{\textit{Tyrosine hydroxylase}} \text{DOPA} \xrightarrow{\textit{DOPA decarboxylase}}$$
$$\text{Dopamine} \xrightarrow{\textit{Dopamine-}\beta\textit{-hydroxylase}}$$
$$\text{Norepinephrine} \xrightarrow{\textit{Phenylethanolamine N-methyl-transferase}}$$
$$\text{Epinephrine}$$

102. In Question 101, which is the rate-limiting enzyme?

Answer: d. Tyrosine hydroxylase.

103. A 28-year-old man has a history of schizophrenia for which he has been receiving dopamine-blocking antipsychotics. He has a history of intravenous drug abuse. He comes to the emergency room because he has developed involuntary spasmodic muscle contractions in his left arm. He has a deep skin infection in his left forearm. His examination is otherwise normal. Which condition is most likely responsible for the left arm movements?
   a. Localized neuroleptic-induced dystonia
   b. Partial status epilepticus
   c. Conscious attempt to secure drugs
   d. A reaction to a toxin elaborated by an infection

Answer: d. The localized form of tetanus occurs in individuals, especially drug addicts, who have partial immunity from distant or ineffective immunizations. The generalized form of tetanus, which develops in individuals who are not immunized, causes the muscles of the entire body to have contractions and the jaw to close forcefully (trismus).

104. Which condition is the least frequent manifestation of Alzheimer's disease?
   a. Delusions
   b. Suicide ideation
   c. Hallucinations
   d. Anxiety

Answer: b. With the onset of dementia, Alzheimer's disease patients typically develop anxiety. Delusions and hallucinations are symptoms of moderate-to-severe dementia. Remarkably few Alzheimer's disease patients have suicidal ideation.

105. Which three of the following conditions are associated with spasticity?
   a. MS that affects only the spinal cord
   b. Parkinson's disease
   c. Cerebellar degeneration
   d. Poliomyelitis
   e. HTLV-1 myelitis
   f. Myotonic dystrophy
   g. Neuroleptic-induced parkinsonism
   h. Middle cerebral artery occlusion

Answers: a, e, h. Spasticity—increased muscle tone resulting in an increased resistance to stretching—is a sign of injury to the upper motor neurons of the corticospinal tract. The injury can affect the corticospinal tract in the cerebrum, brainstem, or spinal cord. Spasticity is characteristic of MS affecting the brain or the spinal cord, HTLV-1 myelitis (spinal cord infection), strokes, and many other conditions. In contrast, muscle rigidity—inflexibility of muscle—is a sign of basal ganglia disorders, such as naturally occurring

or neuroleptic-induced parkinsonism, or dystonia. Cerebellar degeneration leads to muscle hypotonia. Poliomyelitis is an infection of the lower motor neurons that leads to muscle flaccidity and atrophy. Myotonic dystrophy induces myotonia, which is delayed muscle relaxation after a contraction or after percussion.

106. In the preceding question, which three of the choices are associated with clonus?

Answers: a, e, h. Clonus, like spasticity, is a manifestation of to the upper motor neuron injury.

107. Which of the following structures represents the beginning of the lower motor neuron?
   a. Spinal cord
   b. Cauda equina
   c. Anterior horn cells of the spinal cord
   d. Neuromuscular junction
   e. Corticospinal tract
   f. Cervical-medullary junction

Answer: c. The corticospinal tract, which consists of upper motor neurons, terminates on the anterior horn cells of the spinal cord to synapse with lower motor neurons.

108. Where do the corticobulbar fibers terminate?
   a. Anterior horn cells of the spinal cord
   b. Cranial nerve nuclei I to XII
   c. Lower cranial nerve nuclei
   d. Autonomic nervous system pathways

Answer: c. The corticobulbar tract, which is analogous to the corticospinal tract, conveys motor information to the motor nuclei of the brainstem. It contains upper motor neurons and innervates nuclei of cranial nerves that supply muscles of the jaw, face, nasopharynx, and tongue.

109. Which of the following is an example of pseudoneurotoxic disease?
   a. *n*-hexane neuropathy
   b. Nitrous oxide-induce myelopathy
   c. Multiple chemical sensitivity syndrome
   d. Ciguatera fish poisoning

Answer: c. Pseudoneurotoxic diseases are neurologic or psychiatric conditions that develop or worsen coincident with exposure to a neurotoxin, but the neurotoxin neither causes nor worsens the underlying disorder. Studies have shown that multiple chemical sensitivity syndrome, the most famous, has no physiologic basis. The other disorders represent neurotoxins affecting the PNS myelin (*n*-hexane neuropathy), B_{12} metabolism (nitrous oxide-induced myelopathy), and voltage-gated sodium channels in nerves and muscles (ciguatera fish poisoning).

110. Which one of the following conditions is not characterized by neurofibrillary tangles?
a. Alzheimer's disease
b. Down syndrome
c. Dementia pugilistica
d. Huntington's disease

Answer: d. Neurofibrillary tangles are paired helical filaments that are associated with amyloid plaques and neuron loss. They are closely associated with Alzheimer's disease where they correlate with the severity of the dementia. In addition, they are found in several other conditions that cause dementia, such as Down syndrome, dementia pugilistica, and progressive supranuclear palsy. To a limited extent, they appear in normal individuals older than 65 years. Most important, neurofibrillary tangles are not pathognomic of Alzheimer's disease.

111. Which structure forms the roof of the lateral ventricles?
a. Caudate nuclei
b. Corpus callosum
c. Pons
d. Medulla
e. Cerebellum

Answer: b. The corpus callosum forms the roof of the lateral ventricles. The cerebellum forms the roof of the fourth ventricle. The caudate nuclei form the lateral walls of the lateral ventricles.

112. Match the structures (1–10) with their location (a–e).
1. Oculomotor
2. Trochlear
3. Abducens
4. Trigeminal motor
5. Vagus motor
6. Hypoglossal
7. Locus ceruleus
8. Substantia nigra
9. Red nucleus
10. Facial nerve
a. Midbrain
b. Pons
c. Medulla
d. Cerebral hemisphere
e. Cerebellum

Answers: 1-a, 2-a, 3-b, 4-b, 5-c, 6-c, 7-b, 8-a, 9-a, 10-b.

113. A veteran sustained a gunshot wound that transected the thoracic spinal cord 10 years before death. This is a sketch of an upper level of his cervical spinal cord. It has been treated with a stain that blackens normal myelin. Identify the demyelinated tracts.

Answer: Following an injury, neurons in the downstream section of a tract undergo Wallerian degeneration. Those tracts lose their myelin and ability to absorb standard histologic stains. The salient feature in this case is that certain ascending tracts, which are sensory, are unstained and presumably demyelinated because of the spinal cord injury. The spinothalamic tract, which is anterolateral, and the spinocerebellar tract, which is posterior-lateral and also peripheral, are both mostly unstained. The medial portion of the posterior column, the fasciculus gracilis, is also unstained. In contrast, the lateral segment of the posterior column, which consists of the f. cuneatus, is stained. The difference occurs because the f. gracilis originates in the legs and was interrupted by the gunshot wound. Thus, it is unstained; however, the f. cuneatus remained undamaged and its myelin is normally stained. This man's deficits included paraplegia, incontinence, and loss of all sensory modalities in his trunk below the umbilicus and in his legs.

114. Which substance is absent in biopsies of voluntary muscles of Duchenne's dystrophy patients?
a. Dystrophin
b. ACh
c. Ion channels
d. Insulin

Answer: a.

115. A patient who has sustained a left cerebral embolus has left-right confusion, finger agnosia, and agraphia. Which other neuropsychologic abnormality is expectable?
a. Alexia
b. Dementia
c. Acalculia
d. Amnesia

Answer: c. Gerstmann's syndrome, which is usually caused by a dominant parietal lobe lesion, consists of left-right confusion, finger agnosia, agraphia, and acalculia; however, all four components are rarely found together in a single patient, and each component may be incomplete, such as dysgraphia and dyscalculia rather than agraphia and acalculia.

116. In the limbic system, which tract conveys impulses between the hippocampus and the mamillary bodies?
a. Mamillothalamic tract
b. Cingulate gyrus
c. Fornix
d. None of the above

Answer: c. The sequence in the limbic system is hippocampus and adjacent amygdala, fornix, mamillary bodies, mamillothalamic tract, anterior nucleus of the thalamus, cingulate gyrus.

117. Which chromosome contains the gene for β-amyloid?
a. 4
b. 14
c. 21
d. X

Answer: c. Chromosome 21 contains the gene for β-amyloid and is triplicated in most cases of Down syndrome (trisomy 21).

118. At birth, a male infant is found to have a delicate sac-like protrusion at the base of his spine. His legs have flaccid, areflexic paraplegia, and urine dribbles continually from his penis, which never has erections. What condition is present?
a. Cerebral diplegia
b. Meningomyelocele
c. Dandy-Walker malformation
d. Arnold-Chiari malformation
e. Spina bifida

Answer: b. The baby most likely has a meningomyelocele. This congenital abnormality consists of a deformed spinal cord or cauda equina protruding through a defective spinal canal. Meningomyeloceles cause paraplegia with bladder, bowel, and sexual dysfunction. They have been attributed to maternal exposure to environmental toxins, such as potato blight, and medications, particularly valproic acid and carbamazepine. Taking folic acid and other supplements before and during pregnancy may prevent the malformation.

119. Narcolepsy patients are deficient in the peptide neurotransmitters hypocretin 1 and 2, also known as orexin A and B. Which of the following statements about them is untrue?

a. The lateral hypothalamus is completely or almost completely devoid of hypocretin-producing cells in narcolepsy patients.
b. Hypocretin inhibits NREM sleep.
c. Hypocretin inhibits REM sleep.
d. Hypocretin promotes wakefulness.
e. Hypocretin stimulates the appetite.

Answer: b. Hypocretin inhibits REM sleep. In a model of narcolepsy, REM sleep intrudes into daytime wakefulness and causes flaccid, areflexic paralysis and attacks of sleep.

120. Which of the following is not a feature of ataxia-telangiectasia?
a. Deficiency in IgA and IgE
b. Autosomal dominant inheritance
c. Onset of ataxia in childhood
d. Dilated vessels on the conjunctiva
e. Death from sinus or respiratory infection

Answer: b. Ataxia-telangiectasia is a neurocutaneous disorder that is inherited in an autosomal recessive pattern. Children with this disorder have telangiectasia of conjunctival blood vessels, ataxia, and, most important, potentially fatal IgA and IgE deficiencies. They may also have cognitive impairment.

121. Which medicine has not been associated with hyponatremia?
a. Carbamazepine
b. Oxcarbazepine
c. Valproate
d. Lithium
e. SSRIs

Answer: c. Use of numerous medications may be complicated by hyponatremia and its consequences, including delirium and seizures.

122. Which two of the following areas of the brain are most vulnerable to chronic alcoholism?
a. Cerebellar hemispheres
b. Optic nerves
c. Cerebellar vermis
d. Corpus callosum
e. Mammillary bodies

Answers: c, e. Although alcohol may damage any of these areas, chronic alcoholism is most likely to cause atrophy of the cerebellar vermis, which in turn causes gait ataxia. Repeated bouts of alcohol consumption lead to damage of the mammillary bodies and other areas of the limbic system.

123. A 66-year-old hypertensive businesswoman had the sudden painless onset of left-sided hemiparesis. She remains fully alert, comfortable, oriented, and with good memory and judgment. In addition, she has right-sided ptosis, the right pupil is dilated, and the right eye is laterally deviated. Which of the following events probably developed?

a. Periaqueductal petechial hemorrhages
b. Subdural hematoma with herniation
c. Midbrain arterial thrombosis
d. Cerebral hemorrhage

Answer: c. She sustained a right-sided midbrain infarction that damaged her third cranial nerve and adjacent corticospinal tract (Weber's syndrome). Because midbrain, pons, and medulla lesions are distant from the cerebrum, cognitive functions are almost always preserved. Of the other possible answers, periaqueductal petechial hemorrhages are indicative of Wernicke's encephalopathy, a condition in which patients have memory impairment, nystagmus, and ataxia, as well as oculomotor paresis. Subdural hematoma with herniation causes brainstem compression that leads to stupor or coma and decerebrate posturing. A cerebral hemorrhage may cause stupor and a third cranial nerve palsy by its mass effect herniating downward to compress the nerve and necessarily the brainstem.

124. What is the most caudal extent of the central nervous system (CNS)?

a. Foramen magnum
b. Occipital-cervical junction
c. Thoraco-lumbar junction
d. Sacrum
e. Neuromuscular junction

Answer: c. The CNS terminates at the junction of vertebrae T12-L1. At this point, the spinal cord gives rise to the cauda equina.

125. Having suffered from well-documented partial complex epilepsy since late childhood, a 29-year-old woman computer programmer was having a seizure every 2 to 3 months. Most seizures disabled her for at least a day and some had placed her in danger. She had dutifully taken her third regimen of two AEDs. Over the years, she had tried many AEDs singly or in pairs. Her serum AED concentrations were always in the therapeutic range. She had few friends and no boyfriend, despite her wishes. She consulted a psychiatrist for depression. Indeed, the consultant found her depressed. Which would be the best overall strategy?

a. Adding a third AED
b. Adding an antidepressant to the AED regimen
c. Changing one of the conventional AEDs to a mood-stabilizing AED (such as valproate)
d. Seeking consultation regarding epilepsy surgery

Answer: d. She has refractory epilepsy. Adding a third AED has about an 8% chance of suppressing the seizures and it will impose a neuropsychologic burden. Surgical resection of an identifiable cortical focus is her best chance for controlling the epilepsy. In fact, that strategy would even have been appropriate years before—after briefer trials of two AEDs. Successful surgery, which will allow reduction if not elimination of her AEDs, will also probably alleviate her depression and improve her cognitive function. An SSRI and psychotherapy may provide additional help. In general, for depression comorbid with epilepsy, seizure control should be the primary treatment for depression. Epilepsy surgery is routine, highly effective, and reasonably safe.

126. After a lifetime of being underweight and having been accused of having an eating disorder, a 19-year-old woman seeks neurologic evaluation when, several months after starting college, she loses more weight (to the point of appearing cachectic), experiences bloating and abdominal distension after meals, develops diarrhea, and, most disturbing to her, develops numbness in her feet. Her neurologic examination shows mild lower leg weakness and sensory loss and absent ankle DTRs. Routine blood tests are normal. Electrical tests confirm a clinical suspicion of a peripheral neuropathy. Which should be the next procedure?

a. Glucose tolerance test
b. Urine porphyrin measurement
c. Anti-transglutaminase antibody determination
d. Skin tests for tuberculosis
e. Pregnancy tests

Answer: c. She has celiac disease, which is usually an autoimmune disorder, in which patients develop an intolerance of rye and barley. They develop malnutrition with weight loss, abdominal bloating, and diarrhea. Eventually they develop complications in various organ systems, including the CNS and PNS. The most frequent neurologic complications of celiac disease are peripheral neuropathy and ataxia. Switching to a gluten-free diet usually resolves most symptoms. Diabetes can cause many of the symptoms, but the normal routine blood tests exclude it. Acute intermittent porphyria is an intermittent disorder characterized by abdominal pain and neuropathy but not signs of malnutrition. Tuberculosis can cause cachexia, but usually as one of several symptoms of a serious, systemic illness. Pregnancy might be considered as a cause of nausea and vomiting but not peripheral neuropathy.

127. Which four of the following are more characteristic of sleep terrors than nightmares?
    a. Occur in deep NREM sleep
    b. Are actually frightening dreams
    c. Are associated with sleepwalking
    d. Follow a partial awakening
    e. Have contents that are often recalled on awakening
    f. Are accompanied by sweating and tachycardia
    g. Are associated with epileptiform EEG activity

Answers: a, c, d, f. Sleep terrors are a variety of parasomnia, but nightmares are dreams with a frightening content. Seizures often develop during sleep, and sometimes they arise exclusively during sleep.

128. After a minor physical alteration with her boyfriend, a 21-year-old waitress develops left hemiparesis. In the emergency room, she is alert but distraught. Her visual fields, facial strength, sensation, and deep tendon and plantar reflexes are normal. When the neurologist asks her to elevate and then abduct her left leg against his resistance, the leg has no movement. However, when the neurologist asks her to abduct her right leg, she pushes outward with both legs. What does this demonstration signify?
    a. Peripheral nerve rather than CNS injury
    b. Spinal cord injury
    c. Muscle injury
    d. Cauda equina injury
    e. None of the above

Answer: e. Her left leg, which seems to have no strength, reflexly abducts when she forcefully abducts the right leg. This disparity, the abductor sign, indicates psychogenic weakness. The abductor sign is comparable to the Hoover sign, which entices the leg with psychogenic paresis to either forcefully push downward or elevate when the patient's efforts are directed toward moving the unaffected leg.

129. On several occasions, a 21-year-old college student has been unable to rise from bed on awakening in the morning. He becomes terrified, and twice he found himself having visual hallucinations. He is otherwise in good mental and physical health. Which one of the following conditions is the most likely cause of his symptoms?

    a. Incipient psychosis
    b. A paroxysm of spikes and waves from the mesial temporal cortex
    c. An intrusion or persistence of REM sleep into wakefulness
    d. Cerebral artery vasospasm

Answer: c. He is probably having sleep paralysis and sleep hallucinations. Although other aspects of narcolepsy should be sought, sleep deprivation and alcohol abuse should be considered.

130. During withdrawal from chronic cocaine use, a patient describes having vivid, frightening dreams. Which is the most likely explanation for his dreams?
    a. Emergence of psychosis
    b. Drug-seeking behavior
    c. Nocturnal seizures
    d. REM rebound

Answer: d. Marijuana and cocaine, as well as numerous medicines, suppress REM sleep. During withdrawal from chronic use, patients have a compensatory increase in REM sleep, that is, REM rebound.

131. Six weeks after a cardiac arrest with asystole, a 48-year-old man opens his eyes, but he is mute and unresponsive to verbal and gestured requests. Although he breathes normally, he has flexion of his limbs, cannot eat or swallow food that is placed in his mouth, and is incontinent of urine. An EEG shows slow, low-voltage, disorganized activity. An additional month passes and he does not improve. What is his condition?
    a. Persistent vegetative state
    b. Coma
    c. Stupor
    d. Locked-in syndrome

Answer: a. He is in a persistent vegetative state with no consciousness or ability to feel pain. He has no cognitive capacity or purposeful movements. His prognosis for a functional recovery is less than 1 in 1000.

132. At 6 months after surviving a stroke in which his basilar artery was occluded, a 75-year-old retired merchant seaman remains quadriplegic, mute, unable to follow verbal or gestured requests, and unable to breathe, eat, or swallow. However, through eyelid blinks, he can communicate using Morse code, which he had used in the Navy. An EEG often shows 10-Hz activity over the occipital area. What is his condition?
    a. Persistent vegetative state

b. Coma

c. Stupor

d. Locked-in syndrome

Answer: d. In contrast to the prior case, this man has intact cognitive capacity. Damage to the base of the pons and medulla impairs his breathing, swallowing, speaking, and movement of his limbs.

133. Match the cell type (a–e) with its function (1–6).

a. Microglia

b. Astrocytes

c. Oligodendrocytes

d. Schwann cells

e. Ependymal cells

1. Generate myelin for the central nervous system

2. Serve a chemical and physical supportive role for neurons

3. Phagocytosis

4. Generate myelin for the peripheral nervous system

5. Line the ventricles

6. Basic element of the nervous system

Answer: a-3, b-2, c-1, d-4, e-5.

134. Which of the following is most likely to allow malignant pain to become "refractory"?

a. Failure to use tricyclic antidepressants in conjunction with analgesics

b. Administering doses of opioids that suppress respirations

c. Undertreatment with opioids

d. Patients having personality disorders

Answer: c. Undertreatment, especially failure to prescribe opioids, is probably the most common physician deficiency in controlling malignant pain. Generous doses of opioids are clearly indicated in most forms of acute and chronic malignant pain. They may also be indicated in some forms of chronic benign pain.

135. Which of the following is the most common cause of coma in the United States?

a. Cerebral hemorrhage

b. Subarachnoid hemorrhage

c. Seizures

d. Drug overdose

e. Subdural hematoma

Answer: d. Drug overdose, not cerebral mass lesions, is the most common cause of coma in the United States.

136. Which of the following neurologic infections is caused by a spirochete?

a. AIDS encephalitis

b. Meningococcal meningitis

c. Herpes simplex encephalitis

d. Lyme disease

Answer: d. Lyme disease, which is an infection by spirochete *Borrelia burgdorferi*, can cause meningitis, encephalitis, facial nerve injury (which mimics Bell's palsy), or a polyneuropathy.

137. Which three of the following individuals might have an EEG showing electrocerebral silence?

a. A 10-year-old boy who drowned in an icy pond

b. A 60-year-old man who took a massive overdose of barbiturates

c. A 55-year-old woman with the locked-in syndrome

d. A 65-year-old man with profound Alzheimer's disease dementia

e. A 17-year-old boy with massive head trauma from a motor vehicle accident

f. A 79-year-old man in a persistent vegetative state

Answers: a, b, e. EEG electrocerebral silence, a "flat" EEG, usually indicates brain death. Head trauma in a candidate to be an organ donor is the most common circumstance when an EEG is performed to confirm a clinical diagnosis of brain death. On the other hand, an EEG showing electrocerebral silence cannot be interpreted as confirming brain death in either individuals who have hypothermia, such as occurs in children who have drowned in icy ponds, or individuals who have taken a barbiturate overdose. Although these individuals often have no clinical sign of brain activity and have EEGs with electrocerebral silence, they often make a full recovery.

138. Which three of the following are effects of caffeine?

a. Headaches

b. Bradycardia

c. Prolonged sleep latency

d. Sleep fragmentation

e. Urinary retention

f. Tremor

Answers: c, d, f. Although one of the world's most widely consumed drugs, caffeine impairs sleep, induces diuresis, provokes a tremor in susceptible individuals, and causes tachycardia, palpitations, and other cardiac disturbances. Its mental effects sometimes mimic anxiety. On the other hand, caffeine withdrawal, such as results from missing a customary morning coffee, produces headache and anxiety.

139. Which four of the following headaches occur predominantly in the morning?
    a. Muscle contraction headaches
    b. Sleep apnea
    c. Brain tumors
    d. Chronic obstructive lung disease
    e. Sleeping in a warm room with no fresh air
    f. Trigeminal neuralgia

Answers: b, c, d, e. Increased carbon dioxide blood levels from pulmonary dysfunction or absence of circulating air leads to painful cerebral vasodilation. At their onset, brain tumors cause increased intracranial pressure when the patient is recumbent.

140. Insert the proper substrates (a–e) into the synthesis and metabolism of dopamine.

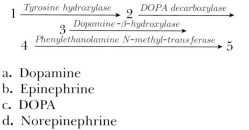

    a. Dopamine
    b. Epinephrine
    c. DOPA
    d. Norepinephrine
    e. Tyrosine

Answers: 1-e, 2-c, 3-a, 4-d, 5-b.

$$\text{Tyrosine} \xrightarrow{\textit{Tyrosine hydroxylase}} \text{DOPA} \xrightarrow{\textit{DOPA decarboxylase}}$$
$$\text{Dopamine} \xrightarrow{\textit{Dopamine-}\beta\text{-hydroxylase}}$$
$$\text{Norepinephrine} \xrightarrow{\textit{Phenylethanolamine N-methyl-transferase}}$$
$$\text{Epinephrine}$$

141. Complete the indolamine pathway.

Answer:

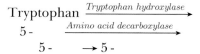

$$\text{Tryptophan} \xrightarrow{\textit{Tryptophan hydroxylase}}$$
$$5\text{-hydroxytryptophan} \xrightarrow{\textit{Amino acid decarboxylase}}$$
$$5\text{-hydroxytryptamine (serotonin)} \rightarrow$$
$$5\text{-HIAA}$$

142. Which one of the following statements regarding anosmia is false?
    a. Compared to age-matched controls, individuals with schizophrenia have an increased incidence of anosmia.

b. Patients with neurodegenerative illnesses, particularly Alzheimer's and Parkinson's diseases, characteristically have a very high incidence of inability to identify certain smells.
    c. In Alzheimer's disease patients, the olfactory bulbs, as well as the cerebral cortex, have plaques and tangles.
    d. Loss of olfactory acuity—inability to identify smells—is a risk factor for Alzheimer's disease.
    e. The small branches of the olfactory receptors are well protected as they pass through the cribriform plate of the skull.

Answer e. The twigs of the nerve's receptors are fragile and liable to be sheared by trauma. They are also susceptible to common viral infections and tobacco smoke. Olfactory nerve dysfunction and pathology are linked to cerebral changes in Alzheimer's disease.

143. A neurologist examined a 70-year-old man who sustained a right cerebral infarction resulting in left hemiplegia. As the neurologist was washing her hands at a bedside sink, the patient pointed to his own left arm and asked her, "Doc! Did you forget your arm?" What disturbance probably gave rise to that question?
    a. Inappropriate humor
    b. Dementia
    c. Anosognosia
    d. A psychogenic disturbance

Answer: c. Patients with nondominant hemisphere lesions, unable to comprehend their left hemiplegia, often disown their body parts and assign them to others. Patients with anosognosia commonly use projection and other defense mechanisms.

144. Which of the following tastes is based on L-glutamate?
    a. Sweet
    b. Sour
    c. Salty
    d. Bitter
    e. Umami

Answer: e. Umami, the fifth taste, is the detection of L-glutamate, which people perceive as "richness." Thus, foods flavored with monosodium glutamate (MSG) and those with high-protein content, such as meat, taste flavorful and satisfying.

145. During which period of gestation is the neural tube formed?
    a. First trimester
    b. Second trimester
    c. Third trimester

d. Variable time

e. At the moment of conception

Answer: a. During the third and fourth weeks of gestation, the dorsal ectoderm invaginates to form a closed, midline neural tube that eventually gives rise to the spinal cord and other elements of the neural tube. This is an intricate maneuver that is susceptible to disruption by medications, including AEDs and toxins. Improper neural tube closure leads to neural tube defects, such as the Arnold-Chiari malformation, spina bifida, and meningomyelocele.

146. Match the medication category with its potential adverse reaction or side effects.

1. β-Blocker
2. Phenytoin
3. Caffeine
4. Anticholinergics
5. SSRIs with MAO inhibitors
   a. Agitation, myoclonus, fever, diarrhea
   b. Blurred vision, urinary difficulty, forgetfulness
   c. Palpitations, tachycardia, anxiety
   d. Exfoliative dermatitis, especially at mucocutaneous boarders
   e. Bradycardia, orthostatic hypotension, fatigue

Answer: 1-e, 2-d (Stevens-Johnson syndrome), 3-c (caffeinism), 4-b, 5-a (serotonin syndrome).

147. Which characteristic distinguishes dementia from toxic-metabolic encephalopathy?

a. Permanence
b. Development only in adults
c. Development only in individuals with normal intelligence
d. Inattention
e. Being alert
f. Disorientation

Answer: e. Depending on the etiology, both dementia and toxic-metabolic encephalopathy, which is also called delirium, can be reversed. Dementia and toxic-metabolic encephalopathy develop in children, young adults, and individuals who are mentally retarded. Both dementia and toxic-metabolic encephalopathy share many clinical features, including inattention and disorientation. However, patients with toxic-metabolic encephalopathy are typically lethargic or stuporous, although sometimes they are overly vigilant and characteristically have a fluctuating level of consciousness. In contrast, individuals with dementia are alert. Complicating this distinction, patients with dementia are much more susceptible to toxic-metabolic encephalopathy than normal individuals. When patients with Alzheimer's disease develop pneumonia, for example, they often manifest a confusing combination of dementia and delirium.

148. A 40-year-old woman reported having chronic fatigue, memory impairments, and inattention to her internist and psychiatrist. Except for an elevated Lyme titer, a thorough internal medical evaluation, neurologic examination, CT, MRI, and other blood tests were normal. She underwent a 3-week course of intravenous antibiotics. When her symptoms persisted, her internist administered a second course of intravenous antibiotics. Afterward, although her Lyme titer reverted to normal, she still reported having no change in her symptoms. When seeking consultation from a multidiscipline team of physicians, she felt strongly that she had chronic Lyme disease and insisted on an additional course of treatment but with a different antibiotic. What would be the best response regarding the value of her proposed strategy?

a. In seropositive, but not seronegative, cases, a third course of antibiotics often reverse the neurocognitive symptoms of chronic Lyme disease.
b. In seronegative as well as seropositive cases, a third course of antibiotics often reverses the neurocognitive symptoms of chronic Lyme disease.
c. In neither seronegative nor seropositive cases will a third course of antibiotics reverse the neurocognitive symptoms of chronic Lyme disease.
d. None of the above.

Answer: c. The etiology of persistent neurocognitive impairments, mood disturbances, and chronic fatigue following adequate treatment of Lyme disease remains unclear; however, additional courses of antibiotics do not reverse those symptoms.

149. A 19-year-old female college student, who seemed to have developed a chronic, noninfectious hepatitis the preceding year, begins to have a subtle decline in her grades, and develops dysarthria, tremor, and depression. Except for abnormal liver function tests, routine laboratory testing and also CT, MRI, CSF, and EEG reveal no abnormalities. Which test should be ordered next?

a. HIV
b. HTLV-1
c. Mononucleosis spot test
d. Antistreptolysin O titer

e. Serum ceruloplasmin

f. MS evaluation

Answer: e. This patient has hepatic dysfunction, cognitive impairment, depression, tremor, and dysarthria. She may have Wilson's disease (hepatolenticular degeneration), in which case the sooner the diagnosis is made and the sooner treatment is instituted, the better the prognosis. A low serum concentration of ceruloplasmin, the copper-carrying serum protein, is indicative of Wilson's disease. This illness, which is transmitted as an autosomal recessive condition, may affect only the liver, but when it has neurologic complications, a slit lamp examination of the cornea may reveal a Kayser-Fleischer ring. Other causes of hepatic dysfunction and mental changes include mononucleosis, alcoholism, and other substance abuse. MS is unlikely in view of the progressive course, early onset of cognitive impairment, and normal MRI.

150. Match the spinal cord tract with its function.

a. Pyramidal

b. Spinothalamic

c. Fasciculus gracilis

d. Spinocerebellar

e. Fasciculus cuneatus

1. Ascends as in the spinal cord to the cerebellum to assist with coordination

2. Descends as the corticospinal tract to innervate the anterior horn cells

3. Ascends to convey pain sensation to the brain

4. Transmits position sense from the upper extremities

5. Transmits position sense from the lower extremities

Answers: a-2, b-3, c-5, d-1, e-4.

151. Which five characteristics indicate that facial weakness is more likely due to a seventh cranial nerve lesion than a cerebral lesion?

a. Only flattening of the nasolabial fold

b. Loss or alteration of taste sensation

c. Inability to close the eyelid muscles and to smile on the same side of the face

d. Hyperacusis or tinnitus ipsilateral to the facial weakness

e. Aphasia

f. Mastoid pain

g. Pain in the mastoid area before the facial weakness

Answers: b, c, d, f, g. Weakness of upper as well as lower facial muscles and the disruption of hearing and taste sensations characterize a cranial nerve VII injury. When the nerve is inflamed, pain is referred to the mastoid region.

152. A 35-year-old woman who has difficulty describing her symptoms seems to have, several times yearly, a several-hour episode of monocular visual obscuration followed by a throbbing, generalized headache. A general medical and neurologic evaluation and CTs with and without contrast infusion are normal. Which one of the following conditions is most likely?

a. Migraine without aura (common migraine)

b. Transient ischemic attacks (TIA) from basilar artery stenosis

c. Migraine with aura (classic migraine)

d. Transient ischemic attacks (TIA) from carotid artery stenosis

e. An AVM

f. MS

g. Tension headaches

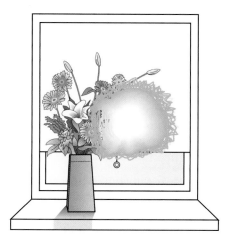

Answer: c. Transient loss of vision (amaurosis fugax) in one eye may result from TIAs of the ophthalmic artery, the first branch of the internal carotid artery. The visual impairment usually lasts for less than 20 minutes and has no accompanying headache. Basilar artery TIAs typically cause bilateral visual changes accompanied by vertigo and ataxia although no headache. MS may cause episodes of unilateral visual loss and pain in or around the eye (optic neuritis), but the symptoms have a duration of several days to weeks and usually are accompanied by other neurologic deficits. AVMs may cause repeated bouts of homonymous hemianopsia and headache, but they are almost always evident on CT or MRI. Visual loss or hallucination may precede a headache or occur as a separate entity in migraine with aura (classic migraine). Tension headaches are frequently episodic, but not accompanied by visual symptoms.

153. Which two are common side effects of dopamine precursor or agonist treatment for Parkinson's disease?

a. Dyskinesias

b. Vivid dreams
c. Neuroleptic malignant syndrome
d. Seizures
e. Elevated serum prolactin concentration

Answers: a, b. When dopamine precursors or agonists—dopaminergic medications—lead to excessive dopamine activity, they routinely cause dyskinesias and vivid dreams. Dopamine agonists may also lead to sleep attacks. Dopamine precursors or agonists suppress serum prolactin concentration, but that change causes no symptoms. Abrupt withdrawal of dopaminergic medications occasionally leads to the neuroleptic malignant syndrome. However, dopaminergic medications do not cause seizures.

154. A 17-year-old woman, found at birth to have phenylketonuria (PKU), was treated successfully with a strict phenylalanine-free diet. However, as a teenager, she frequently deviated from her diet, particularly by drinking diet sodas. She also engaged in antisocial behavior and recently conceived. Her boyfriend, who is the father, is not a carrier of PKU. Which of the following statements regarding the fetus is false?
    a. The fetus will be heterozygote for the PKU gene.
    b. In affected individuals, the blood tyrosine level is low and phenylalanine levels elevated.
    c. Although the mother may sustain brain damage by her deviation from the diet, the fetus, which has normal metabolic enzymes, will be unharmed.
    d. PKU infants appear normal at birth.

Answer: c. Because PKU is an autosomal recessive disorder, the mother carries two abnormal genes, but the father has none. All offspring will be heterozygote. Even though the fetus is heterozygote, the affected mother's excessive phenylalanine intake can overwhelm the fetus' metabolic capacity and produce excessive concentrations of phenylalanine and its metabolic products, which are toxic to the brain. In other words, PKU women must strictly adhere to the diet when they are pregnant.

155. Which six varieties of tremor may be suppressed with β-blocker medication?
    a. Essential
    b. Performance anxiety
    c. Resting
    d. Lithium-induced
    e. Benign
    f. Cerebellar
    g. Hyperthyroid
    h. Psychogenic

Answers: a, b, d, e, g, h. β-blockers suppress the tremor associated with excessive autonomic nervous system activity that may result from anxiety, medications, or genetic factors. The resting tremor in as many as 10% of Parkinson's disease patients responds somewhat to β-blockers.

156. Match the lesion (a–g) with the movement disorder (1–6).
    a. Atrophy of the caudate nuclei heads
    b. Lewy bodies
    c. Depigmentation of the substantia nigra
    d. Infarction of the contralateral subthalamic nucleus
    e. Compression of the seventh cranial nerve by an aberrant vessel
    f. Depigmentation of the locus ceruleus
    g. DYT1 gene
    1. Parkinson's disease
    2. Huntington's disease
    3. Early onset primary (torsion) dystonia
    4. Hemifacial spasm
    5. Meige's syndrome
    6. Hemiballismus

Answers: a-2, b-1, c-1, d-6, e-4, f-1, g-3.

157. Several days after an automobile accident, in which he sustained a whiplash injury, a 16-year-old boy begins to notice progressively worsening neck pain and weakness in his fingers. He has loss of pin sensation in a shawl pattern over his shoulder, upper arms, and hands but intact joint position and vibration sensation. DTRs in his arms are diminished, but those in his legs are brisk. Plantar reflexes are equivocal. Which one of the following processes may be developing?
    a. Worsening of the whiplash symptoms
    b. Development of a herniated cervical intervertebral disk
    c. Bleeding into the center of the spinal cord
    d. Emergence of poststress symptoms

Answers: c. Hematomyelia, bleeding into the center of the spinal cord, which usually occurs in the cervical portion of the spinal cord, may follow neck injuries from motor vehicle, trampoline, horseback riding, or diving accidents. Stretching the crossing fibers of the lateral spinothalamic tract, cervical hematomyelia impairs pin and temperature sensation in the arms. The expanding lesion also compresses the anterior horn cells of the cervical spinal cord, which contain lower motor neurons that innervate the arms and hands, and the corticospinal tracts, which cause long tract motor signs in the legs. Syringomyelia (syrinx), the congenital, nontraumatic variety of this disorder, develops more insidiously, but the findings are similar.

158. Which Parkinson's disease medicine diverts dopamine metabolism, in part, to amphetamine or amphetamine-like substances?
a. Levodopa-carbidopa
b. Deprenyl
c. COMT inhibitors
d. Tocopherol

Answer: b. Deprenyl (selegiline) is an inhibitor of MAO-B. Although it retards dopamine metabolism, it channels some metabolism into amphetamine or amphetamine-like by-products. COMT inhibitors have no such effect.

159. The family of a 55-year-old man, who has a history of cluster headaches and depression, brings him to the emergency room with the report that over 3 months he has developed progressively greater cognitive impairment. His medications included lithium, which he used to treat both the cluster headaches and depression. The physicians found him to be alert but dull and unable to answer questions regarding his orientation, memory, and judgment. The physicians noticed that he had myoclonus. Which of the following tests would be least likely to help in the diagnosis?
a. Serum HIV
b. An EEG
c. CSF 14-3-3 protein
d. Serum lithium level

Answer: a. The patient seems to have developed Creutzfeldt-Jakob disease because of the cognitive impairment and myoclonus. An EEG and a CSF 14-3-3 protein determination would confirm that diagnosis. In addition, various metabolic aberrations, such as lithium or bismuth intoxication, can cause delirium with myoclonus. HIV dementia rarely develops in such an explosive fashion and rarely does it cause myoclonus.

160. An 8-year-old girl has episodes of confusion and headaches lasting between 1 and 2 days. She has no abnormal movements during the attacks. Between attacks her neurologic examination and all routine blood tests, head CT, and head MRI were normal. During EEG-CCTV monitoring for epilepsy, the EEG showed no epileptiform discharges during three episodes. Also, her serum prolactin level, blood, and electrolytes remained normal during the episodes; however, her lactic acid levels rose fourfold. A muscle biopsy showed ragged red fibers, a proliferation of mitochondria, and absence of respiratory enzymes. Which should be the next test?

a. Glucose tolerance test
b. Chromosome analysis for trinucleotide repeats
c. Analysis of her mtDNA
d. Polysomnography

Answer c. She probably has a mitochondrial encephalopathy in view of her episodes of confusion with lactic acidosis and the muscle biopsy's showing characteristic changes. Other causes of episodic confusion—migraines, epilepsy, sleep disorders, and TIAs—might be considered. However, the elevation of the lactic acid suggests only a mitochondrial encephalopathy.

161. A 40-year-old man was struck on the back of his head with a baseball bat. He sustained a skull fracture and was rendered comatose for 2 days. When he became conversant, he confabulated about visitors and often wrongly identified people. He seemed to have marked visual impairment, but he denied it. His pupils were round and reactive to light. Funduscopy revealed no abnormalities. Extraocular movements were normal. What is the nature of his visual impairment?
a. Retinal detachments
b. Ocular trauma
c. Ocular blindness
d. Cortical blindness
e. Anosognosia

Answer: d. Trauma of the visual cortex has led to cortical blindness. Despite having this variety of blindness, his eyes, optic nerves, oculomotor nerves, and midbrain—which form the light reflex arc—characteristically remain normal. His denial of blindness and tendency to confabulate about questions that depend on sight (Anton's syndrome) is a variety of anosognosia. Anton's syndrome, which usually follows sudden loss of vision, may result from occlusion of either posterior cerebral arteries or occipital lobe trauma.

162. Match the system (a–d) with the associated structures (1–4).
a. Cholinergic
b. Serotonergic
c. Noradrenergic (norepinephrine-containing)
d. Dopaminergic
1. Nucleus basalis of Meynert
2. Dorsal raphe nucleus
3. Locus ceruleus
4. Mesolimbic and mesocortical tracts

Answers: a-1, b-2, c-3, d-4.

163. What is the cardinal feature of conduction aphasia?
    a. Patients cannot name objects.
    b. Patients cannot follow simple requests.
    c. Patients cannot repeat.
    d. Patients have diffuse cognitive impairment.

Answer: c. In conduction aphasia, a lesion interrupts the perisylvian language arc and severs the connection between Wernicke's and Broca's areas. Thus, patients characteristically cannot repeat what they hear.

164. Which one of the following conditions is not a disconnection syndrome?
    a. Alexia without agraphia
    b. Conduction aphasia
    c. Split brain syndrome
    d. Gerstmann's syndrome
    e. Ideomotor apraxia

Answer: d. All conditions except Gerstmann's syndrome are disconnection syndromes. Another distinction is that all the conditions, except for the split-brain syndrome, usually result from dominant hemisphere lesions.

165. Which part of the body is most commonly involved in tardive akathisia?
    a. Head
    b. Arms
    c. Legs
    d. Trunk

Answer: c. Although tardive akathisia may involve the trunk, head, neck, and arms, it most frequently and most severely involves the legs. When akathisia is extensive, it resembles chorea.

166. Which are the two most common movements in tardive akathisia?
    a. Walking or marching in place
    b. Tremor of legs
    c. Crossing or rapidly adducting and abducting the legs
    d. Periodic flexion at the hip and ankle, especially when asleep

Answers: a, c.

167. Which statement is false in regard to most cases of neuropathy associated with AIDS?
    a. It is distal and symmetric.
    b. The sensory symptoms, including painful dysesthesias, are more bothersome and more pronounced than motor symptoms, such as weakness and ankle DTR loss.
    c. It is associated with depression.
    d. It develops early in the course of the illness.

Answer: d. Neuropathy associated with AIDS usually occurs late in the course of AIDS, when patients have other medical complications, a high viral load, and low CD4 count. It is typically a painful, distal sensory neuropathy.

168. A neurologist is consulted for a 37-year-old woman who has inability to move her left arm and leg that developed over the previous 3 weeks. Although she has gait impairment and has become unable to use utensils with her left hand, she remains blasé. Her face is symmetric and her visual fields intact. Her DTRs are symmetric and she has no Babinski sign. When asked to abduct her legs against the examiner's hands, the right leg abducts against the force of the examiner's hand. At the same time, the examiner's hand meets considerable resistance when trying to push the left leg medially. Then, the patient is asked to abduct her left leg against the examiner's hand. That leg fails to abduct and, at the same time, the right leg exerts so little force that the examiner easily pushes it medially. Which two of the following statements concerning this case are false?
    a. This patient's abductor test suggests a psychogenic basis.
    b. Her lack of obvious concern is strong evidence of a psychogenic basis.
    c. Patients with left-sided neglect or hemiparkinsonism have left-sided akinesia that might reasonably be mistaken for hemiparesis.
    d. Recent studies have confirmed that psychogenic hemiparesis much more often affects the left than right side.

Answers: b, d. Recent studies have failed to confirm earlier observations that psychogenic hemiparesis is associated with *la belle indifférence* or that it is found much more often on the left than right side. If this patient has psychogenic hemiparesis, she would probably also have a Hoover's sign. Physicians should consider conditions, such as neglect or hemiparkinsonism that cause immobility but not corticospinal tract abnormalities. Patients with those conditions will not have hyperactive DTRs or Babinski signs.

169. By which pathway do almost all lung cancers spread to the brain parenchyma?
    a. Hematogenous dissemination
    b. Lymphatic spread
    c. CSF seeding
    d. Bony extension

Answer: a. Lung cancers metastasize widely by hematogenous dissemination. Some cancers spread through the lymphatic system but not to the brain because it does not have a lymphatic supply. Sometimes cancers spread to the meninges and cause carcinomatous meningitis.

170. A 55-year-old woman and her twin brother, who live hundreds of miles apart, have each developed insomnia that has not responded to several medications. An examination of the siblings reveals inattentiveness and mild confusion, labile hypertension and tachycardia, and myoclonus. MRIs show atrophy of the thalamus. Which illness has developed?
    a. A prion disease
    b. Alzheimer's disease
    c. Lewy body disease
    d. Vascular dementia
    e. Manic-depressive illness

Answer: a. They have developed fatal familial insomnia, a prion illness, because of a genetic susceptibility. This rapidly fatal illness is characterized by refractory insomnia, cognitive and personality changes, autonomic and endocrine system hyperactivity, and motor changes, including myoclonus.

171. What is the lowermost level of the body at which upper motor neurons are found?
    a. Foramen magnum
    b. Medulla
    c. Beginning of the spinal cord
    d. First lumbar vertebrae (L1)

Answer: d. The spinal cord contains upper motor neurons, which are carried in the corticospinal tract. Because the spinal cord terminates by giving rise to the cauda equina at L1, that level is the lowermost extent of upper motor neurons. Thus, neurologists can perform spinal taps at the L2-3 and lower levels and avoid striking the spinal cord.

172. A patient has been under treatment with a tricyclic antidepressant for painful diabetic neuropathy. Shortly after increasing the dose, he developed abdominal distention and other clinical indications of intestinal obstruction. CT of the abdomen showed a paralytic ileus but no mass lesion or focal obstruction. What would be the best medication to correct the problem?
    a. Neostigmine
    b. ACh
    c. Milk of magnesia
    d. Cascara

Answer: a. The patient has developed pseudo-obstruction from the anticholinergic side effects of the tricyclic antidepressant. Neostigmine, an acetylcholinesterase (AChE) inhibitor, will restore ACh activity and bowel motility.

173. Of the following, which is the most significant risk factor for strokes?
    a. Type A personality
    b. Race
    c. Hypertension
    d. Obesity

Answer: c. Of the numerous risk factors for strokes, hypertension and advanced age are the two greatest. Other risk factors, including obesity, diabetes, race, and elevated cholesterol levels, are so closely associated with each other and hypertension that their individual effect is difficult to assess. Psychologic factors carry no significant risk.

174. A 50-year-old man has noticed diplopia on looking to the left. The right pupil is dilated and poorly reactive to light. He has right-sided ptosis. Which injury is most likely to have occurred?
    a. Left sixth cranial nerve palsy
    b. Right third cranial nerve palsy
    c. Right transtentorial herniation
    d. Left third cranial nerve palsy
    e. Left transtentorial herniation
    f. Myasthenia-induced paresis

Answer: b. Although diplopia on left lateral gaze might be attributable to either a left sixth or right third cranial nerve palsy, his signs of a third cranial nerve palsy indicate that the right third cranial nerve is responsible. Patients with herniation are stuporous or comatose: They are not alert enough to be able to express any symptom, except perhaps headache. Myasthenia does not affect the pupil.

175. Which finding is most closely associated with tremor on intention?
    a. Dysdiadochokinesia
    b. Rigidity
    c. Bradykinesia
    d. Ataxia of gait
    e. Tremor at rest

Answer: a. Tremor on intention and other limb coordination problems, such as dysdiadochokinesia (impaired rapid alternating movements), are associated with cerebellar hemisphere injury. Tremor at rest is a feature of Parkinson's disease. Ataxia of gait is related to injury of the midline cerebellum (vermis) or the entire cerebellum.

176. Which medicines are appropriate in the treatment of painful diabetic neuropathy?
   a. AEDs, such as gabapentin
   b. Duloxetine
   c. Tricyclic antidepressants
   d. Opioids
   e. All of the above

Answer: e. Many conditions involving neuropathic pain, such as thalamic pain syndrome, diabetic neuropathy, and postherpetic neuralgia, respond to the same set of medicines. These medicines include tricyclic antidepressants, opioids, and some AEDs. Although SSRIs usually produce little analgesia, duloxetine, a norepinephrine as well as a selective serotonin reuptake inhibitor, is helpful.

177. Which of the following medications does not lower the seizure threshold?
   a. Maprotiline (Ludiomil)
   b. Diazepam (Valium)
   c. Clomipramine (Anafranil)
   d. Chlorpromazine (Thorazine)

Answer: b.

178. The family of a 75-year-old man brought him for evaluation for depression because he seemed apathetic, inattentive, and unresponsive to them. The psychiatrist found that he had marked memory problems and impairments in two other cognitive domains. The psychiatrist also elicited a history of vivid hallucinations at night and during the day. The patient had been in good health and taking no medicine. Several months ago, a neurologist had offered a tentative diagnosis of early Parkinson's disease because he found that the patient had a slow, shuffling gait, but, because the signs were subtle, he started no anti-Parkinson's disease medicine. What is the most likely underlying condition?
   a. Depression
   b. Alzheimer's disease
   c. Dementia with Lewy bodies
   d. Medication-induced hallucinations

Answer: c. The patient has the major features of dementia with Lewy bodies: dementia, fluctuating levels of consciousness, hallucinations, and parkinsonism. Hallucinations complicate Parkinson's disease only in its later stages and when patients are taking substantial doses of dopaminergic medicines.

179. Videotaped monitoring of seizure patients is useful in determining which of the following?
   a. The variety or frequency of the seizures
   b. The presence of psychogenic seizures
   c. The site of the origin of seizures
   d. Correlation of seizures with AED blood levels
   e. All of the above

Answer: e.

180. A 30-year old man has developed neck pain and loss of dexterity of his hands 6 months after a motor vehicle accident in which he sustained a fracture of C4. The neurologist finds that he has atrophy as well as weakness of intrinsic hand muscles. The biceps, triceps, and brachioradialis DTRs are absent, but DTRs in his legs are normal. Plantar reflexes are flexion. He has decreased sensation to pin and temperature in both arms and hands and from the middle of his neck to his upper chest; however, vibration and position sensations are preserved. Of the following, which is the most likely diagnosis?
   a. Spinal cord transection
   b. Syringomyelia
   c. Brown-Séquard syndrome
   d. Whiplash injury
   e. Herniated intervertebral disk

Answer: b. He has a cervical post-traumatic syringomyelia or hematomyelia (syrinx). This disorder follows serious trauma, but it often develops spontaneously in the cervical spinal cord of teenagers and young adults. He presents with classic symptoms and signs: neck pain, areflexic weakness and atrophy of the upper extremity muscles, and a *suspended* sensory loss to pain but not position. A spinal cord transection would have caused quadriplegia or quadriparesis, hyperactive DTRs and other upper motor neuron signs, and sensory loss to all modalities. Brown-Séquard syndrome, which results from a lateral transection of the spinal cord at any level, consists of weakness with hyperactive DTRs and position sense loss of the limbs on the side ipsilateral to the injury and loss of pain and temperature sensation on the contralateral side. Whiplash injury would not have caused nerve injury. Herniated disks would have caused pain, areflexic DTRs, and loss to all modalities in the distribution of only one or two cervical nerve roots.

181. Which of the following medications inhibits HIV reverse transcriptase?
   a. Trimethoprim-sulfamethoxazole (Bactrim, Septra, and others)
   b. Pyrimethamine (Daraprim)
   c. Ganciclovir (Cytovene)
   d. Zidovudine (Retrovir)
   e. Pentamidine

Answer: d. Previously known as AZT and often given when HIV infection is first detected, zidovudine has increased median survival after diagnosis. Side effects include myopathy, headache, fatigue, malaise, and confusion. Trimethoprim-sulfamethoxazole and pentamidine are each effective for *Pneumocystis carinii* pneumonia (PCP). Pyrimethamine (Daraprim) is the treatment of choice for cerebral toxoplasmosis. Ganciclovir (Cytovene) is useful for cytomegalovirus (CMV) infections, especially CMV retinitis and colitis.

182. Which condition constitutes a risk factor for dementia following head trauma?
   a. Blood type A
   b. APOe-4
   c. Rheumatoid arthritis
   d. Periodontal disease

Answer: b. Carrying two alleles of APOe-4 predisposes individuals sustaining traumatic brain injury to post-traumatic dementia. Periodontal disease is a risk factor for stroke.

183. Which of the following areas of the brain is most susceptible to anoxia?
   a. Medulla
   b. Wernicke's area
   c. Globus pallidus
   d. Hippocampus

Answer: d. Although the entire cerebral cortex is sensitive, the hippocampus is exquisitely sensitive. The globus pallidus is damaged not only with anoxia but also with carbon monoxide poisoning.

184. Which two features would indicate that seizures were partial complex rather than petit mal?
   a. Impaired consciousness
   b. Fluttering eyelids
   c. Symptoms that might constitute an aura
   d. Childhood onset
   e. Duration of 5 seconds
   f. Tendency toward retrograde amnesia, personality change, or sleep after the seizure

Answers: c, f (see Table 10-4).

185. Which laboratory abnormality characterizes cyanide poisoning?
   a. Marked serum lactic acidosis
   b. Arterial methemoglobin
   c. Urinary porphyrins
   d. Arterial marked carbon dioxide elevation

Answer: a. Cyanide poisons cellular respiratory enzymes. The interruption of aerobic metabolism leads to marked elevations in lactic and pyruvate acids along with death of highly metabolically active cells, particularly those in the brain. Carbon monoxide poisoning causes arterial methemoglobin. Acute intermittent porphyria leads to excretion of porphyrins. Patients with chronic obstructive pulmonary disease characteristically retain carbon dioxide. At high enough levels, carbon dioxide causes coma.

186. What is the mechanism of action of botulinum toxin when used to treat focal dystonias, such as spasmodic torticollis?
   a. Like curare, botulinum blocks ACh neuromuscular receptors.
   b. Botulinum impairs ACh presynaptic release at the neuromuscular junction.
   c. Botulinum depletes dopamine.
   d. Like pyridostigmine (Mestinon), botulinum enhances ACh activity.
   e. Like nerve gas, botulinum creates a depolarization of the postsynaptic ACh receptor site.
   f. ACh strength is increased because its reuptake is blocked by botulinum.

Answer: b. Botulinum inhibits dystonic muscle contractions by impairing ACh release from the presynaptic neuron at the neuromuscular junction. Although botulinum may cause some weakness, the dystonia is greatly reduced. Curare and many nerve gases block the ACh neuromuscular receptors and thus induce lethal paralysis. In contrast to the activity of dopamine and many other neurotransmitters whose action is partly terminated by reuptake, ACh activity is terminated entirely by cholinesterase metabolism.

187. Match the area of the nervous system (a–i) with its location (1–4).
   a. Anterior horn cells
   b. Corpus callosum
   c. Locus ceruleus
   d. Bulb
   e. Vermis
   f. Cranial nerve nuclei for swallowing
   g. Origin of phrenic nerve
   h. Heschl's gyrus
   i. Hippocampus
      1. Cerebrum
      2. Cerebellum
      3. Brainstem
      4. Spinal cord

Answers: a-4, b-1, c-3, d-3, e-2, f-3, g-4, h-1, i-1.

188. Match the brainstem region (a–l) with its location (1–5).
   a. Cranial nerve nucleus that innervates the jaw muscles
   b. Cranial nerve that adducts each eye
   c. Trochlear nerve

d. Cranial nerves that move eyes laterally
e. Beginning of the nigrostriatal tract
f. Cranial nerves that innervate the tongue muscles
g. Cranial nerves that govern speech and swallowing
h. Thalamus
i. Hypothalamus
j. Locus ceruleus
k. Crossing of the pyramids
l. Cranial nerve that innervates the upper and lower face muscles
   1. Diencephalon
   2. Midbrain
   3. Pons
   4. Medulla
   5. None of the above

Answers: a-3, b-2, c-2, d-3, e-2, f-4, g-4, h-1, i-1, j-3, k-4, l-3.

189. Which two statements concerning syphilis or neurosyphilis are true?
   a. In an appropriate clinical setting, a positive CSF-VDRL test confirms the diagnosis of neurosyphilis.
   b. A dramatic increase in the incidence of syphilis has occurred in conjunction with the AIDS epidemic.
   c. A negative CSF-VDRL test is strong evidence against a diagnosis of neurosyphilis.
   d. A positive serum VDRL or RPR at a dilution of 1:2 is strong evidence of syphilis.

Answer: a, b. A large proportion of patients with neurosyphilis—40% in one study—have a negative CSF-VDRL. One the other hand, a positive CSF-VDRL is strong evidence that a patient has neurosyphilis. False-positive serum results, which are generally 1:4 or less, are attributable to other infection, rheumatologic diseases, drug addiction, and changes in serum proteins found with old age. False-negative serum results may be found when the disease is "burnt out," the infectious activity is low, or in rare cases when the antibody concentration is so great that a visible reaction is prevented (prozone inhibition).

190. Match the skin lesions (a–k) with their associated neurologic disorders (1–11).
   a. Adenoma sebaceum
   b. Kaposi's sarcoma
   c. Vaginal chancre
   d. Congenital facial angioma in the distribution of the first division trigeminal nerve
   e. Acute eruption of vesicles in the distribution of the first division trigeminal nerve
   f. Café au lait spots
   g. Protuberance of hair tuft, skin, and soft tissue over the lumbar spine
   h. Erythema migrans
   i. Anesthetic, depigmented patches on the coolest regions of the face and body
   j. Dermatitis, diarrhea, and dementia
   k. White lines across the nails (Mees' lines)
      1. Possible later development of treponema in the CNS
      2. Round growths in the brain that cause dementia and seizures
      3. Two layers of calcified cerebral cortical angioma that causes seizures
      4. Development of cerebral lymphoma
      5. Neurofibromas
      6. Lancinating pain in the distribution of the skin lesion
      7. Impotence and leg weakness
      8. Pellagra
      9. Bell's palsy-like facial weakness
      10. Leprosy
      11. Arsenic poisoning

Answers: a-2, b-4, c-1, d-3, e-6, f-5, g-7, h-9, i-10, j-8, k-11.

191. Identify the structures (1–6) on this MRI of a normal brain.

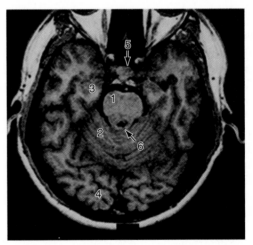

a. Mesial temporal lobe
b. Third ventricle
c. Upper portion of the fourth ventricle
d. Midbrain
e. Pons
f. Medulla
g. Pituitary gland
h. Occipital cortex
i. Cerebellum

Answers: 1-e, 2-i, 3-a, 4-h, 5-g, 6-c.

192. Regarding the MRI in the preceding question, which view of the brain is portrayed?
a. Axial
b. Lateral
c. Coronal
d. Sagittal

Answer: a. This view is the traditional axial or trans-axial image.

193. Match the neurotransmitter (a–d) with the area of the brain where it is formed (1–4).
a. Norepinephrine
b. Dopamine
c. Serotonin
d. ACh
   1. Nucleus basalis of Meynert, which is inferior to the globus pallidus in the basal forebrain
   2. Raphe nucleus, which runs throughout the brainstem
   3. Substantia nigra in the midbrain
   4. Locus ceruleus, which is in the pons

Answers: a-4, b-3, c-2, d-1.

194. Which two of the following are associated with meningomyeloceles?
a. Mental retardation
b. Hydrocephalus
c. Neurofibromatosis
d. Intravenous drug abuse

Answer: a, b. Meningomyeloceles, which are lower neural tube closure defects, are associated with abnormalities of the upper end of the neural tube, particularly hydrocephalus and mental retardation.

195. About 10 days after beginning treatment with phenytoin, a 10-year-old child develops blister-like lesions on the conjunctiva, mouth, and other mucocutaneous regions. Which condition is most likely?
a. Meningococcal meningitis
b. Child abuse
c. Allergy
d. Seizure associated trauma

Answer: c. The child has developed the Stevens-Johnson syndrome, which is a rare, life-threatening, allergic reaction. It has a predilection for mucocutaneous regions but may involve the entire skin.

196. Which AED has a chemical structure that most closely resembles a tricyclic antidepressant?
a. Phenytoin
b. Phenobarbital
c. Carbamazepine
d. Valproic acid

Answer: c. Carbamazepine closely resembles imipramine.

197. Which is the best study in attempting to locate mesial temporal sclerosis?
a. CT
b. MRI
c. EEG
d. Routine x-rays

Answer: b. MRI provides better resolution than CT. Also, with the MRI, the skull does not create artifacts.

198. Which cell transmits congenital illnesses attributable to mitochondria defects?
a. The egg and the sperm in equal proportion
b. The egg exclusively
c. The sperm exclusively
d. The amniotic fluid

Answer: b. The egg carries all the mitochondria for the embryo. The tail of the sperm contains all of its mitochondria. After propelling the sperm to the egg, its tail drops off.

199. In testing a 35-year-old man who had developed gait impairment, the neurologist asked him to stand with his feet together with his eyes open and then closed. With his eyes open, the patient was stable, but when his eyes were closed, the patient began to topple. To avoid falling, he separated his feet to catch himself. In which two regions of the nervous system would damage most likely cause this test result?
a. Peripheral nervous system
b. Cerebellum
c. Posterior columns of the spinal cord
d. Labyrinthine system
e. Corticospinal tracts

Answers: a, c. The neurologist has subjected the patient to the Romberg test, in which a positive (abnormal) result consists of inability to stand erect with closed eyes and the feet held closely together. The explanation is that a stable standing position relies on vision and joint position sensation. An intact system permits continual sensory monitoring and, if necessary, compensatory motor adjustments. Closing the eyes eliminates visual input and forces patients to rely on joint position sensation, which is normally conveyed through peripheral nerves to the posterior columns of the spinal cord to the brain. The Romberg sign is present in peripheral neuropathies, such as diabetic neuropathy, and diseases that damage the posterior columns of the spinal cord, such as MS, combined system disease (B_{12} deficiency), tabes dorsalis, and certain spinocerebellar ataxias. Attempting to elicit a Romberg sign is inappropriate for individuals with cerebellar or labyrinthine disease because they are generally unable to stand with their feet together even with their eyes open.

200. A 50-year-old woman, who recently arrived from the Caribbean, developed a gait impairment characterized by stiffness and mild weakness. Tests of her mental status, cranial nerves and upper extremities showed no abnormalities. However, in her legs, the DTRs were abnormally brisk, and she had spasticity, clonus, and Babinski signs. She had no sensory loss. MRIs of her brain and spinal cord were normal. Which of the following serologies is most likely to be positive?
   a. HTLV-III (human T-lymphotropic virus type III)
   b. Anti-parietal cell and anti-intrinsic factor antibodies
   c. HTLV-I (human T-lymphotropic virus type I)
   d. RPR (rapid plasma reagin)

Answer: c. Her lower extremity spasticity and mild paraparesis indicate that she has a myelopathy. In her case, it is probably due to HTLV-I infection, which is called tropical spastic paraparesis or HTLV-I associated myelopathy. This condition, which is sexually transmitted, occurs in clusters in a world-wide swath straddling the equator, with the Caribbean islands being endemic areas. In contrast, anti-parietal cell and anti-intrinsic factor antibodies are signs of B_{12} deficiency and its associated combined system disease, which is characterized by posterior column sensory loss as well as spasticity. Positive tests for RPR would indicate syphilis. Although one of tertiary syphilis' neurologic complications, tabes dorsalis, also produces gait impairment and posterior column sensory loss, it almost always causes Argyll-Robinson pupils and areflexia in the lower extremities. HTLV-III is an older name for HIV, which causes AIDS. HIV can infect the spinal cord, but it produces a clinical picture similar to combined system disease. HTLV-I associated myelopathy mimics multiple sclerosis (MS) and the CSF in both conditions contains oligoclonal bands, but MS usually develops more rapidly, affects the body in more than one area and in an asymmetric pattern, and uncommonly develops in citizens of Caribbean islands.

201. The parents of a 5-year-old boy report that after a normal first 5 years of growth and development, their son has been withdrawing from them and has begun to flap his hands. During a preliminary evaluation, he seems to have below average intelligence and pronounced loss of language skills but not mental retardation. He has spasticity. Which of the following illnesses are least likely?
   a. Autism
   b. Rett syndrome
   c. Angelman syndrome
   d. Cerebral palsy
   e. Lesch-Nyhan syndrome

Answer: d. Except for cerebral palsy, which is evident by late infancy, all the conditions have symptoms that appear in childhood and include abnormal hand movements. Although Rett syndrome typically develops in girls, cases of this disorder have been reported in boys.

202. Of the following, which is the most common form of inherited mental retardation?
   a. Alzheimer's disease
   b. Rett syndrome
   c. Trisomy 18
   d. Fragile X syndrome
   e. Turner's syndrome
   f. Trisomy 21

Answer: d. Of the choices, the fragile X syndrome is the most common cause of inherited mental retardation. The fragile X syndrome causes retardation in 1 boy in 1000 to 1500. These boys tend to have a long, thin face, large ears, and large testes. In 1 girl in 2000 to 2500, the fragile X syndrome causes retardation that is milder. Although fragile X may cause features suggestive of autism, it has no specific signs. DNA analysis, the definitive test, demonstrates excessive trinucleotide repeats on the X chromosome. Trisomy 21 (Down syndrome), although a genetic disorder, is not an inherited condition because neither parent is affected. The incidence of Down syndrome births is falling because of prenatal testing.

203. Why is carbidopa administered along with L-dopa (levodopa) in the treatment of Parkinson's disease?
   a. Carbidopa is a decarboxylase inhibitor that retards the metabolism of CNS L-dopa.
   b. Carbidopa maximizes the nigrostriatal L-dopa concentration.
   c. Carbidopa is a MAOI.
   d. Carbidopa is a dopa agonist.

Answer: b. Carbidopa is a decarboxylase inhibitor that is administered in fixed combinations with L-dopa (Sinemet). Because carbidopa does not cross the blood–brain barrier, it slows only systemic L-dopa metabolism and maximizes nigrostriatal L-dopa concentration. Because small doses of L-dopa are effective when administered with carbidopa, patients have fewer L-dopa side effects.

204. In evaluating a 68-year-old woman who has begun to have problems walking and performing her activities of daily living, the neurologist asks the patient to remain in place while being pulled backward by the shoulders. On one test, the patient involuntarily takes at least six steps backward. On another test, she seems to fall backward "en bloc" (see the figure below). What is the significance of the patient's reaction?

a. She has paresis of all her limbs, as though she had bilateral cerebral infarctions.

b. She has lost cerebellar function.

c. She has impaired postural reflexes.

d. Although the CNS may be normal, the labyrinthine system has been damaged.

Answer: c. She first had retropulsion and then a positive pull test, which are both manifestations of basal ganglia dysfunction impairing postural reflexes. The pull test (pictured below) is positive in both Parkinson's disease and use of dopamine-blocking neuroleptics.

205. Match the treatment of Parkinson's disease (a–d) with its mechanism of action (1–4).

a. Ropinirole

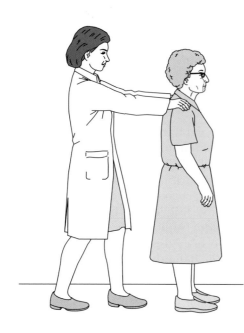
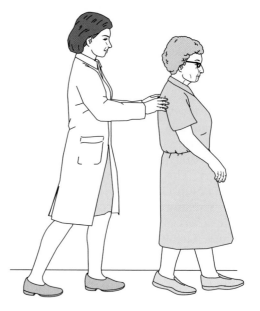
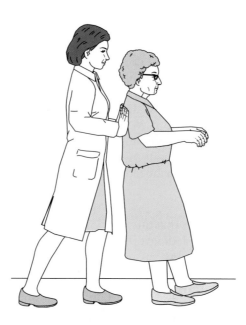

b. L-dopa
c. Selegiline
d. Pramipexole
   1. A dopamine precursor
   2. A dopamine agonist
   3. A MAO-A inhibitor
   4. A MAO-B inhibitor

Answers: a-2, b-1, c-4, d-2.

206. With which condition(s) is violent (directed, aggressive) behavior associated?
a. Epilepsy, all forms
b. Partial complex seizures
c. Episodic dyscontrol syndrome
d. Mental retardation
e. Males with the genotype XYY

Answer: c. Violent ictal behavior may occur, but it is not directed or thoughtful.

207. A 68-year-old man who previously had been in good health experienced a 20-minute episode of aphasia and right hemiparesis 2 days before an evaluation. He has a bruit over the right carotid artery, but otherwise he has normal general and neurologic examinations. An EEG, MRI of the head, and routine blood tests are normal. An angiogram discloses 50% stenosis of the left common carotid artery at its bifurcation. Which is the best course of treatment?
a. Investigate the right carotid artery.
b. Suggest a daily aspirin.
c. Refer him for left carotid surgery.
d. Continue to follow him but add no treatment.

Answer: b. Studies indicate that in patients who have had a TIA (symptomatic patients), carotid endarterectomy was preferable to aspirin in reducing strokes when carotid stenosis was at least 70% and the surgical center had a low complication rate. Because carotid bruits often are detectable over a nonstenotic carotid artery, bruits do not necessarily indicate carotid stenosis. Carotid bruits may be due to blood turbulence from minor atherosclerotic changes or greater blood flow through a normal artery because its counterpart is stenotic. They can also result from stenosis of the external carotid artery.

208. Of the following, which pathologic feature is most closely associated with Alzheimer's disease?
a. Cerebral atrophy
b. Senile plaques
c. Neurofibrillary tangles
d. Pick bodies

Answer: c. Although the initial studies indicated that plaques were the abnormality most closely associated with dementia, recent work indicates that the tangles are even more closely associated. Because tau is the major constituent of neurofibrillary tangles, neurologists often refer to Alzheimer's disease as a tauopathy. Cerebral atrophy is an age-related change.

209. Which is the most commonly occurring brainstem infarction?
a. Midbrain infarction
b. Pontine infarction
c. Lateral medullary syndrome
d. Medial medullary syndrome

Answer: c.

210. Which of the following conditions is indicated by a positive response to the Tensilon (edrophonium) test?
a. Muscular dystrophy
b. Myasthenia gravis
c. Myotonic dystrophy
d. None of the above

Answer: b. Tensilon (edrophonium) is a cholinesterase inhibitor that prolongs the effectiveness of ACh at the neuromuscular junction. This test temporarily reverses ocular and facial weakness in an individual with myasthenia gravis.

211. Which two of the following neurotransmitters project from the brainstem to the spinal cord?
a. Norepinephrine
b. Dopamine
c. Serotonin

Answers: a, c. Projections of norepinephrine and serotonin extend the length of the spinal cord. Dopamine tracts may be extensive, but they are confined to the brain.

212. Which of the following neurotransmitters is not a catecholamine?
a. Norepinephrine
b. Dopamine
c. Serotonin
d. Epinephrine

Answer: c. Serotonin is an indole, which is a five-member ring containing nitrogen joined to a benzene (six-member) ring. Catecholamines have a benzene ring with two hydroxyl groups and one amine group.

213. Which of the neurotransmitters in the preceding question is not derived from tyrosine?

Answer: c. Tryptophan is the precursor for serotonin. Tyrosine is the precursor for the others.

214. Which EEG pattern does benzodiazepines induce?
   a. α
   b. β
   c. θ
   d. Δ

Answer: b. Benzodiazepines induce β activity. Its presence may indicate surreptitious benzodiazepine use.

215. Where does the corticospinal tract cross as it descends?
   a. Internal capsule
   b. Base of the pons
   c. Pyramids
   d. Anterior horn cells

Answer: c. The crossing of the corticospinal tract in the pyramids gives rise to their alternative name, pyramidal tract.

216. Which artery supplies Broca's area and the adjacent corticospinal tract?
   a. Anterior cerebral
   b. Middle cerebral
   c. Posterior cerebral
   d. Basilar

Answer: b. The left middle cerebral artery supplies these areas and the underlying internal capsule.

217. Which group of illnesses is suggested by the presence of spasticity, hyperactive DTRs, and Babinski signs?
   a. Poliomyelitis, strokes, spinal cord trauma
   b. Bell's palsy, strokes, psychogenic disturbances
   c. Spinal cord trauma, strokes, congenital cerebral injuries
   d. Brainstem infarction, cerebellar infarction, neuropathy
   e. Parkinson's disease, generalized dystonia, cerebellar infarction

Answer: c. These signs reflect corticospinal (pyramidal) tract injury, which would be found in central nervous system diseases. They would not be found in diseases of the (1) peripheral nerves (neuropathy), (2) cranial nerves outside the brainstem (including Bell's palsy), (3) cerebellum, or (4) extrapyramidal system (including Parkinson's disease and dystonia).

218. Patients with which group of illnesses usually have muscles that are paretic, atrophic, and areflexic?
   a. Poliomyelitis, diabetic peripheral neuropathy, traumatic brachial plexus injury
   b. ALS, brainstem infarction, psychogenic disturbance
   c. Spinal cord trauma, strokes, congenital cerebral injuries
   d. Brainstem infarction, cerebellar infarction, spinal cord infarction
   e. Parkinson's disease, strokes, cerebellar infarction
   f. Guillain Barré syndrome, MS, and uremic neuropathy

Answer: a. These signs reflect lower motor neuron injury, including diseases of the anterior horn cell (e.g., poliomyelitis), peripheral nerves, and their plexuses.

219. A 73-year-old woman has had the sudden onset of the following signs: right-sided limb ataxia, dysarthria, lack of facial sensation on the right face and left side of the body, and a right-sided Horner's syndrome. To which side will the palate deviate when she attempts to say "ah"?
   a. Right
   b. Left
   c. Both
   d. Neither

Answer: b. She has a right-sided lateral medullary syndrome. The lesion encompasses the right nucleus ambiguus, which leads to paresis of the right palate. When muscles of the palate contract, right-sided palate paresis allows it to deviate to the left.

220. Which is the most characteristic change in Huntington's disease?
   a. D_2 dopamine receptors are hypoactive.
   b. D_2 dopamine receptors are hyperactive.
   c. ACh receptors are reduced in the nucleus basalis of Meynert.
   d. Gamma-aminobutyric acid (GABA) concentrations are reduced to less than 50% of normal in the corpus striatum.

Answer: d. GABA concentrations are reduced to less than 50% of normal in the caudate nuclei, which is one of the major components of the corpus striatum. In Alzheimer's disease, ACh receptors are reduced in the nucleus basalis of Meynert.

221. Of the following, which two tests provide the most reliable confirmation of the clinical diagnosis of MS when it is in a quiescent state?

a. MRI of the head
b. VERs
c. CSF studies for oligoclonal bands
d. CSF studies for myelin basic protein
e. CT of the head

Answers: a, c. The multiplicity of tests indicates that no single test is definitive. Moreover, most may be abnormal in non-MS demyelinating conditions, chronic CNS infections, and inflammatory diseases. MRI portrays plaques as hyperintense white patches that gadolinium infusion may enhance. It allows distinction between acute and chronic plaques, determination of total lesion load, and estimation of disease activity. Oligoclonal bands in the CSF are only suggestive of the illness. Although large doses of contrast and delayed studies increase the sensitivity of CT, it is too insensitive for diagnostic purposes. The CSF myelin basic protein concentration may be elevated in an acute attack of MS, but other inflammatory conditions and infectious illnesses may also increase its concentration. When MS is quiescent, the concentration of CSF myelin basic protein is usually normal.

222. Which of the following descriptions best characterize the MRI changes of MS?
    a. Multiple, white areas scattered in the cerebrum
    b. Conversion of the cerebral hemisphere white matter to gray
    c. Loss of the myelin signal throughout the corpus callosum
    d. Periventricular, high-intensity abnormalities

Answer: d. The MRI typically shows large, white, hyperintense lesions in the periventricular region. It may also reveal lesions in the optic nerve or spinal cord. However, numerous bright, small, or punctate intracerebral lesions, called "unidentified bright objects" or "UBOs," may result from cerebrovascular disease, migraine, and other non-MS diseases.

223. When is MS most likely to be exacerbated?
    a. During pregnancy
    b. During times of stress
    c. In adolescence
    d. After trauma
    e. During the first 3 postpartum months

Answer: e. Although pregnancy is associated with reduction in attacks, women frequently experience MS exacerbations during the first 3 postpartum months. The other factors are unproven precipitants of MS exacerbations.

224. When contemplating having a second child, a young mother who had developed MS during the postpartum period of her first delivery inquires about the effect of a second or third pregnancy on her MS. Which two statements reflect current thinking?
    a. Deliveries are almost always more complicated when the mother has MS.
    b. MS worsens in a stepwise pattern with each succeeding pregnancy.
    c. The number of pregnancies has little or no effect on the ultimate outcome of MS.
    d. Her offspring, compared to the general population, will have an increased risk of developing MS.
    e. Fetal malformations are more common with parents with MS than in the general population.

Answers: c, d.

225. Which MS features are associated with cognitive impairment?
    a. Paraparesis and blindness
    b. Chronicity of the illness
    c. Enlarged cerebral ventricles
    d. Corpus callosum atrophy
    e. Area and volume of cerebral plaques visualized by MRI
    f. Decreased glucose metabolism on positron emission tomography
    g. All of the above

Answer: g.

226. After being comatose for 2 weeks after an attempted strangulation, a 35-year-old woman babbles incoherently. She seems to repeat conversations that take place around her. She sits and eats if given assistance. Although she does not seem to see the television, she repeats the dialogue. She does not respond to visual stimulation. Her pupils are equal and reactive to light. Which is the best description of her condition?
    a. Coma
    b. Psychosis
    c. Vegetative state
    d. Locked-in syndrome
    e. Isolation aphasia, dementia, and cortical blindness from watershed infarctions
    f. None of the above

Answer: e. She has isolation aphasia because of her ability only to repeat. She also has cortical blindness because she cannot see, but her pupil function is spared. She is not comatose because she has interaction with her environment and possesses verbal and motor activity. In the vegetative state and the locked-in syndrome, patients cannot vocalize, eat, or sit.

227. Which of the following are characteristics of the N-methyl-D-aspartate receptor?
   a. It is usually called the NMDA receptor.
   b. It regulates calcium channels.
   c. Excitatory neurotransmitters, such as glutamate, bind onto this receptor.
   d. Overstimulation of the receptor leads to cell death by calcium flooding.
   e. The NMDA receptor may be excitotoxic in strokes, epilepsy, and Huntington's disease.
   f. All of the above.

Answer: f.

228. Which one of the following is not a characteristic of carpal tunnel syndrome?
   a. It results from compression of the median nerve at the wrist.
   b. Tinel's sign indicates carpal tunnel syndrome.
   c. Repetitive stress injury causes the carpal tunnel syndrome.
   d. It results in pain and weakness of the forearm extensor and supinator muscles.
   e. It is typically worse at night.

Answer: d. Carpal tunnel syndrome results from compression of the median nerve at the wrist. Trauma, fluid retention, pregnancy, and repetitive movements are risk factors or direct causes. Tinel's sign is indicative of the disorder. In contrast, "tennis elbow," which consists of pain and weakness of the forearm extensor and supinator muscles, results from bursitis, muscle swelling, or entrapment of branches of the radial nerve. Paradoxically, the most common cause of tennis elbow is not tennis but occupational injury.

229. What is the pattern of innervation of the anal and urinary bladder sphincters?
   a. An internal sphincter is innervated by the peripheral nervous system, and an external sphincter is innervated by the autonomic nervous system.
   b. An internal sphincter is innervated by the autonomic nervous system, and an external sphincter is innervated by the peripheral nervous system.
   c. An internal sphincter is innervated by the central nervous system, and an external sphincter is innervated by the autonomic nervous system.
   d. An internal sphincter is innervated by the peripheral nervous system, and an external sphincter is innervated by the central nervous system.

Answer: b. In both sites, the autonomic nervous system innervates the internal sphincter, and the peripheral nervous system innervates the external sphincter. Thus, the internal sphincter is under involuntary control, but the external sphincter is under voluntary control. The internal sphincter is stronger than the external sphincter.

230. A 49-year-old man under treatment for alcohol withdrawal seizures becomes progressively more stuporous. Which three conditions might explain the deterioration?
   a. Hypoglycemia
   b. AED intoxication
   c. Bleeding from the small intracranial veins
   d. Alcoholic stupor
   e. All of the above

Answers: a, b, c. Chronic alcoholism leads to cirrhosis that depletes stored glycogen. Unless glucose is supplied continuously, hypoglycemia may cause seizures. Inadvertent excessive treatment with AEDs is relatively common, especially if a cirrhotic liver cannot metabolize them. Bleeding from cerebral small veins, which characteristically leads to a subdural hematoma, is common in alcoholics because they tend to sustain head trauma and have impaired coagulation ability. Another possibility in alcoholic patients is that hepatic encephalopathy has developed.

231. Through which structure is CSF normally absorbed?
   a. Spinal cord
   b. Inner surface of the lateral ventricles
   c. Choroid plexus
   d. Arachnoid membrane
   e. Cerebral hemisphere tissue

Answer: d. CSF is normally formed in the choroid plexus and absorbed through the arachnoid layer of the meninges, predominantly at the base of the brain. When meningitis or subarachnoid hemorrhage inflames the arachnoid membrane, CSF absorption is impaired and communicating or normal pressure hydrocephalus may develop. In those conditions, CSF may pass through the inner surface of the ventricles.

232. A 75-year-old woman developed vertigo, nausea, and diplopia after she underwent vigorous hair washing at her local beauty parlor. She has ataxia and nystagmus. A CT shows no abnormalities. What is the most likely cause of her disturbance?
   a. Cerebral infarction
   b. Brainstem ischemia
   c. A chemical in the hair wash
   d. Labyrinthitis

Answer: b. Elderly individuals typically have osteophytes that press against their vertebral arteries as they pass upward through the cervical spine. If their neck is hyperextended, as may occur during hair washing, constriction of the vertebral arteries may interrupt blood flow and lead to brainstem ischemia.

233. A 35-year-old psychiatrist in her last trimester of pregnancy has painful tingling in most of her hands and all of her fingers. She also finds that small objects seem to drop from her fingers. The symptoms are worse in the late afternoon and early morning hours. She has no objective abnormalities. Percussion of the wrist re-creates the paresthesias. What is the cause of her problem?
   a. Entrapment of the median nerve in each wrist
   b. Peripheral neuropathy
   c. Cervical spondylosis
   d. Guillain-Barré syndrome
   e. Lyme disease

Answer: a. She has bilateral carpal tunnel syndrome, which is median nerve compression or entrapment at the wrist. The usual distribution of the median nerve is the palmar surface of the thumb, adjacent two fingers, and the lateral portion of the palm, but many people with carpal tunnel syndrome have sensory disturbances that do not strictly conform to the textbook's map. Paresthesias in the median nerve distribution produced by tapping the flexor surface of the wrist—Tinel's sign—are virtually pathognomonic.

Carpal tunnel syndrome usually results from fluid accumulation in the carpal tunnel, as occurs during pregnancy, before menses, and after trauma to the wrist, including "repetitive stress injuries," such as typing, wrist exercising, and sometimes excessive driving. Nerve conduction velocity studies that demonstrate slowing across the flexor surface of the wrist may confirm a clinical diagnosis.

This patient's carpal tunnel syndrome will probably resolve as fluid accumulation resolves after delivery. Most patients respond to wrist splints, diuretics, or change in activities. Individuals who do not respond to these conservative measures may benefit from steroid injections into the carpal tunnel or surgery.

234. Shortly after her hospitalization for dyspnea, a 19-year-old student at a small New England college developed ascending, flaccid, and areflexic weakness of her legs, trunk, and then arms. MRIs of her head and cervical spine were normal. Her CSF contained 10 lymphocytes/mm^3 and a glucose concentration of 55 mg/dL and protein concentration of 105 mg/dL. She developed ocular, facial, and pharyngeal weakness. She had periods of agitation, for which the intensive care unit physicians solicited a psychiatry consultation. Which of the following conditions is the most likely cause of her disorder?
   a. MS
   b. Conversion disorder
   c. Poliomyelitis
   d. Guillain-Barré syndrome
   e. Botulism

Answer: d. Her extensive, rapidly advancing peripheral neuropathy and the albumino-cytologic disassociation in the CSF indicate that she has the Guillain-Barré syndrome (also called "acute inflammatory demyelinating polyradiculoneuropathy [AIDP]"). In contrast, MS produces signs of corticospinal tract paresis, poliomyelitis is asymmetric and does not involve ocular motility, and botulism begins with bulbar palsy. Moreover, those illnesses do not cause albumino-cytologic disassociation in the CSF. On the other hand, many infectious illnesses—*Campylobacter jejuni* infection, mononucleosis, Lyme disease, AIDS, hepatitis, and porphyria—can cause the Guillain-Barré syndrome. Although several of these illnesses may affect the CNS as well as the PNS, physicians should first assume that hypoxia rather than direct cerebral involvement causes periods of agitation. After they secure proper ventilation, then the physicians can search for the underlying etiology.

235. Which three of the following statements about CNS and PNS myelin are true?
   a. The same cells produce CNS and PNS myelin.
   b. Oligodendrocytes produce CNS myelin and Schwann cells produce PNS myelin.
   c. Both CNS and PNS myelin insulate electrochemical transmissions.
   d. The same illnesses affect both CNS and PNS myelin.
   e. The optic nerves are covered by CNS myelin.

Answers: b, c, e.

236. If a neurologist examines an individual who sustained left lateral geniculate body damage, which will be the most prominent finding?
   a. Loss of the ipsilateral pupillary light reflex
   b. Loss of the contralateral pupillary light reflex
   c. Impaired ipsilateral hearing
   d. Impaired contralateral hearing
   e. None of the above

Answer: e. The lateral geniculate body damage is the origin of the geniculocalcarine tract. The patient will have a contralateral homonymous hemianopsia.

237. Which structure connects the hippocampus to the mamillary bodies?
   a. Cingulate gyrus

b. Mamillothalamic tract
c. Fornix
d. Amygdala

Answer: c.

238. Following vigorous treatment with dopamine-blocking antipsychotic agents for a recurrence of schizophrenia with psychotic behavior, a 29-year-old man lapses into stupor. His temperature rises to 104°F and his pulse increases to 130 bpm. Neurologists find axial and appendicular rigidity. Which one of the following strategies would be least helpful?
a. Treatment with dopamine agonists, such as bromocriptine
b. Administration of intravenous fluids
c. Excluding infectious causes of fever, particularly meningitis
d. Administration of muscle relaxants, such as dantrolene
e. Administration of dopamine precursors, such as L-dopa with carbidopa
f. Halting further administration of antipsychotic agents

Answer: e. Although other causes could be considered, the patient probably has developed the neuroleptic malignant syndrome. Treatments aim at immediate correction of the dopamine depletion, dehydration, fever, and muscle rigidity. Some physicians have advocated electroconvulsive therapy (ECT).

239. Which two of the following statements are true regarding ACh?
a. It is a neurotransmitter at the neuromuscular junction.
b. It is a neurotransmitter in the CNS.
c. Like GABA, ACh is an inhibitory neurotransmitter.
d. ACh is deactivated as much by reuptake as metabolism.

Answers: a, b.

240. Which condition is characterized by absence of dystrophin on a muscle biopsy?
a. Myotonic dystrophy
b. Becker's dystrophy
c. Duchenne's dystrophy
d. Diabetic neuropathy

Answer: c. Absence of dystrophin, the normal muscle cell membrane protein, is virtually diagnostic of Duchenne's dystrophy. In Becker's dystrophy, a variant of Duchenne's dystrophy, dystrophin is reduced or abnormal. Genetic testing has supplanted muscle biopsies for these and many other conditions.

241. Against which site are antibodies directed in myasthenia gravis?
a. ACh nicotinic postsynaptic receptors
b. ACh muscarinic postsynaptic receptors
c. ACh quanta
d. AChE

Answer: a.

242. If an EEG shows "K complexes," in which state of consciousness is the patient?
a. Coma
b. Deep sleep
c. Light sleep
d. Dreaming
e. Alert
f. In a metabolic encephalopathy
g. Beset by a generalized seizure
h. Beset by a partial complex seizure
i. Pretending to be unresponsive
j. Sedated by medications or drugs

Answer: c. K complexes are indicative of stage 2 NREM sleep, which is relatively light sleep.

243. Which two conditions produce areflexic quadriparesis?
a. Hypokalemia
b. REM activity
c. Hyponatremia
d. Cocaine

Answers: a, b. Hypokalemic periodic paralysis, cataplexy, and REM periods during normal sleep cause episodic areflexic quadriparesis. Hyponatremia, when severe, causes stupor and seizures but not areflexic quadriparesis.

244. Regarding mitochondrial DNA (mtDNA), which statement is true?
a. Ragged red fibers in muscles are virtually pathognomonic of an mtDNA abnormality.
b. An individual's mtDNA is inherited exclusively from the mother.
c. mtDNA is not inherited in the chromosomes.
d. mtDNA abnormalities are not inherited in a classic Mendelian pattern.
e. mtDNA abnormalities often produce combinations of myopathies, lactic acidosis, and progressively severe encephalopathies.
f. All of the above.

Answer: f.

245. Several hours after a romantic fish dinner in a Caribbean resort, a couple developed abdominal cramps, diarrhea, nausea, vomiting, and fever.

They also reported to the local physician that they were beset with painful sensations in their fingers and toes. On direct questioning, they recalled that immediately before the onset of the nausea and vomiting, cold objects, such as the ice water glasses, felt warm to the touch and they had tingling of their lips. Which is the most likely cause of their illness?
a. Guillain-Barré illness
b. *Salmonella* poisoning
c. Chemical poisoning
d. Malaria

Answer: c. The couple has consumed a large reef fish, such as grouper or red snapper that had eaten smaller fish contaminated with a food poison, ciguatoxin. Such fish poisoning, common in the Caribbean, increases nerve and muscle cell permeability to sodium by relaxing voltage-gated sodium channels in nerves and muscles. Its primary symptoms, besides headache, nausea, and vomiting, are an acute painful neuropathy and a "heat-cold" reversal. Patients often also describe depression for several weeks following ciguatoxin poisoning.

246. Which description of myotonic dystrophy is false?
a. Females as well as males are susceptible to the illness.
b. It is a dystrophinopathy.
c. In successive generations, the disease appears at a younger age because of anticipation.
d. In successive generations, the disease is more severe because of anticipation
e. Like other dominantly inherited nervous system disorders—Huntington's disease, early onset primary (torsion) dystonia, tuberous sclerosis, and neurofibromatosis—myotonic dystrophy is not associated with storage of a particular metabolic product.

Answer: b. Because myotonic dystrophy, which is transmitted as an autosomal dominant disorder, results from an excessive trinucleotide repeat defect, it causes symptoms at an earlier age and with greater severity (anticipation) in successive generations. Its defect consists of abnormal ion permeability and is therefore labeled a channelopathy. In contrast, Duchenne's and Becker's dystrophies are characterized by defects in the muscle membrane protein dystrophin, they are labeled dystrophinopathies.

247–251. What is the mechanism of action of the following poisons?
247. Poison gases
248. Tetanus
249. Botulism

250. Cyanide
251. Carbon monoxide
a. Blocks the release of glycine and GABA, inhibitory neurotransmitters
b. Poisons the respiratory energy pathway
c. Interferes with the oxygen-carrying capacity of hemoglobin
d. Inactivates AChE, which causes excessive ACh activity
e. Blocks the release of ACh from the presynaptic membrane of the neuromuscular junction
f. Blocks the release of ACh from the presynaptic membranes in the brainstem

Answers: 247-d, 248-a, 249-e, 250-b, 251-c.

252–257. Match the lifestyle (252–257) with its consequences (a–e). If appropriate, use more than one letter for each number.
252. Steroid injections for bodybuilding
253. Deer hunting in Connecticut
254. Using tryptophan-containing products as a hypnotic
255. Alcoholism
256. Eating undercooked game.
257. Excessive pyridoxine (vitamin B_6) consumption
a. Myositis
b. Eosinophilia-myalgia syndrome
c. Upper and lower facial nerve paresis
d. Hypertrophied muscles, excessive facial hair, amenorrhea
e. Peripheral neuropathy

Answers: 252-d.
253-a, c, e. Tics in Connecticut are vectors for Lyme disease, which may cause facial paresis or a peripheral neuropathy.
254-b. Substances that cause eosinophilia and myalgia contaminated tryptophan preparations.
255-e. Alcoholism, probably through the associated nutritional deficiency, causes peripheral neuropathy.
256-a. *Trichinella.* Undercooked venison may contain *Trichinella*, which causes trichinosis.
257-e. Taking excessive pyridoxine (vitamin B_6) causes a peripheral neuropathy.

258. The parents of a 24-year-old man, who has a history of substance abuse, found him standing in the local high-school football field dressed only in short pants, at midnight in the middle of the winter. Although standing upright in the emergency room with his eyes open, he was mute and unresponsive to physicians' questions and requests. He drooled and only stared at his parents and physicians. His blood pressure was elevated and his pulse rapid. On examination, he had intermittent three-direction nystagmus. His muscle tone was so great that it made him rigid. Which one of the following substances is most likely to have caused his condition?

a. Alcohol
b. Cocaine
c. Methamphetamine
d. Phencyclidine (PCP)

Answer: d. His abnormal behavior and mental status, chiefly the "wide awake coma," in combination with the nystagmus and muscle rigidity, is characteristic of PCP intoxication. Wernicke-Korsakoff syndrome causes nystagmus but not muscle rigidity or mutism.

259. A 25-year-old right-handed patient underwent a commissurotomy for intractable seizures. It was successful, but he describes not being able to express himself fully. Which is the most likely explanation?

a. Aphasia is a complication of the procedure.
b. Commissurotomy patients lose cognitive function.
c. Emotions generated in the left hemisphere are not as readily verbalized as those generated in the right hemisphere.
d. Emotions generated in the right hemisphere are not as readily verbalized as those generated in the left hemisphere.

Answer: d. Information generated in the right hemisphere can no longer cross the corpus callosum for verbal expression utilizing the language circuit.

260. Of the following illnesses, which four are most likely affecting this kindred?

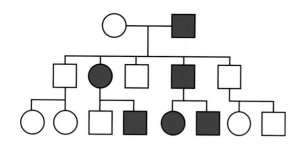

a. Duchenne's muscular dystrophy
b. Myotonic dystrophy
c. Hemophilia
d. Sickle cell disease
e. Wilson's disease
f. Huntington's disease
g. Alzheimer's disease
h. Early onset primary (torsion) DYT1 dystonia
i. PKU

Answers: b, f, g, h. As in the standard portrayal of genetic information, circles represent females and squares represent males. Shaded forms indicate affected individuals. In this and subsequent questions, paternity is assured, parents are unrelated by blood, and parents who are not pictured are free of the illness. This kindred illustrates an autosomal dominant disease that has affected both males and females. Myotonic dystrophy, Huntington's disease, and early onset primary (torsion) dystonia are all autosomal illnesses but with different penetrance rates. Alzheimer's disease is usually a sporadic illness, but occasional families, such as those carrying the presenilin gene, are affected by an autosomal dominant inheritance. A recessive disorder, such as sickle cell disease or PKU, is unlikely because the female in generation 1 and two spouses in generation 2 (not represented) would each have to be a carrier.

261. The individual in this kindred developed a genetic illness that was fatal in childhood. Which three of the illnesses listed in Question 260 might likely have been responsible?

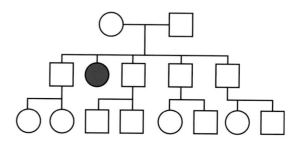

Answers: d, e, i. Her illness was autosomal recessive because neither parent had been affected. Because the patient was a girl, she could not likely have had Duchenne's muscular dystrophy or hemophilia, which are both x-linked recessive illnesses.

262. In this kindred, what is the chance that, if the woman in generation 2 were to have another son, he would have the illness that has affected his two older brothers?

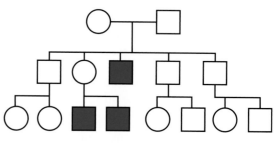

a. 100%
b. 75%
c. 50%

d. 25%

e. 0%

Answer: c. The illness is an x-linked disorder because the only family members with the illness are male. The woman with two affected sons has one normal and one abnormal gene. Only 50% of her future sons will inherit an abnormal gene.

263. Of the illnesses listed in Question 260, which one is most likely to have affected the three individuals in Question 262?

Answer: a. Duchenne's muscular dystrophy

264. In this kindred, five individuals are affected by a genetic illness that became fatal at the ages designated by the numerals. Of these illnesses, which one is most likely to be responsible?

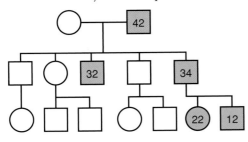

a. Duchenne's muscular dystrophy
b. Myotonic dystrophy
c. Hemophilia
d. Sickle cell disease
e. Wilson's disease
f. Huntington's disease
g. Alzheimer's disease
h. Early onset primary (torsion) dystonia

Answer: f. The illness is an autosomal dominant disorder that becomes apparent and fatal at a relatively young age. Although myotonic dystrophy and early onset primary (torsion) DYT1 dystonia become apparent in children and young adults, neither is usually fatal at that time. Familial Alzheimer's disease becomes apparent before sporadically developing cases, but usually not until at least late middle age.

265. In Question 264, the disease becomes apparent at a younger age in successive generations. In which illnesses listed in Question 260 is that pattern characteristic?

Answers: b, f. Anticipation, the tendency of individuals in successive generations to show signs of a genetic illness at a younger age, which is attributable to the instability of abnormal DNA, is a characteristic of myotonic dystrophy, Huntington's disease, and other illnesses associated with trinucleotide repeats.

266. A family with four generations is plagued by an illness that affects multiple members of both sexes in each generation. The illness involves weakness but has variable other features. Symptoms appear between infancy and age 40 years with variable degrees of severity. Which inheritance pattern does the viable phenotype and this family tree (see below) indicate?
a. Autosomal dominant
b. Sex-linked dominant
c. Autosomal recessive
d. Sex-linked recessive
e. None of the above

Answer: e. The family tree shows that, although both sexes develop the illness, only the mothers transmit it. That pattern indicates that mtDNA transmits the illness. Mitochondrial transmission is also fully consistent with the variable phenotype because it involves the threshold effect and organs being affected differently, but usually in proportion to their energy requirements.

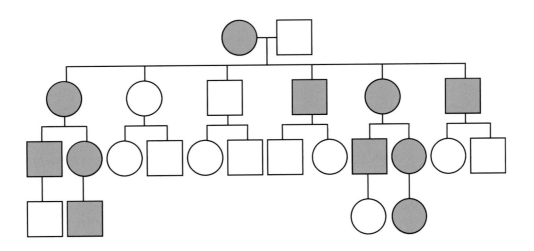

267. Which of the following is a disconnection syndrome?
   a. Nonfluent aphasia
   b. Conduction aphasia
   c. Fluent aphasia
   d. Isolation aphasia
   e. Dementia
   f. Global aphasia

Answer: b. Disconnection syndromes generally refer to neuropsychologic disorders in which connections between the primary neuropsychologic centers are severed, but the centers themselves are intact and capable of functioning. Conduction aphasia consists of the separation of Wernicke's and Broca's areas. Other disconnection syndromes are the split-brain syndrome and alexia without agraphia.

268. Which two forms of communication are based, like speech and hearing, in the dominant hemisphere's perisylvian language arc?
   a. Reading and writing
   b. Melody for most people
   c. American Sign Language
   d. Cursing
   e. Prosody
   f. Body language

Answers: a, c.

269. What is the common neurologic term for the zone of cerebral cortex between branches of the major cerebral arteries?
   a. Watershed area (border zone)
   b. Limbic system
   c. Cornea
   d. Arcuate fasciculus

Answer: a.

270. Which condition is caused by hypoperfusion of the watershed area?
   a. Alexia without agraphia
   b. Fluent aphasia
   c. Hemiparesis
   d. Isolation aphasia

Answer: d. The perisylvian language arc is well-perfused by relatively large branches of the middle cerebral artery. The more distal cortical regions, the watershed areas, have a tenuous blood supply from distal branches of the anterior, middle, and posterior cerebral arteries. With hypotension, the watershed areas often receive insufficient blood supply and develop ischemia; however, the language arc generally continues to receive an adequate supply. When the perisylvian language arc survives but the outlying cortex is damaged, language function is isolated. It will be devoid of cognitive input, and the patient will be able only to perform repetition.

271. Which cerebral artery perfuses the cerebral motor cortex for the contralateral leg?
   a. Anterior cerebral artery
   b. Middle cerebral artery
   c. Posterior cerebral artery

Answer: a.

272. A retired concert violinist sustained a stroke that produced left-sided sensory loss but little or no paresis. During an unremarkable recovery, his left hand began to make involuntary, small exploratory movements. The patient, initially unaware of the hand movements, alternately described the hand in derogatory terms, ignoring it, and claiming that it was his roommate's hand. Which condition best describes the situation?
   a. Hemiballismus
   b. Alien hand syndrome
   c. Dementia
   d. Aphasia
   e. Anosognosia
   f. Occupational dystonia

Answer: b. The alien hand syndrome, which may be a component of the nondominant parietal lobe syndrome, is the perceptual disorder that the hand is independent of the patient or acts under another person's control. Anosognosia and other symptoms of nondominant parietal lobe damage may accompany the alien hand syndrome. Patients often employ various defense mechanisms in response to their problem, but sometimes they become irrational and agitated.

273. Which of the following apraxias is most closely associated with dementia and incontinence?
   a. Ideational
   b. Dressing
   c. Ideomotor
   d. Buccofacial
   e. Oral
   f. Gait

Answer: f. In normal pressure hydrocephalus (NPH), patients have gait apraxia, urinary incontinence, and dementia. The apraxia is the most characteristic feature. It is also the feature most readily responsive to treatment by insertion of a ventriculo-peritoneal shunt.

274. A 40-year-old woman had migraine headaches as a teenager, but they were replaced by tension headaches once she married and had two children. During the past 5 years, the headaches evolved into a pattern of dull, symmetric, non-throbbing pain present throughout every day. She has come to rely on prescription medications but not opioids. However, when she has a flare-up of her headaches, which is about once a month, she visits an emergency room, where physicians give her opioid injections. Further evaluation reveals no underlying neurologic or serious psychiatric disorder. How should this problem be classified?

a. Chronic daily headaches
b. Tension headaches
c. Status migrainous
d. Obsessive-compulsive disorder

Answer: a. This woman has a distinct entity, chronic daily headache (CDH), which typically evolves from migraine and superimposed tension headaches. Medication abuse or at least daily use of analgesic or vasoconstrictor medications predispose patients to CDH. Occasionally patients are addicted to opioids, sedatives, or anxiolytics before or during CDH. In some patients, depression leads to CDH, but in many others, depression results from it. Patients with CDH also take medication to avoid "rebound" headaches and withdrawal symptoms. CDH is a major diagnostic problem because patients request medication for their headaches, but the symptom is medication-induced.

275. Patients often perceive migraine pain in or behind their eye (i.e., in the periorbital or retro-orbital location) even though the abnormality is in the meninges or extracranial vessels. What accounts for this discrepancy?

a. Intraocular pressure rises during migraines.
b. Changes that occur in the ocular circulation produce pain.
c. The trigeminal nerve innervates the meninges and the pain is referred.
d. Nerve receptors for pain in the brain misperceive the location of pain.
e. None of the above.

Answer: c. The trigeminal nerve innervates the meninges, as well as the eye and its orbit. The brain itself has no pain receptors. Thus, neurosurgeons can operate on the brain without using anesthesia, and the patient can remain awake during certain neurosurgical procedures. In migraines and cluster headaches, pain is referred to the eye, which is supplied by the first division of the trigeminal nerve.

276. A despondent farmworker impulsively ingests a nearby, common organophosphorous insecticide poison. He becomes confused, dysarthric, and ataxic. He has bradycardia, miosis, excessive salivation, sweating, and muscle weakness with fasciculations. Which of the following is the best antidote?

a. Atropine
b. Neostigmine
c. Physostigmine
d. None of the above

Answer: a. The farmworker poisoned himself with an AChE inhibitor, which is the active ingredient of common organophosphorous insecticide poisons. He thus developed acetylcholine (cholinergic) toxicity, which is characterized by miosis, bradycardia, and fasciculations. The antidote to the CNS effects is typically atropine, an anticholinergic medication that crosses the blood–brain barrier. Often physicians must also administer other medications, such as pralidoxime, to reverse the cholinergic toxicity at the neuromuscular junction.

277. After a self-prepared meal, a novice plant lover develops excitation, restlessness, euphoria, dilated pupils, an uncomfortable dry mouth, and an intense thirst. Which of the following would be the best antidote?

a. Atropine
b. Neostigmine
c. Physostigmine
d. None of the above

Answer: c. This question is the counterpart of the preceding question. This patient has atropine poisoning, which is characterized by excitement, dry mouth, and dilated pupils. The excessive anticholinergic activity must be counteracted by an AChE inhibitor that crosses the blood–brain barrier. A general rule is that atropine and physostigmine counteract each other.

278. Which two of the following statements are true regarding saccades?

a. Their speed is about 30/s.
b. Their speed is rapid and can reach 700/s.
c. They are governed by supranuclear centers.
d. Abnormalities in saccades characterize the onset of Alzheimer's disease.

Answers: b, c. Cerebral conjugate gaze centers generate saccades, which are high-velocity conjugate gaze movements. Abnormal saccades are one of the first physical findings in Huntington's disease and are also found in schizophrenia.

279. Which one of the following statements is false regarding pursuit eye movements?

a. They are the smooth, steady tracking movements used to follow moving objects.

b. They are abnormal in Huntington's disease.

c. They are governed by supranuclear centers.

d. They are abnormal in many patients with schizophrenia.

Answer: c. Pontine conjugate gaze centers generate pursuits, which are relatively slow, smooth conjugate gaze movements. They are abnormal, slow, and irregular in schizophrenia and, to a lesser extent, in affective disorders, as well as in basal ganglia disorders.

280. In which four conditions might combinations of unilateral miosis, ptosis, and anhidrosis be found?

a. Pancoast tumors

b. Cluster headache

c. Migraine with aura

d. Lateral medullary syndrome

e. Midbrain infarction

f. Chiropractic neck manipulation

Answers: a, b, d, f. Ptosis, miosis (small pupil), and anhidrosis (lack of sweating) constitute Horner's syndrome. Its most common cause is injury of the sympathetic supply of the face and eye. The combination of miosis and ptosis, usually without the anhidrosis, is a classic sign of cluster headaches. Vigorous chiropractic neck manipulation may lead to dissection of the vertebral artery, which causes posterior inferior cerebellar artery (PICA) occlusion and the lateral medullary (Wallenberg) syndrome. Those conditions also cause most or all of the signs of Horner's syndrome. Pancoast tumors produce all the elements of Horner's syndrome because these tumors invade sympathetic ganglia in the chest.

281. To which four vision-impairing conditions are the elderly particularly susceptible?

a. Cataracts

b. Glaucoma

c. Strabismus

d. Amblyopia ex anopia

e. Macular degeneration

f. Temporal arteritis

g. Psychogenic visual loss

Answers: a, b, e, f. Strabismus is congenital extraocular muscle weakness. If uncorrected, the affected eye will become blind from disuse (i.e., amblyopia ex anopia).

282. A neurologic examination of a 75-year-old man shows no abnormality of cognitive or physical function except for impairment of vibration sensation in both great toes. Pain and temperature sensations are preserved. Ankle DTRs are absent. Plantar reflexes are flexor. Which is the most likely explanation for the findings?

a. Combined system disease

b. Alzheimer's disease

c. MS

d. Diabetes

e. None of the above

Answer: e. He merely has age-related peripheral nervous system changes, which include loss of DTRs and sense of vibration. Combined system disease and MS cause spasticity and Babinski signs (extensor plantar reflexes). Diabetic neuropathy, which develops several years after the onset of the illness, is associated with loss of pain and temperature.

283. A 14-year-old boy with pronounced mental retardation has repetitive, stereotyped movements. He has a large forehead, large lobulated ears, and large testicles (macro-orchidism). His sister is reportedly physically normal but slow in school. His mother, who is 43 years old, is planning on remarrying and conceiving. Which two of the following statements is true?

a. The boy probably has the fragile X chromosome.

b. Because her son's condition is rare, the mother's next pregnancy has no greater risk than that of other women of her age.

c. The sister probably is, as the mother says, merely a mediocre student and does not need to be evaluated further.

d. Because she is 43 years old, close evaluation is indicated in future pregnancies.

Answer: a, d. The boy has the fragile X syndrome, which is the most frequent causes of inherited mental retardation and accounts for about 10% of all cases of mental retardation. A faulty X chromosome gene, which consists of excessive trinucleotide repeats, transmits fragile X syndrome. This mother must be concerned because she not only carries the fragile X gene but because she is 43 years old and might conceive a child with trisomy 21 (Down syndrome).

In addition, because in girls fragile X occasionally appears in a modified form—only mild mental retardation—his younger sister should undergo evaluation. She could have a modified form of the fragile X syndrome or carry the disorder.

284. A 17-year-old boy has a dozen light brown, flat "birthmarks," which are each larger than 3 cm by 1 cm, and axillary "freckles." He inquires about some nodules that have been developing on his arms and face. Which two statements concerning these new lesions are true?

a. They represent von Recklinghausen's disease or neurofibromatosis.

b. They are closely associated with bilateral acoustic neuromas.

c. His siblings and parents ought to be examined because one of them is likely to have the same condition.

d. They are adenoma sebaceum (angiofibromas), which is the cutaneous manifestation of tuberous sclerosis.

Answers: a, c. He has von Recklinghausen's disease or neurofibromatosis type 1 (NF1), which is a common inherited neurocutaneous disturbance characterized by a triad of six or more café au lait spots and nodules (neurofibromas) on peripheral nerves that become apparent in adults. NF1 patients tend to develop meningiomas. About 50% of patients acquire the disorder through inheritance. The other 50% apparently acquire it by mutation.

In contrast, the related disorder, previously also called von Recklinghausen's disease and now called neurofibromatosis type 2 (NF2), causes bilateral acoustic neuromas and sometimes several café au lait spots. NF1 and NF2 are transmitted on different autosomal chromosomes: NF1 is transmitted on chromosome 17 and NF2 on 22.

Tuberous sclerosis, a completely different inherited neurocutaneous disorder, consists of a combination of nodules on the malar surface of the face and tubers in the brain. It causes seizures and mental deterioration. Depending on the gene, tuberous sclerosis is transmitted on chromosome 9 or 11. Tuberous sclerosis and NF1 provide the clinician with an excellent opportunity to make a diagnosis by inspection.

285. A 68-year-old man was brought to the emergency room after he called his wife to say that he had become lost while visiting his customers in neighboring towns. Because he was agitated, a psychiatrist was asked to consult. She calmed him and then determined that his primary problem was memory impairment for recent events, such as where he had traveled and whom he had visited. He retained basic, personal knowledge, such as his name, telephone number, and even his Social Security number. He could not recall more than 3 of 6 digits. She also established that he recognized his impairment and that he had no physical neurologic deficits. A head CT and routine blood tests were normal. By the end of several hours, the problem cleared. Which of the following conditions is the least likely diagnosis?

a. Transient global amnesia (TGA)

b. Partial complex seizure

c. Psychogenic amnesia

d. An anticholinergic medication

Answer: c. The cardinal feature of this several hour episode of amnesia is the preservation of personal, deeply seated ("overlearned") information. He most likely had TGA. As in this case, TGA causes amnesia, particularly for recently acquired information, which contradicts the implication that the amnesia encompasses all memory. Moreover, despite its name, the amnesia in TGA is not really *global*. Partial complex seizures and medications with anticholinergic side effects are reasonable alternative explanations; however, these conditions generally cause a clouding of the sensorium. The least likely possibility is dissociative amnesia, previously called psychogenic amnesia, because it is associated with the patients' inability to recall important personal information. Another unlikely possibility is dissociative fugue, previously called psychogenic fugue, because this disorder requires travel away from home or work, as well as inability to recall important personal information.

286. A 4-year-old girl's parents notice that she has begun to lose her clear voice and ability to converse easily with them and other adults. Moreover, she has developed a habit of incessantly playing with her hands. She seems to be washing them or clapping for hours at a time. The neurologist cannot keep her attention. He finds the child's eyes to be blue, her hair blonde, and her head circumference relatively smaller compared to her height and age. Which disorder may be misdiagnosed, in this setting, as autism?

a. Down syndrome

b. PKU deficiency

c. Mental retardation

d. Rett syndrome

e. Nonspecific mental retardation

Answer: d. The child probably has Rett syndrome, which causes mental retardation and autism. This condition is diagnosed on clinical criteria: young girls with acquired microcephaly who lose their verbal abilities and begin to perform repetitive, purposeless hand movements (stereotypies). Its main features are often present, in retrospect, by age 2 years; however, the diagnosis is usually not made until age 5 years. If she had had untreated PKU, which produces blue eyes and blonde hair, it would have caused severe mental retardation since infancy.

287. Which one of the following structures is an intranuclear inclusion?

a. Cowdry body

b. Neurofibrillary tangle

c. Pick body

d. Lewy body

e. Negri body

f. Psammoma body

Answer: a. Cowdry bodies are intranuclear inclusions found in SSPE. Psammoma bodies are macrocytic calcified, whorled, meningeal cells characteristic of meningiomas. Negri bodies are intranuclear inclusions found in rabies.

288. A 17-year-old high school student begins to fall asleep in class. Despite being warned to get more sleep at night, she continues to fall asleep not only in class but also during more exciting activities, such as watching football games. A complete evaluation shows that she is otherwise in good health. After being assured that she gets at least 6 hours of sleep a night but still has excessive daytime sleepiness (EDS), what should be the physician's next two steps?

    a. Delaying the sleep phase

    b. Additional blood tests

    c. PSG (polysomnography) or MSLT (multiple sleep latency test)

    d. EEG

Answer: b then c. Teenagers vary between excessive sleepiness and reluctance to go to bed. Although they often normally have EDS, sleeping in class and during exciting events is abnormal. If she seems to sleep 6 to 8 hours at night, her physician should consider common causes of EDS in teenagers: depression, mononucleosis and other medical illnesses, and drug and alcohol use. Then, narcolepsy and sleep apnea should be considered. A PSG and particularly a MSLT will reveal sleep onset REM periods (SOREMPs) in narcolepsy. The EEG is not suitable for detecting the onset of sleep or the presence of REM.

Narcolepsy is often overlooked in teenagers despite its onset before age 25 years in 90% of cases. Only after several years do patients with narcolepsy develop the dramatic cataplexy. Overall, only 10% of patients with narcolepsy have the complete narcolepsy-cataplexy tetrad: narcolepsy, cataplexy, sleep paralysis, and sleep hallucinations.

Delayed sleep phase syndrome, which causes EDS and typically occurs in teenagers, is associated with a full, restful 6 to 8 hours of sleep but at the "wrong" time. Individuals with this disorder remain awake until late at night and, if possible, sleep late into the next day. Because this teenager had at least 6 hours of sleep, she should have been rested.

289. A 77-year-old man develops EDS at age 75 years. He takes no medications, does not use alcohol, and is in good health. During the night, his wife reports, he has violent movements of his whole body. She does not know if her husband's sleep is restful, but her own sleep is not. Which one of the following should be the next step?

    a. Delaying the sleep phase

    b. Additional blood tests

    c. PSG

    d. EMG

    e. MSLT

Answer: c. People with potentially injurious movements during sleep should be tested with a PSG. An MSLT is unnecessary because narcolepsy is unlikely in view of the lack of daytime naps. Several disorders cause nocturnal movements in 77-year-old individuals: periodic limb movements, restless legs syndrome (RLS), sleep apnea, seizures, and REM sleep disorder. All these conditions interrupt sleep—the bed partner's as well as the patient's—and cause EDS.

290. Which four effects can be attributed to benzodiazepines?

    a. Increase in total sleep time of 10%

    b. Increase in total sleep time of 33%

    c. Increase in total sleep time of 67% or more

    d. Reduced sleep fragmentation

    e. Increase in slow-wave NREM sleep

    f. Hip fractures from an increased tendency to fall

    g. Weight gain

    h. Lowered seizure threshold

    i. Anterograde amnesia

Answers: a, d, f, i.

291. From which structures do most subdural hematomas arise?

    a. Lacerated middle meningeal arteries

    b. Ripped bridging veins

    c. Lacerated great vein of Galen

    d. Aneurysms of the middle or anterior cerebral arteries

Answer: b. Meningeal arterial bleeding leads to epidural hematomas. Aneurysms lead to bleeding that is predominantly subarachnoid. Venous bleeding, which is often so slow that it may be called "oozing," leads to subdural hematomas.

292. Which three of the following are closely associated with spastic cerebral palsy?

    a. Necrotic areas in the white matter around the ventricles, periventricular leukomalacia

    b. Kernicterus

    c. Hyperactive DTRs and clonus

    d. Foreshortened, spastic limbs

    e. Thalidomide

Answers: a, c, d. Kernicterus, basal ganglia bilirubin staining, is associated with choreoathetotic cerebral palsy. Thalidomide causes congenital limb deformity (phocomelia).

293. Which one of the following is most closely associated with neonatal periventricular leukomalacia?
    a. Athetosis
    b. Spastic cerebral palsy, all varieties
    c. Spastic diplegia
    d. MS

Answer: c. Neonatal periventricular white matter necrosis leads to spastic diplegia. MS typically causes periventricular white matter changes.

294. One hour after a grilled tuna fish dinner in a fancy Chicago restaurant, a 29-year-old previously healthy physician develops profound nausea and vomiting. Colleagues find that she has beet-red skin and hypotension, but a temperature of only 100°F. In addition to general supportive measures, which one the following is the best treatment?
    a. Antibiotics
    b. Antidiarrhea medication
    c. Antihistamines
    d. Antiparasitic medications

Answer: c. Even when eaten raw, tuna fish and most other deep-water fish are usually safe. However, if these fish are not refrigerated, bacteria in their gut and gills may proliferate and produce histidine. The histidine, which resists cooking, is transformed into histamine in the human intestine. As in this case, victims develop histamine poisoning that responds to antihistamine treatment. Antidiarrheal medications for fish poisons are ineffective and counteract the body's natural protective reaction to expel toxins.

295. Which one of the following is false regarding the Glasgow Coma Scale (GCS)?
    a. It measures only three clinical parameters: eye opening, verbal response, and motor response.
    b. A high score indicates a greater depth of coma.
    c. GCS scores can be correlated with post-traumatic amnesia.
    d. GCS scores do not correlate with post-traumatic headaches.

Answer: b. GCS scores range from 3 to 15. Patients with low scores are less responsive, have deeper coma, and are more likely to die. If they survive, they have longer post-traumatic amnesia. Notably, GCS scores cannot be correlated with post-traumatic headaches or whiplash injury.

296. Which one of the following statements is false regarding the relationship of alcohol to traumatic brain injury (TBI)?
    a. Alcohol is a frequent contributory factor in motor vehicle, diving, and other accidents that result in TBI.
    b. Alcohol withdrawal may complicate recovery from post-traumatic coma.
    c. Alcohol use in patients surviving TBI increases the incidence of seizures.
    d. Alcohol is a good sedative and minor tranquilizer in patients who have survived minor TBI.
    e. Alcohol may precipitate violence in patients with post-traumatic episodic dyscontrol syndrome.

Answer: d. Alcohol induces insomnia, irritability, and excessive daytime sleepiness and is neither a good sedative nor minor tranquilizer in patients who have survived TBI. Excessive alcohol use, which occurs in many TBI patients, impairs memory and judgment. Post-traumatic insomnia and anxiety may require specific medications, possibly antidepressants. Physicians should assess TBI patients with prolonged anxiety and insomnia for cognitive impairment.

297. When confronted with patients who have sustained acute multiple trauma, emergency room physicians sometimes direct their attention exclusively at head injuries. However, the trauma, extraction, transportation, or examination of the patient may have exacerbated a cervical injury that could cause spinal cord injury. Which of the following are complications of cervical spine injury?
    a. Respiratory failure
    b. Quadriplegia or paraplegia
    c. Herniated intervertebral disks
    d. Urinary retention
    e. Carotid artery dissection
    f. All of the above

Answer: f. Acute cervical spinal cord injury is sometimes overshadowed by head injury. Facial and scalp lacerations, which bleed profusely, are compelling and distracting. Manipulation of the head and neck can be disastrous. Combined head and neck injuries occur in motor vehicle accidents in which the face or forehead strikes the windshield and the neck snaps backward. This type of injury also occurs in diving accidents in which people strike their head in a shallow pool and compress their cervical spine.

298. A 22-year-old Marine, who survived a penetrating frontal lobe shrapnel injury, has episodes of violent, aggressive, destructive behavior. These episodes occur when he drinks only one or two beers and are precipitated by little provocation. Neurologic examination reveals hyperreflexia on the left side and a Babinski sign on the right. His MRI shows bilateral frontal lucencies. An EEG shows intermittent sharp waves that are phase reversed in the left temporal lobe and intermittent slowing when he is drowsy. Which one of the following should a consultant psychiatrist first recommend?
a. Further neurologic evaluation
b. Psychotherapy
c. Use of an AED
d. Use of a minor or major tranquilizer
e. None of the above

Answer: a. He probably has episodic dyscontrol syndrome, which is violent behavior—often with aggression (directed violence)—that typically follows TBI. Patients often have abnormal reflexes and minor, nonspecific EEG abnormalities. Although AEDs may ameliorate the outbursts, the disorder is not epilepsy. In his case, the sharp waves on the EEG might indicate seizures apart from the violence. Before treatment with an AED, he should undergo EEG-TV monitoring that would determine if he has seizures. In addition, he should undergo neuropsychologic testing.

299. A 68-year-old woman loses her accuracy in her relatively complicated assembly-line job. Her family brings her for evaluation for depression and dementia. Soon after the interview begins, she becomes upset and attempts to put on her coat. She tries to put both hands through the left sleeve. She becomes confused and frustrated. Then she puts the coat on backward. Finally, she is perplexed as to how to extricate herself. Which condition is she displaying?
a. Dementia
b. Apraxia
c. Dressing apraxia
d. Left-right confusion
e. Neglect
f. Anosognosia
g. Inattention

Answer: c. Dressing apraxia, a dramatic manifestation of nondominant hemisphere injury, particularly of the parietal lobe, consists of inability to clothe oneself due to a combination of visual-spatial impairment, somatotopagnosia, and motor apraxia. Like other apraxias, dressing apraxia is more than inattention, visual loss, or lack of sensation on one side of the body. Patients with dressing apraxia are befuddled or stymied when attempting to put on a coat, shirt, or hospital robe. Unlike patients with anosognosia, those with dressing apraxia are aware of their problem and are frustrated.

Examiners wishing to demonstrate the phenomenon might ask patients to dress in a hospital robe with one sleeve turned inside-out. Even when warned about the sleeve's being reversed, patients will be unable to dress. Not appreciating the problem or being unable to solve it, they tend to change the normal

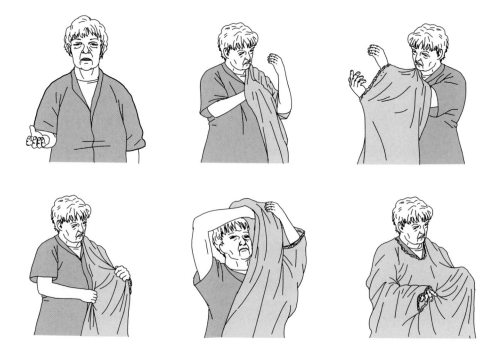

sleeve into an abnormal sleeve, reverse any of their corrections, put both arms through the same sleeve, or drastically misalign the two sides.

In this case, a glioblastoma in the parietal lobe caused the dressing apraxia.

300. Which three of the following tumors originate from glial cells?
   a. Astrocytomas
   b. Glioblastoma multiforme
   c. Oligodendrogliomas
   d. Lymphomas
   e. Meningiomas

Answers: a, b, c.

301. A 31-year-old right-handed waiter has had partial complex seizures since he was 16 years old. His seizures have been refractory to AEDs, except in intoxicating doses. They prevent him from working, traveling, or entering relationships. CCTV documented that his seizures originate in a right-sided temporal lobe focus. MRI showed atrophy of the right hippocampus. Which of the following is probably the best therapy?
   a. Partial right temporal lobectomy
   b. A commissurotomy
   c. Adding an antidepressant
   d. None of the above

Answer: a. Surgery that removes the focus has been a major medical advance that, in skilled hands, benefits about 75% of selected epilepsy patients. A preoperative Wada test or fMRI may reliably predict if the proposed surgery will lead to aphasia. A commissurotomy, which would block the spread to seizures through the corpus callosum, has limited usefulness.

302. Which statement regarding EEG changes that follow ECT is false?
   a. Unilateral ECT is associated with predominantly unilateral β-activity.
   b. Bilateral ECT induces generalized theta and delta activity.
   c. Greater post-ECT slowing is associated with greater antidepressant effect.
   d. Greater post-ECT slowing is associated with greater amnesia.

Answer: a. Unilateral ECT is associated with unilateral EEG slowing (theta and delta activity).

303. What portion of the skull lies immediately medial and anterior to the mesial surface of the temporal lobe?

   a. The temporal bone
   b. The occiput
   c. The sphenoid wing
   d. The petrous pyramid
   e. The nasopharynx

Answer: c. The mesial surface of the temporal lobe is immediately adjacent to the sphenoid wing. Insertion of nasopharyngeal EEG electrodes places them as close as possible to the mesial surface of the temporal lobe. Scalp EEG electrodes, which are placed over the temporal bones, overlie the temporal lobe's lateral surface.

304. In which of the following diseases is apoptosis the mechanism of cell death?
   a. ALS
   b. Head trauma
   c. Huntington's disease
   d. Strokes

Answers: a, c. Apoptosis is programmed, energy-requiring cell death that does not elicit a cellular response from surrounding tissue. It occurs in some aspects of normal development, such as closure of the patent ductus arteriosus and involution of the thymus gland, as well as in many neurodegenerative disorders.

305. In which of the following diseases is necrosis the mechanism of cell death?
   a. ALS
   b. Head trauma
   c. Huntington's disease
   d. Strokes

Answers: b, d. Necrosis is death from catastrophic failure of structure or metabolism. It typically results from anoxia and physical trauma. With the death of cells, surrounding tissue provide a mononuclear cell infiltrate that removes the cellular debris.

306. Which structure is immediately medial and superior to the hypothalamus?
   a. Thalamus
   b. Corpus of Luysii
   c. Corpus callosum
   d. Third ventricle

Answer: d.

307. When a 60-year-old man, who was being evaluated for dementia, was asked to copy the sequence of figures on the top row, he reproduced the sequence on the bottom. When he realized his error, he crumpled the paper, grasped it tightly, laughed uncontrollably, and then urinated. Which of the following conclusions can most reliably be drawn from his copying and behavior problems?

a. He has apraxia for figure copying, which is indicative of nondominant parietal lobe dysfunction.

b. He has dementia, but the problems are nonspecific.

c. These problems are indicative of the subcortical dementias.

d. They are typical of frontotemporal dementia.

Answer: d. The patient perseverated. He could not "switch sets" from drawing squares to circles. Then he demonstrated labile, impetuous behavior, possibly a grasp reflex, and loss of inhibition (the laughing and urinating). These are all signs of frontal lobe impairment.

308. In which condition would the results of evoked potentials be least helpful?

a. Depression

b. Psychogenic blindness

c. MS

d. Optic neuritis

e. Deafness in uncooperative patients

f. Auditory capacity in autistic children

Answer: a. Brainstem auditory evoked responses (BAERS), visual evoked responses (VERs), and somatosensory evoked responses can provide an objective measurement of the function of the auditory, visual, and sensory systems.

309. Which two statements are true regarding the relationship of interictal violence to epilepsy?

a. Violent behavior is no more prevalent among patients with partial complex seizures than other seizures.

b. The consensus among neurologists is that epilepsy does not cause crime. Instead, epilepsy, head trauma, and other brain injuries lead to conditions, such as poor impulse control and lower socioeconomic status that predispose people to crime.

c. Interictal violence is associated with childhood onset seizures.

d. Interictal violence can be reduced with benzodiazepines.

Answers: a, b.

310. In which two patients might brain biopsies reveal Lewy bodies?

a. A 78-year-old person who had encephalitis as a young adult, with tremor, rigidity, and bradykinesia

b. A 70-year-old person who presents with 6 months of dementia, rigidity, and bradykinesia

c. A 40-year-old retired boxer with slurred speech, festinating gait, mild dementia, and resting tremor

d. A 30-year-old former intravenous drug abuser with tremor, rigidity, and bradykinesia

Answers: a, b. Lewy bodies are found in the substantia nigra in Parkinson's disease, especially in the postencephalitic variety (Patient *a*). They are also found in dementia with Lewy body disease, which causes dementia and mild parkinsonism (Patient *b*). However, they are not found in dementia pugilistica (Patient *c*) or MPTP-induced parkinsonism (Patient *d*).

311. Called to evaluate a 63-year-old man who demands to be released from the oncology service of a general hospital, a psychiatrist finds the patient to be relatively calm, oriented, and aware that he has "a melanoma that will be fatal in the near future." Physical examination and laboratory tests reveal no major abnormalities; however, the patient seems to fall to his left and be inattentive to friends and family who stand on his left side. Which of the following tests should the psychiatrist request before attempting to make a determination of the patient's competence?

a. Serum calcium determination

b. EEG

c. Mini-Mental Status Examination

d. CT or MRI of the brain

e. Liver function tests

Answer: d. Melanomas tend to spread widely by blood-borne dissemination. Although the patient seems to be making a rational decision, his left-sided inattention and motor difficulties suggest anosognosia. MRI would be the best test to detect metastases in the nondominant parietal lobe and elsewhere. Whether or not a lesion were present, the psychiatrist would have to judge whether his degree of anosognosia rendered him incompetent.

312. A 67-year-old woman, who has just been admitted with the sudden onset of left hemiparesis, was asked to bisect a line. Which is the most likely result?

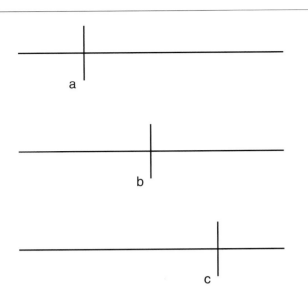

a

b

c

Answer: c. She undoubtedly sustained an extensive right cerebral insult, most likely a stroke. Patients with this perceptual disorder do not appreciate the leftward extent of the horizontal line. They are also likely to be unaware of their left hemiparesis, that is, have anosognosia.

313. Of the following, which is the single most frequent risk factor for falls in the elderly?
   a. Transient ischemic attacks
   b. Use of sedatives or hypnotics
   c. Cardiac arrhythmias
   d. Alzheimer's disease

Answer: b.

314. A psychiatrist is asked to see a 25-year-old methadone-maintenance patient, hospitalized after his first seizure, for agitated, belligerent behavior. MRI performed 3 days before showed a single small, ring-enhancing lesion in the right frontal lobe. Physicians administered phenytoin and anti-toxoplasmosis medications and continued his methadone. Of the following, which is the most likely cause of his behavior?
   a. Cerebral toxoplasmosis
   b. AIDS dementia
   c. Phenytoin-enhanced hepatic metabolism
   d. Anti-toxoplasmosis medications

Answer: c. Phenytoin induces hepatic enzymes that metabolize other medications, including methadone. Thus, instituting phenytoin in methadone patients precipitates withdrawal. Individuals in methadone-maintenance programs are often HIV positive because of prior or concomitant intravenous drug abuse. Many of them have AIDS. This patient may have cerebral toxoplasmosis, but a single small lesion in the right frontal lobe is unlikely to cause his behavioral disturbances.

315. Which are two characteristics of neurosyphilis in AIDS patients?
   a. Neurosyphilis often yields false-positive results.
   b. The diagnosis may be obscured by negative serologic tests.
   c. Treatment with penicillin may be deleterious.
   d. Neurosyphilis occurs rarely in AIDS patients.
   e. The usual doses of penicillin may be inadequate.

Answers: b, e.

316. Which two are the greatest risk factors for dementia in AIDS patients?
   a. The CD4 count below 1000 cells/mm^3
   b. Being HIV positive
   c. Anemia
   d. Depression
   e. Weight loss

Answers: c, e. Dementia is a late manifestation of AIDS. It occurs when immunodeficiency is pronounced and anemia and systemic symptoms have developed. A low CD4 count is an early consequence of AIDS and long precedes dementia in almost all cases. Only a pronounced CD4 depletion, typically below 200 cells/mm^3, is a risk factor for AIDS dementia.

317. Although the distinction's value has been questioned, many neurologists continue to divide dementia into cortical and subcortical varieties. Which of the following illnesses are considered examples of cortical (c) or subcortical (sc) dementia?
   a. AIDS dementia
   b. Alzheimer's disease
   c. Huntington's disease
   d. Normal pressure hydrocephalus
   e. Parkinson's disease
   f. Frontotemporal dementia, including Pick's disease

Answers: a-sc, b-c, c-sc, d-sc, e-sc, f-c. The distinction is arbitrary and fallible because several of these illnesses have overlapping features. The dementia in both AIDS and Huntington's disease, for example, has cortical as well as subcortical features.

318. Which one of the following statements concerning hallucinations in Alzheimer's disease is false?
   a. Hallucinations are mostly visual but are sometimes auditory or olfactory.

b. They are associated with a rapid decline in cognitive function.

c. They have little prognostic value.

d. They are associated with clearly abnormal EEGs.

Answer: c. They are clearly indicative of a poor prognosis.

319. If a man is 45 years old, in which decade of life is he?
    a. Third
    b. Fourth
    c. Fifth
    d. Sixth

Answer: c. The man has entered his fifth decade. This nomenclature is often a source of confusion.

320. Which statement most closely describes the gate control theory of pain control?
    a. Descending pathways inhibit pain.
    b. Endogenous opioids suppress pain.
    c. Large-diameter, heavily myelinated fiber activity inhibits pain transmission by small, sparsely myelinated fibers.
    d. Substance P and serotonin, carefully balanced, regulate pain transmission.

Answer: c.

321. Which one of the following statements is true regarding the periaqueductal gray matter?
    a. Stimulation of the periaqueductal gray matter produces analgesia by liberating endogenous opioids.
    b. Hemorrhage into the periaqueductal gray matter is associated with thiamine deficiency.
    c. The periaqueductal gray matter surrounds the aqueduct of Sylvius, which is the passage for CSF between the third and fourth ventricles.
    d. The periaqueductal gray matter is in the midbrain.
    e. All of the above.

Answer: e.

322. Which is not a characteristic of enkephalins?
    a. They are peptides.
    b. They are neurotransmitters.
    c. Naloxone inhibits enkephalins.
    d. Serotonin inhibits enkephalins.

Answer: d.

323. Which of the following substances serves as a neurotransmitter for pain?
    a. Enkephalins

b. Serotonin
    c. Substance P
    d. Endogenous opioids

Answer: c.

324. In regards to their analgesic strength, NSAIDs can be as potent analgesics as opioids. In which other way are NSAIDs similar to opioids?
    a. They are addictive.
    b. They produce greater analgesia with increasingly higher doses with no limit.
    c. They promote tolerance to their analgesic effect.
    d. Most cause gastrointestinal bleeding.
    e. None of the above.

Answer: e. Unlike opioids, NSAIDs are not addictive and do not induce tolerance. In addition, at a certain dose, their analgesic effect reaches a maximum. With their "ceiling effect," further increases in the dose of NSAIDs do not produce additional analgesia. Moreover, additional medication will expose patients to side effects, particularly gastrointestinal bleeding.

325. What is the primary mechanism of action of NSAIDs?
    a. They inhibit prostaglandin synthesis.
    b. They enhance serotonin activity.
    c. They enhance opioid activity.
    d. They cause opioid-like psychologic side effects.
    e. All of the above.

Answer: a.

326. Which two of the following features are included in a syndrome in 3- to 6-year-old girls that mimics autism?
    a. Stereotypical hand wringing movements
    b. Acquired microcephaly
    c. Low-set, large ears
    d. Fair skin and eczema
    e. Simian palm crease
    f. Seizures

Answers: a, b. Rett syndrome, which has prominent autistic features, is characterized by repetitive hand movements and acquired microcephaly in young girls. Boys with mental retardation caused by fragile X syndrome have large, low-set ears and large testicles. The simian palm crease is a characteristic of trisomy 21. Fair skin and eczema are features of PKU.

327. A first-grade boy runs with his left hand fisted. When asked to walk on the sides of his feet, the left thumb tends to flex toward the palm, as though he were starting to make a fist. Which three other stigmata of neurologic injury can be expected?

a. Hyperactive DTRs in the left arm
b. Mental retardation
c. Clumsy movements with the left arm
d. Spasticity of the arm
e. Hypoactive DTRs in the left arm
f. Athetosis

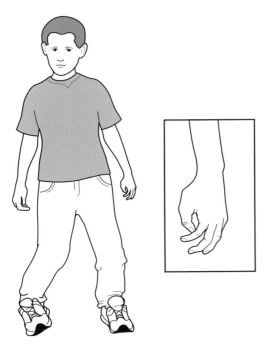

Answers: a, c, d. He is displaying a "cortical thumb." This sign usually indicates congenital corticospinal tract injury that, in turn, would also cause hyperactive DTRs, spasticity, and clumsiness. In cases of unilateral involvement, the affected thumb, fingers, or entire arm may be smaller than the unaffected counterpart. A unilateral cortical thumb and other soft signs suggest (contralateral) congenital cerebral injury. Adults may develop a cortical thumb after a cerebral infarction or trauma.

328. Match the enzyme with the illness that its deficiency produces.
1. Hypoxanthine guanine phosphoribosyl transferase
2. Tyrosine hydroxylase
3. Phenylalanine hydroxylase
4. Arylsulfatase
   a. Phenylketonuria
   b. Lesch-Nyhan syndrome
   c. Metachromatic leukodystrophy
   d. Parkinson's disease

Answers: 1-b, 2-d, 3-a, 4-c.

329. When a vagus nerve stimulator is implanted in an attempt to suppress seizures, where do the impulses first enter the CNS?

a. Temporal lobe
b. Diencephalon
c. Midbrain
d. Pons
e. Medulla

Answer: e. The vagus nerves' afferent fibers terminate in the solitary nucleus of the medulla. Impulses are relayed to the cerebral cortex, as well as to more rostral portions of the brainstem.

330. Match the speech pattern (a–c) with the disorder (1–3).
a. Strained and strangled
b. Hypophonic and monotonous
c. Scanning
   1. MS affecting the cerebellum
   2. Parkinson's disease
   3. Spasmodic dysphonia

Answers: a-3, b-2, c-1.

331. Which finding is compatible with brain death?
a. Slow-wave activity on the EEG
b. Ocular movement artifact on the EEG
c. Presence of oculocephalic reflexes
d. Babinski signs and hyperactive Achilles reflexes

Answer: d. Spinal reflexes, such as Babinski signs and hyperactive Achilles reflexes, may be preserved in brain death. In contract, EEG and clinical signs of brainstem activity, such as pupillary light and oculocephalic reflexes, indicate brainstem function and preclude a determination of brain death.

332. Why is succinylcholine used in conjunction with ECT?
a. It makes the brain more susceptible to the beneficial effects of ECT because it lowers the seizure threshold.
b. It paralyzes muscles by binding to the neuromuscular junction ACh receptors.
c. It reduces subsequent amnesia.
d. It is given to enhance ECT effect, but its usefulness has never been established.
e. It reduces oral secretions that the patient could aspirate.
f. It interferes with cerebral ACh and induces amnesia for the event.

Answer: b. Succinylcholine blocks the neuromuscular junction. It paralyzes muscles and prevents ECT-induced muscle contractions that can cause fractures and other bodily injuries. Succinylcholine does not cross the blood–brain barrier and thus does not affect the seizure threshold or memory pathways. Atropine reduces secretions.

333. The family of a 32-year-old woman brings her to the emergency room. They have not seen the patient in 3 years. The psychiatrist and neurologist find that she has slow and disordered thinking, word-finding difficulties, bilateral weakness and spasticity (but left-sided more than right-sided), and dysarthria and dysphagia. A noncontrast CT of the head and CSF analysis reveal no abnormalities, but an MRI shows numerous, large abnormal areas in the cerebral white matter. Which disorder need not be considered?
a. Toxoplasmosis
b. Adrenoleukodystrophy
c. Toluene (volatile substance) abuse
d. Progressive multifocal leukoencephalopathy (PML)
e. MS

Answer: b. Her neurologic signs—aphasia, pseudobulbar palsy, bilateral corticospinal tract signs, and possibly dementia—indicate diffuse cerebral injury. All the disorders could eventually cause these signs. Also, except for toxoplasmosis, all are demyelinating diseases that can be detected by MRI but not CT. The least likely possibility is adrenoleukodystrophy because it is an X-linked recessive disorder that would develop only in males. Because toxoplasmosis and PML are usually complications of AIDS, she should have an HIV test, as well as a routine evaluation.

334. To which parts of the brain do the letters (A–E) refer? If appropriate, use more than one number for each number.

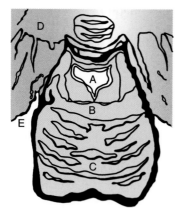

1. Lateral ventricle
2. Third ventricle
3. Aqueduct of Sylvius
4. Fourth ventricle
5. Midbrain
6. Pons
7. Medulla
8. Cerebellum
9. Cerebrum
10. Corticospinal tracts
11. Cerebellar tracts
12. Bulbar cranial nerves
13. Oculomotor cranial nerves
14. Cerebellopontine angle cranial nerves

Answer: The sketch shows the pons (B-6), which is the bulky portion of the brainstem, and the inferior aspect of the cerebellum (D-8). The fourth ventricle (A-4) is located in the uppermost portion of the pons. Corticospinal and cerebellar tracts (C-10 and 11) cross through the base of the pons. Cranial nerves 5, 7, and 8 (E-14) emerge from the cerebellopontine angle.

335. Which four clinical features are more characteristic of frontotemporal dementia than Alzheimer's disease?
a. Dementia
b. Familial tendency
c. Oral exploration
d. Personality disturbances
e. Age-proportional incidence
f. Disinhibition
g. Language disturbances
h. Impaired spatial orientation

Answer: c, d, f, and g. Although the clinical features of frontotemporal dementia and Alzheimer's diseases overlap, frontotemporal dementia is more apt to cause pronounced behavioral and personality disturbances, including elements of the Klüver-Bucy syndrome and lack of inhibition (disinhibition) but preserved spatial orientation.

336. Which one of the following MRI abnormalities is most closely associated with chronic treatment-resistant schizophrenia?
a. Cerebellar atrophy
b. Corpus callosum atrophy
c. Symmetry of the planum temporale
d. Enlargement of the lateral ventricles

Answer: d. Schizophrenic patients with chronic, progressive deterioration resistant to treatment have large lateral ventricles accompanied by a large third ventricle and cerebral cortical atrophy. In addition, the amygdala and hippocampus are decreased in volume and the planum temporale is unlikely to show the normal symmetry.

337. Which visual field cut is associated with alexia without agraphia?

Answer: b. A right homonymous hemianopsia is associated with alexia without agraphia. In fact, a right homonymous hemianopsia is virtually a prerequisite for the condition.

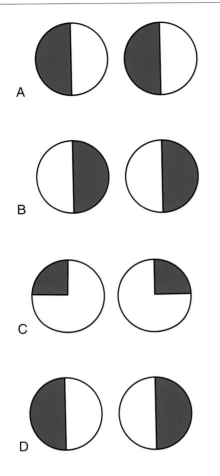

A

B

C

D

1. Front-to-back or head-on
2. Top-down view
3. Side view

Answers: a-2, b-1, c-3.

340. During the Vietnam War, numerous soldiers were exposed to Agent Orange. Which of the following neurologic problems has been found in rigorous scientific studies to be attributable to Agent Orange exposure?
   a. Brain tumors
   b. Peripheral neuropathy
   c. Cognitive impairment
   d. Neuropsychologic deficits
   e. None of the above

Answer: e. No reliable evidence has linked Agent Orange exposure to these neurologic problems.

341. In which two regions of the brain are pathologic changes most pronounced in Alzheimer's disease?
   a. Primary motor cortex
   b. Occipital cortex
   c. Association areas, such as the parietal-temporal junction
   d. Olfactory lobe
   e. Limbic system, especially the hippocampus

Answers: c, e. These regions are especially atrophic and contain dense concentrations of plaques and tangles.

342. Which three of the following medications elevate the serum prolactin concentration?
   a. Thorazine
   b. Bromocriptine
   c. Haloperidol
   d. Clozapine
   e. Pergolide
   f. L-dopa
   g. Risperidone

Answers: a, c, g. Dopamine and dopamine agonists inhibit the release of prolactin by acting on the tubero-infundibular tract. In contrast, dopamine-blocking neuroleptics trigger prolactin release and produce elevated serum concentrations. Prolactin concentration is also elevated for about 20 minutes after most generalized and partial complex seizures. Prolactinomas, a common pituitary adenoma, secrete prolactin. Bromocriptine, a dopamine agonist, can suppress prolactinomas and obviate surgery.

338. Which one of the following results from sequential mental status tests indicates Alzheimer's disease?
   a. A precipitous decline over 6 months
   b. A decline over 6 months and then a plateau for 3 years
   c. A borderline score in a well-educated individual
   d. An uneven decline interrupted by several plateaus lasting 12 to 18 months

Answer: d. An uneven decline, including some plateaus, is typical of Alzheimer's disease. A precipitous decline suggests a rapidly progressive illness, such as Creutzfeldt-Jakob disease, AIDS, or a glioblastoma. A plateau of more than 2 years is unusual for Alzheimer's disease. A borderline score in well-educated individuals is a common diagnostic dilemma. Such individuals might not have been very intelligent in the first place; they could have developed other problems, such as alcoholism; or they could have depression instead of, or comorbid with, dementia.

339. Match the view (a–c) with its common description (1–3).
   a. Transaxial
   b. Coronal
   c. Sagittal

343. Which two of the following nuclei constitute the corpus striatum?
   a. Caudate

b. Putamen
c. Globus pallidus
d. Subthalamic
e. Substantia nigra

Answers: a, b.

344. In hepatolenticular degeneration, to which two structures does "lenticular" refer?
a. Caudate
b. Putamen
c. Globus pallidus
d. Subthalamic
e. Substantia nigra
f. Corticospinal tract
g. Thalamus
h. The liver
i. The cornea

Answers: b, c. Forming a pie-shaped or lens-like structure, the putamen and globus pallidus form the lenticular nuclei (see Fig. 18-1A). In hepatolenticular degeneration (Wilson's disease), copper deposits damage these basal ganglia, the liver, and other organs. Deposits in the cornea form the characteristic Kayser-Fleischer rings.

345. Which three of the following findings indicate a deliberate head injury in an infant?
a. Retinal hemorrhages
b. Discrepancy between history and injuries
c. An Arnold-Chiari defect
d. CT or MRI showing dural hemorrhages of varying ages
e. Absence of the corpus callosum
f. Subconjunctival hemorrhages

Answers: a, b, d. Blood of varying ages in the face, retinae, subdural spaces, and brain of an infant indicates deliberate trauma (i.e., the "shaken baby syndrome"). Absence of the corpus callosum and Arnold-Chiari defects are congenital malformations. Subconjunctival hemorrhages usually result from minimal, accidental trauma, minor illnesses, and bleeding disorders, but retinal hemorrhages strongly suggest trauma.

346. With which phenomenon does the day's lowest body temperature coincide?
a. Intense REM sleep
b. Intense slow-wave sleep
c. Sleep onset
d. 12 noon
e. 4:00 PM

Answer: a. In the early morning, when REM activity is most likely to be present, the body's temperature reaches its daily low point (nadir).

347. A family brings their 72-year-old patriarch for the evaluation of dementia that has developed along with mild rigidity and bradykinesia during the past several months. His course has been particularly troubled by visual hallucinations. What might the brain show?
a. Plaques and tangles in the hippocampus
b. Lewy bodies in the cerebral cortex
c. Lewy bodies in the substantia nigra
d. Atrophy of the head of the caudate

Answer: b. He probably has dementia with Lewy bodies. Lewy bodies in the substantia nigra characterize Parkinson's disease, which does not cause dementia at its onset. Alzheimer's disease causes plaques and tangles in the cerebral cortex and especially the hippocampus, but it usually does not present with either pyramidal or extrapyramidal signs. Huntington's disease characteristically causes atrophy of the head of the caudate nuclei.

348. In the treatment of Parkinson's disease, which dopamine receptors do dopamine agonists stimulate?
a. D_1
b. D_2
c. Both
d. Neither

Answer: b. All commercially available dopamine agonists stimulate D_2. They may either stimulate or inhibit D_1.

349. A 25-year-old man with AIDS has hyperactive DTRs in his legs and impaired posterior column sensations. Which of the following is the most likely problem?
a. AIDS myelopathy
b. AIDS neuropathy
c. HTLV1 myelopathy
d. Combined system disease

Answer: a. HIV infection of the spinal cord causes a pattern similar to combined system disease; however, administration of B_{12} does not alleviate the problem. HTLV1 myelopathy causes spasticity with little or no posterior column impairment.

350. A 50-year-old architect's hand forms a painful cramp several minutes after he begins work. Early in his career, he would develop similar cramps only after many hours of nonstop work. Which condition is responsible for forcing his hand into this position?

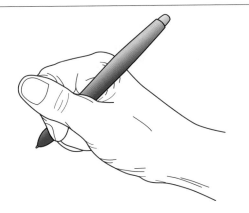

a. Psychogenic disturbance
b. Age-related disturbance
c. Motor neuron disease
d. Focal dystonia
e. Exercised-induced cramp

Answer: d. He has developed writer's cramp, which is an occupational or work-related dystonia. This disorder is a focal dystonia, not a psychologic reaction or an exercise-induced muscle cramp. After several decades, musicians, writers, architects, and other workers who use their hands in a repetitive fashion sometimes develop such focal dystonias. His writer's cramp might respond to botulinum toxin injected into the muscles that spasm. Other body parts used repetitively can also develop occupational dystonias. For example, professional French horn players may develop dystonia of their lip muscles.

351. A 60-year-old man has been developing involuntary contractions of all the facial muscles. The contractions, which begin around the eyes, are bilateral and symmetric. They accumulate to have a duration of several seconds and prevent him from seeing. He remains conscious during the contractions. His jaw, tongue, and ocular muscles are unaffected. Which type of illness is the most likely cause?

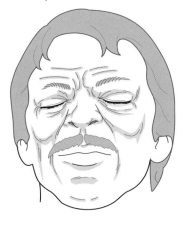

a. Seizure disorder
b. Iatrogenic illness

c. Cranial dystonia
d. Psychogenic condition

Answer: c. He has cranial dystonia, which neurologists often call Meige's syndrome, that is more extensive than blepharospasm because it involves the lower as well as the upper face muscles. Most individuals with this and other cranial dystonias have no history of psychiatric illness or exposure to neuroleptics. When the oral-buccal-lingual form of tardive dyskinesia involves facial muscles, it is usually entered on the tongue and jaw muscles. Cranial dystonias respond to botulinum injections. However, neurologists cannot safely inject the tongue because if it weakens the tongue, it might fall back and occlude the airway. Also, if the injections were to cause bleeding, tongue swelling would also occlude the airway.

352. Which five illnesses result from trinucleotide repeats?
a. Huntington's disease
b. Spinocerebellar atrophy
c. Wilson's disease
d. Dystonia
e. Fragile X syndrome
f. Duchenne's muscular dystrophy
g. Myotonic dystrophy
h. Friedreich's ataxia

Answers: a, b, e, g, h.

353. In which three ways does juvenile Huntington's disease differ from the common adult variety of the illness?
a. Unlike the DNA in the adult variety, the DNA in juvenile Huntington's disease typically has more than 60 trinucleotide repeats.
b. The juvenile variety has a greater tendency toward anticipation in successive generations.
c. The juvenile variety usually results from the father's unstable, abnormal DNA.
d. The juvenile variety tends to cause rigidity rather than chorea.
e. The juvenile variety affects girls more often than boys.

Answers: a, c, d.

354. Which nuclei are most atrophied in Huntington's disease?
a. Lenticular nuclei
b. Corpus striatum
c. Subthalamic nuclei
d. Mamillary bodies

Answer: b. Atrophy of the head of the caudate nuclei is characteristic of Huntington's disease.

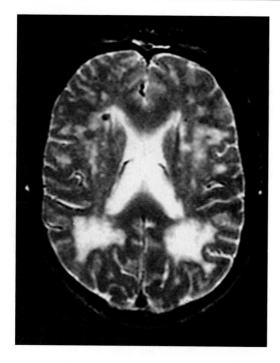

355. A 33-year-old man with AIDS develops vision impairment, confusion, and word-finding difficulties. His MRI is shown above. Which process is causing his symptoms?
   a. HIV encephalitis
   b. MS
   c. Toxoplasmosis
   d. Progressive multifocal leukoencephalopathy (PML)
   e. Lymphoma

Answer: d. The MRI shows two large, hyperintense lesions in the white matter of the occipital lobes. Similar, scattered lesions are located in the dominant hemisphere (on the right side of the MRI). The occipital lesions have caused the visual difficulties. The dominant hemisphere lesions have caused the language problems.

Unlike most intracerebral mass lesions, PML regions are not surrounded by edema and do not exert a mass effect, such as a shift of midline structures or compression of adjacent ventricles. HIV encephalitis does not cause discrete lesions. Although MS attacks white matter, its lesions are typically periventricular. Toxoplasmosis, a common complication of AIDS, causes multiple mass lesions that are not restricted to the white matter. Cerebral lymphomas in AIDS patients are usually large, single mass lesions.

356. A 60-year-old man, who had been in excellent health, developed apathy, inattention, and a flattened affect during a 3-week vacation. His MRI results are shown in the next column. Which is the most likely diagnosis?

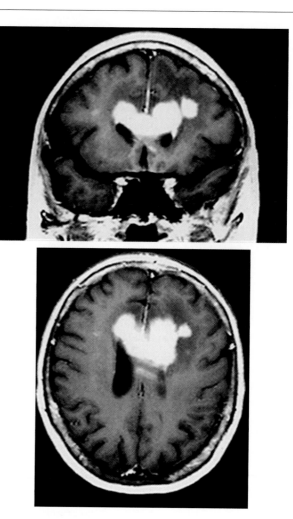

   a. A frontal lobe glioblastoma
   b. MS
   c. Lymphoma
   d. PML

Answer: a. The MRI view on the left is coronal, and the right is transaxial or axial. The patient's symptoms reflect frontal lobe dysfunction. The MRI study shows a large hyperintense lesion in both frontal lobes that has spread through the corpus callosum in a "butterfly" pattern. The rapid course, clinical features, and MRI indicate that he is harboring a bilateral frontal lobe glioblastoma, which is a relatively common tumor in this age group. His age, absence of preceding episodes, and lack of risk factors virtually exclude MS, lymphoma, and PML. Metastatic carcinoma is a possibility, but metastases are usually multiple, surrounded by edema, and do not spread through the corpus callosum.

357. Which of the following is a relay nucleus on the hearing pathway?
   a. Lateral geniculate body
   b. Medial geniculate body
   c. Medial lemniscus
   d. Substantia gelatinosum

Answer: b. The medial geniculate body is an important relay nucleus in the hearing circuit. The lateral geniculate body is a relay station for visual impulses. The medial lemniscus conveys position and vibration sensations. The substantia gelatinosum relays pain sensation from the spinal dorsal nucleus to the lateral spinothalamic tract.

358. An examination by an audiologist determines that a 74-year-old man has bilateral impairment of speech discrimination, particularly for consonants. His hearing loss particularly affects high frequencies. Which is the most likely explanation?
   a. He has NF2.
   b. He has occupation-related hearing loss.
   c. Acoustic neuromas have developed bilaterally.
   d. Age-related changes have developed.

Answer: d. He has normal, age-related changes, presbycusis. NF2 is characterized by the development of bilateral acoustic neuromas.

359. Which of the following is not a normal, age-related change?
   a. Small pupils
   b. Decreased olfaction and taste sensation
   c. Increased proportion of slow-wave sleep
   d. Decreased vibration perception in the toes and ankles
   e. Inability to perform tandem gait
   f. Loss of speech discrimination

Answer: c. Elderly individuals have all of these changes except that they also have a decrease in the proportion of slow-wave sleep, that is, stages 3 and 4 of NREM sleep.

360. Which three of the following involuntary movements are typically preceded by an urge to move?
   a. Periodic limb movements
   b. RLS
   c. Stereotypies
   d. Akathisia
   e. Chorea
   f. Tics

Answers: b, d, f. Patients with classic movement disorders, such as Parkinson's disease, tremor, chorea, and hemiballismus, have no underlying psychologic component that compels them to move. Their movements are entirely subconscious. In contrast, patients with certain movement disorders, such as RLS, akathisia, and tics, typically have a compulsion or urge to move. Their movements provide some psychologic relief; however, more strikingly, suppressing the movements leads to anxiety and a rebound in the movements when they stop suppressing them.

361. Which two conditions typically produce brief, random, involuntary movements accompanied by motor impersistence that develop over several days in a 10-year-old child?
   a. Tourette's syndrome
   b. Lyme disease
   c. Mononucleosis
   d. Sydenham's chorea
   e. Neuroleptic-induced dystonia
   f. Withdrawal emergent dyskinesia

Answers: d, f. The child has chorea that—depending on the history—indicates either Sydenham's chorea or withdrawal emergent dyskinesia. Tourette's syndrome evolves slowly and produces stereotyped tics. Neuroleptic-induced dystonia usually produces extension of the head and neck (retrocollis) and is rare in children. Lyme disease and mononucleosis, which both occur in children, do not regularly produce chorea.

362. Which one of the following children is most apt to have a mitochondria disorder?
   a. A 10-year-old boy who develops dystonia of one foot that begins to spread to the ipsilateral hand
   b. An 8-year-old boy who has had a head toss intermittently for 2 years and then develops an intermittent cough for which there is no pulmonary explanation
   c. A 6-year-old girl who develops polyuria and polydipsia
   d. An 11-year-old autistic girl
   e. A 9-year-old boy with mild mental retardation
   f. A 9-year-old boy who is short and mildly mentally retarded and has repeated hospitalizations for lactic acidosis

Answer: f. The lactic acidosis indicates a systemic metabolic impairment, which reflects a mitochondrial disorder. Curiously, the disorder becomes symptomatic on an intermittent basis.

363. Deficiency of which one of the following vitamins causes CNS demyelination?
   a. Niacin
   b. Pyridoxine (vitamin B_6)
   c. B_{12}
   d. Citric acid (vitamin C)

Answer: c. Vitamin B_{12} deficiency causes demyelination in the posterior tracts of the spinal cord, cerebrum, and other areas of the CNS. It also causes a peripheral neuropathy. Niacin deficiency causes pellagra. Pyridoxine deficiency causes a neuropathy and seizures. Citric acid deficiency causes scurvy.

364. A 64-year-old man with the recent onset of memory loss then became loquacious, overly friendly,

and inappropriately jocular. When the psychiatrist introduced herself, he kissed her "hello." During the examination, in addition to memory impairment, he had minor problems in language comprehension, repetition, and naming. Although he copied line drawings, he incorporated erotic sketches in them. He had no hemiparesis or other overt physical neurologic deficits. If his brain could be examined, which two features would it likely show?
a. Ventricular dilation
b. Caudate lobe atrophy
c. Severe generalized atrophy
d. Atrophy predominantly of the frontal and temporal lobes
e. Intraneuronal argentophilic inclusions
f. Plaques and tangles
g. Spirochetes
h. None of the above

Answers: d, e. In view of the prominent behavioral and personality changes, disinhibition, and aphasia, the most probable diagnosis is frontotemporal dementia. Cases of frontotemporal dementia associated with silver-staining (argentophilic) inclusions in neurons are a subgroup termed Pick's disease.

365. An 18-year-old suburban high school student, with newly developing social and academic difficulties, begins to have rapid, involuntary facial movements and a continual cough. The neurologist finds an otherwise normal neurologic examination, including cognitive function, MRI, EEG, HIV, serum ceruloplasmin, Lyme titer, and syphilis tests. She concludes that the patient has no primary neurologic illness and refers him for a psychiatry consultation. During the course of a psychiatric evaluation, which three other tests should be performed as soon as possible?
a. A complete family history
b. IQ and other academic-psychologic testing
c. Therapeutic trial of haloperidol
d. Testing for MS
e. Other testing

Answers: a, b, e. The neurologist is "half right." The development of tics occurs before age 13 years in 90% of patients. Therefore, the development of tic—vocal or respiratory as well as motor—in a teenager should prompt evaluation for use of cocaine and other stimulants. MS does not usually cause movement disorders because it is a white matter disease. (The basal ganglia are composed of gray matter.) Sydenham's chorea would be unlikely without a pre-existing streptococcal infection or carditis; however, physicians should consider Sydenham's chorea in this situation because it may represent a life-threatening illness.

366. Which two features are present in the involuntary neck movements of tardive dystonia but absent in idiopathic spasmodic torticollis?
a. Response to botulinum injections
b. Movements being predominantly retrocollis
c. Hypertrophy of the neck muscles
d. Accompanying oral-buccal-lingual movements

Answers: b, d. Both varieties of involuntary neck movements respond to botulinum toxin, but neither responds consistently to anticholinergic or other oral medications. Tardive dystonia is usually accompanied by other tardive dyskinesias.

367. Which one of the following substances has an unpaired electron?
a. Monoamines
b. Free radicals
c. Dopamine
d. Choline acetyl transferase (ChAT)

Answer: b. Free radicals are unstable atoms or molecules because they contain a single, unpaired electron. They seize electrons from adjacent atoms or molecules, which oxidizes them. Methylphenylpyridinium (MPP^+), which is the metabolic product of MPTP, is the best-known example of a free radical.

368. Which one of the following does not occur during sleep?
a. Periodic leg movements
b. RLS
c. Parkinson's disease tremor
d. Apnea
e. Palatal myoclonus
f. Generalized seizures
g. Partial seizures
h. Migraines

Answer: c.

369. A 19-year-old student has developed progressively severe intellectual impairment during the preceding year. Examination reveals a resting tremor, dysarthria, and rigidity. The cornea has a brown-green discoloration in its periphery. Liver function tests are abnormal. Which of the following is most likely to be found on further evaluation?
a. Trinucleotide repeats
b. Atrophy of the caudate nucleus
c. History of drug abuse
d. Decreased concentration of the serum protein that transports copper

Answer: d. He has Wilson's disease. His serum would contain insufficient ceruloplasmin, the copper-carrying protein. Trinucleotide repeats and atrophy of the caudate nucleus indicate Huntington's disease.

Although not the explanation in this case, physicians should consider drug abuse in teenagers and young adults with progressive cognitive impairment.

370. In the cholinergic system in Alzheimer's disease, which receptor shows the greatest impairment of binding?
    a. Muscarinic, presynaptic
    b. Muscarinic, postsynaptic
    c. Nicotinic, presynaptic
    d. Nicotinic, postsynaptic

    Answer: a. The presynaptic muscarinic receptor has the greatest reduction in ACh binding.

371. Regarding nicotinic and muscarinic ACh receptors, which statement is false?
    a. Neuromuscular junctions rely on nicotinic receptors.
    b. Atropine and scopolamine block muscarinic receptors.
    c. Nicotinic receptors are blocked by curare.
    d. The CNS has both ACh receptors, but those in the cortex are predominantly nicotinic.

    Answer: d. ACh receptors in the cortex are predominantly muscarinic. Thus, administering atropine or scopolamine produces an Alzheimer-like memory impairment.

372. Following cocaine use that led to small bilateral temporal-parietal hemorrhages, a 28-year-old man has visual difficulties. He has a left homonymous hemianopsia but 20/25 visual acuity bilaterally. He claims that he cannot name similar items unless he can "experience" them. For example, he cannot identify a dog and cat unless he can feel and smell them. Also, he cannot distinguish between a pen and pencil unless he writes with each. Similarly, unless he speaks with family members, rather than just seeing them, he cannot identify them. Nevertheless, he can name and state the use of all objects that he touches, repeat long and complicated phrases, and follow two- and three-step requests. Which is the best description of his visual impairment?
    a. Cortical blindness
    b. Aphasia
    c. Hemi-inattention
    d. Visual agnosia
    e. A psychogenic disturbance
    f. Toxic-metabolic encephalopathy

    Answer: d. A perceptual problem, visual agnosia, prevents him from identifying similar objects despite knowing their name and use. He also has prosopagnosia, a variety of visual agnosia, in which the patient cannot identify familiar faces. These conditions probably result from lesions, as in this case, that are anterior to the occipital visual cortex and impair its communication with the parietal association areas. He does not have blindness because his visual acuity is 20/25, aphasia because he has normal language, hemi-inattention because he brings the objects into his consciousness through tactile routes, or toxic-metabolic encephalopathy because he remained alert enough to complete the testing.

373. A 35-year-old alcoholic man with mild, chronic cirrhosis is brought to the emergency room because of agitation and belligerent behavior. Examination reveals disorientation, slurred speech, and asterixis. He has no nystagmus, extraocular paresis, pupillary abnormality, or lateralized signs. Laboratory data include the following: mildly abnormal liver function tests, 26% hematocrit, and blood in the stool. Which condition is the most likely cause of his behavioral disturbances and confusion?
    a. Wernicke's encephalopathy
    b. Alcohol-induced hypoglycemia
    c. Hepatic encephalopathy
    d. Subdural hematoma
    e. Delirium tremens (DTs)

    Answer: c. Hepatic encephalopathy from gastrointestinal bleeding is the most likely explanation. People with cirrhosis or other causes of hepatic insufficiency will develop encephalopathy when gastrointestinal bleeding results from esophageal varices or gastric ulceration. Sometimes encephalopathy follows a high-protein meal. In both cases, protein breaks down in the intestine to form ammonia or other toxins. Mental status changes and asterixis often occur, as in this case, before liver function tests become markedly abnormal. Physicians should avoid prescribing psychotropic medications that require hepatic metabolism to patients with hepatic insufficiency.

    Physicians should consider Wernicke's encephalopathy, alcohol-induced hypoglycemia, and subdural hematomas in alcoholics with mental status changes. Even without particular indications of these diagnoses, treatment might include intravenous thiamine and, after blood tests are drawn, intravenous glucose.

374. All of these conditions cause weakness. Which three of them result from impaired presynaptic ACh release?
    a. Lambert-Eaton syndrome
    b. Myasthenia gravis
    c. Botulism
    d. Tetanus
    e. Insecticide poisoning
    f. Botulinum treatment

Answers: a, c, f. Lambert-Eaton syndrome, a remote effect of cancer on the neuromuscular junction, slows release of ACh packets. Similarly, botulism and botulinum toxin injections impair ACh release. In contrast, myasthenia gravis results from defective ACh postsynaptic receptors. Anticholinesterase insecticides cause paralyzing, continual postsynaptic receptor stimulation. Tetanus results from loss of normal spinal cord inhibition from impaired GABA activity.

375. After a several-day binge of cocaine and other drug use, a 33-year-old woman presents with hyperactivity of the hands and feet. She describes a "need" to move. She cannot sit still or stand "at attention." When walking, her gait is jerky. Of the following, which one is the most likely cause of her movements?
   a. Drug-induced psychosis
   b. Akathisia
   c. Sydenham's chorea
   d. Excessive dopamine activity
   e. Alcohol withdrawal

Answer: d. Each of these conditions can cause chorea or similar hyperactive movements, particularly of the legs, as if in response to an urge to move. Cocaine and similar illicit drugs increase dopamine activity to toxic levels. The involuntary leg movements represent "crack dancing," which should subside spontaneously over 1 to 3 days. Until then, if necessary, small doses of dopamine-blocking neuroleptics may suppress the involuntary movements.

376. With which receptor does glutamate bind to create toxic reactions?
   a. NMDA
   b. Muscarinic ACh
   c. Nicotinic ACh
   d. Dopamine
   e. Glutamate
   f. None of the above

Answer: a. Glutamate-NMDA interactions are excitotoxic in Huntington's disease and possibly also in epilepsy and strokes.

377. Which four of the following nuclei are pigmented?
   a. Locus ceruleus
   b. Oculomotor
   c. Dorsal motor X
   d. Trigeminal motor
   e. Substantia nigra
   f. Nucleus basalis Meynert
   g. Red nucleus
   h. Abducens

Answers: a, c, e, g. The four pigmented nuclei are one *red* (red nucleus, Fig. 4–8), one *blue* (locus ceruleus), and two *black* nuclei (substantia nigra and dorsal motor X).

378. A 45-year-old man is brought to the emergency room where he is initially belligerent and then stuporous. He is jaundiced, anemic, and has signs of a recent gastrointestinal hemorrhage superimposed on chronic cirrhosis. A neurologic examination shows asterixis and bilateral Babinski signs but equal pupils and no hemiparesis. A CT of the head was normal. What would an EEG most likely reveal?
   a. α activity
   b. Electrocerebral silence
   c. Triphasic waves
   d. 3-Hz spike-and-wave activity

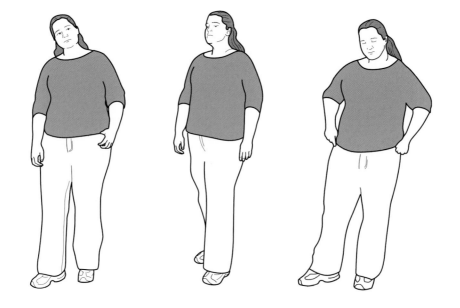

Answer: c. The patient has hepatic encephalopathy in which the EEG typically contains triphasic waves. EEG α activity is found in normal, alert individuals who have their eyes closed. They must be free of anxiety and not concentrating. Electrocerebral silence is found in brain death, and 3-Hz spike-and-wave activity characterizes absence seizures.

379. A 60-year-old man with Parkinson's disease was under treatment with deprenyl and L-dopa-carbidopa. When depression developed, SSRI treatment was initiated. Two days later, he began to be agitated, confused, febrile (temperature 100°F), diaphoretic, rigid, and tremulous and have myoclonus. His CPK was 120 U/L. Which syndrome has probably developed?
   a. Dopamine intoxication
   b. Neuroleptic malignant syndrome
   c. Serotonin syndrome
   d. None of the above

Answer: c. The serotonin syndrome is characterized by mental status changes, autonomic disturbances, and muscle abnormalities. It follows the administration of various medications that increase serotonin activity to toxic levels. It is a rare condition with features similar to the neuroleptic malignant syndrome; however, its fever and CPK elevations are not as pronounced. The serotonin syndrome has been described following administration of SSRIs; MAO inhibitors, including deprenyl; other antidepressants, including the heterocyclics and tricyclics; and the serotoninergic migraine medication, sumatriptan.

380. Which one of the following illnesses results from an RNA-containing infectious agent?
   a. Creutzfeldt-Jakob disease
   b. Bovine spongiform encephalopathy
   c. Scrapie
   d. AIDS-dementia

Answer: d. HIV, which is an RNA retrovirus, causes AIDS-dementia. The other conditions are caused by prions, which contain neither RNA nor DNA. Scrapie is a prion disease of sheep.

381. A 76-year-old woman survived a nondominant cerebral hemisphere stroke but has residual left hemiparesis and sensory impairment. She sometimes finds that at night her left hand moves about and touches her leg or trunk. Sometimes the woman jolts upright, fearful that the hand, which she believes is not hers, is groping at her. Similarly, during the daytime, she jokes that the hand feels like her late husband's. What is the most likely explanation?

   a. Narcolepsy, with hallucinations
   b. Panic attacks
   c. Nocturnal epilepsy
   d. Alien hand syndrome
   e. A delusion
   f. None of the above

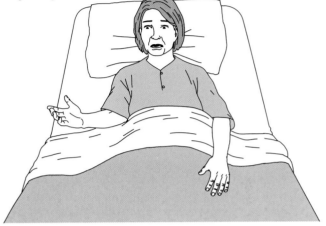

I was frightened, very frightened! In the middle of the night the hand began to grab me all over!

Answer: d. In the alien hand syndrome, which typically follows a nondominant hemisphere stroke, a patient's hand retains some rudimentary motor and sensory functions. Patients feel that their hand is physically and psychologically detached. Moreover, someone else (the alien) governs the movements.

382–389. In assigning a value to a biologic test for a disease, what will be the effect of the following changes (Q382–Q389) on the test's sensitivity and specificity (a–i)?
   a. Sensitivity and specificity will both increase.
   b. Sensitivity and specificity will both decrease.
   c. Sensitivity and specificity will remain unchanged.
   d. Sensitivity will increase and specificity will decrease.
   e. Sensitivity will decrease and specificity will increase.
   f. Sensitivity will increase.
   g. Sensitivity will decrease.
   h. Specificity will increase
   i. Specificity will decrease.

382. Technical changes in the test that increase false-negative results.

383. Technical changes that increase true-positive results.

384. Using the test on a population in which the disease is less prevalent.

385. Technical changes that increase false-positive results.

386. Technical changes that increase true-negative results.

387. Lowering the cut off point of the test results so that both true- and false-positive results increase.

388. Changing the cut off point of the test results so that both true- and false-negative results increase.

389. Testing for a disease in which individuals with and without the disease can be more readily identified.

Answers: 382-g, 383-f, 384-c, 385-i, 386-h, 387-d, 388-e, 389-a.

Sensitivity is defined as the proportion of true-positive results. It equals true-positives / (true-positives + false-negatives). This formula is equivalent to true-positives / all positives. A highly sensitive test will detect almost all individuals with a disease; however, depending on its sensitivity, the test may also incorrectly identify individuals who do not actually have the disease.

Specificity is defined as the proportion of valid negative results. It equals true-negatives / (true-negatives + false-positives). Specificity increases either when true-negatives increase or false-positives decrease, but it is not directly proportional to true positives. In other words, if a highly specific test is positive, the patient is highly likely to have the illness; however, a negative result may not exclude it.

Tests proposed for Alzheimer's disease must be highly specific and sensitive because the clinical diagnosis is approximately 90% accurate.

390. Which of the following AEDs inhibit the hepatic cytochrome P-450 oxidases?
a. Valproate (valproic acid/divalproex) (Depakote)
b. Carbamazepine (Tegretol)
c. Phenytoin (Dilantin)
d. Gabapentin (Neurontin)
e. Phenobarbital

Answer: a. Valproate is the only commonly used AED that inhibits the P-450 enzyme system. Carbamazepine, phenytoin, and phenobarbital all induce the enzyme system. Thus, these AEDs reduce the effectiveness of oral contraceptives and other medications. Gabapentin, lamotrigine, and vigabatrin have little or no effect on the enzyme system.

391. Which of the following AEDs induces its own metabolism?
a. Valproate (valproic acid/divalproex) (Depakote)
b. Carbamazepine (Tegretol)
c. Phenytoin (Dilantin)
d. Gabapentin (Neurontin)
e. Phenobarbital

Answer: b. Carbamazepine autoinduces its own metabolism. Thus, physicians must rapidly increase the dosage of carbamazepine at the start of treatment.

392. During her initial visit for a contact lens prescription, an ophthalmologist finds that a 17-year-old high school student's left pupil is 6 mm and, with bright light, constricts slowly and incompletely. Her right pupil is 3 mm and constricts briskly and completely to bright light. Lenses correct her vision to 20/20 bilaterally. She has no diplopia, ptosis, headache, or other ophthalmologic symptom or sign, but she has no patellar reflexes. Which would be the appropriate test?
a. Nerve conduction studies
b. CT or MRI of the head
c. Tensilon test
d. Instillation of dilute (0.1%) pilocarpine eye drops

Answer: d. Instillation of dilute (0.1%) pilocarpine eye drops will not affect the right (normal) pupil, but will probably cause constriction of the dilated, left pupil. A pupil's constricting from the dilute solution indicates that its constrictor muscles have denervation supersensitivity. That abnormality, an Adie's pupil, results from ciliary ganglia damage. Loss of patellar reflexes often accompanies an Adie's pupil. Although she has dysfunction of parasympathetic innervation of the left pupil and absent patellar reflexes, she has no indication of a peripheral neuropathy that would be detectable by nerve conduction studies. She has no symptoms or signs of a cerebral mass lesion, such as headache, stupor, or Babinski signs, that might cause transtentorial herniation and an oculomotor nerve palsy. A Tensilon test, useful in detecting myasthenia gravis, would be superfluous. Myasthenia gravis does not affect the pupils and she has none of its usual symptoms, such as diplopia, ptosis, dysarthria, and face weakness.

393. A psychiatrist is asked to consult for a 23-year-old woman with the emergence of dementia following approximately 2 months of painful paresthesia in her legs and depression. She had previously been in good health and had no family history of neurologic disease. Her neurologic examination showed subtle myoclonus but no lateralized signs or indications of increased intracranial pressure. The MRI showed increased signal intensity in the posterior thalamus (the pulvinar) but no mass lesions. The EEG was nonspecifically abnormal. The spinal fluid, on routine testing, showed a mildly elevated protein but normal cell count, glucose, and tests for

syphilis, cryptococcal antigen, and HIV. Which should be the next test?
a. Repeat the LP for CSF test for 14–3-3 protein.
b. Send serum for tests for paraneoplastic antibodies.
c. Send serum for a bismuth level
d. Inquire further about sleep patterns.
e. The physician should perform all of the above.

Answer: e. The problem is the rapid onset of dementia in a young adult without the usual causes, such as a mass lesion, prior illness, or HIV disease. These tests concern vCJD and its sister illness, fatal familial insomnia; paraneoplastic limbic encephalopathy; and toxins, particularly bismuth. The prominent sensory changes and the MRI findings, despite the absence of periodic sharp-wave complexes, which is expectable, indicate that vCJD is the most likely diagnosis.

394. A 2-year-old boy with mental retardation has dislocated ocular lenses, pectus excavatum, and an increased length for his age. An increased concentration of homocystine in his urine leads to a diagnosis of homocystinuria. Which of the following is the most common complication of the illness?
a. Dementia
b. Strokes
c. Autism
d. Epilepsy

Answer: b. Approximately 50% of individuals with homocystinuria suffer thromboembolic events. One third of them have strokes. Unlike individuals with trisomy 21, individuals with homocystinuria do not have progressive cognitive impairment. Although homocystinuria patients often have behavior disorders, obsessive-compulsive symptoms, and personality disturbances, they do not show features of autism.

395. In the previous question, which treatment will best lower the homocystine level?
a. A methionine-free diet
b. A homocysteine-free diet
c. Administration of folate and vitamins B_6 and B_{12}
d. L-dopa

Answer: c. Folate and vitamins B_6 and B_{12} will reduce serum homocystine levels. Administered to asymptomatic infants, they will also reduce the incidence of mental retardation and strokes.

396. Deficiency of which enzyme causes homocystinuria?
a. Cystathionine synthase
b. Tyrosine hydroxylase
c. Hypoxanthine-guanine transferase (HGPRT)
d. Phenylalanine hydroxylase

Answer: a. Cystathionine synthase metabolizes homocysteine to cystathionine. Its absence leads to an accumulation of homocysteine. An elevated serum level of homocysteine, as occurs in homocystinuria or for unknown reasons in the adult population, is a risk factor for stroke.

397. Neurosurgeons often perform temporal lobe resection (lobectomy) to alleviate refractory epilepsy. Of the following, which is the most likely potential complication of this procedure?
a. Dementia and delirium
b. Amnesia and aphasia
c. Increase in seizures
d. Neuroleptic malignant syndrome

Answer: b. Resection of temporal lobe tissue containing the hippocampus, especially if the contralateral region is defective, may produce amnesia or the Klüver-Bucy syndrome. Resection of the dominant temporal lobe may cause language impairment. In addition, transient depression can complicate such surgery. However, surgeons may remove the entire nondominant lobe and an anterior portion of the dominant hemisphere with impunity. Complications of epilepsy surgery occur rarely and the potential benefits of surgery greatly outweigh its risks.

398. Emergency Medical Services brings in a young man to the emergency room after he swallowed almost an entire bottle of pills of an unknown medication. He is agitated, confused, combative, and unable to provide a coherent history or cooperate with the examination. His temperature is 104°F and pulse 101 bpm. His skin is hot and dry. His pupils are large but reactive. He moves all his limbs, which have no tremor, rigidity, or increased tone. His bladder is distended and he has no bowel sounds. Which is the most likely category of medical intoxication?
a. Opioid
b. Serotonin reuptake inhibitor
c. Anticholinesterase
d. Anticholinergic

Answer: d. Anticholinergic medicines, such as scopolamine, cause agitated delirium and suppress parasympathetic activity. Thus, they cause hot, dry skin and suppress bowel and bladder function. They also allow excessive sympathetic activity, which leads to tachycardia and mydriasis. Opioids cause small pupils and, with overdose, pulmonary edema. Some anticholinesterase medicines, such as pyridostigmine, do not cross the blood–brain barrier and do not alter mental status. Anticholinesterase medicines (cholinesterase inhibitors) that cross the blood–brain barrier, such as physostigmine and donepezil, do not cause agitated delirium, but they can cause abdominal cramping and diarrhea from gastrointestinal hyperactivity.

399. Which of the followings statements regarding prions is false?
   a. Inoculation may occur through non-neurologic as well as neurologic portals.
   b. The usually short incubation period lengthens with transmission.
   c. Individuals with a defective gene on chromosome 20 are susceptible to prion infections.
   d. The infection strikes the brain predominantly or exclusively.

Answer: b. The incubation period is usually long, but it shortens with both intraspecies and interspecies transmission. Prions enter the host through non-neurologic portals, such as when animals have eaten CNS scraps of infected animals, as well as neurologic portals, as when infected CNS tissue is injected into host animal's brain. Individuals with a mutant PRNP gene, which is encoded on chromosome 20, are susceptible to Creutzfeldt-Jakob disease and vCJD. The brain remains the target organ; however, the olfactory nerves and lymphatic tissue of the ileum also show signs of infection.

400. Of the following MRI abnormalities associated with MS, which is most closely associated with cognitive impairment?
   a. Total lesion area or volume
   b. Enlarged cerebral ventricles
   c. Corpus callosum atrophy
   d. Periventricular white matter demyelination

Answer: a. In MS, cognitive impairment is more closely associated with total lesion area or volume visualized on MRI ("the lesion load") than other MRI abnormalities. Cognitive impairment is also associated with physical disability, duration of the illness, and, as portrayed on PET, cerebral hypometabolism.

401. During the evaluation of a 66-year-old man for the onset of dementia, the physician asked the patient to copy a sequence of four sets, each of three squares followed by a circle. After completing one set, the patient copied only the squares. When he was unable to complete the task, he shouted, cursed, and broke the pencil. An MRI showed generalized cerebral atrophy, especially in the frontal lobes. Of the following, which is the most likely underlying pathology?
   a. Plaques and tangles
   b. Spirochetes in gummas
   c. Intraneuronal argentophilic inclusions
   d. Intraneuronal eosinophilic intracytoplasmic inclusions

Answer: c. As in Question 307, this patient showed perseveration, easy frustration, emotional outburst, decrease in verbal output, and lack of inhibition. These symptoms indicate frontal lobe dysfunction. The underlying problem could be either vascular dementia or, more likely, frontotemporal dementia. Many cases of frontotemporal dementia, which are labeled Pick's disease, are characterized by intraneuronal argentophilic inclusions. Spirochetes in gummas are found in neurosyphilis. Intraneuronal eosinophilic intracytoplasmic inclusions are Lewy bodies, which are a sign of dementia with Lewy bodies.

402. The police bring a 17-year-old boy to the emergency room when, following a verbal fight with his parents, he seems to have developed quadriparesis and blindness. Nevertheless, his motor tone, DTRs, plantar reflexes, and cranial nerves are intact. His pupils are 4 mm, round, and reactive to light. In addition, when rotating a drum with vertical stripes in front of him, his eyes repetitively follow the stripes and then snap back, but again follow the stripes. What is the implication of his ocular movements?
   a. He has ingested PCP or related toxin.
   b. He should be given thiamine.
   c. His opticokinetic nystagmus is intact.
   d. He has sustained a traumatic injury to his occipital lobe.

Answer: c. He has intact opticokinetic nystagmus, which is a normal, irresistible ocular motility reflex. It indicates that his visual and ocular motility pathways are intact. Its presence in someone who seems to be blind suggests that the "visual loss" has a psychogenic basis. Other tests can also indicate that a visual loss has a psychogenic basis. A simple one is for the physician to smile, make ridiculous faces, or hold attractive pictures in front of a patient. Alternatively, the physician might hold a mirror in front of the patient: If people can see, they cannot resist following their image. An EEG will show occipital alpha rhythm in physiologically normal individuals when they are at rest with closed eyes; however, when they open their eyes, the alpha rhythm disappears: Thus, people with psychogenic blindness will lose their alpha activity when they open their eyes. Normal visual evoked responses also indicate an intact visual pathway.

403. A psychiatrist hospitalized a 38-year-old woman for agitated depression with dangerous psychotic features. Despite treatment with antipsychotic and antidepressant medication, she remains agitated. She continually paces and, when sitting, has rhythmic, continual adduction and abduction leg movements. Which is the least likely explanation for the leg movements?

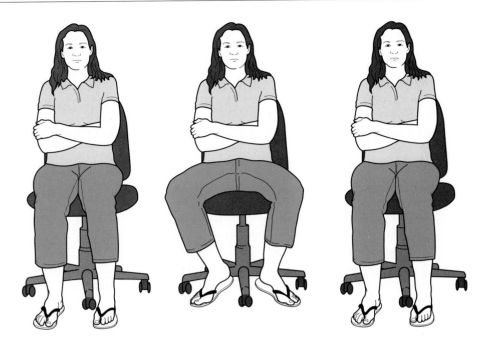

a. Prolonged effect of an illicit drug, such as cocaine
b. Akathisia
c. Undertreatment of the agitated depression
d. Chorea

Answer: d. The possibilities in this situation include the paradox of undertreatment failing to suppress symptoms and overtreatment causing iatrogenic akathisia. Alternatively, cocaine or other stimulant use may cause psychologic and physical agitation. Chorea does not cause agitation and the movements are not rhythmic.

404. Which statement is true concerning Angelman's syndrome?
   a. Angelman's syndrome occurs exclusively in girls.
   b. Children with Angelman's syndrome have imprinted behavior, as described by Konrad Lorenz.
   c. Angelman's syndrome's phenotype is determined by genetic imprinting.
   d. An Angelman's syndrome boy is likely to have a sister with Prader-Willi syndrome.

Answer: c. In Angelman's syndrome and its counterpart, Prader-Willi syndrome, the condition's phenotype depends on which parent transmitted the defective gene (genetic imprinting). Konrad Lorenz described behavioral imprinting among social animals, which is a quite different phenomenon. His theories won him a Nobel Prize in 1973.

405. Which one of the following statements is true regarding adults with ADHD?

a. Although stimulants may be effective therapy in children with ADHD, they are usually ineffective in adults with ADHD.
b. Most cases of childhood ADHD persist in adults.
c. Adults with ADHD usually benefit from phenobarbital.
d. ADHD adults are liable to develop antisocial personality disorder.

Answer: d. Stimulants are effective in adult as well as childhood ADHD. About 15% of children with ADHD grow into adults with ADHD. Phenobarbital and other sedatives are apt to cause paradoxical hyperactivity in both ADHD children and adults. ADHD adults are liable to develop antisocial personality disorder, substance abuse, and other problems.

406. Which change in second messenger characterizes dopamine D_1 receptors?
   a. Adenyl cyclase
   b. Acetyl choline
   c. COMT
   d. NMDA

Answer: a. Increased activity of dopamine D_1 receptors increases AMP production through increased adenyl cyclase.

407. Match the sign (a–g) with its closest implication (1–6).
   a. Babinski
   b. Lhermitte
   c. Romberg

d. Tinel
e. Lasègue's
f. Hoover
g. Abductor
1. Irritation of a lumbar nerve root
2. Spinal cord posterior column impairment
3. Corticospinal tract injury
4. Cervical spinal cord irritation
5. Psychogenic leg paresis
6. Compression of the median nerve

Answer: a-3, b-4, c-2, d-6, e-1, f-5, g-5.

408. In assessing a highly accomplished physician for dementia, in the absence of prior neuropsychologic testing, which of the following is the *least* reliable indication of cognitive decline?
   a. Results of a current neuropsychologic battery
   b. Scores obtained on a current Scholastic Achievement Test (SAT) compared to those in high school
   c. Comparison of current to high school mathematical ability
   d. Job performance, regardless of the results on the neuropsychologic tests

Answer: c. Mathematical ability is an isolated cognitive function that does not reflect overall cognitive capacity. Even in highly successful, intellectual individuals, mathematical ability may not have been well developed during childhood. Moreover, with lack of use, mathematical skills atrophy. In contrast, vocabulary and reading skills, which are deeply ingrained ("overlearned"), are highly resistant to cognitive impairment.

409. Which medication produces the lowest relapse rate in chronic alcoholics?
   a. Naltrexone
   b. Disulfiram
   c. SSRIs
   d. Lithium

Answer: a.

410. On a neurologic examination, a 10-year-old boy, with 6 months of behavioral and academic difficulties, has clumsiness, Babinski signs, and inability to walk "in tandem" (one foot in front of the other [heel-to-toe walking]). The MRI showed extensive cerebral demyelination with surrounding inflammation. In retrospect, an older brother had the same illness but succumbed to adrenal failure before it was diagnosed. Which one of the following statements is false?
   a. The patient's urine will probably contain metachromatic granules.

   b. Adrenal replacement therapy will correct the adrenal insufficiency but not the neurologic deterioration.
   c. This condition can mimic MS; however, it typically occurs in children, leads to death in approximately 5 years, and is characterized by adrenal failure.
   d. This condition results from defective peroxisomes.

Answer: a. He and his brother have had adrenoleukodystrophy (ALD), which is an X-linked leukodystrophy that begins in childhood. Because ALD, like MS, is a leukodystrophy, the MRI in both conditions shows a similar loss of white matter. Unlike MS, however, ALD typically presents with behavioral, emotional, and cognitive difficulties. Soon afterward corticospinal tract and cerebellar signs develop and predominate. At the same time, the adrenal glands fail. ALD results from the accumulation of very long chain fatty acids because of defective peroxisomes, which are intracellular organelles.

Metachromatic granules in the urine indicate metachromatic leukodystrophy (MLD). This illness is another CNS demyelinating disease that usually presents in childhood, but often not until the young adult years. Unlike ALD, MLD is inherited in an autosomal recessive pattern and does not cause adrenal insufficiency.

411. In normal sexual arousal, what is the role of nitric oxide?
   a. It leads to vasoconstriction.
   b. It promotes the production of cGMP-phosphodiesterase.
   c. It promotes cGMP activity.
   d. It leads to amnesia.

Answer: c. Nitric oxide promotes cyclic guanylate cyclase monophosphate (cGMP) activity, which leads to vasodilation. The vasodilation leads to genital engorgement.

412. What is the mechanism of action of sildenafil (Viagra)?
   a. It increases cGMP activity.
   b. It enhances cGMP-phosphodiesterase.
   c. It promotes the production of cyclic guanylate cyclase monophosphate (cGMP).
   d. It provokes the release of nitric oxide (NO).

Answer: a. Sildenafil (Viagra) increases cGMP activity by inhibiting its metabolic enzyme (cGMP-phosphodiesterase).

413. A 40-year-old woman developed burning and prickly sensations in her feet when trying to fall asleep. She had less pronounced symptoms during the daytime. The sensations caused her, she felt, to have irregular movements of her legs and feet. They compelled her to pace around her bedroom for one hour before being able to sleep. Once asleep, she had regular dorsiflexion of her feet and ankles. General medical, neurologic, and psychiatric evaluations revealed no serious abnormalities. Which test should be performed next?

a. PSG
b. MRI
c. EEG
d. Routine blood chemistry and complete blood count
e. MSLT
f. None of the above

Answer: d. She has RLS, which, in 80% of cases, is associated with periodic leg movements. Although the features overlap, she does not have akathisia. Causes of RLS include ischemic, diabetic, and uremic polyneuropathy, iron deficiency, and pregnancy—conditions that should be detectable on a general medical examination or routine blood tests. Although PSG studies might confirm periodic movements, they are unnecessary in RLS because that diagnosis is usually obvious.

414. Which of the following statements concerning melatonin is false?

a. Tryptophan is the amino acid from which melatonin is synthesized.
b. Its primary metabolic product is serotonin.
c. Selective serotonin reuptake inhibitors can increase plasma serotonin concentration.
d. Tryptophan deficiency reduces melatonin plasma concentration.
e. Melatonin is an indolamine.

Answer: b. Melatonin is synthesized through the following synthetic pathway:

$$\text{tryptophan} \rightarrow \text{serotonin} \rightarrow$$
$$N\text{-acetyl-serotonin} \rightarrow \text{melatonin}$$

415. Which of these statements concerning melatonin is false?

a. The suprachiasmatic nucleus of the hypothalamus contains receptors for melatonin.
b. Melatonin is synthesized and secreted from the pineal gland during darkness.
c. Bright light enhances melatonin synthesis and secretion.
d. Melatonin is probably the method by which light-dark cycles regulate circadian hormonal secretion.

Answer: c. Bright light suppresses melatonin synthesis and secretion. Darkness enhances its synthesis and secretion from the pineal gland. Melatonin receptors on the suprachiasmatic nucleus probably allow melatonin to influence circadian hormone rhythm and the sleep-wake cycle.

416. A 26-year-old woman consults a neurologist for 6 weeks of recurring headaches. She had no history of migraine or tension headache, trauma, infections, or risk factors for AIDS. She had irregular menses. She is obese. She has florid papilledema and bilateral abducens nerve palsies. She is fully alert and able to ambulate. She has no ataxia. Of the following, which should be the next diagnostic step?

a. Perform tests for AIDS.
b. Obtain a head CT or MRI.
c. Perform an LP, which will be therapeutic as well as diagnostic.
d. None of the above.

Answer: b. This patient's age, obesity, menstrual irregularity, and absence of focal findings indicate that she has idiopathic intracranial hypertension (pseudotumor cerebri). Before performing an LP to confirm the diagnosis, she should undergo either a CT or MRI to exclude tumor, obstructive hydrocephalus, and other causes of increased intracranial pressure. Some studies indicate that obstructed intracranial venous sinuses underlie some cases of this disorder.

417. In the preceding question, what is a CT most likely to reveal?

a. Normal brain and ventricles
b. Dilated ventricles
c. Small or "slit-like" ventricles
d. Transtentorial herniation

Answer: c. As if the brain were simply swollen from its interstitial edema, the ventricles are compressed. The cerebral swelling also stretches and impairs the function of the sixth cranial nerves, which produces the abducens nerve palsies.

418. What is the effect of dopamine's stimulating D_2 receptors?

a. The interaction increases adenyl cyclase activity.
b. The interaction decreases adenyl cyclase activity.
c. The interaction has no effect on adenyl cyclase activity.

Answer: b. Dopamine-D_1 receptor interaction increases adenyl cyclase activity, but dopamine-D_2 receptor interaction reduces adenyl cyclase activity.

419. A 6-year-old boy begins to have inward turning of his left foot that is most pronounced after school is finished at 3:00 PM. One trick that he shows his parents—he has no friends—is that when he walks backward, the foot assumes a normal position. The boy's pediatrician conceded that the boy probably had sustained a subtle congenital cerebral injury ("cerebral palsy"). When the neurologist evaluated the boy at 4:00 PM, he had intermittent, sustained, inward turning of both legs and rotation of the lower trunk. DTRs were normal. The next morning, the neurologist saw no such movements. Which of the following will be least productive?

a. Inquire as to the ethnicity, as well as the health, of the boy's parents and grandparents.
b. Prescribe a therapeutic trial of L-dopa.
c. Restrict phenylalanine-containing foods.
d. Check for the DYT1 gene.
e. Determine the serum ceruloplasmin concentration.

Answer: c. The diurnal fluctuation of dystonia in children indicates dopamine-responsive dystonia (DRD). Other affected family members should be sought. Tricks that temporarily abolish dystonia—walking backward, skipping, dancing, or applying pressure to the involved limb—confirm a diagnosis of dystonia. Other causes of dystonia in childhood include early onset primary dystonia, which is found predominantly in Ashkenazi Jews and identified by the DYT1 gene, and Wilson's disease. None of them produces a diurnal fluctuation. Phenylketonuria, which would be treated by restricting phenylalanine-containing foods, becomes apparent in infancy and is characterized by mental retardation but not dystonia.

420. Which term is applied to cell death that is programmed, sequential, and energy requiring?
a. Necrosis
b. Apoptosis
c. Anoxia
d. None of the above

Answer: b.

421. Which one of the following is not a characteristic of apoptosis?
a. It is the mechanism of cell death in Huntington's disease and ALS.
b. In Huntington's disease, inflammatory cells surround dying cells.
c. Some organs, such as the thymus gland, mature through apoptosis.
d. Apoptosis is often referred to as "programmed cell death."
e. Apoptosis requires energy.

Answer: b. In apoptosis, which is the mechanism of cell death in Huntington's disease, cell death does not provoke an inflammatory response. In contrast, necrosis elicits a prominent inflammatory response.

422. Which of the following statements concerning the tissue oxidation is false?
a. Free radicals are oxidants.
b. Oxidants have one or more unpaired electrons and seek to acquire electrons.
c. Oxidation is fatal to tissue.
d. Normal cellular metabolism produces oxidants that are detoxified by mitochondria.
e. Tissue oxidation leads to lactic acidosis.

Answer: e. Mitochondrial disorders lead to lactic acidosis. According to the oxidative stress theory of Parkinson's disease, oxidants are incompletely removed by defective mitochondria and the ensuing tissue oxidation destroys basal ganglia.

423. Which of the following characteristics is responsible for paramagnetic agents, such as gadolinium, being able to increase the signal of cerebral lesions during MRI studies?
a. They cross the intact as well as the permeable blood–brain barrier.
b. They attenuate ionizing radiation.
c. They alter the time for protons to resume their alignment after RF signals have been applied.
d. They release photons.

Answer: c. Paramagnetic agents used in MRI do not cross the intact blood–brain barrier. However, when tumors, abscesses, and other lesions disrupt the barrier, these agents penetrate into surrounding brain. Paramagnetic agents alter the time for protons to resume their alignment in magnetic fields. CT depends on ionizing radiation. Radioligands used in PET and SPECT release photons.

424. Which of the following statements regarding radioligands in PET and SPECT is true?
a. These radioligands have a half-life that typically exceeds 7 days.
b. In PET, the radioligands release positrons, which interact with electrons. The reaction annihilates both particles. Their masses are converted into 2 photons.
c. In PET, radioligands produce an anatomic image that has the same resolution as CT.
d. PET radioligands are specific enough to diagnose Alzheimer's disease.

Answer: b. PET produces a relatively gross anatomic image. It can suggest Alzheimer's disease and frontotemporal dementia but not with the specificity required by a clinician.

425. A 33-year-old man with MS has paraparesis and a left-sided visual impairment. He says that the neurologist's red tie appears maroon when he uses only his left eye, but red when he uses only his right eye. Which is the most likely explanation for his visual perception problem?
   a. He has color blindness.
   b. The MS has affected his occipital cortex.
   c. He has a persistent ocular migraine.
   d. He has color desaturation.
   e. He has developed a psychogenic disturbance.

Answer: d. He has color desaturation, which is a common manifestation of optic neuritis. Color blindness, especially the red-green variety, is a sex-linked genetic disorder that affects both eyes and is detectable in childhood. MS can affect the occipital cortex, but lesions there would cause hemianopsia and not affect color perception in this manner. Ocular migraines can cause a unilateral scotoma but not color perception impairments.

426. PET and SPECT use ligands that produce photons. Which of the following does not describe the general composition of ligands?
   a. Organic molecules bound to a radioisotope
   b. Organic molecules bound to a central metal ion, such as hemoglobin
   c. Organic molecules bound to an inorganic molecule
   d. Organic molecules bound to a tracer element

Answer: c.

427. This is the MRI of a 23-year-old man who had noticed that he had been losing hearing ability in his left ear for one year. The MRI was performed during infusion of gadolinium. Where is the lesion located?

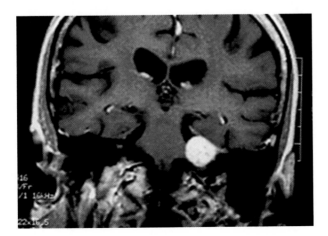

   a. Lateral to the pons
   b. In the pons
   c. In the temporal lobe
   d. None of the above

Answer: a. The lesion arises from the acoustic nerve, which can be seen as a bright streak above and medial to the lesion. The lesion is located in the cerebellopontine angle.

428. The man described in the previous question undergoes surgery. Most of the lesion is removed. Facial strength and most of his hearing are preserved. What is the most likely histology of the lesion?
   a. Glioblastoma
   b. Medulloblastoma
   c. Neuroma
   d. Meningioma

Answer: c. Although a meningoma is possible, he most likely has an acoustic neuroma. Glioblastomas and medulloblastomas are intra-axial.

429. The man described in the previous two questions recovers from surgery. He is found to have no abnormalities except for three small *café au lait* spots. He remains asymptomatic for several years, but then the hearing in his right ear begins to fail. An MRI shows a lesion on the right side similar to the initial, left-sided one. What is the most likely underlying diagnosis?
   a. Toxoplasmosis
   b. Neurofibromatosis
   c. Metastatic carcinoma
   d. A mitochondrial disorder

Answer: b. Bilateral acoustic neuromas indicate that he has the "central type" of neurofibromatosis (NF2), which is inherited on chromosome 22 in an autosomal dominant pattern. Unlike the more common "peripheral" variety of neurofibromatosis (NF1), NF2 produces few neurofibromas or café au lait spots.

430. Which of the following abnormalities is least likely to be found in a 66-year-old man with hypertension who suddenly developed left hemiparesis 2 days before an examination?
   a. Inability to recognize sadness in the face of family members
   b. Inability to draw a simple house
   c. Flattened affect in his speech and facial expression
   d. Tendency to use nonsensical or incorrect words

Answer: d. He has sustained a nondominant stroke, which would cause aprosody, flattened affect, and inability to perceive the emotions of others. He would also have constructional apraxia, which would impair his ability to copy or draw simple figures, such as a clock or a small house. However, he would not make paraphasic errors, which is a feature of aphasia.

431. An 85-year-old retired millionaire is brought to the hospital by his lifelong butler. The patient, who had a 10-year history of Parkinson's disease complicated by dementia, had experienced a seizure. His psychiatrist has been prescribing haloperidol at bedtime because of nocturnal hallucinations, delusions, screaming, and a tendency to wander; however, neither haloperidol nor other antipsychotic controlled his bizarre thinking or abnormal behavior. A CT showed a small acute and larger chronic subdural hematoma. After neurosurgeons drained the subdural hematomas, the patient returned to his usual state. One month later, the patient was readmitted with a fracture-dislocation of his cervical spine and quadriparesis. What is the most likely cause of the repeated hospitalizations?
    a. Falls due to the wandering
    b. Other forms of trauma
    c. Adverse reactions to medications
    d. Age-related deterioration

Answer: a or b. The first admission probably resulted from a combination of acute traumatic bleeding superimposed on a chronic subdural hematoma. The second admission was due to a fall or deliberate trauma that included hyperextension of the head and neck. Physicians should suspect elder abuse in patients with dementia who sustain repeated trauma.

432. A 73-year-old woman was admitted to the hospital immediately after the sudden onset of left-sided hemiparesis. A head CT, performed within two hours, was normal. The neurologists infused tissue plasminogen activator (tPA). During the next 3 days, she became agitated and belligerent. She accused the staff of keeping her in the hospital even though nothing was wrong with her. What is the most likely cause of her feeling that "nothing is wrong"?
    a. The tPA has caused a delirium.
    b. A new stroke developed on the third day of hospitalization.
    c. Anosognosia became manifest.
    d. She has developed dementia.

Answer: c. The thrombolytic agent, tPA, has some potentially serious side effects, such as intracerebral bleeding, but delirium is not one of them. Patients with anosognosia often do not appreciate their situation and reject assistance and medical regimens.

433. As part of a re-evaluation of the patient in the preceding question, this CT was obtained on the fifth hospital day. What does it reveal?

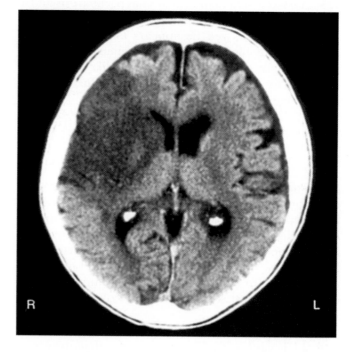

    a. A right middle cerebral artery stroke
    b. A right cerebral tumor
    c. A left middle cerebral artery stroke
    d. Occlusion of the right internal carotid artery
    e. Occlusion of the left internal carotid artery

Answer: a. In keeping with the convention, this CT displays the patient's right side on the left: note the markings. The CT shows a classic pattern of a middle cerebral artery stoke from occlusion of the artery. The tPA failed to dissolve the clot. The middle cerebral artery region is darker than the normal brain because it is necrotic: It has been deprived of relatively radiodense blood. CTs performed within the 2 days after a stroke are often normal because necrosis has not as yet fully developed. In this scan, the right anterior horn of the lateral ventricle is compressed by stroke-induced swelling. In contrast, the regions supplied by the anterior and posterior cerebral arteries are spared. The lesion is not a tumor because the initial CT would have been abnormal; the mass effect on this CT would have been greater, and the lesion does not contain any sign of a mass lesion.

434. During the previous 8 years, a 35-year-old woman has had progressively severe gait impairment, dysarthria, and then cognitive impairment. Her general medical evaluation and routine blood tests were normal. Her neurologic examination revealed signs of dementia, pseudobulbar palsy, optic atrophy, corticospinal tract

impairment, and cerebellar dysfunction. A CT showed only mild cerebral atrophy. Based on her MRI, which portion of the nervous system has been affected?

a. The gray matter
b. CNS myelin
c. All parts of the CNS
d. The ventricular system

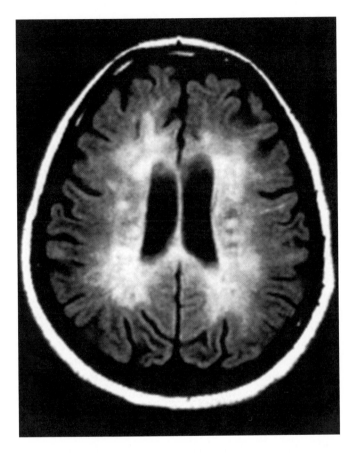

Answer: b. The MRI shows confluent regions of demyelination surrounding the lateral ventricles. It also shows cerebral atrophy. As this case illustrates, MRI is superior to CT in detecting white matter abnormalities.

435. In regard to the patient in the previous question, which of the following illnesses would be least likely to have caused her neurologic symptoms?

a. MS
b. Adrenoleukodystrophy
c. PML
d. Toluene abuse

Answer: b. Each of these conditions, which could cause her symptoms, produces demyelination. However, adrenoleukodystrophy is a sex-linked disorder that usually appears in male infants and children.

When adrenoleukodystrophy affects young men, it causes mania, dementia, and gait impairment accompanied by signs of adrenal insufficiency. Death usually ensues within 2 years after such symptoms appear.

436. A 25-year-old woman has an enlarged and irregular pupil. It remains large when a light is shown into it and has almost no constriction with accommodation. She has no ptosis and no paresis of any extraocular muscle. After a physician instills eyedrops of a dilute solution (0.1%) of pilocarpine, which would not affect a normal pupil, her pupil promptly constricts to smaller than a normal size. What is the etiology of her pupil's enlargement?

a. Sympathetic denervation
b. Parasympathetic denervation
c. Self-induced anisocoria
d. Argyll-Robertson

Answer: b. She has a benign condition that results from parasympathetic denervation, called an Adie's or tonic pupil. The lack of parasympathetic innervation allows the unopposed sympathetic innervation to dilate the pupil and prevents a reaction to light. In addition, the loss of parasympathetic innervation leads to denervation hypersensitivity, which causes the affected pupil to respond unusually rapidly and forcefully to the stimulation of cholinergic agents. In contrast, pupils with sympathetic denervation, such as in Horner's syndrome, are small and react briskly to sympathomimetic agents.

437. Which of the following statements regarding the actions of serotonin receptors in migraines is false?

a. Sumatriptan is a 5-HT$_{1D}$ agonist.
b. Sumatriptan-5-HT$_{1D}$ receptor interactions produce vasoconstriction.
c. Dihydroergotamine (DHE), which is also a vasoconstrictor, produces the same effect as the triptans.

Answer: c. Both the triptans and DHE produce cerebral vasoconstriction and alleviate the headache; however, the triptans, but not DHE, alleviate a migraine's autonomic nervous system symptoms.

438. Which is the phenotype of untreated infants with congenital absence of phenylalanine hydroxylase?

a. Mental retardation, deafness, and epilepsy
b. Episodes of encephalopathy and lactic acidosis
c. Self-mutilation, mental retardation, hyperuricemia, dystonia, and spasticity

d. Mental retardation, eczema, and fair complexion

e. Rigidity, dystonia, and gait impairment that occur in the late afternoon

Answer: d. Infants with congenital absence of phenylalanine hydroxylase have phenylketonuria (PKU), which causes mental retardation, eczema, and lack of pigment in the hair and eyes. Mental retardation, deafness, and epilepsy suggest a congenital rubella infection. Episodic encephalopathy and lactic acidosis suggest a mitochondrial DNA disorder. The combination of mental retardation, self-mutilation, hyperuricemia, dystonia, and spasticity indicates Lesch-Nyhan syndrome. Rigidity, dystonia, and gait impairment that occur in the late afternoon indicate dopamine-responsive dystonia.

439. In which chromosome is amyloid precursor protein (APP) encoded?
   a. 4
   b. 17
   c. 21
   d. X
   e. O

Answer: c.

440. A 60-year-old woman reports having had several episodes, each lasting several days, of incapacitating dizziness. The dizziness develops suddenly and is associated with nausea, but not tinnitus or hearing loss. The physician determined that the dizziness is actually vertigo and that it is present only when her head changes position. During the examination, when she is supine, with her head and neck hyperextended and her head rotated 45 degrees to the right, she develops vertigo and nystagmus. The rest of her neurologic examination, audiometry, and an MRI scan of her brain are normal. Which is the best treatment?
   a. Neurosurgery for an acoustic neuroma
   b. Canalith repositioning maneuvers
   c. ASA for basilar artery TIAs
   d. An SSRI for panic attacks

Answer: b. The maneuver that led to nystagmus (the Dix-Hallpike Test) indicates that she has benign positional vertigo. Recent evidence indicates that this disorder results from dislodged debris in a semicircular canal (otoliths). Canalith repositioning is a therapeutic maneuver that consists of the physician's hyperextending and then rotating the patient's head, which moves the otoliths from the semicircular canal to the utricle.

441. Which of the following antidepressants is most likely to cause priapism?
   a. Fluvoxamine

   b. Fluoxetine
   c. Bupropion
   d. Trazodone
   e. Paroxetine

Answer: d.

442. During the past year, a 10-year-old boy has developed a progressively severe involuntary tendency for his left foot to turn inward when he walks. However, the movement does not occur when he walks backward, dances, or sleeps. His neurologic examination, including cognitive function, is otherwise normal. A serum ceruloplasmin, MRI of his head, EEG, and routine studies were normal. A trial of L-dopa produced no benefit. Which statement is correct?
   a. The gait abnormality's pattern, with a normal evaluation, is indicative of a psychogenic disturbance.
   b. He probably has Sydenham's chorea.
   c. His ethnicity is paramount.
   d. He should have an immediate orthopedic evaluation.
   e. He should have an MRI of the spine.

Answer: c. A gait impairment that is abolished by walking backward, skipping, dancing, or running may be due to a psychogenic disturbance; however, it much more likely represents a "trick" that individuals with dystonia unconsciously employ to suppress or circumvent an involuntary movement. He should be evaluated for early onset dystonia, which is due to the DYT1 gene and is usually confined to Ashkenazi (Eastern European) Jews. The course is too long for Sydenham's chorea.

443. Match each description (a–n) with the region (1–9) on the illustration below. If appropriate, use more than one letter for each number.

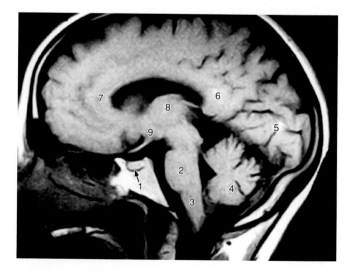

a. Structure where the optic nerves' nasal fibers cross

b. Cortex where the optic tracts terminate

c. Structure that secretes ACTH

d. Structure where face and body pain tracts synapse

e. Structure where the fasciculus gracilis and f. cuneatus terminate

f. Structure damaged when patients have alexia without agraphia

g. Contains nuclei for cranial nerves VI, VII, and VIII

h. Contains the dorsal raphe nuclei

i. Structure injured when patients have crossed hypalgesia and Horner's syndrome ipsilateral to facial numbness

j. Structure contains caudal raphe nuclei

k. Structure contains the locus ceruleus

l. Its midline region is the vermis

m. The site of the crossing of the fibers conveying position and vibration sensation

n. Derives from the Greek, *knee*, as in *genuflect*, to bend at the knee in worship

Answers:

1-c. The *pituitary gland* secretes ACTH and other hormones. Note that it is inferior to the optic nerves and chiasm.

2-g, k. The *pons* not only contains the nuclei for cranial nerves VI, VII, and VIII but also the motor division and most of the sensory divisions of cranial nerve 5. The dorsal raphe nuclei, which gives rise to serotonin-generating neurons, are based primarily in the pons but extend into the midbrain. In addition, the pons contains the locus ceruleus, which gives rise to norepinephrine-generating neurons.

3-i, j, m. When patients have crossed hypalgesia and Horner's syndrome ipsilateral to facial numbness, they probably have infarctions in the *medulla* causing the lateral medullary syndrome. The medulla also contains the caudal raphe nuclei, which gives rise to serotonin-generating neurons. Tracts from the caudal raphe nuclei descend into the spinal cord to promote analgesia. Ascending sensory tracts for position and vibration (fasciculus gracilis and f. cuneatus) cross (decussate) in the medial lemniscus, which is located in the medulla.

4-l. The vermis is the inferior, medial structure of the *cerebellum*. In alcoholics, it characteristically undergoes atrophy.

5-b. The optic (the geniculocalcarine) tract terminates in the visual cortex of the *occipital lobe*.

6-f. Tracts conveying written language information from the right occipital lobe to the language centers in the dominant, left cerebral hemisphere must pass through the *splenium of the corpus callosum*.

7-n.

8-d, e. Tracts that convey pain from the face and body—the trigeminal nerve's sensory divisions and the spinothalamic tract, respectively—synapse in the *thalamus*. From there, sensation is widely disbursed to the cerebral cortex, reticular activating system, limbic system, and other areas. The f. gracilis and f. cuneatus, which convey proprioception from the lower and upper extremities, respectively, also terminate in the thalamus. Those sensations are also conveyed to the cortex, particularly the postcentral gyrus.

9-a. The optic nerves' nasal fibers cross at the *optic chiasm*. An optic nerve can be seen anterior and inferior to the hypothalamus.

444–446. A wife sent her 63-year-old husband for psychiatric consultation because of inappropriate behavior. The psychiatrist, finding that the patient had headaches, cognitive impairment, and a mild left-hemiparesis, requested an MRI.

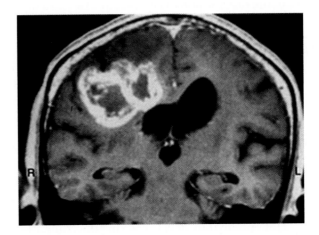

444. Which view has been displayed?

a. Transaxial

b. Axial

c. Sagittal

d. Coronal

e. None of the above

Answer: d.

445. In which region of the brain is the lesion localized?

a. Right frontal-parietal

b. Left frontal-parietal

c. Right temporal

d. Left temporal

e. Right occipital
f. Left occipital

Answer: a. The lesion is in the right cerebral hemisphere (note the letters superimposed on the lateral portion of the skull). It is above and lateral to the lateral ventricle and well above the Sylvian fissure, which separates the temporal lobe from the overlying frontal and temporal lobes.

446. Based on the MRI, which of the following is the most likely etiology?
    a. Hemorrhagic stroke
    b. Thrombotic stroke
    c. Meningioma
    d. Glioblastoma multiforme
    e. MS
    f. PML

Answer: d. The lesion is most likely a glioblastoma multiforme because it is a multilobulated mass that arises from the white matter. It compresses the adjacent lateral ventricle and shifts midline structures. MS plaques and PML, which also arise from the white matter, do not create mass effect. Strokes usually conform to the distribution of cerebral arteries and do not cause mass effect.

447. A psychiatrist is called to evaluate a 13-year-old girl who, after receiving successful treatment for status epilepticus, remains withdrawn, depressed, and amnestic for all events that occurred during the several weeks before the episodes. She had no history of seizures, drug abuse, or other neurologic problem; however, she had had multiple recent admissions for abdominal pain, a spiral humerus fracture, and headaches. The EEG was normal, but a head CT showed a linear, nondepressed skull fracture. Her phenytoin level was in the therapeutic range. Her routine blood tests and toxicology screens were all unremarkable. Which would be the best course of action for the psychiatrist?
    a. Use a tricyclic antidepressant
    b. Use a SSRI
    c. Change her AED
    d. Stop all AEDs
    e. None of the above

Answer: e. In view of the spiral limb fracture, as well as the skull fracture, the psychiatrist should suspect child abuse. Sexual abuse as well as physical abuse is common in children with pseudoseizures.

448. During the previous 2 years, this 7-year-old boy has been developing a progressively severe gait impairment that is most pronounced in the afternoon and evening. During those periods of the day, physicians find that he has a positive pull test and rigidity in all his limbs. When he awakes in the morning, his gait is entirely normal. He has had no cognitive decline, behavioral disturbances, or personality change. There is no family history of this disorder or any other neurologic illness. Which of the following is the most likely cause of his gait impairment?
    a. Dopa-responsive dystonia
    b. DYT1 dystonia
    c. Adrenoleukodystrophy
    d. Athetotic cerebral palsy
    e. Wilson's disease
    f. Huntington's disease

Answer: a. This boy has involuntary movements of all his limbs (as pictured) and a positive pull test, which signifies basal ganglia pathology. Of all the illnesses, only dopa-responsive dystonia has a diurnal fluctuation. Nevertheless, each of these illnesses can appear in childhood and present with gait impairment. Subtle clinical differences can separate some of them.

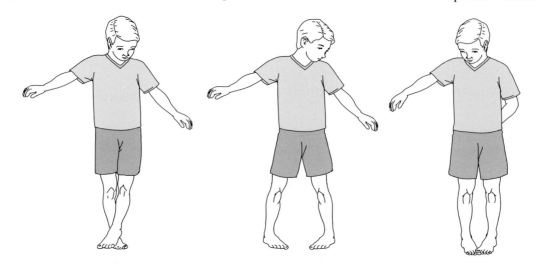

Adrenoleukodystrophy causes spasticity rather than involuntary movements in boys. Athetotic cerebral palsy appears by age 4. The childhood variant of Huntington's disease causes rigidity and, almost simultaneously, cognitive or personality changes. The duration of the illness, as well as the diurnal fluctuation, excludes Sydenham's chorea.

449. Which is the best test for the patient described in the previous question?
  a. MRI
  b. Serum ceruloplasmin
  c. Small doses of L-dopa
  d. Genetic testing
  e. None of the above

  Answer: c. Administering small doses of L-dopa to patients suspected of having dopamine-responsive dystonia serves as a reliable therapeutic trial. In addition, because the manifestations of these illnesses are similar and a delay in diagnosis may lead to irreversible brain damage, children presenting with such a movement disorder should undergo MRI, serum ceruloplasmin determination, and, in many cases, genetic testing.

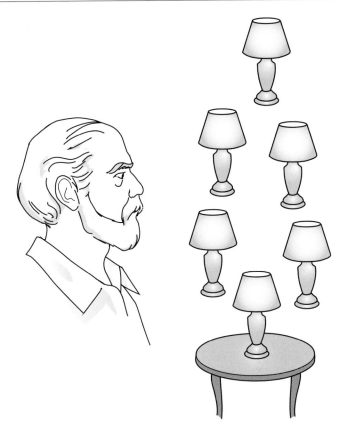

450. A 60-year-old man, who was recently placed in a nursing home, requested a psychiatric consultation because he began to experience episodes of visual hallucinations. A typical hallucination consisted of multiple glowing lamps in the left visual field that were reproductions of a table lamp located in the right side of his room. The most remarkable aspect of the hallucinations, he explained, were that they occurred entirely in his left visual field, which had been rendered blind by a stroke the previous year. The stroke had also caused left-sided sensory loss and mild hemiparesis. Another aspect of the hallucinations was that they consisted of single or multiple replications of objects that he had recently seen in his intact right visual field. The episodes lasted for only several minutes and occurred once or twice daily. During them, he remained fully alert but mesmerized. At almost all other times, he was despondent, discouraged about his health, and unable to sleep restfully. Of the following, which will be the most likely treatment?
  a. Tricyclic antidepressant
  b. SSRI
  c. AED
  d. Psychotherapy
  e. Removal of one of his medications

  Answer: c. The patient is experiencing palinopsia. This disorder, which is also called visual perseveration, consists of recurrent images within an area of visual loss. These visual hallucinations typically occur in a left homonymous hemianopsia. They are usually duplications of individuals or objects in the intact right visual field. Although palinopsia has resulted from depression, hallucinogens, other toxins, and metabolic aberrations, most cases result from recurrent partial seizures from right occipital strokes, neoplasms, or other lesions. When strokes lead to depression, the lesion is usually situated in the frontal lobes (left more often than right) or deeper structures but usually not in an occipital lobe.

451. Which mode of inheritance does the genotype on p. 644 suggest?
  a. Autosomal dominant
  b. Autosomal recessive
  c. Sex-linked dominant
  d. Sex-linked recessive
  e. None of the above

  Answer: e. The inheritance is strictly maternal. It is indicative of a mitochondrial DNA mutation, such as MELAS and MERRF.

452. The emergency medical service workers brought a middle age woman to the emergency room because over the previous 12 hours she developed headache, confusion, and amnesia. She was febrile and had nuchal rigidity. Several 30-second

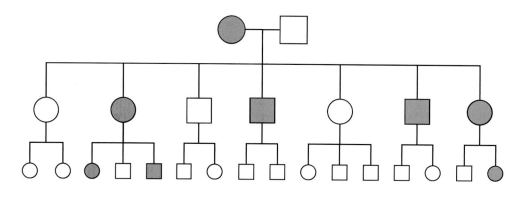

to 2-minute episodes of unresponsiveness with lip-smacking interrupted further examination. The MRI showed hemorrhagic regions in both temporal lobes. The EEG showed sharp waves emanating from the left temporal lobe. The CSF showed 80 WBCs and 400 RBCs per mm^3, glucose of 30 mg/dL, and protein of 90 mg/dL. Of the following, which would be the most appropriate treatment?

a. Penicillin
b. Famciclovir or acyclovir
c. Antituberculous medicines
d. Antiretroviral drugs

Answer: b. In view of the indications of a viral infection, she probably contracted herpes simplex encephalitis, which is the most common nonepidemic encephalitis. A predilection for the temporal lobes, partial complex seizures, and a hemorrhagic aspect in the CSF and MRI characterized this form of encephalitis. An antiviral medication would be the most appropriate treatment. However, neurologists often provide broader antibiotic coverage until the results of specific tests confirm the diagnosis.

Not only does the acute phase of Herpes simplex encephalitis cause distinctive symptoms and laboratory abnormalities, survivors are prone to a variety of neuropsychologic sequelae. Because the temporal lobes, and to a lesser extent the frontal lobes, suffer necrosis, the damage often causes memory impairments (amnesia), partial complex seizures, and Klüver-Bucy syndrome.

453. Which two of the following disorders are considered tauopathies?
a. Alzheimer's disease
b. Frontotemporal dementia
c. Dementia with Lewy bodies
d. Parkinson's disease

Answers: a, b. Neurologists consider Alzheimer's disease and frontotemporal dementia as tauopathies. They consider dementia with Lewy bodies and Parkinson's disease as synucleinopathies.

454. Which of the following AEDs does not enhance age-related osteoporosis?
a. Valproate
b. Phenytoin
c. Carbamazepine
d. Phenobarbital
e. Lamotrigine
f. Primidone

Answer: e. Several AEDs accelerate demineralization and leave epilepsy patients, especially women and those receiving little sunlight, vulnerable to osteoporosis.

455. In the preceding question, which AED does not induce cytochrome P-450 enzymes?

Answer: a. Unlike the other AEDs, valproate does not induce cytochrome P-450 enzymes, but it still accelerates bone loss.

456. A physician caring for a patient with epilepsy, under treatment with valproate 750 mg/day, added lamotrigine. The patient developed fatigue and clumsiness. What was the most likely effect of the addition of lamotrigine?
a. Valproate serum concentrations doubled.
b. Lamotrigine serum concentrations doubled.
c. The combination lowered the seizure threshold.
d. The addition produced no interaction.

Answer: a. The addition of even small doses of lamotrigine to valproate doubles its serum concentration, which reaches toxic levels. In contrast, carbamazepine, phenytoin, phenobarbital, or primidone—inducers of cytochrome P-450 enzymes—reduce lamotrigine serum concentrations by about 40%.

457. Which condition is not associated with hyponatremia?
a. Use of carbamazepine
b. Use of oxcarbazepine
c. Use of valproate

d. Addison's disease

e. Adrenoleukodystrophy

f. Compulsive water drinking

Answer: c.

458. When used to alleviate excessive daytime sleepiness in narcolepsy patients, modafinil creates several effects. Which of the following statements is false?

a. Modafinil acts as an α-1 adrenergic agonist and probably stimulates hypocretin-synthesizing cells.

b. It promotes wakefulness without causing excitation or night-time insomnia.

c. It suppresses narcolepsy but not cataplexy.

d. Stopping modafinil leads to a rebound in sleep.

Answer: d. Unlike stopping amphetamines and other stimulants, stopping modafinil does not lead to sleep rebound.

459. After a vigorous day of training and a fitful night, a 19-year-old Marine recruit suddenly developed a temperature of 103°F and then stupor. In the emergency room, medics find that he has nuchal rigidity. Which three therapies and diagnostic tests should the medical staff perform as soon as possible?

a. Intravenous fluids and electrolytes

b. Oral AEDs

c. Thiamine (50 mg IV)

d. LP

e. Penicillin or penicillin in combination with another antibiotic

Answers: a, d, e. Small epidemics of meningitis frequently erupt in groups of children or young adults brought together from different geographic locations. Clusters of meningitis develop in kindergartens, colleges, and military recruit barracks. Acute bacterial meningitis is usually fatal unless treated promptly with intravenous antibiotics. In this patient, fever, stupor, and nuchal rigidity indicate meningitis. Examination of the spinal fluid by the LP can diagnose subarachnoid hemorrhage, which is an alternative diagnosis, as well as meningitis.

460. A 30-year-old man has a long history of aggressive behavior and other antisocial activities. His electroencephalogram (EEG) shows an isolated, phase-reversed spike focus intermittently over the left frontal lobe. Which single statement is valid?

a. In retrospect, partial complex seizures had been the cause of the behavioral disturbances.

b. The EEG has absolutely no bearing on the case.

c. The EEG of individuals with antisocial personality almost always shows specific EEG abnormalities.

d. Both the EEG and the behavior may reflect cerebral damage.

Answer: d. Although the EEG indicates an area with epileptic potential in the left frontal lobe, that area probably does not actually cause seizures because the EEG shows no paroxysmal activity and the patient has no stereotyped behavior. Depending on the circumstances, further testing might be appropriate. Individuals with antisocial personality disorder have a higher frequency of EEG abnormalities than the general population, but the abnormalities are minor, inconsistent from person to person, and nonspecific.

461. During the course of evaluation for dementia, a 68-year-old patient's CT reveals a small, calcified lesion, without surrounding edema or mass effect, arising from the right parietal convexity. The lesion does not compress the underlying brain. Which two of the following symptoms would this lesion likely cause?

a. Dementia

b. Aphasia

c. Absence seizures

d. Partial seizures without secondary generalization

e. Partial seizures with secondary generalization

Answers: d, e. The lesion is probably a small meningioma. These tumors, which occur commonly, are typically small, slowly growing, and extra-axial. Although they usually do not exert a mass effect, as in this case, they may irritate the underlying cortex and cause seizures. This meningioma may irritate the adjacent parietal cortex and produce seizures involving the left side of the body. In addition, the seizures may undergo secondary generalization. However, small meningiomas do not cause dementia. Especially in the elderly, they need not be removed.

462. Which one of the following patients is most likely to have a seizure?

a. A 65-year-old man with left Bell's palsy

b. A 70-year-old woman with a right third cranial nerve palsy and left hemiparesis

c. A 55-year-old woman with rapidly progressive paresis and sensory loss in her left arm and more so her left leg, which has hyperactive DTRs and a Babinski sign

d. A 40-year-old man who, after an upper respiratory tract infection, develops ascending flaccid, areflexic weakness of both legs

Answer: c. This patient has a lesion involving the right cerebral cortex that could cause seizures. She may have a glioblastoma, abscess, or parasagittal (parafalcine) meningioma. Lesions located outside of the cerebral cortex—such as the left seventh cranial nerve (a), right midbrain (b), or peripheral nerves, such as the Guillain-Barré syndrome (d)—are unlikely to cause seizures.

463. Which two of the following conditions are inherited in an autosomal recessive pattern?
    a. Duchenne's dystrophy
    b. Hemophilia
    c. Sickle cell disease
    d. Phenylketonuria
    e. Homocystinuria
    f. Red-green color blindness
    g. Wilson's disease

Answers: c and g. Duchenne's dystrophy, hemophilia, and red-green color blindness are x-linked.

464. After a prolonged but eventually successful resuscitation from a cardiac arrest, a 70-year-old man has apathy and psychomotor retardation. He says only a few simple words. However, he repeats many long, complex phrases, and he accompanies singers on the radio. He can move all his limbs, but he is too weak to walk. What is the nature of this patient's language impairment?
    a. Nonfluent aphasia
    b. Fluent aphasia
    c. Frontal lobe dysfunction
    d. Isolation (transcortical) aphasia

Answer: d. Isolation of the perisylvian language arc—Broca's area, the arcuate fasciculus, and Wernicke's area—from the remaining cerebral cortex produces isolation (transcortical) aphasia. Anoxia, as occurs with cardiac arrests and carbon monoxide poisoning, is the most common cause of this variety of aphasia. Although patients are able to repeat words, phrases, and songs because the language arc itself remains intact, they are unable to utilize other intellectual functions because anoxia has damaged the rest of the cerebral cortex. In addition, they may have cortical blindness.

465. Below are six sketches of spinal cords portrayed with normal myelin stained black, demyelinated areas white (*unstained*), and central gray areas crosshatched. Match the sketches (A–F) with the descriptions of the clinical associations (1–6).
    1. During 4 years, a 45-year-old man has had progressively severe intellectual and personality impairment. He has loss of vibration and position sensation, absent reflexes in the legs, and a floppy-foot gait. His pupils are miotic. They constrict to closely regarded objects but not to light.
    2. A 65-year-old man, who underwent a complete gastrectomy 4 years ago, now has dementia, hyperactive DTRs, bilateral Babinski signs, and loss of vibration sensation in the legs.
    3. During the previous 4 months, a 70-year-old woman has developed weakness of her left leg, right arm, and neck muscles. She has atrophy of limb muscles. The physician sees fasciculations in her tongue and several atrophic muscles. Despite her disability, she has normal cognitive function. Anticipating her need for artificial ventilation and imminent death, she requests physician-assisted suicide.
    4. A 35-year-old man has optic neuritis, internuclear ophthalmoplegia, and gait impairment from ataxia and spasticity.

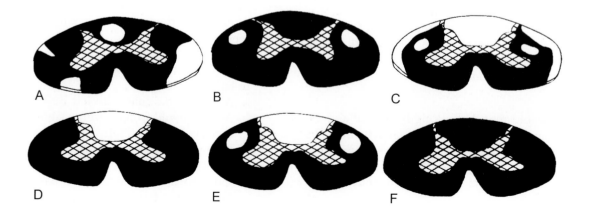

5. A 40-year-old woman and her sister have pes cavus, intention tremor on finger-to-nose testing, and loss of position and vibration sensation.

6. A 47-year-old man who has confusion, nystagmus, and bilateral abducens nerve palsy.

Answers

A-4: The spinal cord shows multiple areas (plaques) of demyelination (sclerosis). The patient has signs of optic nerve, brainstem, and spinal cord dysfunction. Both the clinical and pathologic information indicate MS.

B-3: The spinal cord shows demyelination of the lateral corticospinal tracts and loss of the anterior horns, which contain the motor neurons. This is the typical picture of ALS, the most common form of motor neuron disease, in which both the upper and lower motor neuron systems degenerate but cognitive function remains intact.

C-5: The spinocerebellar, posterior column, and corticospinal tracts have undergone demyelination. Their loss would cause intention tremor, position and vibration sense loss, and a foot deformity (pes cavus). This clinical and pathologic pattern indicates a spinocerebellar ataxia.

D-1: The spinal cord shows demyelination of the posterior columns. Loss of these tracts impairs position sensation and forces patients to walk with a high, uncertain, and awkward pattern (a steppage gait). This patient also has Argyll-Robertson pupils. This is a case of neurosyphilis of the brain and spinal cord (tabes dorsalis).

E-2: The spinal cord shows demyelination of the posterior columns and the lateral corticospinal tracts. This pattern, combined system disease, is associated with B_{12} deficiency from pernicious anemia or surgical removal of the stomach because both conditions remove intrinsic factor. In addition, B_{12} deficiency is associated with prolonged exposure to nitrous oxide because it oxidizes the cobalt in B_{12} (cobalamine) to an inactive form. Combined system disease causes dementia, paraparesis, hyperactive DTRs, and position and vibration sense loss. These findings are similar to those of tabes dorsalis with dementia; however, although combined-system disease causes hyperactive DTRs and Babinski signs, tabes dorsalis causes hypoactive DTRs and Argyll-Robertson pupils but neither spasticity nor Babinski signs.

F-6: The spinal cord remains normal despite Wernicke's encephalopathy.

466. Which of the following is not a complication of lithium toxicity?
a. Cerebellar damage
b. Excessive secretion of antidiuretic hormone
c. Hypothyroidism
d. Tremor
e. Symptoms and signs that mimic Creutzfeldt-Jakob disease

Answer: b. Lithium toxicity inhibits antidiuretic hormone. The deficiency of the hormone causes a concentration defect that leads to hypernatremia. At very high levels, lithium toxicity causes irreversible cerebellar damage, but the other complications recede as the lithium concentration falls.

467. A 50-year-old worker in a battery factory, which had poor ventilation, developed excitability, memory loss, insomnia, and then delirium. On neurologic examination, he had poor handwriting, tremor on finger-to-nose and heel-to-shin testing, and gait ataxia. His gums each had developed a black horizontal line. Which is the most likely industrial intoxication?
a. Toluene
b. Ethanol
c. Mercury
d. Lead
e. Arsenic

Answer: c. In addition to his cognitive and personality changes, this man has cerebellar dysfunction. That combination is attributable to several illnesses, particularly alcoholism. However, mercury intoxication, which may result from inhalation of mercury vapors in industrial settings, is the only one that characteristically leads to a black "gum line." Excessive exposure to toluene, ethanol, and, in adults, lead usually causes a peripheral neuropathy.

468. Despite some false-positive and false-negative results, neurologists often relate several CSF abnormalities to certain neurologic illnesses. Match the CSF abnormality to the disease that it frequently indicates.
a. Oligoclonal bands
b. 14–3-3 protein
c. Increased levels of tau
d. Myelin basic protein
e. Anti-measles antibodies
f. Albumino-cytologic disassociation
g. Anti-GAD antibodies
  1. Alzheimer's disease
  2. Multiple sclerosis
  3. Creutzfeldt-Jakob disease
  4. Guillain-Barré syndrome
  5. SSPE
  6. Stiff-person syndrome

Answers: a-2, b-3, c-1, d-2, e-5, f-4, g-6.

469. One evening, the emergency health service workers bring a disheveled, gaunt man to the psychiatry emergency room. He has alcohol on his breath, lice in his hair, and a thick, burn-like rash on his hands and around his neck. He has loose, watery bowel movements. On examination, he fluctuates between inattention and lethargy. When responsive, he cannot state the month, year, or place. He has poor memory, judgment, and language use. However, eye movements are full and without nystagmus. He has no paresis or ataxia. His reflexes are hypoactive. Which is the most specific immediate treatment?
   a. Thiamine
   b. Referral to Alcoholics Anonymous
   c. Pyridoxine
   d. Niacin

Answer: d. His dermatitis, diarrhea, and delirium (the "3D's") indicate that he has pellagra ("rough skin," from the Italian, *pelle,* skin and *agro,* rough). A necklace-like rash is characteristic. Pellagra, which was endemic in rural southeastern United States in the early 1900s, results from absence of niacin in the diet. In addition to nutritional deprivation from starvation, inadequate diet, or alcoholism, use of isoniazid can cause this disorder. When the result of nutritional deprivation, Wernicke-Korsakoff disease may be co-morbid with pellagra. The treatment is niacin, usually combined with thiamine.

470. The family of a 30-year-old woman, with a history of partial complex epilepsy refractory to AEDs and surgery, found her in a car with its engine running in a closed garage and brought her to the emergency room. She is stuporous but has round, equal, and reactive pupils. Her extraocular movements are intact. Although she has Babinski signs, she has no hemiparesis. Staff members call her skin color pink or cherry-red. Which of the following findings will probably be absent?
   a. Elevated concentration of carbon monoxide in the blood
   b. Elevated concentration of methemoglobin in the blood
   c. Toxic concentrations of an AED
   d. Hypoxia

Answer: c. Depression and suicide are frequent complications of partial complex epilepsy, especially when it is refractory. In this case, the patient made a suicide attempt by exposure to carbon monoxide. Although the pink or cherry-red skin color indicates carbon monoxide poisoning, the distinctive coloration occurs in less than 10% of cases and also follows cyanide poisoning. Carbon monoxide displaces oxygen from hemoglobin and thereby causes methemoglobin. The treatment is hyperbaric oxygen.

471. A 25-year-old woman with Wilson's disease, which occurs in 1 person in 40,000, wants to have a child with her perfectly well husband, who she met through RandomSelection.com. Assuming that no DNA tests are available, what is the approximate risk that they will have a child with the illness?
   a. 0.5%
   b. 1.0%
   c. 2.0%
   d. 25%
   e. 50%

Answer: a. If she is the 1 person in 40,000 who has Wilson's disease, which is an autosomal recessive illness, she caries two mutant genes (ww). Therefore, two individuals among 200 will carry one mutant gene, that is, 1% of the population will be heterozygotes (Ww) (see below). Even if her husband were a heterozygote, the child has only a 50% chance of receiving the mutant gene (w) rather than the wild gene (W). Then there is only a 0.5% chance of her husband passing on the mutant gene. If he were to pass on that gene, and she must necessarily pass on a mutant gene, the child would have a 0.5% chance of developing the illness. Fortunately, genetic tests can detect asymptomatic carriers and, if the disease were detected, treatment before the onset of symptoms.

	W	w
W	WW = 1 ^	Ww = 1/200 *
w	Ww = 1/200 *	ww = 1/40,000 +

If the frequency of individuals with the illness (ww) is 1/40,000, that frequency is equivalent to the square of the frequency gene of the mutant gene (1/200).
^ WW = Homozygous wild type (no illness), approximately 1.
* Ww = Heterozygotes (asymptomatic carriers) 1/200 + 1/200 = 2/200 = 1%.
+ ww = Homozygous mutant (individuals with the illness) = 1/40,000.

Index

Page numbers followed by t and f indicate figures and tables, respectively.

A

Abducens nerves, 29–34, 31f, 32f, 33f, 281, 282f
Ablative procedures, for Parkinson's disease, 414
Absence seizures, 220–221, 221f, 222t
Abuse
  child, visual disturbances and, 269–270, drug, 511–524
  elder, TBI due to, 543
Accommodation reflex, 268, 269f
ACE (angiotensin-converting enzyme), 361
Acetaminophen (Tylenol), 184, 189, 320, 320t
Acetazolamide, 38
Acetylcholine. See ACh
ACh (acetylcholine), 87, 88, 89–90, 371, 439, 491
  anatomy relating to, 517, 517f
  receptors, 517
  reduced activity
    in CNS, 517–518
    at neuromuscular junction, 517, 518t
  synthesis and metabolism of, 516–517
Acoustic nerves, 38–40, 38f, 158
Acoustic neuroma, 465t, 503f
Acquired immunodeficiency syndrome. See AIDS
ACTH (adrenocorticotropin), 320, 472
Acupuncture, 324t
Acute dyskinesias
  acute dystonias, 436–437, 436f
  akathisia, 437, 437f
  Parkinsonism and Parkinson-hyperpyrexia syndrome, 436
Acute dystonias, 436–437, 436f
Acute inflammatory demyelinating polyradiculoneuropathy. See AIDP
Acute intermittent porphyria. See AIP
Acute therapy, for headaches, 183
Acyclovir (Zovirax), 327
ADAS (Alzheimer's Disease Assessment Scale), 115–116, 117f
ADHD (attention deficit hyperactivity disorder), 165, 303, 306, 308, 434, 542
Adjuvants
  AEDs, 323
  antidepressants, 323
α-Adrenergic antagonists, 358
β-Adrenergic blockers, 430–431
Adrenocorticotropin. See ACTH
Adrenoleukodystrophy. See ALD
Adults
  tics in, 432
  young, Parkinsonism in, 412
Advil. See Ibuprofen

AEDs (antiepileptic drugs), 38, 66, 184, 190, 203, 205, 210, 211, 213, 214, 215, 216, 223, 225, 298
  for brain tumors, 469
  for epilepsy, 217–219, 217t
  mental side effects of, 218
  for pain, chronic, 323, 325, 327
  physical side effects of, 218
  pregnancy and, 218–219
  surgery and, 219–220
Agent Orange, 91
Aggrenox. See Dipyridamole
Aging
  mental changes relating to, 67–68
  normal, 112–114
  normal sleep relating to, 113, 375–376
  sexual function, changes in, relating to, 359
  sleep disorders relating to, 375–376
Agnosia
  color, 273
  prosopagnosia relating to, 274
  simultanagnosia relating to, 274
  visual, 273
Agraphia alexia, 165, 165f, 171, 502f
AIDP (acute inflammatory demyelinating polyradiculoneuropathy), 64
AIDS (acquired immunodeficiency syndrome), 13, 69–70, 91, 131, 192, 210, 268, 269, 326, 466, 485, 494f, 553. See also HAD
AIDS-induced cerebral lesions, 136–137
AIP (acute intermittent porphyria), 70
Akathisia, 437, 437f
  tardive, 440
Alcohol, 10, 13, 25, 225, 375, 387
Alcoholics, dementia in, 129–130
ALD (adrenoleukodystrophy), 345
Alexia, agraphia relating to, 165, 165f, 171, 502f
Alien hand syndrome, 167–169
Allodynia, 61
Alpha tocopherol, 414
ALS (amyotrophic lateral sclerosis), 34, 41, 43, 71–73, 72f, 99, 248, 340, 347, 553
Altered levels of consciousness, 251–254
Altered mental states, 98
Altered states of awareness, 207
Alzheimer's disease, 3, 7, 27–28, 30, 341, 363, 388
  amyloid deposits relating to, 121–122, 121f
  clinical features of
    cognitive decline, 118–119
    neuropsychiatric manifestations, 119
    physical signs, 119–120, 121f

dementia relating to, 408
genetic causes of, 122–123, 124t
imaging studies for, 485, 487, 491, 492
other symptoms of, 124–125
pathology of, 120–121
resource for, 553
risk factors for, 122–123
tests for, 120, 556
treatment of, 123–124
Alzheimer's Disease Assessment Scale. See ADAS
Amantadine, 339, 414, 440
Ambidextrous, 158
Amitriptyline, 323
Amnesia, 111–112
  transient, 111–112, 112t
Amphetamines, 98, 193, 375, 514, 522
Amyloid deposits, 121–122, 121f
Amyotrophic lateral sclerosis. See ALS
Anafranil. See Clomipramine
Analgesia. See also PCA
  stimulation-induced, 324, 324t
Analgesic pathways, of pain, 319–320, 319t
Analgesics
  nonopioid, 320–321, 320t
  opioids, 321t
Anatomic nervous system. See ANS
Anencephaly, 299
Anesthetic agents, for pain, chronic, 323–324, 327
Angiotensin-converting enzyme. See ACE
Angle-closure (closed-angle or narrow-angle) glaucoma, 271f, 272
Anosmia, 27, 28
Anosognosia, 169–170
ANS (anatomic nervous system), 360, 371
  parasympathetic division of, 355
  sympathetic division of, 355
Anterior cerebral artery syndrome, 171
Anterior horn cells, 61, 73
Anticholinergic poisoning, 98
Anticholinesterases, 87
Antidepressants, 66, 190, 323, 371. See also TCA
Antiemetics, 189, 469
Antiepileptic drugs. See AEDs
Antihistamines, 469
Antipsychotics, 66, 323, 412
Anton's syndrome, 272–273
Aphasia, 6, 38, 250, 468
  classification of, 160t
    fluent, 162–164
    nonfluent, 160–162